P9-AFD-944

RESEARCH METHODS
IN HEALTH PROMOTION

RESEARCH METHODS IN HEALTH PROMOTION

Richard A. Crosby
Ralph J. DiClemente
Laura F. Salazar

Editors

Foreword by Lawrence W. Green

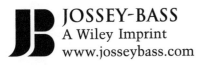

JOSSEY-BASS
A Wiley Imprint
www.josseybass.com

Published by Jossey-Bass
A Wiley Imprint
989 Market Street, San Francisco, CA 94103-1741   www.josseybass.com

Jossey-Bass books and products are available through most bookstores. To contact Jossey-Bass
directly, call our Customer Care Department within the U.S. at 800-956-7739 or outside the U.S.
at 317-572-3986, or fax to 317-572-4002.

Jossey-Bass also publishes its books in a variety of electronic formats. Some content that appears in print
may not be available in electronic books.

This publication is designed to provide accurate and authoritative information in regard to the subject
matter covered. It is sold with the understanding that the publisher is not engaged in rendering
professional services. If professional advice or other expert assistance is required, the services of a
competent professional person should be sought.

Library of Congress Cataloging-in-Publication Data

Research methods in health promotion / Richard A. Crosby, Ralph J.
    DiClemente, Laura Francisca Salazar, editors.
        p. ; cm.
    Includes bibliographical references and index.
    ISBN-13: 978-0-7879-7679-8 (alk. paper)
    ISBN-10: 0-7879-7679-2 (alk. paper)
    1. Health promotion—Research—Methodology.   I. Crosby, Richard
A., 1959-   .   II. DiClemente, Ralph J.   III. Salazar, Laura Francisca,
1960-   .
    [DNLM: 1. Health Promotion.   2. Research—methods.   WA 590
R432 2006]
    RA427.8.R46 2006
    613'.072—dc22   2005016228

Printed in the United States of America
FIRST EDITION
HB Printing   10 9 8 7 6 5 4 3 2 1

CONTENTS

PART TWO: RESEARCH DESIGN 73

PART THREE: MEASUREMENT, SAMPLING, AND ANALYSIS 227

FIGURES, TABLES, AND BOXES

Figures

Tables

Boxes

FOREWORD

Much that has been written on research methods misses the mark for students of the health professions because academic authors tend to emphasize research methods that will meet scientific needs rather than practitioner needs. They often start with theory or research questions from more basic disciplines and ask what opportunities or challenges clinical, school, or community health situations offer to test those theories. It seems too often that preprofessional students are being trained to turn their practices into community laboratories to serve the cause of science and theory testing, rather than using science and theory to solve their problems in practice. The editors of this volume have challenged their contributing authors (and themselves, with the many chapters they have written) to show how their research methods can answer the questions that practitioners are asking. They acknowledge the growing demand for evidence-based practice and theory-based practice, but they demonstrate that these will come most effectively when we have more practice-based evidence and practice-based theory.

Rather than starting with theories and asking what practice situations can offer to test them, practice-based research starts with problems in practice and asks what research and theory can offer to solve them. It is that twist that sets this book apart from the usual emphasis of textbooks often used in professional preparation programs.

Each chapter offers applied examples from health promotion that illustrate the key concepts or research methods presented in that chapter. The chapters present a series of pros and cons for the methods presented, and case studies that challenge readers to apply what they have learned. Another added value of this book as distinct from the numerous textbooks available on research methods for each of the cognate disciplines (for example, epidemiology, psychology, sociology, anthropology, political science, economics) underpinning health promotion practice, is that this book seeks the multidisciplinary blending of methods necessary to understand, predict, and address the several ecological levels at which causation happens and change must occur. Any of the excellent research methods books from other disciplines would deal only with a relatively narrow slice of the multilayered reality that health promotion must address. Research methods in health promotion must blend methods from psychology and sociology, for example, to encompass the ecological reality of reciprocal determinism between individual behavior and environment.

While integrating these several complexities of multiple methods and multiple levels of analysis, the editors have strived to give cohesiveness to varied research methods by maintaining a consistent theme that "research involves a predetermined series of well-defined steps." They revisit these steps throughout in a common sequential format. They seek to present a cohesive understanding of the role of science in public health and, more specifically, in health promotion. At the same time that they are ecumenical in their admission of the methods from various disciplines, they are critical in evaluating their use and their limitations in health promotion research, and the ethical issues surrounding some methods of experimental design, sampling, and randomization in the health promotion context.

The editors have drawn on their considerable academic experience in teaching students of health promotion, and their field experience in practice-based research in HIV/AIDS, school health, reducing health disparities, and numerous other areas of public health, to represent research methods specifically for students in health promotion.

November 2005　　　　　　　　　　　　　　　　　　　　　Lawrence W. Green
Adjunct Professor, Department of Epidemiology and Biostatistics
School of Medicine and Comprehensive Cancer Center
University of California at San Francisco

ACKNOWLEDGMENTS

We would not have been able to produce this volume without our contributors. Each contributor spent a great deal of time, effort, and careful thought in organizing and clearly presenting his or her subject.

Furthermore, we extend our thanks to Becky Flannagan for her superb editorial acumen as well as her stellar figures and tables; to Justin Wagner for his original artwork and conceptualization of Dincus and Mincus; and to Dr. Roger Bakeman, for his helpful review and insightful comments on the statistics chapters.

Also, we wish to acknowledge our Jossey-Bass editor, Andy Pasternack, who has been instrumental in producing this volume. He has been diligent in guiding its preparation, thoughtful in conceptualization of the format, understanding of our needs, and helpful in ways uncountable. He has become a dear friend and a valued resource. The editorial team at Jossey-Bass has been tremendous. Seth Schwartz, Catherine Craddock, Susan Geraghty, and David Horne have made the process enjoyable and have contributed greatly.

Finally, we wish to acknowledge all scholars who aspire to make the world a safer and healthier place to live and those students who will shape and guide the future of health promotion research and practice.

Thanks to my family for their continued inspiration, and especially
to my wife for her love, support, and perseverance in my years
of growth as a scholar.
—R.A.C.

To my lovely wife, Gina, and beautiful daughter, Sahara Rae,
for their love, support, patience, and encouragement.
They are always in my thoughts.
—R.J.D

I would like to thank my wonderful husband, Chuck,
whose support and love sustained me through the process,
and my amazing children, who inspire me every single day.
—L.F.S.

THE EDITORS

Richard A. Crosby is an associate professor in the Department of Health Behavior in the College of Public Health at the University of Kentucky. Crosby received his B.A. degree (1981) in school health education from the University of Kentucky and his M.A. degree (1984) in health education from Central Michigan University. His Ph.D. degree (1998) is in health behavior and is from Indiana University.

Crosby was formerly an assistant professor at the Rollins School of Public Health, and previous to that appointment he was a Fellow of the Association of Teachers of Preventive Medicine. He currently teaches graduate courses in public health and research methods. Crosby's research interests include development and application of behavioral theory to health promotion, particularly in adolescent and young adult populations. He is primarily involved in health promotion practice and research that contributes to reducing the incidence of sexually transmitted diseases, especially infection with the human immunodeficiency virus. Also affiliated with the Rural Center for AIDS and STD Prevention, Crosby has published numerous journal articles that report empirical findings relevant to the sexual risk behaviors of adolescents and adults.

Ralph J. DiClemente is Charles Howard Candler Professor of Public Health and associate director, Emory Center for AIDS Research. He holds concurrent appointments as professor in the School of Medicine, the Department of Pediatrics, in the Division of Infectious Diseases, Epidemiology, and Immunology;

the Department of Medicine, in the Division of Infectious Diseases; and the Department of Psychiatry. He was recently chair, the Department of Behavioral Sciences and Health Education at the Rollins School of Public Health, Emory University. DiClemente was trained as a health psychologist at the University of California, San Francisco, where he received his Ph.D. degree (1984) after completing an S.M. degree (1978) in behavioral sciences at the Harvard School of Public Health and his B.A. degree (1973) at the City University of New York.

DiClemente's research interests include developing decision-making models of adolescents' risk and protective behaviors. He has a particular interest in the development and evaluation of theory-driven HIV/STD-prevention programs for adolescents and young adult women. He has published numerous books and journal articles in the fields of adolescent health and HIV/STD prevention. He currently teaches a course on adolescent health and serves on numerous editorial boards and national prevention organizations.

Laura F. Salazar is currently an assistant research professor in behavioral sciences and health education at the Rollins School of Public Health at Emory University. Salazar completed her B.S. degree (1982) in business management from the State University of New York at Buffalo. After a brief career in business, and raising a family, she pursued an M.A. degree (1996) and a Ph.D. degree (2001) in community psychology at Georgia State University in Atlanta, Georgia.

Salazar's research interests focus on examining the societal, community, and institutional influences of certain health risk behaviors, such as sexual risk behavior and violence against women. She also holds a keen interest in examining the intersection of these two health risks and how they should be addressed simultaneously through the development of innovative programs. She currently teaches graduate courses in theory and applied research methods. She has published many scientific articles in peer-reviewed journals related to these health issues, and is also the author of numerous book chapters.

THE CONTRIBUTORS

Katherine A. Atwood, Sc.D., is an assistant professor in the Department of Health Behavior of the College of Public Health at the University of Kentucky in Lexington, Kentucky.

Richard R. Clayton, Ph.D., is the chairperson and a professor in the Department of Health Behavior of the College of Public Health at the University of Kentucky in Lexington, Kentucky.

Pamela K. Cupp, Ph.D., is project director for the Institute for HIV, Other STDs, and Pregnancy Prevention and research assistant professor in the Department of Communication at the University of Kentucky in Lexington, Kentucky.

David R. Holtgrave, Ph.D., is professor and vice-chair in the Department of Behavioral Sciences and Health Education at the Rollins School of Public Health at Emory University.

Michelle C. Kegler, Dr. PH., M.P.H., is an associate professor in the Department of Behavioral Sciences and Health Education at the Rollins School of Public Health, and deputy director of the Emory Prevention Research Center at Emory University.

John F. Santelli, M.D., M.P.H., is professor and chairperson in the Heilbrunn Department of Population and Family Health at the Mailman School of Public Health, Columbia University in New York City.

Nancy Thompson, M.P.H., Ph.D., is an associate professor in the Department of Behavioral Sciences and Health Education at the Rollins School of Public Health at Emory University.

Rick S. Zimmerman, Ph.D., is a professor in the Department of Communication at the University of Kentucky in Lexington, Kentucky.

RESEARCH METHODS
IN HEALTH PROMOTION

PART ONE

FOUNDATIONS OF HEALTH PROMOTION RESEARCH

CHAPTER ONE

KEY STEPS IN THE RESEARCH PROCESS

Richard A. Crosby, Ralph J. DiClemente, and Laura F. Salazar

Health promotion has become a cornerstone of efforts designed to prevent morbidity and premature mortality (Smedley and Syme, 2000). Indeed, many nations have embraced health promotion as an approach to enriching and extending the lives of their people. Core tasks of health promotion include the primary and secondary prevention of disease and health-compromising conditions. These tasks are reflected in two overarching goals established by the United States Department of Health and Human Services: to "increase the quality and years of healthy life" and to "eliminate health disparities" (Department of Health and Human Services, 2000). Of course, the broad scope of these tasks presents an enormous challenge to the discipline of health promotion. This challenge demands that the efforts and resources of health promotion practitioners must be firmly grounded in the context of research findings.

To begin, then, it is important to state that health promotion research is the harbinger of effective health promotion practice. Thus, a great deal of time and attention should be devoted to research agendas before health promotion programs are designed and widely implemented. In turn, successful research endeavors must ensure rigor. Rigor may best be viewed as the hallmark of science.

Rigor is properly thought of as a quantity—it exists (or fails to exist) in varying degrees. Although no study can be "perfect" in rigor, studies can have a high degree of rigor. As rigor increases, confidence in the findings also increases. Therefore, rigorous studies have great potential to shape health promotion practice.

Although this book focuses on the application of research methods to health promotion, there are at least two frameworks that address a number of other issues relevant to the conceptualization, design, implementation, evaluation of programs. In particular, an emerging framework, RE-AIM (Glasgow, Vogt, and Boles, 1999) can be used as both a design and an evaluation tool for health promotion planning. Also, the PRECEDE-PROCEED Model (Green and Kreuter, 2005) is a comprehensive framework for organizing the health promotion planning process from its inception to its widespread implementation and ongoing evaluation.

Illustration of Key Concepts

As was ancient Rome, rigor is built "one brick at a time." Fortunately, clear blueprints exist for building rigorous studies. In fact, successful research can be characterized by a series of well-defined steps. Although some of these steps may appear tedious, they are all essential. Following the steps sequentially is equally important. In this chapter we provide an overview of the process and then illustrate each of the essential and sequential steps in detail.

Discovery

Without question, one of greatest rewards of health promotion research is the excitement generated by evidence-based conclusions. Health promotion research is a process that reveals insights into human behavior as it pertains to health and wellness. This exploration into people's lives should never be taken for granted; indeed, the opportunity provides health promotion practitioners a partial blueprint for the design, implementation, and justification of behavioral and structural interventions.

The process of discovery in health promotion research is iterative. Each time a research question is addressed successfully, several new questions emerge. The diversity of potential research questions in any one aspect of health promotion creates an unending challenge (see Chapter Four for more detail regarding potential research purposes and questions). Research questions can be appear quite humble, yet demand rather complex and intense investigation efforts. Consider, for example, a question as simple as determining why people consume large amounts of saturated fats despite widespread awareness that these fats cause heart disease. An investigator could pursue cognitive reasons (for example, "those foods taste really good" or "those foods are satisfying"), social reasons (such as "most party foods are not healthy, but having fun is more important"), cultural reasons (for instance, "those foods are a tradition in our house"), or economic reasons (for example, "fatty foods are usually more filling and less expensive than healthy foods"). An investigator could also approach the question based on perceived vulnerability of the study participants to the multiple forms of disease associated with a diet high in saturated fats (such as heart disease, stroke, obesity, and some forms of cancer). Obviously then, the seemingly humble research question is actually an entire research career. In fact, successful researchers typically devote themselves to only one or two areas of inquiry. This focus enables them to use the findings from one study as a platform to formulate subsequent research questions for the next study, and so on.

MINCUS "DISCOVERS" HIS RESEARCH IDEA.

Because health promotion research is a discovery process it is also a public venture. Conclusions from health promotion research often have a direct impact on public health (for example, "evidence suggests that people who wear sunscreen are less likely to develop skin cancers") or an indirect impact on public health through changes in health promotion practice and policy (for example, the practice of providing same-day results for HIV testing is based on empirical findings that indicated low return rates for people testing positive). As a public venture, then, discovery through health promotion research is an indispensable contribution to maintaining the health and well-being of society. In the next section, we illustrate the discovery process using tobacco as the public health issue.

◆ ◆ ◆

In a Nutshell

As a public venture, then, discovery through health promotion research is an indispensable contribution to maintaining the health and well-being of society.

◆ ◆ ◆

Vignette: Preventing Tobacco Dependence

Globally, the use of tobacco is a behavior that leads to multiple forms of *morbidity* (incidence of disease in a given population) and premature *mortality* (incidence of death due to a particular disease in a given population). Thus, health promotion programs designed to prevent tobacco dependence among young people are strongly warranted. A substantial number of these programs seek to prevent youths from initial experimentation with tobacco. These approaches certainly have value; however, research suggests that among young people tobacco dependency may be an extended process, which may be amenable to intervention even after their initial use of the substance. Imagine, then, that you have been asked to determine the *efficacy* (that is, the ability to produce the desired effect) of providing behavioral interventions to youths who have recently begun to use tobacco, but have yet to develop a physical dependence.

A Nine-Step Model

The research process can easily become unwieldy. Even seemingly simple research questions may lead an investigator to wonder if he or she is "on the right track" with regard to the process. To streamline the thinking and actions involved in rigorous research, we have created a nine-step model that may be helpful.

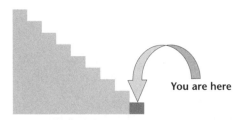

Step 1: Defining the Research Population. Given that the elimination of health disparities is a priority, health promotion research typically seeks solutions to problems that disproportionately exist among members of a defined population. Because *population* is a broad term and can be defined in many different ways, it is up to the researcher to specify the parameters that will describe the target population. For example, the researcher may define the population as "low-income youths, thirteen to nineteen years of age, residing in rural, tobacco-producing states."

Moreover, the process of defining the target population is far from arbitrary. Ideally, selecting the target population should be based on known *epidemiology* (the scientific discipline studying the distribution of disease in human populations) of the disease or health risk behavior under consideration. Generally speaking, health promotion programs should be delivered to epidemiologically defined populations on a prioritized basis (in other words, those with the greatest degree of burden—often expressed as the rate of disease per 100,000 people—are served first).

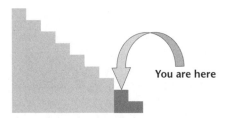

Step 2: Defining the Research Goal and Specifying the Exact Research Questions. This second step is a turning point for the remainder of the research process. As a rule, narrow and precisely defined goals and questions are far more amenable to rigorous research designs than broadly defined goals and questions. At times, new researchers propose goals and questions that are far too broad to be addressed with ample rigor. An effective strategy to avoid this pitfall is to thoroughly review the recent and relevant empirical literature. This can be a

time-consuming process, but is nonetheless time well spent. Engaging in this process will inevitably yield a clear picture of gaps in the existing research. For new investigators, these gaps represent an opportunity to build on and extend the research literature, and should be a logical focus of their subsequent research.

◆ ◆ ◆

In a Nutshell

As a rule, narrow and precisely defined goals and questions are far more amenable to rigorous research designs than broadly defined goals and questions.

◆ ◆ ◆

Although conventional standards do not exist, from a practical standpoint many researchers restrict their review of the literature to the past five years. On-line search engines such as Medline® and PsychInfo® are invaluable assets to the review process. A thorough review should include articles directly related to the topic and those that are related tangentially. Articles directly related, for example, could include those that report findings from research designed to prevent tobacco dependence in new smokers. Indirectly related articles could include those involving different populations (for instance, middle-class urban high school students) and address broader issues such as use of other substances like alcohol or marijuana. When interpreting your review, it is important to assign a higher priority to directly related articles, whereas articles that are indirectly related should be applied judiciously.

Once the literature review is complete, a research goal can be formulated. The research goal is a general statement that conveys the purpose of the planned study. The following statement, "to determine the efficacy of providing behavioral interventions for youths who have recently begun to use tobacco" is the research goal as stated in the vignette. The goal provides an overview of purpose and scope, but it lacks precision and specificity. Rather, it is the research questions that provide the precision and specificity. Research questions are based on the research goal. In the given vignette, samples of a few appropriate research questions may be as follows.

- Will a twelve-hour small-group intervention promote tobacco cessation among a greater percentage of youths than a brief version (six hours) of the same program?
- Will a twelve-hour small-group intervention promote tobacco cessation among a greater percentage of youths as compared to youths who receive no program at all?
- Will a six-hour small-group intervention promote tobacco cessation among a greater percent of youths as compared to youths who receive no program at all?

Please notice that each question is a derivative of the overarching research goal. Thus, each research question should provide information that serves the research goal. This derivative approach to research questions ensures that research efforts are accurately directed. Research questions should be centered upon a common purpose: the research goal. This practice sets the stage for the next step.

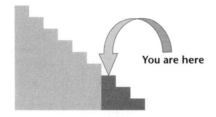

Step 3: Determining Whether the Research Should Be Observational or Experimental. Briefly stated, *observational research* refers to research in which variables are observed as they exist in nature—no manipulation of variables occurs. Observational research asks questions pertaining to "why people do what they do." This form of research *does not involve* treatment or intervention.

Experimental research, however, *does involve* manipulation of a variable (this could include education, policy changes, or changes in the environment). Thus, it builds upon observational research by asking, "How can we help people achieve positive change?" Experimental research is always concerned with the essential question of whether a given intervention program can produce outcomes of statistical significance and, more important, practical significance.

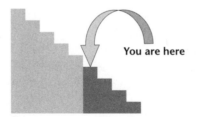

Step 4: Selecting a Research Design That Provides a Rigorous Test of the Research Questions. The choice of research designs ranges from simple observational studies (requiring relatively little time and generally manageable resources) to complex experimental studies (requiring several years to complete and the use of extensive resources).

The guiding principle in making the selection is parsimony. Parsimony implies that the need (that is, investigating the research questions) is met by a tool (that is, research design) that does the job well, without going beyond that which is necessary.

FIGURE 1.1. A TRAJECTORY OF RESEARCH IN HEALTH PROMOTION.

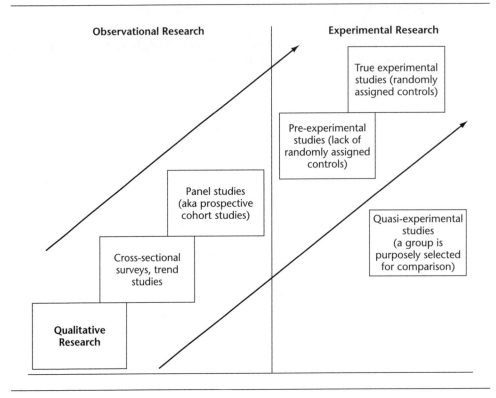

Figure 1.1 shows a trajectory of research designs that accommodate various forms of health promotion research. These designs are described in greater detail in Chapter Four. At the left and lower end of this trajectory, relatively simple research designs can be identified. Examples include qualitative studies and cross-sectional studies. As the level of complexity increases, the trajectory includes designs that necessitate the maintenance of a *cohort* (a cohort being a sample of research participants) over multiple assessment periods. A *cohort study* is synonymous with the terms *panel study, longitudinal study,* or *prospective study* and is located mid-level along the trajectory. Similarly, various levels of complexity exist among experimental designs, which are located toward the upper right end of the trajectory. The phrase "randomized, controlled, trial (RCT)" denotes a true experimental design located at the peak of the trajectory. Figure 1.1 also shows that quasi-experimental designs are located further along on the trajectory, but do not achieve the same "gold standard" status as the true experimental designs.

Quasi-experimental designs, however, are often necessary in health promotion, as certain intervention programs or structural-level interventions limit the ability to randomize (Murray, 1998).

As a rule, research should be constructed with designs that approximate the trajectory shown in Figure 1.1. That is, designs located to the left end of the trajectory serve as the building blocks for subsequent research questions that can then be addressed by progressively more complex designs.

◆ ◆ ◆

In a Nutshell

Designs located to the left end of the trajectory serve as the building blocks for subsequent research questions that can then be addressed by progressively more complex designs.

◆ ◆ ◆

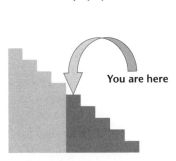

Step 5: Determining the Variables That Must Be Measured. First and foremost, the immediate goal is to be absolutely sure that every *variable* required for a rigorous study is identified. A variable is anything that changes, meaning it must assume a range of values. The research question and the literature review will inform variable selection. For example, suppose that the literature review indicated that efficacy of other tobacco-dependence programs was a function of participants' family environment (in other words, programs may work better for youths with a supportive family). Given even a remote chance that this same dynamic may operate in our hypothetical planned study of low-income youths residing in rural areas, it is incumbent upon the researchers to measure participants' perceived level of family support in addition to other critical variables.

The way in which the variables are measured is equally important. Indeed, rigor is dependent upon the selection of reliable and valid measurement instruments. Like research, measurement is a process. It involves identifying appropriate measures, or adapting existing measures to your unique research question, or creating new measures. Chapter Nine provides details about measurement issues in health promotion research.

Some variables may be measured directly using a physical instrument (for example, a sphygmomanometer for blood pressure, or a scale for weight), whereas other variables such as level of skill applying a condom to a penile model can be measured directly through observation. In health promotion research most variables are measured indirectly using participants' self-reports (See Chapter Ten for more detail regarding the use of self-report measures). In this case, a mode of administration (for example, paper and pencil, face-to-face interview, or computer-assisted self-interview) must be selected based upon previous knowledge of the research population and the nature of the previously identified research questions.

The process concludes with pilot testing designed to ensure that measures are appropriate for the planned study population. The pilot test also allows researchers to evaluate the psychometric properties of the self-report measures that purport to represent a *construct*. Constructs are defined concepts that would otherwise be considered abstractions. Examples of constructs used in health promotion research include self-esteem, depression, and self-efficacy.

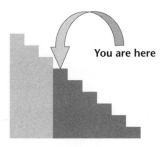

You are here

Step 6: Selecting the Sampling Procedure. As in other aspects of the research enterprise, there are numerous sampling procedures that can be used in health promotion research. Sampling exists across a continuum of complexity and rigor. The sampling procedure employed is one of the most critical determinants of *external validity. External validity* refers to the ability to generalize study findings to the population of individuals with similar characteristics represented in the study sample. It should be noted, however, that not all research studies need to use a sampling procedure that yields high external validity.

Sampling should also include specifying the number of study participants. This number is selected based on a *power analysis*. Stated simply, a power analysis is the estimated ability of a statistical test to find true differences between variables or between groups of study participants. Although a study's power is determined by multiple factors, sample size is one of the most important determinants. Planned sample sizes that provide inadequate power are crippling to the overall study. In the vignette, for example, a power analysis may suggest that each of the three study conditions should have one hundred participants. Having fewer participants in each condition could severely jeopardize the power of the study. More detailed descriptions of sampling procedures are presented in Chapter Eleven.

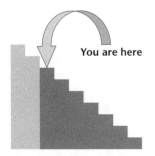

Step 7: Implementing the Research Plan. A basic requirement of *internal validity* is consistency in the implementation of all study protocols. *Internal validity* implies that the study is not confounded by design, measurement, or poor implementation of study procedures. Protocols spell out key procedures such as the sampling procedure to be used, how participants will be assigned to intervention conditions, when and where assessments will occur, who will provide the assessments, what participants will be told or not told about the research study, and how reticent participants will be enticed to return for follow-up programs or assessments. Because protocols are generally quite detailed, subtle departures from these detailed plans can be a common problem. Over time, however, this "drift" can amount to substantial changes in the way late-entry participants are treated as compared with those enrolling earlier in the study.

As an example of drift, consider the study of preventing tobacco dependence outlined in this chapter. The protocol specifies that teens will be "randomly assigned to either (1) the twelve-hour condition, (2) the six-hour condition, or (3) the no-treatment condition. Furthermore, assume that the protocol states that, "random assignment will be achieved by drawing colored marbles from an opaque container. Blue marbles signify assignment to the twelve-hour group, green marbles signify assignment to the six-hour group, and yellow marbles signify assignment to the no-treatment group. One hundred blue, one hundred green, and one hundred yellow marbles are placed in the container as the study begins. A dedicated research assistant has been charged with the implementation of this procedure.

In the first three months of the study, the research assistant performs flawlessly. Subsequently, however, the assistant learns that teens are benefiting from the twelve-hour and six-hour conditions. This perception leads the assistant to invite some teens (those who blindly pulled a yellow marble) to return the marble and "draw again." Repeated over time, this drift can create a systematic bias with respect to the composition of teens assigned to the three conditions.

Other common forms of drift include departure from the planned intervention (perhaps the health educator for the six-hour program develops an "improved" method), deviations in how assessments are administered (perhaps research assistants change the way they perform interviews), and departure from sampling protocols. Fortunately, drift can be averted by vigilant attention to an established set of quality-assurance procedures. Ultimately, then, the principle investigator is the one person who must be accountable for implementing these procedures, thereby ensuring that drift does not occur.

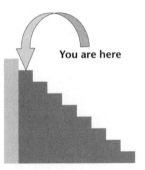

You are here

Step 8: Analyzing the Data. Once all the assessments have been conducted, a data set can be established. The data set consists of the variables measured for each participant. The data set is, of course, quite valuable, as it can subsequently be used to answer the research questions that were formulated in step 2. After the data are checked for logical inconsistencies (called "cleaning"), the research process becomes dependent on the statistical skills of the research team. Again, parsimony is important at this step—the goal is *not* to perform a sophisticated analysis; instead, the goal is to perform an analysis that provides a rigorous and fair test of the research questions while avoiding the introduction of artificially imposed procedures.

In the tobacco-dependence vignette, a parsimonious analysis would be to simply compare the mean number of cigarettes smoked in the past week in each group, assessed at a designated point in time after the interventions have been completed. Suppose the means are (1) 8.3 for the twelve-hour condition, (2) 12.1 for the six-hour condition, and (3) 17.2 for the no-treatment condition. The means can be compared using a very simple test (a one-way analysis of variance), which answers an essential question: Are the differences between means a function of the interventions or are they a function of chance? Analyses, however, can become quite complex when considering logically occurring questions such as: (1) Do intervention effects differ based on gender of the participant? (2) Do effects differ based on age of the participant? (3) Do effects differ based on the baseline assessment of tobacco use? Of course, these questions are vitally important, and each takes the analysis a necessary step farther away from simply comparing means. Chapters Twelve and Thirteen provide a more detailed discussion of data analysis.

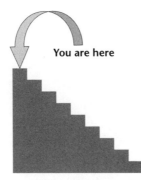

You are here

Step 9: Disseminating the Findings. Rigorous research clearly warrants widespread dissemination. Indeed, this step elevates the project from a work in progress to science. Like each of the previous eight steps shown in this chapter, step 9 is also a process unto itself. The rudimentary starting point in this process is transforming the analytic results (numbers) into carefully articulated findings.

◆ ◆ ◆

In a Nutshell

The rudimentary starting point in this process is transforming the analytic results (numbers) into carefully articulated findings.

◆ ◆ ◆

Findings are answers to the research questions that are generated by the data analysis. Next, the findings must be considered within the context of related research by showing how they strengthen or extend previous work. At this juncture, it is important to know that nonsignificant findings can be just as important

FIGURE 1.2.   SCHEMATIC ILLUSTRATION OF THE NINE-STEP RESEARCH PROCESS.

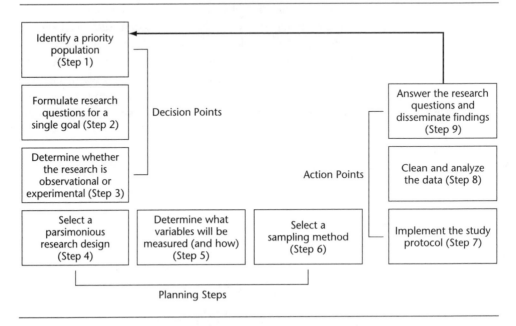

as significant findings with respect to building the research base. The caveat to this statement, however, is that the study should have a high degree of rigor.

Moreover, the findings may raise additional questions that bring the research process back to its origin. Figure 1.2 illustrates this point. Inspection of the figure shows that research is an iterative process. Every time a research question is asked and answered another question (or set of questions) becomes apparent. New researchers should be aware that their research debut (initial entry into this iterative process) is likely to be difficult, but that repeated cycles become progressively less difficult. In fact, this observation may explain why health promotion researchers often tend to specialize in a narrowly defined field of study (such as prevention of adult-onset diabetes, prevention of HIV infection among women, or promoting Pap testing among Latinas).

After the researcher (or research team) has successfully answered the research questions, the remaining task is to prepare written and visual (that is, tables and figures of study results) summaries of the research process (steps 1 through 8). Recall from step 2 that research is a collective process; therefore disseminating the results adds to the larger empirical knowledge base. Fortunately, the preparation of written and visual summaries does not have to be a daunting task. In fact, when rigor is high, this task can be very satisfying and enjoyable. The task is primarily a historical account of the rationale underlying the research questions and the protocols used to answer these questions. Researchers customarily bring the task to a close by suggesting subsequent research questions that could be investigated to further strengthen and expand the research base.

Dissemination of the research findings is widely embraced as a key part of the scientific process. The written and visual records can then be disseminated through multiple channels. Oral presentation of the findings at professional meetings is generally a first step. These presentations create opportunities for informal peer review of the research and study conclusions—peer review is a valued and vital aspect of science. Submission of the written summary to an appropriate professional journal provides opportunity for formal peer review.

◆ ◆ ◆

In a Nutshell

Dissemination of the research findings is widely embraced as a key part of the scientific process.

◆ ◆ ◆

Returning to the vignette, suppose the conclusions have been written and appear as follows:

> In this study of three hundred low-income teens residing in rural, tobacco-producing states, we found that a twelve-hour tobacco-dependence prevention program was equally efficacious compared to a similar program lasting only six hours. The mean number of cigarettes smoked (in one week) for teens in the twelve-hour program and in the six-hour program was significantly lower relative to the number of cigarettes smoked by teens who did not receive either program. Findings suggest that these small-group interventions may be an important strategy for interrupting the formation of tobacco dependence among members of the study population. Further research should continue to investigate the efficacy of this program among teens residing in largely metropolitan states.

Peer review may help identify the strengths and weaknesses of the study and its conclusions. For example, a reviewer might ask, "Do the results truly indicate interruption of dependence?" Another reviewer might ask, "How were rural, tobacco-producing states defined?" Questions derived from the peer-review process can help researchers identify the limitations of the study and its contribution to the health promotion literature base.

When steps 1 through 8 have been thoroughly addressed, and the peer-review process has been successfully navigated, the final product will generally take the form of a published journal article (Chapter Fourteen provides more details related to the publishing of research findings). In health promotion, however, publication of a journal article is *not* the endpoint in the research process. At least two other obligations exist. First, media relations should be cultivated and used to disseminate findings to the public. Second, successful health promotion programs should be made widely available. The process of translating science into practice is ongoing and labor intensive, but is also the cornerstone of health promotion practice.

◆ ◆ ◆

In a Nutshell

The process of translating science into practice is ongoing and labor intensive, but is also the cornerstone of health promotion practice.

◆ ◆ ◆

The Context of Health Promotion Research

The research process occurs in a context characterized by scholarship, grantsmanship, and vigilant attention to ethics. These three principles are highly valued and cherished in the profession. Scholarship implies that the researcher possesses an inherent curiosity regarding the research questions and a dedication to expanding the knowledge base in health promotion. Integrity is a key feature of scholarship. Like rigor in the research process, integrity in the researcher ensures a fair test of the research questions. Integrity implies that any preconceived desire to prove or disprove study hypotheses is not allowed to interfere with the research process. The research process is quite eloquent in that it forces objectivity; however, adherence to the process is based on self-report of the researcher (making integrity vital).

Grantsmanship is also a vital part of the research process. Rigor is often expensive, and obtaining funds for health promotion research is typically a competitive process. In addition to other factors (for example, quality of the research proposal, the importance of the topic and the population, and so on), grant awards, to some extent, are given based on the current degree of engagement in the iterative process shown in Figure 1.2.

Vigilant attention to ethics is the most critical of the three concerns briefly described here (see Chapter Three). Just as practitioners of medicine take the Hippocratic Oath, health promotion researchers must adopt the principle, "First, do no harm." Moreover, health promotion research is highly regulated by local and federal organizations that protect the rights of research participants. The nature of health promotion research demands studies of humans, and these studies are oftentimes directed at very personal (and therefore protected) behaviors.

Applied Example

A study published in the *American Journal of Public Health* provides a good illustration of the nine-step model. Hagan and colleagues (2001) selected a priority population for the prevention of infection with hepatitis C: injection drug users (step 1). Their research question was firmly grounded in the context of previous research. They noted that shared use of drug preparation equipment, in the absence of self-injection with a used syringe, had not been investigated as a source of transmission for the hepatitis C virus (HCV). Their primary research question was to assess the risk of HCV infection incurred by sharing cookers, cotton filters, and water used to rinse drug-injection syringes (step 2).

The study was strictly observational (step 3). A panel study design (with a one-year follow-up) was used. This design is relatively advanced with respect to its location on the trajectory of research shown in Figure 1.1. Only persons initially testing negative for HCV were included in the study. This approach allowed the investigators to compare drug equipment sharing behavior—in the ensuing year—between those who tested positive (seroconverted) and those who tested negative for HCV at the one-year follow-up assessment (step 4). Selected variables included the assessment of race, age, sex, homelessness, sexual behaviors, types of drugs injected, and a battery of measures related to drug equipment sharing behaviors. HCV was assessed through a reliable and valid blood assay (step 5).

The sample comprised a subset of 507 people who were drawn from a larger sample of injection drug users from nine locations in Seattle, Washington. At each location, a random-numbers table was used to select a representative portion of eligible participants (step 6). Unfortunately, procedures used for quality assurance of the data-collection process were not described (step 7). Data were analyzed separately for persons who reported injecting with previously used syringes and those not reporting this form of risk. Among those reporting this risk, persons sharing cookers or cotton were 3.8 times more likely to acquire HCV over the observation period of one year. This difference was significant (that is, not attributable to chance). Significant differences with respect to shared cleaning water were not observed (step 8).

The research team concluded by suggesting that HCV infection may be commonly transmitted by sharing cookers and filtration cotton. This conclusion squarely addressed the research question and provided a valuable extension to the research base. The high degree of rigor, combined with an important research question, yielded findings that contributed to health promotion practice (the initial portion of step 9). From a practice perspective, the finding suggests that injection drug users can benefit from health education efforts that create awareness of HCV risk as a consequence of cooker and cotton sharing. Dissemination of the written report in the *American Journal of Public Health* made this information available to thousands of journal subscribers, untold numbers of media organizations, and (via electronic posting on engines such as Medline) to most anyone with access to the Internet (step 9).

Summary

Health promotion practice and policy should be based on rigorous research. This chapter has provided a thumbnail sketch of the research process as it applies to health promotion. This sketch can be used as a platform to gain competence and proficiency in each of the nine steps described. Competence and proficiency in scholarship, grantsmanship, and ethics should be an equally high priority. The remainder of this volume is devoted to expanding this thumbnail sketch into a more complete primer of health promotion research methods.

Issues to Consider

1. An overriding issue is whether health promotion practice should always be grounded in research. Consider, for example, the emergence of the AIDS epidemic in the United States. By the mid-1980s, the rapid escalation of HIV infection demanded an immediate and escalated public health response (Garrett, 1994). Unfortunately, from a health promotion perspective, research chains specifically pertaining to behavioral intervention of HIV transmission had barely begun to form. In lieu of best practices based on research findings, health promotion programs were created to increase awareness of risk and provide people with essential prevention messages. In retrospect, the efficacy of these initial approaches to prevention may be questionable. Alternatively, the urgency of the epidemic demanded a response. An unfortunate reality of the research process is that it moves slowly. Given the inherent urgency, then, should practice perhaps sometimes proceed without research?

2. The research process as described in this chapter is designed to create objectivity in the investigation of any given research question. Suppose that a study high in rigor (and therefore objectivity) is funded by a drug company (Company Y). The study investigates behavioral compliance with an arthritis medication that typically caused temporary side effects. Furthermore, suppose that the findings indicates that compliance was extremely low due to a nearly universal physical intolerance among study participants for the drug. The research team proceeds to step 9 and is informed by Company Y that dissemination should not occur. Considering the principles of scholarship and ethics, how should the research team respond?

3. The term "publication bias" has often been used to describe a tendency of journals to preferentially accept research reports that find significant results (meaning the data supported a proposition that can add to the quality of health promotion practice). Conversely, studies with nonsignificant findings only provide insight on "things that won't work"; thus, these studies may be less attractive for publication. While nonsignificant findings are admittedly less exciting, they may nonetheless be based on important research questions and stem from rigorously conducted research. Yet, despite a high degree of importance and rigor, nonsignificant findings have very little practical meaning for anyone other than persons investigating questions in the same research chain. How can this seemingly irresolvable problem be addressed?

For Practice and Discussion

A philanthropic organization has asked you to design and conduct a study that can benefit the health of women by promoting regular Pap testing and annual mammography among post-menopausal women. After reviewing the surveillance data relevant to cervical cancer and breast cancer, you conclude that Hispanic women are a priority population for intervention (step 1). Next you develop a single but important research question: What are the cultural and economic barriers that preclude post-menopausal Hispanic women from receiving regular Pap tests and annual mammograms? (step 2). Having resolved steps 1 and 2, you begin to think about the planning phase of the study. Thus, you consider steps 4, 5, and 6. Please think each of these steps through carefully and create a rigorous plan to investigate this research question (if you have trouble with this, please try the exercise again after you have read the remaining chapters in this book).

References

Department of Health and Human Services. (2000). *Healthy people 2010.* Available on-line at
www.health.gov/healthypeople. Accessed June 30, 2001.

Garrett, L. (1994). *The coming plague: Newly emerging diseases in a world out of balance.* New York:
Farrar, Straus, and Giroux.

Glasgow, R. E., Vogt, T. M., and Boles, S. M. (1999). Evaluating the public health impact of
health promotion interventions: The RE-AIM framework. *American Journal of Public Health,
89,* 1322–1327.

Green, L. W., and Kreuter, M. W. (2005). *Health program planning: An educational and ecological
approach* (4th ed.). Boston: McGraw Hill.

Hagan, H., Thiede, H., Weiss, N. S., Hopkin, S. G., Duchin, J. S., and Alexander, E. R.
(2001). Sharing of drug preparation equipment as a risk factor for hepatitis C. *American
Journal of Public Health, 91,* 42–45.

Murray, D. M. (1998). *Design and analysis of group randomized trials.* New York: Oxford
University Press.

Smedley, B. D., and Syme, S. L. (Eds.). (2000). *Promoting health: Intervention strategies from social
and behavioral research.* Washington, DC: National Academy Press.

CHAPTER TWO

PHILOSOPHY OF SCIENCE AND THEORY CONSTRUCTION

Laura F. Salazar, Ralph J. DiClemente, and Richard A. Crosby

Health promotion research, in general, comprises some or all of the nine steps that were delineated in Chapter One and that are undertaken to investigate health-related behaviors. The overarching goal is to understand better ways in which we can influence health behaviors and ultimately health by first identifying the behavioral risk factors for a particular disease. By first understanding and then affecting behaviors that contribute to health, health promotion researchers can have a substantive impact on the associated morbidity and mortality. When conceptualizing and undertaking health promotion research, however, in addition to knowing the research process, it is also important to understand the underlying philosophy.

Derived from the Latin word *scientia*, the literal meaning of *science* is knowledge. Yet, science can also be viewed as a process. The process entails the systematic gathering of seemingly disparate facts and then organizing them into an interconnected whole. Science is the process of acquiring knowledge for the purpose of having knowledge. Why is science important, and why do we hold science in such reverence? Because science is knowledge, and knowledge is the source of empowerment. Creating a body of knowledge regarding myriad subjects such as the properties of matter and energy (physics), the structure of matter (chemistry), living organisms (biology), human behavior (psychology), or human societies (sociology), to name a few scientific disciplines, can benefit greatly the human experience and provide insight into how nature works and how we as human beings function within nature and with each other. Think of science as an indispensable tool much like the wheel that can take us where we want to go by aiding us in our understanding of, and in our attempt to control, our environment.

◆ ◆ ◆

In a Nutshell

Derived from the Latin word scientia, *the literal meaning of* science *is knowledge. Yet, science can also be viewed as a process. The process entails the systematic gathering of seemingly disparate facts and then organizing them into an interconnected whole.*

◆ ◆ ◆

Health promotion research also involves a process. In Chapter One, we referred to this as a discovery process. Interestingly, if health promotion research is the process through which knowledge on health-related behaviors is "discovered," and science equals knowledge, then health promotion research must be considered a science, right? To answer this question fully and accurately, we first provide an overview of what constitutes science and describe key concepts from its related discipline—the philosophy of science. Philosophy is from the Greek word *philosophia*, meaning love (*philo*) and the pursuit of knowledge (*sophia*). Philosophy of science, therefore, pertains to the structure, principles, and components of the scientific process—the framework lovingly used for the pursuit of knowledge.

Another important and related term used often when discussing the philosophy of science is *epistemology*. Epistemology is the branch of philosophy that studies knowledge and attempts to answer the basic question: what distinguishes true (adequate) knowledge from false (inadequate) knowledge? There are different ways of acquiring knowledge, some of which will be described in more detail later in this chapter. As a health promotion practitioner or researcher you may be called upon to evaluate different types of health information. Learning to distinguish valid health-related information from false information will be an important skill.

Illustration of Key Concepts

The goals of this chapter are to introduce the various epistemological positions taken in pursuit of knowledge, such as authority, tenacity, logic, and, of course, scientific inquiry. Once you have built a solid foundation in epistemology, you may then be in the position to ascertain whether or not specific instances of health promotion research constitute science. Of course, you will also be able to ascertain whether other field's inquiries can be considered science, "junk science," or neither. Consequently, you will also acquire insight about how science generates knowledge.

Epistemology: Ways of Acquiring Knowledge

Given that science is a process in which we gather knowledge and organize that knowledge systematically, does the way or method in which the knowledge is collected determine whether or not the process can be called science? The way in which knowledge is generated determines whether or not it should be deemed science and therefore added to an overall scientific body of knowledge. Just because an effort is conducted "in the name of science" does not necessarily make it science. Second, although *science* literally means knowledge, in the modern sense it refers more to a specific process that adheres to standards and methods of generating knowledge. Thus, it matters greatly indeed, for there are many different ways in which we come by our knowledge regarding the world. Some ways in which we gather knowledge may contribute to science, whereas other ways may appear to be scientific, but, in reality, are not considered science in the technical sense. Regardless of the method, knowledge is conveyed (although it may vary in value). Thus, not all knowledge is created equal. It is most important to know the different ways or methods in which we accrue knowledge so that the quality of the knowledge can be judged appropriately and the implications for choosing one method over another can be determined.

In the following section, we describe various ways of knowing such as authority, tenacity (sometimes called tradition), and logic and reason, which are not considered as science in the modern sense, but nevertheless provide new ideas and suggestions. In addition, we describe scientific inquiry as a way of knowing. The former methods (authority, tenacity, and logic) are ways in which knowledge is derived, so they are important to know. By understanding these alternative epistemologies you will better understand science. Consequently, you may embrace scientific inquiry as the most important way of knowing. As you will see, these ways must be evaluated rather subjectively and contrast sharply with scientific inquiry as a way of knowing because science is able to provide both a body of knowledge and a specific method in which to evaluate that knowledge.

Unfortunately, in some instances, science may not have yet contributed to a specific research goal and thus may not be an available source of knowledge. For example, in the early 1980s before the HIV virus was discovered, researchers did not know what caused the decline in the immune system condition (AIDS) or how it was being transmitted. The other ways of knowing (authority, tenacity, and logic) were the only sources of knowledge available. In essence, scientific inquiry is the only epistemology that requires data-driven conclusions. Other epistemologies exist regardless of whether data are available or whether people choose to consider the data. The challenge in those instances is to examine the underlying source of the knowledge and make the best determination regarding its accuracy.

Authority. Albert Einstein dubbed Galileo "the father of modern physics— indeed of modern science altogether" (Sobel, 1999, p. 326). Most everyone is familiar with the historical account of the renowned mathematician and scientist Galileo and his quest to advance the field of science, which up to that point in history was based mostly on the philosophy of Aristotle. Galileo sought to move beyond an understanding of why *phenomena* occur to how they occur. By phenomena, we mean events or circumstances evident to the senses and possible to describe scientifically. For Galileo, mathematics was one of his scientific tools:

> "Philosophy is written in this grand book the universe, which stands continually open to our gaze. But the book cannot be understood unless one first learns to comprehend the language and to read the alphabet in which it is composed. It is written in the language of mathematics, and its characters are triangles, circles, and other geometric figures, without which it is humanly impossible to understand a single word of it; without these, one wanders about in a dark labyrinth" [quoted in Drake, 1957, p. 237].

Although most scientists concur that Galileo's greatest contribution to science is his application of mathematics to the study of motion, he has been immortalized for his defense of Copernicus's theory that posited the sun rather than the Earth is the center of the cosmos. This sun-as-center-of-the-universe perspective was not only contrary to the Aristotelian perspective (that is, the Earth is the center of the cosmos), but more important, it contradicted the teachings and beliefs espoused by the Catholic Church. Interestingly, the Church also based its views on the Aristotelian perspective.

During this period in history, the Catholic Church was the moral and philosophical authority. If the Catholic Church said it was so, then most people accepted it for fact. Most people did not understand the order of the universe at this time. Thus, it was easier for people to defer to some authority, one who held some degree of knowledge regarding an issue. People during this era mostly obtained their knowledge through authority because there were not many other sources. This approach has a major shortcoming, however; the authority in question can be wrong, as was the case with the Church. Unfortunately, because Galileo went against the most powerful authority of his time, he was tried by the Church in front of the Inquisition. Because he would not recant his beliefs, he was sentenced to life imprisonment, which was later reduced to house arrest (Sobel, 1999).

In his search for knowledge Galileo truly believed that, "the authority of a thousand is not worth the humble reasoning of a single individual" (Redondi, 1987, p. 37). Even in our modern times, this quote should still apply. Yet, many of us still rely upon authority for facts and guidance. For example, many of us look up to our religious leaders as well as our politicians, physicians, and professors. Reliance on authority is not always problematic. Yet, not taking the time to evaluate the validity of an authority's ideas, suggestions, or comments may be problematic. Of course, an evaluation of the knowledge would require knowing what evidence (if any) the authority is using. For example, when a politician describes our current state of the union, we must consider whether or not the description is based on scientific evidence (such as gathering of key economic indicators, scientific surveys, archival data, and so on) or on anecdotal evidence from a few people, or, even worse, is not based on any evidence but is simply rhetoric. Furthermore, when a physician instructs someone to drink eight eight-ounce glasses of water per day, the person can ask if this recommendation is based on scientific evidence or if the recommendation is based on tenacity with no real basis (see Box 2.1, which describes an investigation into the origins of the health recommendation to drink eight glasses of water per day). Even with your professors (including the one teaching this course), you should question knowledge presented in class and inquire about the epistemology. These are only a few ways in which

Box 2.1. The "8 × 8" Recommendation

Valtin (2002) conducted a review of the scientific literature to determine the origin of the advice to "drink at least eight eight-ounce glasses of water per day." He found no scientific studies in support of the "8 × 8" health belief, and he could not find its origins in the scientific literature. In fact, he found evidence to suggest that such large amounts of water are not necessary in *healthy* adults, who live in temperate climates and are largely sedentary. Moreover, his review of a large body of related research suggested that the human body's osmoregulatory system maintains water balance naturally. Thus, it would appear that the ubiquitous "8 × 8" water recommendation is without scientific merit, but persists as a modern myth that is viewed as medically beneficial.

MINCUS TAKES DR. DINCUS'S ADVICE FOR GOOD HEALTH.

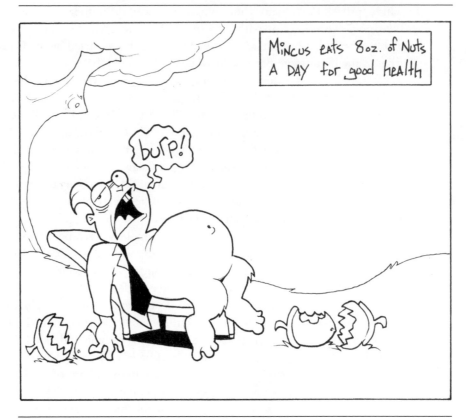

Copyright 2005 by Justin Wagner; reprinted with permission.

to question authority, but as health promotion researchers and purveyors of knowledge, you should learn to question the knowledge that is presented to you. Moreover, you have an obligation to employ scientific inquiry regardless of the prevailing epistemologies. As with Galileo, however, your research may not be popular or readily accepted by society. Yet, as Albert Einstein stated, "A foolish faith in authority is the worst enemy of truth" (quoted in Calaprice, 2000, p. 303).

Tenacity or Tradition. Even in this postmodern age of technology, it is interesting that many health beliefs that have been around for a very long time and are sometimes referred to as "wives' tales" remain firmly entrenched in our minds and culture and continue to influence our health behaviors. For example, were you told that it is dangerous to swim unless you wait an hour after eating? Were you scolded for going outside as a child with wet hair because it would cause you to catch a cold? Did your mother stress to you that you should eat all of your carrots because it will improve your eyesight? Or certainly you have heard the expression, "an apple a day helps keep the doctor away"? Do you still believe that chocolate causes acne? Are you familiar with the notion that oysters are an aphrodisiac? Many young women maintain that they cannot get pregnant while breast-feeding or the very first time they have vaginal intercourse. A more recent health belief that has become somewhat entrenched in modern society is that the flu vaccine will cause you to get the flu. Not surprising, some of these health beliefs may be rooted in truth, which may explain their longevity. For example, eating vegetables high in vitamin A (for example, carrots) is good for maintaining healthy eyesight; however, more than the recommended daily requirement will not improve your eyesight. What is surprising is that some of these health beliefs continue to persist despite the fact they have been proven false—hence the term *tenacity.* For example, many people still believe that going out in cold weather with wet hair will cause them to catch a cold, even though science has shown it is exposure to a virus that causes a cold.

Why do these beliefs persist even though they are false? Many of these beliefs have been handed down from one generation to the next through storytelling, through printed material, and presently through other forms of media. For many cultures, these beliefs become their traditions, and as traditions they tend to provide people with an acceptable way of exerting control over certain unavoidable events. Thus, accepting traditional beliefs as a way of knowing at a very basic level may serve to help people understand and exert control over their environment.

Health beliefs based on tradition, whether true or not, may also contribute to the cohesiveness of a cultural group. For example, unified cultures are grounded in their acceptance of similar beliefs and traditions. It is for these reasons that there may be problems with using only tenacity as a valid way of knowing: if the beliefs are erroneous, then there will be great difficulty in changing or discrediting them once they have been accepted widely and are entrenched within a culture. It may be useful for you to think about different health beliefs you have accepted and consider whether or not they are based on tradition, evidence, or truth.

Logic and Reasoning. The term *logic* is derived from the Greek word *logos,* which traditionally means "word," "thought," "principle," or "speech." *Logos* has been used among both philosophers and theologians and embodies both human reason (that is, intellect, capacity to discern and distinguish) and universal intelligence (that is, the Divine). Although philosophers are undoubtedly concerned with both

aspects of *logos,* as health promotion researchers we are concerned mainly
with the human-reason aspect for this construct. Reason, along with its cousin
term *logic,* is the foundation of philosophy and is still in use today as a way of
knowing.

In modern terms, *logic* can be defined as the science of reasoning, proof, thinking, or inference. Logic is useful in that it allows you to analyze arguments or a
piece of reasoning and determine whether or not they are accurate or "illogical."
Although logic is considered a science, knowing the basics of logic and reasoning can assist you in spotting which arguments are invalid and which conclusions are false.

As previously stated, the Catholic Church based much of its beliefs and knowledge on another authority—Aristotle. Because Aristotle concerned himself with
the investigation of natural phenomena, he was able to make many observations
about the world. He then used logic and reasoning to define, analyze, and sys-
tematize his observations to make sense of what he observed. Logic and reasoning were his tools; thus, in the absence of science, logic and reasoning were the
accepted standards of the time.

Specifically, Aristotle used an approach called a *syllogism,* which means an
argument of a very specific form consisting of two premises and a conclusion, to
amass his knowledge. Generating knowledge regarding the Earth and the cosmos,
Aristotle used the following syllogism:

> Again, everything that moves with the circular movement, except the first
> sphere, is observed to be passed, and to move with more than one motion. The
> earth, then, also, whether it move about the centre or as stationary at it, must
> necessarily move with two motions. But if this were so, there would have to be
> passings and turnings of the fixed stars. Yet no such thing is observed. The
> same stars always rise and set in the same parts of the earth [Aristotle, 350 B.C.
> (2004), part 14, paragraph 1].

Using this syllogism, Aristotle concluded that "the earth, spherical in shape, is at
rest in the centre of the universe" (Aristotle, 350 B.C. (2004), part 14, paragraph 4).
Of course, it was later ascertained that Aristotle's conclusion was inaccurate.
His syllogism contained a *fallacy.* In logic, the term *fallacy* has a very specific meaning: a fallacy is a technical flaw which makes an argument unsound or invalid.
In this instance, the premises of Aristotle's argument were not true. Although
his conclusion was sound, it was based on false premises and was therefore false.
There are many other types of fallacies that occur quite frequently, such as a fallacy
called *cum hoc ergo propter hoc* ("with this, therefore because of this"), which is to assert

that because two events occur together, they must be causally related. An example for this type of fallacy would be

Teenagers eat a lot of chocolate.

Teenagers have acne.

Therefore, eating chocolate causes acne.

Another fallacy is called *converse accident* or *hasty generalization* and is the reverse of the fallacy of *accident*. The former occurs when you generalize to an entire group based on a few specific cases, which aren't representative of all possible cases. For example, "Professor Dincus is eccentric. Therefore all professors are eccentric."

The latter fallacy (accident) is also referred to as a sweeping generalization and occurs when a general rule is applied to a particular situation, but the features of that particular situation mean an exception to the rule should be made. For example, "College students generally like junk food. *You* are a college student, so you must like junk food." Finally, one last fallacy is called *post hoc ergo propter hoc* (after this, therefore because of this), which occurs when a cause-and-effect relationship is assumed because one factor occurred temporally before the other factor. For example, "After receiving his flu vaccine, Rick came down with the flu. Therefore, we must avoid the flu vaccine because it *caused* him to get the flu."

In present times, people still rely upon information that is derived from logic and reasoning, especially if there are not alternative ways of knowing. Yet, much information derived from logic and reasoning is based on arguments that may contain fallacies. Another issue with this way of knowing is that arguments cannot determine whether a statement is correct. Thus, as a way of knowing, logic and reasoning are useful but only if the arguments presented do not contain fallacies and if there are alternative ways to verify the conclusions. The challenge is to critique any arguments or information presented to you and to attempt to uncover any fallacies.

Scientific Inquiry as Epistemology

Scientific inquiry or research is conducted as a means to test ideas, to evaluate questions, and to determine how things work. Generally speaking, the goal is to generate knowledge regarding the nature of our universe. The nature of our universe can range from knowing and understanding weather patterns to knowing and understanding people's exercise patterns. Scientific inquiry is simply another way of knowing, but as you will discover, it is quite different from the other epistemologies that were described previously. For one thing, "research is a disciplined way we come to know what we know" (Bouma and Atkinson, 1995, p. 9). It involves a process as described in Chapter One, but it also posits certain structures or components to that process. Concepts and structures such as *empiricism, data, theory, hypothetico-deductivism,* and *falsification* are the main building blocks of scientific inquiry and constitute the foundation of modern science. Furthermore, it is because of these concepts and structures that scientific inquiry as an epistemology is considered more reliable and valid than other methods of inquiry.

◆ ◆ ◆

In a Nutshell

Concepts and structures such as empiricism, data, theory, hypothetico-deductivism, *and* falsification *are the main building blocks of scientific inquiry and constitute the foundation of modern science.*

◆ ◆ ◆

Empiricism. From its inception, science began as a process that was viewed as objective and *empirical.* From the Greek word *emperirikós* meaning experienced or skilled, empirical is a concept that denotes observation and experimentation and is therefore linked literally to the concept of scientific inquiry. Moreover, the term *empiricism* represents the philosophical position that true knowledge is a product of sensory perceptions gleaned from observation. The strength of adopting this position is that many important research questions can be answered objectively through the collection of empirical *data.*

Data. Data are essentially concrete facts, records, or collections of information regarding some aspect of our universe that take on meaning when applied to a research question. Data are plural; datum is singular. For example, does Brand X cholesterol-lowering drug reduce LDL cholesterol more effectively than Brand Y drug? is a research question for which there is an answer that can be derived from empirical data. In this instance, empirical data collected to answer this question are the LDL cholesterol levels of people before taking the drugs and after taking the drugs. A limitation of adopting empiricism is that some questions cannot be answered in this manner because the answers cannot be derived from empirical data. For example, is Brand X cholesterol drug's name better than Brand Y cholesterol drug's name? is a question for which there is not empirical data available. Of course, we could modify the question into an empirical question by asking, do women aged forty-five to seventy-five who have high cholesterol judge

Brand X's name to be better than Brand Y's name? We could then survey women in this age category who have high cholesterol and ask them which name they prefer. The survey responses would constitute the empirical data. Thus, when conducting research to answer a health-related question, it is critical that the research question is constructed so that it is an empirical question from the beginning.

◆ ◆ ◆

In a Nutshell

Data are essentially concrete facts, records, or collections of information regarding some aspect of our universe that take on meaning when applied to a research question. Data are plural; datum is singular.

◆ ◆ ◆

Theory. If science were a movie, then theory would be the screenplay. No matter how talented the actors are, a good screenplay is still necessary to provide the framework in which the actors showcase their talents. Without the screenplay, they are simply improvising. For some talented actors, improvisation may work; however, for the majority of actors, a cohesive and intriguing plot coupled with realistic dialogue is critical. In science, theories play a major role as well because they provide an understanding of phenomena. In other words, they organize relationships among "characters" (that is, observations) into a coherent picture of what it all means. They provide a starting point for making future predictions as well. Furthermore, theories guide the research question.

◆ ◆ ◆

In a Nutshell

If science were a movie, then theory would be the screenplay.

◆ ◆ ◆

What exactly constitutes a scientific theory? How are theories generated? And how does a theory contrast with a hypothesis? Many people use the term *theory* interchangeably with *hypothesis,* and you will read instances in textbooks and research articles that use *theory* when they mean *hypothesis;* however, theory expands upon simple hypotheses and considers sets of relationships. *Hypotheses* are statements that specify the nature of the relationships between variables, whereas a *theory* is much more involved and provides order and structure to sets of relationships. For example, "obesity is related to increased risk of breast cancer among postmenopausal women" is a hypothesis that could be tested by comparing incidence of breast cancer among postmenopausal women who are not obese to incidence among postmenopausal women who are obese. A theory, however, would account for differences in breast cancer rates by describing the causative interaction of physiological, environmental, and psychological variables.

It is important to note that the phenomena involved in a theory must also be verifiable, meaning we can measure them or observe them either directly or indirectly. Once phenomena are measured or observed, understanding them translates into two types of theoretical explanations: *phenomenological* and *explanatory*. Phenomenological is when the phenomena are described and generalized, but without specific reference to causal mechanisms. In contrast, an explanatory theory identifies and explains the underling causal mechanisms.

Most theories used in health promotion research are phenomenological theories that specify which variables are involved in health-related behaviors and how the various variables interact to determine the behavior. For example, the Health Belief Model (HBM) is a theory of behavior developed in the 1950s by a group of social psychologists who wanted to better understand the widespread failure of people to participate in programs to prevent or to detect disease (Janz, Champion, and Strecher, 2002). The HBM is depicted in Figure 2.1 and posits that three major components, individual perceptions, modifying factors, and likelihood of action influence behavior. The HBM has been applied to the understanding of health behaviors where much research has generated support for the theory. Such behaviors include flu inoculations, breast self-examination, high blood pressure screening, seatbelt use, exercise, nutrition, smoking, and regular checkups. Other types of behavior that have been tested also include compliance with drug regimens, diabetic regimens, and weight loss regimens.

Given the critical role of theory in science, how are theories generated initially before they are widely implemented? In the case of the HBM, the theory grew out of the academic backgrounds of the theorists and the other theories to which they were exposed. Although there are several strategies for developing theories, such as intuition, previous knowledge, and personal observation, only two main strategies will be described in this section: *Baconian Inductivism* and *hypothetico-deductivism*. Both methods were conceptualized centuries ago and are still in use today. Each has its own strengths and weaknesses, but determining which method to use depends greatly on the domain or scope in which the theory will apply.

If Galileo was the father of modern science, Francis Bacon (1561–1626) was its champion. During the time Galileo was honing new methods to study

FIGURE 2.1.   HEALTH BELIEF MODEL COMPONENTS AND LINKAGES.

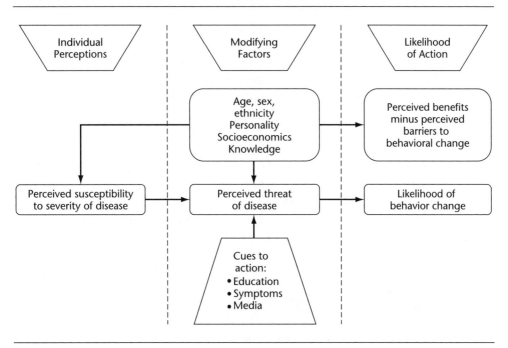

phenomena, Francis Bacon was a philosopher (among other professions) who "proposed an entirely new system based on empirical and inductive principles and the active development of new arts and inventions, a system whose ultimate goal would be the production of practical knowledge for 'the use and benefit of men' and the relief of the human condition" (Internet Encyclopedia of Philosophy, n.d., paragraph 1). His system or method was later called Baconian Inductivism, and it comprised four steps:

- Observation and classification of relevant facts
- Generalization by means of inductive reasoning
- Construction of a theoretical framework that allows one to deduce predictions from its laws and postulates
- Verification of the predictions

Although much improved over other nonscientific methods for generating knowledge, Baconian Inductivism has two major flaws: it cannot be used to derive theories regarding phenomena that are unobservable (for example, gravity), and its validity depends on a large number of observations under varying conditions.

Consequently, it did not emerge as an accepted standard for conducting scientific research and was not embraced widely. In certain instances, however, there may be no other alternative. For example, in the beginning stage of the U.S. AIDS epidemic, two physicians in Los Angeles observed that typically harmless opportunistic bacterial and viral infections among several young, gay male patients were making them extremely sick. Simultaneously, other similar observations were being noted among young, gay men in other cities. It was the emergence of these early anomalous observations that prompted scientists to convene and infer that a serious health issue was looming. From these early irregular observations general hypotheses emerged to explain these data. (See Box 2.2, which describes the various hypotheses that emerged from the data collected during the onset of the AIDS epidemic in the early 1980s.) Of course, many of the early hypotheses were flawed because they were based on a small number of observations and did not consider other varying conditions (e.g., observations from people who contracted the syndrome and were not gay).

Box 2.2. Early AIDS Hypotheses

In the beginning of the epidemic, AIDS was referred to as GRID—Gay-related immunodeficiency disease. The name was not changed to Acquired Immune Deficiency Syndrome until 1982. These are some of the early AIDS "theories" (which actually should be viewed as hypotheses) that were inferred from the available data (Garrett, 1994).

- A virus called "cytomegalovirus" or "CMV superinfection" is the root, where repeated exposures to the virus result in the deadly syndrome.
- Gay men have been exposed to too many microbes and have "microbial overload," causing the immune system to self-destruct.
- The recreation drug called "poppers" (amyl nitrites) plays a critical role in the deadly syndrome along with other gay lifestyle practices such as "fisting," "rimming," or steroid skin creams.
- AIDS is caused by some new variety of the HTLV virus, the virus that causes immune system disruptions and cancer.
- AIDS is an opportunistic infection causing disease only in persons who are already immuno-compromised from other microbes or conditions.
- AIDS is a new manifestation of the hepatitis B virus.
- AIDS is caused by an unknown contaminant of the hepatitis vaccine (early experimental trials of the vaccine had been conducted with gay men).
- AIDS is caused by African swine fever.

Following Bacon in the late 1600s, Sir Isaac Newton (1642–1727) developed a scientific method later termed "hypothetico-deductivism," which was essentially the opposite of Baconian Inductivism. His method entailed beginning with a hypothesis or statement of general principles and then subsequently using deduction to make predictions for a specific event. The predictions could be tested through empirical observation and verified. If the hypothesis is not verified then, it may be modified or rejected.

The strength of hypothetico-deductivism lies in the ability to test any hypothesis and confirm its validity through empirical observation. For example, using this method, Newton was able to test his theory of gravitation. Newton used his theory of gravitation to guide him in deducing specific predictions for which he was then able to make observations that supported or verified his theory. Thus, as a method, hypothetico-deductivism was much improved over inductivism and emerged as the new method for generating reliable and valid knowledge.

However, hypothetico-deductivisim is not without its problems. Research conducted with the main purpose of confirming a theory may, over time, become irrelevant as the theory is modified and perhaps rejected. Moreover, a set of data cannot irrevocably confirm or prove that a theory is valid because different theories can be supported by the same set of data.

◆ ◆ ◆

In a Nutshell

Research conducted with the main purpose of confirming a theory may, over time, become irrelevant as the theory is modified and perhaps rejected. Moreover, a set of data cannot irrevocably confirm or prove that a theory is valid because different theories can be supported by the same set of data.

◆ ◆ ◆

Falsification. Sir Karl Popper (1902–1994), considered one of the most influential twentieth-century philosophers of science, asserted that for a theory to be science, a necessary condition is that the theory consist of hypotheses that could be falsified. According to Popper, *falsification* is the best approach for testing scientific theories and contrasts sharply with the verification approach. The theory must be organized in a way such that its assertions can be refuted. This necessity for a scientific theory to be falsifiable is known as the *demarcation criterion*. Advocating the use of falsifiability as a scientific method to test theories, Popper therefore rejected inductivism, because falsification dictates that you must begin with falsifiable hypotheses before observations are made. Then, you collect data to refute them—not verify them. As noted earlier, it is easy for the same set of data to support or verify many different theories simultaneously. Thus, falsification provides more rigor and confidence in the conclusions.

Integration with the Research Process

Integrating the research process with these underlying scientific principles will provide a better understanding of health phenomena. To accomplish this integration, health promotion research should undertake the nine steps delineated in Chapter One while interjecting scientific structure to those steps. For example, theory should be used to aide in the development of the research question (step 2) and in the choice of variables to be measured (step 5). The research questions should be empirical questions formulated from theory and falsifiable. Moreover, the research design should allow for the falsification of the proposed hypotheses (step 4). The variables chosen also have to allow for empirical measurement. And finally, data analysis (step 8) should go beyond whether or not the data confirm or support the hypotheses to include the falsification of hypotheses. If the research process incorporates these scientific principles, then health promotion as a field will continue to expand and garner the respect of a true scientific discipline.

Summary

Over the centuries, science has revolutionized its sources of knowledge, moving from authority, tenacity, and logic and reason to an elegant arrangement encompassing principles of empiricism, data, theory, deduction, and falsification. As science is considered a process that aids in our understanding of our world, throughout time, numerous scientific disciplines pertaining to specific aspects of our world have emerged. Health promotion can be considered one of the more modern scientific disciplines, but only if it adheres to sound scientific principles. In this chapter, we reviewed the philosophy of science from its origins to better understand the underlying concepts and the importance of science to health promotion research. We noted that one of the most critical scientific principles is the generation and rigorous testing of theory. As health promotion researchers investigating health-related behaviors, most of what we do should be grounded in theory. Theory constitutes the basic structure of our scientific inquiries for two reasons: theory guides the design of basic research studies and theory can be used to design a health promotion program that targets risk factors deemed modifiable and that are related to health-related outcomes.

Issues to Consider

1. In 2001, the Department of Health and Human Services assembled a panel of experts to determine whether condoms are effective in protecting against sexually transmitted diseases. Their conclusion was that the evidence was generally insufficient to support condom effectiveness. The Centers for Disease Control later retracted their fact sheet about condoms from their Website. What are the epistemologies that apply here?

2. Because behavior cannot be isolated (like a pathogen) to determine its causes, what are some scientific issues to consider when generating theories of behavior? Also, given that human behavior, especially health-related behaviors, is complex and multifaceted, how confident would you be in attributing a specific cause to a specific behavior such as smoking?

3. A theory in the scientific sense goes beyond simple hypotheses and provides order and structure to sets of relationships. A theory must also be verifiable either directly or indirectly. Given this definition of theory, what arguments would you present in debating whether or not Creationism should be considered a scientific theory taught in high school science classes?

For Practice and Discussion

You can get a better idea of the different ways we gather knowledge and the implications of choosing one way over another by the following hypothetical example. Say, for instance, that you have been given funds to design a program to prevent heart disease. Before you decide what type of program you would like to conceptualize and implement, you determine there are several possible ways in which you can make your decision. What are all of the different sources you can turn to that will help you conceptualize your program? Will you base your decision on what a cardiologist thinks is the best approach (use authority)? If you are to use logic and reason, what are your premises and conclusion? (for example, men who make more than $100,000 per year are Type A personalities; men with Type A personality will develop heart disease; therefore, men who make more than $100,000 per year are at risk for heart disease). Are there health beliefs related to heart disease that you already know are true? (for example, an apple a day keeps the doctor away). Which approach would you base your decision on and why? How would you examine the underlying sources of the nonscientific approaches?

References

Aristotle. (350 B.C.). *On the heavens.* J. L. Stocks (trans.). Retrieved November 19, 2004, from http://classics.mit.edu/Aristotle/heavens.2.ii.html.

Bouma, G. D., and Atkinson, G.B.J. (1995). *A handbook of social science research.* New York: Oxford University Press.

Calaprice, A. (Ed.). (2000). *The expanded quotable Einstein.* Princeton, NJ: Princeton University Press.

Drake, S. (1957). *Discoveries and opinions of Galileo.* Garden City, NY: Doubleday Anchor Books.

Garrett, L. (1994). *The coming plague: Newly emerging diseases in a world out of balance.* New York: Farrar, Straus, and Giroux.

Internet Encyclopedia of Philosophy. (n.d.). Francis Bacon. Retrieved November 19, 2004, from www.iep.utm.edu/b/bacon.htm.

Janz, N. K., Champion, V. L., and Strecher, V. J. (2002). The health belief model. In K. Glanz, B. K. Rimer, and F. M. Lewis (Eds.), *Health behavior and health education* (3rd ed., pp. 45–66). San Francisco: Jossey-Bass.

Redondi, P. (1987). *Galileo: Heretic.* R. Rosenthal (trans.). Princeton, NJ: Princeton University Press.

Sobel, D. (1999). *Galileo's daughter: A historical memoir of science, faith, and love.* New York: Walker and Co.

Valtin, H. (2002). "Drink at least eight glasses of water a day." Really? Is there scientific evidence for "8 × 8"? *American Journal of Physiology—Regulatory Integrative and Comparative Physiology, 283*(5), R993–R1004.

CHAPTER THREE

ETHICAL ISSUES IN HEALTH PROMOTION RESEARCH

John F. Santelli

Ethical conduct should be intrinsic to health promotion research. Protections for research subjects are essential to prevent harm and maximize benefit. High ethical standards also apply to health promotion practice; however, specific requirements of the federal research regulations do not. Many professional associations have ethical codes of conduct that address the professional practice for the members of the association. Ethical practice in research is guided by core ethical principles including respect for persons, beneficence, and justice. Researchers receiving funds from the U.S. federal government are bound by a specific set of federal regulations designed to protect human subjects, commonly referred to as 45 CFR 46. The federal regulations incorporate special protections for vulnerable populations such as children and prisoners. These research regulations cover all biomedical and behavioral research that is federally funded; however, research institutions commonly extend these protections to participants in non–federally supported research.

I would like to thank Shelly Makleff for her timely assistance with manuscript preparation.

Ethical considerations when designing and implementing health promotion programs and research should be paramount. In fact, one author has questioned the philosophy and corresponding ethical issues underlying the practice of health promotion (Buchanan, 2000). Others have written about ethical concerns in very specific areas of health promotion practice. For example, a recent journal article covers specific ethical issues involved in conducting community-based participatory research (Minkler, 2004) and a book chapter described ethical issues relevant to community-based intervention studies (Glanz, Rimer, and Lerman, 1996). Alternatively, this chapter reviews the essential and most commonly encountered ethical issues related to health promotion research, including the ethical underpinnings of current federal regulations, differences between health promotion research and health promotion practice, regulatory requirements for research, special protections for vulnerable populations, professional codes of conduct, collaboration with communities, and common ethical issues that arise in health promotion research. It concludes with practical suggestions for working with Institutional Review Boards and ensuring that research subjects are protected. Although processes such as ethical review and informed consent are important in the protection of persons involved in health promotion research, ultimately, subjects' protection is dependent upon informed and conscientious investigators.

Illustration of Key Concepts

"Sometimes, with the best intentions, scientists and public officials and others involved in working for the benefit of us all, forget that people are people. They concentrate so totally on plans and programs, experiments, statistics—on abstractions—that people become objects, symbols on paper, figures in a mathematical formula, or impersonal 'subjects' in a study, not human beings."

THE ATLANTA CONSTITUTION, JULY 27, 1972, AS QUOTED IN JONES, 1993.

Research is essential to the advancement of health. Research can provide knowledge that leads to the creation of new health promotion programs (HPPs), and evaluation research can lead to improvement in the practice of health promotion. For specific populations (minorities, women, children, and adolescents) to receive the full benefits of research, it is critical for them to participate in health research. Unfortunately, the story of research ethics begins with episodes of terrible lapses in ethical conduct by researchers (Beecher, 1966; Lederer and Grodin, 1994).

The potential for abuse by researchers became widely understood after World War II with revelations of the atrocities committed by Nazi researchers on unwilling concentration camp inmates. Such abuse was often considered an aberration by the medical community. Yet Beecher, a Boston physician, in 1966 documented twenty-two cases in which investigators endangered "the health or the life of their subjects." All of Beecher's examples included studies that had been published in leading medical journals. One such study involved purposeful infection of severely mentally retarded residents of the Willowbrook State School with the hepatitis virus in order to study the natural history of hepatitis. Abuses have more often been documented in biomedical research, but one of the most notorious examples, the Tuskegee Syphilis Study, involved public health.

The experience of poor, African American men in the Tuskegee Study is especially instructive. The Tuskegee Study was a forty-year (1932–1972) natural history study of untreated syphilis in African American men living in Macon County, Alabama (Jones, 1993; Thomas and Quinn, 1991). It started as a demonstration project for testing and treatment of syphilis, but the Great Depression intervened and resources for treatment became scarce. The U.S. Public Health Service then converted the study into a natural history study. From a research ethics viewpoint, Tuskegee had many problems. Informed consent was not obtained from the men, who were also deceived about the purpose of certain medical procedures conducted for the research. Moreover, when penicillin became widely available for the treatment of syphilis in the mid-1940s, it still was not given to the men. In fact, investigators colluded with the local and state boards of health and with the local draft board so that they would not receive treatment. It was only after the details of the study were highlighted in the press coupled with the resulting Congressional pressure that the Public Health Service halted the study.

The public outrage to the Tuskegee Study along with other serious research abuses led directly to development of the National Commission for the Protection of Human Subjects in Biomedical and Behavioral Research, which wrote the Belmont Report, a key document in research ethics, and created many of the current federal regulations on research. Although the Tuskegee Study was finally stopped in March of 1972, it created profound distrust within the African American community regarding research and researchers. Such distrust has had a negative impact on the current research environment for AIDS, including prevention research in the African American community (Thomas and Quinn, 1991). The Tuskegee Study poignantly demonstrated the potential for initially well-intentioned researchers to fail in their ethical obligations to research subjects.

Researchers should understand this history of research abuse. Such knowledge will help them understand the stringent regulation of research. Understanding this history should motivate them to avoid repeating past mistakes. Finally, a careful understanding of this history teaches that good intentions are not sufficient to protect research subjects.

Ethical Principles from the Belmont Report

The Belmont Report, published in 1979, provides an ethical foundation for the conduct of research in the United States (U.S. Department of Health, Education, and Welfare, 1979). This short document is very readable and is an excellent primer on research ethics. Professional groups have used the ethical principles in the Belmont Report in establishing standards for the proper conduct for researchers and clinicians. The Belmont Report emphasizes three basic ethical principles: respect for persons, beneficence, and justice. Health promotion researchers should understand these principles and incorporate these into their research activities.

Respect for persons means treating people as autonomous beings and not as a means to an end. It also means honoring the capacity of individuals (whose judgment is *not* impaired) to make decisions that are in their own best interests. From the principle of respect for persons flows the notion of full disclosure and free choice for research participants. This means that research participation must be voluntary and given knowing the fundamental goals and aspects of the research. Moreover, freedom from undue persuasion to participate does not end with the start of the research but continues throughout the research study. Respect for persons also demands that special protections be extended to groups with diminished autonomy when they are included in research studies. This includes persons with diminished capacity for informed consent, such as children and those who are cognitively impaired, and those who are unable to exercise free choice such as prisoners. For these groups, certain types of research are not permitted. With children, informed consent processes are tailored to their specific circumstances and abilities. Most children attain adult cognitive capacity during early adolescence. While younger children may not be capable of understanding all the details of an informed consent form, they generally understand salient risks and benefits. Researchers should provide information that is developmentally appropriate and understandable to children. Given that teenagers have cognitive capacity similar to adults, the informed consent process for teenagers should include similar information found in adult consent forms.

Beneficence is the ethical obligation to do good and to avoid harm. In research this means maximizing benefits and minimizing risks. Federal policies to extend the benefits of research to women, minorities, children, and adolescents by promoting their inclusion in research studies are motivated by this principle of beneficence.

Beneficence provides the ethical basis for conducting research that seeks to improve the health and well being of participants. It provides a general guideline that helps determine the acceptability of a research study by creating a balance of the predicted benefits against the predicted risks. Researchers must consider what the potential benefits and risks may be to individual research participants and to groups, and precludes researchers from causing harm to any research participant regardless of the benefit to others.

When considering the benefits of a proposed research study, it is first important to consider *what* the benefits are; however, it may be virtually impossible to truly estimate all the potential benefits. If all the benefits were known, then there would be no point in conducting the research. Nevertheless, an assessment of potential benefits must be made in order to judge the ethics of the proposed research.

The second thing to consider is *who* benefits. The proposed research may have important benefits to individuals, specific groups such as women at risk of HIV infection, specific ethnic communities, or all of the above. For example, research on school-based programs to reduce HIV-related risk behaviors may benefit not only the young people who receive the curriculum but also future generations of teenagers. Thus, there is a concept of benefits accruing directly for the participants involved while also providing indirect benefits for future generations. However, survey research to understand HIV risk behaviors may accrue no direct

MINCUS AGREES TO PARTICIPATE IN DR. DINCUS'S DNA STUDY.

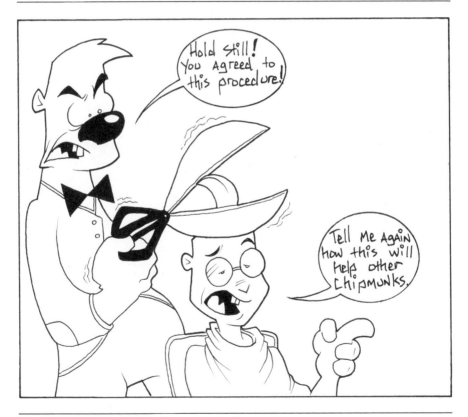

Copyright 2005 by Justin Wagner; reprinted with permission.

benefit to the participants but may provide significant benefits to others at risk of HIV if the research is applied in the design of targeted and effective intervention programs.

Justice entails a fair distribution of the benefits and burdens of research. The principle of justice demands a fair sharing of both risks and benefits and is important in the selection of research participants. The interests of justice demand that specific communities or specific groups not be exploited for the benefits of others, nor should they be excluded from participation in research that may have direct or indirect benefit to them. Research should not be conducted with groups or communities who are unlikely to benefit from the findings. For example, HIV treatment research conducted overseas by U.S. researchers has been questioned, when citizens of those countries are unlikely to benefit directly from the new treatments that are being tested. Likewise, promoting participation by groups that historically have been excluded from research is founded on the principle of justice. If certain groups of persons are systematically excluded from participation in research, then these groups may not share in the beneficial results of that research. For example, if women are not included in cardiovascular prevention trials, clinicians cannot be sure that interventions that are tested will be effective with women.

◆ ◆ ◆

In a Nutshell

The principle of justice demands a fair sharing of both risks and benefits and is important in the selection of research participants.

◆ ◆ ◆

Federal Inclusion Policies

Federal inclusion policies are motivated by the ethical principles outlined in the Belmont Report. The principles of the Belmont Report, given historical research abuses, are focused on protecting individuals from harmful research. These same principles are also used to weigh the potential benefits with the potential risks of research participation. Such an understanding has fostered the development of policies designed to promote a policy of inclusiveness in research. Such thinking and policies represent a fundamental shift in ethical thinking and federal regulatory approaches, in which the focus is still on *protection* but there is now an added emphasis on *access* (Levine, 1995). Such policies suggest that participation in research is essential if individuals and groups are to accrue the full benefits of research. During the 1990s, children and adolescents, women, and minority groups won rights to increased access to participation in research. AIDS activists, women, and minority health advocates led successful campaigns demanding access to research which led to the enactment of the National Institutes of Health (NIH) Revitalization Act of 1993. The *NIH Policy and Guidelines on the Inclusion of Women and Minorities as Subjects in Clinical Research* (promulgated in 1994 and revised in 2001) were intended "to ensure that all future NIH-supported biomedical and behavioral research involving human subjects will be carried out in a manner sufficient to elicit information about individuals of both genders and the diverse racial and ethnic groups and, in the case of clinical trials, to examine differential effects on such groups" (National Institutes of Health, 2001).

In 1998, given concerns about exclusion of children from research, the NIH issued the *NIH Policy and Guidelines on the Inclusion of Children as Participants in Research Involving Human Subjects* (National Institutes of Health, 1998). The goal of this policy was to increase the participation of children in research so that adequate data will be developed to support the treatment modalities for disorders and conditions that affect adults and may also affect children (National Institutes of Health, 1998). This policy specifies that children must be included in all human subjects' research, conducted or supported by the NIH, unless there are scientific and ethical reasons not to include them. Although much of the impetus for inclusion policies was fair access to clinical trials, notions of inclusion have also been applied to health promotion research.

Policies promoting inclusion in research are rooted in the principle of justice and the concept of nondiscrimination. Research has been "transformed" from being perceived as a fundamentally dangerous activity from which persons must be protected, to being seen as entailing a balance of risk and benefit. Although research may entail risk, it holds the potential of bringing much benefit. Demands for increased participation of women, minorities, and children in research have occurred due to a changing societal understanding about the risks and benefits of participation in research. Health promotion researchers will need to address both inclusion and protection.

◆ ◆ ◆

In a Nutshell

Health promotion researchers will need to address both inclusion and protection.

◆ ◆ ◆

Codes of Ethical Conduct

Although specific federal regulations govern research, professional codes of conduct are designed more broadly to set standards of conduct for both research and practice. A code of ethics is designed to reflect the profession's collective conscience and to promote ethical behaviors based on the collective experiences and traditions of the scientific discipline (Frankel, 1992). A code can be used to evaluate the behavior of individual professionals as well as to create a collective responsibility within a profession. A profession's code of ethics may also contribute to the socialization of new professionals by providing guidance on and standards of expected behavior. Finally, a code of ethics establishes standards that may be used by legislative, administrative, and judicial bodies in adjudicating allegations of misconduct (Frankel, 1992). Thus, the ethical principles found in the Belmont Report, while intended to govern research, also provide a basis for ethical conduct in professional practice.

What Is Health Promotion Research, and What Is Health Promotion Practice?

It is important to understand the distinctions between research and practice within the context of ethical principles and federal regulatory guidelines. The Belmont Report provides guidance on the boundaries between practice and research (U.S. Department of Health, Education, and Welfare, 1979). Similarly, public health researchers have attempted to distinguish between public health practice and public health research (Snider and Stroup, 1997). These documents may be helpful in understanding key differences between health promotion *research* and the *practice* of health promotion. As stated previously, there are ethical standards that apply to health promotion practice; however, it is important to understand that the specific regulatory requirements that apply to *research* do not apply to health promotion *practice*.

Health promotion research includes activities designed or *intended* to contribute to generalizable knowledge. The critical word here is *intended*; research is defined by the intentions of the researchers. Research is often expressed in terms of theory, principles, and statements of relationships (U.S. Department of Health, Education, and Welfare, 1979). Results are often published in research journals. In research, there may be benefits to the individual, but a primary objective is to provide benefits to others via enhanced understanding or knowledge. An experimental evaluation of a new drug prevention curriculum compared to standard health education would generally be considered research. Likewise, a school survey to explore potential new risk factors for drug use among adolescents would be research under this definition. The intention of the survey is to enhance knowledge.

Health promotion practice refers to interventions designed solely to help the individual or group; such interventions are generally recognized as being beneficial or efficacious (U.S. Department of Health, Education, and Welfare, 1979). Health promotion practice may include health education, behavioral interventions such as counseling, and data collection designed to monitor or improve existing programs and policies to enhance health. Publication of results in a research journal is generally not a goal. For example, delivery of a well-evaluated drug prevention curriculum in a public school would generally be considered health promotion practice. Process evaluation to see that the program is well delivered would generally be considered health promotion practice, as the primary benefit is for those receiving the intervention. Likewise, routine, periodic public health surveillance of adolescent drug use via school surveys to assess the need for drug prevention programs and to monitor prevention activities would also be considered practice. There is no intention to contribute to generalizable knowledge; rather the intention is to directly improve prevention practices in these schools.

Practitioners have responsibilities to individual program participants. Researchers have responsibilities to individual participants but also to the integrity of the research. These responsibilities may be in conflict and such conflicts may not be readily apparent to the researcher. Given these dual responsibilities and the potential for harm to research participants, a higher level of scrutiny is required for research than practice. Such scrutiny generally requires review by an Institutional Review Board (IRB).

An IRB is regulated and controlled by the federal government, specifically the Office for Human Research Protections (OHRP). The OHRP provides leadership and oversight on all matters related to the protection of human subjects participating in research conducted or supported by the U.S. Department of Health and Human Services (DHHS). The OHRP helps ensure that such research is carried out in accordance with the highest ethical standards and in an environment where all who are involved in the conduct or oversight of human subjects research understand their primary responsibility for protecting the rights, welfare, and well-being of subjects (U.S. Department of Health and Human Services, 2005).

In addition to human subjects' protection, the regulations also provide standards for the membership of each institution's IRB. An IRB must have at least five members, with varying backgrounds, to ensure adequate ethical review for research activities commonly conducted by the institution. Considerations include the experience and expertise of IRB members, sensitivity to the community, and diversity in terms of race, gender, and cultural backgrounds. The IRB must be capable of reviewing proposed research studies in terms of scientific knowledge, institutional commitments and regulations, applicable law, and standards of professional conduct. IRB members should be knowledgeable in these various aspects of the research endeavor. If an IRB commonly reviews research that involves vulnerable subjects, such as children or prisoners, then the IRB should consider including individuals who are knowledgeable about and experienced in working with these groups. The IRB membership must include at least one scientist member, one nonscientist, and one member not otherwise affiliated with the institution. The regulations require initial review by the IRB and annual review while the research is ongoing.

◆ ◆ ◆

In a Nutshell

An IRB must have at least five members, with varying backgrounds, to ensure adequate ethical review for research activities commonly conducted by the institution.

◆ ◆ ◆

Federal Regulations on Research

U.S. regulations on research (U.S. Department of Health and Human Services, 2005) provide for a nationwide system of IRBs located within specific research institutions and regulated by the OHRP in the DHHS. Institutions conducting research provide an "assurance" to OHRP regarding their capability to comply with the federal regulations by creating a written set of institutional standards on how they will review research in order to protect human subjects. Once the assurance is accepted by the federal government, an assurance number is issued. Federal assurance is contingent on periodic review of the institution's IRB procedures. An institution can lose its federal assurance to conduct research if it fails to meet high standards. OHRP over the past several years has publicly revoked the federal assurances at prominent research universities, stopping all federally funded research (Levine, 2001). Researchers must understand and follow these regulations in all their research activities.

An institution's IRB provides ethical review and approval for all research funded by the U.S. federal government and involving human participants unless the study is determined to be *exempt* (in other words, IRB review is not required). Most institutions in the United States extend the protections of the federal regulations to all research conducted within the institution, including non–federally funded research. For each study, the appropriate IRB must assess the risks and benefits to human participants, ensure proper informed consent procedures, and provide special protections for vulnerable populations. Special safeguards cover pregnant women and the fetus, prisoners, and children. Special sections of the regulations, called subparts, address special protections for specific vulnerable populations. Pregnant women, human fetuses, and neonates are covered under Subpart B; prisoners under Subpart C; and children under Subpart D (U.S. Department of Health and Human Services, 2005). Other populations such as persons who are disabled, who have impaired cognitive capacities, or who are poor and socially disenfranchised do not have special sections in the regulations per se, but nonetheless receive special consideration. The U.S. federal regulations also cover many practical aspects of ethical review including the composition of IRBs, how often research must be reviewed, IRB records, the elements of informed consent, circumstances under which informed consent may be waived, and categories of exempt research.

Certain categories of research are considered exempt from IRB review because they represent little or no risk to human participants (see Table 3.1). Most research institutions require a review by the IRB office to verify an exempt status. As shown in the table, the categories of exempt research that commonly apply to health promotion research are category 2, which involves certain types of interviews and surveys, and category 4, which involves data that are publicly available or where persons cannot be identified. Notably, exemption category 2 does not apply to surveys and interviews with children.

Likewise, certain research requires IRB review that is considered *expedited* (that is, can be reviewed by a single IRB board member such as the chairperson). Expedited research can present no more than minimal risk to human subjects. For a current list of categories of research that can be reviewed in an expedited fashion, see the Department of Health and Human Services Website: www.hhs.gov/ohrp/humansubjects/guidance/expedited98.htm (retrieved March 8, 2005). Expedited categories relevant to health promotion research include certain research employing surveys, interviews, oral histories, focus groups, and program evaluation; and continuing review of research previously approved by the convened IRB.

Consistent with the Belmont Report, the regulatory definition of research is "a systematic investigation, including research development, testing and evaluation, designed to develop or contribute to generalizable knowledge" (U.S. Department of Health and Human Services, 2005, section 46.102). This definition and the federal regulations on research apply no matter what the specific mechanism

TABLE 3.1. CATEGORIES OF EXEMPT RESEARCH IN THE U.S. FEDERAL REGULATIONS.

Exact Language of the Federal Regulations	Common Interpretations and Examples
(Category 1) Research conducted in established or commonly accepted educational settings, involving normal educational practices, such as (i) research on regular and special education instructional strategies, or (ii) research on the effectiveness of or the comparison among instructional techniques, curricula, or classroom management methods.	This applies to education research. It generally does not include health research conducted in schools.
(Category 2) Research involving the use of educational tests (cognitive, diagnostic, aptitude, achievement), survey procedures, interview procedures or observation of public behavior, unless: (i) information obtained is recorded in such a manner that human subjects can be identified, directly or through identifiers linked to the subjects; and (ii) any disclosure of the human subjects' responses outside the research could reasonably place the subjects at risk of criminal or civil liability or be damaging to the subjects' financial standing, employability, or reputation.	This includes focus groups, health surveys, and interviews if they are not sensitive or conducted anonymously. Importantly, exempt research in this category does not cover research involving children, such as school surveys.
(Category 3) Research involving the use of educational tests (cognitive, diagnostic, aptitude, achievement), survey procedures, interview procedures, or observation of public behavior that is not exempt under paragraph (b)(2) of this section, if: (i) the human subjects are elected or appointed public officials or candidates for public office; or (ii) Federal statute(s) require(s) without exception that the confidentiality of the personally identifiable information will be maintained throughout the research and thereafter.	This is not a commonly used category. It is similar to category 2, but involving public officials or candidates, or federal statutes providing for confidentiality of personally identifiable information.
(Category 4) Research involving the collection or study of existing data, documents, records, pathological specimens, or diagnostic specimens, if these sources are publicly available or if the information is recorded by the investigator in such a manner that subjects cannot be identified, directly or through identifiers linked to the subjects.	This applies generally to research on existing data that is publicly available or where subjects cannot be identified.

TABLE 3.1. (*Continued*)

Exact Language of the Federal Regulations	Common Interpretations and Examples
(Category 5) Research and demonstration projects which are conducted by or subject to the approval of Department or Agency heads, and which are designed to study, evaluate, or otherwise examine: (i) Public benefit or service programs; (ii) procedures for obtaining benefits or services under those programs; (iii) possible changes in or alternatives to those programs or procedures; or (iv) possible changes in methods or levels of payment for benefits or services under those programs.	This applies to research involving public benefit or service programs that is approved by federal department or agency heads.
(Category 6) Taste and food quality evaluation and consumer acceptance studies, (i) if wholesome foods without additives are consumed or (ii) if a food is consumed that contains a food ingredient at or below the level and for a use found to be safe, or agricultural chemical or environmental contaminant at or below the level found to be safe, by the Food and Drug Administration or approved by the Environmental Protection Agency or the Food Safety and Inspection Service of the U.S. Department of Agriculture.	This applies to certain kinds of research on food preferences.

Source: U.S. Department of Health and Human Services, 2005, section 46.101.

for federal funding. For example, a federally funded public service program (such as Head Start) may be deemed primarily as nonresearch but may practice activities that would be considered research. These activities would then be subject to the U.S. federal regulations.

The purpose of the federal regulations is to protect human subjects participating in research. The federal regulations define *human subject* as "a living individual about whom an investigator (whether professional or student) conducting research obtains (1) data through intervention or interaction with the individual, or (2) identifiable private information" (U.S. Department of Health and Human Services, 2005, Section 46.102). This definition excludes information on deceased persons. Caution should be exercised, however. Health information about a deceased person, such as his or her HIV status, may have important implications for the privacy of living persons.

The federal regulations provide specific criteria for IRB approval of a research protocol. These criteria require that

- Risks to subjects are minimized.
- Risks to subjects are reasonable in relation to anticipated benefits, if any, to subjects, and the importance of the knowledge that may reasonably be expected to result.
- Selection of subjects is equitable.
- Informed consent is sought from each prospective subject or the subject's legally authorized representative.
- Informed consent is appropriately documented.
- When appropriate, the research plan includes adequate provision for monitoring data collection to ensure the safety of subjects.
- When appropriate, adequate provisions are in place to protect the privacy of subjects and to maintain the confidentiality of data.

Informed consent is a central practice for protecting human subjects, and the federal regulations define specific requirements for the process of obtaining informed consent and the specific content of the informed consent document. Informed consent, as described in the Belmont Report, includes three key elements: full information, adequate comprehension, and free choice. Consent is generally obtained from the research subject, although permission may be sought from a guardian or surrogate for individuals or classes of persons, such as children, who are unable to consent for themselves. The criteria for informed consent in the federal regulations are found in Figure 3.1. A sample of an informed consent form is provided in the appendix to this chapter.

◆ ◆ ◆

In a Nutshell

Consent is generally obtained from the research subject, although permission may be sought from a guardian or surrogate for individuals or classes of persons, such as children, who are unable to consent for themselves.

◆ ◆ ◆

Although informed consent and documentation of informed consent by the person's signature on a consent form are general requirements for research, under certain circumstances an IRB may waive requirements for informed consent

FIGURE 3.1.   GENERAL REQUIREMENTS FOR INFORMED CONSENT (45 CFR 46.116).

1. A statement that the study involves research, an explanation of the purposes of the research and the expected duration of the subject's participation, a description of the procedures to be followed, and identification of any procedures which are experimental

2. A description of any reasonably foreseeable risks or discomforts to the subject

3. A description of any benefits to the subject or to others which may reasonably be expected from the research

4. A disclosure of appropriate alternative procedures or courses of treatment, if any, that might be advantageous to the subject

5. A statement describing the extent, if any, to which confidentiality of records identifying the subject will be maintained

6. For research involving more than minimal risk, an explanation as to whether any compensation and an explanation as to whether any medical treatments are available if injury occurs and, if so, what they consist of, or where further information may be obtained

7. An explanation of whom to contact for answers to pertinent questions about the research and research subjects' rights, and whom to contact in the event of a research-related injury to the subject

8. A statement that participation is voluntary, refusal to participate will involve no penalty or loss of benefits to which the subject is otherwise entitled, and the subject may discontinue participation at any time without penalty or loss of benefits to which the subject is otherwise entitled

Additional elements of informed consent. When appropriate, one or more of the following elements of information shall also be provided to each subject.

1. A statement that the particular treatment or procedure may involve risks to the subject (or to the embryo or fetus, if the subject is or may become pregnant) which are currently unforeseeable

2. Anticipated circumstances under which the subject's participation may be terminated by the investigator without regard to the subject's consent

3. Any additional costs to the subject that may result from participation in the research

4. The consequences of a subject's decision to withdraw from the research and procedures for orderly termination of participation by the subject

5. A statement that significant new findings developed during the course of the research which may relate to the subject's willingness to continue participation will be provided to the subject

6. The approximate number of subjects involved in the study

and documentation of informed consent. For example, IRBs commonly waive documentation of written informed consent for telephone interviews when it would be impractical to obtain a signature. Similarly, an IRB may waive informed consent for review of existing health records when obtaining consent would be impractical and the risk is minimal. Criteria for granting these two kinds of waivers are found in sections 46.116 and 46.117 of the federal regulations.

For example, under section 46.117 a signature is not always required. Although this may seem counterintuitive at first, consider a study that is said to be anonymous. Unlike with confidential studies, an anonymous study does not involve the collection of names. The anonymous nature of the study may be important to potential volunteers, and often recruitment efforts will feature the point that "your participation is entirely anonymous." Given such a pledge to volunteers, imagine what their reaction would be if they were asked to sign an informed consent form. Thus, an IRB can grant the study permission to obtain verbal rather than written consent. In this case, volunteers may be provided with formalized, written information about the study. Of course, the informed consent form (minus the signature blanks) can serve this purpose well.

Yet another key point regarding the informed consent document is the question of what qualifies as a potential benefit to the participant. First, it is important not to confuse compensation with benefit. Compensation is typically a cash payment (or its equivalent) that is used to formally recognize that volunteers have given their time to the study. Their time is considered valuable, and thus payment is made to compensate them for this time. It is not a benefit. Second, there may be instances in which there is no direct benefit to the participant, and this should be stated in the consent form. Third, accurately describing the level of potential benefit is important because the level of risk and the level of benefit will ultimately be weighed by the IRB to determine approval or disapproval of the protocol. Thus, the following guidelines are offered to help you think about potential benefit.

- Receipt of an effective education program is a potential benefit.
- A question and answer session following an assessment is a potential benefit of study participation.
- Having free screening tests (for example, tests for a disease) is a potential benefit.
- Any treatment provided in the context of the study, that would not otherwise occur, is a potential benefit.
- Providing referral services to study participants is a potential benefit.

Any explanation of the potential benefits that could reasonably be anticipated must also be accompanied by an explanation of potential risks. Likelihood of risk and magnitude of risk are both important; common risks and potential serious risk should be included in the consent form. Risk can pertain to physical problems or disorders and to a host of emotional, mental, and social problems that could potentially occur as a result of study participation. Guidelines for thinking about risk in health promotion research are provided in the following list.

◆ ◆ ◆

In a Nutshell

Risk can pertain to physical problems or disorders and to a host of emotional, mental, and social problems that could potentially occur as a result of study participation.

◆ ◆ ◆

- Potential risk exists if the study records of the volunteer are identifiable and contain sensitive information.
- If the assessment process could lead to emotional or mental distress then that risk should be disclosed.
- If participation in the intervention could cause emotional, mental, or social distress then that risk should be disclosed.
- For some studies, simply being in the study may cause emotional, mental, or social distress when friends, family members, or sex partners of the volunteer discover that the volunteer is participating. This risk should be anticipated and disclosed.
- Physically invasive procedures, even those that are routine (such as a Pap test), may entail risk, and this risk should be disclosed.

Another critically important aspect of the informed consent document is that it must be written in language that is comprehensible to the study volunteers. This means that the choice of terms and the overall reading level must be appropriate to the people who will compose the sample (Hochhauser, 2003). Many IRBs require that informed consent forms be graded for reading level. For example, typically IRBs require the consent for general U.S. populations to be at an eighth grade reading level. For research presenting significant risk, the research team should check for understanding before consent is obtained.

Regulation of Research Involving Vulnerable Populations

As noted previously, the federal regulations provide special protection for several populations, including children, prisoners, pregnant women, human fetuses, and neonates. These special protections commonly require a higher level of scrutiny by the IRB, restrictions or prohibitions on particular kinds of research (for instance, research involving greater than minimal risk), and alternative procedures for obtaining informed consent, such as requesting the permission of a parent or guardian. Certain research with pregnant women requires the permission of both the pregnant woman and the father of the fetus. In this section we detail some of the specific requirements for research with prisoners and children, including adolescents.

Requirements for Research with Prisoners. Prisoners are afforded special consideration when they are the subjects of research. Some of the worst abuses in the history of human subjects' maltreatment involved Nazi prisoners during World War II. Even where penal systems are not inherently malevolent, incarceration severely limits the ability of prisoners to make voluntary decisions about research participation. The inherently coercive nature of prison implies that full voluntary informed consent may be precluded. Subpart C of the federal regulations describes additional duties of IRBs in reviewing research involving prisoners. When reviewing prisoner research, the IRB must include at least one board member who is a prisoner or a prisoner representative who is sensitive to the circumstances of prisoners. Research involving prisoners may require review by the Secretary of the DHHS and publication in the Federal Register. Research with prisoners is limited to four categories as found in section 46.306 and shown in Box 3.1

Requirements for Research with Children, Including Adolescents. Special protections for children, including minor adolescents, are covered in Subpart D. Within this context, children are defined as persons who have not attained the legal age for consenting to treatments or procedures involved in the research. Under this subpart, a hierarchy of risk and benefit is used in defining the specific protections required. The four categories of research involving children are research that

- Involves no more than minimal risk
- Involves more than minimal risk, but there is a potential for direct benefit to individual research subjects
- Involves a minor increase over minimal risk without direct benefit, but research is likely to yield generalizable knowledge about the subject's disorder or condition
- Is not otherwise approvable but presents an opportunity to understand, prevent, or alleviate a serious problem affecting the health or welfare of children

Minimal risk is defined as follows: "The probability and magnitude of harm or discomfort anticipated . . . are not greater . . . than those ordinarily encountered in daily life or during the performance of routine physical or psychological examinations or tests" (U.S. Department of Health and Human Services, 2005, section 46.102).

Box 3.1. Research with Prison Populations, Section 46.306

A. Study of the possible causes, effects, and processes of incarceration, and of criminal behavior, provided that the study presents no more than minimal risk and no more than inconvenience to the subjects

B. Study of prisons as institutional structures or of prisoners as incarcerated persons, provided that the study presents no more than minimal risk and no more than inconvenience to the subjects

C. Research on conditions particularly affecting prisoners as a class (for example, vaccine trials and other research on hepatitis which is much more prevalent in prisons than elsewhere; and research on social and psychological problems such as alcoholism, drug addiction, and sexual assaults) provided that the study may proceed only after the Secretary has consulted with appropriate experts including experts in penology, medicine, and ethics, and published notice, in the Federal Register, of his intent to approve such research

D. Research on practices, both innovative and accepted, which have the intent and reasonable probability of improving the health or well-being of the subject. In cases in which those studies require the assignment of prisoners in a manner consistent with protocols approved by the IRB to control groups which may not benefit from the research, the study may proceed only after the Secretary has consulted with appropriate experts, including experts in penology, medicine, and ethics, and published notice, in the Federal Register, of the intent to approve such research.

Source: Department of Health and Human Services, 2005, Section 46.306.

Specific requirements exist for each category of risk and benefit. All four categories require the *assent* of the child and the *permission* of one or both parents. Assent is the child's affirmative agreement to participate in research, whereas permission is the agreement of parent(s) or guardians to their child's or ward's participation in research. The federal regulations use the terms *permission* and *assent* to distinguish these processes from the usual informed consent process. Parents are not the research subjects and generally do not experience risks or benefits from the research. Children may lack the intellectual capacity or judgment to make decisions about research, although the concept of assent recognizes the emerging developmental capacity of children to provide informed consent. By the recommendations of the National Commission, assent is commonly obtained from children who are aged seven and older. For minor adolescents who are more cognitively developed (that is, beginning at twelve to fourteen years of age), the content of assent forms may closely resemble that for consent forms used with adults. In some instances, when obtaining parental consent is problematic, the federal regulations governing research dictate that the IRB may waive parental permission.

IRBs may determine that parental permission would not be appropriate because of the nature of the topic under investigation, for example, research involving confidential health care when adolescents may legally receive treatment without parental consent and research involving mature minors, that is, those capable of making a good decision about participation (Society for Adolescent Medicine, 2003). Section 46.408 states

> In addition to the provisions for waiver contained in 46.116 of Subpart A, if an IRB determines that a research protocol is designed for conditions or a subject population for which parental permission is not a reasonable requirement to protect subjects (e.g., neglected or abused children), it may waive consent requirements provided an appropriate mechanism for protecting the children who will participate as research subjects is substituted and provided the waiver is not inconsistent with federal, state, or local law [U.S. Department of Health and Human Services, 2005].

Similar to the protections provided to prisoners, special protections are also provided to children who are wards of the state (for example, those in foster care).

Research in Schools

When health promotion research is conducted in schools additional regulatory requirements are covered by two federal laws: the Family Educational Rights and Privacy Act (FERPA) and the Protection of Pupil Rights Amendment (PPRA). FERPA addresses the privacy of student educational records and the circumstances under which educational records may be accessed, amended, or disclosed. PPRA specifically addresses surveys administered in schools. PPRA requires that written parental permission be obtained for students who are not emancipated prior to participation in surveys or evaluations, funded partially or fully by the U.S. Department of Education (DOE), that collect information about eight specific topics: mental health and psychological problems; sexual behaviors or attitudes; illegal, antisocial, self-incriminating, or demeaning behaviors; critical appraisals of individuals with whom respondents have close family relationships; religious practices, affiliations, or beliefs; political affiliations or beliefs; income; and legally recognized privileged relationships such as those with physicians, lawyers, or ministers. Surveys not funded by the DOE that address any of these eight topics may be conducted after parental notification and after allowing parents an opportunity to opt their child out of participation. Parents have a right to inspect questionnaires and instructional material used in conjunction with surveys, analyses, or evaluations. Local education agencies must notify parents at least annually about school policies regarding these rights and any upcoming surveys. These rights transfer to students when a student becomes an adult or is emancipated. Additional information can be found at www.ed.gov/policy/gen/guid/fpco/ index.html and at www.ed.gov/policy/gen/guid/fpco/hottopics/ht10-28- 02.html?exp=0 (retrieved March 4, 2005).

Health Insurance Portability and Accountability Act

The Health Insurance Portability and Accountability Act of 1996, commonly known as HIPAA, is designed to ensure the confidentiality of medical records and private health information. HIPPAA requirements may come into play in health promotion research that is conducted in health care delivery settings. HIPAA provisions also address patients' access to their own medical records and privacy protections that govern both clinical care and research. HIPAA addresses privacy rights of children and adolescents. A full review of HIPAA is beyond the scope of this chapter. Additional information can be found at www.hhs.gov/ocr/hipaa/ (retrieved March 8, 2005).

Risks and Benefits of Health Promotion Research

Health promotion research, like other research, offers the potential for health benefits and presents specific risks. Health promotion research commonly includes intervention programs to reduce harmful behaviors and to increase protective behaviors, as well as projects designed to improve understanding of the factors influencing health-related behaviors. Such research commonly collects data on personal behaviors and behavioral determinants, including sexual practices, alcohol and other drug use, mental health concerns, and perceived support for prevention practices. In contrast to biomedical research, health promotion research generally presents minimal risk to participants. Principal risks may include invasion of privacy, embarrassment, stress and discomfort, loss of self-esteem, and potential loss of confidentiality regarding private information and personal behaviors. Loss of privacy resulting from health promotion research is generally a rare phenomenon. Although the risks of participating in health promotion research may be minimal or even trivial compared to those in biomedical research, the potential risks still must be weighed against the potential benefits to justify the research. Health promotion research may benefit the individuals or groups by improving understanding of adverse health outcomes, by reducing involvement in health risk behaviors, and in the prevention of both. Moreover, completion of surveys may increase self-understanding of one's own risk, and by raising such understanding, survey research may facilitate the process of seeking care. Potential benefits from the informed consent process may include an increased sense of self-control and increased decision-making capacity.

Improving Ethical Practice: Working with Communities

Communities may view the intentions of researchers with skepticism, and these perceptions are not without justification. The legacies of Tuskegee and other abusive research projects have given rise to a mistrust of researchers in many communities (Thomas and Quinn, 1991). Communities may fear direct harm to community members or indirect harm such as when unflattering research findings stigmatize their community.

The involvement of community may enhance human subjects' protection and improve the scientific quality of health promotion research (Melton, Levine, Koocher, Rosenthal, and Thompson, 1988; Quinn, 2004; Society for Adolescent Medicine, 2003; and Sieber and Stanley, 1988). Community consultation provides a context for research findings and may help the researcher to better understand the meaning of behaviors. Community involvement may provide insight into the underlying forces influencing health and may lead to stronger programs that serve to improve health. Community advice on the acceptability and feasibility of study approaches can save resources. Early dissemination of research findings to the community may increase confidence in the research process and help community members understand the potential benefits from research. Likewise, community involvement can assist in the dissemination of health practices and programs shown to be effective. When communities partner with researchers, they learn useful skills and obtain knowledge that can enhance their ability to advocate for community programs and services. Community advisory boards can make communities integral partners in health promotion research.

Practical Guidance

To assist researchers, here is some practical advice for ensuring the ethical conduct of health promotion research:

- The IRB, the informed consent process, and the researcher all have important roles in protecting human subjects. Before submitting a protocol to the IRB, make sure you've considered all potential risks and protections for human subjects. Work with the IRB in helping it understand your research aims, risks and benefits, and your plan to protect human subjects.
- In writing a research protocol for IRB review, explain and justify your plans for human subjects' protection in terms of ethical principles and the specific

requirements of the regulations. For example, if you are requesting an alteration to or waiver of informed consent, provide an ethical rationale for this change and justify this change according to the specific requirements of the federal regulations.

- Strive to understand research involvement from the viewpoint of the research subject. Informed consent documents should address the concerns of the subject and provide them the information needed to make a free and informed decision. Strive to make the informed consent form readable and easily understood.
- IRBs are made up of busy people who have an important mission to protect human subjects. Do your part to create an attitude of mutual respect and openness. Be clear in your written communications to the IRB.
- Make sure that the confidentiality of data is maintained throughout the process of data collection and analysis. Remove identifiers from the data when they are no longer needed.
- Work with the community in preparing the research protocol, conducting the research and disseminating results. Understand community concerns and incorporate these into your research plan.

Remember that the ethical conduct of an informed investigator is the ultimate mechanism for protecting human subjects.

Applied Example

As noted previously in this chapter, Appendix A displays a sample informed consent document. Careful inspection of this document can be quite informative. For example, you will see that the study is a cross-sectional survey designed to assess people's feelings about being screened for colorectal cancer. The survey is estimated to take from forty-five to sixty minutes to complete. The study procedures are outlined for potential volunteers to read. However, it is critically important to remember that the event of obtaining informed consent is viewed as a platform for having a dialogue with potential volunteers about the study procedures.

The informed consent form is intentionally simple. Note that the language used in the form is basic and unsophisticated. It is written at a reading level appropriate for someone in seventh grade. Note also that the sentences are rather short (compound sentences are avoided) and that the document avoids giving potential volunteers an abundance of information. Instead, the document simply provides people with basic information pertaining to the study and describes the likely risks and benefits of participation. It should also be noted that the $20 compensation is mentioned but not emphasized in any way. After reading the form people should have an opportunity to clarify any questions they may have.

Finally, the document shown in Appendix A also provides an example of the principles outlined in the Belmont Report. *Respect for persons,* for example, is demonstrated throughout the document and should be adhered to throughout the informed consent process. The essential spirit of the document and process is to allow people to autonomously decide whether they want to take part in the study. Note that the document specifically informs that such a decision can be revoked at any time, without giving a reason. *Beneficence* is also apparent in the document. The benefits described are benefits to the volunteers. Although the document does state that "we [doctors, researchers and scientists] may learn new things that will help prevent cancer deaths," it does so only after listing personal benefits and then specifically stating that other personal benefits will not occur. Finally, the principle of *justice* may be apparent to students of public health practice. The challenge of promoting colorectal cancer screening has been a long-standing question in health promotion practice and the study apparently seeks data from people who will also ultimately benefit from any applied practice resulting from the brief intervention program.

Integration with the Research Process

Ethical considerations should be at the forefront of your mind from the inception of a research project until the last paper has been published. Thus, each step of the nine-step model shown in Chapter One should be taken in harmony with the ethical considerations described in this chapter. Steps 1 and 2, for example, address the principle of justice. The question must be asked, is this an important research question for this particular population? Unless the answer is clearly "yes," the research may be unlikely to meet the principle of beneficence. In other words, when you tell someone, "Your participation in this study will help others," the statement should be true to form and not simply a vacuous phrase designed to inspire volunteerism.

◆ ◆ ◆

In a Nutshell

Each step of the nine-step model shown in Chapter One should be taken in harmony with the ethical considerations described in this chapter.

◆ ◆ ◆

As you continue to read the remaining twelve chapters of this book, you will begin to see that every aspect of the research process is linked to ethics. This is the case when selecting a study design, conducting program evaluation, or even analyzing data. Thus, you can expect to see the concepts outlined in this chapter implicitly represented within the topics yet to be presented. In many chapters that follow you will find that ethical issues are posed quite frequently. Consequently, you are invited at this juncture to begin thinking with a "critical eye" about research and to thoughtfully deliberate about its obligation to protect volunteers from harm. In addition, Internet resources are available to help you develop a critical eye (see Figure 3.2).

FIGURE 3.2. INTERNET RESOURCES ON HUMAN SUBJECTS' PROTECTION.

Federal Code of Regulations (45 CFR 46)

Federal Policy for the Protection of Human Subjects (Basic DHHS Policy for Protection of Human Research Subjects). The policy applies to all research involving human subjects conducted and supported by any Federal Department or Agency. www.hhs.gov/ohrp/humansubjects/guidance/45cfr46.htm

The Belmont Report

The document that serves as the basis for the Federal Regulations for protecting human research participants (45 CFR 46). Published in 1979 as a result of the Belmont Commission, this report was the culmination of a presidential commission established to set ethical guidelines for protecting human research subjects in federally funded research.
www.hhs.gov/ohrp//humansubjects/guidance/belmont.htm

National Institutes of Health (NIH), Bioethics Resources of the Web

Resources are available to individuals with an interest in bioethics and the responsible conduct of research, especially when involving human participants in studies. http://www.nih.gov/sigs/bioethics/
NIH Policy and Guidelines on the Inclusion of Children as Participants in Research Involving Human Subjects. http://grants.nih.gov/grants/guide/notice-files/not98-024.html

CDC Guidelines for Defining Public Health Research and Public Health Nonresearch

This document sets forth CDC guidelines on the definition of public health research conducted by CDC staff irrespective of the funding source (in other words, whether provided by the CDC or by another entity). This document provides guidance to state and local health departments and other institutions that conduct collaborative research with CDC staff or that are recipients of CDC funds. The guidelines are intended to ensure both the protection of human subjects and the effective practice of public health. http://www.cdc.gov/od/ads/opspoll1.htm

Public Responsibility in Medicine and Research

A national nonprofit organization dedicated to educating the medical and legal professions, industry, and the public about the ethical, legal, and policy dimensions of appropriate and ethical research. http://www.primr.org/

Summary

Ethical treatment of human subjects is essential in health promotion research. This chapter addressed the general principles used to guide health promotion research. The intent was not to provide an exhaustive review of all the ethical issues involved in conducing health promotion research; however, the most critical issues were presented. Researchers should be knowledgeable about the history of research abuse, core ethical principles, federal inclusion policies, and federal regulations regarding research protections and should incorporate such understanding into their research plans and personal conduct within the research setting. Specific regulations guide research involving children and prisoners and research conducted in schools and involving health care information. Working with communities can improve the quality of health promotion research and the protection of human subjects involved in that research.

Issues to Consider

1. As noted in the Belmont Report, respect for the person is a paramount principle in research ethics. This principle clearly implies that coercion or undue influence to gain assent or consent from potential study volunteers is not ethical. It must be noted, then, that coercion is "in the eye of the potential volunteer" rather than being an objective entity. Thus, an important issue to consider is whether any of the potential volunteers could possibly perceive even minor levels of pressure when making their decision about enrolling in the study. Several factors may contribute to this perception, including
   • Offering compensation amounts that exceed customary payment levels for the people in the population
   • Situations in which the potential volunteer is a student enrolled in a class taught by the investigator
   • Situations in which the potential volunteer's decision may reflect upon the decision of a third party such as a parole board or prison officials
   • Clinical trials that would provide treatment to subjects who could otherwise not afford medical care
   • The perception that the decision to volunteer is somehow linked to the quality of care that people may receive at a given clinic
2. An important issue is the ethics of neglecting to include people from all appropriate populations when conducting research. While it is often easy to limit the study sample to a homogenous population, the cost of excluding populations who otherwise stand to benefit from the research should be carefully

considered. If a research question for a population is truly important then one could make the case that choosing not to include that population in the research constitutes an ethical violation. For example, consider a study designed to investigate the efficacy of a health promotion program aimed at improving the dietary intake of iron, folic acid, and calcium among pregnant women. The proposed study is to be conducted in a community comprising predominantly white, middle-class women. Although African American women and Latinas are not specifically excluded from participation, the selection of the recruitment sites unfortunately will yield a sample that, for all practical purposes, excludes minority participation.

For Practice and Discussion

Box 3.2 provides several realistic scenarios designed to challenge your thinking regarding ethics. Please complete each question in writing. Then, find a colleague who has completed the same exercise and compare your answers to his or hers. For items where there is disagreement, engage in debate until a consensus answer is achieved.

In each of the following ethical case studies, identify risks and benefits, importance of inclusion versus exclusion from the study, specific regulatory requirements, and means of obtaining informed consent

Maria, a fifteen-year-old Hispanic female, is making her first prenatal visit to a university hospital clinic in California and is invited to join a longitudinal study. The study is looking at social and physical environmental exposures during pregnancy and early childhood and the effect of these on child and adolescent health (such as effects on early puberty). She receives a consent form that describes the purposes of the study, the number of follow-up visits, the number of questionnaires and their consents, who to call for questions about the study and who to call at the IRB, and other standard consent language. The research involves several different questionnaires and blood and urine specimens, repeated on a periodic basis. The research assistant also wants to review Maria's medical record. At the first visit, she meets with a clinical social worker who asks her to complete a psychosocial risk assessment. These assessments reveal that she is eighteen weeks pregnant and in generally good health. She has a history of a chlamydia infection a year ago and says that she uses condoms, but not always. She reports that abortion is not an option for her because she could never "kill her baby." She has recently stopped smoking. She is currently repeating ninth grade and getting B's and D's in school. She is living with her parents in an inner city neighborhood. Her parents immigrated from Mexico ten years ago. Maria reports that her father is "very angry" with her about getting pregnant. She initiated intercourse at age

Box 3.2. Scenarios for Ethical Consideration

Is it an ethical violation if

- The amount of financial compensation is so high that people feel they "can't afford" to say no?
- A study is promoting STI prevention but teenagers under the age of 18 are not included?
- The same study includes only African Americans?
- A study is designed in a way that does not provide a fair test of the study hypotheses?
- The data obtained from the study are not disseminated by presentation or publication?
- The data obtained from the study are disseminated but only after a lengthy delay?
- People are recruited in groups (such as in a classroom setting)?
- A member of the research staff urges someone to complete "all" of the questions (even though people have a right to "pass")?
- The intervention program leads people to engage in behaviors that may place them at-risk (for example, a program designed to motivate women to negotiate condom use with men could unintentionally cause negative effects from the male partners including abuse)?
- Participation in the study leads to the diagnosis of conditions or diseases that would otherwise go undetected *and* treatment is not provided?
- Participation in a study is the only way to receive education and treatment about HIV infection?
- Recruitment occurs in a setting where perceptions of coercion may be inherently impossible to avoid (for example, prisons)?
- The control condition is known to be of very little value
- Study participants are led to believe that compensation will not be provided to them unless they complete all aspects of the study?
- Medical records from a local hospital are used to recruit patients with HIV infection into a health promotion study?
- The study concludes by asking people to take part in yet another study?

fourteen with her current boyfriend, Ramon, who is eighteen. She denies physical abuse by her family or Ramon. Ramon hopes to join the Army and Maria hopes to finish school, after she has the baby.

Estelle, a sixteen-year-old white female, is visiting an adolescent health clinic for acne. Per clinic routine she is offered a comprehensive biopsychosocial health assessment, based on the AMA's *Guidelines for Adolescent Preventive Services.* Per the clinic routine, she was enrolled in the clinic by her mother but her mother does not always accompany her to the clinic. There is no specific consent-assent form for the health assessment. Per the assessment, Estelle is currently in tenth grade, is getting A's and B's, but doesn't like school sports or clubs. She began smoking at age eleven and reached menarche at age twelve. She has had several boyfriends but has not initiated sexual intercourse; her current boyfriend is eighteen. She likes to drink wine coolers and admits to blacking out a number of times while drinking. She lives with her parents, and says they don't know much about her smoking and drinking. The clinic is conducting a natural history study of HPV and other viral STDs. She is eligible for the study because she has not initiated sexual intercourse. Participants would be randomized to one of two counseling interventions. A risk assessment would be completed on a laptop computer, using headphones. Repeat study visits would occur every three months and involve collection of blood, urine, and vaginal samples. Male partners would be recruited.

APPENDIX A. SAMPLE INFORMED CONSENT DOCUMENT.

Consent to Be a Research Subject

Title: Cancer Screening

Principal Investigator: Dr. Feel Good

Introduction/Purpose:
You are being asked to volunteer for a research study. The purpose of the study is to learn about your feelings toward screening tests for cancer of the colon. If you join, the study will ask you questions about why you might or might not be tested for this type of cancer. The questions ask about side effects, safety, and how good the test is for finding cancer.

Procedures:
You will be asked to take part in a face-to-face interview. A staff member will give the interview. It will last forty-five to sixty minutes. After you are done the staff member will discuss questions you might have. The interview will be taped. The tape will be erased after written versions of the interview have been made. You may refuse to answer any of the questions.

Risks:
Some people may feel a little nervous when thinking about cancer. If the questions cause you a lot of stress, you may end the interview.

Benefits:
Taking part in this study could provide some benefit to you. You will have a chance to discuss cancer with a staff member. Also, the study might increase your awareness of cancer screening. Other benefits to you will not occur. However, we [doctors, researchers, and scientists] may learn new things that will help prevent cancer deaths.

Confidentiality:
The information you give will be kept private. Your name will not appear on any document that also shows the answers you gave. Agencies that make the rules about how research is done, and those that pay for the research, have the right to review records of research subjects. Agencies that have the right to look at records from this research include the Human Investigations Committee at Hip Hop University. If an outside review occurs, your records will be kept private to the extent allowed by the law. Your name will not be used in any report nor will it be used on study records. Only an I.D. number will be used in the study records.

Compensation/Costs:
$20 will be given to you for being in the study for your time and effort. There are no costs to you. If you are injured as a result of this research, medical care will be available. The study will not pay for the cost of this care. If you believe

that you have been injured by this research, please contact Dr. Feel Good at 403-712-5997.

Contact Persons:
If you have any questions about this study, contact Dr. Feel Good at 403-712-5997. If you have any questions or concerns about your rights as a person in this study, contact the Chairman of Human Investigations Committee at 403-783-5649.

Voluntary Participation:
Participation in this study is completely voluntary, and you have the right to refuse to join. You can stop at any time after giving consent, and you can skip any question in the interview. This decision will not affect you in any way nor will you be penalized. The interviewer may stop you from taking part in this study at any time if it is in your best interests or if you do not follow instructions.

New Findings:
If anything new is learned during the study that we believe is important to you, we will tell you about it.

You will be given a copy of this consent form to keep.

I agree to participate for this research study.

_____	_____	_____
Volunteer's signature	Date	Time
_____	_____	_____
Person obtaining consent	Date	Time

References

Beecher, H. K. (1966). Ethics and clinical research. *New England Journal of Medicine, 274,* 1354–1360.

Buchanan, D. R. (2000). *An ethic for health promotion.* New York: Oxford University Press.

Frankel, M. S. (1992). Professional societies and responsible research conduct. In *Responsible science: Ensuring the integrity of the research process.* Vol. II (pp. 26–49). Washington, DC: National Academy of Sciences, National Academy of Engineering, and Institute of Medicine.

Glanz, K., Rimer, B. K., and Lerman, C. (1996). Ethical issues in the design and conduct of community-based intervention studies. In S. S. Coughlin and T. L. Beauchamp (Eds.), *Ethics and epidemiology* (pp. 156–177). New York: Oxford University Press.

Hochhauser, M. (2003). Concepts, categories, and value judgments in informed consent forms. *Institutional Review Board, 25*(5), 7–10.

Jones, H. S. (1993). *Bad blood: The Tuskegee syphilis experiment.* New York: Free Press.

Lederer, S. E., and Grodin, M. A. (1994). Historical overview: Pediatric experimentation. In M. A. Grodin and L. H. Glanz (Eds.), *Children as research subjects: Science, ethics, and law.* New York: Oxford University Press.

Levine, R. J. (1995). Adolescents as research subjects without permission of their parents or guardians: Ethical considerations. *Journal of Adolescent Health, 17*(5), 286–296.

Levine, R. J. (2001). Institutional review boards: A crisis in confidence. *Annals of Internal Medicine, 134,* 161–163.

Melton, G. B., Levine, R. J., Koocher, G. P., Rosenthal, R., and Thompson, W. C. (1988). Community consultation in socially sensitive research. Lessons from clinical trials of treatments for AIDS. *American Psychologist, 43,* 573–81.

Minkler, M. (2004). Ethical challenges for the "outside" researcher in community-based participatory research. *Health Education & Behavior, 31*(6), 684–697.

National Institutes of Health. (1998). *NIH policy and guidelines on the inclusion of children as participants in research involving human subjects.* March 6, 1998. Retrieved April 7, 2005, from grants1.nih.gov/grants/guide/notice-files/not98-024.html. National Institutes of Health.

National Institutes of Health. (2001, October). *NIH policy and guidelines on the inclusion of women and minorities as subjects in clinical research.* Retrieved March 8, 2005, from grants.nih.gov/grants/funding/women_min/guidelines_amended_10_2001.htm.

Quinn, S. C. (2004). Ethics in public health research: Protecting human subjects: The role of community advisory boards. *American Journal of Public Health, 94*(6), 918–922.

Sieber, J. E., and Stanley, B. (1988). Ethical and professional dimensions of socially sensitive research. *American Psychologist, 43,* 49–55.

Snider, D., and Stroup, D. (1997). Defining research when it comes to public health. *Public Health Reports, 112,* 29–32.

Society for Adolescent Medicine. (2003). *Guidelines for adolescent health research.* A position paper of the Society for Adolescent Medicine. Prepared by J. S. Santelli, A. S. Rogers, W. D. Rosenfeld, and others. *Journal of Adolescent Health. 33*(5), 396–409.

Thomas, S. B., and Quinn, S. C. (1991). The Tuskegee syphilis study, 1932 to 1972: Implications for HIV education and AIDS risk education programs in the black community. *American Journal of Public Health, 81,* 1498–1504.

U.S. Department of Health and Human Services, National Institutes of Health, Office for Protection from Research Risks. (2005, June 23). Code of Federal Regulations: Title 45-Public Welfare; Part 46: *Protection of Human Subjects.*

U.S. Department of Health, Education, and Welfare. (1979). *The Belmont report: Ethical principles and guidelines for the protection of human subjects of research.* Washington, DC: U.S. Government Printing Office, DHEW publication no. (OS) 78–0012.

PART TWO

RESEARCH DESIGN

CHAPTER FOUR

CHOOSING A RESEARCH DESIGN

Laura F. Salazar, Richard A. Crosby, and Ralph J. DiClemente

The research design of a study is the *strategy* the investigator chooses for answering the research question. The research question directs the type of design chosen. Other factors may play a significant role as well in deciding what type of research design will be applied. Ethical issues, cost, feasibility, and access to the study population will undoubtedly influence the design of the study in addition to the research question. It is critical for the investigator to choose the most appropriate design as this will have an impact on the success of the research project. Each design has its own strengths and limitations, some of which will determine the conclusions that may be drawn from the research.

Illustration of Key Concepts

In this chapter, we will provide an overview of the research process. This will entail a description of the two overarching stages of research. We will identify general purposes of health promotion research that fall within these two stages, and delineate appropriate research designs that are used to achieve each purpose. Examples from the health promotion research literature will be interjected to illustrate the respective purposes and designs.

FIGURE 4.1.   THE CHAIN OF RESEARCH IN HEALTH PROMOTION.

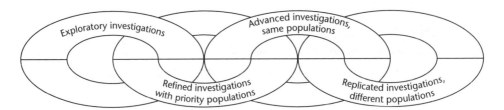

Exploratory investigations generate (rather than test) specific research questions.
Refined studies initially test a given set of research questions, and priority
populations are defined through surveillance and epidemiological studies.
Advanced investigations are built on findings from previous tests of research questions.
After the research questions have been adequately addressed in a priority
population, investigations should be replicated with a second priority population.

Two Stages of the Research Process

In general, scientific inquiry can be conceptualized as an interlocking chain—with
each link being a precursor of the other. The first link in the chain represents *exploratory research,* and the subsequent links represent varying levels of *conclusive research.* The model shown in Figure 4.1 can be applied to health promotion research.

As shown, exploratory research is often conducted because the health issue
has not been clearly defined, or a scientific basis for inquiry has not been established. In other words, hardly anything is known about the topic. In this early stage,
observations are needed to provide investigators with data to define health issues, to begin to understand the etiology of those health issues, to formulate theories, to reveal relevant factors, and to identify potential relationships. The research
conducted in this early stage is regarded as preliminary research and serves as the
basis for future conclusive research efforts. Some examples of exploratory research
questions would include

- Are college students being harassed online?
- What does "using condoms" mean for Latino immigrants?
- What are the factors contributing to obesity among toddlers in the U.S.?
- Does intimate partner violence affect HIV risk for men who have sex with men?
- Is intimate partner violence related to women's health-seeking behaviors?

As these examples indicate, the research question involves investigations that will
describe the issue. Depending on the outcomes, this type of research usually is
viewed as a springboard for further inquiry.

Box 4.1. Prevalence Versus Incidence

Prevalence and incidence are different ways of measuring a disease's occurrence and two very important concepts in health promotion research. *Prevalence* of a condition equates with the total number of people who currently have the condition, whereas *incidence* refers to the annual number of people who have been diagnosed with the condition. These two measures are very different. A chronic incurable disease such as AIDS can have a low incidence but high prevalence. A short-duration curable condition such as a bacterial sexually transmitted disease (STD) can have a high incidence but low prevalence because many people get a STD each year, but few people actually have a bacterial STD at any given time.

Conclusive research, as the term suggests, provides information that is useful for reaching conclusions or in making decisions. Research in this phase generally has five overarching purposes: (1) to document the scope of the issue (see Box 4.1 for common public health indicators of scope), (2) to test causal or etiological theories, (3) to identify the sequelae of disease or health conditions, (4) to evaluate measurement instruments, (5) and to evaluate treatments or interventions (Salazar and Cook, 2002). Take the issue of HIV/AIDS for example; at the onset of the epidemic in the early 1980s, the research conducted was exploratory in nature. Little was known about the issue. Now that we are in the third decade of research and there has been much knowledge generated, most of the research is conclusive research. To glean a better idea of what types of research purposes would be considered as conclusive research, a sample of questions pertaining to HIV/AIDS research from each of these five research purposes is provided:

- How many new cases of HIV infection occurred among men who have sex with men (MSM)?
- How many new cases of AIDS were diagnosed among injection drug users in the Northeastern United States?
- What are the risk factors for HIV infection among African American women?
- What are the psychological and psychosocial effects of HIV diagnosis among adolescents?
- Does social support protect against negative effects of HIV diagnosis among homeless women?
- How well does a sexual risk-reduction program reduce unsafe HIV-related behaviors as compared with an abstinence program?
- What are the long-term side effects of Highly Active Anti-Retroviral Therapy?
- What are the side effects of an HIV vaccine among black men?

As these examples illustrate, conclusive research has clearly defined research questions. In comparison with exploratory research, the process is more formal and structured. Findings inform hypothesis testing and decision making.

Both exploratory and conclusive research can be further subdivided into two major categories of research purpose: *descriptive* and *causal research*. *Descriptive research* provides data describing the "who, what, when, where, and how" of a health issue, not what caused it. Therefore, studies that reveal who either is at risk or has a particular health issue or condition; that document incidence, prevalence, or both; that examine risk factors; that look at the effects of having the health issue; and that assess scale properties designed to measure a construct related to a health issue would be categorized as descriptive research. The main limitation with descriptive research is that it cannot assess what *caused* the health issue. This is where causal research steps in. Determining a cause-and-effect relationship is imperative in situations in which the investigator must reveal the true cause(s) of a particular disease or when evaluating whether or not a program caused the observed changes.

◆ ◆ ◆

In a Nutshell

Determining a cause-and-effect relationship is imperative in situations in which the investigator must reveal the true cause(s) of a particular disease or when evaluating whether or not a program caused the observed changes.

◆ ◆ ◆

Descriptive Research

Descriptive research, whether exploratory or conclusive, uses *observational designs* to achieve its objectives. The term *observational research designs* refers to research in which variables are observed as they exist in nature—no manipulation of variables occurs. Furthermore, observational research can involve both *qualitative* methods and *quantitative* methods. Observational research that uses qualitative methods does not entail the use of specific research designs per se; rather, depending on the research question, different strategies are used (Morse, 1994). A few qualitative strategies are phenomenology, ethnography, and grounded theory. Observational research that uses quantitative methods would entail the use of *cross-sectional designs, successive independent samples design,* and *longitudinal designs* (as noted in Chapter One, these also include prospective cohort designs and panel studies).

Qualitative research methods and strategies are described in greater depth in Chapter Seven; however, in simple terms, qualitative data consists of observations that do not take the form of numbers. For example, conducting interviews with people is one type of qualitative method used. The data collected consist of verbal responses to either structured or semistructured questions. These responses may be audiotaped and then transcribed. The investigator would conduct an analysis by reviewing the transcriptions and identifying themes that emerged. All results are conveyed through description. An example of a qualitative study that used grounded theory as the strategy and face-to-face interviews as the method was conducted by Melville and others (2003). They conducted interviews with twenty-four participants who had a positive herpes simplex virus type 2 (HSV-2) serology by western blot to assess the emotional and psychosocial responses to receiving a positive diagnosis. They identified three categories of themes: short-term emotional responses (for example, denial, surprise), short-term psychosocial responses (for example, fear of telling sex partner, anger at sex partner), and perceived ongoing responses (for example, feeling socially stigmatized, feeling sexually undesirable). The results were used to conceptualize a complex model involving these themes as interrelated constructs that could be tested quantitatively in the future.

Conversely, the nature of quantitative data involves numerical values. Data can be frequency of responses or occurrences, or the data can entail a process whereby participants' verbal or written responses are quantified by transforming them into numerical values. Analyses of quantitative methods require the use of statistical procedures. One example of a quantitative approach would be a surveillance study. For example, the Centers for Disease Control and Prevention (CDC) is interested in knowing how many adolescents engage in certain health risk behaviors. The Youth Risk Behavior Surveillance System (YRBSS) monitors six categories of priority health-risk behaviors among youths and young adults— behaviors that contribute to unintentional injuries and violence; tobacco use; alcohol and other drug use; sexual behaviors that contribute to unintended pregnancy and sexually transmitted diseases (STDs), including human immun-odeficiency virus (HIV) infection; unhealthy dietary behaviors; and physical inactivity plus being overweight. Some results from the 2003 national Youth Risk Behavior Survey (YRBS) demonstrated that among the high school students surveyed, 30.2 percent had ridden with a driver who had been drinking alcohol; 17.1 percent had carried a weapon; 44.9 percent had drunk alcohol; and 22.4 percent had used marijuana (Centers for Disease Control and Prevention, 2004).

Observational Research Designs

In Chapter Five, you will find specific details of *how* to conduct observational research. In this section, we describe what is considered observational research by providing an overview of the different types of observational research designs with examples drawn from the published literature.

One of the most commonly used research designs in health promotion is the *cross-sectional design*. The hallmark of this design is that time is fixed (it does not move). One or more samples are drawn from the population at one time point. Most survey-research designs are cross-sectional; however, types of research other than survey research can use cross-sectional designs.

Survey research constitutes a field of scientific inquiry in its own right and is best defined as a scientific method to help understand the characteristics of a population. By *characteristics,* we mean people's thoughts, opinions, feelings, and behaviors. Surveys are conducted for myriad reasons and are used not only by public health professionals, but also by political scientists, psychologists, sociologists, and of course marketing researchers. Moreover, surveys can vary according to their mode of administration. Surveys can be conducted over the telephone or in person. They can be self-administered using paper and pencil in a classroom or using a computer. Some surveys are administered via mail and some are administered via the Internet.

As an example of survey research, consider a study conducted by the Family Violence Prevention Fund. This organization conducted a national telephone survey of a thousand men and women over eighteen years of age living in the United States to investigate public opinion on the issue of domestic violence (Klein, Campbell, Soler, and Ghez, 1997). Respondents were given a fixed set of explanations of why a man would beat a woman (for example, "he gets drunk," or "he wants to control her"). They were then asked to choose which explanation was closest to their own view. The results showed that 20 percent of respondents indicated drinking was involved, 23 percent said that it stemmed from the man being beaten as a child, 34 percent indicated it was to control the woman. In another example, a study conducted by Finn (2004) administered a survey on-line to male and female college students. The goal was to gather data regarding the extent of on-line harassment. Among 339 respondents, 10 to 15 percent reported receiving repeated e-mail or Instant Messenger messages that were threatening, insulting, or harassing; more than half reported receiving unwanted pornography. Although the mode of administration differed, both of these studies sampled the population at one time point and the goal was to describe certain characteristics of the population sampled.

Although there is one criterion to a cross-sectional design (that is, measurement is conducted at one time point), research that uses a cross-sectional design can have more than one purpose. For example, cross-sectional designs can be used to document the prevalence of a health issue. DiClemente and colleagues (2004) used a cross-sectional design to describe the prevalence of sexually transmitted diseases (STDs) among a sample of pregnant African American adolescent females attending a prenatal clinic in the southeast. They found that, overall, approximately

24 percent tested positive for one of four STDs: Chlamydia trachomatis, Neisseria gonorrhoeae, Trichomonas vaginalis, or Treponema pallidum. In another example, Varma and colleagues (2004) also used a cross-sectional design to estimate the prevalence of ocular hypertension and open-angle glaucoma (OAG) in adult Latinos. They found that among 6,142 Latinos, forty years of age or older who lived in the Los Angeles area, and who underwent a complete ophthalmologic examination, approximately 5 percent were diagnosed with OAG and almost 4 percent had ocular hypertension. Moreover, Varma and colleagues made comparisons by age and gender. They found no gender differences, but significantly higher prevalence rates for both conditions were found in older Latinos than in younger Latinos.

In addition to assessing prevalence of disease, cross-sectional designs can be used to estimate levels of knowledge about any given health threat or health protective behavior, and health-related attitudes, beliefs, opinions, and behaviors. For example, Lapidus and colleagues (2002) conducted a mail survey among pediatric primary care physicians to determine rates of screening practices for domestic violence (DV)—the behavioral outcome in this study. Twelve percent of the respondents reported routinely screening for DV at all well-child care visits, 61 percent reported screening only certain patients, and 30 percent said they did not screen for DV at all.

◆ ◆ ◆

In a Nutshell

It is the manner in which you collect the data and not the statistical technique that allows one to make causal inferences.

◆ ◆ ◆

Another function addressed by cross-sectional designs is the ability to assess the relationships among variables for a given population. When investigating relationships among variables, the research is often referred to as *correlational,* but a distinction must be made between the statistical technique and the design. Using a cross-sectional design to investigate the relationship between two variables by applying statistical correlational techniques (for instance, Pearson product moment correlation coefficient) precludes the ability to infer causal relationships. In a correlational relationship, changes in one variable accompany changes in another; however, it cannot be said that one variable influences another when the two variables were measured using observational methods. Conversely, an exception would be made if the data were collected

MINCUS ITERATES THAT CORRELATION DOES NOT MEAN CAUSATION.

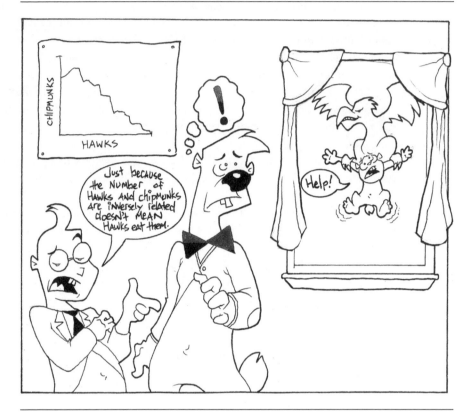

Copyright 2005 by Justin Wagner; reprinted with permission.

using experimental methods. Then, in this scenario, a correlation between two variables may imply a causal relationship. This is an important distinction that needs to be made: **It is the manner in which you collect the data and not the statistical technique that allows one to make causal inferences.** For example, it has been observed that crime rates and ice cream consumption tend to be correlated (because more crimes are committed in warm weather and more ice cream is eaten in warm weather). Yet, you would not conclude that eating more ice cream causes crime rates to increase. This is the classic *third-variable problem*, in which there is another unmeasured variable affecting both of the measured variables and causing the two variables to appear correlated with each other. Although cross-sectional designs are used frequently in correlational research, the design is limited in inferring causation. The design is also unable to establish directionality. Consider the significant inverse correlation (as one variable increases, the other variable decreases) between depression and self-esteem found frequently in the literature as another example. It is unclear whether depression leads to low self-esteem or whether low-esteem leads to depression. In reality, both propositions are equally plausible; thus, a correlational design is incapable of distinguishing cause from effect. An experimental design is necessary for causality to be determined. In an example from the published research, Salazar and others (2004) were able to demonstrate a significant correlation between African American adolescent girls' self-concept (including self-esteem, body image, and ethnic identity) and the frequency in which they refused unsafe sex. However, there was no way of determining with certainty whether or not self-concept *influenced* unsafe sex refusal, or whether the reverse was true. It is also possible that neither variable influenced or caused the other. This is one of the major limitations of conducting correlational research, especially research that uses cross-sectional designs.

◆ ◆ ◆

In a Nutshell

Although cross-sectional designs are used frequently in correlational research, the design is limited in inferring causation. The design is also unable to establish directionality.

◆ ◆ ◆

Nonetheless, we continue to conduct observational research using cross-sectional designs as it provides the necessary foundation for more elaborate studies that improve upon the limitations of a cross-sectional design. Also, in many instances, it is not feasible or ethical to conduct an experimental research study when manipulation of the variable is impossible, or it is unethical to do so (for instance, you cannot assign a person to any condition that entails risk). Furthermore, cross-sectional correlational studies are also useful to identify correlates of behavioral variables, but not necessarily variables that have a cause-and-effect relationship. For example, Hall, Jones, and Saraiya (2001) conducted a cross-sectional study to determine the correlates of sunscreen use among U.S. high school students. They found that among a nationally representative sample ($N = 15,349$) of students, infrequent use of sunscreen was associated with other risky health behaviors such as driving after drinking, riding in a car with a drinking driver, cigarette smoking, being sexually active, and being physically inactive. Clearly, the authors of this study were not attempting to imply a cause-and-effect relationship, but rather, they were trying to reveal a cluster of health risk behaviors to address comprehensively in a health promotion program.

A *successive independent samples design* improves upon the time limitation of cross-sectional designs by incorporating a series of cross-sectional studies conducted over a period of time. Each cross-sectional survey is conducted with an independent sample, which means that a new sample is drawn for each of the successive cross-sectional surveys. This design is used to assess change in a population characteristic (for example, tobacco use, condom use, pregnancy rates) over time and is also referred to as a *trend study*.

As health promotion researchers for example, we may want to document the change in certain health risk behaviors or the prevalence of disease for a given population over a period of time. This would be very important information to have and could inform programs and policy. In fact, this type of design is used quite often in *epidemiology*—the discipline studying the incidence, distribution, and control of disease in a population.

The CDC conducts and sponsors many studies using the successive independent samples design. One example is the CDC's serosurveillance system, which is used to monitor the prevalence of human immunodeficiency virus type 1 (HIV-1) in the United States. In collaboration with state and local health departments, surveys were conducted in selected sites from 1988 through 1999. Populations that were included ranged from low risk (for instance, military, blood donors) to high risk (such as injection drug users and men who have sex with men (MSM)). The objectives of the serosurveillance system are (1) to provide standardized estimates of HIV prevalence among the selected populations, (2) to describe the magnitude and changes over time of HIV infection in these populations, (3) to recognize new or emerging patterns of HIV infection among specific subgroups of the U.S. population, and (4) to assist in directing resources and in targeting programs for HIV prevention and care. The results showed that in general, prevalence was higher among survey participants who were in the older age categories and, with the exception of Job Corps entrants, among those who were male. For most of the surveillance populations included in the report, prevalence by region, race or ethnicity, and age group either decreased or remained stable from 1993–1997. For the MSM population, these results are depicted in graph form and show trends in HIV prevalence by region (Figure 4.2) and race or ethnicity (Figure 4.3).

The CDC also uses this type of design to track changes in behaviors over time. For example, Serdula and others (2004) examined trends in fruit and vegetable consumption among adults living in the United States from 1994 to 2000. Using

FIGURE 4.2.   HIV PREVALENCE AMONG MEN WHO HAVE SEX WITH MEN, AT SEXUALLY TRANSMITTED DISEASE CLINICS, BY REGION (1993–1997).

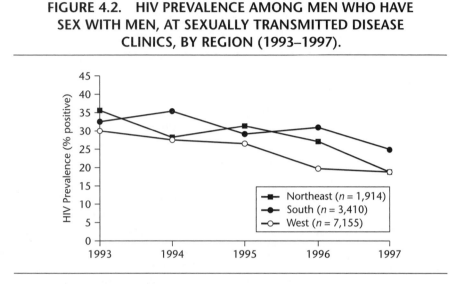

FIGURE 4.3.   HIV PREVALENCE AMONG MEN WHO HAVE SEX WITH MEN, AT SEXUALLY TRANSMITTED DISEASE CLINICS, BY RACE OR ETHNICITY (1993–1997).

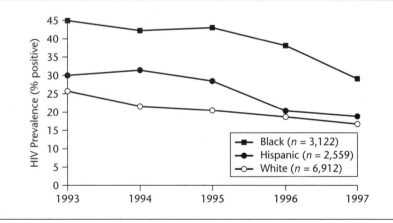

Note: Standardized to 1993 STD clinic population by region and age group.

random-digit-dialing procedures, a method in which each household that has a telephone has an equal probability of being selected, they sampled 434,121 adults in total. Each sample of adults was surveyed at four different time points: 1994, 1996, 1998, and 2000. The results showed that the mean frequency of fruit and vegetable consumption declined over time, although the proportion of respondents who consumed fruit or vegetables five or more times per day remained stable.

Although an improvement over the cross-sectional design, successive independent samples design also suffers from limitations. It is very useful for measuring changes over time for a characteristic such as disease; however, for other characteristics such as behavior, attitudes, or opinions, the researcher cannot determine with certainty the extent to which the population truly changed because the results are based on different samples of people. In order to attribute documented changes to the time factor, the same group of people needs to be followed and surveyed over time.

Longitudinal designs, however, are capable of determining changes in behavior, attitudes, or opinions over time. The defining characteristic of a longitudinal design is that the same participants are followed over a period of time and interviewed more than once during the time period. The time period could range from months to years. In such a study, sometimes referred to as a *cohort study, prospective study,* or *panel study,* the analysis of data usually involves estimation of rates of disease or behavior in the cohort during a defined period of observation. Traditionally, the term *cohort* refers to the part of the population born during a particular period (for instance, baby boomers) and whose characteristics such as causes of death and those still alive can be ascertained as it enters successive time and age periods. The term *cohort study* describes an investigation of any designated group of persons that are followed over a period of time.

The analysis of data typically involves estimation of rates of disease or behavior change during the observation period. Newly diagnosed cases (incidence) of a disease for a cohort would be calculated for an observation period that is measured in years of observation time per person (in other words, person-years). Thus, if you have a cohort of 2000 people who are followed for a period of 30 years, then the incidence of disease would be the ratio of newly diagnosed cases to a denominator equal to 2000×30 years. This ratio would typically be expressed in terms of 100,000 person-years.

Longitudinal designs improve vastly on some of the limitations of cross-sectional designs and of the successive independent samples design. For example, by following the same cohort over a long period of time you may be able to establish the temporal order of occurrences and you may be able to attribute change to the time factor. Also, you may be able to ascertain the effects of naturally occurring events. For example, if within the time frame of your longitudinal study an event such as a natural disaster, a divorce, or heart attack occurs, you could investigate whether or not there were any differences between those in the cohort who experienced the event and those who did not. If significant differences were found, then you could reasonably attribute them to the event. Of course, one major problem with longitudinal studies is *attrition*. Also referred to as *mortality*, attrition is the loss of participants from the research study and can bias the results. Severe attrition can be dealt with statistically by comparing those who returned for follow-up interviews (or completed follow-up questionnaires) with those who did not and determining critical differences between the two groups. For example, in sex research, if those lost to attrition had baseline indicators of more frequent risky sexual activity than those who remained in the study, then the loss to follow-up could bias the study conclusions.

◆ ◆ ◆

In a Nutshell

Longitudinal designs improve vastly on some of the limitations of cross-sectional designs and of the successive independent samples design.

◆ ◆ ◆

An example of a longitudinal study that examined behaviors was conducted by Repetto, Zimmerman, and Caldwell (2004). They were able to determine the correlational relationships between depressive symptoms and alcohol use among a cohort of 456 black high school students. The students were interviewed every year during high school and for three years following the transition to adulthood. The researchers were able to document the temporal order of depressive symptoms, alcohol use, and life changes associated with adulthood.

In another study that used a longitudinal design, Finnish researchers Huurre, Aro, and Jaakkola (2004) identified incidence of asthma and allergic rhinitis. They recruited a cohort of 2,269 that was followed from birth to thirty-two years of age. They estimated the incidence rate of asthma and allergic rhinitis during the full time period, while also estimating the prevalence rates for the diseases at three ages: sixteen, twenty-two, and thirty-two years of age. The overall incidence rate of asthma was 2.1 new cases per 1000 person-years and the overall incidence rate for allergic rhinitis was approximately 12 new cases per 1000 person-years. They found changes in prevalence rates of asthma from 3 percent to 5 percent as the cohort moved from sixteen years of age to thirty-two years old. Prevalence rates of allergic rhinitis also changed significantly from 17.5 percent to 26 percent for the same age ranges.

The *cohort-sequential design* is essentially a hybrid of cross-sectional and longitudinal designs. Starting with an initial cohort and following it over a period of time, another cohort or cohorts are then added at varying intervals within that time period. Changes over time for the first cohort can be assessed while also being able to make cross-sectional comparisons among the different cohorts at specific time points.

An example of cohort-sequential design was conducted by Chassin, Presson, Rose, and Sherman (2001). They reported the results from a study designed to assess age-related changes in health-relevant beliefs from the middle school years through age thirty-seven. Participants were initially recruited between 1980 and 1983, and the sample comprised sixth through twelfth graders in a county school system. Participants completed a survey each year. The final sample included the participation of ten cohorts (that is, the graduating classes of 1980–1989). Follow-up surveys were conducted in 1987, 1993, and 1999 with retention rates of 73 percent, 73 percent, and 71 percent respectively. The results showed systematic age-related changes in the perceived risks of cigarette smoking.

Causal Research

As compared with descriptive research, causal research transcends the natural order of things through manipulation and provides an ability to make cause-effect statements. Thus, causal research employs *experimental designs* so that causal inference can be made with a high degree of certainty, and in some instances *quasi-experimental designs*. Experimental designs entail the manipulation of a variable to test the effects of the manipulation on some outcome. Quasi-experimental designs approximate experimental designs but do not use randomization. Why should we care about making cause-effect statements? Making cause-effect statements provides both theoretical and practical benefits. For example, by isolating the cause of a condition or disease, we may begin work on devising a cure. In addition, causal research allows us to find out if a particular program is helpful in solving a problem. This type of research is usually conducted in controlled settings with small groups of people. If the treatment or program is *efficacious*, meaning it had the ability to produce the desired effect, then it can be applied to a larger group in real-life settings. Within the context of health promotion research, causal research allows us not only to predict, understand, and control behavior, but also to change behavior.

The two main defining characteristics of experimental research designs are the manipulation of an *independent variable* and control over *extraneous variables*. The independent variable is the variable chosen by the investigator to determine its effect on the *dependent variable* and is manipulated or controlled by the investigator. If the investigator is manipulating only one factor, then the design is a single-factor design; if more than one factor, it is called a factorial design. The number of independent variables equates with the number of factors in the design. The dependent variable is the outcome variable of interest and is measured by the investigator. Extraneous variables are not directly related to the hypothesis being tested, but may nevertheless have an effect on the dependent variable. You may *control* the effects of extraneous variables either by holding them constant or by randomizing their effects across treatment levels. To the extent that extraneous variables provide alternative explanations or rival hypotheses for the findings, the *internal validity* of the study will be threatened.

The internal validity of the study is the ability of the design to test the hypothesis it was designed to test. Internal validity can be thought of as the approximate truth about inferences regarding cause-effect or causal relationships. Seven common threats to internal validity have been identified and deserve consideration when designing your study: history, maturation, testing, instrumentation, statistical regression, biased selection of subjects, and experimental mortality (Campbell and Stanley, 1966). These threats to internal validity are defined in Box 4.2. Common threats that may seriously threaten internal validity must be addressed prior to conducting your study so that alternative hypotheses can be ruled out.

Before the different types of experimental designs are discussed, an important and related factor to understand when planning health promotion research is that conducting experiments in a controlled laboratory with pathogens is markedly different from conducting experiments with human subjects in the real world. Although controlling for extraneous variables is critical to the integrity of an experiment, the level of control may vary widely when the experiment takes

---

Box 4.2. Common Threats to Internal Validity

1. History—results might be due to an event that occurred between observations.
2. Maturation—results might be due to participants growing older, wiser, stronger, or more experienced between observations.
3. Testing—results might be due to the number of times responses were measured.
4. Instrumentation—results might be due to a change in the measuring instrument between observations.
5. Statistical regression—results might be due to the selection of participants based on extreme scores, and when measured again, scores move back to an average level.
6. Selection bias—results might be due to differences that existed between participants in groups before treatment occurred.
7. Mortality—results might be due to the differential loss of participants from groups.

place in a real-world setting (such as a classroom or community) as opposed to a laboratory or other "controlled setting" (for instance, an isolated room), and the subjects compose a heterogeneous group. Having a lower level of control over environmental factors and human subjects' factors threatens internal validity and may introduce *error variance. Error variance* refers to the variability in the dependent variable that *cannot* be attributed to the independent variable, but rather is attributed to extraneous variables or to variability among human subjects. Thus, reducing or controlling error variance is an important matter to consider as error variance may affect the ability to attribute observable effects to the manipulation of the independent variable. Furthermore, different types of designs handle error variance differently and should be a consideration when choosing an appropriate design.

To illustrate these two main experimental concepts of manipulation and control, consider the research question What are the side effects of a hepatitis vaccine on black men? The independent variable would be the administration of the hepatitis vaccine. There must be at least two levels to an independent variable or it is not a variable. In this instance, manipulation of the independent variable could be using two vaccines qualitatively different, such as a surface antigen vaccine as one and a *placebo* (an inactive substance that may look like medicine but contains no medicine, a "sugar pill" with no treatment value) or a different type of hepatitis vaccine as the second. Moreover, different levels of the independent variable could be quantitatively different when the same vaccine type was used, but in different dosages. The latter scenario is referred to as a dose-ranging study, in which two or more doses (starting at a lower dose and proceeding to higher doses) of a vaccine are tested against each other to determine which dose works best and has acceptable side effects. The dependent variable in this hypothetical study would be the "side effects" and could include measures of fatigue, quality of life, and nausea.

To achieve a high level of control in this study, there are two main issues to consider: first, control related to subject selection and assignment; second, control related to the type of experimental design chosen. Control over extraneous variables through the use of experimental designs increases the confidence that observed outcomes are the result of a given program, treatment, drug, or innovation instead of a function of extraneous variables or events and greatly enhances internal validity. Given these two important issues, the first issue to consider would be the method in which the potential participants will be sampled from the population of black men. A *random selection* procedure such as the use of a random numbers table would ensure a high degree of control in that each potential participant would have an equal chance of being selected. This procedure helps to control variables that could be introduced into the selection process and could cause not only low *generalizability* but also *selection bias.* Generalizability is the degree to which the research findings can be applied to the population under study (for example, black men). Using random selection helps to increase the representativeness of the sample thereby enhancing generalizability. As indicated in Box 4.2, selection bias results when groups differ from each other. Differences could be on either measured or unmeasured characteristics. Selection bias also occurs when the sample is not representative of the population. If random selection is used, then selection bias should not be an issue unless the response rate or the rate in which participants agreed to be in the study was extremely low. Furthermore, if random selection is not possible, then a nonrandom sampling technique such as *convenience sampling* (using individuals who are convenient to access) or *snowball sampling* (using recruited participants to identify others) would have to be used and would not reduce selection bias in the sample. Thus, if participants differ in ways that affect the dependent variable (side effects of HIV vaccine), then the results might be attributed to these differences rather than to the vaccine.

Once the sample is recruited, the next factor to consider is how to assign the subjects into the two groups. Other sources of error variance involving the subjects such as socioeconomic status, age, and education level, to name a few, need to be controlled. One method that would control (in this instance, by "control" we mean hold the effects of these variables constant) these sources of error variance would be to use *random assignment* (a.k.a. randomization) as the method to assign participants into respective groups. Randomization entails assigning participants by chance to one of two or more groups. There are different methods, such as using a random numbers table, using a software program, or even flipping a coin. Randomization minimizes any differences between or among groups by equally distributing subjects with particular characteristics between or among all the trial arms. Randomization rules out many threats to internal validity, but not all of them.

◆ ◆ ◆

In a Nutshell

Randomization entails assigning participants by chance to one of two or more groups. There are different methods, such as using a random numbers table, using a software program, or even flipping a coin. Randomization minimizes any differences between or among groups by equally distributing subjects with particular characteristics between or among all the trial arms.

◆ ◆ ◆

The second and probably the most important issue of control is the specific experimental design chosen. There are different ways in which this specific research question could be answered. The various designs that are used to conduct causal research vary in quality of evidence they provide for making causal inference and in the level of control. Moreover, there are distinctions between experimental designs, "true" experimental designs, and quasi-experimental designs that further influence the level of control and the ability to attribute changes in the dependent variable to the manipulation of the independent variable.

In the remaining section of this chapter, we will describe the various experimental and quasi-experimental research designs that make up causal research along with examples drawn from the scientific literature. We will provide an overview of the related concepts and terminology. Because the focus of this book is on the research methods used in health promotion and practice, we describe designs and methods related to health promotion. For example, research concepts or methods used in the study of pathogen isolation (such as Koch's Postulates), albeit important, are outside the scope of this text and will not be covered.

Experimental Research Designs. In health promotion research, much research can be considered *controlled trial* research, in which human volunteers are recruited to answer specific health questions. For example, controlled trials in health promotion would involve testing the efficacy of prevention programs for reducing health risk behaviors, disease, or the effects of disease. When conceptualizing and evaluating controlled trials, a common experimental design employed is the *between-subjects design*. In this type of experimental design, different groups or *arms* (that is, a group of participants in a clinical trial all of whom receive the same treatment) are exposed to the different levels of the independent variable. Furthermore, if you randomly assign subjects to the different arms, then you have a randomized between groups design. In health promotion research, this type of design is referred to as a randomized controlled trial (RCT) and is considered the "gold standard" of experimental designs.

Although the criteria of an experiment are manipulation and control, there is a distinction between a "true" experimental design and an experimental design. According to Campbell and Stanley (1966), a true experimental design must include more than one group, common measured outcome(s), and random assignment. Thus, because the RCT is a between-subjects design that uses random assignment it is considered a true experiment. The specific details of how to conduct an RCT are provided in Chapter Six. Most health promotion researchers concur that the RCT is the most effective and rigorous design for testing the efficacy of a program or treatment because it allows for causal inference and has the highest level of control possible in a real-world setting.

The number of levels of the independent variable dictates the number of arms to be employed in an RCT. For example, if you were examining the efficacy of an HIV-preventive intervention relative to a general health intervention, then you would require two groups; if you were examining the efficacy of an HIV-preventive intervention and an HIV-preventive intervention with booster sessions relative to the general health intervention, then you would need three groups. An example of a two-arm RCT was a study conducted by Shrier and others (2001), in which they evaluated a theory-driven safer-sex intervention for high-risk girls with cervicitis or pelvic inflammatory disease ($N = 123$). The clinical trial took place in an urban children's hospital adolescent clinic and inpatient service. The intervention was administered by trained female health educators during the time when the adolescents received STD treatment. The adolescent participants were not randomly selected to participate, but they were randomly assigned to the intervention group or to the control group. The intervention included topics such as STD transmission, secondary abstinence, and the female condom. Difference between groups on the behavioral outcomes was not statistically significant at the $P < .05$ level (likely due in part to small sample size).

Another type of between-subjects design, which may be useful in health promotion research, is the *matched groups design*. This design is employed when the researcher is aware of a particular subject characteristic that is strongly associated with the dependent variable. Using randomization, the characteristic may not get equally distributed between groups. Thus, to ensure that the characteristic is distributed equally, subjects are matched on the characteristic prior to random assignment. Depending on the number of groups in the experiment, subjects are matched with other subjects as close as possible to form pairs (two groups), triplets (three groups), or even quadruplets (four groups). Then, taking each set, subjects are assigned at random into groups. The main advantage of this design is significant reduction of the effect of the matched characteristic on the dependent variable. One example would be matching adolescents enrolled in a two-arm sexual-risk-reduction intervention on alcohol and drug use prior to randomization into groups. In this instance, prior to randomization, subjects would be measured on their alcohol and drug use. Subjects who reported similar behavior would be paired together. Each subject would be randomly assigned to one of the two conditions.

Within health promotion research, often the use of this design involves the site versus individual subjects as the unit of assignment (for instance, school, community, workplace, and so on). For example, Emmons, Linnan, Shadel, Marcus, and Abrams (1999) evaluated a multiple-risk-factor health intervention to determine its effectiveness in increasing physical-activity levels, increasing nutritional value of food intake, and smoking cessation among employees. The study employed a randomized matched-pair design in which the worksite was the unit of assignment. Twenty-six manufacturing worksites were matched on characteristics that were thought to be strongly associated with the study outcomes. The matching characteristics were whether or not there was a smoking policy and a cafeteria, size of the worksite, gender distribution, blue or white collar worker status, and the response rate to the baseline survey. Among the final sample of 2,055 participants who completed all three assessments, significant differences in the hypothesized direction were found between treatment conditions in exercise behavior and consumption of fruits, vegetables, and fiber. No differences by condition were found for percentage of calories from fat consumed or smoking cessation. A similar design was used in an evaluation of a community-based health promotion in India (Bhandari and others, 2003). The intervention was an educational program designed to promote exclusive breastfeeding for six months. Eight communities in India were matched on socioeconomic indicators, child mortality rates, recent morbidity, and the prevalence of wasting (the breakdown of body tissue such as muscle and organ for use as a protein source when the diet lacks protein) and stunting prior to randomization into either the intervention or control group. At three-month follow-up, exclusive breastfeeding rates in the intervention condition (79 percent) were significantly higher than the control condition (48 percent). Diarrhea prevalence was also lower in the intervention group than in the control group.

The *within-subjects design,* or *repeated-measures design,* is another experimental design that is also effective in reducing error variance due to human subject differences. In this design, the same subjects are exposed to the different levels of the independent variable. Thus, the same subjects form the different groups for comparisons. For example, if there are two levels of the independent variable, condition one is formed when subjects are exposed to the first level; condition two is formed when subjects are exposed to the second level. Although matching in a between-groups design reduces error variance due to individual differences to a large degree, the within-subjects design is more effective because the same subjects are exposed to the different treatments. Thus, error variance due to subject differences is significantly reduced or eliminated. With this level of reduction in error variance, the ability to detect the effects of the independent variable is greater than in other designs. Although the within-subjects design is classified as an experimental design because of manipulation and control, it is important to note that because this design does not have random assignment, it cannot be considered a true experimental design.

In health promotion research that involves a behavioral intervention, the within-subjects design is rarely used mainly because of *carryover effects,* which occur when exposure to the first treatment (in this instance it could be an educational intervention) affects the subjects' performance during subsequent treatments. Depending on the carryover effect, performance can be enhanced or reduced. For example, subjects may learn a skill in the first treatment that may enhance the observed outcomes after subsequent treatments; however, the observed change in outcome may be from the first treatment and not the second. This effect is called *learning.* Other types of carryover effects include *fatigue* (deterioration in performance due to being tired from the first treatment), *habituation* (repeated exposure to stimulus leads to reduced responsiveness), *sensitization* (stronger responses to stimuli stemming from initial exposure to a different stimulus), and *adaptation* (adaptive changes to a stimulus lead to a change in outcome).

A specific form of the within-subjects design used quite often in drug efficacy trials is called a *crossover trial.* In this type of design, the same group of subjects is exposed to all levels of the independent variable, but the order in which groups of subjects are exposed is varied. Thus, for every possible order combination, there is a group formed. For example, if researchers wanted to examine the efficacy of a drug on reducing pain, then using a crossover trial, they could randomly assign half the subjects to receive the drug first and then the placebo, while the other half receives the placebo first and then the drug. When each group of subjects switches from the first treatment condition to the next, this is the point at which they "crossover." By random assignment into the "groups" in this way, the more simple within-subjects design can be classified as a true experiment.

A randomized crossover trial design was used in a sexual health promotion study conducted among women attending an urban, reproductive health clinic in the southeastern United States to assess their acceptability and use of male and female condoms (Kulczycki, Kim, Duerr, Jamieson, and Macaluso, 2004). The sample of women was randomly assigned to one of two groups: the first group used ten male condoms first followed by a crossover to using ten female condoms; the second group was the reverse order. An intervention was also administered and consisted of a nurse providing instruction in correct condom usage and was given to all women. Overall, the results indicated that regardless of order, women preferred male condoms to female condoms and judged them to be superior.

Many studies in health promotion use *combined* or *mixed designs* in which there are independent groups (that is, an indicator of a between-groups design) that are assessed at multiple time points (in other words, an indicator of a within-subjects design). In this instance, the within-subjects factor is "time" with the number of levels corresponding to the number of time points. This is slightly different from the within-subjects design described previously, in which the within-subjects factor was the administration of all possible levels of the treatment to the same group of subjects. Thus, in a mixed design, comparisons can be made not only between groups and within groups, but also for the interaction of the two factors.

The RCT is considered a mixed design when subjects are assessed at multiple time periods. For example, in simplest terms, implementation of an RCT would involve (1) assessing subjects at baseline, (2) randomizing subjects into groups, (3) exposing subjects to the respective treatment, (4) assessing subjects after completion of the treatment (could be immediately following or at a follow-up period), and (5) assessing them again at subsequent follow-up period(s). Analysis goals for this design could include determining overall differences between groups (main effect for group), overall differences within groups (main effect for time), or whether or not subjects in the treatment group changed differentially over time as compared with subjects in the control group (an interaction of group and time).

St. Lawrence, Wilson, Eldridge, Brasfield, and O'Bannon (2001) applied a mixed design to test the efficacy of an HIV-preventive intervention based on the theory of gender and power, an HIV-preventive intervention based on social learning theory, and an HIV-preventive intervention based on cognitive behavioral principles relative to a wait-list control condition. The population for the evaluation study was disadvantaged African American women, and the sample of 445 was drawn from several community venues. Women were given baseline assessments and then randomly assigned into one of four groups: one of the three theoretically derived programs or the wait list control. Thus, this study had four levels of the first factor. Assessments were also made at postintervention and at a one-year follow-up period indicating three levels of the second factor. The results showed that at one-year follow-up, although there was no difference in condom use among the three treatment groups, in all of the three treatment conditions, condom use increased relative to the wait list control group.

Quasi-Experimental Designs. The word *quasi* means as if or almost; thus, a quasi-experiment approximates a true experiment. Quasi-experiments are similar to true experiments in that there is a treatment of some kind to examine and there are outcome measures; the main difference is that quasi-experiments do not use random assignment to create the groups necessary for comparison on the outcome measures. Many times, conducting health promotion research precludes using random assignment into groups or conditions because it may not be feasible, possible, ethical, or legal. For example, withholding a drug treatment or critical health program from vulnerable populations such as prisoners or pregnant women would be unethical or illegal in some instances if one group benefits and one group is deprived. For school-based health educational programs, resources may dictate that only one designated school receives the program, and it may be cost prohibitive to incorporate another school as a comparison. Although there are myriad reasons underlying the choice to use a quasi-experimental design, especially when conducting field research, it is important to understand that quasi-experiments are considered causal research, but the ability to rule out alternative explanations is much more limited than when using an experimental design. Furthermore, within the category of quasi-experimental designs, there is variability among the different designs as far as level of control and the ability to infer causation.

The *nonequivalent control group design* (NCGD) is used often in health promotion research, as it offers more control than some quasi-experimental designs by including a comparison group. Although similar in concept to the matched-pairs between-groups design, the nonequivalent control group design deviates from the matched-subjects design in that there is no randomization of the matched subjects, sites, workplaces, or communities into respective groups. Because the investigator does not control the assignment to groups through randomization, this design is deemed as having "nonequivalent groups." In the NCGD, a group is matched as closely as possible to the experimental group and is used as a comparison group; however, the groups may be different prior to the study. Because of this nonequivalence of groups at the start, the NCGD is especially susceptible to the selection threat to internal validity. Any prior differences between the groups may affect the outcome of the study. Under the worst circumstances, this can lead us to conclude that our health promotion program did not have an effect, when in fact it did, or that the program did have an effect, when in fact it did not.

◆ ◆ ◆

In a Nutshell

Because of this nonequivalence of groups at the start, the NCGD is especially susceptible to the selection threat to internal validity.

◆ ◆ ◆

Two main types of designs fall under the general category of NCGD: the nonequivalent group, posttest only and the nonequivalent group, pretest-posttest. The nonequivalent, posttest-only design consists of administering an outcome measure to two groups such as a program-treatment group and a comparison group or possibly two program groups, each receiving a different version of the program. For example, one group of students at a high school might receive an abstinence-only program while students at another school receive a comprehensive sexual-risk-reduction program. After twelve weeks, a test measuring sexual debut and risky sexual behaviors can be administered to see which program was more effective. A major problem with this design is that as stated previously the two groups might not be necessarily the same before the program takes place and may differ in important ways that may influence the outcomes. For instance, if it is found that the students in the abstinence-only program reported a delay in sexual debut and less engagement in sexual risk behavior, there is no way of determining if they were less likely to engage in those behaviors even before the program or whether other factors (for example, level of parental monitoring or parental communication about sex) may have influenced their sexual behavior.

The nonequivalent group, pretest-posttest design improves on a major limitation of the nonequivalent group, posttest-only design by allowing the researcher to empirically assess differences in the two groups prior to implementation of the program. If the researcher finds that one group performs better than the other on the posttest, then initial differences (if the groups were in fact similar on the pretest) can be ruled out as explanations for the differences. Furthermore, if in fact the groups did differ on the pretest measure, then the researcher could potentially control for these differences statistically.

Bastani and others (2002) used a longitudinal nonequivalent control group design to evaluate the effects of a systems-level intervention that sought to increase cervical cancer screening among underserved women attending one of several clinics composing the second largest County Health Department in the United States. The intervention consisted of multiple strategies that involved physician education, physician feedback, patient education, policy interventions, and expanding the capacity to serve women better. The authors stated that "logistical constraints, limited resources, and other practical consideration in the County health care system largely dictated the choice of this design. Intervention and control sites were selected in consultation with our partners in the County Health Department. The system did not include sufficient sites to allow for randomization to intervention and control conditions. Likewise, the structure of the health care system made it impossible to randomize the intervention to only a portion of the women receiving care at any one site" (Bastani and others, 2002, p. 893). Intervention sites were a hospital, a comprehensive health center (CHC), and three public health centers (PHCs) and were matched on size, patient characteristics, and a range of services provided to another hospital, a CHC, and three PHCs. Intervention effects were observed at the hospital and the CHC, where there was a significant increase in cervical cancer screening.

The *interrupted time series design* (ITSD) is the strongest quasi-experimental approach for evaluating the longitudinal effects of interventions. It involves collecting data at multiple instances over time before and after a treatment of some kind. The treatment can be a health promotion program, implementation of a new health policy, or a naturally occurring event. Data used in a time series design can range from individual behavior to cumulative incidence of sexually transmitted diseases. It does require knowledge about the specific time in which the program or intervention occurred in the time series. An advantage of collecting a series of observations both before and after the treatment is that a reliable picture regarding the outcome of interest can be gleaned. Thus, the time series design is sensitive to trends in performance. The aim is to determine whether or not the intervention had an effect over and above any trend present in the data. For example, the data collected prior to the treatment may reveal several trends in the data such as a maturational trend (in which observations involve human subjects who are changing their behavior as they age) or a seasonal trend (in which observations are influenced by the season in which data are collected). These trends can be identified and assessed, and treatment effects ascertained. A treatment effect is demonstrated only if the pattern of posttreatment responses differs significantly from the pattern of pretreatment responses. That is, the treatment effect is demonstrated by a discontinuity in the pattern of pretreatment and posttreatment responses. For example, an effect is demonstrated when there is a change in the level or slope of the posttreatment responses as, or both, compared with the pretreatment responses.

The most basic of the ITSDs is the simple interrupted time series, in which there is only one experimental group. This design can be diagrammed as follows:

$$O_1 \quad O_2 \quad O_3 \quad O_4 \quad \text{Treatment} \quad O_5 \quad O_6 \quad O_7 \quad O_8$$

The greatest threat to the internal validity of this design is history, although other threats such as instrumentation and selection can occur.

Adding a nonequivalent control group to the simple interrupted time series will improve on some of the limitations mentioned. This design, called an interrupted time series with a nonequivalent control group time series, is diagrammed as follows:

$$O_1 \quad O_2 \quad O_3 \quad O_4 \quad \text{Treatment} \quad O_5 \quad O_6 \quad O_7 \quad O_8$$

$$O_1 \quad O_2 \quad O_3 \quad O_4 \qquad\qquad\qquad O_5 \quad O_6 \quad O_7 \quad O_8$$

As shown, a series of observations are collected both prior to and following the administration of the treatment for the experimental group; during this same time period, a series of observations are also collected for a comparison group. This design allows the researcher to control for history effects, as a historical event would most likely affect both treatment and control groups equally. What may be problematic, however, is when one group experiences a unique set of events. This type of threat is deemed an interaction between selection and history and is called a selection-history effect. It is important to note that for a historical event to pose a threat to internal validity, the event must occur at the same time as the intervention or treatment. Other threats to the internal validity are similar to the basic NCGD, with selection being the greatest threat and the interaction of selection with threats other than history such as selection-maturation, selection-instrumentation, and selection-regression.

Wong, Chan, and Koh (2002) used a simple ITSD to examine the impact of a sexual-risk-reduction program that encouraged condom use for oral sex among female brothel-based sex workers in Singapore. The study observed two outcomes: condom use trends and the pharyngeal gonorrhea trends. Comparisons on the two study outcomes were made across four time periods that corresponded to different phases of the intervention: a preintervention period of two years; an intervention phase of two years; a postintervention phase of one year when activities were withdrawn; and a follow-up period of one year when activities were resumed and incorporated into the brothel's health education policy for its sex workers. The results indicated that for the preintervention phase, consistent condom use for oral sex was stable at below 50 percent. Following the intervention, condom use increased significantly. During the postintervention phase of one year, when activities were withheld from brothels, condom use leveled off and decreased to 79.7 percent. In the last year, when activities were institutionalized, condom use increased significantly to 89.9 percent. The significant changing trend in condom use was mirrored by changes in pharyngeal gonorrhea incidence rates. Preintervention, pharyngeal gonorrhea incidence rates were stable and remained high (12.4 to 16.6 per 1000 person-months). During the two-year intervention phase, the pharyngeal gonorrhea incidence rate significantly decreased to 3.3 per 1000 person-months, but was followed by an increase when program activities were withdrawn. This increase was in tandem with the decrease in condom use during this same phase. During the final phase, when condom use increased significantly, there was also a major decline in the pharyngeal gonorrhea incidence rate, from 14.4 to 4.0 per 1000 person-months.

Integration with the Research Process

Choosing an appropriate research design is a critical part of the overall research process and may depend to a large degree on the nature of the research question; however, there are other issues to consider that may influence the overall process. For example, the stage of the research process, either exploratory or conclusive, will influence greatly many aspects of the research. For example, if a research field is in the exploratory stage, then this may affect the ability to fulfill step 1 (identify a priority population) in the nine-step model described in Chapter One. Consequently, identifying specific populations that require priority because of their risk status may be the goal of the research, especially if previous research has not determined which populations are most at risk. Moreover, the stage of the research process will influence the nature of the research question (step 2). If still the exploratory phase, research questions will be geared toward a better understanding of the phenomena involved or perhaps toward identifying what the problem is. If the field has moved to the conclusive stage, research questions will be more clearly defined involving testable hypotheses with important implications. Once the research question is formulated, it is equally important to identify the main goal or purpose associated with that research question (step 3). That is, is the research purpose to describe salient risk factors associated with a health issue or to determine who is most at risk for a health issue (that is, descriptive purpose), or is it to identify cause-and-effect relationships or test the efficacy of health programs (that is, causal purpose)? The research purpose in turn will affect the selection of a parsimonious research design (step 4). Finally, once an appropriate research design is selected, this defines the appropriate statistical technique to be employed for data analysis (step 8).

Making good decisions in the first three steps of the process will have a positive impact on the latter steps in the process, whereas unwise decisions may negatively affect the latter steps. Specifically, having an understanding of all potential research issues will enhance the planning of the research (steps 4–6). For example, an important practice is to consider whether an HPP might inadvertently produce negative effects of any kind. Indeed, an emerging framework in health promotion suggests that negative, unanticipated outcomes should be measured (Glasgow, Vogt, and Boles, 1999). Also, thinking ahead about research issues may greatly facilitate the implementation of the research (step 7), and, consequently, assist in the testing of the research hypotheses and the dissemination of the results (step 9).

Summary

All of the designs described in this chapter have associated strengths, limitations, and varying levels of rigor. The important thing to know is the strengths and limitations of each research design, and how these may affect the study results and the interpretation of those results. Thus, perhaps the most important decision to make is the selection of a research design. This decision should be examined carefully by every member of the research team, and the pros and cons of each option should be weighed with great attention to rigor. Many of these pros and cons were outlined in this chapter. It may be useful to begin by defining whether the research is exploratory or conclusive, and then asking whether it is descriptive or causal. From that point, it is critical to consider what resources are available to the project so that the selected study design is not only functional but also feasible. In addition, although implicit in this chapter, it is important to remain vigilant regarding your obligation to design research studies that are ethical in nature and that do not violate the rights or well-being of the participants. Finally, it is imperative that your research design optimizes the ability to provide a rigorous and valid test of the research question(s) because your work may have great potential to shape health promotion practice and policy and contribute another link in the chain of research.

Issues to Consider

1. Early in the HIV/AIDS epidemic, researchers wanted to ascertain the effectiveness of giving antiretroviral therapies (ARTs) to HIV-positive women who were pregnant, to prevent the transmission of the virus to their unborn child. At the time, this was considered a risky treatment, and the safety of this drug treatment on the unborn child was not known. Using an experimental design to randomly assign pregnant women who are HIV-positive to receive ART or to receive a placebo would be the most rigorous design with a high degree of control and internal validity. On the one hand, using an experimental design could provide definitive evidence of the effectiveness of the treatment; on the other hand, some women would not receive the treatment, which

could benefit them greatly and prevent HIV infection in their baby. Was there an alternative design that could have been used in this instance? What are the ethical considerations of using an experimental design with a placebo-control group?

2. The value of the cross-sectional study is not always recognized among researchers. At one extreme, researchers might say that "cross-sectional studies are only good for hypothesis generation." At the other extreme, researchers might say that "cross-sectional studies could be very useful, even to the point of supporting causal relationships." Because such a large volume of health promotion research is based on data collected using cross-sectional research designs, this issue of "value" is indeed an important one. Thus, perhaps a critical question to ask is, Under what circumstances can findings from a cross-sectional study be used to test a hypothesis?

3. Earlier in this chapter it was noted that within-subjects designs (also known as the repeated-measures design) actually has less within-subject error variance than a between-groups design. Alternatively, it was noted that the lack of a control group implies that the within-subjects design is not a true experimental design. Given that the use of a control group may not always be feasible (due to limited research funds) or ethical (due to the potentially highly effective nature of the HPP and the lack of any acceptable attention-control condition), could a within-subjects design ever be preferable? If so, under what conditions would this be so? Also, what types of research questions would be the *most* appropriate for this design? Conversely, what types of research questions would be the *least* appropriate for this design?

For Practice and Discussion

1. A research question asks about the relationship of Internet health seeking to the health of infants among first-time parents. The researcher suspects that new parents who vigilantly seek health information on the Internet pertaining to the infants will provide better health care (and preventive care) to their infants as opposed to parents who rarely or never seek this type of information. Assume that sufficient evidence exists to conduct conclusive research. Given that your research funding is only sufficient for an *observational study*, please select the study design you would employ and provide a rationale for your selection to a colleague who is also completing this same exercise. Allow the colleagues to challenge your selection and then "trade places" by asking the colleague to allow you to challenge his or her selection.

2. Please repeat the exercise outlined in number 1, but this time assume that you have sufficient funds to conduct an experimental study.

3. Working with at least one colleague, please consider (and list) the advantages and disadvantages of random assignment. Please rank each advantage on a scale from one to five (with five being the most extreme level of concern). Similarly, please rank each disadvantage on a scale from one to five (with five being the most extreme level of "gain" resulting from randomization). Next, please find another pair of colleagues who have completed this same exercise and compare the two sets of lists and rankings.

4. For each research goal listed below, please select the best research design that could be applied to most effectively address the goal. Parsimony is an important criteria. Be prepared to defend your answer.

A. To determine the efficacy of a three-session intervention program designed to promote the consumption of a diet low in saturated fats among cardiac rehabilitation patients

B. To test the hypothesis that childhood activity levels predict obesity in early adulthood

C. To determine the relationship of sleep to depression in college students

D. To explore the role of self-efficacy in the decision to enroll in a smoking cessation course

E. To test the hypothesis that fewer high school students are engaging in sex in 2004, compared with high school students in the 1980s

F. To assess whether a media program can promote the use of infant car seats

G. To identify the effectiveness of an alcohol use awareness program (note: you have a strong suspicion that the assessment instrument used for alcohol awareness is also likely to foster awareness—you would like to test this suspicion as well)

References

Bastani, R., and others. (2002). Increasing cervical cancer screening among underserved women in a large urban county health system: Can it be done? What does it take? *Medical Care, 40*(10), 891–907.

Bhandari, N., and others. (2003). Effect of community-based promotion of exclusive breastfeeding on diarrhoeal illness and growth: A cluster randomized controlled trial. *Lancet, 361*(9367), 1418–1423.

Campbell, D. T., and Stanley, J. C. (1966). *Experimental and quasi-experimental designs for research.* Chicago: Rand McNally.

Centers for Disease Control and Prevention. (2004, May 21). Surveillance Summaries. *Morbidity and Mortality Weekly Report, 53*(SS-2).

Chassin, L., Presson, C. C., Rose, J. S., and Sherman, S. J. (2001). From adolescence to adulthood: Age-related changes in beliefs about cigarette smoking in a Midwestern community sample. *Health Psychology, 20*(5), 377–386.

DiClemente, R. J., and others. (2004). A descriptive analysis of STD prevalence among urban pregnant African-American teens: Data from a pilot study. *Journal of Adolescent Health, 34*(5), 376–383.

Emmons, K. M., Linnan, L. A., Shadel, W. G., Marcus, B., and Abrams, D. B. (1999). The Working Healthy Project: A worksite health-promotion trial targeting physical activity, diet, and smoking. *Journal of Occupational & Environmental Medicine, 41*(7), 545–555.

Finn, J. (2004). A survey of online harassment at a university campus. *Journal of Interpersonal Violence, 19*(4), 468–483.

Glasgow, R. E., Vogt T. M., and Boles, S. M. (1999). Evaluating the public health impact of health promotion interventions: The RE-AIM framework. *American Journal of Public Health, 89,* 1322–1327.

Hall, H. I., Jones, S. E., and Saraiya, M. (2001). Prevalence and correlates of sunscreen use among U.S. high school students. *Journal of School Health, 71*(9), 453–457.

Huurre, T. M., Aro, H. M., and Jaakkola, J. J. (2004). Incidence and prevalence of asthma and allergic rhinitis: A cohort study of Finnish adolescents. *Journal of Asthma, 41*(3), 311–317.

Klein, E., Campbell, J., Soler, E., and Ghez, M. (1997). *Ending domestic violence: Changing public perceptions/Halting the epidemic.* Thousand Oaks, CA: Sage.

Kulczycki, A., Kim, D. J., Duerr, A., Jamieson, D. J., and Macaluso, M. (2004). The acceptability of the female and male condom: A randomized crossover trial. *Perspectives on Sexual & Reproductive Health, 36*(3), 114–119.

Lapidus, G., and others. (2002). A statewide survey of domestic violence screening behaviors among pediatricians and family physicians. *Archives of Pediatrics 7 Adolescent Medicine, 156*(4), 332–336.

Melville, J., and others. (2003). Psychosocial impact of serological diagnosis of herpes simplex virus 2: A qualitative assessment. *Sexually Transmitted Infections, 79,* 280–285.

Morse, J. (1994). Designing funded qualitative research. In N. K. Denzin and J. S. Lincoln (Eds.), *Handbook of qualitative research* (pp. 220–235). Thousand Oaks, CA: Sage.

Repetto, P. B., Zimmerman, M. A., and Caldwell, C. H. (2004). A longitudinal study of the relationship between depressive symptoms and alcohol use in a sample of inner-city black youth. *Journal of Studies on Alcohol, 65*(2), 169–178.

Salazar, L. F., and Cook, S. L. (2002). Violence against women: Is psychology part of the problem or the solution? A content analysis of psychological research from 1990 through 1999. *Journal of Community and Applied Social Psychology, 12,* 410–421.

Salazar, L. F., and others. (2004). Self-concept and adolescents' refusal of unsafe sex: A test of mediating mechanisms among African American girls. *Prevention Science, 5*(3), 137–149.

Serdula, M. K., and others. (2004). Trends in fruit and vegetable consumption among adults in the United States: Behavioral risk factor surveillance system, 1994–2000. *American Journal of Public Health, 94*(6), 1014–1018.

Shrier, L., and others. (2001). Randomized controlled trial of a safer sex intervention for high-risk adolescent girls. *Archives of Pediatrics and Adolescent Medicine, 155*(1), 73–79.

St. Lawrence, J. S., Wilson, T. E., Eldridge, G. D., Brasfield, T. L., and O'Bannon, R. E. III. (2001). Community-based interventions to reduce low-income, African American women's risk of sexually transmitted diseases: A randomized controlled trial of three theoretical models. *American Journal of Community Psychology, 29*(6), 937–964.

Varma, R., and others. (2004). Prevalence of open-angle glaucoma and ocular hypertension in Latinos: The Los Angeles Latino Eye Study. *Ophthalmology, 111*(8), 1439–1448.

Wong, M. L., Chan, R. K., and Koh, D. (2002). Promoting condoms for oral sex: Impact on pharyngeal gonorrhea among female brothel-based sex workers. *Sexually Transmitted Diseases, 29*(6), 311–318.

CHAPTER FIVE

CONDUCTING OBSERVATIONAL RESEARCH

Richard A. Crosby, Laura F. Salazar, and Ralph J. DiClemente

As described in Chapter One, observational research is an important link in the chain of research evidence. Whether as a forerunner to randomized controlled trials (RCTs) or as a definitive form of study, observational research is very much the "bread and butter" of evidence in health promotion. Indeed, observational research constitutes the vast majority of early- and mid-level work in any chain of research evidence. Given the low cost and relatively short time commitments of some forms of observational study, graduate students and entry-level researchers are particularly likely to take on a project that is observational rather than experimental.

◆ ◆ ◆

In a Nutshell

Whether as a forerunner to randomized controlled trials or as a definitive form of study, observational research is very much the "bread and butter" of evidence in health promotion.

◆ ◆ ◆

Of course, the ultimate caveat with observational research is that rigor must be high. Several textbooks have provided a litany of conceptual issues that must be addressed to ensure this rigor (for example, Huck and Cormier 1996; Shi, 1997; Sim and Wright, 2000). Unfortunately, the "nuts and bolts" of conducting observational research (that is, the steps that can and should be taken to avoid these conceptual problems) have often been neglected. Indeed, the process of conducting observational research is far from straightforward, and the number of potential pitfalls is endless. Therefore, this chapter will address multiple concerns relevant to the conception, design, and implementation of observational research in health promotion.

Illustration of Key Concepts

Researchers typically confront four distinct types of issues when conducting observational research. The first is gaining access to a sample. Access alone, however, is not enough; thus, effective recruitment strategies are paramount. Next, issues related to assessment are critically important to the preservation reservation of rigor. Finally, studies that follow people over time must have built-in mechanisms to ensure that attrition in the cohort is minimal.

Gaining Access to a Sample

As noted in Chapter One, the first step in the research process is to define the study population. This task, however, is highly dependent on accessibility to the targeted population. For example, imagine that you have identified runaway youths as the study population. You have two options. You could hire staff to recruit youths from various street locations, or you could centralize the process by working in a shelter for runaway youths. The first option may be quite labor intensive, given that you would need to efficiently intercept and screen a massive number of youths on the streets to find even a few (with luck) who are runaways. The second option seems more attractive, yet this option requires something that may be difficult to secure: administrative "buy in" from the shelter. Whether the point of access is a shelter or a public venue, there are *gatekeepers* (in other words, people who are in positions to grant or deny access) who are controlling access. Research ideas may often be looked at with great suspicion among gatekeepers. Thus, gaining their approval to conduct the study may be a challenging (and ongoing) process. The goals of the research and the goals of the gatekeepers may be not only quite different but also incompatible. For example, the shelter for runaway youths may view its primary goal as providing a temporary, safe haven where youths can receive referrals to social services.

Given this mission, concerns about the proposed observational research may arise and could include

- How will kids who take part in this study benefit from participating?
- What assurances do you have to offer that kids will not feel coerced into participating?
- What type of questions will you be asking? Will these questions be personally invasive?
- Will your assessments be anonymous?
- How will your study help us? How will it help the community?

Naturally, addressing these issues in a satisfactory manner is a prerequisite to gaining access to the population; however, this could be a complicated response not addressed easily. For example, in responding to how youths will benefit, one problem is that you are not providing a health promotion program (HPP) (that is, a program that promotes health and well-being). Also, you cannot guarantee that youths will *not* perceive the "offer to participate" as coercive. Furthermore, your research questions necessitate assessing substance abuse and sexual behaviors and may be considered invasive. If your study is prospective, then you will need to ask youths for contact information so you can locate them again in about thirty days (thus, anonymity is not possible). Finally, the expected findings from your study may have very little relevance to the provision of services.

How can these problems be brought to a successful resolution? The answer lies within the second step of the research process (formulating the research question), the fifth step (determining what variables should be measured), and potentially the sixth step (sampling). For example, you may need to include a research question that addresses a unique need of the shelter or the immediate community. This does not diminish your original intent in any way; instead, it simply adds to the magnitude of your project. Next, you may need to either justify or remove planned measures from your assessment. Removing measures may diminish the quality and scope of your research, however.

To illustrate this point further, consider this real-world example. The Centers for Disease Control and Prevention (CDC) conducts a cross-sectional survey of U.S. high school students every two years called the Youth Risk Behavioral Surveillance System (YRBSS) that assesses health risk behaviors. Questions about sexual behaviors, which were to be included in the questionnaire, raised red flags among certain people who had the authority to grant or deny access to the population of high school students. In the 1999 survey year, twenty states either did not participate in the survey or denied the CDC permission to ask questions related to adolescents' sexual risk behavior. Three states (North Dakota, Vermont, and Maine) agreed to ask some of the questions pertaining to sex, but not others (Crosby, Holtgrave, DiClemente, Wingood, and Gayle, 2003). Of note, none of the sexual behavior questions were necessarily "invasive" beyond the level of asking kids if they ever had sex, if they had had sex in the past three months, if they had used a condom or contraceptive at last intercourse, and if they had ever been (or caused) a pregnancy. Questions about oral and anal sex were not included. Thus, in this example, the quality and scope of the research was compromised to gain access to a population. Some states agreed to ask the majority of the questions, but not those related to sex. Other states decided to select which questions they would allow in relationship to assessing sexual behavior.

Based on a delicate balance between gaining access and asking the "right" questions in the assessment, researchers must be prepared to make compromises, but only to a point. The point at which the required compromises jeopardize the ability of the research process to generate rigorous findings is the terminal point of the negotiation. It may be preferable to identify a different population rather than conduct a study that does not meet your needs. Indeed, the search for a population to access may be a time-consuming and labor-intensive task.

◆ ◆ ◆

In a Nutshell

The point at which the required compromises jeopardize the ability of the research process to generate rigorous findings is the terminal point of the negotiation.

◆ ◆ ◆

Finally, gaining access may require compromise in the sampling plan. For example, shelter administrators may insist that youths be recruited into the study only during the daytime hours on Saturday and Sunday (they may feel strongly that other times of the week are "just too busy"). Furthermore, they may insist that only kids aged sixteen and older can participate. Again, the research team needs to respect the negotiation and make every effort to accommodate these requests, but requests that are perceived by the team to jeopardize the rigor and scope of the research should *not* be met. Providing decision makers with a carefully delivered explanation of the sampling needs may go a long way toward achieving a successful resolution.

Recruiting

Chapter One described the importance of rigor. Rigor is lost in small, sometimes seemingly unimportant, aspects of a study. Recruitment is a good example of an opportunity for rigor to decrease substantially. The primary concern is that a low *participation rate* (sometimes called a *cooperation rate*) may lead to *participation bias,* also called *selection bias* (in other words, the sample is not representative of the population). This problem is not a consequence of the selected sampling technique; rather, it stems from poor planning or poor implementation of a recruitment protocol. Incidentally, a criterion for defining "low" participation rate does not exist.

Understanding two key principles can set the stage for successful recruitment in health promotion research: (1) strategies have been devised to promote effective (that is, high participation rate) recruiting, and (2) recruiting efforts should always be systematic. The importance of *effective* and *systematic* recruiting cannot be overstated. Chapter Eleven will describe a number of sampling options that are commonly applied to health promotion research. Sampling plans (also known as sampling protocols) are the direct result of carefully matching a sampling option with the research question(s). Unfortunately, the best laid plans may fall apart if a large number of those eligible (that is, people who were sampled and met the inclusion criteria) do not enroll in the study. This problem may be a direct consequence of ineffective recruiting. Furthermore, plans may fall apart if some of the eligible "would-be" volunteers are recruited more vigorously than others. This problem may be a direct consequence of recruiting efforts that are not systematic.

Effective Recruiting. Although research methods are used to answer health promotion research questions, studies of the various methods employed (that is, research about conducting research) have been neglected. For example, it would be quite enlightening to know the relative importance of three factors involved in the recruitment process: (1) the amount of financial incentive being offered, (2) the effect of timing and the setting on recruitment success, and (3) the effect of the recruitment approach on recruitment success. Unfortunately, empirical evidence addressing these questions is scarcely found in the published literature. In this instance, we rely on anecdotal evidence (from our own studies and studies conducted by colleagues) to provide guidance in effective recruiting.

First, incentives are important. These can take the form of cash, vouchers, gift cards, or tangible goods. The value of the incentive should be commensurate with the amount of time and effort required to fulfill the requirements of the study. For example, spending three to four hours to answer a lengthy questionnaire should have a much larger incentive as compared with taking a fifteen-minute survey. The amount of compensation may be established in part by local standards. In addition to being considered coercive, high-value incentives may create participation bias.

Second, timing is important because it can influence recruitment efforts. For example, people may be more receptive to participating when they are not under stress and when they have "time on their hands." Also, people attending a medical clinic may be more easily recruited while they are in a waiting room and are essentially a "captive audience" rather then when they have finished their appointment. Thus, timing of when people will be approached is everything. In fact, the lead author of this chapter achieved high participation rates (90 percent) in studies of men attending sex resorts by recruiting during the daytime hours (near a swimming pool) rather than in the evenings and nights when a primary concern of the men was engaging in sex (Crosby and DiClemente, 2004).

Third, the recruiting approach can be an important determinant of success. Of course, a "one size fits all" approach does not exist. The best approach is one that matches the needs and perceptions of the potential volunteers. For example, in a CDC-sponsored cross-sectional survey of men who have sex with men, the lead author of this chapter and his colleagues achieved high participation rates, which may be attributable to a recruiting appeal. Men were informed that the study was designed to help researchers learn more about the prevention of HIV and AIDS among men who have sex with men. Given that this population of men has been hit particularly hard by the AIDS epidemic, the study was appealing to men for personal reasons. Indeed, the nature of the study (combined with how it is explained during the recruitment encounter) may be the most important factor in terms of producing a high participation rate.

Recruiting approaches can also be deemed as *active* or *passive*. Active recruiting occurs when investigators seek out participants, whereas passive recruiting is when participants seek out investigators as a result of some advertisement (flyers, radio and television announcements, newspaper ads, newsletters, and Internet banner ads). Box 5.1 displays an example of a recruitment brochure. Active recruiting is necessary when the number of eligible study participants is expected to be low. For example, we collaborated with colleagues to examine the psychological and psychosocial effects of receiving a positive herpes diagnosis among asymptomatic clinic patients. Patients were referred to our study by their health care provider, who had conveyed the diagnosis (Melville and others, 2003). A methodological benefit of this approach is determining a true participation rate and refusal rate, and in some instances, if data are available, then comparisons can be made between those who participate and those who refuse.

Alternatively, passive recruitment relies on the assumption that an ample number of people are eligible, and also that a large number of eligible people will be exposed to the advertisements. A contemporary example of passive recruitment

Box 5.1. Example of a Recruitment Brochure

You're Invited!

You are invited to participate in a study that will investigate concerns people may have about accepting an AIDS vaccine if one ever became available for use in the United States. To be eligible you must

- Be 18 years of age or older
- Be able to read and understand English
- Not knowingly be positive for HIV (the virus that causes AIDS)

Enrollment in the study means that you will agree to participate in a one-hour interview (on the day of enrollment) and another one-hour interview two months after the first. After each interview, you will be provided with $35 to compensate you for your time. All information that you provide will be confidential.

If you would like to learn more about this study, please contact:

Study Director
402 Main Street, Room 390
Washington, MO 30111
Phone: (234) 555-1234

---

can be found in conjunction with federally funded research designed to test potential AIDS vaccines in human volunteers. Recruitment protocols for these studies require a passive approach (using multiple forms of media to promote the study to massive numbers of people). In contrast to active recruitment, passive recruitment does not allow for the computation of a true participation rate because the total number of people exposed to the solicitation is unknown. Passive recruitment methods also do not allow for making comparisons between participants and those who do not participate.

Systematic Recruiting. A rigorous study will follow a strict recruiting protocol. All potential volunteers should be treated in the same manner. This "sameness" is as equally important as the content of the protocol. One common practice to ensure consistency is to provide research staff with recruitment scripts. Scripts should be short enough that staff can recite the script naturally versus artificially and long

MINCUS AND DINCUS USE PASSIVE RECRUITMENT FOR THEIR STUDY.

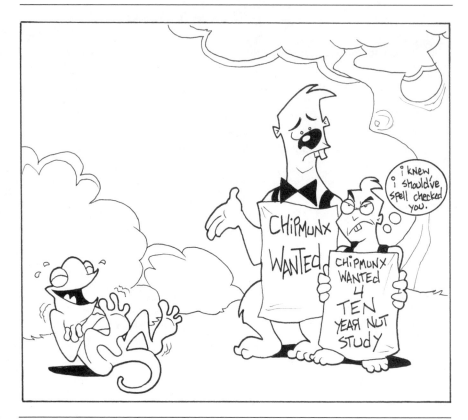

Copyright 2005 by Justin Wagner; reprinted with permission.

enough so that they accurately portray the study. Box 5.2 displays several examples of recruitment scripts applied to health promotion research. One of the best examples of this kind of commitment to a protocol can be found in phone surveys—in these protocols research staff are reciting recruitment lines verbatim. To ensure that staff do not drift from the script, supervisors should intermittently monitor (and correct) staff performance. The importance of this supervision cannot be overstated.

Keeping Recruitment and Retention Records

As described in Chapter Fourteen, a rigorous study will need to document (1) how many people were screened for eligibility, (2) how many were eligible,

Box 5.2. Examples of Recruitment Scripts

"We are conducting a study that will help us learn about the HIV prevention needs of African American women. Would you be willing to provide us with thirty minutes of your time?"

"The Wyoming State Department of Health has commissioned a study of farm injury prevention. Part of that study involves interviewing the teenage children of farm families. You qualify to participate in the study. If you are interested, I can explain the process to you in detail."

"I am recruiting study volunteers who are willing to help me and others who work with me to learn about the reasons why men do not always use condoms. Because you have been diagnosed with an STD today, you qualify to be in the study. Are you interested in helping us? The information you provide could be very useful in the eventual design of an education program."

"To improve the quality of our health care services, we are asking clients to consider volunteering for a two-year study. We would ask you some questions today and then contact you by phone three times during every six months. The questions and phone calls are intended to provide us with data regarding how you make decisions whether or not to be seen by a doctor in our clinic. We are trying to improve our services as much as possible. Would you consider helping us out?"

and (3) how many participated. In prospective studies, it is equally important to include (4) how many returned to the first planned follow-up assessment, and (5) how many returned to the second planned follow-up assessment, and so on. Maintaining these records is, of course, labor intensive. Ideally, a study director (someone who is always "on duty") should keep these records by using a daily diary. However, the records may also require the use of forms. If the local Institutional Review Board (IRB) permits it, documentation could include asking people who refused to participate why they refused and also collecting basic demographic data (age, gender, race) to compare nonvolunteers to volunteers. Some local IRBs, however, may prohibit any data collection among nonvolunteers. The ultimate goal of this data collection is to build a table that empirically addresses the potential for participation bias. Table 5.1 provides an example of this type of evidence.

Notice that the table provides a head-to-head comparison of volunteers and nonvolunteers. The data make clear that volunteers were significantly less likely

TABLE 5.1.   A COMPARISON OF VOLUNTEERS AND NONVOLUNTEERS.

Characteristic	Number (%) Volunteers (*N* = 1,000)	Number (%) Nonvolunteers (*N* = 400)
Age		
18–29	90 (9.0)	40 (10.0)
30–39	450 (45.0)	160 (40.0)
40–49	410 (41.0)	160 (40.0)
50 and older	50 (5.0)	40 (10.0)
Race		
American Indian or Alaskan Native	12 (1.2)	12 (3.0)
Alaskan or Pacific Islander	95 (9.5)	40 (10.0)
Black or African American	**455 (45.5)**	**200 (50.0)**
White	**438 (43.8)**	**148 (37.0)**
Ethnicity		
Hispanic	290 (29.0)	120 (30.0)
Non-Hispanic	710 (71.0)	280 (70.0)
Employment		
Full-Time	770 (77.0)	320 (80.0)
Part-Time	70 (7.0)	30 (7.5)
Unemployed	**110 (11.0)**	**6 (1.5)**
Retired	**50 (5.0)**	**44 (11.0)**
Sex		
Male	490 (49.0)	210 (52.5)
Female	510 (51.0)	190 (47.5)

Note: Bold entries represent differences that are significant at $P < .05$.

than nonvolunteers to be black or African American and significantly more likely to be white. Also, volunteers were significantly more likely than nonvolunteers to be unemployed and significantly less likely to be retired.

Assessment

Chapter Nine will describe methods of assessment in great detail. For now, it is sufficient to note that the selected assessment method must be implemented with great fidelity. Just as a sampling plan can be foiled by poor recruiting, an assessment method can be compromised by poor implementation. Three key issues are paramount: (1) avoiding response bias, (2) avoiding undue respondent fatigue, and (3) facilitating accurate recall.

◆ ◆ ◆

In a Nutshell

Just as a sampling plan can be foiled by poor recruiting, an assessment method can be compromised by poor implementation.

◆ ◆ ◆

Avoiding Response Bias. Response bias can take on several forms. One common concern is that study participants will "play to" or "play against" their perception of the study hypotheses. For example, if a male participant suspects that the study is designed to test whether people are more likely to be abusive toward a sex partner during periods of intoxication, then his hunch may knowingly or even unknowingly skew his responses to the questions. He may answer in a way that falsely supports the hypothesis or in a way that falsely fails to support the hypothesis. One strategy that is sometimes used to avoid this form of bias is not to provide information to participants about the hypotheses. IRBs will occasionally approve consent forms that do not fully disclose the purpose of the study. Of course, the recruitment script and even the questions being asked should be constructed to avoid bias. Most important, however, research staff must be skilled in the art of responding to any questions volunteers may ask without appearing impolite or unconcerned when they do not directly answer questions that would betray the hypotheses.

Another common form of bias stems from social desirability. This form of bias is easy to understand for anyone that has ever been sitting in a dental chair and been asked, "How often do you floss?" Most people are tempted to inflate their answer to "please" the hygienist or dentist and to create the impression that they practice excellent dental hygiene. In observational research that addresses health behavior, study volunteers may experience a similar need to please the person conducting the interview. Fortunately, this problem can be addressed by informing participants that the "best answer" is an honest answer. Although this seems simple enough, it requires a completely nonjudgmental atmosphere (especially in face-to-face interviews). For example, if someone is asked, "How many sex partners have you had in the past three months" and the answer provided is "about three dozen," then the person conducting the interview must not react any differently to this response than if the response had been "two."

Avoiding Undue Respondent Fatigue. Although research is the backbone of science, conducting research with people also requires simple attention to their needs. One important principle to keep in mind is that the research and the questions are probably not as interesting to the study participants as they are to the researchers. In fact, the questions may be perceived as tedious. Apart from constructing clear questions and devising interesting response formats (see Chapters Nine and Ten), the people conducting the assessment must be attuned to the energy and interest-level of the respondents. Are people attentive during the entire assessment period or does their attention wane after the first ten minutes? If their attention does wane, then what can be done to get them back on track? Do people need a break at some point during the process? Does providing food help? Attending to these questions is the responsibility of the research staff and is similar to being a good host who ensures the comfort and enjoyment of his or her guests. The goal is to create an environment that is comfortable and ask people to complete a reasonable task without undue constraints.

Simultaneous with the process of alleviating fatigue, the research staff also must engage in a form of quality assurance. One of the worst fates suffered by a data set is the absence of answers—to any number of questions—from a substantial proportion of the participants. Depending on the arrangements agreed upon in the consent process, members of the research staff may, for example, review completed questionnaires before respondents leave the setting. A polite request to "please consider providing responses to questions 76 through 89 on the last page" (for example) may be met with cooperation. This small task may make the difference between including and excluding the participant's data from the final analysis. Less forward strategies include asking participants—before they leave—to please be sure they have answered all of the questions except for those that don't apply or those they purposefully chose not to answer. Of course, participants should also be informed (perhaps at several points in the assessment process) that the research staff would be happy to clarify any of the questions that may be confusing or problematic to answer. This offer, though, must never be taken lightly by the research staff because "clarification" can easily become a source of bias if the staff member strays from the written, spoken, or recorded question. Defining words and modestly paraphrasing questions are two practices that may be safe.

◆ ◆ ◆

In a Nutshell

A polite request to "please consider providing responses to questions 76 through 89 on the last page" (for example) may be met with cooperation. This small task may make the difference between including and excluding the participant's data from the final analysis.

◆ ◆ ◆

Facilitating Accurate Recall. Health promotion research often asks people to re-call past events. Infrequent events that have high salience generally do not pose a problem (for example, events that occurred on September 11, 2001). Generally it can be expected that events with high saliency and low frequency facilitate the most accurate recall. As an example in health promotion, consider someone who has had sex (high salience) twice in the past six months. Recalling the details of these two events may be relatively easy. Conversely, someone who has had more than a hundred sexual events in the past six months may be challenged to recall with a high degree of accuracy any details of these one hundred events. Other events may be frequent but lack salience, leading to low accuracy in recall. For example, asking study participants who regularly eat eggs to recall the number of eggs they have consumed (low salience) in the past thirty days would probably lead to inaccuracies in recall. The most challenging scenario occurs when the behavior under study is low in salience and is relatively frequent. Such a challenge may require the use of shortened recall periods, calendars marked with key dates, and verbal "probes" if the assessment is given in a face-to-face format.

◆ ◆ ◆

In a Nutshell

The most challenging scenario occurs when the behavior under study is low in salience and is relatively frequent.

◆ ◆ ◆

Short recall periods may be extremely useful. It is not at all unusual for health promotion research studies to use a one-day recall period (for example, "what are the foods that you consumed yesterday?") or a last-event recall period (for exam-ple, "the last time you ate out at a restaurant, what did you order?"). Of course, the risk of this truncated assessment period is that the "one day" or "last event" may not represent the true nature of the health behavior of the person being assessed.

Research staff might also increase accurate recall by starting each assessment with a large calendar. In settings where the staff member can interface with par-ticipants individually, the session can begin by helping participants fill in key dates. To illustrate, imagine asking questions designed to assess how many alcoholic bev-erages people consume in a typical month. To facilitate accurate recall, a staff member might ask, "Have you had any special events in the past month that were celebrated by having a party?" Another question might be, "In the past month, there were four weekends (show these by pointing at the calendar). On any of these weekends (if so, which ones) did any sporting events occur that you watched while drinking?" Another example might be, "In the past month, was there a time in your life when you were extremely stressed or depressed? Can you please indicate those days on the calendar for me?" Any affirmative answer can be followed up to elicit a date which is then recorded on the calendar. This entry may serve as a benchmark for the person when asked to recall how many drinks had been consumed. Notice that the questions are not the issue here; instead, the goal is to train research staff in the "art" of conducting an assessment that will maximize the odds of accurate recall from the participants.

◆ ◆ ◆

In a Nutshell

The goal is to train research staff in the "art" of conducting an assessment that will maximize the odds of accurate recall from the participants.

◆ ◆ ◆

Finally, in face-to-face interviews, verbal probes can greatly facilitate accurate recall. For example, to assess how many sex partners someone had over the past six months, the interview would begin with the basic question and proceed with probes if the initial answer is somewhat unclear. A hypothetical example follows:

Interviewer: In the past six months, how many different people have engaged in sexual intercourse with you? (Sexual intercourse means that the penis is placed into the mouth, vagina, or rectum of another person.)
Participant: Uhhh, umhh, I would have to say between ten and twelve people. On second thought, umhh, make that fifteen.
Interviewer: This kind of counting can be difficult—I noticed you initially said "ten" and finally said "fifteen." Please think about why you raised your answer—did you raise it too much—or perhaps not enough?

Maintaining the Cohort

The advanced version of recruitment is retention. In prospective observational studies, retention is so vital that complete failure of the study may easily occur if the rate is low. Prospective data are complete only when at least two time points have been covered by the study. A baseline assessment alone will not answer research questions that are prospective in nature. Thus, the attrition of any one participant negates the value of his or her baseline assessment. Of course (as described previously in this chapter and elsewhere in this book), as attrition rates grow, rigor shrinks.

◆ ◆ ◆

In a Nutshell

In prospective observational studies, retention is so vital that complete failure of the study may easily occur if the rate is low.

◆ ◆ ◆

Unfortunately, attrition is inevitable: in general, the longer the follow-up period the greater attrition. To minimize attrition, a number of tracking procedures have proven effective. These procedures include (1) hiring a full-time recruitment-retention coordinator to track participants; (2) requesting friendship contacts—participants are required to provide the name, telephone numbers, and addresses of two confidants; (3) providing monetary compensation for completing follow-up assessments; (4) ensuring confidentiality of data and identifying information (in other words, all data will be maintained, offsite, in a locked cabinet that is limited to access by key staff only, with only code numbers used on data forms); (5) providing appointment cards indicating the time and date of the follow-up assessments; (6) providing reminder phone contacts a week before as well as forty-eight hours prior to their scheduled follow-up assessment; (7) mailing "thank you" cards to participants for attending their follow-up assessments; and (8) mailing "touching-base cards" such as birthday cards and holiday cards (there are many holidays throughout the year that provide an opportunity to maintain contact with participants). There are a range of strategies designed to maintain the study cohort. Implementing them in a timely fashion, treating participants with courtesy and respect, providing assurances of confidentiality, and maintaining frequent contact to identify changes in locator information will enhance retention. We will discuss two of these strategies in greater detail.

Phone Contacts. The type of "maintenance contact" that occurs between research staff and study participants will be a function of the agreement with the IRB. The telephone is an essential tool for contact; therefore, gaining permission from the IRB to ask volunteers for a reliable phone number is clearly important in prospective studies. After the baseline assessment is complete, research staff members have two essential obligations: (1) collect accurate contact information and (2) provide any promised incentives for study participation. Both tasks can be performed with one goal in mind: to establish a rapport with participants in order to inspire them to come back! Merely asking for a phone number would be wasting an opportunity to build rapport. The occasion should, instead, be used to learn when and how to contact participants. An example follows.

◆ ◆ ◆

In a Nutshell

The telephone is an essential tool for contact; therefore, gaining permission from the IRB to ask volunteers for a reliable phone number is clearly important in prospective studies.

◆ ◆ ◆

Staff Member: I would like to call you a few times before we meet again in three months. It would be very helpful to me if you would let me know what time of day is good for me to call you.

Participant: I work the night shift so the best time is just before I leave for work, usually around ten P.M.

Staff Member: Great, thanks. Is that every weeknight or do you have to work on weekends sometimes?

Participant: Luckily, I never have to work on weekends—just Monday through Friday.

Staff Member: Okay, thanks. What phone number should I use when I call you around ten o'clock?

Participant: My home number, 345-1733, would be fine, but the problem is I don't want my spouse or anyone else that may be at my house to know that I'm in this study.

Staff Member: I understand—I will ask for you by name, and I will not leave a message if you are not home. If someone else answers and that person asks who I am, what would you like me to say?

Participant: Just tell them that you are trying to sell me something and hang up after that.

Staff Member: Sounds fair—I will be polite if that happens.

When making phone contact with a participant it is important to "talk" rather than run through a scripted agenda. The staff member should have and show a genuine interest in the person. This interest may result in potentially important information being conveyed. For example, the staff member might ask, "When we talked last you were living an apartment that you hated; have you had any luck getting a better one?" This question may yield a new address (information that may also be critical to keeping the retention rate high).

Mail Contacts. Birthday cards, holiday cards, and postcards can all be efficient ways to keep the study and the staff member relatively "fresh" on the minds of participants. Sending cards requires thoughtful use of the time between when participants complete the baseline assessment and when participants are given their promised incentive. If the birth date was not collected in the assessment, then it can be requested during this time. Honesty is important—simply tell participants that you want to send them a birthday card! Similarly, it easy enough to think about upcoming holidays and then to ask participants whether or not they celebrate these.

Although birthday and holiday cards may be hit or miss, every participant should be sent a postcard if possible. Postcards are an informal way of keeping in touch with someone, and their use can be casual—almost anonymous. The word "anonymous" is important because it may be that the study involves a sensitive topic (sex, drugs, disease) and the participant does not want his or her involvement disclosed. Thus, the postcard should be from a place not a person, and the "place" should be generic rather than specific. For example, it may come from "The Greater Chicago Board of Health" rather than from the "Substance Abuse Prevention Center of Greater Chicago." To promote recognition of this communication, the staff member could actually show a blank postcard to the respondent and say, "I would like to send one of these to you before we meet again—if that is okay with you, then what address should I use?" The postcard should only be a greeting—it should not be personalized to the point where the participants' involvement in the study is disclosed in any way. Postage for this card should include a guarantee that it will be returned to the sender if needed. This is an important way for a staff member to know that someone in the cohort has moved without leaving a forwarding address. This event necessitates immediate attempts to make phone contact.

A critical aspect of promoting retention is to assign one staff member only to "track" any given participant. This should be the same staff member who performs the baseline assessment and, more important, interfaces with the participant to collect contact information (phone and address) and provides the incentive payment. At this time, the assigned staff member should make it clear that he or she will be the only person making the interim contact, and that one purpose of the contact is to ensure that the follow-up assessment occurs on the day and time planned. Naturally, planning this day and time should be a very deliberate process—one that is guided by the needs of the participant only (research staff *should not* be under the illusion that data collection must occur between nine A.M. and five P.M. Monday through Friday). Once the day and time are planned, a brightly colored appointment card should be provided to the participant. The card should also clearly indicate how the participant can contact the staff member. If time allows, then the staff member should run the card through a lamination machine to give it some durability and to make it stand out. Reminding participants about their appointment should occur only by phone, and it should occur close in time to the agreed-upon date.

Attrition bias is naturally a prime concern. If, for example, people who drop out do so for a variety of practical reasons (for example, change of residence, employment schedule conflicts with appointment times, lack of transportation to the appointment) then odds of developing a biased final sample are relatively low. Alternatively, if people drop out based on lack of interest in the study or personal conflicts with the nature of the research questions, then odds of developing a biased final sample go up substantially. Indeed, the final sample might comprise people who really like the study topic and who are not in conflict with the topic in any way. In health promotion research, this "one-sided" sample may rarely reflect reality. Here are just a few of many possible examples of topics that may create this problem:

- Sex and sexuality research
- Research on eating disorders
- Vaccine-acceptance research
- Substance abuse prevention research
- Drunk driving prevention research
- Cancer prevention research
- Research on compliance with exercise and diets to improve cardiovascular health

Experimental Studies

These key concepts apply to observational studies; however, each concept also applies to the larger and more challenging task of conducting experimental studies. Chapter Six will use the material covered in this chapter as a starting point for a detailed description of planning and implementing experimental research from a "nuts and bolts" perspective.

Applied Example

A study published in *Cancer Nursing* provides a good example of recruitment and retention strategies applied to a difficult-to-reach population: women diagnosed with lung cancer. Cooley and colleagues (2003) conducted a prospective study of women with lung cancer to assess their quality of life. Sites in five cities participated in the study. To be eligible, women had to have been diagnosed with lung cancer at least six months previous to the potential enrollment date, but the diagnosis also had to be less than five years old.

Three of the five sites reached agreement with their IRBs to use active as well as passive recruitment methods. In this case, a member of the research team made direct contact with potential participants by phone or in person. The contact was initiated by the researcher. Passive approaches (used at all five sites) included distributing brochures, mailing letters, hanging up flyers and posters in key locations, and advertising in newspapers or by radio. The researchers also used the media to promote community awareness of the study. Once potential study participants initiated contact, a member of the research team used a phone script to recruit these individuals into the study.

Screening and enrollment rates were monitored on a monthly basis. Overall, 435 women were screened and 364 were deemed eligible. Of these 364 women, 230 (63 percent) were enrolled. Enrollment success rates varied by site (this could be due to differences in populations by site or to different practices by recruiters at each site). Of great interest, the success rate for passive recruitment was 92 percent compared to 61 percent for active recruitment. The finding is quite logical given that passive recruitment begins with people who already have enough interest in the study to initiate contact, whereas active recruitment does not "screen out" the people who are clearly disinterested.

The article displayed a table enumerating reasons for attrition from the prospective study. Attrition rates varied by site and by method of recruitment (active versus passive). The overall attrition rate was 24 percent. Again, passive recruitment produced better results in that attrition was more likely (33 percent) among those recruited actively as opposed to passively (22 percent). Detailing the reasons for attrition was clearly important, especially given that a substantial number of women experienced severe relapse (with some deaths). Efforts to keep attrition low included the provision of a pleasant baseline assessment (including breaks during the interview) and measures designed to promote contact between the research staff and participants between the first and second assessments. These methods included birthday cards, holiday cards, periodic phone calls, and a $25 cash incentive provided after each interview.

Integration with the Research Process

Just as one defective O-ring can cause an entire space shuttle to come crashing back to earth, a study designed without adequate attention to the daily activities of the project director and research staff is likely to fall apart. Thus, the planning steps (steps 4 through 6) in the nine-step model of Chapter One should always be pursued with great attention to detail. Major barriers to effective recruitment, retention, and assessment (for example) can sometimes be averted through the exercise of foresight and caution when selecting a study design (step 4), crafting an assessment plan (step 5), and choosing a sampling method (step 6). However, implementing the research protocol (step 7) is ultimately the last chance a study has to permanently gain or lose rigor. Note that data analysis can be repeated over and over again, but planning and implementation steps occur at discrete points in time and cannot be "reversed."

◆ ◆ ◆

In a Nutshell

Data analysis can be repeated over and over again, but planning and implementation steps occur at discrete points in time and cannot be "reversed."

◆ ◆ ◆

Summary

Although observational research is often a forerunner to experimental research, it may also constitute the terminal point of evidence in the research chain. Either way, rigor in observational research is essential. This chapter has described some of the key concepts that ensure this rigor. An initial concern is gaining access to the desired population followed by the creation and implementation of a successful recruitment protocol. Assessment, the main activity in observational research, is important in its own right and is also related to whether volunteers return for scheduled follow-up interview sessions. Given the importance of using prospective designs in health promotion research, multiple steps can and should be taken to ensure an optimally high retention rate. Ultimately, constant attention to the everyday operation of observational research is vital to ensuring a high degree of rigor. This attention includes careful record keeping, thorough training of research staff, and periodic monitoring of all recruitment and retention procedures. The successful study will be one that is planned in great detail and implemented with fidelity.

◆ ◆ ◆

In a Nutshell

The successful study will be one that is planned in great detail and implemented with fidelity.

◆ ◆ ◆

Issues to Consider

1. In observational studies, it is not uncommon for researchers to differentiate between refusal rates and dropouts before the first assessment. In essence, people may be recruited (and agree to enroll) at a discrete point in time that precedes the first scheduled assessment. This may be particularly likely when assessments are conducted in groups rather than on an individual basis. Thus, people who agree to participate may not "show up" for assessment. For example, imagine that 900 people were eligible. Of these, 810 (90 percent) agreed to enroll in the study with the understanding that an initial assessment would occur during the first Saturday of the following month. Of the 810 who agreed, 630 (70 percent of those eligible) showed up on the appointed Saturday. Is the participation rate 90 percent or is it just 70 percent? Also, when does enrollment occur? Does it occur upon agreement to participate or when the person actually provides data? (Please keep in mind that the researcher has discretion over when informed consent will be provided—the only requirement is that it must occur before assessment.)

2. The relationship of the research question(s) to the design implementation of the observational research study protocol should also be considered. Without question, the research question should be the sole driving force behind the design of any study. During planning, any level of compromise that impinges on the scope of the research question should be avoided. However, it may become sadly apparent during this phase that the logistical complications of implementing the necessary protocol will unfortunately produce low participation and retention rates. Upon reaching this conclusion, should the researcher abandon the project? Would your answer be different if the study had been federally funded and money would have to be returned to the federal treasury?

3. Given that active recruitment is sometimes a necessity, it is important to keep in mind that this procedure may yield lower success rates than a passive procedure. However, active recruitment may actually provide more information about the relationship of the sample to the population. For example, imagine that the research question involves the study of people newly diagnosed with genital herpes. In a relatively small community it might be logical to assume that only a few health care providers perform this test and therefore these providers could (conceivably) provide a fairly complete count of the number of community residents diagnosed with genital herpes during any given period of time. Developing these relationships with the providers would easily lead to the next step—active recruitment of those testing positive during a given time frame. Conversely, passive recruitment techniques would be "blind" to the number of potentially eligible participants. Thus, an important issue to consider is whether active or passive recruitment is better suited for any particular study.

For Practice and Discussion

1. A search to find standards for acceptable participation rates and acceptable retention rates would be endless and produce multiple answers. Two explanations for this problem are apparent. First, as noted earlier in this chapter, research about conducting research has been neglected. Although having a defensible number (for example, 70 percent) available for judging the likelihood of participation bias (or attrition bias) would be ideal, an empirically derived value does not exist. Second, it can be argued that a universal standard for participation and attrition rates should not be applied to health promotion research. The argument would be based on the concept that these rates are inevitably a function of (1) the selected population and (2) the nature of research. Please consider each of these explanations and then select one to defend in conversation with a colleague who is completing the same exercise.

2. Much of the material contained in this chapter is intimately connected with ethical issues and principles as described in Chapter Three. Due to this intimacy, several conflicts could occur. For example, a perceived need to have a high participation rate may lead research staff to present skewed versions of the consent process—leaving out or under-emphasizing aspects of the study that may be less appealing. Working with a colleague who is completing this same exercise, please identify at least two additional conflicts between ethical principles and achieving goals described by the key concepts outlined in this chapter. Take a position on each conflict that you identify (for instance, what is the solution?).

References

Cooley, M. E., and others. (2003). Challenges of recruitment and retention in multisite clinical research. *Cancer Nursing, 26,* 376–386.

Crosby, R. A., and DiClemente, R. J. (2004). Use of recreational Viagra among men having sex with men. *Sexually Transmitted Infections, 80,* 466–468.

Crosby, R. A., Holtgrave, D. R., DiClemente, R. J., Wingood, G. M., and Gayle, J. (2003). Social capital as a predictor of adolescents' sexual risk behavior: A state-level exploratory study. *AIDS and Behavior, 7,* 245–252.

Huck, S. W., and Cormier, W. H. (1996). *Reading statistics and research.* New York: Longman.

Melville, J., and others. (2003). Psychological impact of a serological diagnosis of herpes simplex virus type 2: A qualitative assessment. *Sexually Transmitted Infections, 79,* 280–285.

Shi, L. (1997). *Health services research.* Albany, NY: Delmar Publishers.

Sim, J., and Wright, C. (2000). *Research in health care: Concepts, designs, and methods.* Salisbury, Wiltshire, UK: Stanley Thrones (Publishers) Ltd.

CHAPTER SIX

DESIGNING RANDOMIZED CONTROLLED TRIALS IN HEALTH PROMOTION RESEARCH

Ralph J. DiClemente, Laura F. Salazar, and Richard A. Crosby

As noted in Chapter Five, much of the research in health promotion has been observational in nature. However, the very definition and, indeed, the identity of the discipline of health promotion are predicated on the premise of designing programs that "promote health." As such, a mainstay of health promotion is the development and implementation of programs that have as their expressed purpose enhancing the health of human populations.

At this juncture, perhaps it would be useful to define health promotion programs (HPPs). By HPPs, we imply any intervention, whether it's a new school smoking-cessation curriculum, a new exercise-enhancement class at a community-based organization, or an HIV-prevention program. Broadly defined, an HPP can be any intervention that has as its expressed purpose changing a person's health-related attitudes, beliefs, intentions, and behavior so as to enhance his or her health.

The focus of this chapter will be on describing how to design and conduct experimental research. Although experimental research is used in many fields, in health promotion we focus mainly on evaluating whether HPPs are effective in enhancing health-protective behaviors (or health-protective attitudes, beliefs, knowledge, and intentions). There are many different types of evaluation strategies applicable for these assessments (see Chapter Eight); however, in this chapter we focus on a *true experimental research design* because it is the optimal research design in health promotion and indeed, in any discipline involving human populations.

Illustration of Key Concepts

This chapter describes key concepts in the design of the randomized controlled trial. This is not an exhaustive treatment of this area of methodology. We do, however, describe the essential concepts that form the cornerstone of the randomized trial design and discuss the importance of these concepts in enhancing the validity of health promotion research.

What Is an Experiment in Health Promotion Research?

An experiment in health promotion research involves the manipulation of an *independent variable* (something that is intentionally altered by the research team). In this case, the HPP would be the independent variable. It is altered by randomly allocating some people to receive the HPP and others not to receive the HPP. Then the effects of this manipulation can be measured by assessing the designated outcome variables (for example, weight, blood pressure, depressive symptoms, and so on) over some specified period of time. In the parlance of experimental research, the outcome measure is called the *dependent variable.*

To illustrate, an investigator (you, for example) has developed an innovative approach designed to motivate adolescents to increase their consumption of vegetables. Essentially, the HPP comprises five group sessions that describe the health benefits associated with higher vegetable consumption. You have decided to develop this program based on evidence derived from numerous studies, which observed significant decreases in adverse health outcomes (such as heart disease and some cancers) for people with higher vegetable consumption.

You recruit about two hundred teens from the local Boys and Girls Club. You ask them to complete a baseline questionnaire that assesses their consumption of vegetables. Then you randomly assign them to either your innovative HPP or to a group that does not receive any health promotion intervention (this could be some other program that does not include any focus on enhancing vegetable intake). Next, you present the program comprising five sessions and then follow all the teens (from both groups) over time, let's say twelve months. You ask them to return and complete a follow-up questionnaire that again assesses their intake of vegetables. This time, however, you ask them about their vegetable consumption over the past twelve months. You hypothesize (and hope) that the teens in the HPP report more consumption of vegetables over the past twelve months relative to the teens in the control. This would be an indication that the program was successful (effective) in enhancing vegetable consumption. You have just conducted an experimental research study! This is a simplified illustration; of course, there are other design nuances that need to be considered in your study.

The Advantages of Experimental Research

The major advantage of experimental research over observational research is the strength of *causal inference* it offers. *Causal inference* implies that a fair conclusion can be made regarding the effect of an independent variable on a dependent variable (for example, a change in X will create a corresponding change in Y). It is the best research design for controlling potential confounding influences. As we'll see in more detail later in this chapter, in experimental research casual inference is based on comparing the outcomes observed among the teens in the HPP (for instance, the amount of their vegetable consumption) relative to the teens not in the program. Thus, in this example, manipulating the independent variable, randomization into groups, and then observing differences in outcomes for those exposed to the HPP and those who were not exposed represent a "true" experiment.

Types of Experimental Research Designs

Experimental research designs, like ice cream, come in multiple flavors. There are a number of choices. We suggest you see Campbell and Stanley (1963) for a more detailed discussion. Rather than try to review all the available designs (see Chapter Four), this chapter will focus on what is commonly referred to as *between-groups experimental research design*. Between-groups research design compares the outcomes observed in two or more groups of people that receive different interventions. Between-groups designs are commonly used in health promotion research. One between-group design, the *randomized controlled trial* (RCT) is often described as the "gold standard" for evaluating HPPs (or, for that matter, any intervention). In this experimental design participants are assigned, by chance alone, to either receive or not receive the HPP. This is not to say that other experimental designs are methodologically weak, just that the RCT is considered the optimal design.

Given the importance of methodological rigor for accurately evaluating HPPs, this chapter will focus exclusively on the RCT. There are, of course, numerous variations of this design. We will, however, restrict our discussion to describing the basic research structure of the RCT. Readers interested in more detailed presentations are referred to Piantadosi (1997) and Pocock (1993).

FIGURE 6.1.   A SCHEMATIC ILLUSTRATION OF A RANDOMIZED
CONTROLLED TRIAL (RCT).

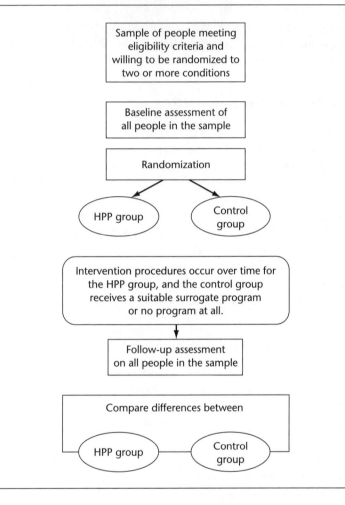

Conceptualizing a Randomized Controlled Trial

We have graphically represented a basic RCT in Figure 6.1. Although the research design shown may appear basic, do not be fooled. This is a very powerful evaluation design.

There are a number of key steps that are necessary to consider when designing and implementing any RCT. We provide a step-by-step approach to designing an RCT. These steps include

1. Defining the sample
2. Conducting a baseline assessment
3. Randomizing participants
4. Implementing the health promotion program
5. Following the sample over time

Step 1: Defining the Sample

The first step is to decide who will be in the study and how best to recruit them to participate. There are numerous sampling strategies that can be used to identify a target sample. (See greater detail about sampling in Chapter Eleven.) There are also a number of effective strategies that can be used to recruit the sample into the study (see Chapter Five). Whatever the sampling and recruitment strategy employed, it is important when defining the sample to establish a set of inclusion and exclusion criteria that specify the target population and are appropriate to the research question the study purports to answer. These criteria, sometimes referred to as *eligibility criteria*, establish the parameters for determining who is able to participate (*inclusion*) and who is not able to participate in the study (*exclusion*).

For example, consider an HPP for preventing dating violence among adolescents. First, it is important to define the characteristics of those adolescents who will be selected and recruited to participate in the study. The HPP to be implemented will be tailored by gender (that is, designed for young men) and will focus on preventing perpetration (the key outcome). Thus, inclusion criteria would be that participants have to be male, between fourteen and eighteen, and actively dating. Because this is a primary prevention program, the exclusion criterion would be previous perpetration. There is no magic formula for defining the inclusion and exclusion criteria. It is based on understanding the HPP that is to be evaluated: understanding the key outcomes of interest, and weighing the competing concerns of *internal validity* (the extent to which the study evaluates the hypotheses) and *external validity* (the extent to which the results of the study can be extended beyond the sample used in the study). Once the sample is defined, selection of the sample and recruitment can begin.

Step 2: Conducting a Baseline Assessment

Once the sample has been selected and recruited, the next step is to "characterize" the sample. This involves assessing the characteristics of the sample at baseline (before they are randomized to either receive or not receive the HPP). The purpose of characterizing the sample is to obtain measurements of key outcome variables prior to the HPP that will provide a baseline for measuring anticipated change in those key outcomes for those randomized to the HPP condition relative to those in the control condition. Another important aspect of characterizing the sample is to test for group differences after randomization. The groups should theoretically be identical, implying that randomization worked. This is a critical step to ensuring the internal validity of the study. If there are significant differences, for example, on sociodemographic characteristics (age, gender, race, SES, and so on) or outcome variables (behaviors, attitudes and beliefs), then these differences may confound the results. Significant differences between groups on these characteristics should be further explored and possibly controlled for in statistical analyses.

DINCUS'S SIMPLE RANDOMIZATION PROCEDURE.

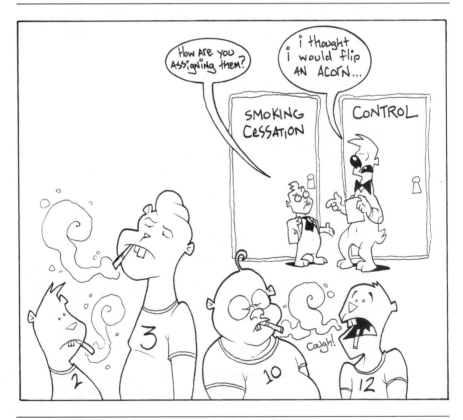

Copyright 2005 by Justin Wagner; reprinted with permission.

Step 3: Randomizing Participants

Once participants have completed baseline assessments, the next step is to randomize them to either receive or not receive the HPP. Randomization is one of the most critical aspects of the RCT. By randomization, we mean that participants are assigned to receive or not receive the HPP by chance alone. Randomization has a number of advantages in experimental research. Foremost, randomization comparably distributes subject characteristics that were assessed at baseline across groups. Moreover, randomization provides an efficient strategy for also distributing characteristics that were not measured. Often, for a variety of reasons (such as prohibitive cost, time, participant burden) the baseline assessment cannot reasonably measure all variables that may potentially affect the relation between exposure to the HPP and key outcomes.

◆ ◆ ◆

In a Nutshell

Foremost, randomization comparably distributes subject characteristics that were assessed at baseline across groups. Moreover, randomization provides an efficient strategy for also distributing characteristics that were not measured.

◆ ◆ ◆

How to Randomize Participants. Because randomization is so critical to an RCT, it is important that it be conducted properly. In general, there are two main features to consider when randomizing participants to study conditions; first, implementing a valid randomization procedure, and second, establishing procedures to safeguard the integrity of the randomization procedure so that unintentional or intentional biases do not influence the allocation process. We discuss both aspects in turn in this section.

◆ ◆ ◆

In a Nutshell

There are two main features to consider when randomizing participants to study conditions; first, implementing a valid randomization procedure, and second, establishing procedures to safeguard the integrity of the randomization procedure so that unintentional or intentional biases do not influence the allocation process.

◆ ◆ ◆

Implementing randomization requires reliable procedures that create comparability between groups. As with many other aspects of research, there are numerous randomization procedures that could be effectively and efficiently employed in an RCT. One common way is to manually use a table of random numbers to assign participants to groups. In this case, the investigator could consult a statistics textbook or even the Internet. How exactly does this work? Participant 1 (P_1) has just completed the baseline assessment and is now ready to be randomized. Opening a random numbers table, begin reading down the column of numbers, paying particular attention to the last digit in the sequence. Read down the column until you come to a number sequence that has either a "1" or a "0" as the last digit. If the number has a "1," then P_1 would be assigned to the HPP group. Now, the next participant completes the baseline assessment (P_2). Starting from where you ended, again read down the column of numbers until you come to a number sequence that has a "1" or "0" as the last digit. This time, suppose the next number has a "0" as the last digit. Then P_2 would be assigned to the control group. Continue this process until all participants have been assigned to either the HPP or the control group. Although this randomization strategy is effective, it can be time-intensive and does not guarantee an equal number of participants in each group. Fortunately, computer programs are now available to conduct randomization. These programs provide an equivalent randomization process, and they may be more efficient for larger numbers of participants.

Safeguarding the Integrity of the Randomization Procedure. The second concern in implementing randomization is to safeguard the integrity of the randomization procedure so that unintentional or intentional biases are avoided. This is essential to reduce potential confounding effects associated with bias. In terms of health promotion research, this means designing randomization procedures so that members of the research team who have contact with the participant cannot influence the assignment of the participant to the HPP or the control group. Sometimes, given the nature of the HPP, a team member involved in the randomization procedure may tacitly decide that a particular participant could benefit from being in the HPP group. This person may assign that participant to the HPP group without adhering to the established randomization procedure. In this instance, the participant did not have an equal chance of being in either the HPP or control group. In effect, the randomization procedure has been subverted.

To avoid subverting the randomization procedure, participants could be assigned to study conditions using *concealment of allocation procedures.* (See Schulz, 1995, Schulz and Grimes, 2002, and Schulz, Chalmers, Hayes, and Altman, 1995, for a thoughtful discussion of concealment of allocation in randomized controlled trials and for a more detailed account of subverting randomization.) Essentially, prior to beginning study enrollment, an investigator could generate the allocation sequence using a random numbers table. Thus, all the participants who are to be randomized would adhere to this pregenerated sequence. In practice, this procedure would operate as follows. The randomization sequence (that is, 0 or 1) is written on a piece of paper and placed in sealed opaque envelopes. As participants are ready to be randomized they are either given or asked to draw the envelope from the top of the stack of envelopes containing the randomization sequence. The investigator (or the participant if he or she drew the envelope) opens the envelope and displays the group to which the participant has been allocated. Although this is an effective procedure to protect the randomization process, it is critical that the randomization sequence be determined beforehand, and that only the principal investigator or the project statistician be involved in constructing the stack of envelopes. Minimizing the involvement of other staff and having a predetermined randomization sequence that is concealed from other research team members will guard the integrity of the randomization procedure.

◆ ◆ ◆

In a Nutshell

Although this is an effective procedure to protect the randomization process, it is critical that the randomization sequence be determined beforehand, and that only the principal investigator or the project statistician be involved in constructing the stack of envelopes.

◆ ◆ ◆

Step 4: Implementing the Health Promotion Program

Implementing an RCT requires particular attention to a number of methodological issues that revolve around the HPP. Four key issues to consider are (1) blinding, (2) designing the control condition, (3) ensuring fidelity of HPP implementation, and (4) enhancing participation in the HPP.

Blinding. Blinding is a research procedure that prevents participants from knowing whether they have been assigned to the experimental or control condition. This procedure effectively avoids problems known collectively as *demand characteristics.* Demand characteristics occur when participants behave differently as a consequence of knowing they are being "studied." In essence, they may selectively change their behaviors or distort their reports of behaviors upon assessment.

◆ ◆ ◆

In a Nutshell

Demand characteristics occur when participants behave differently as a consequence of knowing they are being "studied." In essence, they may selectively change their behaviors or distort their reports of behaviors upon assessment.

◆ ◆ ◆

Furthermore, if the research staff is aware of the study hypothesis, their behavior could affect study outcomes. This phenomenon is called *experimenter bias*. To control for this bias, a *double-blind* procedure can be implemented. For example, in medical trials, particularly studies designed to evaluate the differential effectiveness of medication, double-blind trials are often designed. In a double-blind trial, neither the investigator nor the participant is aware of whether the assigned condition is experimental or control.

Finally, the person conducting data analysis could be biased by knowing which participants' data come from experimental and control conditions. Thus, a study could be *triple-blinded*. In this case, the participants, investigators, and persons conducting data analysis are all unaware of whether the assigned condition is experimental or control.

Although an effective procedure, blinding is difficult to implement in the context of HPP. Typically, participants and group facilitators are aware of (or surmise) what program they have been assigned. For example, in a dating-violence-prevention program, it would be difficult (if not impossible) to adequately blind the participants and group facilitators who are, respectively, receiving and administering the intervention. Indeed, the facilitators are often involved in developing the HPP and thus blinding on this level would be impractical.

Not all forms of bias are remedied by blinding. For example, one common form of a demand characteristic is known as the *Hawthorne effect*. This effect was named after a study conducted in the town of Hawthorne, Illinois. The study assessed changes in employee productivity as a hypothesized consequence of additional lighting. Productivity increased when lights were made brighter, but also when they were dimmed! The conclusion was that simply knowing they were being observed caused employees to increase their productivity. This form of bias can be minimized by the use of a *structurally comparable control group* (in other words,

Box 6.1. A Control Group Is Not the Same as a Comparison Group

A simple and important rule to keep in mind is that a control group can only be formed through random assignment. Because people are randomly assigned to the control group, it is reasonable to anticipate equivalence between groups before the intervention begins. Often, however, forming a control group is not feasible. For example, imagine that the research question asks, "Does a community-level intervention, designed to reduce risk of cardiovascular disease, produce behavior change that is maintained for at least five years?" The question implies that the HPP is delivered to an entire community (perhaps using mass media and working with local health agencies). Thus, one key step in the planning process will be gaining support from key members of the community. Given that this process can be quite time consuming, it may not be feasible to garner support from several communities and then randomly allocate only half of these to receive the HPP. Instead, it makes sense to assign all of the communities to receive the HPP and to carefully select communities that "match" the HPP communities with respect to basic demographic profiles. Because the communities are not selected randomly, they are termed a comparison group rather than a control group. This difference is used to classify experimental designs apart from quasi-experimental designs. Thus, random assignment produces a control group, making the design experimental. Alternatively, nonrandom assignment produces a comparison group, making the design quasi-experimental.

a randomly assigned group of people who do not receive the HPP). See Box 6.1 for a full discussion. The control group would be similar to the HPP with respect to time, frequency of meetings, intensity of activities, and enjoyment of intervention activities. In the dating violence example, the experimental intervention could be four hours in duration (time) and four sessions (frequency), and could use interactive role-play techniques to enhance learning. A comparable control condition would therefore have to mirror these same conditions. This provides a suitable remedy to the Hawthorne effect, although this increases the cost of conducting the study, as additional staff is needed to develop and implement the comparable control group.

Designing the Control Condition. There are three types of control groups. One type is to have the control condition receive no intervention or attention. This is referred to as a "true control" group. Essentially, participants who are assigned to the control group following baseline assessment would return to complete follow-up assessments roughly on the same time schedule as participants randomized to the HPP group. Participants in a true control group would not receive any additional intervention. Sometimes, if the study is conducted in a clinical setting that routinely offers treatment and counseling, the control group would receive the "usual care or standard-of-care treatment or counseling" that would normally be provided. A second type is to have the participants assigned to the control group enter into the HPP following a wait period. There may be ethical issues involved that require every participant to receive the HPP. (See Chapter Three for more details.) In this type of control group, referred to as a *wait-list control group*, participants follow the same schedule of assessments as the HPP group. After all assessments are completed, they enter the HPP. The third type has been discussed and involves having a structurally similar attention control group that does not receive information or education hypothesized to affect the study outcome variables but does receive different health promotion messages (sometimes this is referred to as a "comparison group" because they are receiving some form of intervention, although the intervention selected is not thought to affect the study outcomes).

When using a structurally similar attention control condition, create a program that can be relevant and valuable to the participants. Be careful that the control program does not provide information or skills that are relevant to the goals of the HPP (sometimes referred to as "bleeding"). This could potentially compromise the validity of the RCT and produce artificial null findings.

◆ ◆ ◆

In a Nutshell

Be careful that the control program does not provide information or skills that are relevant to the goals of the HPP.

◆ ◆ ◆

Ensuring Fidelity of HPP Implementation. In any RCT it is imperative that implementation of the HPP be monitored regularly to safeguard against *drift* (that is, deviation from the established protocol). Drift can occur when persons delivering the intervention unintentionally or intentionally deviate from the intervention protocol. At times, they may interject personal experiences or anecdotes into a given HPP that clearly deviate from the HPP curriculum. In addition, they may perceive that the situation or circumstances in a particular group necessitate presenting information that is not included in the scripted curriculum.

Implementation drift can affect the internal validity of the RCT and reduce the ability to detect effects of the HPP on study outcomes. Internal validity may be compromised because the intervention is delivered differently by different staff members, or may be delivered differently by the same staff member throughout the course of the study. Thus, evaluation of the "HPP" is problematic because it may have assumed several forms throughout the trial.

To minimize implementation drift it is always critical to develop an implementation monitoring or assurance protocol. This is the protocol that governs what can and cannot be done in delivering the HPP. The protocol should be sufficiently detailed, and include (1) specification of each activity, (2) the goal and objectives for each activity, (3) who will implement the activity, and (4) the time allocated to each activity. Investigators and research staff need to be acutely aware of all aspects of the protocol and taught to adhere to it diligently. Although a detailed training program can be useful, continual monitoring of implementation is also needed to ensure that drift is avoided. And, if drift does occur, then it can be promptly detected and rectified.

Detecting drift requires constant monitoring by HPP implementation staff. To this end a number of procedures have proven useful. In our own research, we use a *dual-assurance methodology*. First, we ask participants to rate the health educators after each HPP group session. The health educators are blind to the participants' ratings, as these are collected by other staff members and placed in unmarked envelopes. Identifying information is not requested on the rating forms. The form asks participants to check off all the activities that were covered in the HPP group session that day. Thus, the investigators have an objective determination of the HPP activities that participants report being exposed to during the group session. This record is then checked against the implementation manual. Inconsistencies can then be addressed in meetings with the health educators.

Our second method of assessing fidelity of implementation is to have a rater assigned to each and every HPP intervention group session and also to each and every comparison group session. The rater completes a checklist much like the participants' rating form. The rater's checklist is significantly more detailed and requests not only whether particular HPP activities were implemented but also the amount of time spent on each activity and whether they were correctly implemented. These assurance methods can be used to quickly identify a health educator who is not compliant with the HPP manual and help to minimize the adverse effects of poor implementation fidelity.

Enhancing Participation in the HPP. In any multisession HPP there exists the potential that some proportion of participants will not complete the full HPP program. It is critical to develop strategies designed to minimize participant loss during the implementation of the HPP. For example, consider a study designed to test whether yoga exercises, conducted during a one-hour session for thirty consecutive days, help reduce blood pressure. Unfortunately, nearly 36 percent of the participants in the HPP (yoga) group do not attend all thirty sessions. Thus, they have not received the "full dose" of the HPP.

Dropping out before completing the full HPP can result in reducing the likelihood that HPP effects will be detected. To remedy the situation, it may be tempting to discard or eliminate data from participants who do not complete the full intervention. To do so would be inappropriate. Once participants have been randomized to their respective treatment groups, they are analyzed within those groups, regardless of whether they complete all required procedures. A common phrase that captures this rule is, "once randomized, always analyzed." This is referred to as an *intent-to-treat analysis*. This approach is critically important because it avoids what would otherwise result in a *self-selected sample*. In essence, eliminating those with incomplete attendance to the HPP changes what had initially been a randomized group. A second aspect of the intent-to-treat analysis is that it should be applied when issues arise relative to missing follow-up assessments (or key items within those assessments). Again, the initial temptation may be to delete people from the analysis. Doing so, however, would introduce further bias into the findings. A substantial number of techniques have been devised to deal with missing data and should be used when appropriate. For a discussion of these techniques please consult Graham and others, 1997, or Schafer, 1999.

◆ ◆ ◆

In a Nutshell

Once participants have been randomized to their respective treatment groups, they are analyzed within those groups, regardless of whether they complete all required procedures. A common phrase that captures this rule is, "once randomized, always analyzed."

◆ ◆ ◆

Because statistical solutions to missing data are not as desirable as design-based solutions, it is important to consider how best to ensure full participation in the HPP and follow-up assessments. A number of strategies have been designed to reduce barriers to attending health promotion interventions. First, although compensation to participants for attending HPP may not be permissible by certain funding agencies, it is permissible to provide compensation for completing assessments. Typically, assessments are administered at baseline and subsequent follow-up time points, which occur after the completion of HPP activities. Thus, it is important to build in brief assessments that coincide with HPP intervention sessions. One example would be to provide compensation to participants for completing the rating form of each HPP session. Another example would be to provide compensation for child care, if necessary. Also, providing compensation for transportation to and from the HPP sessions could be effective in reducing barriers to accessing the HPP and enhancing participation. Finally, designing an HPP that is perceived by participants as valuable, enjoyable, and engaging, and having health educators (that is, group facilitators) who are perceived as caring, knowledgeable, and dedicated are critical features of any HPP.

Step 5: Following the Sample over Time

Maintaining the cohort over protracted periods of time may be one of the most formidable challenges in conducting an RCT. Several problems can easily occur. Here we describe some of the problems that are unique to RCTs. Chapter Five provides more detail about procedures that can be used to maintain cohorts over time.

Conducting the Follow-Up Assessment. Follow-up is critical to capturing data assessing the effectiveness of the HPP. After participants complete an HPP, we need to follow them over time and ask them to return for another assessment (follow-up assessment), so that we can measure any changes in attitudes, beliefs, intentions, behaviors, or health indices. A number of issues are related to participant follow-up.

One issue associated with the follow-up assessment is to decide who will collect the follow-up data. Health educators involved in administering the HPP should not be involved in conducting the follow-up assessments. Health educators have established a relationship with participants, which may influence the way in which participants respond to questions. Likewise, health educators may subtly influence participants' responses. Thus, using a person not known to the participants may reduce this form of bias. A related issue involves the mode of administration of the assessment instrument. Face-to-face interviews may create greater potential for bias, as participants may respond in socially desirable ways (in other words, providing answers they think the assessor wants to hear). Furthermore, this bias may be even greater if the assessor is also the facilitator who administered their HPP. This potential for bias may be minimized, although not entirely eliminated, with computer-assisted techniques to administer the assessments (Turner and others, 1998). The most effective strategy to reduce this potential bias is to maintain a strict distinction between HPP implementation staff (interveners) and the data collection staff (assessors).

◆ ◆ ◆

In a Nutshell

Health educators involved in administering the HPP should not be involved in conducting the follow-up. Health educators have established a relationship with participants, which may influence the way in which participants respond to questions. Likewise, health educators may subtly influence participant responses.

◆ ◆ ◆

Blinding of Data Collectors. Though it is difficult to blind the participants and interveners, it is not as difficult to blind the data collectors so that they are unaware of the participants' group assignment (that is, whether participants are in the HPP group or the control group). Unblinded assessors, knowledgeable about the participants' group assignment, may differentially probe or assess participants during the follow-up interview, thus resulting in interviewer bias. Again, new advances in technology, such as computer-assisted and audio-computer-assisted data collection procedures are available that avoid this potential bias. Self-administered surveys are also less susceptible to this bias.

Applied Example

In this section we describe a recently published RCT that was designed to test an HPP. Our aim is to use this example as a heuristic strategy to illustrate some of the key concepts previous described and discussed.

A Health Promotion Program for Stroke Survivors

A study published in the *American Journal of Preventive Medicine* provides an example of an RCT designed to test an HPP for recent survivors of stroke (Rimmer and others, 2000). The HPP comprised thirty-six sessions delivered over twelve weeks (three sessions per week). The HPP was designed to achieve multiple goals:

- Improve lipid profiles
- Increase peak oxygen uptake
- Increase muscular strength and flexibility
- Reduce obesity

- Increase physical activity
- Reduce dietary fat intake
- Increase life satisfaction
- Reduce depression

To test the efficacy of this HPP the research team employed a pretest, posttest design using a wait-list control group. Recruitment occurred by provider referrals. Sixty-two people met the following eligibility criteria: (1) the person was thirty to seventy years of age, (2) the person was able to walk at least fifty feet without a mechanical aid, (3) at least six months had elapsed since the person had had a stroke, (4) the person served as his or her own guardian, (5) the person resided within a one-hour commute of the intervention site, and (6) the person's primary care physician provided written medical permission for the person to participate. Thirty-eight of these sixty-two people were then randomly selected to enroll in the study. Of these, thirty-five agreed to participate.

The HPP was described in detail. Each session included fitness instruction, exercising, nutrition education (including cooking instruction), and education designed to improve health behaviors. Persons performing the education were well qualified, including an exercise physiologist, psychologists, a social worker, and postdoctoral research assistants.

Of interest, the research team identified several barriers (for instance, lack of transportation) that might have precluded participation in the thirty-six-session HPP. Efforts were then made to eliminate these barriers (for example, providing free transportation to and from the intervention site). The overall attendance rate for the thirty-six sessions was 93 percent.

Eighteen persons were randomly assigned to receive the HPP, with the remainder being placed in the wait-list control group. Findings included (1) a significant decrease in total cholesterol serum levels for HPP group members versus an increase for those in the control group, (2) a significant loss of weight for HPP group members but not for the control group, (3) a significant improvement in "time to exhaustion" among HPP group members but not the control group, and (4) improvement in several indicators of life satisfaction and depression for HPP members but not for the control group.

Several points deserve mention. For example, the research team was quite successful in ensuring optimal attendance to the thirty-six sessions. In addition to eliminating barriers, such as transportation issues, the HPP actively involved participants in learning (for example, cooking classes, exercise sessions, group discussions), and this high level of interaction may have inspired people to return. (Note: people were not financially compensated to participate in this study.) Also, the wait-list control group was used for ethical reasons, as the research team did not want to withhold a potentially beneficial program from any of the study volunteers. It should also be noted that the small sample size should not be counted as a "strike" against the study. Indeed, the authors provided evidence suggesting that the statistical power for the study was adequate to detect a medium effect size. (See Chapter Eleven for a more in-depth discussion of power and effect size.) Most important, it should be noted that (with some exceptions) the HPP was effective (it worked!). Without conducting the RCT, evidence to support the efficacy of the HPP would not exist; thus, the RCT served as a way to validate and justify the continuation of the HPP for stroke survivors.

Integration with the Research Process

This chapter has focused on a single but highly important research design, namely, the randomized controlled trial. Recall that in step 3 of the nine-step research process (Figure 1.2), the task is to determine whether the research question necessitates the use of observational or experimental research designs. Although other types of experimental designs exist (see Chapter Four), the RCT provides evidence that is widely accepted as rigorous and valid. As a tool, the RCT is an indispensable part of research in health promotion practice. The design requires attention to two distinctly different activities. First, all of the rules and procedures of conducting an RCT (as described in this chapter) must be followed. Equally important, however, is that an HPP must be developed and implemented with great fidelity in order to create a "treatment." Unlike drugs that are tested by RCTs, the HPP is not a tangible entity and therefore it cannot be easily or readily dispensed. To the contrary, the HPP requires constant attention to ensure consistent delivery of a treatment throughout the course of the study.

A final note is offered as a word of caution. Findings from even the most rigorous RCT should never be generalized beyond the population in which it was conducted. For example, in the study of stroke survivors the majority of participants were low-income African Americans residing in an urban area. Whether the HPP would be comparably effective for a population of middle-class Caucasians can only be determined by repeating the RCT with an entirely different sample. This cautionary note speaks to a general principle of the RCT: internal validity does not guarantee external validity.

Summary

The aim of this chapter was to provide fundamental information to help guide the design of randomized controlled trials assessing the effectiveness of HPPs. One limitation of this chapter is its inability to cover all aspects of RCT design.

A second limitation is the inability to provide an in-depth discussion of the issues presented. Notwithstanding these limitations, the chapter has provided a broad overview of key issues to be considered in designing and implementing an RCT. In addition, we emphasized how these issues affect the validity of the study and the interpretation of the findings. And finally, we proposed practical solutions. Given the importance of HPPs and the cost and time associated with designing and implementing these programs, it is critical that we also consider how best to evaluate their effectiveness. The RCT, carefully designed and implemented, represents a rigorous methodological approach to assessing the effectiveness of health promotion interventions.

Issues to Consider

1. As noted in this chapter, deciding what kind of "treatment" will be provided to control group participants is often a difficult task. The research team must weigh two competing concerns. On one hand, it is imperative that the control condition does not provide participants with information, motivation, or skills that could predispose them to improvement on the outcome measure(s). On the other hand, an ethical and moral responsibility exists to help people at risk of any negative health outcome to avoid continued or escalated risk. Thus, several questions arise. Is a wait-list control group an ethical alternative to a do-nothing control group? If so, will the quality of the HPP be equal and highly monitored when delivered to the wait-list control group even though the study has ended? If a placebo-attention control group is used, what constitutes a reasonably interesting and valuable HPP that does not confound the study design?

2. An unresolved issue in RCTs involves the provision of monetary compensation to study participants. From a research perspective, the core issue becomes whether the amount of compensation creates an artificial incentive to participate in the HPP. Stated differently, would people attend the HPP if they were not being paid? Would they be equally motivated to learn if they were not being paid? In essence, any suspicions that answer either question with a "no" should lead to doubts about the external validity of the RCT. Thus, in an "ideal" RCT, compensation would not be provided. We suspect, however, that an RCT without participant compensation would be very difficult to conduct, given the potentially low participation rate and (in all likelihood) a high attrition rate. Not providing compensation to study participants for their time and effort also presents an ethical issue in that the intervention is "experimental" and, thus, of unproven value.

3. Finally, an important question to consider is "Are RCTs always the logical end-point of the research chain?" Do some research questions require evidence that cannot be provided using an RCT? We feel compelled at this juncture to refer you to a recent commentary published in the *British Medical Journal*. The authors suggested (with a great deal of wit) that the protective value of para-chutes has never been established by an RCT (Gordon and Pell, 2003). The satire of this work is as informative as it is entertaining.

For Practice and Discussion

1. Imagine that you accessed a population of low-income Hispanic women who are at high risk of cervical and breast cancer. Your intent is to test an HPP designed to promote regular Pap testing and mammography. The HPP is a nine-hour program delivered in three sessions. Women will be paid $50 to complete a baseline assessment and another $50 to complete a follow-up assessment. All women will be asked to provide permission for study investi-gators to track their medical records for the next five years. Because these women would not otherwise have any education designed to promote Pap test-ing or mammography use, you decide to use a do-nothing control group for your RCT. Provide a defense of this decision. Then assume that the defense is not sufficient and provide an alternative plan that can be defended on the basis of rigor alone (excluding ethical concerns from your argument).

2. This chapter emphasized the importance of using an intent-to-treat analy-sis for RCTs. Unfortunately, a rather large number of articles reporting RCTs have been published that do not employ the intent-to-treat principle. Consider a hypothetical scenario in which 140 women were randomized to the HPP condition and 110 women were randomized to an attention control condition. Baseline measures were collected on all 250 women. In the ensu-ing six weeks, women were expected to attend a two-hour intervention on each Saturday afternoon. By the end of the sixth week, 90 percent ($n = 126$) of the women in HPP condition remained in the study (that is, they attended the sessions as required). By contrast, only 50 percent of the women in the control group ($n = 55$) remained in the study. How might failure to use an intent-to-treat analysis influence the study findings? Keep in mind that the influence is a form of bias, and that bias can favor the null hypothesis (the HPP did not work) or the alternative hypothesis (the program worked). Provide and be prepared to defend an answer that takes all of the possibili-ties into account.

References

Campbell, D. T., and Stanley, J. C. (1963). *Experimental and quasi-experimental designs for research.* Chicago: Rand McNally College Publishing Company.

Gordon, C. S., and Pell, J. P. (2003). Parachute use to prevent death and major trauma related to gravitational challenge: Systematic review of randomized controlled trials. *British Medical Journal, 327,* 1459–1461.

Graham, J. W., Hofer S. M., Donaldson, S. I., MacKinnon, D. P., and Schafer J. L. (1997). Analysis with missing data in prevention research. In K. Bryant, M. Windle, and S. West (Eds.), *The science of prevention: Methodological advances from alcohol and substance abuse research* (pp. 325–366). Washington, DC: American Psychological Association.

Piantadosi, S. (1997). *Clinical trials: A methodologic perspective.* New York: John Wiley & Sons.

Pocock, S. J. (1993). *Clinical trials.* New York: John Wiley & Sons.

Rimmer, J. H., Branschweig, C., Silverman, K., Riley, B., Creviston, T., and Nicola, T. (2000). Effects of a short-term health promotion intervention for a predominately African-American group of stroke survivors. *American Journal of Preventive Medicine, 18,* 332–338.

Schafer, J. L. (1999). Multiple imputation: A primer. *Statistical Methods in Medical Research, 8,* 3–15.

Schulz, K. F. (1995). Subverting randomization in controlled trials. *Journal of the American Medical Association, 274,* 1456–1458.

Schulz, K. F., and Grimes, D. A. (2002). Blinding in randomized trials: Hiding who got what. *Lancet, 359,* 696–700.

Schulz, K. F., Chalmers, I., Hayes, R. J., and Altman, D. G. (1995). Empirical evidence of bias: Dimensions of methodological quality associated with treatment effects in controlled trials. *Journal of the American Medical Association, 273,* 408–412.

Turner, C. F., Ku, L., Rogers, S. M., Lindberg, L. D., Pleck, J. H., and Sonenstein, F. L. (1998). Adolescent sexual behavior, drug use and violence: Increased reporting with computer survey technology. *Science, 280,* 867–873.

CHAPTER SEVEN

QUALITATIVE RESEARCH STRATEGIES AND METHODS FOR HEALTH PROMOTION

Laura F. Salazar, Richard A. Crosby, and Ralph J. DiClemente

As iterated throughout this book, the overarching purpose of scientific inquiry is to generate knowledge. In the context of health promotion, scientific inquiries are undertaken to generate knowledge specifically regarding prevalence and incidence of disease, risk factors for disease and health-risk behaviors, etiologic factors, theoretical perspectives, and effectiveness of health promotion programs, to name a few. The long-term goal of these scientific inquiries is to prevent morbidity and premature mortality. Conceptualizing and implementing these scientific inquiries entails embarking on a journey through a nine-step research process (see Figure 1.2).

As with any journey, however, there are always many decisions to make and myriad options from which to choose. To some degree, each leg of this research journey will have consequences (both good and bad), and, depending on the path taken, may result in reaching a crossroad or even reaching a dead end. Thus, it is important to consider each decision point and plan your journey carefully. Of course, because you may not have been on this type of journey before, we don't expect you to travel alone. We have attempted to be your tour guide for this journey, walking you through the research process, helping to identify salient points of interest, and issuing warnings of any potential dangers. In the spirit of being the best tour guides possible, however, we must acknowledge that so far we have taken you on this journey using only one mode of transportation. Let's assume that for this analogy you have been primarily traveling by plane. As you can imagine, traveling cross-country by plane will provide quite a different experience than going by train. Therefore, because we want you to have the fullest experience possible, it is time to deplane and see how the countryside looks from the seat of a passenger train.

In this journey analogy, the mode of transportation refers to the methodological *paradigm* applied to the research process. From the Greek word *paradeigma*, *paradigm* literally means model, pattern, or example; however, this rather simple definition can be expanded to encompass a "worldview" that may be influential in shaping the development of a discipline. A methodological paradigm is a discipline's view of which research techniques and practices are promoted and should be practiced. A discipline's methodological paradigm has strong implications for how the discipline as a whole will progress. Thomas Kuhn, a twentieth-century professor in philosophy and history of science, is credited with popularizing the term *paradigm*. He wrote a provocative book titled *The Structure of Scientific Revolutions*. In it, he describes science as "a series of peaceful interludes punctuated by intellectually violent revolutions" (Kuhn, 1970, p. 10), which can change profoundly the existing view and result in a paradigm shift. He articulated the importance of paradigms in shaping and guiding a scientific discipline:

> A shared commitment to a paradigm ensures that its practitioners engage in the paradigmatic observations that its own paradigm can do most to explain. Paradigms help scientific communities to bind their discipline, in that they help the scientist create avenues of inquiry, formulate questions, select methods with which to examine questions, define areas of relevance, and establish or create meaning. A paradigm is essential to scientific inquiry [Kuhn, 1970, p. 142].

◆ ◆ ◆

In a Nutshell

A methodological paradigm is a discipline's view of which research techniques and practices are promoted and should be practiced. A discipline's methodological paradigm has strong implications for how the discipline as a whole will progress.

◆ ◆ ◆

The approaches, methods, designs, and perspectives described thus far mostly fall under a paradigm termed *positivism*. Positivism is the view that serious scientific inquiry should not search for ultimate causes deriving from some outside or unidentifiable source, but rather must confine itself to the study of relations existing between facts, which are directly accessible to observation. Science or knowledge is based on the exploration of natural phenomena, in which properties and relations are observed and are verifiable. Consequently, positivism involves the use of methods that should be objective and involves testing theories through the generation and falsification of hypotheses in order to assemble "facts" (see Chapter Two for more details). In the end, relations can be supported, disconfirmed, or falsified. As you can extrapolate from this description of positivism, positivistic inquiries lend themselves to the use of quantitative modes of inquiry.

Given that the research questions, designs, and methods described thus far can be labeled as positivistic, if we stopped and did not go any further, then we would have presented a skewed view of health promotion's paradigm. It would ostensibly appear that health promotion research was ideologically bound by research methods (for example, experimental designs, random sampling, quantitative data, inferential statistics) that many of us have been conditioned to view as the epitome of rigor and as "real" research (Glesne and Peshkin, 1992). Although much health promotion research uses these methods, designs, and data justifiably, as a discipline we are not *bound* by them. Indeed, much health promotion research uses epistemologies that are supported by an *interpretivist* paradigm (Glesne and Peshkin, 1992).

In contrast to positivism, interpretivism views the world as a multiplicity of realities where each individual perceives, understands experiences, and makes meaning of that reality in different ways; thus, reality is socially constructed. Research in this paradigm focuses on studying individuals' lives and their significance. The overall aim within this paradigm is to understand others' experiences and relate them to one's own reality (Colangelo, Domel, Kelly, Peirce, and Sullivan, 1999). Thus, an interpretivist paradigm is supported through the use of qualitative modes of inquiry. Just as positivism and interpretivism differ, because they are supported mainly through two different modes of inquiry, their modes of inquiry also differ. Quantitative and qualitative modes of inquiry differ in the assumptions made about the generation of facts, in their purposes, in their approaches, and in the role of the researcher. These differences are highlighted in Table 7.1.

In viewing Table 7.1, is it important to note that there is no judgment attached to the underlying assumptions of the two modes and there shouldn't be; rather, differences are illuminated to assist in making decisions regarding the research process. One approach is not necessarily better than the other in this instance, and one approach should not be considered more scientific or more rigorous than the

TABLE 7.1. PREDISPOSITIONS OF QUANTITATIVE AND QUALITATIVE MODES OF INQUIRY.

Quantitative Mode	Qualitative Mode
Assumptions	
Social facts have an objective reality	Reality is socially constructed
Primacy of method	Primacy of subject matter
Variables can be identified and relationships measured	Variables are complex, interwoven, and difficult to measure
Etic (outsider's point of view)	Emic (insider's point of view)
Purpose	
Generalizability	Contextualization
Prediction	Interpretation
Causal explanations	Understanding of perspectives
Approach	
Begins with hypotheses and theories	Ends with hypotheses and grounded theory
Manipulation and control	Emergence and portrayal
Uses formal instruments	Researcher as instrument
Experimental	Naturalistic
Deductive	Inductive
Component analysis	Searches for patterns
Seeks consensus, the norm	Seeks pluralism, complexity
Reduces data to numerical indices	Makes minor use of numerical indices
Abstract language in write-up	Descriptive write-up
Researcher Role	
Detachment and impartiality	Personal involvement and partiality
Objective portrayal	Empathic understanding

Source: From C. Glesne and A. Peshkin, *Becoming Qualitative Researchers: An Introduction,* copyright © 1992. Published by Allyn & Bacon, Boston. Copyright © by Pearson Education. Reprinted by permission of the publisher.

other—just different. There are some similarities as well. We strongly advocate that both are compatible and that each approach provides a different perspective and reveals additional information that allows us to gain a fuller understanding of whatever it is we are trying to know. Nevertheless, it is important to learn how the two modes differ along the dimensions presented in Table 7.1.

Illustration of Key Concepts

In this chapter, we will provide an overview of several qualitative research strategies, methods, and analyses so that you can glean a better understanding of how to conduct a qualitative inquiry. We will describe what constitutes qualitative research and several major purposes within health promotion for which qualitative inquiry is conducive. We also identify the methods most appropriate for health promotion research. Last, we provide a basic approach to data analysis. Keep in mind as you read through this chapter that unlike traveling by plane, this train trip requires no seat belt. So, relax and enjoy your trip!

What Constitutes a Qualitative Mode of Inquiry?

Essentially, there are five aspects of qualitative research that make it "qualitative": it is naturalistic, the data are descriptive, there is concern with process, it is inductive, and meaning is the goal (Bogdan and Biklen, 1998). In any one given qualitative research study it is not necessary to have all five features weighted evenly to signify that the research is qualitative, or to even have all five of the features. For example, imagine that a qualitative researcher studying homeless women wants to understand the circumstances of their lives and what led them to become homeless. He or she may collect descriptive data, be concerned with the process, and be focused on revealing the meaning of the participants' experiences. Yet, he or she may conduct in-depth interviews with the women in a coffee shop rarely visited by homeless women. Some qualitative research will emphasize certain features more so than others, but for practical purposes, ideally, qualitative research should attempt to encompass all five features.

◆ ◆ ◆

In a Nutshell

Essentially, there are five aspects of qualitative research that make it "qualitative": it is naturalistic, the data are descriptive, there is concern with process, it is inductive, and meaning is the goal.

◆ ◆ ◆

Naturalistic. Qualitative research is *naturalistic* as opposed to observational or experimental. Naturalistic and experimental differences can be quite distinct; however, distinctions between naturalistic and observational are more subtle. Although both designs involve a lack of manipulation or control, naturalistic signifies that the data are collected in the natural setting such as a person's home or school, whereas observational research can occur in an artificial setting. Furthermore, it is the setting in which the research takes place that provides the data, and it is the researcher who serves as the mode for data collection. Thus, the data are collected in a manner that is also natural (such as observing or conversing). Because qualitative research is concerned with contextualizaton, naturalistic approaches provide a high level of context. In a study of women seeking drug treatment, for example, one researcher went to a methadone clinic where he observed women in various areas of the clinic and interviewed them onsite (Fraser, 1997). Although we cannot say for certain, had the researcher attempted to bring the women into a different setting such as a university, conducting the interviews in an artificial setting could have had an impact on the results.

Descriptive Data. Qualitative research uses data that are descriptive (Bogdan and Biklen, 1998). Qualitative data can take several different forms such as words, pictures, video, notes, charts or records, and narratives. Data are not represented in numerical terms. If some numerical interpretation is provided, it is usually minor and may be presented to emphasize a pattern in the data. Written results may contain participants' quotes, interview transcripts, field notes, photos, and so on and provide a rich, in-depth analysis centering on interpretation. This approach, of course, contrasts with a quantitative mode in which data are expressed in numerical forms and statistical analyses are performed to describe the data and to test hypotheses. The results are then presented in statistical terms with little or no context.

Melville and colleagues conducted a qualitative research study of patients visiting a sexually transmitted disease clinic to determine the emotional and psychosocial impact of receiving a positive genital herpes diagnosis (Melville and others, 2003). In-depth interviews were conducted with twenty-four clinical patients onsite. A sample of the "data" is provided in Box 7.1 and a sample of the write-up from the published article is provided in Box 7.2. As shown, the data are words composing the transcription of the interview, and the results represent the researchers' interpretations and understanding of the participants' words.

Process-Focused. Qualitative research entails a focus on the process rather than on the outcomes (Bogdan and Biklen, 1998). Again using the research study of homeless women as an example, one focus of the research could be to understand the process through which women came to be homeless. How did these women become homeless? What happened in their lives that brought them to this point? Other examples from health promotion could be, how do young women negotiate condom use with their partners? What processes do they go through to protect themselves? And, why do some young women think they are overweight? How do they come to view themselves in this way? What is the impact of thinking they are overweight? Yu-Jen, Yiing-Mei, Shuh-Jen, and Mei-Yen (2004) conducted semistructured interviews with five young women to investigate their experiences with body image and weight control, and other researchers (Johnson, Kalaw,

Box 7.1. Text Transcribed Verbatim from an Interview with a Patient from an STD Clinic

I: Thinking back to when you first found out you had genital herpes, how did you feel at the time? This would have been not when you and I talked the other day, but when you first heard your results. And I'm assuming you talked to them on the phone, is that correct?

P: Yeah, I called in. How did I feel? Uh . . . I don't . . . can you stop this for a second?

I: Sure.

P: Okay.

(Tape stops.)

I: So you're not even sure how you actually felt?

P: I knew I had something, but in a way I was relieved to find out what it was, because as bad as it could be . . .

I: Right, I understand that.

P: And I guess a part of me could move on now. I could figure out what I needed to do.

I: As opposed to someone saying, "No no you don't have anything." And yet you know you have these weird symptoms?

P: Yeah.

I: Okay. So part of you was relieved and part of you was . . . ?

(Pause)

P: You know I think I had a little bit of anger too, because I think I know who it was. I remembered back to this whole incident and I'm pretty sure, so I had a little bit of anger with that. So relief and I don't know . . .

I: Herpes is a source of stress for some people but not for others. Did your discovering that you had herpes cause you enough stress to affect your daily behavior, for example your work, friends, and relationships? If so could you please explain in as much detail as possible?

P: No it hasn't really. It hasn't changed. The relationship a little bit. I'm putting off . . . I have a girlfriend but I'm putting off going over to her house. I know I need to tell her, but I'm not sure exactly how to go about that. So that's stressful, that could be classified as stressful. But as far as work goes, no.

I: But it sounds like from what you said before though that part of it was confirming and a relief to hear that you had something. That would be a relief of some kind of stress as opposed to creating stress. And having to tell someone about it—that's a whole different category that needs to be addressed at some point.

P: And as far as my life goes, I've been through a lot and I'm used to rolling with what comes at me. So I don't really feel all that much stress.

I: Maybe this is minor compared to some other things?

P: Yeah.

I: Self-concept is broadly defined as how you view yourself as a person. Did any of the feelings you experienced when you first discovered you had herpes change your self-concept in any way?

P: Wow. I think it makes me feel like, How am I going to get something going in a relationship as far as being with somebody? I don't understand how I could talk to someone about this, I really don't. I think in a way it's closed me—I'm already pretty closed as it is—but I think it's closed me a little bit more. Out of fear—I guess bottom-line rejection.

I: Do you recall if the discovery affected your daily moods at all?

P: I don't really recall. Maybe it'd be better if you had a list of questions—I'd get a chance to think about them before I came in.

(Laughter)

No. I don't think so.

I: Did it affect your feelings of body image and sexual attractiveness?

P: Maybe body image. I'm not sure about sexual attractiveness. That's really a mind thing I think. I think attractiveness is really a mind thing. I think it's the same.

I: Has it affected your sex drive?

P: No.

I: Has it affected your desire for long-term sexual relationships?

P: Has it affected my desire for long-term sexual relationships? I don't know. I still have that desire, it's just what am I going to do with this?

I: After the tape is off, we can talk more about this and your sex partners.

P: Okay.

I: Has it affected your ability to relate to your partner?

P: Yes.

I: Yeah, you mentioned that you haven't gone to her house.

P: Yeah, I'm staying away. I have to tell her, I can't just . . .

I: How long have you been with her?

P: Uh, two months, three months.

I: Some of the initial affects experienced by people who newly discover they have herpes change with the passage of time. Can you compare the answers that you just gave me to the feeling you have today? For example, how do you feel about learning that you were positive for herpes type 2?

P: How do I feel?

I: Well for example when you first heard your results part of you felt relieved because you suspected and now it was confirmed. And another part of you was angry because you were thinking who gave it to you and it brought that up. So now that you've had some time since you first heard your results what are your feelings now? Are they different from that day?

P: Yeah, I think now I'm more, not resigned but like resigned to move on. There's not really anything I can do about that now. It's water under the bridge. But I need to move on.

I: That's the impression I have too. So in terms of stress affecting your daily behavior, that sounds like it's still just affecting your relationship with your girlfriend?

P: Yeah work is going, it's really going well.

I: Has there been any change in your self-concept in any way?

P: Well I have a pretty good self-concept for someone who just did a lot of time. But I think as far as—I don't understand the question. I'm trying to ramble on.

I: Since finding out that you have herpes you talked about how initially it did affect your self-concept a little bit. But I'm hearing from the way you are talking about things, it's probably not affecting you as much anymore. In fact if I could put forth what I'm picking up is that maybe in the beginning it was something you thought about a lot, but now it's on the back burner and it comes up when you think about seeing your girlfriend because then you have to talk about it. But otherwise it's not really bothering you.

P: Very good, very good!

I: Is that where you are?

(Laughter)

P: Yeah. Part of me puts it off into the back and then when the opportunity arises when she'll call me up and I'll make excuses.

I: Oh good. We're going to have a lot to talk about when the tape is off.

P: Okay okay.

I: For many people, having herpes causes problems at some points in life but not at other times. After you knew you had herpes up till now, do you recall specific situations that may have intensified any negative feelings attached to your having herpes?

P: Something negative that is attached?

I: Yes.

P: I would think that outbreaks would be negative. That would be a hard time to deal with it. But I can't really think of anything else.

Box 7.2. Sample Results Write-Up

"Fear of telling a current partner was a frequent psychosocial response associated often with fear of rejection, present even for participants who knew that their current sex partner had herpes. One man (32, STD) said, 'I thought she was going to freak out and run away from me. Scared that she was going to run off and leave me forever.' Another man (37, STD) reported that his initial thought was, 'Oh my gosh, I'm positive, and if I tell him, he probably, you know, might reject me for this. Then I thought, oh no he's had herpes so he's certainly not going to do this to me. But there's always the possibility. So there was this little thinking that went on subconsciously. . . . I waited a couple of days and then told him, because I think I had to go through my own little process of dealing with that.'"

Source: From Melville and others (2003). "Psychosocial Impact of Serological Diagnosis of Herpes Simplex Virus Type 2: A Qualitative Assessment," *Sexually Transmitted Infections, 79,* p. 282.

Lovato, Baillie, and Chambers, 2004) have used a qualitative approach to examine the process youths undergo to regain control over their smoking. In each instance, the focus was on the process rather than the outcome of "being overweight" or "smoking."

Inductive Approach. Qualitative research is inductive. As you may recall from Chapter Two, inductive logic involves deriving general patterns from your observations that may eventually become hypotheses or that may constitute a theory. This approach contrasts with deductive logic, which involves testing specific hypotheses that were derived from general ideas and is the approach most often used in quantitative inquiries. The process underlying qualitative research is considered inductive because in very simple terms you begin by making observations and gathering data, then you describe the data, and finally, an attempt is made to interpret the data. The interpretation typically involves putting the pieces together so that they make an understandable "whole." This process is ongoing, dynamic, and emerging. After making initial observations and deriving initial patterns, you might go back and gather more observations, and you might even revise your initial conclusions. In this sense, the process is inductive, but you may at times use deduction within this process. Not surprisingly, considering this type of research process, qualitative research has been compared to patchwork quiltmaking and filmmaking (Sterk and Elifson, 2004).

Finding Meaning Is the Goal. Essentially, the task of qualitative research is to find meaning in the observations and experiences of the participants, which brings us to the fifth feature of qualitative research. The perspective of the participants is the main concern. For example, Miller-García (2004) wanted to understand the *meaning* of condoms for Mexican couples. Through in-depth interviews with five couples, she found that condoms meant "preventing pregnancy" and "being responsible." Her interpretation of the data is provided in Box 7.3.

Box 7.3. Meaning of Condom Use

Condoms as Contraception

All participants were asked what using a condom means to them. The overwhelming response among both women and men is that using a condom means preventing pregnancy. In fact, four of the five couples were in agreement that this was the primary meaning that condom use has for them. The fifth couple also said that using condoms means prevention of pregnancies to them, but only second to the prevention of illnesses and infections—this couple, however, has never used condoms.

For one woman, using condoms to prevent pregnancy is very important to her. She explained that while she is here in Atlanta working with her husband to save money and pay off debt, their two small children live in Mexico with her mother-in-law: "No, I can't get pregnant. Supposedly, one comes here to work, and so I am the one who says, 'I don't want to get pregnant because I don't want my children to feel betrayed . . . if I go back to Mexico with another baby in my arms.'" Another woman, in addition to the primary meaning of pregnancy prevention, expressed that condom use has a more global meaning for her: "To me, using condoms means fewer unwanted children in the world, fewer abortions, fewer illnesses, and fewer submissive women."

Condoms as Responsibility

Several men's explanation of what condom use means to them extended beyond contraception. For one man, using condoms means taking precautions, and for another, using condoms is "something special, something necessary." Another explained that for him, using condoms means being responsible: "It means being responsible. As a responsible person, I prefer to have to wrinkle up my nose a little so that, well, you have to use a condom to be together for a while or else you get the surprise of another baby."

Source: Miller-García, 2004. *Gender, Power, and the Meaning of Condom Use: A Qualitative Assessment of Condom Use Among Latino Couples.* Unpublished master's thesis, Rollins School of Public Health, Emory University, Atlanta.

Understanding the perspective of the participants in their natural surroundings in some way that is meaningful is the main goal of qualitative research. Although ostensibly this may seem like an easy task, interpreting the experiences of other people is rather difficult. As with any research, qualitative or quantitative, researchers bring their own experiences, values, and biases with them that may color or influence the interpretation. The main difference (refer to Table 7.1), however, between providing meaning to qualitative research and quantitative research is that in the former, the researcher typically acknowledges his or her values and biases and also understands that the process is subjective. Conversely, in quantitative research, an assumption of objectivity is made by the researcher when collecting and interpreting the data. This implies that the researcher is detached and impartial for all aspects of the research including the interpretation. You may want to consider whether or not researchers truly detach themselves from the process just because they are implementing an experimental design, administering quantitative measures, and performing statistical analyses.

Purposes for Which Qualitative Mode of Inquiry Can Be Used

Although there may be an infinite number of purposes for which qualitative inquiry can be used and should be used in health promotion research, we shall focus on four major purposes. Qualitative inquiry is useful for conducting exploratory research where little is known about a particular health issue. Qualitative inquiry should also be used when conducting formative research to develop a health promotion program (HPP). In this instance, qualitative inquiry can be combined with quantitative approaches. Qualitative research should also be viewed in certain instances as a complement or supplement to quantitative inquiries. Program evaluation is one such instance. Finally, qualitative inquiry can be used as an alternative when other methods are precluded.

Exploratory Research. As you may recall from Chapter Four, investigations of certain health phenomena generally evolve through a two-stage process, exploratory and conclusive. The exploratory stage entails research questions that will shed light on an issue for which little is known. "In this early stage [of the process], observations are needed to provide investigators with data to define health issues, to begin to understand the etiology of those health issues, to formulate theories, to reveal relevant factors, and to identify potential relationships." Thus, there is purpose to exploratory research, and its purpose corresponds highly with a qualitative mode of inquiry.

Because not much is known yet during the exploratory stage, it would be difficult to develop any hypotheses a priori that warrant testing. It may not be prudent at this stage to launch a large-scale research study using large samples and geographically diverse locations. Thus, exploratory research lends itself quite nicely to a qualitative mode in which you could begin to gather observations using a naturalistic approach within a limited geographical context, and data collected are not structured and formalized but descriptive. Interpretation of the data would center on defining the patterns grounded in the data and making sense of it all. Perhaps preliminary hypotheses or even a theory could emerge from the data at this point. Let's illustrate this point by referring back to the research study involving patients with herpes who were asymptomatic. At the time the study was conceptualized there was little known about how varied asymptomatic people's reactions would be to receiving a positive herpes diagnosis. Also, the serological test (western blot) used to detect antibodies to herpes simplex virus was becoming readily available and was emerging as a useful screening tool for diagnosing large numbers of people. The researchers felt that it was important to understand the emotional and potential psychosocial responses people may have to receiving a diagnosis, so that counseling strategies could be devised that would address these responses. Thus, a qualitative study was conducted to ascertain a relatively small number (twenty-four) of people's responses to receiving a positive diagnosis. The results suggested a theory of both short-term and ongoing responses and their relations as well as the influence of other factors (such as social support or knowledge about herpes) on those responses—both negatively and positively. The theory that Melville and others (2003) generated from the data is graphically depicted as a model in Figure 7.1. In viewing the model one can see the nature of the relationships between the variables and that the variables are such that measurements could be derived; thus, a quantitative mode could be employed to test the model on a larger scale. Thus, this example of exploratory research helped to advance the field to the next stage so that conclusive research could be conducted.

Referring back to Table 7.1, we can see that qualitative inquiry's purposes, which are parallel to that of exploratory research's, are contextualization, interpretation, and understanding of perspectives. Contextualization means that the research seeks to provide an understanding based on the experiences of the participants in a *particular* social setting. Whether or not the interpretation of those experiences will generalize to others is not the goal. Once an understanding of perspectives is reached, depending on the situation, future research can use other modes of inquiry to see whether these experiences generalize to others. Suppose, for example, that you are interested in understanding better the role parents may play, beyond the genetic component, in contributing to the obesity of their children. You could choose a setting such as small, rural town or even a particular school district that may have unusually high rates of obesity for the inquiry. Your approach in understanding the daily lives of the families who reside in the setting could entail not only observing, interviewing, and interacting with them

FIGURE 7.1.   MODEL OF PSYCHOLOGICAL RESPONSES TO A SEROLOGICAL HSV-2 DIAGNOSIS.

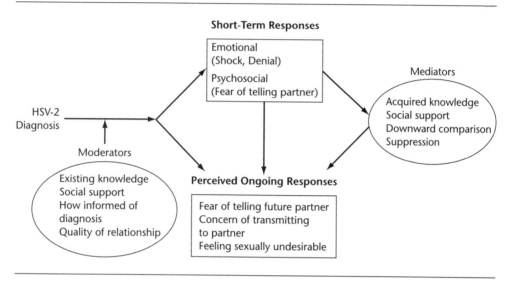

and trying to determine how they view their lives, but also identifying the historical, social, political, and environmental influences that interact and shape their reality. Once meaning is derived and a complex picture of the phenomena is obtained, then perhaps a larger-scale study that is more on the "conclusive" side can be justified and implemented.

When using a qualitative mode of inquiry, another caveat may be in order: this process is one of complexity, and trying to reduce or simplify the complexity of people's lives is not the goal. The researcher must "do justice to that complexity, to respect it in its own right" (Glesne and Peshkin, 1992, p. 7). Thus, for researchers using qualitative mode of inquiry, it helps if they immerse themselves and take an insider's point of view (that is, emic) and use multiple methods such as interviewing, observation, focus groups, and so on. The end result will reveal the complex nature of the phenomena in question and help to identify relevant qualities, interactions, and relationships. Consequently, new theories may result, hypotheses may develop, and hopefully the field will advance to the next stage in the process. Similar to quantitative inquiries, qualitative inquiries can also add yet another link to the research chain.

As Formative Research to Designing and Implementing HPPs. There may be some instances when it will be the research stage or the specific research question that dictates the decision to use either a quantitative or qualitative mode; other times, either mode may be plausible. In these instances, the researcher may have to choose. The decision that the researcher makes more than likely will rest on the personal perspective of the researcher. Each researcher holds a worldview that is shaped by his or her discipline's paradigm, personal experiences, and other socialization processes; thus as researchers our own ideals and values shape our research. More important, however, is that regardless of how or why the decision is made to adopt a certain approach, we do not want to present this decision as a conflict. The two approaches are not necessarily incompatible, and choosing which approach to use in your research does not have to be viewed as an "either-or" decision.

◆ ◆ ◆

In a Nutshell

As researchers our own ideals and values shape our research.

◆ ◆ ◆

Many times in health promotion research both modes are useful, compatible and, indeed, desirable. In fact, as opposed to endorsing or adopting only one approach, researchers should aspire to *triangulation* when planning any research study. Triangulation is a way for researchers to obtain a multidimensional view of phenomena of interest and involves multiplicities in data sources, methods, investigators, or theoretical frameworks (Denzin, 1978). It does not mean that you are limited to "three" types of each, however. Thus, the literal meaning of the word is not used in this context. It does imply that by incorporating both quantitative and qualitative approaches and data sources into any one research study, you can provide a more thorough understanding of phenomena.

◆ ◆ ◆

In a Nutshell

Triangulation is a way for researchers to obtain a multidimensional view of phenomena of interest and involves multiplicities in data sources, methods, investigators, or theoretical frameworks.

◆ ◆ ◆

Designing HPPs is a major goal of health promotion researchers and practitioners. Before programs can be designed, however, we must garner a thorough and complex understanding of the factors contributing to a particular health behavior or disease occurrence. One way is to conduct observational research as described in Chapter Five. For example, observational research using quantitative modes of inquiry is an effective way to document the prevalence and incidence of disease and to identify measurable risk factors; however, qualitative modes of inquiry may be used as an effective way of knowing both *why* a particular disease is prevalent, and also *how* to begin to prevent it. Thus, triangulation is a comprehensive way for health promotion researchers to know as much as possible, so that more effective programs can be derived. Nakkash and others (2003) used triangulation of methods (quantitative and qualitative) and data sources (community members and coalition members) in their development of a cardiovascular disease prevention program. They first conducted a household survey (a quantitative method) using a representative sample from the community (the first data source) in which the program was to be implemented. The survey was designed to assess knowledge, attitudes, and behaviors related to cardiovascular disease and to identify risk factor levels. They also asked participants from the household survey to participate in focus groups (a qualitative method) to identify the facilitators and barriers to achieving healthy lifestyles as well as intervention ideas. A coalition consisting of key informal and formal community leaders (the second data source) was assembled. The researchers conducted natural group discussions (a qualitative method) with the coalition members to understand the relevancy, feasibility, affordability, acceptability, and sustainability of proposed intervention activities. The researchers made the following comments regarding their use of triangulation in developing the community-based program:

> The advantages far outweigh the disadvantages. The intervention activities developed as a result of the triangulation of data methods and sources are community specific, relevant, and affordable. As a result, they are more effective and sustainable. This combination of intervention activities could not have been developed in the absence of any one piece of information. Effective and sustainable interventions are, in fact, cost-effective. Thus, the cost-intense disadvantage is ultimately diminished in an assessment of efficiency. Practitioners are encouraged to obtain information from a variety of methods and sources in the development of community-specific interventions [Nakkash and others, 2003, p. 738].

Although some researchers may admit that carrying out a sophisticated quantitative study while also conducting in-depth qualitative research is rife with challenges and may be difficult for many; essentially all research is rife with challenges. Thus, given the breadth of experiences described by Nakkash and others (2003) and their subsequent endorsement of combining approaches in retrospect, it would be hard to argue that using a combination of approaches should not be attempted or at least considered. If the researcher's perspective endorses more of a quantitative view, then he or she could use triangulation of data sources. Furthermore, if multiple methods are desired, the researcher could use triangulation of investigators (that is, a multidisciplinary approach) and collaborate with researchers who are experts in qualitative methods thereby expanding the methods used. There are myriad ways to use triangulation, but you may have to be creative.

Another way in which qualitative research may be useful is before the HPP is implemented. Methodological issues related to the implementation of the program are best determined beforehand through the use of qualitative research. These include issues such as

- Recruitment strategies (for example, what the best way is to recruit)
- Participants' perceptions of randomization (for example, thoughts of being in a control group)
- Retention of participants (for example, strategies to stay in contact with participants)
- Compensation (for example, the amounts or the type that are appropriate)
- Logistical issues (for example, what the most convenient time is to have the HPP)

Given the time and resources involved in developing an HPP, it would be judicious to conduct some qualitative research to ensure that the program will be well-received and that the research to evaluate it can be conducted successfully. For example, Salazar, Holtgrave, Crosby, Frew, and Peterson (2005) conducted a qualitative research study to examine the attitudes and beliefs toward obtaining a hypothetical AIDS vaccine (in this instance, the vaccine would be considered an HPP) among men who have sex with men (MSM). The purpose of the research was to understand their perceptions and opinions toward vaccination given the commercial availability of an AIDS vaccine, and also to understand the salient issues critical to their decision-making process. Because several AIDS vaccines are currently undergoing Phase II and Phase III clinical trials, understanding the barriers to and facilitators toward getting vaccinated is necessary to ensure widespread uptake of a vaccine that may be approved in the future. For a vaccine to truly protect people there must be widespread acceptance of the vaccine. Limited motivation to obtain vaccination would have a great impact on the success of a vaccine program. Thus, the qualitative inquiry was conducted with twenty-four MSM to better understand their motivation to participate in an AIDS vaccine program. The interviews were transcribed and analyzed. The main issues that emerged from the data are shown in Table 7.2.

TABLE 7.2. EMERGENT THEMES RELATED TO GETTING A FUTURE AIDS VACCINE.

Factors and Description	Illustration
Knowledge Factors	
Vaccine strategy	"Is it made with a piece of the HIV virus?" "Do they actually inject you with HIV?" "What symptoms or damage would it prevent?"
Clinical trial research	"First of all that it's solid and that it works 100 percent." "Very little side effects where it would not affect our daily lives." "How many people were in the study; what was the make of the study as far as males, females; different ethnic groups; what were their sexual practices, were they straight or gay (sexual orientation); and how the long does the study last?" "How does this drug work on different ethnic groups?"
Vaccine attributes	"We have to realize that medicine costs money, and our health has an economic consequence." "Is it something that I would only need to take once?" "Can it be put into a pill?" "I'd like to know who sponsored it and who stands to make a profit." "Does the vaccine have FDA approval?"
Racial differences	"It makes a big difference to me if it was tested in Acorra, Cameroon, where it's all black people, with high HIV percentage rate, or if it was tested on white gay males in Chelsea, in New York."
Encouraging Factors	
Knowledge about AIDS vaccine	"I would be cool with it if there were no side effects."
Perceived high risk	"If I were dating someone who was HIV positive, I may take the vaccine."
Cost	"If all the research states that it works fine, no adverse reactions, I don't see why I would not take it as long as I could afford it."
Discouraging Factors	
Harsh side effects	"I can't really think of a reason why I would not want to take this vaccine other than side effects that would affect my body that would stifle my daily progress or my daily functions in my life."
Low perceived risk	"If I have sex, which might be rarely, it is safe sex and I don't put myself in the situation where I would need the vaccine."
Backlash effect	"Because our people take it and think 'Oh God, it's a cure and let me go throw my rubbers away, I can get back out there and do whatever I want.'"
Cost prohibitive	"Something that was really expensive . . . like $1,500 or $5,000."

Numerous studies have been conducted that have examined patient characteristics such as race, marital status, and age as influencers of enrollment in cancer trials (Roberts, 2002), while other studies have examined barriers to participation such as lack of social support, availability of child care, and transportation concerns (for example, Richardson, Post-White, Singletary, and Justice, 1998), uncertainty of side effects (for example, Barofsky and Sugarbaker, 1979), and even physicians' communication style (for example, Grant, Cissna, and Rosenfeld, 2000). Although these studies have provided much-needed information that is helpful for researchers implementing a randomized controlled trial (RCT) of cancer treatments, Roberts (2002) felt that a clear understanding of *how* trials were being presented to potential volunteers was lacking. She wanted to understand the process that oncologists went through in their presentation of options to potential study volunteers. In other words, she wanted to know what type of information was being presented as well as how it was being presented. She audiotaped interactions between oncologists and their patients who had been diagnosed with breast cancer. The interaction represented the communication between the oncologists and their patients as they discussed the patient's options for adjuvant therapy. She analyzed the transcripts and found much variation in the way oncologists presented information regarding the clinical trial option. Her qualitative analysis suggests that differences in the way physicians present information for the same clinical trial can lead to differential response rates. This information could not have been gleaned using a quantitative mode of inquiry.

When implementing an RCT, equally important to understanding the physician's perspective is understanding the potential volunteer's perspective. How do certain people perceive the details of participating in a trial? Knowing and understanding this viewpoint may provide information needed to ensure adequate enrollment and reduce participation bias. Moreover, ethical guidelines stipulate that patients who participate must be adequately informed, but how do you gauge or measure whether participants have been adequately informed? Not surprisingly, we advocate that qualitative research methods are an appropriate way to answer some of these methodological and ethical questions. Ferguson (2002) used a qualitative approach to explore seventy-eight trial participants' views on the amount of information provided and of their own understanding of that information. The participants' perceptions were that they felt they had been given adequate amounts of information and that they were able to understand the information presented to them.

Featherstone and Donovan (1998) wanted to understand participants' perspective of one of the most critical aspects of the RCT—the randomization process. They conducted in-depth interviews with twenty clinical trial participants and found that they had recalled and were able to describe aspects of the process such as "chance," "comparison of treatments," and "concealed allocation," but relayed some confusion in terminology (for instance, "trial" and "random") and held some misgivings about the procedures used. These results suggest that potential volunteers may need more information regarding the rationale for the RCT and specific terms used by the researchers. Thus, their qualitative study provided information that is useful for implementers of RCTs but most likely could not have been ascertained using a quantitative approach.

Complement or Supplement to Quantitative Inquiry. With the advent of new treatment modalities for combating disease and the need for new behavioral programs to modify a spectrum of high-risk behaviors, trials to evaluate these regimens are critical to moving the field forward and to determining what works and what doesn't. In Chapter Eight, on program evaluation, you will learn the importance of program evaluation and specifically how triangulation (in other words, multiple data sources, methods, and investigators) is often used when designing and conducting a program evaluation. As you may have been able to glean from the phrase "program evaluation," it basically involves some type of HPP and a research plan to evaluate it. Whether it is a large-scale phase III clinical trial involving thousands of participants or a smaller scale pilot study, these evaluation investigations can only benefit from including qualitative research as an adjunct to the methods and data sources constituting the quantitative component.

A specific type of quantitative mode, namely the experimental design, is used quite often to evaluate HPPs and is described in detail in Chapter Six. Thus, the quantitative approach answers whether the HPP was effective. Yet, a quantitative approach may be limited in answering *how* or *why*. Because qualitative research is about the process, it is an excellent mode to use for researchers to learn *how* the intervention worked. What activities resonated to the participants, and what activities did not? Why did the participants change their attitudes or alter their behavior? If the program was not effective, then why did participants think it didn't work? What about the intervention evoked the observed changes? Even if the program was effective, what did they like about it? All of these questions could be asked of the participants and their responses could reveal patterns that would provide researchers with a much more in-depth understanding of their intervention. In fact, a recent textbook has been dedicated to describing various process evaluations that have used qualitative methods and strategies for answering many of these questions (see Steckler and Linnan, 2002). Clearly, it is critical to know whether the program worked, but equally important is to know why and how it worked. Thus, incorporating a qualitative approach into an evaluation will help to supplement, validate, explain, and illuminate or possibly reinterpret the quantitative data gathered from the participants. The result will be more comprehensive and have a multidimensionality that could not otherwise have been achieved without triangulation (Miles and Huberman, 1994).

◆ ◆ ◆

In a Nutshell

Incorporating a qualitative approach into an evaluation will help to supplement, validate, explain, and illuminate or possibly reinterpret the quantitative data gathered from the participants.

◆ ◆ ◆

An Alternative Method When Other Methods Are Precluded. In certain jurisdictions of the United States there are laws that restrict the type and nature of educational programs and subsequent inquiries to evaluate those programs. For example, Box 7.4 highlights a specific piece of legislation from the state of Louisiana that dictates the type of sex education programs that can be implemented in the schools and proscribes the nature of questions students can be asked. As you can see from the bolded text, "Students shall not be tested, quizzed, or surveyed about their personal or family beliefs or practices in sex, morality, or religion." Thus, for health promotion researchers who are interested in prevention of pregnancy and STDs among adolescents in Louisiana, not only must they adhere to abstinence-only education, but also they must restrict their evaluations of these programs to content other than sexual beliefs and behavior.

Clearly, this presents a challenge to program evaluators who are seeking to determine the effectiveness of abstinence-only educational programs in this jurisdiction. Thus, alternative ways of investigating students' experiences with the program must be devised. Of course, this legislation does not preclude the use of surveys or quantitative instruments per se; however, it does limit to a large degree what *can* be surveyed. One alternative in this instance would be for program evaluators to query participants' about their experiences with the program and what value the program had for them. Moreover, they could ask participants their opinions of how the program could be improved. Thus, in this context, a qualitative mode of inquiry may be the best method and even perhaps the only method for gathering these types of information related to the program.

Yoo, Johnson, Rice, and Manuel (2004) implemented a qualitative evaluation of a sexual abstinence program that was implemented in southern Louisiana. They conducted semistructured interviews with principals, teachers, and peer mentors. In addition, they conducted eight gender-stratified focus groups of students who received the program. By using qualitative methods, they were able to garner

Box 7.4. Louisiana State Legislation

RS 17:281 SUBPART D-1. PERMITTED COURSES OF STUDY

281. Instruction in sex education

A.(1) (a) Any public elementary or secondary school in Louisiana may, but is not required to, offer instruction in subject matter designated as "sex education," provided such instruction and subject matter is integrated into an existing course of study such as biology, science, physical hygiene, or physical education. When offered, such instruction shall be available also to nongraded special education students at age-appropriate levels. Except as otherwise required to comply with the provisions of Subparagraph (b) of this Paragraph, whether or not instruction in such matter is offered and at what grade level it is to be offered shall be at the option of each public local or parish school board, provided that no such instruction shall be offered in kindergarten or in grades one through six. Such instruction may be offered at times other than during the regular school day, at such times to be determined by each school board. All instruction in "sex education" shall be identified and designated "sex education."

(b) Effective beginning with the spring semester of the 1992–1993 school year and thereafter, whenever instruction in sex education is offered by any school, such instruction shall be available also to any student in such school, regardless of the student's grade level, who is pregnant or who is a mother or father.

(2) It is the intent of the legislature that, for the purposes of this Section, "sex education" shall mean the dissemination of factual biological or pathological information that is related to the human reproduction system and may include the study of sexually transmitted disease, pregnancy, childbirth, puberty, menstruation, and menopause, as well as the dissemination of factual information about parental responsibilities under the child support laws of the state. It is the intent of the legislature that "sex education" shall not include religious beliefs, practices in human sexuality, nor the subjective moral and ethical judgments of the instructor or other persons. **Students shall not be tested, quizzed, or surveyed about their personal or family beliefs or practices in sex, morality, or religion.**

(3) No contraceptive or abortifacient drug, device, or other similar product shall be distributed at any public school. No sex education course offered in the public schools of the state shall utilize any sexually explicit materials depicting male or female homosexual activity.

(4) The major emphasis of any sex education instruction offered in the public schools of this state shall be to encourage sexual abstinence between unmarried persons and any such instruction shall:

(a) Emphasize abstinence from sexual activity outside of marriage as the expected standard for all school-age children.

(b) Emphasize that abstinence from sexual activity is a way to avoid unwanted pregnancy, sexually transmitted diseases, including acquired immune deficiency syndrome, and other associated health problems.

(c) Emphasize that each student has the power to control personal behavior and to encourage students to base action on reasoning, self-esteem, and respect for others.

B. Notwithstanding any other provisions of law, the qualifications for all teachers or instructors in "sex education" shall be established and the selection of all such teachers or instructors shall be made solely and exclusively by the public local or parish school board.

C. All books, films, and other materials to be used in instruction in "sex education" shall be submitted to and approved by the local or parish school board and by a parental review committee, whose membership shall be determined by such board.

D. Any child may be excused from receiving instruction in "sex education" at the option and discretion of his parent or guardian. The local or parish school board shall provide procedures for the administration of this Subsection.

E. In the event of any violation of the provisions of this Section, the public local or parish school board in charge of administering and supervising the school where said violation has occurred, after proper investigation and hearing, shall correct the violation and take appropriate action to punish the offending party or parties responsible for said violation.

F. No program offering sex education instruction shall in any way counsel or advocate abortion.

G. A city or parish school system may accept federal funds for programs offering sex education only when the use of such funds does not violate the provisions of this Section and only upon approval by the local school board. The acceptance and use of federal funds for sex education shall in no way be construed to permit the use of any federally supplied materials that violate Louisiana law regulating sex education.

H. Notwithstanding any other provision of law, the Orleans Parish School Board may offer instruction in sex education at the third grade level or higher.

"valuable insights for future improvement in abstinence-only programs" (p. 329). For example, they were able to learn that all respondents indicated that the program should be taught in lower grades (the program had been implemented in grades seven through nine) and that responses to the program were mixed: some felt it was of no value and some felt it provided needed information and skills (Yoo and others, 2004). It should be noted, however, that although this inquiry provided participants' opinions toward the program, it still does not provide a behavioral indication of program effectiveness.

As health promotion practitioners and researchers, we must always work within laws and follow policy guidelines as they pertain to program content and the research. Thus, in these instances when certain content cannot be measured or surveyed, a qualitative approach can provide an alternative to quantitative approaches and yield valuable information that would have otherwise been omitted.

Qualitative Research Strategies for Health Promotion Research

Up to this point, we have discussed the features of qualitative research and the instances in health promotion in which qualitative research is warranted; however, we haven't provided a clear discussion of the different types of qualitative research. Essentially, unlike quantitative research, qualitative research does not have specific designs per se; rather, qualitative research has varying strategies that can be thought of as different philosophical orientations providing a general direction for implementing the research. The research strategy can also be thought of as the "tool" for accomplishing a particular research task. These various orientations have historical roots in different disciplines such as anthropology, philosophy, education, zoology, and sociology. The strategy selected is dictated largely by "the purpose of the study, nature of the research question, and the skills and resources available to the investigator" (Morse, 1994, p. 223).

◆ ◆ ◆

In a Nutshell

Qualitative research does not have specific designs per se; rather, qualitative research has varying strategies that can be thought of as different philosophical orientations providing a general direction for implementing the research.

◆ ◆ ◆

Because qualitative strategies are too numerous to describe in great detail, we cover five basic strategies that can be useful for conducting qualitative research in health promotion. Morse (1994) has outlined these five basic qualitative strategies: phenomenology, ethnography, grounded theory, ethnoscience, and qualitative ethology. Each of these qualitative strategies offers "a particular and unique perspective that illuminates certain aspects of reality more easily than others and produces a type of results more suited for some applications than others" (Morse, 1994, p. 223). To illustrate the differences among these strategies, Morse used a hypothetical research scenario involving travelers arriving and departing at an airport. Her conceptualization of each strategy is presented in Table 7.3.

Note the highlighted differences among the five strategies in the nature of the research question, recommended sample sizes, the types of results that could be gleaned, and the types of qualitative methods appropriate for the research question. As we go through each of the strategies in more detail, it may be helpful to apply another hypothetical research example derived from health promotion. For example, a phenomenon that has been highlighted in the literature and

TABLE 7.3. A COMPARISON OF STRATEGIES IN THE CONDUCT OF A HYPOTHETICAL PROJECT: "ARRIVALS AND DEPARTURES: PATTERNS OF HUMAN ATTACHMENT."

Strategy	Research Question or Focus	Participants/ Informants[a]	Sample Size[b]	Date Collection Methods	Type of Results
Phenomenology	What is the meaning of arriving home?	Travelers arriving home; phenomological literature; art, poetry, and other descriptions	≈ six participants	In-depth conversations	In-depth reflective description of the experience of "what it feels like to come home"
Ethnography	What is the arrival gate like when an international plane arrives?	Travelers, families, others who observe the setting, such as skycaps, rental car personnel, cleaning staff, security guards, and so forth	≈ thirty to fifty interviews	Interviews; participant observation; other records, such as airport statistics	Description of the day-to-day events at the arrival gate of the airport
Grounded theory	Coming home: Reuniting the family	Travelers, family members	≈ thirty to fifty	In-depth interviews: Observations	Description of the social psychological process in the experience of returning home
Ethnoscience	What are types of travelers?	Those who observe the setting daily—skycaps, rental car personnel, cleaning staff, security guards, and so forth	≈ thirty to fifty	Interviews to elicit similarities and differences of travelers, card sorts	Taxonomy and description of types and characteristics of travelers
Qualitative ethology	What are the greeting behaviors of travelers and their families?	Travelers and their families	Units—numbers of greetings—one hundred to two hundred	Photography, video, coded	Descriptions of the patterns of greeting behaviors

[a]Examples only.
[b]Number depends on saturation.

Source: From J. Morse (1994), "Designing Funded Qualitative Research," in N. K. Denzin and Y. S. Lincoln (Eds.), Handbook of Qualitative Research, Thousand Oaks, CA, Sage, p. 225. Copyright 1994 by Sage Publications, Inc. Reprinted with permission.

sensationalized in the media is the notion of living on the "down low." *Down low* is a term that has been applied mostly to African American men and refers to their living a heterosexual lifestyle (that is, married to a woman) while engaging in sexual intercourse with other men surreptitiously. Of course, this is not a new phenomenon. Many men in the past have lived double lives or remained in "the closet" for fear of social ostracism. However, there is some evidence to suggest that engaging in sexual intercourse with other men place men at risk for HIV infection, which in turn may place their female partners at risk. Given that blacks compose only 12 percent of the total U.S. population but 40 percent of all cumulative AIDS cases (Centers for Disease Control and Prevention, 2005), conducting qualitative research on the phenomenon of living on the down low may help researchers to understand better men's perspectives of this lifestyle and perhaps devise programs that can lead to a reduction in both types of exposure: heterosexual contact and male-to-male contact.

Phenomenology. Within an interpretivist paradigm, phenomenology refers to an analysis made by phenomenological investigation rather than the typological classification of a class of phenomena. Stemming from the discipline of philosophy, phenomenological investigations focus on interpreting "the meaning of events and interactions to ordinary people in particular situations" (Bogdan and Biklen, 1998, p. 23). The emphasis is on understanding the ways in which people construct their realities; that is, an attempt is made to reveal what perspective they hold and how they interpret events that happen. As a research strategy, it is subjective and relies heavily on trying to understand the participants' point of view. You may be wondering at this point, how can a research approach that is subjective also be considered as scientific research? As we have stated previously, quantitative modes of inquiry attempt to be objective and it is that objectivity that serves as a gauge of methodological rigor. Conversely, in the phenomenological interpretivist approach, subjectivity is treated as "a topic for investigation in its own right, not as a methodological taboo" (Holstein and Gubrium, 1994, p. 264). Thus, within this approach, subjectivity is the underlying mode and is embraced.

The method to accomplish phenomenological inquiries may be in-depth conversations and interviews with participants. For researchers using this strategy, however, gaining access to another person's point of view implies that in doing so the researcher may have some influence on the participant's perspective. Nonetheless, there is great utility in this approach, as it involves the collection of data that can provide an in-depth understanding of a phenomenon. Consequently, we may learn something which in turn may be useful for improving some aspect of the human condition. For example, Moore (2000) conducted a phenomenological study to understand the meaning of severe visual impairment to older women diagnosed with macular degeneration. The research question was "What is the lived experience of severe visual impairment in older women diagnosed with macular degeneration?" Interviews with eight women revealed that severe visual impairment meant "persisting toward unfolding ways of being in the world sparked by personal discoveries amidst enveloping losses" (Moore, 2000).

Applying phenomenology to our example of men living on the down low would be very useful for gaining insight into the lives of these men. Our research question could be "What is the meaning of living on the down low?" and could be approached by engaging men in conversations (if you could find them) about sexual orientation, homosexuality, being an African American man in our society, how they view their lifestyle, and how they make sense of their lifestyle. Our emphasis would be on describing the structures (their opinions, values, beliefs, attitudes) of participants' reality that help to explain and interpret the meaning they have attached to their reality. In this example, one hypothetical result could be the following: "For African American men living on the down low, their secretive behavior means keeping their families intact while fulfilling a sexual fantasy that makes them happy and ultimately a better husband or partner."

Ethnography. Ethnography is a qualitative strategy that has its origins in cultural anthropology, the study of human beings in relation to their social interactions and culture. Derived from the Greek term *ethnos,* meaning a people, a race, or a cultural group, and the term *graphic,* meaning descriptive, ethnography is a social scientific description of a people and the cultural basis of their peoplehood (Peacock, 1986). In this context, culture refers to the "acquired knowledge that people use to interpret experience and generate social behavior" (Spradley, 1979, p. 4). Culture is therefore relative and can be interpreted from more than one perspective, such as an outsider's or an insider's point of view. As a qualitative research strategy, ethnography focuses on providing a detailed and accurate *description* of values, behaviors, practices, and beliefs of a given group of people rather than explanation; however, the description should be in terms of the native's point of view rather than from the researcher's. Yet doing ethnography does not entail only studying people and observing their behavior; rather, the ethnographer must go beyond the gathering of observations and facts and learn what they mean. This experience requires the researcher to immerse herself or himself in the culture under study and not only observe the behavior, artifacts, and emotions but also try to understand the meaning attached to them from an insider's perspective. Thus, because ethnography is also concerned with meaning, it is similar to phenomenology, but differs in that its purpose has a much greater scope and culture is the guiding framework used to interpret and attach meaning to the experiences.

◆ ◆ ◆

In a Nutshell

Because ethnography is also concerned with meaning, it is similar to phenomenology, but differs in that its purpose has a much greater scope and culture is the guiding framework used to interpret and attach meaning to the experiences.

◆ ◆ ◆

To conduct ethnography, researchers should use multiple data collection methods such as naturalistic observation, interviews with natives, gathering of artifacts, and examination of archival data. In this way, they can capture a full description of those aspects of culture that shape people's experiences, behavior, beliefs, and emotions. For example, Reisinger (2004) conducted an ethnographic study of an outpatient adolescent drug treatment program. The purpose of the ethnography was to "understand better the treatment experience from the perspective of the adolescent clients" (Reisinger, 2004, p. 244). She conducted four in-depth interviews with each of twenty-five adolescents who presented for treatment. Researchers also observed seventy group sessions and conducted both formal and informal interviews with clinic staff. Moreover, extensive field notes were compiled.

Getting back to our hypothetical example, if we were to apply ethnography to the study of men living on the down low, we would be interested in describing what life is like for men who live this way. In this situation, we might have to enlist the assistance of an *informant*, someone who could be a source of information to help communicate knowledge regarding the experience and serve as a teacher to the researcher. We could conduct interviews with men and perhaps hang out at a bar where they may go to meet other men while observing and taking notes. We would also want to consider interviewing other relevant participants such as a wife or girlfriend, or other members of the community that may play a cultural role in this lifestyle. We would attempt to describe their lives in a way that is in relation to the culture in which they are embedded. This attempt at description involves a *translation process,* which entails "discovering the meanings of one culture and communicating these meanings to people in another culture" (Spradley, 1979, p. 205). In this example, one hypothetical result could be something like the following:

> African American men, who live on the down low, view being gay as religiously immoral and also as detrimental to a person's standing in the community—as many people in the African American community support the view that

homosexuality is taboo, and gay men are viewed as being less than men. They do not describe themselves as gay, as this would contradict their notion of male identity and upset their lives and their family's lives. Instead, personal and social self-preservation requires that they adhere to the cultural norm of heterosexuality. Thus, they fulfill their need for male sexual contact in secret. They justify this behavior by saying it is only an indulgence in male fantasy; it is not a betrayal nor is it hurtful to their wives because they are not sleeping with other women.

Grounded Theory. Essentially, grounded theory is a general methodology for deriving a theory or theories from data systematically gathered and analyzed (Strauss and Corbin, 1994). Grounded theory has been described as a marriage between positivism and interpretivism. First conceptualized as a strategy by two sociologists, Glaser and Strauss (1967), grounded theory is best used for understanding phenomenal processes (Morse, 1994). By processes, we mean that what is being studied or understood is dynamic and may entail stages or phases but may also involve "reciprocal changes in patterns of action-interaction and in relationship with changes of conditions either internal or external to the process itself" (Strauss and Corbin, 1994, p. 278). Because theory development is the main focus of this qualitative strategy, it differs in its central purpose from other qualitative strategies in which meaning and describing are the core purposes. The brilliance of this qualitative approach lies in its logic: explicitly link empirical data to the creation and elaboration of a theory. As you may recall from Chapter Two, we stated that intuition, previous knowledge, or Baconian inductivism were ways in which theory can be developed. Similar in concept to Baconian inductivism, however, the grounded theory approach is a unique and superior way in which theory development should be approached—through research. "A theory is not the formulation of some discovered aspect of a preexisting reality 'out there' . . . rather theories are interpretations made from given perspectives as adopted or researched by researchers" (Strauss and Corbin, 1994, p. 279).

To use grounded theory as your approach you must gather and analyze data in a systematic way, hence grounded theory possesses some features of positivism. The system entails an iterative process sometimes referred to as *constant comparative analysis,* in which data are used first to generate a theory, and then subsequent data are compared against the initial theory. At the beginning of the process, an assumption is made that the initial theory will be provisional; thus, changes and modifications, if necessary, can be made as new data are generated and analyzed, and new patterns and themes emerge. Key to this process is the use of multiple perspectives when gathering and analyzing the data. If you refer back to Table 7.2, note that approximately thirty to fifty participants are recommended when undertaking this approach. Moreover, a distinction should be made when using this approach as to the type of theory that is trying to be developed. *Substantive theory*, which is theory derived from research in one substantive area (for example, short-term and ongoing psychosocial reactions to herpes diagnosis), and *formal theory*, which is a more general theory with broader applications (such as social cognitive theory), are the two overarching categories of theories. The former typically serves as a springboard to the development of the latter. Both types of theories can be developed using grounded theory; however, the approach is better suited to the development of substantive theory. For example, Canales and Geller (2004) conducted a grounded theory study in which they examined mammography decision making across the breast cancer screening continuum: women who consistently got yearly mammograms, women who were inconsistent or failed to get a mammogram, and breast cancer survivors. They were able to develop a theory titled "Moving in Between Mammography," which described the decision-making process and identified several factors that influenced their behavior (Canales and Geller, 2004). Applying a grounded theory strategy to our hypothetical example, we could use this strategy to develop a psychosocial theory that attempted to explain the psychological, psychosocial, and sociocultural factors that influenced the behavior of men on the down low. Using Canales and Geller's theory as inspiration, we could title our theory, "Between Straight and Gay," and potential influencers could be impulsivity, risk-taking, social anxiety, cultural norms, social support, and religiosity.

Ethnoscience. Ethnoscience is a branch of cognitive anthropology, which focuses on the relation between human culture and human thought. Cognitive anthropology strives to understand how people understand and organize their own reality. This branch of anthropology goes beyond studying the behavior of a particular culture by attempting to identify the culturally derived classification systems people use to make sense of their reality. Each person's classification system comprises cognitive categories that provide some order and understanding to life experiences. The main objective of an ethnoscience inquiry is to reliably represent these cognitive categories; that is, reveal a cogent classification system used by people to process and understand behavior, events, emotions, and things—a taxonomy of sorts. Each culture has its own indigenous classification system. Consequently, people from different cultures will have markedly different perceptions of any given set of behavior, events, emotions, or things. Bottorff and others (1998) conducted a qualitative ethnoscience study to examine breast health practices of South Asian women living in Canada. They conducted in-depth interviews with fifty women, which were analyzed and used to develop a taxonomy that represented relationships among emerging cultural themes and domains.

They found that women held four central beliefs regarding breast health practices that ranged from beliefs about taking care of your breasts to beliefs about accessing services.

In our hypothetical example, an ethnoscience study would focus on developing a reliable classification system that the men use to explain their lifestyle. A taxonomy could be developed that would classify men according to their underlying cultural beliefs. An example of this taxonomy could be several domains of beliefs that represented the explanations of their lifestyle choice, such as "cultural taboos against being gay," "homophobia," and "endorsement of the sexual double standard for men that permits promiscuity and adultery."

Qualitative Ethology. Qualitative ethology has its roots in zoology, which is the study of natural animal behavior and falls under the discipline of biology. Typically, ethology involves naturalistic observation designed to ascertain the significance of some naturally occurring behavior and its relationship to the environment. Applying this strategy to humans entails observing them in their natural environment with goals of revealing the cause(s) of the behavior, seeing how the behavior develops, identifying the biological function of the behavior, or determining whether the behavior has evolved. Thus, the ethologist is not interested in the participant's perspective per se. This strategy contrasts with the other qualitative strategies, in which participants' perceptions of events, beliefs, or practices along with their respective meaning are the focus of the inquiry. In qualitative ethology this is not the main emphasis (Blurton Jones and Woodson, 1979, p. 99). This strategy is most useful when the specific behavior of interest can be readily observed in as unobtrusive a way as possible, and also when the behavior is not well-suited to using other self-report methods (such as interviewing).

If we refer to Table 7.3, qualitative ethology is the strategy used to describe patterns of a naturally occurring behavior (in this case, the greeting behaviors of travelers and their families). Instead of in-depth interviews, video and photography of the travelers are the two data-collection modalities used to capture the behavior. In health promotion research, qualitative ethology could be used in clinical settings to characterize interactions between health care providers and their patients (for example, Bottorff and Varcoe, 1995; Solberg and Morse, 1991), to document the interactions between health educators and intervention participants, or to capture certain health-risk behaviors in a field setting (such as drug use or needle sharing). Behaviors of interest to analyze could be communication patterns, both verbal and nonverbal, with an emphasis on how the participant interacts with the particular environment. For example, Morse and Pooler (2002) used qualitative ethology to examine the interactions of patients' family members with the patients and nurses in the trauma room of an emergency department of a hospital. Video was used to film these interactions. Analyzing 192 videotapes, the authors coded the verbal and nonverbal behaviors and were able to categorize these interactions as "families learning to endure, patients failing to endure, family emotionally suffering and patient enduring, patient and family enduring, and resolution of enduring" (Morse and Pooler, 2002, p. 240).

Applying qualitative ethology to men who live on the down low may not be a viable option. Men on the down low are engaging in sexual behavior with other men in secret. Clearly, their behavior would not be open to observation let alone videotaping. Furthermore, it would be difficult to identify a specific setting in which the behavior would naturally occur. Thus, qualitative ethology may not be the best strategy for investigating this type of behavior.

Qualitative Data-Collection Methods for Health Promotion Research

As we have described five main qualitative strategies of inquiry, you may have noted that each strategy was associated with certain data-collection method(s). Primary data-collection methods can include observations and in-depth interviews as well as personal and official documents, photographs, recordings, drawings, e-mails, and informal conversations. For example, in Table 7.2, phenomenology was associated with in-depth conversations, whereas grounded theory used in-depth interviews and observations. Qualitative ethology used video and photography. Thus, the strategy selected by the investigator is connected to a specific method for data collection (Sterk and Elifson, 2004). In this section, we describe and discuss two data-collection methods widely used to conduct qualitative inquiries: interviewing and participant observation.

Interviewing. In general, interviewing can take several different forms that range from unstructured to structured, and may involve interviewing an individual, a dyad, or a group (that is, a focus group). The first form of interviewing we will discuss is considered the least structured and can be thought of more as an informal conversation than a formal interview. When using this method, there are no specific questions asked; rather, topics emerge and flow from the conversation. Of course, the interviewer must prepare a plan to discuss certain general topics related to the research; however, the process is provisional in that certain topics may not get discussed and there is no set order to the discussion (Babbie, 2004). This form of interview is used frequently in phenomenological investigations or other inquiries in which the investigator is interested in understanding the meaning behind participants' experiences, events, practices, or behavior. Thus, it would be difficult to construct specific questions a priori.

The goal of this type of interview is to explore and to probe the interviewee's responses so that an in-depth understanding of the phenomena can be reached. This process places a major emphasis on the details of the interviewee's life experiences and social behavior. The interviewer attempts to engage the interviewee in conversation about the interviewees' attitudes, interests, feelings, concerns, and values as these relate to the research topic. Because this interview is an interaction, meaning is jointly constructed by the interviewer and the interviewee; meaning is rarely revealed as an epiphany by the interviewee, although it may happen! A skilled interviewer allows participants to describe their experiences and explore their thoughts and opinions about the research topic. Because of this dynamic, it is critical that the interviewer try to establish a rapport with the participant and create a sense of trust; however, building trust and establishing a respectful relationship in which the interviewee feels comfortable may be affected by other issues such as gender and race, which may play a role in this process (Fontana and Frey, 1994).

In conducting this type of interview, interviewees should be given a considerable amount of latitude to expand upon the topics because it is they who are "knowledgeable, have a meaningful perspective to offer, and are able to make this explicit in their own words" (Sterk and Elifson, 2004, p. 137). It truly is a conversation taking place between the interviewer, who is an active participant, and the interviewee. Thus, although there is a predetermined topic of interest, the conversation or interview should be viewed as spontaneous and unstructured. A caveat must be stated, however. Even though the interview should be viewed as a conversation, the interviewer must focus on listening to the interviewee. Rather than trying to appear to *be interesting,* the interviewer should *appear interested in* what the interviewee has to say (Babbie, 2004). In fact, Lofland and Lofland (1995) recommend adopting the role of the "socially acceptable incompetent" when interviewing (p. 56).

It is prudent to begin the conversation with less sensitive, benign topics and then gradually ease the conversation toward more sensitive and complex issues. For example, if a researcher were to have a "conversation" with a man who lives on the down low, he or she would want to start the conversation with a discussion of what it is like to be an African American man in today's society, what his experiences were growing up, and what life is like for him in the present. Because this is a highly personal and sensitive topic, it might be best to consider matching the interviewer's gender and race with those of the interviewee (for example, male and African American). This matching may facilitate the establishment of rapport. Then, once trust has been established (this could take from several hours to perhaps several interview sessions over the course of several days), the conversation could be steered toward more sensitive topics such as sexual behavior. During the interview or the conversation, it is also beneficial if the interviewer is cognizant of any responses that would allow for more in-depth probing. Probing takes many forms, but basically entails an effort either verbally or nonverbally on the part of the interviewer to elicit more details, to guide the dialogue, to iterate the meaning of something said by the interviewee, or to allow the interviewee to feel comfortable in preparing his or her response. Probes perform these functions while also allowing the interviewer to establish a relationship with the interviewee and indicate the desire to understand what the interviewee is saying (Fontana and Frey, 1994). For example, the interviewer could ask a directive question such as "Could you tell me more about your thinking on that?" The interviewer could also use the echo probe, in which he or she repeats what the interviewee has just said. This indicates to the interviewee that the interviewer is listening to what they say. The interviewer could also simply use comments such as "uh huh," "I see," "Yes," or "Mm." Nonverbal probes are also effective and include nods of the head or simply remaining silent to give the interviewee time to reflect or prepare their next thought. In any event, the function of the probes is to motivate the participants to communicate more fully and to help them focus on the general topics while keeping the communication flowing.

◆ ◆ ◆

In a Nutshell

Probing takes many forms, but basically entails an effort either verbally or nonverbally on the part of the interviewer to elicit more details, to guide the dialogue, to iterate the meaning of something said by the interviewee, or to allow the interviewee to feel comfortable in preparing his or her response.

◆ ◆ ◆

A more structured type of interview than the unstructured interview is the semistructured interview. This form of interviewing uses a series of open-ended questions that are typically asked of all participants in a predetermined order. The questions are considered directive and are used to ascertain specific topics related to the research. The interviewer should read the question exactly as it is worded to avoid changing the intent of the question in addition to asking all of the questions that apply. Although the interviewer is encouraged to use probes, the probes should be as neutral as possible to avoid introducing bias into the process. For example, if the interviewer asks a question and the participant says, "I don't know," or "I am not sure," one type of neutral probe, called a "clarification probe," that could be used in this instance is, "There are no right or wrong answers to these questions, we are only interested in finding out how you feel about this."

Although there is more structure to this form of interview, the open-ended questions still allow the participant to elaborate and provide significant details on his or her experiences. Thus, this type of interview is well-suited for grounded theory, ethnography, and ethnoscience strategies, when little is known about a certain issue but the research question has a definite direction. For instance, semistructured interviews were used in a study of fourteen Mexican and Mexican American women staying at a battered women's shelter. The study sought to describe the barriers to the women negotiating condom use with their abusive partners. Themes of physical, psychological, and sexual abuse of the women who requested condom use emerged, as did the influence of power and control exerted over their public, private, and sexual interactions (Davila and Brackley, 1999). The semistructured interview guide used in the study is presented in Box 7.5.

When the interviewer interviews a small group of people at the same time, it is termed a focus group. Focus groups typically involve between six and twelve individuals who are a homogeneous group, but who do not usually know each other. Participants should be chosen specifically on the basis of the research topic. For example, if were we to conduct a qualitative inquiry as formative research to designing an HPP to prevent teen alcohol and drug use, we would choose participants for the focus group that were similar in age, gender, and ethnicity to the targeted intervention population. Focus groups involve a small sample that is usually generated using nonprobability techniques such as convenience sampling (see Chapter Eleven). Although the results may not be generalizable, they can still provide very useful information. In contrast to the one-on-one interview, the emphasis of the focus group is not necessarily on each participant's individual experiences, beliefs, and attitudes; rather it is the interaction between participants that is of interest to the investigator.

Focus groups have been used for a very long time in advertising and marketing research, in which researchers have gathered information about new product ideas, name changes to existing products, or customer's opinions about existing products (Brilhart and Galanes, 1998). In health promotion, focus groups are used quite frequently to provide information about interventions, salient health issues, or health care needs; to identify interests, topics, or concerns of the targeted population; or to develop new scale measures. Focus groups can be unstructured, with the moderator—the person facilitating and conducting the focus group—announcing the topic to be discussed and allowing the participants to respond freely. This should entail participants presenting their own views and then also responding to the views expressed by the other group members. Focus groups can

Box 7.5. English and Spanish Semistructured Interview Guide from a Study of Mexican and Mexican American Women

English

1. Tell me what you know about HIV/AIDS?
   A. How do women and men get it?
   B. What does it do to the body?
   C. Is there a vaccine or cure for HIV/AIDS?
2. What can a person do to keep from getting HIV/AIDS?
   A. What do you do to keep from getting HIV/AIDS?
3. In the past three months, what would you say your chance of being infected with HIV/AIDS has been?
4. In the past three months, how have you protected yourself against HIV/AIDS?
   A. For what reasons have you protected yourself?
   B. For what reasons have you not protected yourself?
5. What do you know about condoms?
6. Tell me what you think or know that is good about condoms?
7. Tell me what you think or know that is bad about condoms?
8. Tell me about your first experience with a condom.
9. Tell me about your last experience with a condom.
10. Tell me about your best experience with a condom.
11. Tell me about your worst experience with a condom.
12. Have you ever asked a male partner to use a condom?
    A. When?
    B. Under what circumstances?
    C. How did you ask him?
13. How does your partner respond when you ask him to use a condom?
14. What additional information would you like to discuss or share related to condom use?

Spanish

1. Dígame lo que usted sabe sobre de VIH/Sida?
   A. ¿Cómo las mujeres y los hombres lo cogen?
   B. ¿Qué le hace al cuerpo?
   C. ¿Hay una vacuna o una cura por el?
2. ¿Qué puede hacer una persona para evitar infección de VIH/Sida?
   A. ¿Qué hace usted para evitar infección de VIH/Sida?
3. ¿En los últimos tres meses, qué piensa ira su peligro de ser infectada con VIH/SIDA?
4. ¿En los últimos tres meses, cómo se ha protegido en contra del VIH/Sida?
   A. ¿Cuál son las razones porque se ha protegido?
   B. ¿Cuál son las razones porque no se ha protegido?

5. ¿Dígame lo qué sabe usted de condones?
6. Dígame que piensa o sabe usted de porque condones son buenos.
7. Dígame que piensa o sabe usted de porque condones son malos.
8. Dígame de su primera experiencia con condones.
9. Dígame de su última experiencia con condones.
10. Dígame de su mejor experiencia con condones.
11. Dígame de su peor experiencia con condones.
12. ¿Usted ha preguntado a su compañero que use condones?
    A. ¿Cuándo?
    B. ¿En qué circunstancias?
    C. ¿Cómo le preguntó?
13. ¿Cómo responde su compañero cuando usted le pregunta que use condones?
14. ¿Qué otra información gustara usted discutir con relacio al uso de condones?

Source: Copyright © 1999 from *Issues in Mental Health Nursing* by Davila and Brackley. Reproduced by permission of Taylor & Francis Group, LLC, www.taylorandfrancis.com.

---

also be semistructured, with the moderator using a guide to cover questions and specific topics presented in some order.

Depending on the topic, there are instances in which the group should be stratified by gender, age, or some other relevant characteristic. For example, Cameron and others (2005) conducted four on-line focus groups (similar in structure to a regular focus group, however, on-line focus groups are conducted in a chat room via the Internet) with Internet-using teens to discover their experiences with, exposure to, and perceptions of sexually oriented Websites and sexually explicit Websites. Because of the sensitive nature of the topic, the researchers stratified each group by gender and age to ensure that participants felt comfortable responding to sexually related content, and to ensure that the topics presented were developmentally appropriate.

One advantage of using a group interview as opposed to conducting individual interviews is the group dynamics. People reacting to each other tend to create a synergy that is much greater than what could be created on an individual basis. Thus, the method is synergistic and holds the potential for generating additional topics and information that might otherwise have been missed. Other advantages include its flexibility, low cost, and speedy results (Krueger, 1988). Yet, there are some disadvantages. At times, there may be one group member who tends to dominate the conversation or who may intimidate other group members. This is a difficult situation that must be addressed skillfully by a trained moderator. Clearly, because there is the group dynamic, the moderator has less control of the situation as compared with individual interviews. There is also the issue of confidentiality. The moderator can assure the participants that whatever is discussed "within the group stays within the group," but the same cannot be said for the participants. If the topic is sensitive, then precautions should be taken such as having participants agree to maintain confidentiality in the informed consent form and also agree to explicit protocol guidelines prior to when the focus group begins (Sterk and Elifson, 2004).

Whether the interviews are semistructured or unstructured, or conducted with an individual or with a group, there are some basic issues for the qualitative researcher to consider. For example, how many participants or focus groups should be conducted? Table 7.2 provides some general guidelines for sample size depending on the research question and the strategy; however, most qualitative researchers agree that these are meant as guidelines and should not be used in the same manner as sample size estimation performed in power analyses. Essentially, the number of participants or the number of focus groups is sufficient when the selected participants represent the range of potential participants in the setting, and at the point at which the data gathered begins to be redundant, that is, when consistent themes are repeated. This latter point of data redundancy and repetition is also referred to as data saturation. It is at this point that the investigator should feel confident in knowing that an adequate sample size has been reached or a sufficient number of focus groups has been conducted.

All interviews and focus groups conducted should be audiotaped with the permission of the interviewee(s). Of course, taping, or in some instances, videotaping, interviews does not preclude the interviewer from taking notes during the interview or writing notes after the interview. Once the interview or focus group is completed, the audiotapes can be transcribed "verbatim" to begin the process of data analysis.

Observation. To emphasize the importance of observation as a research method to the overall research enterprise, one need mention only one name—Charles Darwin. His meticulous attention to detail, copious notes, and commitment to extended and lengthy periods of observation resulted in his formalization of a biological theory of evolution with his assertion that natural selection was the main underlying mechanism. Needless to say, the impact of his research on science, society, religion, education, and politics is immeasurable, and his work is considered by many as scientifically revolutionary. Yet interestingly, rather than study his subjects under controlled settings using manipulation and randomization, Darwin's research method was naturalistic observation. Thus, observation as a scientific method has great utility. In addition to generating new theories, observation can be used to supplement other data-collection methods, such as interviews, to provide an expanded understanding of some phenomenon or to provide "insight into the social context in which people operate" (Sterk and Elifson, 2004, p. 142).

Participant observation is a specific type of naturalistic observation in which the researcher enters the world of the people he or she wants to study. In order to do this, however, the investigator must first identify an appropriate setting and then gain access to that setting. Whether the setting is public or private, there typically is some *gatekeeper*, a person who has the power and authority to control access, with whom the investigator should negotiate to gain access. For public settings, identifying a gatekeeper may be more difficult, or one may not exist. The investigator must also consider the ethics of observing people who are in the public realm without their informed consent. For example, how would you feel if you were out at a coffee shop or at a bar with your friends and you happen to notice a person sitting off in the corner taking notes and watching what you and your friends did? We are not contending that observing people in a public setting is unethical or wrong. In fact, many sociological and anthropological studies of public settings have been conducted in this way (for example, Lofland, 1973; McCoy and others, 1996; Monaghan, 2002; Tewksbury, 2002); however, there are other important issues to consider, and these issues must be weighed against the importance of the research and the balance of ethics and methodological rigor. For example, the investigator must decide what role he or she will adopt when making observations and whether or not to be covert or overt. Gold (1958) outlined four potential roles moving from the more involved and covert to complete detachment and overt.

The first role is that of *the complete participant,* with the researcher allowing the people under study to see him or her as a participant, not as a researcher. Thus, it is considered covert because participants in the setting do not realize this person is researching them. Acting in the role of a participant may also raise methodological problems because the investigator interacts with the participants, which may have an effect on the dynamics of the setting, the participants' behavior, or both. Because of these considerations (ethical and scientific), the decision to adopt the role of the complete participant should be well-justified. In other instances, it may be practical to adopt the second role, that of the *participant as observer.* In the participant-as-observer role, the investigator is overt, in that he or she identifies as a researcher while interacting with the participants in the social process. Thus, this role avoids some of the ethical issues in the complete participant role, but some of the methodological issues remain (for instance, observer effects). The advantage of both roles is they provide a unique insider's perspective that assists in the interpretation of what is being observed.

The third role is that of the *observer as participant,* in which the investigator's main role is that of the observer. She or he identifies as a researcher, but enters

MINCUS AND DINCUS AS "COMPLETE PARTICIPANTS" FOR THEIR CHICKEN STUDY.

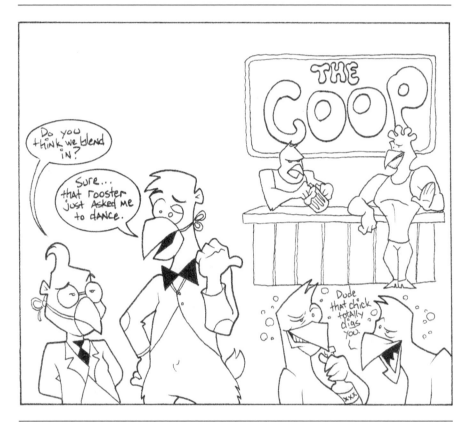

Copyright 2005 by Justin Wagner; reprinted with permission.

the setting periodically and for brief periods of time to conduct the observations. In this role, the ethical issues are rectified; however, because of the higher level of detachment than the first two roles and the lack of involvement in the setting and with the participants, it may be more difficult to garner the perspective of the participants and provide accurate interpretation to the observations. Finally, the fourth role is that of the *complete observer*, in which the researcher observes the social process without ever becoming a part of it. Within this role, there is some variation in the level of detachment. Observations can be made directly by researchers as they passively observe the setting, or there are some instances when researchers may remain completely outside of the setting. In this instance, they may opt to use equipment such as video recorders to make the observations. This role is more along the lines of an "objective" researcher, with ethical issues and observer effects minimized; however, the researcher does not have the benefit of understanding what is going on from the perspective of an insider. Thus, he or she may not interpret the findings in a way that captures accurately the participants' perspectives. Thus, the complete-observer role is more suited to qualitative ethology, in which the participants' perspectives are not the main focus of the inquiry.

Once the researcher has identified the setting, gained access, and worked through the issues of what role to adopt, it is now time to begin observing. How, what, and when you record your observations depend on the nature of the study, whether or not there is freedom to take notes as the observations are being made, and the stage of the research process. Note taking is generally the mode used to record observations. The process of note taking can require some level of expertise and may be approached systematically. In the initial stage of the research process, observations should be more broad and descriptive. These initial observations serve as a guide to identify the key aspects of the setting, people, and behaviors that are of interest. This may involve unstructured note taking in a free form, with the researcher trying to hone in on the most relevant aspects of what is going on and record not only the actual observation but also his or her interpretation of the observation (Babbie, 2004). As the research progresses, the investigator may begin to narrow the focus and record observations of fewer people, interactions, events, times, or processes, but with more detail and elaboration (Adler and Adler, 1994). You may want to try and create a list of key words and participants based on your initial observations, and then use this list to organize and outline your subsequent observations. At this point, field notes should be descriptive as well as reflective about what one has seen, heard, experienced, and thought about during an observation session. You may want to leave wide margins on the page for interpretations or for noting your personal impressions of the event. We cannot emphasize enough the importance of detail when generating field notes. Notes should include at a minimum the date, site, time, and topic. Notes can also include diagrams of setting layout in addition to other pertinent context. To facilitate the process, some researchers create a more structured guide. For example, you could create a form beforehand that allows the recording of essential information regarding participants' characteristics, and their roles, appearances, and interactions.

In addition to knowing how and what to record, the qualitative researcher should be aware of *when* to record. In his study of gay men attending bathhouses, Tewksbury (2002) adopted the role of complete participant. He "entered and spent several hours in the bathhouse, circulated with and among patrons, and carefully observed others, their activities, movements, interactions and the use of the physical features of the environment. Field notes were written during periodic re-treats (usually every 10 to 15 minutes) to one of the private rooms available for rent to patrons" (pp. 84–85). Although it is recommended to take field notes while observing, in this instance because of his covert role, Tewksbury was not at liberty to take field notes while he was observing. Moreover, even if it is possible to take notes while the events are occurring, it may not be feasible to observe everything let alone record everything. To solve this problem, Spradley (1979) recommends using an approach that entails first making a condensed account of what occurs while it is occurring, followed-up with an expanded account in which the researcher fills in the details that were not recorded on the spot. This approach ensures that relevant observations are not missed because of note taking. In addition, Spradley asserted that his "ability to recall events and conversations increased rapidly through the discipline of creating expanded accounts from condensed ones" (p. 75).

Many qualitative researchers also suggest maintaining a fieldwork journal that records feelings, reactions, ideas, fears, and problems that arose during the course of the study. This journal will assist later on in the data analysis and may become an important data source (Spradley, 1979). This process for recording thoughts and ideas is sometimes referred to as "memoing" and can provide a picture of how the study evolved.

Similar to conducting interviews, field notes should be transcribed verbatim on a regular basis. Transcribing the field notes allows the researcher to begin the process of identifying preliminary themes and helps pinpoint the right time to end the study. As was the case with interview data, ending the study should occur at the point of data saturation, when later themes and patterns are consistent with earlier findings and no new themes have emerged.

Qualitative Data Analysis

It is beyond the scope of this chapter to provide an in-depth discussion of qual-itative data analysis. Many texts have been written on the subject and should be consulted (for example, Lofland and Lofland, 1995; Miles and Huberman, 1984, 1994). Yet in this section we thought it would be beneficial to provide a cur-sory overview of the process because the best way to learn how to do qualita-tive data analysis is to actually do it. We realize that the first time it may seem like a formidable task because the data are voluminous and initially unorganized. Therefore, we provide some basic steps for data management and analysis which the novice investigator can draw upon to perform a reasonable qualitative data analysis.

Before data analysis can begin, the data must be processed. This entails revising, deciphering, and editing field notes, and then transcribing notes and audiotaped interviews. Hopefully, this process has been ongoing during the data-collection period. Once all the data have been processed, the first step in analysis is to try to sort the data and impose some type of organization. This process should also be ongoing. You would not want to wait until all data have been collected to begin the process of organization; rather, it should occur parallel to data collection. Some researchers organize their data first by type (for example, interviews, field notes, archival records) and then within each type, an additional sort is done by question, date, people, or places.

Once a system has been created, the next step is to become familiar with the data by reading through it and, if available, reading memos or research journal entries. This will help to identify main concepts or themes and to assist in providing detailed descriptions of the setting, participants, and other activities relevant to the research methods. In addition, researchers may want to continue the method of memoing to record their analytical decisions made and insights into the analysis.

The next step is to create a basic coding scheme. Coding especially in the context of using the grounded theory approach is a multifaceted process. We will consider for the sake of space only three of the main processes: *open coding*, *axial coding*, and *selective coding* (Strauss and Corbin, 1990). Initially one does open coding, in which the data are considered in detail while developing some initial categories. This is the process whereby qualitative data are first categorized. Codes can be descriptive words or short phrases that are attached to units of data (such as a word, a sentence, or a paragraph) and that represent a core concept, central category, or theme. For example, in their study of gay men's acceptance of a hypothetical AIDS vaccine, one of the codes in the researchers' codebook was "sides," and it signified the side effects from taking the vaccine (Salazar, Holtgrave, Crosby, Frew, and Peterson, 2005). A codebook is a complete description of every code used. For each code you must define what the code means and how it relates to your research.

Coding the data is a relatively simple task. As you read through the data, you systematically code with respect to the core concepts in your codebook. You can underline or highlight the units of data that apply to a particular code while placing the assigned code in the margin (Sandelowski, 1995). This is coding by hand. It is important to note that there are myriad qualitative software packages available to facilitate the entire data-analysis process if desired (for example, QSR NUD*IST, Atlas/Ti, or Ethnograph). Keep in mind that as you develop your codebook and code your data, this is an iterative process in which you may add new codes the deeper you delve into the data, while old codes may be removed.

Later, if using the grounded theory strategy, the next process is axial coding, in which data are put together in new ways. The basic premise is to develop a system of coding that seeks to identify causal relationships *between* categories and reveal connections between categories and subcategories. Thus, axial coding serves to begin the process of developing the theoretical framework underpinning your analysis. Finally, selective coding involves the process of selecting and identifying the core category and systematically relating it to other categories. These relationships eventually are integrated and form the basic theoretical structure. This process is about synthesis and interpretation of the meanings. To aid in this process, it is recommended that data displays be used. Displays of the data entail diagrams, any graphics that are useful, concept maps, or simple cartoons that can act as summarizing devices.

The last step in this process is writing your results. This involves describing in detail the central or core categories using direct quotes from the data to illustrate and support. The challenge is to create an engaging narrative that reveals the underlying meaning to the phenomena under study and tells a story. You should also consider using tables and figures. The ultimate objective is to allow the reader to draw similar conclusions based on what has been presented.

◆ ◆ ◆

In a Nutshell

The challenge is to create an engaging narrative that reveals the underlying meaning to the phenomena under study and tells a story.

◆ ◆ ◆

Integration with the Research Process

Ostensibly, qualitative research does not seem to fit with the overall research process as presented in Figure 1.2; however, with some modification to the existing steps, we can propose a process that illustrates a qualitative mode of inquiry. For example, for step 1, imagine the priority population of low-income rural Americans at risk of diabetes. For step 2, imagine that you want to know what having diabetes means to this population or what the psychological and sociocultural processes associated with developing diabetes are. You would then determine that the research would be observational (step 3) and, in fact, naturalistic, as you would want to interview and observe people in their rural setting. Instead of selecting the most parsimonious research design (step 4) as described in Chapter Four, you would want to consider which qualitative strategy (such as phenomenology, grounded theory, and so on) would best serve the research goals. As you approach step 5, you will note that there is not a selection of variables per se; rather, you select the data-collection method, such as observing or interviewing, that can best capture the phenomena under study. To identify and recruit participants into your study (step 6), your sampling techniques are typically limited to nonprobability sampling, such as purposive, snowball, and convenience. The final steps (7 through 9) are similar except that steps 8 and 9 are iterative rather than occurring sequentially.

Summary

This chapter is unique because it is the only chapter in this book that adopts the interpretivist perspective, which should be viewed with great importance and relevance to health promotion research and practice. Qualitative research can address research questions that cannot be addressed by quantitative approaches. Because it is contextual it provides a more thorough understanding of the phenomena that may be missed with a quantitative strategy. Furthermore, one of qualitative research's greatest strengths is that it can be used to generate testable hypotheses, theories, or both. Qualitative research encompasses varying strategies, uses multiple methods (in other words, triangulation), and involves data-collection methods that are integrated with the setting and the researcher. Qualitative data are descriptive and comprise text and images; thus, data analysis cannot be performed using standardized procedures and techniques; rather, the analysis is iterative, subjective, and subject to the researchers' professional intuition and views. Like quantitative research, although there is no manipulation, the nature of qualitative research may still necessitate attention to certain ethical issues. Contrary to what some may believe (qualitative research is "easier" than quantitative research), qualitative research involves a personal commitment and voluminous amounts of data; thus, qualitative research may not be for the faint of heart. Nevertheless, qualitative research has contributed to the overall research enterprise in substantive ways and will continue to do so. Therefore, we recommend highly that you take your next trip by train and see for yourself!

Issues to Consider

1. One of the roles qualitative researchers can adopt when doing field research is that of the complete participant. This role requires that the researcher's goals remain covert. Thus, people involved are not aware that they are being

studied. What if the goal of the research is to reveal, for example, the heterosexual practices of men who frequent nightclubs and bars. What are the ethics involved when a researcher who in the course of the study has sex with female patrons?

2. For the most part, in addition to the relatively small sample sizes, qualitative research uses nonprobability sampling techniques such as snowball sampling, convenience sampling, and so on to recruit participants. Thus, qualitative research is not generalizable; however, there are many quantitative studies that employ nonprobability sampling techniques. Because these studies use data that are quantitative and perform statistical analyses, are they considered more generalizable than qualitative research?

3. As indicated in this chapter, qualitative research is very useful as a formative research to the development and implementation of HPPs, and as a follow-up or adjunct to program evaluations; however, there is a paucity of these types of published studies. Why might this be true? If the HPP showed no significant effects quantitatively, should this be the end of the road research-wise for this program?

For Practice and Discussion

1. Working with a colleague, formulate a research question that lends itself to a qualitative approach. Next, you and your colleague find another pair of colleagues that can perform the same exercise. Then give this other pair of colleagues your research question and ask them to select the most appropriate qualitative strategy conducive to answering the question, and identify the best data-collection technique(s). Have them provide a rationale for why they chose the particular strategy and methods. In turn, you and your colleague should do the same for their research question. Compare and discuss the outcomes.

2. Ask five other students if they would participate in a phenomenological investigation. You could ask them what health promotion *means* to them. Try to take notes of the conversations you have with them and identify any main themes that emerge from these conversations.

3. Visit several venues in your community, such as a local coffee shop, a public health clinic, a courtroom, or a nightclub, and observe for a couple of hours. Your goal is to conduct a qualitative ethology. If possible, record notes while you observe. Try to determine whether people in the venue are exhibiting a pattern of behavior. You may want to create a form beforehand to assist with your observations.

References

Adler, P. A., and Adler, P. (1994). Observational techniques. In N. K. Denzin and J. S. Lincoln (Eds.), *Handbook of qualitative research* (pp. 377–392). Thousand Oaks, CA: Sage.

Babbie, E. R. (2004). *The practice of social research* (10th ed.). Belmont, CA: Wadsworth.

Barofsky, I., and Sugarbaker, P. H. (1979). Determinants of patient nonparticipation in randomized clinical trials for the treatment of sarcomas. *Cancer Clinical Trials, 2,* 237–246.

Blurton Jones, N. G., and Woodson, R. H. (1979). Describing behavior: The ethologist's perspective. In L. Lamb, S. Suomi, and G. Stephenson (Eds.), *The study of social interaction: Methodological issues* (pp. 97–118). Madison, WI: University of Wisconsin Press.

Bogdan, R. C., and Biklen, S. K. (1998). *Qualitative research in education: An introduction to theory and methods* (3rd ed.). Boston: Allyn and Bacon.

Bottorff, J. L., and Varcoe, C. (1995). Transitions in nurse-patient interactions: A qualitative ethology. *Qualitative Health Research, 5*(3), 315–331.

Bottorff, J. L., and others. (1998). Beliefs related to breast health practices: The perceptions of South Asian women living in Canada. *Social Science & Medicine, 47*(12), 2075–2085.

Brilhart, J. K., and Galanes, G. J. (1998). *Effective group discussion* (9th ed.). Boston: McGraw-Hill.

Cameron, K. A., and others. (2005). Adolescents' experience with sex on the Web: Results from online focus groups. *Journal of Adolescence, 28,* 535–540.

Canales, M. K., and Geller, B. M. (2004). Moving in between mammography: Screening decisions of American Indian women in Vermont. *Qualitative Health Research, 14*(6), 836–857.

Centers for Disease Control and Prevention. (2005). *HIV/AIDS among African Americans.* CDC fact sheet. Retrieved March 30, 2005, from www.cdc.gov/hiv/pubs/facts/afam.htm.

Colangelo, L., Domel, R., Kelly, L., Peirce, L., and Sullivan, C. (1999). *Positivist and interpretivist schools: A comparison and contrast.* Retrieved February 16, 2005, from www.edb.utexas.edu/faculty/scheurich/proj2/index.htm

Davila, Y. R., and Brackley, M. H. (1999). Mexican and Mexican American women in a battered women's shelter: Barriers to condom negotiation for HIV/AIDS prevention. *Issues in Mental Health Nursing, 20*(4), 333–355.

Denzin, N. K. (1978). *The research act: A theoretical introduction to sociological methods* (2nd ed.). New York: McGraw-Hill.

Featherstone, K., and Donovan, L. (1998). Random allocation or allocation at random? Patients' perspectives of participation in a randomized controlled trial. *British Medical Journal, 317,* 1177–1180.

Ferguson, P. R. (2002). Patients' perceptions of information provided in clinical trials. *Journal of Medical Ethics, 28,* 45–48.

Fontana, A., and Frey, J. H. (1994). Interviewing: The art of science. In N. K. Denzin and J. S. Lincoln (Eds.), *Handbook of qualitative research* (pp. 361–376). Thousand Oaks, CA: Sage.

Fraser, J. (1997). Methadone clinic culture: The everyday realities of female methadone clients. *Qualitative Health Research, 7*(1), 121–139.

Glaser, B. G., and Strauss, A. L. (1967). *The discovery of grounded theory: Strategies for qualitative research.* Chicago: Aldine.

Glesne, C., and Peshkin, A. (1992). *Becoming qualitative researchers: An introduction.* White Plains, NY: Longman.

Gold, R. L. (1958). Roles in sociological field observations. *Social Forces, 36,* 217–223.

Grant, C.H.I., Cissna, K. N., and Rosenfeld, L. B. (2000). Patients' perceptions of physicians communication and outcomes of the accrual to trial process. *Health Communication, 12*(1), 23–29.

Holstein, J. A., and Gubrium, J. F. (1994). Phenomenology, ethnomethodology, and interpretive practice. In N. K. Denzin and J. S. Lincoln (Eds.), *Handbook of qualitative research* (pp. 262–272). Thousand Oaks, CA: Sage.

Johnson, J. L., Kalaw, C., Lovato, C. Y., Baillie, L., and Chambers, N. A. (2004). Crossing the line: Adolescents' experiences of controlling their tobacco use. *Qualitative Health Research, 14*(9), 1276–1291.

Krueger, R. A. (1988). *Focus groups: A practical guide for applied research.* Newbury Park, CA: Sage.

Kuhn, T. (1970). *The structure of scientific revolutions* (2nd ed.). Chicago: University of Chicago Press.

Lofland, J., and Lofland, L. (1995). *Analyzing social settings* (3rd ed.). Belmont, CA: Wadsworth.

Lofland, L. (1973). *A world of strangers.* New York: Basic Books.

McCoy, C. B., and others. (1996). Sex, drugs, and the spread of HIV/AIDS in Belle Glade, Florida. *Medical Anthropology Quarterly (New Series), 10*(1), 83–93.

Melville, J., and others. (2003). Psychosocial impact of serological diagnosis of herpes simplex virus type 2: A qualitative assessment. *Sexually Transmitted Infections, 79,* 280–285.

Miles, M. B., and Huberman, A. M. (1984). *Qualitative data analysis: A sourcebook of new methods.* Thousand Oaks, CA: Sage.

Miles, M. B., and Huberman, A. M. (1994). *Qualitative data analysis: An expanded source book* (2nd ed.). Thousand Oaks, CA: Sage.

Miller-García, T. D. (2004). *Gender, power, and the meaning of condom use: A qualitative assessment of condom use among Latino couples.* Unpublished master's thesis, Rollins School of Public Health, Emory University, Atlanta.

Monaghan, L. F. (2002). Opportunity, pleasure, and risk: An ethnography of urban males heterosexualities. *Journal of Contemporary Ethnography, 31*(4), 440–477.

Moore, L. W. (2000). Severe visual impairment in older women. *Western Journal of Nursing Research, 22*(5), 571–595.

Morse, J. (1994). Designing funded qualitative research. In N. K. Denzin and J. S. Lincoln (Eds.), *Handbook of qualitative research* (pp. 220–235). Thousand Oaks, CA: Sage.

Morse, J. M., and Pooler, C. (2002). Patient-family-nurse interactions in the trauma-resuscitation room. *American Journal of Critical Care, 11*(3), 240–249.

Nakkash, R., and others. (2003). The development of a feasible community-specific cardio-vascular disease prevention program: Triangulation of methods and sources. *Health Education and Behavior, 30*(6), 723–739.

Peacock, J. L. (1986). *The anthropological lens: Harsh light, soft focus.* New York: Cambridge University Press.

Reisinger, H. S. (2004). Counting apples as oranges: Epidemiology and ethnography in adolescent substance abuse treatment. *Qualitative Health Research, 14*(2), 241–258.

Richardson, M. A., Post-White, J., Singletary, S. E., and Justice, B. (1998). Recruitment for complementary/alternative medicine trials: Who participates after breast cancer. *Annals of Behavioral Medicine, 20*(3), 190–198.

Roberts, F. (2002). Qualitative differences among cancer clinical trial explanations. *Social Science and Medicine, 55,* 1947–1955.

Salazar, L. F., Holtgrave, D., Crosby, R. A. Frew, P., and Peterson, J. L. (2005). Issues related to gay and bisexual men's acceptance of a future AIDS vaccine. *International Journal of STDs and HIV, 16*(8), 546–548.

Sandelowski, M. (1995). Qualitative analysis: What it is and how to begin. *Research in Nursing and Health, 18*, 371–375.

Solberg, S., and Morse, J. M. (1991). The comforting behaviors of caregivers toward distressed postoperative neonates. *Issues in Comprehensive Pediatric Nursing, 14*(2), 77–92.

Spradley, J. P. (1979). *The ethnographic interview.* Orlando: Harcourt Brace Jovanovich.

Steckler, A., and Linnan, L. (Eds). (2002). *Process evaluation for public health interventions and research.* San Francisco: Jossey-Bass.

Sterk, C., and Elifson, K. (2004). Qualitative methods in community-based research. In D. Blumenthal and R. DiClemente (Eds.), *Community-based research: Issues and methods* (pp.133–151). New York: Springer.

Strauss, A. L., and Corbin, J. (1990). *Basics of qualitative research: Grounded theory procedures and techniques.* Thousand Oaks, CA: Sage.

Strauss, A., and Corbin, J. (1994). Grounded theory methodology: An overview. In N. K. Denzin and J. S. Lincoln (Eds.), *Handbook of qualitative research* (pp. 273–285). Thousand Oaks, CA: Sage.

Tewksbury, R. (2002). Bathhouse intercourse: Structural and behavioral aspects of an erotic oasis. *Deviant Behavior, 23*(1), 75–112.

Yoo, S., Johnson, C. C., Rice, J., and Manuel, P. (2004). A qualitative evaluation of the Students of Service (SOS) program for sexual abstinence in Louisiana. *Journal of School Health, 74*(8), 329–334.

Yu-Jen, C., Yiing-Mei, L., Shuh-Jen, S., and Mei-Yen, C. (2004). Unbearable weight: Young adult women's experiences of being overweight. *Journal of Nursing Research: JNR, 12*(2), 153–160.

CHAPTER EIGHT

PROGRAM EVALUATION

Nancy Thompson, Michelle C. Kegler, and David R. Holtgrave

Evaluation uses social science research methods to determine whether programs or parts of programs are sufficient, appropriate, effective, and efficient. Evaluation also generates information about how to improve programs that do not meet these criteria. If a program has unexpected benefits or creates unforeseen problems, evaluation will let us know about this as well (Deniston and Rosenstock, 1970; Thompson and McClintock, 1998). In short, evaluation provides information to serve a variety of purposes:

- Finding out whether proposed program materials are suitable for the people who are to receive them
- Learning whether program plans are feasible before they are put into effect
- Ensuring that a program is conducted as it was designed

- Serving as an early warning system for problems that could become serious if unattended
- Monitoring whether a program or activity is producing the desired results
- Demonstrating whether a program has any unexpected benefits or problems
- Providing program managers with the information needed to improve service
- Monitoring progress toward the program's goals
- Producing data on which to base future programs
- Demonstrating the effectiveness of the program to the target population, the public, those who want to conduct similar programs, and those who are providing the funding [adapted from Tobacco Technical Assistance Consortium, 2005]

There are also indirect benefits that may result from formally evaluating a program. One is that program staff have the opportunity to hear from the people they are trying to serve. In turn, this lets the program participants know that they have a voice in the running of the program, and that the program personnel respect what they have to say. It conveys the message that the program is not being imposed upon them. Evaluation can also improve staff morale by providing evidence either that their efforts have been fruitful, or that leadership is aware of problems and taking appropriate steps. Staff also get to hear the good news about the program in the words of the people served. A third indirect benefit is that the results can demonstrate such an effect that the media may develop an interest, further promoting the program (Thompson and McClintock, 1998).

Evaluation differs from research in that its primary purpose is to provide information to decision makers to help them make judgments about the effectiveness of a program and to help them make improvements to a program. Evaluations are typically guided by the needs of key stakeholder groups and designed in a way that is sensitive to the dynamic and political organizational settings in which programs exist. More so than with pure research, evaluation methods must balance scientific rigor with the need to produce meaningful findings in a timely manner in a way that is minimally disruptive to program operations.

Illustration of Key Concepts

Numerous texts have been written on evaluation (for example, Rossi, Lipsey, and Freeman, 2004; Patton, 1997; Weiss, 1997). This section draws from these foundational sources, as well as from commonly accepted wisdom in the field, to highlight some of the major concepts and issues in evaluation. Topics covered in this section include planning for evaluation, stakeholders, target population, description of the program, logic models, formative evaluation, process evaluation, outcome evaluation, economic evaluation, and evaluation reports.

Evaluation Planning

A frequent error made in developing a program is to add an evaluation after the fact. Evaluation should begin while the program is being created, in fact, as soon as someone has the idea for a program. Once begun, it should continue through the duration of the program, only ending once a final assessment has measured the extent to which the program met its intended goals. The following scenario describes why it is important to start the evaluation process so early. Suppose a health promotion practitioner created a program to provide free bicycle helmets to youths from low-income neighborhoods. To initiate the program, program staff placed posters in grocery stores and flyers in mailboxes throughout the neighborhoods they hoped to reach. The posters invited youths to come to the program location for a free bicycle helmet. Some youths responded but not as many as had been expected. So, to determine why the numbers were low, the health promotion practitioner decided to evaluate. The staff may learn that youths in the area are in after-school programs during the hours the program is open. They may learn that it is the parents who are most interested in seeing that their children obtained a helmet, but that their messages targeted the youths. They may learn that the location is too far for the youths to travel alone. So the staff now need to rewrite the posters and flyers, change the hours, or move the location. Had the health practitioner assessed interest and access to the location before the program began, it would have saved time, money, and the disappointment and frustration of the program staff.

During the course of running the program, any public health program should produce most of the information needed to evaluate its effectiveness in achieving its goals and objectives. Thus, evaluation activities can and should be integrated into the design and operation of the program. If this happens, then evaluation may require little more than analyzing the information collected throughout the operation of the program.

◆ ◆ ◆

In a Nutshell

Evaluation activities can and should be integrated into the design and operation of the program.

◆ ◆ ◆

Failure to evaluate a public health program can be considered irresponsible, and perhaps unethical. Why? It is evaluation that allows us to determine whether a program benefits or harms the people it is designed to serve. We do not use medications that are untested, and we should not use educational, behavioral, or social interventions that have not been tested either. Ineffective programs can discourage people from behavior change, and insensitive programs can build public resentment, causing people to resist future, more effective, interventions (Thompson and McClintock, 1998).

Let's look at another example. Suppose the staff of an injury prevention program invited a fifty-five-year-old with an automobile-acquired spinal cord injury to talk to students about the hazards of driving above the speed limit. The staff hoped that this person's story about speeding at age sixteen, and the subsequent adverse health effects he suffered, would discourage the students from driving above the speed limit. Evaluation might show, however, that many teenagers do not relate to the problems of people over age thirty and are not influenced by what they have to say. Evaluation could also show what type of people the students would listen to—perhaps sports stars or other young people (their peers) who have had difficulty finding a job because of their driving history. It can be nonproductive, and even counterproductive when the wrong person delivers a message, no matter how good the message is.

Budgeting for evaluation is an important part of the planning. The cost of evaluation varies. Operating a program with a design that includes a comparison group or multiple repeated assessments over time is more expensive than operating a service program only, but evaluation should be built into the program design and included in the cost of the program (Thompson and McClintock, 1998). What is more, programs with comparison groups or repeated measures (see Chapter Four for more detail) are better able to demonstrate whether the program is producing the intended result. Typically, programs with good evaluation components have the greatest likelihood of receiving funding. Figure 8.1 presents a listing of some costs that are commonly encountered when conducting an evaluation.

FIGURE 8.1.   COMMON EVALUATION-RELATED COSTS.

Some costs commonly encountered in an evaluation:

- Flyers, press releases, or other recruitment materials
- Meeting or interview space
- Telephone costs for scheduling or conducting interviews or focus groups
- Purchasing, copying, or printing of data collection instruments or questionnaires
- Recording devices
- Audiotapes or videotapes
- Participant or interviewer transportation
- Mailing
- Incentives for participants
- Transcriptionists for taped material
- Computer(s)
- Data entry personnel
- Statistical consultant
- Printing or copying of final report

Source: Adapted from Tobacco Technical Assistance Consortium, 2005.

Stakeholders

One of the first steps in conducting an evaluation is to identify and engage stakeholders in the planning process. Stakeholders include all persons who have an interest in the program being evaluated, the conduct of the evaluation, and the evaluation findings. Stakeholders include program participants; program staff and volunteers; those providing funding to the program or the evaluation; those providing other resources, such as space, for the program; and evaluation personnel. Depending on the program, the stakeholders may also include parents or family members of participants, or all community members, whether or not they participated in the program. Involving major stakeholders in the process of evaluation planning, execution, and analysis ensures that the evaluation results will have value. It also helps to ensure that the results of the evaluation will be used to improve the program.

◆ ◆ ◆

In a Nutshell

Involving major stakeholders in the process of evaluation planning, execution, and analysis ensures that the evaluation results will have value.

◆ ◆ ◆

Describing the Program

Another early step in the evaluation process is to develop a thorough understanding of the program to be evaluated. Key elements include the target population, need for the program, goals and objectives, program components and activities, underlying logic, resources, stage of development, and program context (Centers for Disease Control and Prevention, 1999).

Target Population. The target population is the group the program is intended to serve. The more clearly this population has been defined, the easier it will be to determine whether the population has been reached and whether the program was effective for these people. As a part of evaluation planning, it is important to determine whether the program intended to reach all people in the county, for example, or only those persons who currently use the services of the county health department, or only males between the ages of eighteen and fifty who use the services of the county health department. How you can best reach each of these groups will vary.

Logic Models. An important part of describing a program is to understand the logic underlying it. The evaluation should identify the program's ultimate goal(s) and enumerate clearly the program's activities and how they are expected to lead to the goal. Putting this information together with sufficient detail to be of value can be a difficult task. A logic model is a tool that is designed to help you with this process. A logic model provides a graphic representation of the relationships among three aspects of the program: the resources put into the program, the program activities, and the results.

The five parts of a logic model are

- Inputs
- Activities
- Outputs
- Outcomes
- Impact (Goals)

Figure 8.2 depicts what a logic model should look like. Inputs are the resources that the program must have in order to conduct the program's activities. These include funding, personnel (staff as well as volunteers), equipment, supplies, and space. They also include collaborations with other organizations and people whose interests are consistent with those of the program. Planning, too, is an input that is required in order to conduct program activities.

Activities are the actual events that take place when the program is occurring (Tobacco Technical Assistance Consortium, 2005), or constitute the program itself. Some activities include the educational program, distributing condoms or smoke alarms, or holding support groups. But activities can also include inviting collaborators to a meeting, sending letters to supporters, building relationships with communities to be served, gathering materials for a resource center, maintaining an inventory of resources, responding to telephone inquiries, and disseminating information to interested parties.

Outputs are measures that can be used to demonstrate that the program was conducted as planned, and reveal the *process* the program goes through to achieve its outcomes. These include indicators such as the number of training sessions

FIGURE 8.2.   BASIC LOGIC MODEL COMPONENTS.

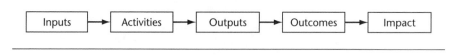

FIGURE 8.3. ABBREVIATED PROGRAM LOGIC MODEL.

Inputs	Activities	Outputs	Outcomes		Impact
			Short-term	Long-term	
Staff	Coalition meetings	Groups attending	Policies adopted	Decrease in smoking	Decrease in tobacco-related cancer
Volunteers	Meetings with legislators	Meetings attended			
Computers		Legislators met with			

held or the number of collaborators in attendance at a meeting. In contrast, outcomes are measures that can be used to demonstrate that program participants *received* what you put out there. Outcomes would include indicators such as an increase in knowledge or changes in attitudes or behavior. In the case of tobacco use prevention programs, outcomes could include an increase in the belief that smoking is dangerous, and a decrease in the rate of smoking.

The impact of a program is the measure of whether or not the overall program goal was achieved and is usually long-term in nature. For health programs, this is usually a measure of decreases in morbidity and mortality. In our smoking example, the program's impact could be a decrease in new cases of lung cancer or deaths from this disease. It could also be a decrease in overall smoking-related mortality, including both cancer and heart disease.

A logic model can be developed for an entire program or for one of its parts, such as a particular activity. Figure 8.3 presents an example of an abbreviated logic model for a program to reduce tobacco-related cancer. Figure 8.4 presents an example of a more detailed logic model for the process portion of a cardiovascular disease prevention program designed to reduce disparities in exercise behavior.

Types of Evaluation

Several typologies exist for the different kinds of evaluations. A common distinction is that between summative and formative. Rossi and colleagues (2004) define summative evaluation as "evaluation activities undertaken to render a summary judgment on certain critical aspects of the program's performance, for instance, to determine if specific goals and objectives were met" (p. 65). They define formative evaluation as "evaluative activities undertaken to furnish information

FIGURE 8.4. LOGIC MODEL WITH DETAILED INPUTS, ACTIVITIES, AND OUTPUTS.

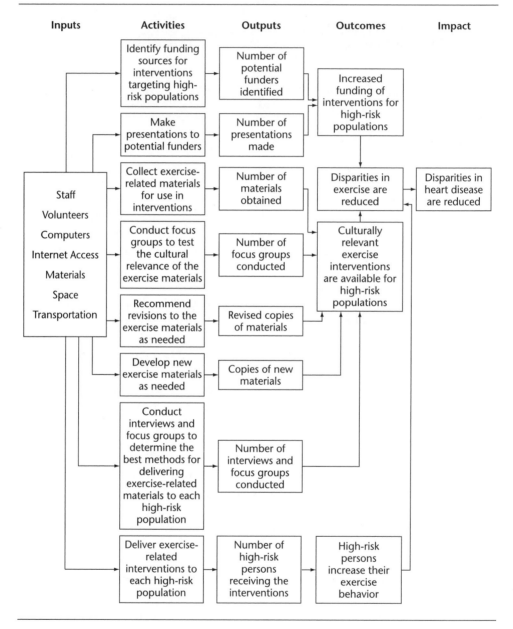

that will guide program improvement" (p. 63). In public health and health promotion, four types of evaluation are widely recognized: formative, process, outcome, and economic. Each of these is described here.

Formative Evaluation. The purpose of formative evaluation is to determine that an element of the program (for example, materials, message, and location) is feasible, appropriate, meaningful, and acceptable to the program's target population (Tobacco Technical Assistance Consortium, 2005). In other words, it tends to focus on the inputs and activities of the program. When we discuss program plans, messages, materials, or strategies with members of the target population before they are put into use, we are conducting formative evaluation. Formative evaluation should be conducted when program materials, messages, and procedures are being developed, before the program begins. It should also be conducted when changes are made, such as revising the materials, adapting the program to a new population or setting, or attempting to resolve problems that occurred with prior materials or procedures.

The methods used in formative evaluation can be qualitative or quantitative. For example, suppose you were working with a program designed to provide diet counseling to citizens of your state in order to reduce deaths from heart attack and stroke. If you needed to find out whether or not it was working to provide the counseling through county health departments, you might use in-depth interviews in a number of ways. For example, you might interview those who have received counseling and those who have not and ask questions such as

- What led you to attend (or not attend) the counseling?
- Was the health department a factor in your decision? If yes, what was its role?
- What do you like about having the counseling through the health department?
- What do you dislike about having the counseling through the health department?

You might also interview the providers of the diet counseling and ask them questions such as

- What works well about the program?
- What does not work well?
- What are the benefits of providing the counseling through the health department?
- What are the problems with providing the counseling through the health department?
- What are some better ways to provide the counseling?

You might interview program administrators and ask

- Why was the health department chosen as the means of providing the counseling?
- What were the perceived benefits of using the health department? Have these benefits been realized?
- What were the perceived drawbacks of using the health department?

You might also interview administrators of the health department and ask

- What do you know about the diet counseling program?
- What are the benefits to the health department associated with this program?
- What are the costs to the health department associated with this program?

Many of these same questions could also be addressed by conducting focus groups with each of these types of program affiliates.

Observation is another qualitative method that can be used for formative evaluation. Suppose you are working with a program designed to provide hypertension screening in rural areas of your state through churches and civic groups and you want to determine whether the civic group screenings were working. An observer at the screening locations could note

- How the facilities are laid out and whether the physical setup works
- What problems participants appear to encounter
- Whether participants appear to know where to go
- How much participants and program personnel interact
- Whether there is any grumbling as people leave

In observing program personnel, the observer could note

- How they set up for the screening
- Who is responsible for what tasks
- How they approach participants
- What steps they take to ensure privacy
- Whether they take time to explain each step
- What feedback they provide to those who were screened

In observing participants, the observer could note

- Do they tend to be of similar ages or social backgrounds?
- Do any people approach and choose not to participate? If so, are their characteristics similar to those of the people who choose to participate?

- How do people respond when approached by program personnel?
- Do they ask questions? What kind of questions do they ask?

Quantitative methods, such as cross-sectional surveys, can also be used to conduct formative evaluation. Suppose, for example, you wanted to assess the effectiveness of your advertising for a screening program such as the one described above. You could query people who did and did not participate in the screening by using a survey similar to that shown in Figure 8.5. Combined with demographic information, the responses to surveys like these could be used to determine for whom the advertising is and is not appropriate and effective.

Process Evaluation. Process evaluation assesses the way the program is being delivered, rather than the program's effectiveness. It documents what is actually being provided by the program and compares that to what was supposed to be provided to determine whether there are any gaps. In other words, process evaluation functions as a form of quality control. It also serves many other purposes, such as providing managers with feedback on the quality of delivery, documenting the fidelity and variability in program delivery across sites and personnel, providing information to assess exactly what components of the program are responsible for particular outcomes, and providing data that can be used to demonstrate how the program affects funders, sponsors, participants, and the public. To serve these purposes, process evaluation focuses on the activities and outputs

FIGURE 8.5. SAMPLE SURVEY.

Please indicate the extent to which you agree or disagree with each of the following statements	Strongly Agree	Agree	Neither Agree nor Disagree	Disagree	Strongly Disagree
There was enough advertising.	SA	A	N	D	SD
The location of the advertising was good.	SA	A	N	D	SD
The ads were easy to understand.	SA	A	N	D	SD
Overall, I liked the ads.	SA	A	N	D	SD

of the program, for example, what was done in each screening, and how many screenings were held. Program context, reach of the program, dose delivered and received, fidelity to the original program plan, implementation, and recruitment are some of the typical components of process evaluation (Linnan and Steckler, 2002).

Common process evaluation questions (adapted from Patton, 1997) include

- What are the program's main characteristics as perceived by major stakeholder groups?
- Who participates in the program, and how do they compare to the intended target population for the program?
- Which components of the program are working as expected? What is not working well? What challenges and barriers have been encountered?
- What do participants and staff like and dislike?
- What has changed from the original implementation design and why?
- What are the startup costs of the program? What are the ongoing costs of implementation?
- What has been learned about the program that might inform efforts elsewhere?

As in formative evaluation, the methods used in process evaluation can be qualitative or quantitative. For example, suppose you were working with a program designed to provide child safety-seat checks and education to caregivers who transport children under the age of seven years in their vehicles. If you wanted to find out how the checks were being conducted, you could use observation. The observer could note whether or not the program technician checked both the installation of the seat and the placement of the child within the seat. The observer could also note whether the technician involved the caregiver in the seat check, whether or not she or he discussed with the caregiver any problems that were identified, and whether or not she or he provided instruction to the caregiver about how to correct the problem.

Quantitative methods can also be used for process evaluation. For example, counts of number of vehicles checked, number of seats checked, and number of caregivers educated could be used to verify the program's output. If the program was advertised through a radio campaign, counts of radio spots developed and taped, stations contacted and stations accepting spots, number of spots aired, frequency of airing per spot, and minutes of airtime would also be elements of process evaluation. Other common data-collection methods in process evaluation include diaries or logs, document review, record abstraction, and monitoring or tracking systems.

Outcome Evaluation. Outcome evaluation is linked to the outcomes in the program's logic model, and often uses experimental or quasi-experimental study designs, along with quantitative methods. Short-term outcome evaluation can measure the short-term effects of the program on a participant immediately after he or she participates. Consequently, it measures outcomes that can change rapidly as a result of an intervention, such as knowledge, attitudes, and intended behavior. Changes in these outcomes are typically assessed with pretest-posttest designs—that is, administering the measures before and after participants take part in the program. Short-term outcome evaluation provides evidence of the degree to which a program is meeting its short-term or intermediate goals, such as increasing participants' awareness of the hazards of secondhand smoke or changing their knowledge, attitudes, and beliefs about secondhand smoke. Surveys, interviews, and observation are common data-collection methods in these kinds of evaluations.

Changes in outcomes such as actual behavior, for example, quitting smoking indoors, usually take longer to manifest themselves. As a consequence, they are usually assessed over longer periods of time, when a follow-up assessment is administered in addition to the standard pretest-posttest assessment. Control or comparison groups are often used to aid in attributing the observed effects to the program. See Chapters Four and Six for more detailed discussion of experimental and quasi-experimental research designs.

The value of outcome evaluation is that it provides an indicator of both program effectiveness and the extent to which a program's objectives are being met. When combined with process evaluation, outcome evaluation can indicate which activities and outputs appear to have the greatest influence, and allow program managers to shift resources from less effective to more effective elements of the program. Demonstrating a program's ultimate impact upon morbidity and mortality, however, can be challenging due to the long-term nature of these outcomes and the multiple influences on them. Program evaluations in public health and health promotion, therefore, often focus on intermediate outcomes rather than on morbidity and mortality.

Economic Evaluation. Part of evaluating a program is determining whether or not the effects it produces are worth the program's costs. Economic evaluation methods are a family of techniques that can answer questions about the affordability of the program, the efficiency of the program, and the standards the program must achieve to be considered cost-saving or cost-effective. Five cost-related evaluation issues are of real interest to decision makers: (1) affordability; (2) assessing costs of unmet needs; (3) performance standard setting; (4) comparing programs within one disease area to each other; and (5) comparing programs in one area to health-related services in other disease areas.

Cost Analysis (Determining Affordability). Consider the following question. "There is a highly effective risk-reduction program that was developed in another state—can we afford to offer the service in my hometown?" To answer this "affordability" question, we need to know the cost of delivering the program activities. This might mean knowing the dollar cost of conducting each activity per participant served, or it might mean simply knowing, in detail, what types of human resources and materials are needed to conduct the activity.

The economic evaluation technique of cost analysis is well-suited to answering the affordability question (Gold, Siegel, Russell, and Weinstein, 1996; Trentacoste, Holtgrave, Collins, and Abdul-Quader, 2004). In a cost analysis of a prevention program, a table is constructed with the categories of resources consumed by the program as the rows (for example, staff time, incentives given to participants, materials distributed, staff travel time) and inputs as the columns of the table. These inputs include (1) a definition of each resource category; (2) a definition of the unit of each resource category; (3) the number of units of each resource category consumed; (4) the dollar value of each resource category; and (5) the product of the number of resource units consumed and the dollar value of each unit for each resource category. Summing these products across all resource categories gives the total cost of the program. Dividing the total cost by the number of clients yields the per-client cost of the program.

Overall, there are seven basic steps in a cost analysis (Gold, Siegel, Russell, and Weinstein, 1996; Gorsky, 1996):

- Choose a time period for the cost-analysis
- Count the clients served during this time period
- Inventory the resources, in specific units, required for all program activities
- Calculate the cost per unit of each resource used
- Count the number of units of each resource used in the time period specified
- Calculate the total costs of the program
- Calculate the expected cost per client served

If a decision maker is interested in questions of the affordability of particular programs, the economic evaluation technique of cost analysis is well-suited to providing answers. Cost analysis can determine the price of delivering a program, and it can provide detailed information about the exact types (and quantities) of resources consumed by the program.

Cost of Unmet Needs Analysis (Assessing Costs of Unmet Needs). Consider yet another question that might be posed by a health professional in a given community. "How much would it cost to run a program that addresses the unmet prevention service delivery needs

DINCUS FORGETS TO DO A COST-UTILITY ANALYSIS BEFORE IMPLEMENTATION.

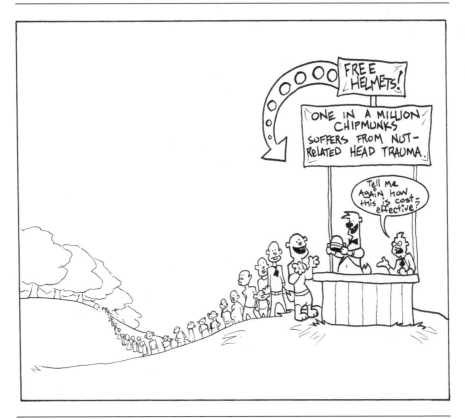

Copyright 2005 by Justin Wagner; reprinted with permission.

of a population?" From time to time, decision makers may need to know how much it would cost to address the unmet needs of any particular population or populations. Cost of unmet needs analysis can answer this question (Holtgrave, Pinkerton and Merson, 2002). A cost of unmet needs analysis has just a few basic steps:

- The number of people in need of a particular activity or service is estimated (for example, using epidemiologic and behavioral information).
- The most effective activities or services for this population are identified (for example, using the published literature or local evaluation information).
- The per-client cost of these activities or services for this population is identified (for example, using the published literature or local cost analyses).

The per-client costs of the programs are multiplied by the number of people needing the programs; this yields the cost of unmet needs for this particular population. Cost of unmet needs analysis can answer cost of unmet needs questions for decision makers, *and* it can also equip decision makers to answer questions from media, state legislators, federal agencies, and others interested in the real cost of unmet needs in a particular locale.

Threshold Analysis (Performance Standard Setting). Another important question might be, "The State Legislature wants to know if it is saving money by preventing disease and averting medical costs. How much disease would this program have to prevent in order to be cost-saving?" In a threshold analysis, we start by taking the cost of a particular program (Holtgrave and others, 1997). Then we divide it by the present value of the lifetime medical care cost of treating one case of the disease the program is designed to prevent. (*Present value* is a technical term meaning, roughly, that we use a 3 percent annual discount rate to bring future health care costs into present value.) The result tells us how many cases of disease would have to be permanently prevented by this program for it to be considered cost-saving. Note that we do not have to know anything about how much disease is actually prevented by this program in order to calculate the cost-saving threshold.

These simple calculations constitute a threshold analysis in its entirety. However, we can go one step further and ask whether the approximate number of cases of disease that might be prevented by a particular program is likely to be above or below the threshold. For instance, if a state does a threshold analysis on its HIV counseling and testing program and finds that only five HIV infections would have to be prevented for the program to be cost-saving, it can try to identify whether there is evidence to suggest that the actual number of infections prevented is above or below five (even if the precise number is unknown). Oftentimes there will be sufficient evidence to determine whether or not it is likely that a threshold is being met, even when the exact level of effectiveness is not known. Identifying whether the number of infections prevented is above or below a threshold can be a much more practical evaluation question to answer, rather than trying to estimate the exact number of infections prevented.

Here, we mention an analysis designed to determine a "cost-saving" threshold. Other, related techniques can be used to determine if an intervention is cost-effective even if not cost-saving.

Cost-Effectiveness Analysis (Comparing Programs Within One Disease Area to Each Other). Again, please consider the following question. "We would like to prevent as many cases of a particular disease as possible given the level of resources that our state has available—how can we do this?" People working in one particular area of disease prevention (for instance, HIV prevention) all desire to avert as many cases of that illness as possible—indeed, that is the very nature of their work. Consequently, they want to give priority to prevention programs that will prevent as many cases of that disease as possible. Of course, a real limitation is the amount of resources available, so, public health personnel have to maximize the cases of disease prevented within those resource constraints.

The technique of cost-effectiveness can help with this decision (Pinkerton, Johnson-Masotti, Holtgrave, and Farnham, 2001). As applied here for illustration, cost-effectiveness analysis estimates the cost-per-case-of-disease-prevented by a given program. Different types of services to prevent that one type of disease could then be compared on a cost-effectiveness basis. For instance, if there were five different types of services to avoid lung cancer, they could be compared on the basis of cost-per-case-of-lung-cancer-prevented.

Cost-Utility Analysis (Comparing Programs in One Area to Health-Related Services in Other Disease Areas). Here, please consider a question posed at the national level. "The Office of Management and Budget in the White House is wondering whether investment in HIV prevention is better than investments in diabetes, cancer, or heart disease. How can we even begin to answer a question like that?" Many public health policymakers must set priorities across disease areas. For instance, appropriations committees in the U.S. Congress must work to make funding decisions across many areas of expenditure, including making health service funding decisions that pit cancer programs versus heart disease programs versus HIV prevention programs versus diabetes control programs (and so on). The Office of Management and Budget in the White House has endorsed cost-benefit and cost-utility analysis as important forms of input into such decision making. (We'll focus here on the more broadly useful cost-utility analysis rather than cost-benefit analysis.)

Cost-utility analysis evaluates a program in terms of the cost-per-quality-adjusted-life-year-saved (or cost per QALY saved, for short) (Gold, Siegel, Russell, and Weinstein, 1996; Pinkerton and Holtgrave, 1998). Note that in the cost-effectiveness analysis discussed earlier, the cost-effectiveness outcomes were in the form of cost per case of a particular disease prevented (for example, case of lung cancer prevented); that outcome form is useful for comparing prevention programs that target the same disease to each other, but is not of use for comparing prevention programs for one disease to those in other disease areas. The cost-utility analysis outcome of cost per QALY saved can be used across disease areas since a quality-adjusted life year saved in one area is (at least theoretically) the same as a QALY saved in another disease area.

Simply put, a cost-utility analysis can show that a program is cost-saving, cost-effective, or not cost-effective. If a cost-utility analysis shows that the costs prevented (usually health care costs prevented) by a program are greater than the cost of delivering the program itself, then the program is said to be cost-saving. Clearly, if a program saves more money than it costs to deliver, it can justifiably be labeled "cost saving."

However, a program may cost more to deliver than it saves but still be quite worthwhile. For instance, kidney dialysis, many forms of surgery, and many medical screening programs cost more than they save, but as a society we readily accept them and invest in them. Although there is no magic cutoff value, very commonly it is cited that programs that are not cost-saving but cost less than $50,000 per QALY saved should be labeled as cost-effective. (Note that some researchers would place the cutoff at $80,000, $100,000, or even $120,000 rather than $50,000.) Programs that cost more than the cutoff value (say, $50,000 per QALY saved) cannot be justifiably labeled as cost-effective.

The Evaluation Report

No matter what type of evaluation is conducted, the results have to be shared with major stakeholders. Generally, the main function of an evaluation report is to provide answers to the questions posed at the beginning of the evaluation and discuss what these answers mean. In evaluation, meaning is often derived through some form of comparison. Patton (1997) discusses comparing program outcomes to outcomes from a similar program, to stated program objectives, to outcomes from the same program in a prior time period, or to external standards of desirability. Other objectives of an evaluation report include providing management with a basis for decisions regarding program changes, soliciting continued funding, providing staff with feedback, making others aware of the program and its contributions, and making recommendations for future action.

The reporting of results is especially important in evaluation, as it becomes the basis for future action. Without an adequate report of the findings, the evaluation is largely worthless. In formulating the report, consider each of the categories of stakeholders, their needs, and their interests. Also consider what actions they might want to take as a result of the report. This will ensure that you provide them with sufficient information to inform their action as fully as possible.

◆ ◆ ◆

In a Nutshell

Without an adequate report of the findings, the evaluation is largely worthless.

◆ ◆ ◆

There are numerous additional issues to consider in reporting evaluation findings. For example, should the report be written or oral? If it is written, options include an executive summary followed by a full report, an executive summary only, press releases, newsletters, or a traditional academic research monograph (Patton, 1997). Other issues to consider include authorship and contributors to the report, as well as whose perspectives are represented. Options range from including only the evaluator's perspective to the evaluator writing the report on behalf of a particular stakeholder group.

Applied Example

Pool Cool is a sun-safety program initially implemented in Hawaii and Massachusetts and currently being disseminated nationwide. Because of its comprehensive evaluation, the Pool Cool program is used here to illustrate many of the key concepts covered in this chapter. Designed as an intervention research study, the project included formative, process, and outcome evaluation. (For a more detailed description of the program and related evaluation findings, please see Glanz, Geller, Shigaki, Maddock, and Isnec, 2002; and Glanz, Isnec, Geller, and Spangler, 2002.)

Stakeholders

Stakeholders are those who have a stake or a vested interest in evaluation findings. This includes individuals who make decisions about a program or simply desire information about the program or its evaluation. For Pool Cool, major stakeholders included the Pool Cool staff (behavioral scientists, health educators, research assistants, and data managers), the aquatics and recreation staff, parents of young children, and children taking swimming lessons at the participating pools. Stakeholders also included those who would ultimately pay medical care expenses for any cases of cancer that might arise in the future. The funding agency is also considered a stakeholder, and for Pool Cool this was the Centers for Disease Control and Prevention (CDC). Patton (1997) advises evaluators to go beyond identification of stakeholders and to develop a strong relationship with at least one primary intended user. This requires evaluators to find strategically located people who are enthusiastic about an evaluation and committed to using the results. For Pool Cool, the project team both designed and evaluated the program. This integration facilitated use of the evaluation findings in making decisions about the program.

Defining the Program

A critical step in designing an evaluation is to develop a thorough understanding of the program to be evaluated. The Pool Cool program uses both behavioral and environmental strategies to prevent skin cancer by improving sun protection behaviors, reducing sunburns, and promoting sun-safety policies and environments at swimming pools (Glanz, Geller, Shigaki, Maddock, and Isnec, 2002). The *target audience* for the Pool Cool program was children who took swimming lessons and their parents, as well as aquatics instructors at the participating pools (Glanz, Isnec, Geller, and Spangler, 2002; Glanz, Geller, Shigaki, Maddock, and Isnec, 2002). Educational strategies included lifeguard and aquatic instructor training, sun-safety lessons to be implemented as part of swimming lessons, a series of interactive activities, and incentives. Environmental strategies included informal consultation on policy change and provision of sunscreen pump bottles, a shade structure (such as a tent, a canvas or tarp cover, or an umbrella), and signage with sun-safe messages.

The Pool Cool program was based on the social cognitive theory, which asserts that behaviors are influenced by the social and physical environment and that people, their behaviors, and the environment have a reciprocal relationship with each influencing the other (Glanz, Geller, Shigaki, Maddock, and Isnec, 2002; Bandura, 1986). The logic underlying the Pool Cool program was relatively straightforward. If knowledge, skills, health beliefs, and social and physical environments can be altered to support sun safety, the prevalence of preventive behaviors will increase among children taking swimming lessons, their parents, and aquatics instructors. An increase in these behaviors will lead to reductions in sun exposure and sunburns among program participants, and in the long-term, reductions in skin cancer. Thus, short-term outcomes included changes in knowledge and skills, health beliefs, social norms, social acceptability, and physical environments. Specific environmental and policy-related outcomes included existence of shade structures and sun-safety signage, and availability of sunscreen at the participating swimming pools. Intermediate behavioral outcomes included use of sunscreen, wearing protective clothing, seeking shade during peak sun hours, and wearing sunglasses. The longer-term outcomes that would, in theory, result from an increase in these preventive behaviors included reduced sun exposure, reduced sunburns, and, ultimately, a lower incidence of skin cancer.

Types of Evaluation

Formative evaluation is usually conducted in the developmental phase of a program to provide input that can be used to modify a program and document the feasibility of program implementation. Data from formative evaluations are useful in crafting and tailoring intervention strategies and messages that effectively reach the target population, resonate with selected audiences, and are culturally appropriate. Planning a successful program requires a solid understanding of the knowledge, attitudes, behaviors, and culture of the target audience (Green and Kreuter, 1999). In Pool Cool, this required learning the culture of the swimming pool environment, and learning about the sun-safety practices and views of lifeguards, aquatics instructors, and pool managers. It also required developing an understanding of sun-safety beliefs and practices of parents and children.

The Pool Cool formative evaluation used multiple data-collection methods (Glanz, Carbone, and Song, 1999; Glanz, Isnec, Geller, and Spangler, 2002). Qualitative evaluation methods included focus groups, discussion groups, and interviews with children, parents, recreation staff, pool managers, aquatics instructors, and lifeguards. Site visits to swimming pools were also completed. Quantitative data were collected through self-administered written surveys. Several issues affecting program design emerged from the formative component of the evaluation.

The process evaluation component of Pool Cool was multifaceted and served several purposes (Glanz, Isnec, Geller, and Spangler, 2002). For example, it assessed the extent of implementation of the educational and environmental program components, how much time was spent delivering the program, exposure to program components, program reach, and how the target audience—lifeguards and children—rated the various aspects of the program. It also was designed to catch any unintended consequences or unexpected circumstances that might influence either program implementation or outcomes.

Three types of data collection were employed in the process evaluation: monitoring forms, observation records, and select items from posttest surveys. The monitoring forms were completed by lifeguards and aquatics instructors and were designed to assess delivery of the eight sun-safety lessons. They were also used to assess the presence of parents at the pools, how well lessons were received, and which components were taught.

Staff logs were used for quality assurance purposes and were completed on site visits to the participating pools. Staff logs helped to document that participation and implementation were affected by the weather. Relevant survey items asked parents about participation, their reactions to the program, and incentives they had received. Overall, the process evaluation findings enabled the project team to feel comfortable that the program was being implemented as planned. Good documentation of the implementation process also shed light on how the program outcomes were achieved. For a more detailed description of the process evaluation, see Glanz, Isnec, Geller, and Spangler (2002).

The outcome evaluation design for the Pool Cool Program was a randomized controlled trial (see Chapter Six for more details on RCTs) with swimming pools as the unit of randomization and analysis (Glanz, Geller, Shigaki, Maddock, and Isnec, 2002). Pools were randomized into either the intervention arm ($n = 15$) or the control arm ($n = 13$), with the latter receiving an attention-matched injury-prevention program. Primary outcome data were collected through self-administered written surveys completed by two cross-sectional samples of parents at the beginning of the summer and eight weeks later. These were parents of children ages five to ten who were taking swimming lessons. Major measures included demographic factors, knowledge about skin cancer and sun protection guidelines, attitudes, policies for sun protection at the pool, parent and child's sun-protection practices, and child's sunburn experiences for the previous summer and the summer when the program took place. Environmental outcomes were assessed through observation at three points in time: the beginning, middle, and end of the summer. Two independent observers completed observations forms to assess availability of sunscreen, shaded areas, sun-safety signage, and lifeguard sun-safety practices.

Results showed significant intervention effects in children's use of sunscreen, staying in shade, and sun-protection habits. Use of sunscreen, wearing a hat, and sun-protection habits also increased among parents. Furthermore, pool sun-protection policies increased in the intervention pools. Environmental results documented greater improvements in availability of sunscreen, posting of sun-safety signs, and lifeguard shirt use in intervention pools relative to control pools. Overall, outcome evaluation results showed a modest, but significant program effect. Evaluation results have been disseminated through publication in peer-reviewed journals. The program is currently being disseminated nationwide. This second phase of the project also included process and outcome evaluations. For a more detailed description of the outcome evaluation, see Glanz, Geller, Shigaki, Maddock, and Isnec (2002).

Integration with the Research Process

Numerous similarities exist between applied research and program evaluation. Both use social science research methods, for example. Both involve developing study questions, selecting a study design, determining what should be measured and how, and sampling decisions. Furthermore, both require attention to reliability and validity of measures, qualitative or quantitative data collection, protection of human participants, data analysis, interpretation of findings, and dissemination of results.

The nine-step model presented in Chapter One can be compared with the framework for program evaluation in public health developed by the Centers for Disease Control and Prevention (1999). The latter model specifies six steps in the evaluation process: engage stakeholders, describe the program, focus the evaluation design, gather credible evidence, justify conclusions, and ensure that evaluation findings are used. Differences in the two models stem largely from the purposes of the two endeavors. In evaluation, the purpose is to provide information to make decisions about a specific program. Common guiding questions include, Is the program meeting its objectives? Is the program effective? Is the program implemented as planned? How can the program be improved? Not surprisingly, the evaluation framework emphasizes attention to stakeholders and the program description, as well as concern with the use of the evaluation findings. These concepts are largely absent in the research model, which makes sense, since the primary purpose of research is to create or discover generalizable knowledge.

◆ ◆ ◆

In a Nutshell

The evaluation framework emphasizes attention to stakeholders and the program description, as well as concern with the use of the evaluation findings.

◆ ◆ ◆

Other, more subtle, differences also exist. Whereas the research process begins with identifying a priority population, identification of a priority population, assessment of needs and assets, and selection of intervention strategies are typically driven by the program planning process in evaluation. Ideally, of course, evaluation planning is fully integrated into program planning, but that is not always the case in practice. The middle steps in the research and evaluation processes are similar, with selecting the design, determining measures, and sampling subsumed under the "focus the evaluation design" and "gather credible evidence" steps of the evaluation framework.

Summary

Evaluation involves the systematic collection of information to answer questions about a program. These questions can be classified into four types of evaluation: formative, process, outcome, and economic (outcome evaluation as a broad category also includes impact evaluation). Formative evaluation is conducted during the developmental phase of a program to determine whether specific components such as materials, message, and learning activities are feasible and acceptable to the program's target population. Both qualitative and quantitative methods are common in formative evaluation. Process evaluation focuses on the internal operations of a program and attempts to provide information that can lead to program improvement. It also uses both qualitative and quantitative methods. In contrast, outcome evaluations usually employ quantitative methods to determine the effectiveness of a program. In other words, Is the program achieving the desired outcomes? As described in this chapter, numerous types of economic analysis can be conducted under the rubric of program evaluation. These include cost analysis, cost of unmet needs analysis, cost-effectiveness, threshold analysis, and cost-utility analysis.

Evaluation is similar to applied research and draws heavily upon social science research methods. It differs from research in its emphasis on stakeholder involvement and its focus on providing information to decision makers to aid them in making judgments about a particular program. Typical steps in the process include engaging stakeholders; describing the program along with its underlying logic; focusing the evaluation design; collecting, analyzing, and interpreting data; and reporting study results. Program evaluation exemplifies how research methods can be applied to real-world situations to make a difference both in how we approach social and public health problems and in people's day-to-day lives.

Issues to Consider

1. An important decision that must be made early on in an evaluation is whether the evaluator should be someone internal to the program or organization being evaluated, or whether he or she should be external to the program or organization (Patton, 1997). External evaluators are typically private consultants, or associated with a university or research organization. They usually conduct evaluations through contracts with the funder or the organizational sponsor of the program. They do not have a long-term relationship with the program and are thus often viewed as more objective and independent than an evaluator who is employed by the program or its organization. Inside evaluators are believed to be more susceptible to organizational pressures to report findings that support a particular point of view. External evaluators, although possibly more objective, often do not understand the program or its context as well as an inside evaluator. Furthermore, the knowledge they gain about the program may not remain with the program once the contract is over. When internal evaluators are used, their knowledge and insights about the program remain

accessible to the organization. Given the pros and cons of internal and external evaluators, which would you generally recommend? Why?

2. In the course of conducting an evaluation, even an external evaluator will develop relationships with program personnel. For an internal evaluator, these relationships can be even stronger. Especially in the case of service programs such as those conducted in public health, evaluators can learn about staff members' motivations and dedication to the program. When volunteers are involved, an evaluator may hear about how these people have given generously of their time for program activities with no compensation. When it comes time to report negative results, it is incumbent upon the evaluator to balance respect for the efforts of program personnel with a clear and truthful accounting of the findings. How would you go about doing that?

For Practice and Discussion

1. You are an evaluator in the State Health Department, and your supervisor approaches you about a new project. It seems that a coalition in one of the cities of your state has received some new funding for its two-year-old program to increase exercise among people with arthritis. The pain associated with arthritis can cause arthritis sufferers not to use their muscles and, as a result, their muscles can atrophy. The goal of the arthritis exercise program has been to increase participants' joint flexibility and aerobic fitness while preventing the loss of their muscle condition. So far, they have served 225 people with arthritis.

    The program planners are excited about the additional funding and the potential to reach more people. The staff has just learned, however, that before the funds will be released, the program must submit a complete evaluation plan to their funder. You are assigned to develop their evaluation plan. How would you begin? Since the program has already been running for two years, what problems might that create in developing the plan? What parts of the plan might be easier to write for an existing program?

2. You have been asked by the director of a local hospital's cardiac rehabilitation department to evaluate a program conducted through the department. In this program, women with a history of myocardial infarction or of coronary artery bypass surgery who exercise regularly are asked to make telephone calls to other women with a similar history who do not regularly exercise. The purpose of the calls is to encourage the nonexercisers to participate in group exercise as a means of providing social support, since studies have found that women who persist in exercising after cardiac rehabilitation are more likely to have social support (Moore, Dolansky, Ruland, Pashkow, and Blackburn, 2003).

Although program evaluations can produce positive findings as well as negative findings, the personnel in charge of the program are not enthusiastic about the evaluation. Specifically, they express fear that it will not show all the good things their program is doing. As the evaluator, what can you do to help the program personnel become invested in your evaluation plan?

3. You have been conducting an evaluation of a state program designed to encourage African Americans to consider becoming organ donors. As a part of the evaluation, television stations in the state aired television spots about the need for organs in the African American community. African Americans in the state were later surveyed, and their knowledge and attitudes about organ donation were compared to those of African Americans in a neighboring state.

After completing the evaluation, you are invited to present your findings at a national meeting. A hepatologist (liver doctor) in the audience complains about your results, saying that you did not randomly assign people to receive the program or not. How would you respond to this person?

References

Bandura, A. (1986). *Social foundations of thought and action: A social cognitive theory.* Upper Saddle River, NJ: Prentice-Hall.

Centers for Disease Control and Prevention. (1999). Framework for program evaluation in public health. *Morbidity and Mortality Weekly Report, 48*(RR-11), 1–40.

Deniston, O. L., and Rosenstock, I. M. (1970). Evaluating health programs. *Public Health Reports, 85*(9), 835–840.

Glanz, K., Carbone, E., and Song, V. (1999). Formative research for developing targeted skin cancer prevention programs for children in multiethnic Hawaii. *Health Education Research, 14*(2), 155–166.

Glanz, K., Geller, A., Shigaki, D., Maddock, J., and Isnec, M. (2002). A randomized trial or skin cancer prevention in aquatics settings: The Pool Cool program. *Health Psychology, 21*(6), 579–587.

Glanz, K., Isnec, M., Geller, A., and Spangler, K. (2002). Process evaluation of implementation and dissemination of a sun safety program at swimming pools. In A. Steckler, and L. Linnan (Eds.), *Process evaluation for public health interventions and research* (pp. 58–82). San Francisco: Jossey-Bass.

Gold, M. R., Siegel, J. E., Russell, L. B., and Weinstein, M. C. (Eds.). (1996). *Cost-effectiveness in health and medicine.* New York: Oxford University Press.

Gorsky, R. D. (1996). A method to measure the costs of counseling for HIV prevention. *Public Health Reports, 111*(supplement 1), 115–122.

Green, L., and Kreuter, M. (1999). *Health promotion planning: An educational and ecological approach* (3rd ed.). Mountain View, CA: Mayfield.

Holtgrave, D. R., Pinkerton, S. D., and Merson, M. (2002). Estimating the cost of unmet HIV prevention needs in the United States. *American Journal of Preventive Medicine, 23*, 7–12.

Holtgrave, D. R., and others. (1997). Setting standards for the Wisconsin HIV counseling and testing program: An application of threshold analysis. *Journal of Public Health Management and Practice, 3,* 42–49.

Linnan, L., and Steckler, A. (2002). *Process evaluation for public health interventions and research.* San Francisco: Jossey-Bass.

Moore, S. M., Dolansky, M. A., Ruland, C. M., Pashkow, F. J., and Blackburn, G. G. (2003). Predictors of women's exercise maintenance after cardiac rehabilitation. *Journal of Cardiopulmonary Rehabilitation, 23*(1), 40–49.

Patton, M. Q. (1997). *Utilization-focused evaluation.* Thousand Oaks, CA: Sage.

Pinkerton, S. D., and Holtgrave, D. R. (1998). Assessing the cost-effectiveness of HIV prevention interventions: A primer. In D. R. Holtgrave (Ed.), *Handbook of economic evaluation of HIV prevention programs* (pp. 33–43). New York: Plenum Press.

Pinkerton, S. D., Johnson-Masotti, A. P., Holtgrave, D. R., and Farnham, P. G. (2001). Using cost-effectiveness league tables to compare interventions to prevent sexual transmission of HIV. *AIDS, 15,* 917–928.

Rossi, P. H., Lipsey, M. W., and Freeman, H. E. (2004). *Evaluation: A systematic approach* (7th ed.). Thousand Oaks, CA: Sage.

Thompson, N. J., and McClintock, H. O. (1998). *Demonstrating your program's worth: A primer on evaluation for programs to prevent unintentional injury.* Atlanta: Centers for Disease Control and Prevention, National Center for Injury Prevention and Control.

Tobacco Technical Assistance Consortium. (2005, January). *The power of proof: An evaluation primer.* Retreived February 6, 2005, from www.ttac.org/power-of-proof/index.html.

Trentacoste, N. D., Holtgrave, D. R., Collins, C., and Abdul-Quader, A. (2004). Disseminating effective interventions for HIV prevention: A cost analysis of a risk reduction intervention for drug users. *Journal of Public Health Management and Practice, 10,* 130–139.

Weiss, C. (1997). *Evaluation: Methods for studying programs and policies.* Upper Saddle River, NJ: Prentice-Hall.

PART THREE

MEASUREMENT, SAMPLING, AND ANALYSIS

CHAPTER NINE

MEASUREMENT IN HEALTH PROMOTION

Richard R. Clayton and Richard A. Crosby

Measurement is everywhere. It is woven in, on, over, around, and through everything we do. As soon as a baby is born the medical personnel determine "vital statistics"— the height, weight, and Apgar score for the newborn—and record the month, day, year, and time of birth. The time lapsed since birth is used to determine when visits to the pediatrician are scheduled and when certain immunizations are administered. At each postnatal visit, medical staff determine and record the baby's weight and height in order to measure "change," and may take the baby's temperature. Temperature is measured in degrees. Throughout an individual's life, his or her birthday is celebrated and used to mark important developmental transitions such as reaching the ages to drive, to vote, and to drink. Over time, while the specific measures taken may change somewhat, virtually everything in an individual's life is measured. For example, when individuals enter school their attendance or absence will be recorded in a student record database as will their test and achievement scores.

Each of the measures taken and recorded has a metric. Temperature is measured in degrees Fahrenheit or Celsius, weight is measured in pounds or grams and kilograms, test scores are measured in actual numbers (as in SAT and GRE scores) or in percentiles. As you may already know, some metrics are more sophisticated than others. For example, metrics for measures range from a nominal scale to an ordinal to an interval to a ratio scale.

If measurement is everywhere and in everything, then measurement should be viewed as an essential element of health promotion strategies, campaigns, and programs. Measurement is central, critical, and absolutely vital to our understanding of health promotion research. In this chapter, the emphasis will be on *who* and *what* is measured in public health, *when, how,* and *where* the measurements occur, and, most important, *why* public health phenomena are measured. We have chosen to use one behavior, tobacco use, and its role in public health to illustrate the key concepts presented in this chapter. We will also address contextual-level influences on health by using the family unit as an example of a key variable, which may pose several challenges to measurement. Specifically, this chapter will focus on step 5 in the nine-step model described in Chapter One. However, because health promotion research is frequently based on the use of self-reported measures, this chapter precedes a chapter (Chapter Ten) that will provide an in-depth analysis of issues relevant to increasing the validity of self-reported measures. Both chapters are dedicated to providing you with up-to-date techniques for assessment in health promotion research.

◆ ◆ ◆

In a Nutshell

Measurement is central, critical, and absolutely vital to our understanding of health promotion research.

◆ ◆ ◆

Illustration of Key Concepts

Perhaps one of the most fundamental aspects of measurement is determining the metric used for variables. A variable is a single measure that, by definition, can take on more than one value. If only one value is possible, then the measure cannot vary and therefore must be a constant. Distinctions between four metrics used to categorize or quantify variables are commonly made. As will be shown in Chapters Twelve and Thirteen, the metric associated with a variable will determine the type of statistical analysis performed.

Metrics

Nominal data are especially common in health promotion research. A nominal metric simply categorizes or groups according to some *attribute*. Attributes constitute the mutually exclusive and exhaustive response categories for a variable and are qualitative in nature versus quantitative. Before you were born, your mother went through carefully and strategically scheduled measurements. One of those measures determined whether she was pregnant. The answer to the pregnancy test had only two categories—Yes or No. Either you are pregnant or you are not pregnant; thus, this metric does not include a more or less dimension. Something that is measured "Yes or No," "zero or one," or "present or not present," is a dichotomy and is a specific form of a nominal scale. Nominal measures may also extend beyond a dichotomy. Race, for example, is a nominal variable that may have many different attributes. Some attributes of a nominal variable for religion may include Christian, Jewish, Muslim, Buddhist, Hindu. Nominal attributes cannot be ranked in any fashion. Sex is another example of a nominal variable (male or female).

The next metric is *ordinal*. As your mother endured labor, the physician, nurse, and perhaps your father or some other family member might have asked your mother to tell them how bad the labor pains were—say on a scale from low to medium to high. This is called an ordinal level of measurement. It is characterized by transitivity, in which it is clear that high is more than medium which is more than low. Thus, the attributes are ranked along a continuum. However, it is worth noting that the distance between ranks is *not* known to be equal. For example, presenting a statement to people and then asking them to indicate their level of agreement on a scale with five responses that range from "strongly disagree" to "strongly agree" is something that is measured on an ordinal scale. From this example you can see how you *cannot* determine with certainty whether the difference between "strongly agree" and "somewhat agree" is exactly the same as the difference between "somewhat agree" and "neither agree nor disagree."

The next metric is *interval*. Like ordinal measures, an interval scale has transitivity; however, the distance between ranks is equal. Moreover, a score of "zero" does not equate with a complete absence of the variable that is being measured; rather, it is arbitrary. One example of a measure that uses this type of metric is temperature measured by the Fahrenheit or Celsius scales.

The final metric is *ratio*. As your mother went through labor the physician, nurse, or midwife used what is called a ratio scale of measurement—the number of centimeters that her cervix had dilated so that you could be born. A ratio scale has not only transitivity and equal distance between ranks, but also an absolute zero point. Common measures in health promotion such as "knowledge of heart disease prevention practices" are measured on a ratio metric. Other examples include number of cigarettes smoked per day, number of times a person attended a smoking cessation class, and the amount of money a person spends on cigarettes in one week. The advantage of having a measure that is a ratio scale of measurement is that it allows for statements about proportions. In other words, thirty cigarettes smoked per day as compared to ten cigarettes smoked per day represents a ratio of 3:1. You are unable to make these ratio statements with the other three types of metrics.

Measuring Constructs

Measuring physical properties such as weight, height, and age is a relatively straightforward process. In essence, it is easy to measure things that are tangible. If all measurement in health promotion research were this easy, then this chapter would be extremely short. Because health promotion research is intertwined with health behaviors and their underlying psychological and psychosocial influences, research questions are frequently centered upon intangibles such as self-esteem, depression, self-efficacy, attitudes, perceptions, and beliefs. Thus, while weight exists as a physical entity, self-esteem does not. Indeed, a concept such as self-esteem is not directly observable or measurable, but rather is hypothetical and may be linked to a particular theoretical orientation. For example, scholars theorize that people develop a sense of their own value and that this overall evaluation of their worth or value is influential in shaping some behaviors. Thus, self-esteem can be viewed as a concept versus an object. The question becomes, how do we measure something that is not tangible? The answer begins with the brief schematic shown below.

Concept → Operational Definition → Construct → Indicators

Because the epistemology of scientific inquiry is built on objectivity, the first step in measuring a *concept* such as self-esteem is to create a formalized definition. In a sense, this *operational definition* will become "the" definition of self-esteem for the purpose of the study being conducted. The definition does not need to be universally accepted, it simply needs to be provided so that consumers of your research can know, without question, what you mean when you use the term *self-esteem*. Once you have operationalized the concept it becomes a *construct*. The construct now requires measurement. It stands to reason that complex constructs such as self-esteem must be measured with multiple questions or items. The questions or items should be designed to be distinct *effect indicators* of the construct. Effect indicators signify that each question or item relating to the construct infers some "effect" or influence on an observable behavior and "taps into" the construct (Streiner, 2003). Rarely will a single-item indicator provide a complete assessment of a construct. Therefore, it is quite common to use multiple indicators to assess one construct.

◆ ◆ ◆

In a Nutshell

Once you have operationalized the concept it becomes a construct.

◆ ◆ ◆

Self-esteem represents a unitary construct for which multiple effect indicators can be used to measure it. In this instance, the measure of self-esteem would be called a *scale*. Specifically, a scale is a measure that is composed of "theoretically correlated items" (Streiner, 2003, p. 217) that are measuring the same construct. Examples of scales include the Rosenberg Self-Esteem Scale (Rosenberg, 1989) and the Beck Depression Inventory (Beck, Ward, Mendelson, Mock, and Erbaugh, 1961). Each of these scales has multiple effect indicators that theoretically relate to how self-esteem and depression would manifest. For example, one item from the Rosenberg Scale is "I am able to do things as well as most other people."

Although you may encounter instances when other terms are used interchangeably in the literature or in other texts to describe a collection of items or questions such as scale, test, questionnaire, index, or inventory, it is important to note that there are specific distinctions between a scale and an *index*. Thus, these two terms should not be used interchangeably, as they mean different things. An index refers to a measure in which the items are considered *causal indicators* because they themselves define the construct and influence the value of the construct (Streiner, 2003). The items in an index typically are heterogeneous and may not necessarily be correlated with each other. The Apgar Scale, mentioned previously in this chapter, specifically rates newborns on several characteristics such as heart rate, respiration, muscle tone, reflex response, and skin color and is an excellent example of an index. As you may be able to extrapolate, items composing indexes are not tapping into a unitary construct. In health promotion research, other examples of indexes are quality-of-life questionnaires, tests that assess levels of physical functionality, and knowledge tests. To illustrate these

Box 9.1. Example of a Scale

Below is a list of the ways you might have felt or behaved. Please tell me how often you have felt this way during the past week.

| Rarely or None of the Time (< than 1 day) | Some or a Little of the Time (1–2 days) | Occasionally or a Moderate Amount of Time (3–4 days) | Most or All of the Time (5–7 days) |

1. I was bothered by things that usually don't bother me.
2. I did not feel like eating; my appetite was poor.
3. I felt that I could not shake off the blues even with help from my family or friends.
4. I felt that I was just as good as other people.
5. I had trouble keeping my mind on what I was doing.
6. I felt depressed.
7. I felt that everything I did was an effort.
8. I felt hopeful about the future.
9. I thought my life had been a failure.
10. I felt fearful.
11. My sleep was restless.
12. I was happy.
13. I talked less than usual.
14. I felt lonely.
15. People were unfriendly.
16. I enjoyed life.
17. I had crying spells.
18. I felt sad.
19. I felt that people dislike me.
20. I could not get "going."

Source: Center for Epidemiologic Studies Depression Scale (CES-D) (Radloff, 1977).

---

distinctions, an example of a scale is shown in Box 9.1 and an example of an index is shown in Box 9.2.

Two key questions about any scale or index are Is this measure reliable? and Is it valid? *Reliability* means that a measure consistently provides the same answer every time it is used. So if one has a yardstick but it is forty-two inches long, it will still consistently provide the same measurement each time you use it. Unfortunately for the person using this "yard" stick, the consistency is always six inches too long. This brings us to the topic of validity. Although this "yard" stick

---

Box 9.2. Example of an Index

Quality of Life—Modified

I want to find out how you feel about various parts of your life. Please tell me the feelings you have in general according to the following responses.

Very Happy	Happy	Mostly Satisfied	Mixed	Mostly Dissatisfied	Unhappy	Very Unhappy

1. How do you feel about your life overall?
2. In general, how do you feel about yourself?
3. How do you feel about your personal safety?
4. How do you feel about the amount of fun and enjoyment you have?
5. How do you feel about the responsibilities you have for members of your family?
6. How do you feel about what you are accomplishing in your life?
7. How do you feel about your independence or freedom—that is, how free do you feel to live the kind of life you want?
8. How do you feel about your emotional and psychological well-being?
9. How do you feel about the way you spend your spare time?

Source: Andrews and Withey, 1976.

---

may be reliable, it is certainly not valid. Validity refers to whether or not the measure is measuring what it is supposed to measure.

Determining the reliability of a measure could be achieved in several ways. First, reliability could be established by administering the index or the scale to a sample at two points in time and looking for a relatively strong correlation in scores for time 1 and time 2. This is known as *test-retest reliability*. Notice that the underlying assumption here is that the construct is stable; therefore, a reliable measure should produce the same score at time 2 that it did at time 1 for each person in the sample. Thus, a principle in establishing test-retest reliability is that the construct must not be one that undergoes dramatic change over time.

Second, reliability can be established by computing the inter-item correlations between all items comprised in the scale. Note that this technique is appropriate for establishing the reliability of a scale because scale items should be tapping into a unitary construct. Thus, they should be intercorrelated. The same is not true for indexes, however. Computing inter-item correlations is not appropriate

MINCUS REVEALS A VALID MEASURE OF CHIPMUNK I.Q.

Copyright 2005 by Justin Wagner; reprinted with permission.

for establishing the reliability of an index (Streiner, 2003). Calculating the inter-item correlations is called assessing the *internal reliability* of the scale.

We can determine the intercorrelations between items on a scale by employing a statistical procedure that yields the statistic Cronbach's alpha. Cronbach's alpha (α) has a range of 0 to 1, with higher scores representing greater inter-item reliability. Although hard-and-fast rules don't exist, an α of .70 or higher is considered sufficient evidence of reliability. It is, however, worth noting that extremely high alphas such as .95 suggest that there may be redundancy among some of the indicators. In effect, a scale with an alpha close to 1.0 could probably be reduced to fewer indicators. Note that inter-item correlation could be used in conjunction with the test-retest technique. Conversely, it is also noteworthy that the inter-item reliability method can be used in a cross-sectional study, whereas the same cannot be said about the test-retest method.

Third, reliability could be established by using the *split-half* method. Like the inter-item reliability method, this test for reliability could be performed in the context of a cross-sectional study. This analytic procedure begins with dividing the scale into two parallel forms of the measure. For example, an eight-item scale would be randomly divided into two four-item measures. These two shortened forms would then be administered to a sample. The correlation between scores for the two halves is calculated and then used in a formula (such as the Spearman Brown) to estimate the reliability of the total measure (Ghiselli, Campbell, and Zedeck, 1981). Similar to inter-item reliability, this method is not appropriate for indexes, as splitting the index into parts would not be meaningful.

As mentioned previously, validity refers to the index or scale measuring exactly what it is supposed to measure. So a yardstick that is forty-two inches long might be reliable, but it is not valid. A valid measure measures what it is supposed to *and* does so consistently. Thus, for a measure to be valid it must also be reliable, whereas a reliable measure is not necessarily valid.

◆ ◆ ◆

In a Nutshell

For a measure to be valid it must also be reliable, whereas a reliable measure is not necessarily valid.

◆ ◆ ◆

Like reliability, validity can be established through the application of several different techniques. Two of the most elementary techniques are *face validity* and *content validity*. Both techniques employ a *jury of experts* (a panel of professionals who possess expertise with respect to the construct(s) under consideration). Face validity is judged by asking the jury, Does the index or scale appear to measure the construct? Content validity, on the other hand, goes a bit further. For scales you would want to ask, Do the items represent the "universe" of all possible indicators relevant for the construct? For indexes, you would want to ask, Do the items represent a census of items underlying the construct? Content validity can be assessed for both scales and indexes, but judgments made regarding the items differ. Scales assume that there is a universe of potential items from which to draw a sample that represents the unitary construct, whereas items composing an index should be viewed more as a census of items and are dependent on the underlying theory of the construct and prior research (Streiner, 2003). Nevertheless, for both types of validity, the support for a measure being valid is a judgment. Because all constructs are measured by self-report, the more sophisticated techniques of establishing validity are an integral part of the next chapter (Chapter Ten), which is devoted to increasing the validity of self-reported measures.

Types of Variables

Variables can be qualitative or quantitative, can have different levels of measurement, and can represent myriad constructs that are not directly observable or measurable. All of these things have an effect on how the variables can be used and analyzed. In addition to knowing these important aspects of variables, it is also important to understand the role variables can adopt given a particular research context. Variables can be classified into several different types based largely on their function in serving the research question. The first level of distinction is whether the research question is descriptive or causal in nature (see Chapter Four for more detail). The second level of distinction is whether the variable is intended as a "causal" element or an outcome.

Variables in Descriptive Research. In health promotion descriptive research, observational designs rather than experimental designs are used, and the variable of interest is typically known as the *outcome measure*. Outcome measures can be physical indicators of morbidity such as lung cancer, atherosclerosis, blood serum cholesterol levels, emphysema, and chronic obstructive pulmonary disease. Outcome measures may also be health-risk behaviors such as smoking cigarettes, using chew tobacco, eating a diet low in cruciferous vegetables, and being exposed to asbestos. An excellent way to gain first-hand knowledge of health promotion outcome variables considered important to the federal government is to review the document *Healthy People 2010* (Department of Health and Human Services, 2000).

In descriptive research, variables presumed to cause or precede specified outcomes are typically known as *predictor variables*. The mark of a good predictor variable is its ability to reduce error when one makes predictions about an outcome. For example, in 1964 the Surgeon General of the United States issued the first report on the relationship between smoking and lung cancer. In essence, knowing whether (and how much) someone has smoked enables a more accurate prediction of the outcome, in this case lung cancer. Does that mean that smoking cigarettes is the only cause of lung cancer? The answer obviously is no. Some individuals who have never smoked get lung cancer. It does mean, however, that smoking behavior can be used as one of many predictors of developing lung cancer. This concept of using predictors to improve the estimate of an outcome is called *proportional reduction in error.*

◆ ◆ ◆

In a Nutshell

The mark of a good predictor variable is its ability to reduce error when one makes predictions about an outcome.

◆ ◆ ◆

One problem in labeling a given variable as a predictor is that there must be a reasonable level of certainty that the predictor is actually preceding the outcome. This certainty is made possible by assessment of the predictor at a point in time before assessment of the outcome occurs. Consider, for instance, a research question that asks whether nonsmoking teens who believe that smoking causes lung cancer are less likely to ever begin smoking. In this study, the predictor variable can be measured before the outcome occurs (as the sample comprised only nonsmokers). Over the next five years or so, many of those nonsmokers are likely to become smokers. If those who believed, during their teen years, that smoking causes lung cancer were statistically less likely to initiate smoking in the next five years, then it is safe to say that the belief preceded the outcome. But what if you don't have the luxury of doing a longitudinal (prospective) study? Instead, imagine that you have funding for only a cross-sectional design. You wisely sample all teens (not just those who are nonsmokers) to ensure variability in your outcome variables: smoking status and belief that smoking causes lung cancer. You are quite satisfied when the results support your research hypothesis. You find that those holding the belief are statistically less likely to smoke than those not holding the belief. The downside of this finding is that you cannot establish a *temporal order* (see Chapter Four). Thus, one could make the reverse argument (that smoking *causes* a person to deny that a connection between tobacco use and lung cancer even exists). Therefore, in a cross-sectional design, the concept of a predictor variable is problematic. Instead, the term *correlate* is used. Within this context, correlate represents a variable hypothesized to precede the outcome.

The discipline of public health is population oriented. Therefore, in public health, correlates and predictor variables are often measured at the macro or population level. One example of a population-level variable is the state excise tax rate for each of the fifty states in the United States. We could obtain the tax rate while also measuring the percentage of the population that reports being a current smoker. The correlate would be the amount of the state excise tax, ordered from the lowest to the highest. The percentage of the population that smokes would be the outcome variable. One hypothesis to consider would be the higher the state excise tax on cigarettes the lower the percentage who report being a current smoker. If there was an association between the correlate (excise tax) and the outcome (smoking behavior), then it would be reasonable to assume that by manipulating the excise tax rate we could influence smoking behavior. Health economists would be very interested in what would happen to the current smoking rate if the excise tax were increased. In such a case, the results might be reported as "a 10 percent increase in the price of cigarettes yielded a 7 percent decrease in the percentage of people who are smokers."

Variables in Causal Research. Causal research in health promotion uses mainly experimental or quasi-experimental designs (see Chapter Four). The *dependent variable* in experimental research designs is the counterpart to the outcome measure in observational research designs. In a randomized controlled trial (RCT) of a health promotion program (HPP) designed to prevent teens from *ever* initiating tobacco use, the dependent variable might be intent to ever smoke. Thus, intent would be assessed at some point after teens complete the program or the equivalent control condition. If the research hypothesis is supported, then those receiving the program will have less intent to smoke than those receiving the control program.

◆ ◆ ◆

In a Nutshell

The dependent variable *in experimental research designs is the counterpart to the outcome measure in observational research designs.*

◆ ◆ ◆

In health promotion research we often are interested in a variety of dependent variables. For example, mass media is used often in health promotion campaigns to influence individual level change. The dependent variables might be (1) awareness of the campaign (yes or no), (2) remembering the central theme or message of the campaign (knowledge beyond mere awareness), (3) a change in knowledge about the content of the campaign, (4) a change in one's attitude about the topic of the campaign, (5) a change in intention to change a behavior pattern that puts one at greater risk for a negative health outcome, or (6) a change in one's behavior thus reducing the risk for a negative health outcome. All of these are desirable outcomes and are related to each other.

Alternatively, in experimental research designs, *independent variables* cannot take on several different forms. Instead, these variables are limited to group assignment in the randomization process. By definition, the independent variable is manipulated by the investigator. Therefore, assignment to condition (the HPP or the control group) is an example of an independent variable.

◆ ◆ ◆

In a Nutshell

By definition, the independent variable is manipulated by the investigator.

◆ ◆ ◆

Mediating Variables. In the smoking–lung cancer relationship example, one might ask, How does smoking actually "cause" lung cancer in some people? This is a question about the mechanisms and processes that occur after the cause and before the effect. These mechanisms are said to *mediate* the observed relationship between smoking and lung cancer. In health promotion, the focus is more often on factors that might, at a population level, cause a reduction in lung cancer. For example, suppose a state embarks on a comprehensive and large-scale campaign to reduce the amount of smoking in that state. The health promotion campaign involves a substantial increase in the state excise tax on cigarettes; a universal prohibition on smoking in restaurants, bars, and other public places; the dissemination of effective prevention programs in schools; and the funding of effective smoking cessation interventions in health insurance plans and in worksites. All of this would be presented as an integrated strategy via a huge public awareness and marketing campaign. On average, it takes about twenty to twenty-five years of chronic smoking for lung cancer to appear, and the ultimate mediating variable for the smoking–lung cancer relationship is gene mutations. However, by reducing the levels of smoking through the use of massive campaigns that involve raising cigarette taxes, reducing environmental tobacco smoke, preventing dependency, and mass media, one might expect the rates of lung cancer and other tobacco-related illnesses and deaths to decline. A targeted outcome of the anti-smoking campaign could be a change in social norms surrounding smoking so that smoking is frowned upon. In this instance, affecting social norms is one mechanism that allows the intent of campaign to be translated into reduced risk for lung cancer. In essence then, mediating variables "come between" the cause (in this case the antismoking campaign) and the effect (in this case the reduction of cigarette use in a population).

Moderating Variables. Moderating variables identify the conditions under which the relationship between two variables might be stronger or weaker. For example, if the relationship between smoking and lung cancer was statistically stronger among whites than among blacks and Hispanics, then race or ethnicity would be considered the moderating variable. If the relation was stronger among those who are from rural rather than suburban and urban areas, then place of residence would be the moderating variable. Social support is a classic example of a moderating variable in the health promotion literature, in which perceptions of high levels of social support serve as a buffer (that is, moderator) against experiencing the negative effects of stress on health outcomes. Furthermore, some variables may moderate the effectiveness of HPPs. One example could be that HPP was effective in reducing smoking, but only for women. For men, it was not effective. Thus, in this example gender serves as the moderating variable. It is important to consider what variables may serve as moderators both of significant relationships between correlates and outcomes and of HPP effectiveness.

◆ ◆ ◆

In a Nutshell

Moderating variables identify the conditions under which the relationship between two variables might be stronger or weaker.

◆ ◆ ◆

Measuring Behavioral Variables

Think about how to measure a rather simple variable, a behavior, such as smoking cigarettes. All of us have seen individuals smoking so we know what the behavior involves or looks like. Some of us are "experts" on smoking because we may have tried smoking cigarettes in the past, or we may be (hopefully not) a current smoker.

Tobacco use is important from a public health perspective because 430,000 deaths each year in the United States are attributable to smoking. This figure is more than the combined deaths from suicide, homicide, automobile accidents, alcohol, drug abuse, and HIV/AIDS. Second, smoking is a leading cause of cardiovascular disease, the leading cause of death in the United States. Third, 90 percent of lung cancer is attributable to smoking. Simply put, there is no other health-related variable as important as smoking in terms of its consequences for society.

Given the enormous consequences from smoking, it is essential that we understand how to measure this behavior so that valid and useful conclusions can be drawn from our research. Therefore, in this section we will review some of the ways that smoking is measured in both observational and experimental studies. In almost all studies individuals are asked to self-report their behavior on either a self-administered questionnaire or to an interviewer.

Lifetime Experience with Smoking. An example of a question designed to measure lifetime experience with smoking specifies that "ever" smoking includes as little as taking even a puff from a cigarette. Consider the following example.

Have you ever tried cigarette smoking, even a puff? (mark one box)

❏ Yes

❏ No

There is nothing inherently wrong with this question. One could presume that a "yes" is different from a "no," and that those who have ever smoked may be different from those who have never smoked. One goal of prevention in tobacco use is to increase the number and percentage of the population that has never tried cigarettes. However, this is a very gross measurement. It tells us nothing about when in a person's life they had this experience. Presumably, those who try cigarettes earlier in their life rather than later may be different on a number of dimensions. Presumably, the earlier that people try cigarettes, the more likely they are to continue. These are hypotheses that require more precise measurement than *ever* versus *never*. The ever-never dichotomy (nominal variable) doesn't tell anything about whether smoking was a transitory behavior or something that continued, perhaps increased, and became a chronic behavior pattern. Yes or no response to "ever tried smoking?" doesn't provide much data, certainly not enough information to guide the design of a health promotion program.

Recognizing the need to understand how long smoking has occurred, one could ask two questions, one about age at the onset of smoking and one about current smoking. In fact, the following question about one's first experience with smoking is also a question about lifetime ever smoking. If they provide an age at onset it means that they have smoked. If they answer that they have never smoked even a puff of a cigarette, then they are a no on ever smoking. There is also a subtle difference between the first question and the one that follows. In the ever-never question, the investigator is assuming that the person answering the question never smoked. In the question below, there is an implicit assumption that the person answering the question has smoked. They are then required to deny the behavior.

How old were you the very first time you smoked even a puff of a cigarette?
(mark one box)

❑ I have never smoked even a puff of a cigarette
❑ 8 years old or younger
❑ 9 years old
❑ 10 years old
❑ 11 years old
❑ 12 years old
❑ 13 years old
❑ 14 years old
❑ 15 years old
❑ 16 years old
❑ 17 years old
❑ 18 years old
❑ 19 years or older

The second question that will help one develop at least a preliminary picture of the extent of smoking asks about current smoking. In the tobacco field, "current" is defined as the past thirty days or past month.

During the past thirty days, on how many *days* did you smoke one or more cigarettes? (mark one box)

❑ 0 days
❑ 1 or 2 days
❑ 3 to 5 days
❑ 6 to 9 days
❑ 10 to 19 days
❑ 20 to 29 days
❑ All 30 days

This question is more precise than the previous questions. It does provide some information about current use of cigarettes. The answers to this question provide an investigator with information about the frequency of use (an ordinal variable).

We assume that current cigarette use is related to a host of other variables measured at the same time. So, from a health promotion perspective, current cigarette use could be a predictor variable that is associated with some other variable (for example, use of alcohol and other drugs, recent respiratory illnesses, or dependence on nicotine). It could be an outcome variable that is associated with epidemiological and demographic variables that have public health relevance (nominal variables such as race or ethnicity, sex, or rural urban residence, or ordinal variables such as attitudes toward tobacco use, stress, and so on).

One of the problems with subjects such as the number of days one smoked in the past thirty days is that some people may not organize their memory around thirty days, some of which may have occurred during the current month and some in the previous month. The month is a much more common organizing framework for memory. However, if the question were about the "past month," what month would we be asking about? If it were March 20, would we be asking about the nineteenth days of March or about the entire month of February? Another problem is the categorization of number of days. Ten to nineteen days covers a lot of time. One might assume that someone who has actually smoked ten days (assuming it is possible to remember accurately this number) may be different from someone who has smoked nineteen days (assuming it is possible to remember accurately this number). Therefore, the preceding question is often coupled with the following question to create a two-question measure of current cigarette use. Some of these issues related to recall are discussed in more detail in Chapter Ten.

On the days that you smoke, how many cigarettes do you typically smoke?
(mark one box)
❏ I have never smoked even a puff of a cigarette
❏ Less than 1 cigarette per day
❏ 1 to 2 cigarettes per day
❏ 3 to 7 cigarettes per day
❏ 8 to 12 cigarettes per day
❏ 13 to 17 cigarettes per day
❏ 18 to 23 cigarettes per day
❏ At least 24 cigarettes per day

This is an interesting way to measure current cigarette use. Think about how cigarettes come packaged. A pack contains twenty cigarettes. Notice that none of the categories are easily translated into one-half a pack or two packs. Regular or heavy smokers may gauge how much they smoke in terms of packs rather than individual cigarettes. Another problem with the question is that it requires the individual answering the question to engage in some mathematical computations. Most of us are not very good at such math. Another major problem with this approach to measuring a simple but evidently complex behavior is the assumption that smokers are consistent from day to day in how much they smoke. This may be true for individuals who have been smoking for some time. For relatively new smokers, however, their pattern from day to day and week to week may be erratic.

These limitations can be seen most clearly in Figure 9.1. Data in the figure come from an adolescent smoker who was asked the two previous questions—number of days smoked and number of cigarettes per day. She reported that she smoked twenty to twenty-nine days and that she smoked eleven cigarettes a day. She was then asked to keep a daily diary of her smoking patterns.

As shown in Figure 9.1, of the thirty days in the month, the subject smoked for nineteen days (thirty minus the eleven days that she didn't smoke at all). So, in terms of the categorization, the appropriate answer would have been that she smoked ten to nineteen days, not twenty to twenty-nine days. She smoked on 63 percent of the days in that thirty-day period. She did accurately report that she smoked eleven cigarettes a day, but for only eight of the thirty days in the month. The average number of cigarettes per day was 4.9.

FIGURE 9.1.   A FEMALE ADOLESCENT'S DAILY SMOKING PATTERN.

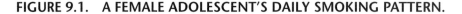

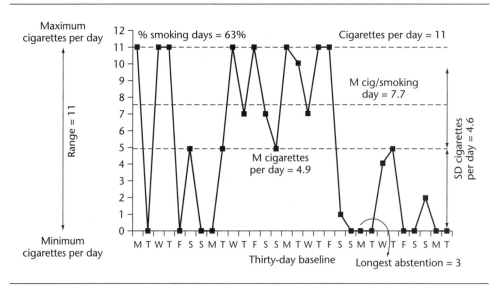

As you can see by now, measurement of a behavior, a behavior with which we are all familiar, a behavior that is based on consumption of a discrete commodity (each cigarette in a pack of twenty cigarettes is not connected to the others in the pack) is not a simple task. From a public health perspective, these examples should make it clear that our traditional approach to measuring this very important health-related behavior is fraught with limitations. In health promotion research it is critical that our measurement be valid. That is, the measures we use should represent the actual behavior as closely as possible. Next, we will attempt to show two less traditional approaches to measurement that may get us closer to understanding this very important behavior. If we are going to be successful in preventing or reducing the consequences of this behavior, it will be necessary for us to do a better job of measuring it.

A Web-Driven Approach. Thirty days is a long time. Smoking occurs in real time—in minutes and hours in a day. The burn time on a cigarette is typically five minutes—three hundred seconds. A smoker typically takes about ten puffs on a cigarette, each of which lasts about three seconds—a total of thirty seconds. This being true, a day is a long time. So, to measure the behavior accurately we have to be more precise.

One of the more modern ways to collect data, and thus measure important variables, is to use a Web-driven approach. Hypothetically, it is possible for individuals involved in a Web-driven study to answer questions at any time of day or night, seven days each week. However, until there is more experience with this approach to measurement, the most common approach is to ask study participants to complete periodic on-line questionnaires.

To illustrate how this approach to measurement works, we will report on a study conducted among 912 members of the freshman class of 2002 at Purdue University. A total of 4,690 in this freshman class completed a short, paper-and-pencil screener questionnaire in the summer during their orientation, when they received their schedule for the fall semester. Of these, 2,001 had some previous experience with cigarettes, somewhere between "just a puff" and much more involvement. These 2,001 were invited to participate in the Web-based study, and 912 agreed to participate.

In addition to completing a forty-five-minute baseline questionnaire, these freshmen participants agreed to provide weekly data (usually on a Sunday) via a secure server once a week for thirty-five weeks. They were asked specifically to report on their use of cigarettes, alcohol, and marijuana for each of the previous seven days. A logical question that you may have is, Why seven days? There are two reasons. The first is that this is a relatively short period of time, less time available for the memory to decay. Second, most people, particularly students,

FIGURE 9.2. CIGARETTES PER DAY AVERAGED OVER EACH WEEK.

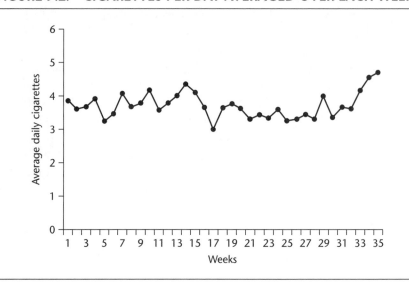

think about their life in terms of weeks. Simply put, the investigators were concerned about the reliability of the data, and a seven-day period of recall seemed reasonable to collect "close to real time" data. Furthermore, because these data were collected on the Web, every response was day and time dated, so it was possible to know when the data were provided and what reference point was being used to report the cigarette use.

> During the past seven days, about how many cigarettes did you smoke each day? If you haven't smoked on a particular day in the last week, enter "0." If you smoked less than a whole cigarette, enter "1."

Figure 9.2 shows the data on cigarettes smoked per day averaged over each of the thirty-five weeks. This is what cigarette use data look like when they reflect a smaller interval. They are still subject to the concerns often raised about self-report data (see Chapter Ten for an in-depth discussion of self-reported data).

The data can be broken down even further to obtain more precision for each week reported. Figure 9.3 indicates the average number of cigarettes per day reported by the sample of 912 freshmen for the period. Every individual in the study who reported smoking had a trajectory of smoking. Therefore, it is possible to show the trajectory for each individual (see Figure 9.1) or, as is the case for Figures 9.2 and 9.3, data are aggregated for the entire sample.

FIGURE 9.3.   CIGARETTES: AVERAGE DAILY NUMBER.

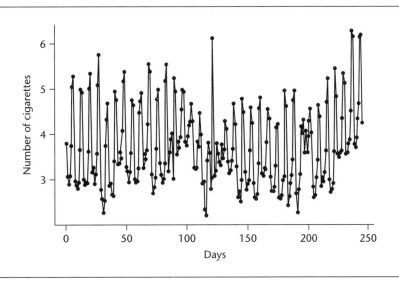

Figure 9.4 breaks the data down even further to show smoking behavior on days when both smoking and drinking occurred. The added dimension of "drinking behavior" provides an interesting context that helps enrich the understanding of smoking. College students will immediately recognize what is happening with these freshmen. Their smoking is mostly low on Sunday, Monday, Tuesday, and Wednesday. However, smoking in this sample is higher on Thursday than on the previous days. The first question that comes to mind is, Is Thursday a weekday or part of the weekend? The second question is, Why the higher rates of use of cigarettes on Friday and Saturday? The answer to this question is simple—this is when students tend to party. As Figure 9.4 indicates, there is a strong connection between smoking and drinking among college freshmen. In fact, a careful examination of the data in Figure 9.4 reveals that over 50 percent of the cigarettes smoked on Friday and Saturday were smoked while students were drinking. Although sophomores, juniors, and seniors were not studied, the data suggest that similar patterns would most likely be found for these students.

In Figure 9.3, the daily smoking data were reviewed for the first thirty-five weeks. Much more precise data allow an investigator to ask a number of questions that are not possible with less precise data. For example, the investigators in the Purdue study asked, What is the highest Thursday with regard to smoking? The answer is Halloween. They also asked about the lowest and highest smoking day for the first semester. You can probably guess the answer. The lowest day was

FIGURE 9.4. AVERAGE PROPORTION OF CIGARETTES SMOKED WHILE DRINKING ON DAYS THAT SMOKING WAS REPORTED.

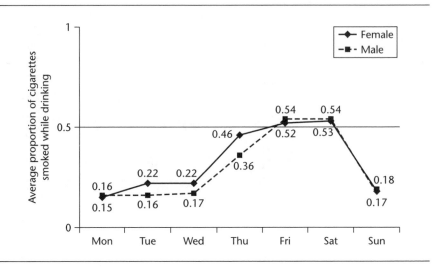

Christmas Day when the students were probably with their parents, who may not know of their smoking. The highest day was seven days later—you guessed it—New Year's Eve.

New Strategies for the Measurement of Behavioral Variables. There is every reason to believe that with improvements in technology there will be a number of new and exciting ways to measure health-related behaviors, which are vitally important to health promotion in particular and to public health in general. One of the more recent developments has been the personal digital assistant (PDA) and the hand-held computer, while there has been a parallel development in observational approaches for data collection known as Ecological Momentary Assessment (EMA). EMA is an outstanding example of an innovative strategy made possible with technological advancements. EMA can greatly improve the reliability and validity of measures pertaining to smoking behavior.

To illustrate the application of EMA to smoking behavior, it is important first to establish several points. The time interval between initially trying cigarettes and becoming a regular user is about two to three years on average. The progression from experimentation to regular use, and often addiction, involves multiple social, psychological, and biological factors, all of which should be measured as reliably and validly as possible. There is evidence that these factors may contribute differentially to stages of transition in smoking. However, this stage categorization may be an artifact of an over-reliance on retrospective questionnaire measures, long periods between observations, and statistical treatment dictums. Only a few studies have examined whether there are differential predictors of stages of smoking. They suggest that stages of transition in smoking may be artificial and that development of dependence on nicotine may be more of a continuum than a switching point. Past research on smoking has usually measured smoking in very gross ways and often on a yearly basis using self-reports of smoking in the past thirty days as "the" measure of smoking. Thus, the lack of precision in some of this research may have contributed to a conceptualization of smoking behavior in "stages" rather than on a continuum.

Although smoking is a behavior exhibited by individuals, smoking among adolescents may occur more frequently within certain contexts. EMA provides a window into the lives of adolescents and serves as a way of examining the influences of specific contexts. EMA is able to capture more accurately than other measurement approaches the frequency, intensity, and tone of social experiences as they occur, as well as the mood associated with those exchanges. EMA data can be collected by PDAs or hand-held computers (Shiffman, 2000). These are used to collect data on adolescents' lives and smoking episodes in real time.

How does EMA work? One study by Mermelstein and her colleagues had the adolescents carry PDAs for seven consecutive days every six months (Mermelstein, Hedegar, and Flay, in press). They were trained to respond to *random prompt interviews* (the PDA or hand-held is programmed to beep randomly, thereby prompting participants to answer questions) and also to self-initiate recordings both of smoking episodes and of no-smoke events (defined as times when the adolescent considers smoking, has an opportunity to smoke, but makes an active decision not to smoke). The interviews took approximately sixty to ninety seconds to complete and asked about mood, activity (what the adolescent was doing), companionship (with whom or alone), presence of other smokers, where they were, and other behaviors (eating, drinking, substance use). At the end of each data-collection week, adolescents underwent an extensive semistructured qualitative interview about their experiences during the week and also reported on their past six-month smoking through a *time-line follow-back interview*. In this type of interview, study participants are asked to recall events as they occurred (that is, in chronological order).

So, do EMAs facilitate adolescents' reporting of their smoking behavior? The average number of random prompts answered during the week of data collection was 33.5. The average number of missed prompts was 5.7. On average, the adolescents answered 85 percent of the random prompt interviews. A total of 89 percent of the prompts were answered within three minutes. There may be times when adolescents can't answer a prompt. In this measurement strategy they can suspend the hand-held computer for up to two hours at a time when it would be difficult to respond. There was, however, some data loss due to damage to the equipment. In follow-up assessments compliance to prompts was about 90 percent.

Compliance with any data-measurement approach is important. Being able to embed the behavioral patterns in situational contexts is also important. We need to know who is doing what with whom, where, how, and of course, why. The *what*, the behavior, can be readily measured in close to real time using EMA, especially if the PDA or hand-held alerts the participant on multiple occasions every day for some specified period. The *who* involves strategic selection of samples that are meaningfully different on important characteristics. The *with whom* and *where* can be measured by simple questions inserted into the computer program. The *why* is also possible by asking specific questions about proximal events and circumstances, such as those that are occurring at the time the PDA or hand-held beeps and asks the participant to provide some answers. For example, Mermelstein and her colleagues were interested in the association of positive and negative mood with smoking (Mermelstein, Hedegar, and Flay, in press). It appears that among adults who smoke, smoking events are more likely to occur in negative-mood situations (depression, anger, anxious). Among adolescents, many of whom are new smokers, the question was whether smoking events were more likely to occur simultaneously with positive rather than negative mood states.

In addition to measuring behaviors and their contextual influences, another application for EMA is with program evaluation. A good example might be the measurement of the influence of certain media events (a health promotion campaign) to see whether people are exposed to the public service announcement by beeping them following the appearance of the PSA on a particular station. By knowing who is watching what programs, it might be possible to more strategically place the health promotion ads and to tailor them for specific types of individuals.

In addition to using EMA with PDAs and hand-helds, consider other new technologies that are either brand new to the health promotion field or close to being tested. For example, in response to the question of *where* certain behavioral events are occurring, it is now possible for the hand-held computer to use a GPS (global positioning system) technology to pinpoint exactly where the person is when he or she is beeped. To determine *with whom* certain behavioral events are occurring, it is now possible to use cameras built into PDAs and hand-helds to get a picture of the space from all four points of the compass. This may create some problems with regard to human subjects' issues, but the limitation is not with the technology. With regard to *why*, there are a host of portable measurement devices that can simultaneously assess heart rate, blood pressure, and a number of other potentially relevant biometric variables.

Finally, think about the fact that every individual is embedded in a variety of contexts. Think about those contexts as if the individual were a pebble dropped in a calm pool or lake. The circles emanating from the pebble (individual) represent the contexts in which he or she is embedded from the most intimate to the most distal. We need better ways of measuring all of the spaces between the various waves coming from the center. This might include, with regard to smoking, the rules and policies present in the home regarding smoking, the rules and policies regarding smoking at school and the programming designed to prevent or treat smoking, laws regarding point of purchase advertising, the rules and policies regarding environmental tobacco smoke, and the laws that vary from state to state about state excise taxes on tobacco products.

Measurement of Contextual Variables

In the previous section we have outlined a host of issues regarding measurement. In addition to understanding how best to measure the behavior of individuals, we also need to measure the contexts within which they are embedded and the influence of certain contextual factors on behavior. This moves us back into the "population"-based world of public health where, in order to change behavior, we have to implement interventions that have broad reach and penetration— interventions that attempt to change behavior through changing the environmental constraints within which individuals live their lives.

In health promotion we are interested in knowing whether and how individuals change their health-related behaviors over time. We also recognize that individuals are embedded in ecological contexts that have a great deal of influence on these health-related behaviors. To understand who and what needs to be changed, it is critical that these contexts be measured reliably and with validity.

There is a plethora of contexts in which individuals may be embedded. This includes families, peer groups, neighborhoods, communities, counties, states, and nations. There is also a variety of organizational contexts such as schools, religious organizations (church-synagogue-mosque), and work organizations (a particular company or a work group within that company) that are potentially important in understanding how and why behaviors change for some and not for other individuals. We will not describe all of the different ways that each of these contexts can be measured. Instead, we will use one of these contexts, the family, to illustrate the difficulties inherent in the measurement of contextual variables.

In studying changes in health behavior it is possible that families exert an influence on the individuals embedded in them to change, or to not change. Think about this for a moment. If we were to treat *family* as a variable to be measured in a health promotion study, how would you measure it? Would you develop a nominal variable? Families have many different dimensions, and as such, it is important to measure these. One of these dimensions is structure. Structure is composed of the different roles that individuals play within families. These roles are mother, father, child, only child, oldest child, second, third, and so on child, youngest child, grandmother, grandfather, aunt, uncle, cousin, and so on. Should we try to create a nominal variable that includes all of the potential structures? If so, then this variable would have too many attributes, rendering the variable impractical for application. In the 1960s Sheppard Kellam and his colleagues began a longitudinal study of first-graders and their families who lived in Wood-lawn, a neighborhood in Chicago. Virtually all of the residents of Woodlawn were African American. Kellam asked a rather simple question of these first-graders and their mothers to obtain a measure of family structure. He asked, Who lives with you? The answer was surprising. While many of the first-graders were living in so-called traditional family structures (mother-father-children, mother-children, father-children), overall, there were close to seventy-five different family structures in that one neighborhood. Many of these structures did not have many people in them, but they were nevertheless each a unique family structure (Kellam, Ensminger, and Turner, 1977).

So, how would a public health researcher characterize family context as a variable in this type of situation? Before we decide how to measure family context, perhaps we could use the research hypothesis to guide us. The hypothesis guiding the Kellam research was that children would be more likely to exhibit psychological well-being and social adaptation if they were in an intact family. Intact was de-fined as living in the presence of both a mother and a father. Family could therefore be a nominal variable—intact or not. However, what could be done to recognize the heterogeneity in the family structure variable? One option is to create *dummy variables* that allow for the comparison of the intact-family category to each of the other seventy-four family categories. Dummy variables are considered nominal variables that distinguish two or more attributes of the variable and can be used to code information concerning group membership into a series of binary distinc-tions (Bakeman, 1992, p. 205). One category (for example, intact-family) would be used as the referent category, and each of the other categories would be compared to it. The referent category would be coded as zero, and every other category (for example, the other family structures) would be coded as 1. A few examples from the Kellam study, which used a dummy variable coding scheme, follow.

Referent category = mother-father-child	coded as	0
Referent category = Mother-child	coded as	1
Referent category = mother-father-child	coded as	0
Referent category = Father-child	coded as	1
Reference category = mother-father-child	coded as	0
Referent category = Mother-grandmother-child	coded as	1

[Kellam, Ensminger, and Turner, 1977]

As shown, in this approach, every structural combination would be compared to the referent category, and thus the influence of each structure on the outcome variables (psychological well-being and social adaptation) could be assessed.

The importance of this approach is apparent from what Kellam and his colleagues found when these first-graders were studied again in their teen years. As teenagers, children who lived with their mother and had another adult present, regardless of who that other person was, were less likely to be involved in drug use and other forms of delinquent behavior. The conclusion was rather dramatic and counter to common beliefs of society at that time. It was that father absence is less important in predicting psychological well-being and social adaptation in children than mother aloneness. We believe this conclusion is profound because Kellam began his study at about the same time that the federal government claimed that the African American family (notice that the government did not recognize the heterogeneity) was in deep trouble because of the absence of the black male in the family. The larger lesson here is that measurement is important because it establishes boundaries and directions for the analysis, which in turn can have profound effects on the findings, interpretation, and implications of the study.

◆ ◆ ◆

In a Nutshell

Measurement is important because it establishes boundaries and directions for the analysis, which in turn can have profound effects on the findings, interpretation, and implications of the study.

◆ ◆ ◆

Applied Example

To apply some of the issues discussed, we have selected an example that pertains to how the Internet might influence certain health behaviors. The study is ongoing and has several components. One important component of the study assesses the feasibility of recording participants' Web use. One of the major strengths of the proposed research is that it measures the effects of exposure to sexual content on the Web by capturing participants' *actual exposure* to sexual content as opposed to relying entirely on self-reported exposure. This approach is possible because all Web pages visited by participants are stored, processed, and viewed electronically. The process of tracking Web usage and screening Web pages for sexual content is automated. Proprietary technology is used to allow the tracking of all the Web sites visited by individuals by running all household Web activity through a proxy server. This technology allows for capturing the URLs of Web sites visited by the study volunteers. A unique and tailored algorithm is employed. It is based on key words and predesignated categorizations to "bucket" Web sites that are coded as "adult," and to reduce the number of Web pages to be coded. This procedure results in a queue to be viewed and content analyzed for sexually explicit and sexually oriented images and text by human coders. All data are recorded using only a unique study identifier. Data are then encrypted and stored on a secured server.

Integration with the Research Process

Although measurement (step 5 in the nine-step model) appears to be a "middle step," it actually permeates decision making in steps 1 and 2. Implicit in this chapter, the measures selected must be tailored to the needs (literacy and culture) of the selected priority population. An index, for example, might have established reliability and validity for use with African American women. Does this mean that the same index will be reliable and valid for white women, Latinas, or African American men? The answer, of course, is no. The degree to which indicators constitute a construct is a function of the study population.

◆ ◆ ◆

In a Nutshell

The degree to which indicators constitute a construct is a function of the study population.

◆ ◆ ◆

The research question should also be selected with a priori attention to the question of measurement. If the research question entails assessment of a behavior such as smoking, then asking, Can I perform a procedure such as EMA? may be wise question before proceeding to set up the research project. As demonstrated in this chapter, a simple retrospective recall assessment of smoking may be far less than rigorous. The point, then, is to ensure that your available resources can match the implied needs of your research question relative to measurement.

This chapter has also shown that measurement decisions potentially can have a dramatic bearing on the research findings. This point should be at the forefront of thought when the findings are being disseminated. Part of disseminating your findings involves listing the limitations of your study (see Chapter Fourteen). Without question, the most common limitations are those related to measurement. This is particularly true with respect to the issue of validity (again, this is also why Chapter Ten addresses the validity of self-reported measures in greater detail).

Summary

Achieving rigor in measurement can be a vast undertaking. Once the level of measurement (nominal, ordinal, interval, or ratio) for any given variable is determined, the task is to decide how the variable will be used. Essentially, the research team must determine what variables will be designated as predictor variables (or correlates if a cross-sectional design has been used), mediating variables, moderating variables, and outcome variables. If the design is experimental, the same question applies, except the terms *independent variable* and *dependent variable* replace *predictor* and *outcome*, respectively. Once all the necessary variables have been identified, the task becomes one of determining how each will be measured. For variables that represent constructs, the additional task is to create an operational definition of the concept being measured. Although variables such as age, gender, income, and education level are relatively easy to measure, the assessment of variables such as smoking frequency or self-esteem may pose tremendous challenges to the research team. This challenge brings several issues to the table. Among these issues are the length of the recall period, the wording of the question(s), the response alternatives, and the technique that will be employed to actually collect the data. Although long-standing techniques such as paper-and-pencil questionnaires may serve the research question well, advances in technology have created a host of new options that may add to the validity of the measure. Moreover, these innovations may be very useful for assessing the context of behavior rather than simply the behavior in isolation.

Issues to Consider

1. Given that *how* a variable is measured can greatly influence the obtained value, it may be critically important to consider how findings from any given study may have been much different based on the use of a different measurement protocol. For example, a descriptive study may conclude that "49 percent of American teens report they have ever smoked a cigarette." Such a finding would result from the use of a question that simply asked teens, Have you

ever smoked a cigarette? The issue to consider is, What value does this type of information have for health promotion research and public health?

2. Suppose that you read a journal article which concludes, "Our findings support the hypothesis that women who have low self-esteem are less likely to eat a balanced diet than women who do not have low self-esteem." The finding is intriguing. But, upon reflection, you remember reading that the inter-item reliability alpha for the measure of self-esteem was .59. You also find no evidence in the article that the measure of self-esteem was validated. Unfortunately, this type of scenario is all too common in health promotion research. The issue, then, is, How can this type of potentially misleading dissemination be avoided?

For Practice and Discussion

1. Please refer back to the first Issue to Consider. You may have answered that the value is quite small because the measure does not capture habitual use. More specifically, the question that is not addressed is, What percentage of American teens smoke cigarettes habitually? Given this research question, how would you proceed to measure "habitual use"?

2. Please return for a moment to the second Issue to Consider. Imagine that you have decided to replicate this study. How would you go about achieving each of the following tasks?
   - Operationalize isolation
   - Identify indicators of isolation
   - Establish reliability of the index
   - Establish face and content validity of the index
   - Collect data from women without recall periods of more than forty-eight hours

3. Please return for a moment to the portion of this chapter that describes EMA. In particular, the data shown in Figure 9.3 are quite striking. These data suggest the possibility that the finely tuned measures may produce results that have previously been masked by the use of less precise measures. While EMA has been applied to the outcome variables of smoking behaviors and sexual behaviors, it is nonetheless a relatively new technology as applied to health promotion research. Please identify at least three other outcome variables (or dependent variables) that you believe would have a much different complexion if they were assessed by EMA rather than traditional retrospective recall methods.

References

Andrews, F. M., and Withey, S. B. (1976). *Social indicators of well-being: Americans' perceptions of life quality.* New York: Plenum.

Bakeman, R. (1992). *Understanding social science statistics: A spreadsheet approach.* Hillsdale, NJ: Erlbaum.

Beck, A. T., Ward, C. H., Mendelson, M., Mock, J., and Erbaugh, J. (1961). An inventory for measuring depression. *Archives of General Psychiatry, 4,* 561–571.

Department of Health and Human Services. (2000). Healthy people 2010. Retrieved March 10, 2005, from www.health.gov/healthypeople.

Ghiselli, E. E., Campbell, J. P., and Zedeck, S. (1982). *Measurement theory for the behavioral sciences.* New York: W. H. Freeman.

Kellam, S. G., Ensminger, M. E., and Turner, R. J. (1977). Family structure and the mental health of children. *Archives of General Psychiatry, 34,* 1012–1022.

Mermelstein, R., Hedegar, D., & Flay, B. (in press). Real-time capture and adolescent cigarette smoking: Moods and smoking. In A. Stone, S. Shiffman, and A. Atienza (Eds.), *The science of real-time data capture: Self-report health research.* New York: Oxford University Press.

Radloff, L. S. (1977). The CES-D scale: A self-report depression scale for research in the general population. *Applied Psychological Measurement, 1*(3), 385–401.

Rosenberg, M. (1989). *Society and the adolescent self-image* (Rev. ed.). Middletown, CT: Wesleyan University Press.

Shiffman, S. (2000). Real-time self-report of momentary states in the natural environment: Computerized ecological momentary assessment. In A. A. Stone (Ed.), *The science of self-report: Implications for research and practice.* Mahwah, NJ: Lawrence Erlbaum.

Streiner, D. L. (2003). Being inconsistent about consistency: When coefficient alpha does and doesn't matter. *Journal of Personality Assessment, 80*(3), 217–222.

CHAPTER TEN

IMPROVING VALIDITY OF SELF-REPORTS FOR SENSITIVE BEHAVIORS

Rick S. Zimmerman, Katherine A. Atwood, and Pamela K. Cupp

The important outcomes in health promotion research and interventions are often behaviors, such as smoking, condom use, and breast self-examination. For a variety of reasons, people often feel a bit uncomfortable about telling the truth in reporting health or risk behaviors, lest they feel they have let their educators or instructors down (for example, what foods they have eaten that they weren't supposed to eat or how often (or little) they came to the gym to work out), or they may not feel comfortable talking about other behaviors at all (for example, about marijuana use or having sex without a condom).

◆ ◆ ◆

In a Nutshell

People often feel a bit uncomfortable about telling the truth in reporting health or risk behaviors.

◆ ◆ ◆

Valid and reliable measurements of sensitive risk behaviors, such as drug use and sexual behaviors, are important for a number of reasons. Accurate measurements of sensitive behaviors allow researchers to estimate their prevalence in the population, which is needed for adequate resource allocation and planning. Careful measurement of these behaviors helps researchers assess the characteristics of the person and the environment associated with risk, and aids in the development of theoretical models of behavior change. In addition, valid and reliable measurements of sensitive behaviors allow for more rigorous evaluation of the very programs designed to reduce their prevalence in the population.

This chapter focuses on how to address threats to validity when measuring sensitive behaviors. For the purposes of illustration, we focus on two sensitive behaviors, drug use and sexual activity. We use these examples to demonstrate how biases can emerge when obtaining estimates of self-reported behaviors and what can be done during the design and administration of surveys to reduce these biases.

Illustration of Key Concepts

We will present the chapter in two sections. First, we present issues to consider related to cognitive processes in improving validity of reports of sensitive behaviors. Second, we present issues to consider related to situational factors in improving validity of these self-reports. We conclude by reviewing evidence about the use of objective or unobtrusive measures to provide additional validation of survey responses.

Validity and Reliability

Let's start by defining what we mean when we talk about validity and reliability and then clarify the focus of this chapter. First, validity has two kinds of possible meanings in research: sometimes we talk about the (internal or external) validity of a study or research design, but we can also talk about validity of a measure. The internal validity of a study or research design is the extent to which we are able to derive clear, causal conclusions from our study; the external validity of a study or research design is the extent to which we are able to generalize to a specific population or other populations beyond those involved in our study.

Our focus in this chapter is on the validity of measures used in health promotion interventions and research. Validity is the degree to which a survey item and its response alternatives measure the phenomenon they are suppose to measure (Bainbridge, 1989). Put differently, it is the extent to which our variables in fact measure the constructs we intend for them to measure. For example, it has been reported that some scientists in the early 1900s believed that one's hat size was associated with intelligence. However, we know that this is not true. So asking about someone's hat size is not a valid measure of intelligence (Bainbridge, 1989). There are several different kinds of validity of measures: two types related to the issues to be discussed in this chapter are *construct validity* and *criterion validity*. Construct validity is defined as the extent to which a measure relates to other measures in theoretically predictable ways. Construct validity can be assessed in studies of adolescent sexual behavior by examining how age of initiation of sexual activity is related to age of initiation of alcohol use, cigarette or marijuana smoking, or frequency of delinquent behaviors, as these behaviors often have been found in previous research to be related to early initiation of sexual activity. A measure can be considered to have strong construct validity when it is significantly correlated with these other variables, or these other factors account for a reasonable proportion of the variance in the sexual behavior measure.

◆ ◆ ◆

In a Nutshell

Validity is the degree to which a survey item and its response alternatives measure the phenomenon they are suppose to measure.

◆ ◆ ◆

Criterion validity is the relationship of a measure to an outcome to which, by the very definition of the measure, it should be related. The SAT (scholastic aptitude test) was created to predict college success; the correlations between the SAT and measures of college success are ways to assess the criterion validity of the SAT. If a self-report measure of condom use were to have high criterion validity, it should be related to a measure of condom sales in the community. If, for people treated for any current STDs, it is unrelated to incidence of new STDs over the next six months, it would be said to have low criterion validity. Both of these types of validity are used by researchers in assessing the validity of measures, and will be referred to throughout the chapter.

Besides validity, the other key dimension for assessing the quality of a measure is reliability. *Reliability* is the degree to which a measure produces stable and consistent results (Bainbridge, 1989). It is important to note that a measure cannot be valid without also being reliable. If a measure of condom use yields different responses every time a respondent answers the measure, how could it possibly be a good, that is, valid, measure of condom use? However, an item can be reliable (give consistent results) and not be valid; asking people how many fingers they have will provide consistent results, though it is probably not a valid measure of number of sexual partners in the past twelve months for most respondents. Because of this relationship between reliability and validity, that reliability is a necessary though not sufficient condition for validity, evidence of reliability can yield greater confidence about the validity of the measure, and so some of the data presented in this chapter concerning validity also references evidence about reliability of measures.

In the section that follows, we discuss the sources of validity problems that may emerge when obtaining self-report data on sensitive behavior. To help organize the discussion about threats to validity, we use Brener and colleagues' definitions of two theoretical perspectives, under which most threats to validity can be organized: (1) cognitive processes and (2) situational processes (Brener, Billy, and Grady, 2003). *Cognitive processes* are defined as the "mental processes underlying self-reported data." These processes are responsible for the inaccurate reporting of events that arise from problems with comprehension of the survey question, recalling relevant events, and placing them in the appropriate time frame (Brener, Billy, and Grady, 2003). *Situational processes* are defined as "problems that arise from factors related to social desirability and interviewing conditions" (Brener, Billy, and Grady, 2003).

Threats to Validity of Self-Report Data Due to Cognitive Processes

The cognitive process of retrieving information from one's memory is said to involve four distinct steps, though more detailed models have been developed to describe this process of retrieval (Oksenberg and Cannell, 1977; Cannell, Miller, and Oksenberg, 1981; Means, Habina, Swan, and Jack, 1992). Threats to validity can occur at each of these steps (Brener, Billy, and Grady, 2003).

Step 1: Comprehension of the Question. The first step involves comprehension of the question. Comprehension is the way in which the respondent understands the question. Understanding involves prior knowledge and experience, how the interviewer interacts with the respondent, perceived goals of the research, and implicit messages communicated by previous survey questions (Means, Habina, Swan, and Jack, 1992).

Step 2: Retrieval of Information. The second step involves retrieval of the information. Retrieval of information requires scanning one's memory and rebuilding the event based on what can be retrieved and then "filling in the gaps" to produce a coherent response (Means, Habina, Swan, and Jack, 1992; Loftus, Smith, Johnson, and Fiedler, 1988). The respondent is often unable to distinguish between what comes directly from his or her memory bank and what has been reconstructed. The process of "reconstruction" allows respondents to provide responses to questions, instead of blurred memories, but can also lead to inaccurate reporting (Loftus, Smith, Johnson, and Fiedler, 1988).

Step 3: Judgment Process. The third step is when one assesses whether the information retrieved is sufficient, referred to as the judgment process. If the information is insufficient, additional retrieval attempts are made. Even after repeated retrieval attempts, the information that is retrieved will not necessarily conform to the parameters of the question. The respondent may use his or her own heuristics (which vary from person to person) to arrive at an estimate, based on the information retrieved (Means, Habina, Swan, and Jack, 1992).

Step 4: Response Generation. The last step is response generation. During this step, the retrieval information is reviewed to assess the extent to which the response is reflective of the respondent's belief system (Brener, Billy, and Grady, 2003) and whether the response meets the needs of the interviewer (see Figure 10.1). Situational factors such as the setting and circumstances of survey administration can affect these four steps of cognitive processing. Brener and colleagues (2003) point out that cognitive and situational factors can overlap or act independently to create bias in survey responses.

Now that we have described the cognitive processes involved in information retrieval and response formulation, let us turn our attention to what can be done when designing surveys to reduce inaccurate reporting of sensitive behaviors.

FIGURE 10.1.   MODEL OF THE COGNITIVE PROCESS OF INFORMATION RETRIEVAL.

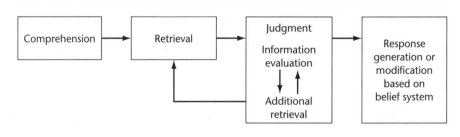

Source: Brener, Billy, and Grady, 2003.

Frequency and Timing. One of the challenges of survey construction is how to word questions about sensitive behaviors to yield accurate responses. The retrieval of information from one's memory is made even more challenging when the behavior involves licit or illicit drug use. A general rule is, the simpler the question, the more accurate the reporting. For example, it is easier to remember whether you have ever engaged in a behavior (such as using a drug or having sexual intercourse) than having to estimate the numbers of times you have engaged in that specific behavior in the past thirty days or in the past year.

◆ ◆ ◆

In a Nutshell

A general rule is, the simpler the question, the more accurate the reporting.

◆ ◆ ◆

When it is necessary to ask more detailed questions about the frequency of a given behavior, estimates are generally more valid when the question asks about the more recent past and shorter time periods (Brener, Billy, and Grady, 2003; Forsyth, Lessler, and Hubbard, 1992). For example, in the substance abuse research, Bachman and O'Malley found that asking high school seniors about the past thirty days of drug use yielded year-long prevalence rates that were approximately three times larger than reports of use in the past year (Bachman and O'Malley, 1981). They reached these estimates by extrapolating twelve months of use from usage over the past thirty days. Their findings were consistent across licit and illicit drugs and different levels of use. In this example it is possible that one of two things were going on: respondents were overreporting their drug use in the shorter time periods, or they were underreporting their use over the past year (Bachman and O'Malley, 1981). It is possible that respondents may overreport behaviors in the past thirty days due to *telescoping*—recollecting events that occur in the past several months and attributing them to the past thirty-day time period. However, researchers tend to concur that as the time from the event increases, the validity of responses deteriorates. This has been found in a wide variety of studies comparing self-report data to external records such as medical records, consumer purchases, and financial statements. For example, in a recent study that examined participants' reports of drug use during sex, fewer inaccuracies were found when the event occurred more recently than when the event occurred in the more distant past (Bell, Montoya, and Atkinson, 2000). In these cases respondents tend not to remember events as well in the distant past as they do in the more recent past.

Although recalling events in the more recent past may improve accuracy, there are some drawbacks to this approach. A thirty-day time period, for example, may not be long enough to capture sufficient numbers of events for meaningful statistical analysis. This is often the case when researching adolescent sexual or drug use behaviors. In these cases, researchers may need to rely on questions that ask about past behaviors over longer time periods.

When surveying substance-using populations, especially treatment populations (in other words, people currently receiving therapy for their addictions), measurement issues can be even more complex. Treatment populations tend to provide more valid estimates of use when the measurement is *more distant* than more recent (Willis, 1997). Substance users are more willing to report past drug use than recent use due to socially desirable responding or fears of reprisal. For example, treatment populations in particular may fear that if they admit to recent drug use certain benefits may be taken away, or others will hold less than favorable opinions about them. Parallel results were found for reports of masturbation, a sensitive sexual behavior which young adult males said they had done as adolescents at much higher rates than they had reported while adolescents (Halpern, Udry, Suchindran, and Campbell, 2000).

Like all elements of designing and implementing research, one must constantly weigh the costs and benefits of certain approaches to survey measurement. For example, in surveys for active drug users, the quality of the information may be compromised when asking about behaviors in the distant past. However, this bias must be weighed against possible invalid reporting of recent drug use if respondents revise their answers to present themselves in a more favorable light.

Retrospective or Longitudinal Assessment of Change.

The way that time is conceptualized and assessed in surveys may affect the validity of self-report data in that respondents are asked to measure their own levels of change. Due to the very nature of cross-sectional surveys (data collection at one time point only), if one is interested in assessing respondents' change in some behaviors or attitudes, one must ask the respondent to *estimate* his or her change over time. However, in longitudinal designs, researchers can assess differences between reports of attitudes or behaviors at two or more time points by calculating differences between those reports given at different times. Which assessment strategy is more valid? Common sense, as well as many studies conducted to assess results of interventions, suggests that people are prone to overreport positive changes when reporting retrospectively, as compared with researchers' calculations of differences between pre- and postintervention change. Some recent research, however, suggests that under certain circumstances, retrospective reports may be more accurate (Stone, Catania, and Binson, 1999).

Placement and the Sequencing of Questions. Decisions about the order of survey questions involve a series of strategic decisions. In some circumstances, such as in face-to-face interviews, when it is important for the interviewer to develop a relationship with the respondent, the placement of questions within the survey may make a difference (that is, whether toward the beginning, in the middle, or near the end). For example, to increase the likelihood that respondents will answer sensitive questions, the optimal place for them is in the middle of the survey. By this time, rapport has been established and respondents will have successfully answered questions about less emotionally charged topics. Conversely, by the end of the survey participants may be experiencing fatigue, boredom, or annoyance with the survey process (Bachman and O'Malley, 1981).

However, in self-administered surveys of college students and young adults, other researchers have found that the placement of questions near the beginning, middle, or end of the survey has little impact on the validity of responses to questions about sexual behaviors (Catania, McDermott, and Pollack, 1986). It has been proposed that it is not so much the placement but the "sequencing" or context of questions (near, before, or after certain other questions) that may affect validity (Catania, Binson, Van der Straten, and Stone, 1995). For example, asking questions about a person's attitudes about a specific behavior first may affect the "social meaning" (Catania, Binson, Van der Straten, and Stone, 1995) of the behavior and reduce socially desirable responding about the behavior. Johnson found that married couples reported higher levels of extramarital affairs when questions about their attitudes about affairs preceded questions about having an affair, as compared to reported levels of infidelity when attitude questions appeared after behavior questions (Johnson, 1970). It is suggested that attitudinal questions implicitly communicate to the respondent that they will not be judged for having attitudes that support these behaviors or for engaging in these behaviors (Catania, Binson, Van der Straten, and Stone, 1995).

Daily Data Collection. Daily data collection is another approach that is used to increase the accuracy of self-report data and reduce measurement error by reducing errors attributable to retrospective recall. Using this method the respondent completes either a daily diary or a phone interview detailing his or her daily behaviors. Those involved in a diary study make notes about their target behaviors and send the diary back to the research team at scheduled intervals (for example, each day or each week). One advantage of daily diaries over the phone interview method is that the respondent has greater flexibility since he or she doesn't have to schedule phone calls with the research team. However, diaries may not be successfully completed and mailed, particularly among higher-risk populations who tend to lead disruptive lives and experience low literacy rates. Another benefit of daily diaries over telephone interviews is that the data may be less affected by socially desirable responding because the diaries are completed privately. Using the phone interview approach, either the interviewer or the respondent initiates a daily call to obtain or provide information about behaviors that occurred since the last call. Having the respondent initiate contact with the research staff leads to increased flexibility for the participant; however if the respondent forgets to call, entire days of recording can be missed (Morrison, Leigh, and Rogers, 1999). The advantage of having the interviewer initiate contact with the respondent is that missing days may be minimized because the burden is left on the interviewer to reach the respondent; however disconnected phones can become a significant problem for transient populations. In addition, the interviewer may call when others are present, introducing further bias if the participant responds differently because of the presence of a third party.

There are significant drawbacks to either of these methods. In each of these approaches, researchers tend to include both sensitive and nonsensitive behaviors (for example, physical activities levels, care use) and to nest hypotheses into a larger questionnaire about health behaviors to reduce socially desirable responding (Morrison, Leigh, and Rogers, 1999). Unfortunately, this leads to longer questionnaires. A final concern is *reactivity*. Reactivity has been described as changes in behavior that occur due to the frequent recording of the behavior and the implicit message that this behavior is nondesirable or merits changing (Fremouw and Brown, 1980; Gillmore and others, 2001). It is problematic if surveys designed to simply *assess* behaviors implicitly encourage *change* in these behaviors. The research literature is mixed regarding the extent to which reactivity affects the validity of data collected using daily collection strategies (Fremouw and Brown, 1980; Gillmore and others, 2001).

In response to some of these concerns, a more innovative method that has been used is the *experience sampling method*. Using this method a respondent is paged, or beeped, at random times during the day, and he or she provides responses at that moment. This method can reduce recall bias and reactivity because respondents are more likely to remember the event, cannot anticipate when they will be contacted, and will have less opportunity to alter or rehearse responses. This method may *not* be useful for behaviors such as sexual intercourse that do not occur at predictable times, nor appropriate for institutional settings, where beeping the respondent may be considered intrusive (Kubey, Larson, and Csikszentmihalyi, 1996). Table 10.1 summarizes the discussion of the past several pages, presenting

TABLE 10.1. ADVANTAGES AND DISADVANTAGES OF APPROACHES RELATED TO COGNITIVE FACTORS.

Survey Construction	Advantages	Disadvantages
1. Frequency and timing	Enhances recall	Problematic for sporadic behaviors
Dichotomous questions	Yields higher prevalence	May over-report due to telescoping
More recent reports	Improves accuracy	Reduces number of events for statistical analysis
2. Retrospective versus longitudinal reports of changes	Not well understood	Not well understood
3. Placement and sequencing	Middle of interview best Appropriate context may yield higher prevalence	
4. Daily data collection	Enhances recall	Significant respondent burden May be inappropriate for sporadic behaviors or less stable populations Increased recall bias if diaries completed days later Reactivity possible

advantages and disadvantages of various survey approaches that relate to cognitive factors in the completion of those surveys.

Threats to Validity of Self-Reports Due to Situational Processes

Situational factors are defined as "characteristics of the external environment" (Brener, Billy, and Grady, 2003). Situational factors are factors related to socially desirable responding and interviewing conditions, such as the real or perceived level of privacy and confidentiality, characteristics of the interviewer, and method of survey administration. Social desirability and fear of reprisal are two forms of bias that may be reduced or exacerbated by situational factors such as the setting and method of survey administration; how privacy and confidentiality are explained, perceived, and adhered to; characteristics of the interviewer; and how research is perceived within the broader community. Socially desirable responding takes place when subjects respond to questions in such a way that their responses will leave a more favorable impression on others (DeMaio, 1984). For example,

MINCUS HAS DOUBTS ABOUT SELF-REPORTED BEHAVIOR.

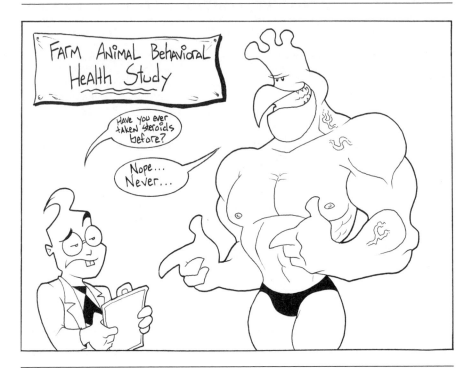

Copyright 2005 by Justin Wagner; reprinted with permission.

respondents may be less inclined to report current drug use if an interviewer administers the survey as opposed to the survey being self-administered.

Fears of reprisal are a second threat to validity that can be affected by situational factors. For example, fear of reprisal may arise when interviewing adolescents or in-treatment populations about illicit drug use; respondents may be concerned that this information could be disclosed to others such as administrators, parents, or teachers. In the following sections we review a variety of situational factors and examine how they may affect the validity of survey responses.

Mode of Survey Administration. Overall, respondents tend to report a higher prevalence of sensitive behaviors when the survey is self-administered—in other words, completed by the subject, rather than by the interviewer. Self-administered questionnaires (SAQ) have been found to yield a higher prevalence for a number of sensitive behaviors including drug and alcohol use, condom use, and number of sexual partners when compared with face-to-face interviews or telephone surveys (Catania, Gibson, Chitwood, and Coates, 1990; Aquilino and LoSciuto, 1990; Gfroerer and Hughes, 1991; Turner and others, 1998; Tourangeau, Jobe, Pratt, and Rasinski, 1997; Boekeloo and others, 1994).

Despite the higher prevalence of sensitive behaviors reported on self-administered questionnaires, there are some advantages to an interviewer-administered survey that should not be overlooked. For example, interviewer-administered questionnaires can significantly reduce the number of missed questions and help to ensure completeness of the interview. If the questionnaire has a more sophisticated design, interviewers also can successfully move the client through the instrument to prevent navigational problems. Many of these former "advantages" of interviews, discussed in reviews and textbooks in the 1960s through the early 1990s, can now be addressed within self-administered surveys using computer-enhanced data-collection techniques.

Computer-Enhanced Data Collection. One of the significant challenges to the validity of self-administered surveys is literacy. Recent developments in computer-assisted and audio-computer-assisted self-interviewing (A-CASI) have helped overcome measurement problems that were due to low literacy levels. These newly emerging technologies have been found to increase perceptions of privacy and reduce social desirability bias, as well as enable respondents to understand both questions and responses and to navigate complex surveys. Computer-assisted software programs have been found to yield higher rates of responding about alcohol, drug use, and sexual-risk behaviors when compared to self-administered paper surveys or interview-administered surveys. In the 1995 National Survey of Adolescent Males, subjects were randomly assigned to an A-CASI ($n = 1,361$) survey condition or self-administered paper survey condition ($n = 368$) (Turner and others, 1998). Males randomized to the A-CASI condition were significantly more likely to report engaging in some type of male-to-male sexual contact (5.5 percent versus 1.5 percent) and in injection drug use (5.2 percent versus 1.4 percent), when compared with those randomized to the paper questionnaire condition (Turner and others, 1998). They were also more likely to report other sensitive behaviors including being drunk or high during sex or having sex with someone who injected drugs. Other researchers have found that while adolescents reported higher rates of drug and alcohol use via computer-assisted assessment, young adults did not (Wright, Aquilino, and Supple, 1998). The observed effects for adolescents varied by level of stigmatization of the drug in question. For example, questions about less sensitive drugs, such as ever smoking a cigarette or ever use of alcohol, were less affected by the mode of survey administration than those about more stigmatized drugs (Wright, Aquilino, and Supple, 1998). The researchers also found that adolescents had fewer concerns about privacy and had more positive attitudes toward computer technology than did older participants (Wright, Aquilino, and Supple, 1998).

While computer-assisted technologies have been heralded as innovative and have allowed for more sophisticated survey design, some classroom-based studies using A-CASI have found no difference in prevalence estimates when compared with self-administered paper surveys (Hallfors, Khatapoush, Kadushin, Watson, and Saxe, 2000). In addition, computer-assisted technologies may be prohibitively expensive and physically cumbersome when surveying large samples. Other considerations include attention to detail in downloading and saving data and, particularly if the research occurs in high-crime areas, issues of safe transport and storage.

Three other computer-enhanced data-collection methods are telephone A-CASI (T-ACASI), touchtone data entry (TTDE), and audio-enhanced personal digital assistant (APDA) technologies. In the T-ACASI methodology, either respondents call in and listen to an interviewing system that asks questions in a standardized, prerecorded way (stopping for responses by use of the touchtone pad), or a human interviewer calls the respondent and then switches over to the recorded interview when the respondent is ready. Unlike typical phone interviews, questions are asked in a standardized way and privacy is provided even if others are in the same room through the use of the telephone touchtone pad. In the TTDE application, human interviewers ask questions over the phone that are responded through use of the touchtone pad. The APDA method involves the use of small, hand-held personal digital assistants (Palm Pilots and similar devices) by students completing surveys in the classroom, with an audio channel via earphones that "reads" the survey to the students. The technology is very similar to A-CASI, but is significantly less expensive, takes up less space, and provides a greater sense of privacy for respondents. Results to date indicate that T-ACASI (Gribble, Miller, Rogers, and Turner, 1999) and TTDE systems (Blumberg, Cynamon, Osborn, and Olson, 2003) yield greater reports of sensitive behaviors than do more traditional telephone interviewing methods, suggesting greater validity of responses. The APDA technology is still in initial testing phases by a small number of researchers, but initial results suggest it can be used effectively, is perceived as providing greater privacy, and yields less missing data than do self-administered questionnaires (Trapl and others, forthcoming). Between the time this chapter was written and the time you are reading it, undoubtedly some of the information about the usefulness of various existing technologies provided here will no longer be accurate, and new technologies not available now will probably be used to improve the validity of self-reported responses of sensitive behaviors.

Internet-Based Data Collection. Increasingly, Internet- (or Web-) based surveys are becoming standard practice. A primary advantage of Web-based surveys involves access to respondents, as researchers clearly have easy access to a variety of populations via the Web that would require more time and resources to recruit elsewhere (from general adolescent and college student populations to marginalized populations such as gay men and transgender individuals). But with that access comes questions about external validity: are those who access and respond to surveys on the Internet different in substantive and meaningful ways from respondents who might have been accessed using more standard or more random sampling procedures? Answers to this question are only beginning to emerge and seem to vary considerably across populations. They are also not directly relevant to the central issue of this chapter, as this chapter is concerned with the validity of measures and not external validity.

More relevant to our concerns here is whether responses to Web-based surveys and surveys completed in other formats (interviews, self-administered paper-and-pencil surveys, or A-CASI surveys) demonstrate comparable validity. The small amount of data available to date suggest that Web-based surveys may produce about the same level of reports of alcohol and illicit substance use as do mail or self-administered questionnaires and yield similar levels of reliability of measures. However, levels of missing data may be greater for respondents to Web-based surveys (Mustanski, 2001; Smith, 2003; McCabe, Boyd, Couper, Crawford, and D'Arch, 2002; Lenert and Skoczen, 2002; and McCabe, 2004).

Interviewer Effects. The effective training of interviewers is a key element in obtaining valid data. Regardless of the shared demographic characteristics or life experiences of the interviewer and the respondent, it is the degree to which the interviewer is able to accomplish the following that is most important: (1) enlist the cooperation of potential research subjects, (2) encourage respondents to answer questions thoughtfully, (3) ask questions in a standardized fashion that does not sway respondents, (4) take his or her time, and (5) be a good listener (Fowler, 1984). For example, if an interviewer rushes through a questionnaire, he or she leaves the impression that the respondent should move quickly, increasing the possibility of error or leaving the impression that the respondent's answers are not important (Fowler, 1984).

Other characteristics that have been assumed to affect validity include the gender, ethnicity, age, or sexual orientation of the interviewer when compared with that of the interviewee. However, it remains an underanswered empirical question as to when and under what circumstances it is necessary to match age, race, sexual orientation, or gender of the respondent and interviewer (Catania, Gibson, Chitwood, and Coates, 1990; Fowler, 1984). Some in the research community believe that both male and female respondents are more likely to report engaging in more stigmatized sexual behaviors to female interviewers than to male interviewers, but these assumptions are based more on anecdotal evidence than recent studies. Recent reviews suggest that the measurement of some sensitive behaviors may in fact yield the most valid responses when interviewers are matched to respondents on demographic characteristics (Catania, 1999).

Setting. The setting where the survey is administered is an additional important situational factor that can affect the validity of self-report data. Some studies suggest that among adolescents there is significant underreporting of sensitive behaviors (including illicit drug use and sexual behaviors) when surveys are completed in the household as compared with school settings (Kann, Brener, Warren, Collins and Giovino, 2002; Gfroerer, Wright, and Kopstein, 1997), although some earlier studies have found no such affects. For example, in an analysis of two national surveys, Kann and colleagues found that of the fourteen behaviors related to alcohol and illicit drug use, students who completed the school-based survey were significantly more likely to report higher levels of alcohol and illicit drug use than were youths responding to the household survey (Kann, Brener, Warren, Collins, and Giovino, 2002). With regard to sexual behaviors, those who completed the school-based survey were significantly more likely to report first intercourse before age thirteen, multiple sex partnerships, and use of alcohol or drugs during their last sexual encounter (Kann, Brener, Warren, Collins, and Giovino, 2002). The comparative analysis did not find differences in prevalence estimates for less stigmatizing behaviors such as physical-activity levels. Kann and colleagues concluded that privacy or perceived privacy is an important element in obtaining valid estimates of stigmatized or illicit behaviors.

When researching substance abuse behaviors among adults in institutional settings, researchers have found that the setting also can have a significant impact on data quality to the extent that respondents perceive that their privacy and confidentiality can or cannot be maintained, with potential fear of reprisal related to significant underreporting in self-report surveys among treatment and incarcerated populations.

Experimental Manipulations to Increase Validity of Self-Reports. A variety of methods to enhance the validity of self-reports have been used by survey researchers using experimental methods, that is, involving significant manipulations beyond such things as word variation and order of questions. Two promising such methods are presented here: the "Bogus Pipeline" procedure and the "Randomized Lists Technique." Information about the first is presented here, and information about the second is presented in Box 10.1.

Box 10.1. The Randomized Lists Technique: A Promising But Experimental Approach to Improving Validity in Surveys

A very interesting, creative, and promising technique to improve the validity of people's self-reports about sensitive behaviors was called by the original author (Miller, 1984) the "Item/Count Paired Lists Technique," and more recently has been called by Zimmerman and Langer (1995) the "randomized lists technique." In this approach the respondent is given a list of behaviors, which includes the sensitive behavior of interest and a set of innocuous (unrelated) items, and is instructed to report the total *number* of activities in the list that he or she has participated in. A second, randomly selected sample of respondents is given a list that is similar in all respects, except that the sensitive behavior has been removed. An estimate of the prevalence of the sensitive behavior is achieved by subtracting the mean count of items reported by respondents who received the list including the sensitive behavior, *minus* the mean count of items reported by respondents who received the list excluding the sensitive behavior. For example, let's say the researcher is interested in how many respondents used marijuana. Half of the sample of respondents then answers how many of the following they have ever done: used marijuana, lied to someone, cheated on a test, kissed someone, or killed someone. The other half indicate how many of the following they have ever done: lied to someone, cheated on a test, kissed someone, or killed someone. If the average number of things done for people responding to the first list is 3.5 and the average number of things done for people responding to the second list is 3.2, the difference of 0.3 (or 30 percent) is then the estimated proportion of people who have used marijuana.

We are aware of six reported studies that have used the technique to assess the prevalence of substance use or sexual behavior. An early test of the technique was promising, but only for young men with less than a higher education who, using this technique, were estimated to have used heroin at a higher rate than when the direct question was asked (Miller and Cisin, 1983); the researchers found little difference between direct and paired lists techniques in prevalence estimates for marijuana and cocaine use in the national household population, however (Miller, Cisin, and Harrell, 1986). Equivocal results were also found in a study conducted by Droitcour and others (1991), which found that prevalence estimates of injecting drug use and receptive anal intercourse were not significantly different from estimates based on direct questions. Some more promising results have been found more recently, however. Wimbush and Dalton (1997) found higher reports for stealing from one's company using the technique than when asking the question directly to respondents. Similarly, Zimmerman and Langer (1995) found higher reports of adolescents having had sex, using marijuana, or having sex with someone of the same gender using this technique than using direct questions, as did LaBrie and Earleywine (2000) when college students were asked about having sex, having had sex without a condom, or having sex without a condom after drinking.

(We think this is a technique that might be used more frequently to assist researchers in obtaining valid prevalence estimates of very sensitive behaviors. We would encourage you to consider using this technique in your own research!)

Researchers, specifically in the smoking-prevention field, have used various forms of the "Bogus Pipeline Procedure" in an effort to increase validity of self-reported use. The Bogus Pipeline Procedure, initially developed by Jones and Sigal (1971), instructs participants that after completion of the survey they will be asked to provide some sort of biologic marker that would presumably verify reported drug use. This procedure is "bogus" because it assures the participant that his or her substance use will be validated by a biologic measure, when it will not. Various "bogus" methods that are used include getting a saliva sample from a cotton swab or having the participant breath into a tube to detect smoking levels. Bogus pipeline procedures must be authentic enough to convince the respondent that the testing procedure can actually verify use (Akers, Massey, Clarke, and Lauer, 1983).

The impact of the Bogus Pipeline Procedure on improving the validity of self-reported data about smoking, alcohol use, and other drug use has been mixed. In many studies, researchers have randomized students either to an intervention condition that includes the Bogus Pipeline Procedure and the completion of a self-reported survey or to a control condition where they complete the self-reported survey only (Campanelli, Dielman, and Shope, 1987). In some cases, students were randomized to a third condition that includes the discussion of the use of the procedure some time in the future but has the students only complete the survey (Werch, Gorman, Marty, Forbess, and Brown, 1987). The purpose of this third condition is to try to answer whether it is the threat of using the procedure or the procedure itself that is associated with increased reporting. Generally, studies have found small or nonsignificant differences in reported levels of drug use, smoking, or alcohol use between these conditions (Werch, Gorman, Marty, Forbess, and Brown, 1987; Akers, Massey, Clarke, and Lauer, 1982). A recent study of the impact of the Bogus Pipeline Procedure on reporting about sexual behaviors found that stereotypical, potentially socially desirable responses reflected in gender differences in reports were smaller in the bogus pipeline condition; this suggests that the Bogus Pipeline Procedure may have yielded more valid responses, in particular involving less overreporting by males and less underreporting by females (Alexander and Fisher, 2003). Table 10.2 summarizes the discussion of the past several pages, presenting the advantages and disadvantages of various survey approaches that relate to situational factors in the completion of those surveys.

TABLE 10.2. ADVANTAGES AND DISADVANTAGES OF APPROACHES RELATED TO SITUATIONAL FACTORS.

	Advantages	Disadvantages
1. Survey mode: Self	Higher prevalence estimates Reduces socially desirable responding Greater privacy	Cannot ensure completeness Cannot prevent navigational problems
2. Technology-enhanced methods A-CASI T-ACASI TTDE APDA	Reduces socially desirable responding Reduces problems due to low literacy Allows for internal consistency checks Allows for sophisticated branching and skip patterns	May be cumbersome and expensive when surveying large samples Safe storage and transport problematic Risks of losing data if not properly saved
3. Internet-based surveys	Easier access to study samples Access to hidden populations On-line data is collected about survey completion process	Representativeness of sample is unknown or low Concerns about identity and eligibility of respondents
4. Interviewer effects: Training important Matching by demographics to respondent	Reduces social desirable responding Increases comfort level and reports about sensitive topics	May be expensive When and for whom this is important is not well understood
5. Setting: School versus household Treatment facilities Criminal justice systems	Higher prevalence estimates Greater perceived privacy Easier to reach target population Easy to reach hardcore drug users Easier to reach high risk populations	May be problematic for longitudinal studies Underreporting due to socially desirable responding Underreporting posttreatment Underreporting due to fears of reprisal
6. Experimental manipulations Bogus Pipeline Procedure Randomized Lists Technique	Possibly reduces socially desirable responding	Small or nonsignificant impact on reporting Respondent burden

Objective Measures

One of the most persistent criticisms of behavioral research, particularly around sensitive behaviors, is whether self-reports are valid. As discussed so far in this chapter, there is a wide variety of approaches researchers can use within their survey designs and implementations to improve the validity of self-reports. However, even when using a number of these methods, behavioral researchers and medical scientists may still be skeptical of self-reports. Other types of data may be required before a conclusion can be made that relationships among variables or effects of interventions have public health or medical significance. To address this criticism, researchers often compare self-reports to more objective measures that are thought to be less influenced by bias, recall, or socially desirable responding. Thus, while assessments of construct validity and reliability (in other words, correlations to other self-report measures and consistency of the self-report measures themselves, respectively) can contribute to increased confidence in these data, criterion validity (association with outcome data beyond self-reports) may afford an even greater level of confidence about these measures and related results. We will briefly discuss two sorts of these objective measures: biologic measures or markers, and unobtrusive measures.

Biologic Measures or Markers. In the substance abuse literature from the early 1980s, it was generally assumed that self-reports of drug use were valid since validity studies comparing self-reported use with urine testing found similar results. However, at that time urine analysis was less sophisticated than it is now and was less likely to detect drug use; therefore self-reports tended to concur with urine testing (for historical review see Wish, Hoffman, and Nemes, 1997). With the advance of more sophisticated hair and urine testing, the validity of self-reported drug use has been called into question. In addition, with the onslaught of the War on Drugs and stiff prison sentences for possession, reporting of drug use has become a high-risk venture, particularly among treatment and criminal justice populations. A recent meta-analysis of twenty-four validity studies published between 1985 and 1996 compared biochemical measures with self-reported drug use among high-risk populations. Overall, 42 percent of those who tested positive for drug use reported drug use in self-report surveys (Magura and Kang, 1996).

Generally, it has been found that underreporting increases with the severity of the drug, with greater underreporting for cocaine and heroin than for marijuana (Fendrich and Xu, 1994; Mieczkowski, Barzelay, Gropper, and Wish, 1991; Magura and Kang, 1996; Dembo, Williams, Wish, and Schmeidler, 1990). In addition, underreporting seems greatest among criminal justice populations. It is presumed that inmates and arrestees are skeptical of assurances of confidentiality and fear disclosure to those in authority (Magura and Kang, 1996). Other studies have delineated differences in underreporting within incarcerated populations. They found that levels of underreporting were greater among those with more severe criminal offenses (Page, Davies, Ladner, Alfassa, and Tennis, 1977). Among substance abusers, rates of underreporting of drug use are greater after drug treatment than at admission (Magura and Kang, 1996; Hinden and others, 1994), inviting concerns about treatment outcome studies. For example, Hindin and colleagues found that at admission to a residential treatment program, 96 percent of heroin-positive and 89 percent of cocaine-positive clients accurately reported their drug use. At posttreatment, 67 percent of heroin-positive and 51 percent of cocaine-positive users accurately reported their drug use (Hinden and others, 1994). Similarly, Wish and colleagues, in a small study of drug treatment clients, found that 96 percent of clients who tested positive for opiate use at intake reported opiate use. Three months after discharge 46 percent of those who tested positive for opiate use accurately reported their drug use (Wish, Hoffman, and Nemes, 1997), with greater discordance among those who were heavier drug users.

Although self-reported data may be imperfect, biologically assessed measures are not without their drawbacks, including possible contamination, false negatives, limited time windows for detecting the presence of a drug, and considerable expense. There are no extant biologic markers or measures related to sexual behavior that serve as the "gold standard" as urine and hair analysis do for substance use. There are no direct biologic measures to assess whether an individual has had sexual intercourse, has used a condom, or has had a certain number of partners over a given interval of time. However, several measures have been used in preliminary tests.

Udry and Morris (1967) assessed the presence of sperm in women's urine and correlated it to their self-report of recent unprotected intercourse, finding concordance between the two in twelve out of fifteen women. For individuals treated for STDs in a clinic setting, contraction of an incident STD over a period of time can be correlated with self-reported condom use to validate the condom self-report measure; Zenilman and others (1995) found a relatively high, but not perfect, correspondence between the two; 15 percent of men and 23 percent of women who reported always using condoms had new STDs at follow-up. STD testing has increasingly become the "silver standard" for assessment of behavioral effects in interventions related to HIV, pregnancy, or STD prevention. Halpern, Udry, and Suchindran, (1998) report on testosterone as a correlate of levels of sexual activity; this may become useful in validating reports of sexual behavior. More recently, Zenilman, Yuenger, Galai, Turner, and Rogers (2005) have developed a measure to detect the recent presence of sperm in the vaginal cavity of women through assessment of the Y chromosome, indicating recent unprotected sexual intercourse.

Unobtrusive Measures. Unobtrusive measures are those that "do not require the cooperation of a respondent and that do not themselves contaminate the response" (Webb, Campbell, Schwartz, and Sechrest, 1966, p. 2). With respect to measures of substance use or sexual behavior, these may include measures such as alcohol consumption at the community level; use of condom vouchers by study participants; STD or teen birth rates in a community to assess the impact of an intervention; reports of others (partners, close friends, or counselors); or arrest or treatment records. However, these methods also have disadvantages. It is not always possible to interview third parties about a participant's substance abuse, causing possible sampling bias if the study is limited only to those who provide a third-party contact. Some studies have suggested that, in fact, third parties and arrest or treatment records may provide less information about drug use behaviors than the actual respondent (Maisto, McKay, and Connors, 1990). Community-level rates of STDs or teen births require reporting in both cases and exclude spontaneous or voluntary abortions in the latter case.

Concluding Thoughts About Objective Measures. As Webb and colleagues persuasively argued nearly forty years ago, "Over-reliance on questionnaires and interviews is dangerous because it does not give us enough points in conceptual space to triangulate. It is only when we naively place faith in a single measure that the massive problems of social research vitiate (bring into question) the validity of our assumptions" (Webb, Campbell, Schwartz, and Sechrest, 1966, p. 34). Use of objective or unobtrusive measures, alongside self-report data, at a minimum provides stronger evidence for the validity of our measures and results than when they are not used. Indeed, in a review of the literature on self-reports of condom use and STDs over thirty-five years later, Fishbein and Pequegnat (2000, p. 110) arrive at a very similar conclusion: "Both behavioral and biological measures are important outcomes for studying the efficacy and effectiveness of behavior-change interventions. However, one measure cannot substitute for or validate the other, and neither serves as a true surrogate for HIV prevalence or incidence." Use of both self-report and objective measures of sensitive behaviors contributes to our understanding of both the behaviors and their relationship to public health or medical outcomes.

Applied Example

In this section we present an in-depth example for heuristic purposes.

National Survey of Adolescent Males

The primary objectives of the National Survey of Adolescent Males (NSAM) are to "obtain information about patterns of sexual activity and condom use among U.S. teenage males 15–19 years old; to assess their knowledge, attitudes, and risk behaviors relative to AIDS; and to conduct analyses which would identify determinants of condom use" (Pleck, Sonenstein, and Ku, 1993). The first survey was conducted with 1,880 young men in 1988, who were followed up in 1991; a new cohort of 1,741 males were surveyed in 1995. Choices made in developing these surveys and in changes made in administering the 1988 survey and that in 1995 are illustrative of a number of the issues we've discussed here (see Pleck, Sonenstein, and Ku, 1993, and Turner, Miller, and Rogers, 1997, for more details about survey development and methodological issues surrounding the survey).

Three days of training were conducted for the 1988 and 1991 surveys and five days of training for the 1995 surveys. Interviewers were trained in not being judgmental and the sensitive nature of the questions. Interviewers also were allowed to choose other surveys to work on if they felt uncomfortable with these topics, and supervisors screened out interviewers who performed at less than ideal levels. The training was one way of improving the *situation* in which the interview took place to reduce potential respondent bias or perceptions of social desirability.

The researchers also spent considerable resources and time on the mode of survey administration. In the 1988 and 1991 surveys, primarily face-to-face interviews were conducted by trained interviewers. In addition, a self-administered questionnaire was used to assess some of the most sensitive behaviors. In the 1995 survey, the newer A-CASI methodology was used for most respondents, based on successful pilot-testing that showed higher reports of sensitive behaviors using A-CASI compared with self-administered questionnaires. Results for the 1995 survey were again supportive, also showing higher rates of reporting of sensitive behaviors for A-CASI than for self-administered questionnaires (Turner and others, 1998).

The researchers reported various methods for clarifying the wording of questions—for example, those related to whether respondents had had sex. At each time point, they conducted focus groups and pretests of small samples of young men to determine questions or words that were not clear. They also opted for a simpler rather than lengthier definition of intercourse, selecting "Have you ever had sexual intercourse (sometimes this is referred to as 'making love,' 'having sex,' or 'going all the way')?" The researchers also focused on the cognitive processes involved in responding to surveys in their decisions about methods for increasing recall. They asked questions first about the most recent partners, with more limited information being collected about the previous four partners, believing that the most accurate information was likely to be recalled about most recent partners. They also asked about various behaviors, including condom use on a partner by partner basis, rather than overall, expecting it to be remembered better this way. Basing their decision on previous data (indicating most fifteen- to nineteen-year-old males had fewer than six partners in the past twelve months, but many had only episodic sexual experiences during that time interval), they decided to collect information about number of partners using a twelve-month interval because a significantly shorter period might have resulted in loss of data about sexual activity for a substantial portion of the sample.

As a final method for assessing and even improving the quality of their data, the researchers have shown correlations between trends in condom use (from their data) to condom sales nationwide and with pregnancies and births reported by males for their female sex partners in the longitudinal sample between their reports in 1988 and 1991. They have also added the collection of biologic markers, specifically using urine samples from respondents over the age of eighteen in their 1995 testing for chlamydia and gonorrhea to further validate reports of behaviors such as condom use and to add further information to the self-report data.

Integration with the Research Process

The issues discussed in this chapter—how to improve the validity of self-reports of sensitive behaviors by considering cognitive and situational factors as well as biologic and unobtrusive measures—are key elements of the research process. Several key questions pertain to step 5 of the nine-step model shown in Chapter One. What type of survey will be administered? Will it involve interviewers, self-administration using paper and pencil, A-CASI, telephone, Internet, or PDA administration? Should the design be cross-sectional or longitudinal? Will other sorts of validating data, such as biologic markers or unobtrusive measures, be used? How can the research questions be answered while placing the least possible burden on the respondent? In particular, the question of "how" is embedded into this step. How will the questions be worded? What time periods should be used in asking about behaviors? Will questions ask about ever engaging in a behavior or frequency of engaging in that behavior? What will the order of questions be?

Consideration of the sample population (step 6 in the nine-step model) is also important. Clearly, the answers to many of the questions posed in the previous paragraph will be contingent on a thorough knowledge of the people who will be included in the study. Finally, step 7: (implement the study protocol with attention to fidelity) is also connected to the issues discussed here. How will interviewers be trained? Will quality controls or observations be conducted to assess their performance or behavior throughout the study? What checks will be implemented within the survey to reduce missing data, inappropriate skips, inconsistency in reporting, or a respondent completing a Web survey multiple times?

Summary

When asking questions about sensitive behaviors one must be acutely aware of potential threats to the validity and reliability of the survey items that are used and the responses that are provided. In this chapter we reviewed drug use and sexual behaviors as examples of sensitive behaviors for which the validity of self-reports is frequently called into question. We describe validity as being affected by two separate factors (1) cognitive factors and (2) situational factors. Factors that affect cognition, or the remembering of events, include how the question and response items are crafted and the ways that the data are collected to enhance the recollection of past events. Situational factors such as who administers the survey, where the survey takes place, who is present, and how research is perceived are external factors that can affect how likely it is that respondents will provide valid answers to questions about sensitive or stigmatized behaviors. Both cognitive and situation factors affect the overall validity of self-report behaviors.

All of these techniques for improving the validity of self-report data have their strengths and their limitations. Constructing surveys and conducting research is a balancing act. Some cognitive approaches, such as daily diaries, can enhance recall of past events but may be too difficult or too burdensome for some higher-risk populations to use. In other cases, situational factors such as the use of brief close-ended questions about highly stigmatized behaviors may provide the data you are interested in, but if you don't build rapport with the respondent or sequence these questions with other attitudinal questions, respondents may provide invalid answers due to socially desirable responding.

This chapter has also reviewed objective measures that are used to externally validate self-report responses, such as urinalysis and STD testing. While these methods allow you to compare self-reports to an outside criterion measure, biologic testing is labor intensive and expensive, and may provide limited time windows when it is possible to validate the behavior. Creating opportunities for assessing the construct validity of survey items, which is being able to compare responses to behavior questions with other behavior or attitude questions in the survey, is a critical method for assessing validity when more laboratory-based measures are not feasible or appropriate.

Issues to Consider

1. As we move away from open-ended, qualitative methods of data collection and move toward more technologically advanced, quantitative data-collection methods, are we losing richness in exchange for improved validity and reliability?

Under what conditions are technologically based quantitative assessments appropriate, and when are more qualitative, open-ended, or interviewed administered research techniques more appropriate? What about areas of research where we don't know very much?

2. Throughout this chapter we have reviewed some of the available evidence regarding the validity of self-reports of sensitive behaviors, particularly when compared with outside criteria such as drug testing or STD testing. What do you conclude about the overall accuracy of self-report data? Is the cup half full or half empty? If you were presenting to a room full of physicians, could you report that you were confident the survey data you collected were accurate? Or would you prefer to present to a room full of prevention and behavioral scientists and enthusiastically support the use of biologic markers whenever possible to validate self-report data? Defend your argument based on the available evidence for drug use and sexual behaviors.

For Practice and Discussion

1. You are writing a grant to study the frequency of unprotected sexual intercourse among adolescents and want to understand the influence of drugs or alcohol use on your target outcome behavior. You are deciding how you want to design and administer the survey to ensure that you can make a link between drug use and the sexual behavior and to ensure valid reporting of the behaviors. Work in groups to define the following: (1) the population and setting of the study; (2) the mode of survey administration (A-CASI, paper and pencil, daily diaries); (3) whether self-administered or interview administered; (4) specific survey questions to measure frequency of the behavior; (5) survey items or other data-collection methods that will provide construct validity; and, finally, (6) whether you will use biologic measures, unobtrusive measures, or both to validate self-reported behaviors. Discuss the advantages and disadvantages of your approach and defend your design decisions based on how they will improve the validity of responses.

2. Use the information learned in this chapter to describe how the issues clearly related to self-reports of *very sensitive* behaviors such as illegal drug use and stigmatized sexual behavior might relate to self-reports of *less sensitive* behaviors, such as assessing exercise behavior as part of an evaluation of an exercise or wellness program in the workplace. To what extent do you think that mode of administration, use of technology-enhanced data-collection techniques, issues of timing and frequency, longitudinal versus retrospective reports, and use of

biologic or unobtrusive measures might be more or less important in the case of exercise behavior as compared with more sensitive behavioral reports?

References

Akers, R. L., Massey, J., Clarke, W., and Lauer, R. M. (1983). Are self-reports of adolescent deviance valid? Biochemical measures, randomized response and the Bogus Pipeline in smoking behavior. *Social Forces, 62,* 234–251.

Alexander, M. G., and Fisher, T. D. (2003). Truth and consequences: Using the Bogus Pipeline to examine sex differences in self-reported sexuality. *The Journal of Sex Research, 40*(1), 27–35.

Aquilino, W. S., and LoSciuto, L. A. (1990). Effects of interview mode on self-reported drug use. *Public Opinion Quarterly, 54,* 362–395.

Bachman, J. G., and O'Malley, P. M. (1981). When four months equal a year: Inconsistencies in student reports of drug use. *Public Opinion Quarterly, 45,* 536–548.

Bainbridge, W. S. (1989). *Survey research: A computer-assisted introduction.* Belmont, CA: Wadsworth.

Bell, D. C., Montoya, I. D., and Atkinson, J. S. (2000). Partner concordance in reports of joint risk behaviors. *Journal of Acquired Immune Deficiency Syndromes, 25,* 173–181.

Blumberg, S. J., Cynamon, M. L., Osborn, L., and Olson, L. (2003). The impact of touch-tone data entry on reports of HIV and STD risk behaviors in telephone interviews. *The Journal of Sex Research, 40*(2), 121–128.

Boekeloo, B. O., and others. (1994). Self-reports of HIV risk factors at a sexually transmitted disease clinic: Audio vs. written questionnaires. *American Journal of Public Health, 84,* 754–760.

Brener, N. D., Billy, J.O.G., and Grady, W. R. (2003). Assessment of factors affecting the validity of self-reported health risk behavior among adolescents: Evidence from the scientific literature. *Journal of Adolescent Health, 33,* 436–457.

Campanelli, P. C., Dielman, T. E., and Shope, J. T. (1987). Validity of adolescents' self-reports of alcohol use and misuse using a Bogus Pipeline Procedure. *Adolescence, 22*(85), 7–22.

Cannell, C. F., Miller, P. V., and Oskenberg, L. (1981). Research on Interviewing Techniques. In S. Leinhardt (Ed.), *Sociological methodology.* San Francisco: Jossey-Bass.

Catania, J. A. (1999). A framework for conceptualizing reporting bias and its antecedents in interviews assessing human sexuality. *The Journal of Sex Research, 36*(1), 25–38.

Catania, J. A., Binson, D., Van der Straten, A., and Stone, V. (1995). Methodological research on sexual behavior in the AIDS era. *Annual Review of Sex Research, 6,* 77–125.

Catania, J. A., Gibson, D. R., Chitwood, D. D., and Coates, T. J. (1990). Methodological problems in AIDS behavioral research: Influences on measurement error and participation in studies of sexual behavior. *Psychological Bulletin, 108*(3), 339–362.

Catania, J. A., McDermott, L., and Pollack, L. (1986). Questionnaire response bias and face-to-face interview sample bias in sexuality research. *Journal of Sex Research, 22,* 52–72.

DeMaio, T. (1984). Social desirability and survey measurement: A review. In C. Turner and E. Martin (Eds.), *Surveying subjective phenomena* (pp. 257–282). New York: Russel Sage Foundation.

Dembo, R., Williams, L., Wish, E. D., and Schmeidler, J. (1990). Urine testing of detained juveniles to identify high-risk youth. In *National Institute of Justice: Research in Brief.* Washington, DC: National Institute of Justice.

Droitcour, J., and others. (1991). The item count technique as a method of indirect questioning: A review of its development and a case study application. In P. P. Biemer, R. M. Groves, L. E. Lyberg, N. A. Mathiowetz, and S. Sudman (Eds.), *Measurement errors in surveys* (pp. 185–210). New York: Wiley.

Fendrich, M., and Xu, Y. (1994). The validity of drug use reports from juvenile arrestees. *International Journal of the Addictions, 29*(8), 971–985.

Fishbein, M., and Pequegnat, W. (2000). Evaluating AIDS prevention interventions using behavioral and biological outcome measures. *Sexually Transmitted Diseases, 27,* 101–110.

Forsyth, B. H., Lessler, J. T., and Hubbard, M. L. (1992). Cognitive evaluation of the questionnaire. In C. Turner and J. Lessler (Eds.), *Survey measurement of drug use: Methodological studies* (pp. 13–52). Rockville, MD: National Institute of Drug Abuse, Division of Epidemiology and Prevention Research.

Fowler, F. J., Jr. (1984). *Survey research methods.* Thousand Oaks, CA: Sage.

Fremouw, W. J., and Brown, J. P. (1980). The reactivity of addictive behaviors to self-monitoring: A functional analysis. *Addictive Behaviors, 5,* 209–217.

Gfroerer, J. C., and Hughes, A. L. (1991). The feasibility of collecting drug abuse data by telephone. *Public Health Reports, 106*(4), 384–394.

Gfroerer, J., Wright, D., and Kopstein, A. (1997). Prevalence of youth substance use: The impact of methodological differences between two national surveys. *Drug and Alcohol Dependence, 47*(1), 19–30.

Gillmore, M. R., and others. (2001). Daily data collection of sexual and other health-related behaviors. *Journal of Sex Research, 38*(1), 35–43.

Gribble, J. N., Miller, H. G., Rogers, S. M., and Turner, C. F. (1999). Interview mode and measurement of sexual behaviors: Methodological issues. *Journal of Sex Research, 36,* 16–24.

Hallfors, D., Khatapoush, S., Kadushin, C., Watson, K., and Saxe, L. (2000). A comparison of paper vs. computer-assisted self-interview for school, alcohol, tobacco and other drug surveys. *Evaluation and Program Planning, 23*(2), 149–155.

Halpern, C. T., Udry, J. R., and Suchindran, C. (1998). Monthly measures of salivary testosterone predict sexual activity in adolescent males. *Archives of Sexual Behavior, 27*(5), 445–465.

Halpern, C. T., Udry, J. R., Suchindran, C., and Campbell, B. (2000). Adolescent males' willingness to report masturbation. *Journal of Sex Research, 37,* 327–332.

Hays, R. D., and Huba, G. J. (1988). Reliability and validity of drug use items differing in the nature of their reponse options. *Journal of Consulting and Clinical Psychology, 56*(3), 470–472.

Hinden, R., and others. (1994). Radioimmunoassay of hair for determination of cocaine, heroin, and marijuana exposure: Comparison with self-report. *International Journal of Addiction, 29,* 771–798.

Johnson, R. (1970). Extramarital sexual intercourse: A methodological note. *Journal of Marriage and Family, 32,* 279–282.

Jones, E. E., and Sigal, H. (1971). The Bogus Pipeline: A new paradigm for measuring affect and attitude. *Psychological Bulletin, 76,* 349–364.

Kann, L., Brener, N. D., Warren, C. W., Collins, J. L., and Giovino, G. A. (2002). An assessment of the effect of data collection setting on the prevalence of health risk behaviors among adolescents. *Journal of Adolescent Health, 31*(4), 327–335.

Kubey, R., Larson, R., and Csikszentmihalyi, M. (1996). Experience sampling method applications to communication research questions. *Journal of Communication, 46,* 99–118.

LaBrie, J. W., and Earleywine, M. (2000). Sexual risk behaviors and alcohol: Higher base rates revealed using the Unmated-Count Technique. *Journal of Sex Research, 37,* 321–326.

Lenert, L., and Skoczen, S. (2002). The Internet as a research tool: Worth the price of admission? *Annals of Behavioral Medicine, 24,* 251–256.

Loftus, E. F., Smith, K. D., Johnson, D. A., and Fiedler J. (1988). Remembering "when": Errors in the dating of autobiographical memories. In M. Gruneberg, P. Morris, and R. Sykes (Eds.), *Practical aspects of memory* (pp. 234–240). Chichester, UK: John Wiley and Sons.

Magura, S., and Kang, S-Y. (1996). Validity of self-reported drug use in high-risk populations: A meta-analytical review. *Substance Use & Misuse, 31*(9), 1131–1153.

Maisto, S. A., McKay, J. R., and Connors, G. J. (1990). Self-report issues in substance abuse: State of the art and future directions. *Behavioral Assessment, 12,* 117–134.

McCabe, S. E. (2004). Comparison of Web and mail surveys in collecting illicit drug use data: A randomized experiment. *Journal of Drug Education, 34,* 61–72.

McCabe, S. E., Boyd, C. J., Couper, M. P., Crawford, S., and D'Arch, H. (2002). Mode effects for collecting alcohol and other drug use data: Web and U.S. mail. *Journal of Studies on Alcohol, 63,* 755–761.

Means, B., Habina, K., Swan, G. E., and Jack, L. (1992). Cognitive research on response error in survey questions on smoking. *Vital and Health Statistics, 6*(5) (DHHS Pub. No. PHS 89–1076). Washington, DC: Government Printing Office.

Mieczkowski, T., Barzelay, D., Gropper, B., Wish, E. (1991). Concordance of three measures of cocaine use in an arrestee population: Hair, urine, and self-report. *Journal of Psychoactive Drugs, 23*(3), 241–249.

Miller, J. D. (1984, July). *A new survey technique for studying deviant behavior.* Unpublished dissertation. Dissertation Abstract: 1984-56841-001. *Dissertation Abstracts International, 45*(1-A), 319.

Miller, J. D., and Cisin, I. H. (1983). *The item-count/paired lists technique: An indirect method of surveying deviant behavior.* Unpublished manuscript. Washington, DC: George Washington University, Social Research Group.

Miller, J. D., Cisin, I. H., and Harrell, A. V. (1986). A new technique for surveying deviant behavior: Item-count estimates of marijuana, cocaine, and heroin. Paper presented at the annual meeting of the American Association for Public Opinion Research, St. Petersburg, Florida.

Morrison, D. M., Leigh, B. C., and Rogers, G. M. (1999). Daily sata collection: A comparison of three methods. *Journal of Sex Research, 36*(1), 76–82.

Mustanski, B. S. (2001). Getting wired: Exploiting the Internet for the collection of valid sexuality data. *Journal of Sex Research, 38,* 292–301.

Oksenberg, L., and Cannell, C. (1977). Some factors underlying the validity of response in self-report. *Bulletin of the International Statistical Institute, 48,* 325–346.

O'Malley, P. M., Bachman, J. G., and Johnston, L. D. (1983). Reliability and consistency in self-reports of drug use. *International Journal of Addictions, 18*(6), 805–824.

Page, W. F., Davies, J. E., Ladner, R. A., Alfassa, J., and Tennis, H. (1977). Urinalysis screened versus verbally reported drug use: The identification of discrepant groups. *International Journal of the Addictions, 12*(4), 439–450.

Pleck, J. H., Sonenstein, F. L., & Ku, L. (1993). Changes in adolescent males' use of and attitudes toward condoms, 1988–1991. *Family Planning Perspectives, 25,* 106–110.

Smith, T. W. (2003). An experimental comparison of knowledge networks and the GSS. *International Journal of Public Opinion Research, 15*, 167–179.

Stone, V. E., Catania, J. A., and Binson, D. (1999). Measuring change in sexual behavior: Concordance between survey measures. *The Journal of Sex Research, 36*(1), 102–108.

Tourangeau, R., Jobe, J. B., Pratt, W. F., and Rasinski, K. (1997). Design and results of the Women's Health Study. (1997). In L. Harrison and A. Hughes (Eds.), *The validity of self-reported drug use: Improving the accuracy of survey estimates* (NIDA Monograph Series No. 97-4147, pp. 344–365). Rockville, MD: National Institute of Drug Abuse.

Trapl, E. S., and others. (forthcoming). *Use of audio-enhanced personal digital assistants for school-based data collection.* Manuscript under review.

Turner, C. F., Miller, H., and Rogers, S. M. (1997). Survey measurement of sexual behavior: Problems and progress. In J. Bancroft (Ed.), *Research Sexual Behavior* (pp. 37–60). Bloomington, IN: Indiana University Press.

Turner, C. F., and others. (1998). Adolescent sexual behavior, drug use, and violence: Increased reporting with computer survey technology. *Science, 280*(5365), 867–874.

Udry, R. J., and Morris, N. M. (1967). A method for validation of reported sexual data. *Journal of Marriage and the Family, 29*, 442–446.

Webb, E. J., Campbell, D. T., Schwartz, R. D., and Sechrest, L. (1966). *Unobtrusive measures: Nonreactive research in the social sciences.* Chicago: Rand-McNally.

Werch, C. E., Gorman, D. R., Marty, P. J., Forbess, J., and Brown, B. (1987). Effects of the Bogus Pipeline on enhancing validity of self-reported adolescent drug use measures. *Journal of School Health, 57*(6), 232–236.

Willis, G. B. (1997). The use of the psychological laboratory to study sensitive survey topics. In L. Harrison and A. Hughes (Eds.), *The validity of self-reported drug use: Improving the accuracy of survey estimates* (NIDA Research Monograph Series No. 97-4147, pp. 416–438). Rockville, MD: National Institute of Drug Abuse.

Wimbush, J. C., and Dalton, D. R. (1997). Base rate for employee theft: Converge of multiple methods. *Journal of Applied Psychology, 82*, 756–763.

Wish, E. D., Hoffman, J. A., and Nemes, S. (1997). The validity of self-reports of a drug use at treatment admission and at follow-up: Comparisons with urinalysis and hair assays. In L. Harrison and A. Hughes (Eds.), *The validity of self-reported drug use: Improving the accuracy of survey estimates* (NIDA Research Monograph Series No. 97-4147, pp. 344–365). Rockville, MD: National Institute of Drug Abuse.

Wright, D. L., Aquilino, W. S., and Supple, A. J. (1998). A comparison of computer-assisted and paper and pencil self-administered questionnaires in a survey on smoking, alcohol, and drug use. *Public Opinion Quarterly, 62*, 331–353.

Zenilman, J., Yuenger, J., Galai, N., Turner, C. F., and Rogers, S. M. (2005). Polymerase chain reaction detection of Y chromosome sequences in vaginal fluid: Preliminary studies of a potential biomarker for sexual behavior. *Sexually Transmitted Diseases, 32*, 90–94.

Zenilman, J. M., and others. (1995). Condom use to prevent incident STDs: The validity of self-reported condom use. *Sexually Transmitted Diseases, 22*(1), 15–21.

Zimmerman, R. S., and Langer, L. M. (1995). Improving estimates of prevalence rates of sensitive behaviors: The Randomized Lists Technique and consideration of self-reported honesty. *Journal of Sex Research, 32*, 107–117.

CHAPTER ELEVEN

PRINCIPLES OF SAMPLING

Richard A. Crosby, Laura F. Salazar, and Ralph J. DiClemente

Ultimately, the utility of a research project is a function of its generalizability. In turn, generalizability is a function of how well the sample represents the selected priority population. Sampling is a science unto itself; one that is used to predict winners of political elections before the polls even close, and one that may someday be used in place of a "head by head" count for the U.S. census. In health promotion research, sampling methods can be divided into two main categories: (1) methods that are admittedly weak in generalizability (nonprobability sampling methods) and (2) methods that yield high generalizability (probability methods). Despite its limitations, the former category is often very useful in the early stages of the research chain or when the nature of the selected population precludes the application of probability methods. The latter category, although far more rigorous, is often problematic to apply, as it depends on the existence of a sampling frame.

Indeed, asking the question, Does a *sampling frame* (a listing of people in the population) exist? is the most effective way to determine if a nonprobability sample or a probability sample should be used. Because this basic decision about sampling is so critical, this chapter is devoted to an in-depth discussion of the nonprobability and probability sampling techniques that are most often used in health promotion research.

Illustration of Key Concepts

The Sampling Goal

As with most endeavors, the key aspect of successful sampling is a great deal of attention to planning. Planning, in a sense, is the "art" of sampling; it requires creativity and cautious optimism regarding possibilities. At the foundation of this planning, the researcher is formulating an operationally defined goal. Three vital decisions are needed to formulate this goal: (1) What is the sampling element? (2) Is a sampling frame accessible? and (3) What type of sampling technique should be employed?

Sampling Elements. The goal of any sampling technique is to maximize the *generalizability* of the sample to the population. In this sense, the term *population* refers to all possible *elements* of a defined group. An element, in turn, can be people (as is usually the case) or well-defined units (or clusters) that have importance in public health (such as emergency care centers, schools, and homeless shelters). When people are the sampling element, the research questions are centered on the person (for example, Do outpatients from cardiac care centers consume a healthy diet?). Conversely, when elements compose well-defined units the research questions will involve "behavior" of an entire system such as, How effectively do cardiac care centers teach outpatients to consume healthy diets? Thus, an initial step in defining the sampling goal is to determine whether the research questions necessitate investigation of individual-level behavior or the collective behavior of an organized system. Table 11.1 presents several examples of health promotion research questions shown by this essential division in purpose.

◆ ◆ ◆

In a Nutshell

An initial step in defining the sampling goal is to determine whether the research questions necessitate investigation of individual-level behavior or the collective behavior of an organized system.

◆ ◆ ◆

TABLE 11.1. EXAMPLES OF RESEARCH QUESTIONS DISPLAYED BY LEVEL OF ANALYSIS.

Person-Level Research Questions	System-Level Research Questions
How does condom availability influence teens' use of condoms?	What factors influence school systems to adopt condom distribution programs?
Is religiosity associated with lower rates of domestic violence?	Do churches actively teach couples and families conflict-resolution skills?
Are first-time parents able to properly install infant car seats?	Do hospitals offer first-time parents training in the installation of car seats?
Do women residing in low-income nursing homes consume diets adequate in fiber?	Do low-income nursing homes provide women with diets that are adequate in fiber?
Is affiliation with social organizations associated with decreased substance abuse?	To what extent do urban social organizations provide teens with alternatives to substance abuse?
Do people with adult-onset diabetes practice the consistent and correct use of insulin?	What is the extent of postdiagnostic education provided to adults newly diagnosed with diabetes in state-funded health clinics?

Sampling Frame Accessibility. Once the type of element has been identified, the next question that presents itself is whether a *sampling frame* exists (or can be created). A sampling frame can be loosely defined as an exhaustive list of elements. The word *exhaustive* is critical here because the list must represent every element in the population. For example, imagine that the research question is, Are unemployed men residing in rural counties more likely to be heavy smokers than unemployed men residing in urban counties? At first, the existence of a sampling frame seems intuitive—unemployed men are "listed" by offices that provide government assistance (that is, unemployment benefits). Ignoring for a moment whether such lists would even be made available, the researcher needs to ask the question, Is this frame exhaustive of the population?

An unfortunate reality of sampling is that very few sampling frames are truly exhaustive of the population. For example, do all unemployed men collect government assistance? Even seemingly clear-cut cases of an effective sampling frame can be problematic. A classic example of this is the use of telephone directories as a sampling frame. The directory is not exhaustive because it will not include people who use cell phones exclusively, people who cannot afford phone service, people who pay extra for an unlisted number, or people who have recently moved into the listing area. Thus, the question, Is this frame exhaustive of the population? is answered by degree rather than by a simple "yes" or "no." ("No" would almost always be the answer.) Table 11.2 displays examples of sampling

TABLE 11.2. SAMPLING FRAMES WITH HIGH AND LOW DEGREES OF GENERALIZABILITY.

Higher Generalizability	Lower Generalizability
Research Question:	Research Question:
Is parental monitoring associated with health risk behavior among boys thirteen to sixteen years of age from low-income homes?	Are cancer patients who remain optimistic likely to survive longer than those who lose hope?
Sampling Frame:	Sampling Frame:
Boys enrolled in reduced-cost lunch programs at public schools	People diagnosed with cancer at publicly funded medical offices.
Note: Findings could be generalized to low-income boys attending public schools, but not to those who have dropped out or been placed in an alternative setting (including juvenile detention)	*Note:* Publicly funded medical offices may represent only a very small portion of the locations where cancer is diagnosed—thus generalizability is quite low.
Research Question:	Research Question:
Are women who receive WIC benefits at risk of rapid repeat pregnancy?	What behavioral factors predict iron-deficiency anemia among pregnant women?
Sampling Frame:	Sampling Frame:
Women enrolled in WIC programs	Women receiving prenatal care
Note: In this scenario, the sampling frame and the research question "line up" perfectly! Thus, generalizability would be optimal.	*Note:* The key question to consider is what portion of pregnant women do not receive prenatal care. To the extent that pregnant women in any given setting may not receive this care, generalizability decreases.
Research Question:	Research Question:
To what extent do hospital-based pediatricians meet guidelines for children's vaccination schedules?	Are low-income elderly women less likely than their male counterparts to exercise on a regular basis?
Sampling Frame:	Sampling Frame:
Hospital registry of pediatricians with privileges	Women and men receiving Medicare benefits
Note: Again, the sampling frame and the research question appear to line up quite nicely. Thus, potential for generalizability is high.	*Note:* Here, it is important to realize that all low-income elderly people may not receive Medicare benefits. Further, not all people receiving Medicare benefits are likely to be low-income and many may not perceive themselves to be "elderly." Thus, generalizability is likely to be quite low.

frames that adequately represent the population (providing a higher degree of generalizability) and those less likely to represent the population (providing a lower degree of generalizability).

Careful scrutiny of Table 11.2 will reveal two important points. First, note that none of the examples involves units as the sampling element. In each example, including the one regarding pediatricians, the research question is about behavior at the individual level. The question here is, Why weren't examples provided for elements defined by well-defined units? The answer is that, with some exceptions, well-defined units typically have a sampling frame that will offer a high degree of exhaustion. As a principle, exhaustion is generally far more likely when the sampling element is defined by a unit rather than by people. The difference is that social structures and law often protect individual identities, whereas group identities are often made public by intention. For example, churches, voluntary health agencies, schools, and neighborhood organizations are units that, by design, can be easily identified. Hospitals, soup kitchens, youth organizations, and drug treatment centers are just a few other examples of potential elements that are amenable to sampling for research questions at the system level.

Second, deeper scrutiny of the left-hand column in Table 11.2 raises an essential question: Can these sampling frames be accessed? Access to lists of pediatricians with hospital privileges may be possible; however, one can easily imagine "lists" that could not be obtained (for example, people receiving psychotherapy, convicted felons, persons living with tuberculosis, people who have survived cancer). This key concern leads to compromise between two competing conditions: (1) the need for the sample to be generalizable to the target population, versus (2) the practical reality of obtaining sampling frames that list people.

This compromise is often inevitable, and it may shape the research question. For example (from Table 11.2), imagine that the initial research question is to investigate the relationship of parental monitoring to health risk behavior among low-income boys attending public schools. That the sampling frame exists is not in question, but whether this list will be provided to a researcher is another question entirely. Thus, compromise occurs by altering the research question to accommodate the sampling frame that is accessible. For example, the question could become, What is the relationship of parental monitoring to health risk behavior among boys attending public schools? Note that the slightly altered research question no longer includes the term *low-income*. Because of privacy regulations, disclosing a comprehensive list of boys who qualify for a reduced or free lunch is problematic, whereas disclosing a comprehensive list of *all* boys may be acceptable. Moreover, the advantage of this inclusive sampling frame is that the original research question could still be evaluated. For example, the study questionnaire could ask all boys, Do you qualify for a free or reduced-price lunch at school? Then the analysis could compare low-income boys (defined by the "lunch" criterion) to remaining boys. In fact, such a comparison could lead to a more elaborate version of the initial research question: What is the relationship of parental monitoring to health risk behavior among low-income boys attending public schools compared with boys not classified as low income? Thus, when sampling is being considered, the art of planning research requires that you understand the reciprocal relationship between framing the research question and accessing a sampling frame. Research planned with rigor has little value if access to the sampling frame is not practical or feasible.

Sampling Techniques. Effective sampling from the sampling frame referred to as the selection process is predicated on a thorough understanding of techniques. The overarching goal of this selection process is to maximize the *representativeness* of the sample with respect to the sampling frame and ultimately the population that is represented by the sampling frame. This goal is ostensibly simple and has been illustrated in Figure 11.1.

The extent to which the sample, denoted by the small circle, mirrors the exact composition of the population, depicted by the larger circle shown in Figure 11.1, will increase the degree of representativeness. Because gauging the representativeness of the sample relies on determining the extent to which the sample mirrors the population, an important consideration is, How do you determine the exact composition of the population? It must be stated that it is not possible to know

FIGURE 11.1.   THE RELATIONSHIP OF A SAMPLE TO A POPULATION.

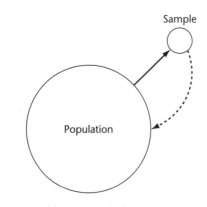

A sample is selected from a population (⎯⎯►)
Inferences about a population are based on findings from the sample (⎯ ⎯ ⎯►)

with certainty the infinite parameters of any given population. Thus, the best we can do in science is to use rigorous sampling techniques that enhance the likelihood that the sample represents the population.

◆ ◆ ◆

In a Nutshell

It must be stated that it is not possible to know with certainty the infinite parameters of any given population. Thus, the best we can do in science is to use rigorous sampling techniques that enhance the likelihood that the sample represents the population.

◆ ◆ ◆

The lack of correspondence between the sample and the population *not* attributed to chance represents the sampling bias in a research study. Because chance alone cannot be controlled, it is critically important to eliminate other factors that may introduce sampling bias. As with other forms of bias in research, sampling bias may yield inaccurate results that are not generalizable. Thus, choosing the most rigorous and appropriate sampling technique will ensure that sampling bias is reduced to as close to "zero" as possible. Reducing sampling bias provides the ability to *extrapolate* the findings to the population. Extrapolation implies making an inference based on the quality of the sampling technique. These inferences are an accepted and expected product of the research process. Indeed, health promotion research is very much about achieving large-scale change, and it is therefore necessary to think far beyond the relatively small numbers of people who make up the sample.

Common Probability Sampling Techniques

Several textbooks can be obtained that provide extensive discussion of probability sampling techniques (for example, Babbie, 2001; Shi, 1997). In the behavioral and social sciences, this category of sampling techniques is the most rigorous because the sampling strategies employ a *random selection* technique (a technique that ensures that each element has an equal probability of being selected), which greatly reduces the probability of sampling bias. Random selection is key to minimizing sample bias and therefore enhancing generalizability of the findings. A word of caution: random selection should not be confused with random assignment! (see Chapter Six for description of random assignment). The different types of probability sampling techniques are described in the following section.

Simple Random Sampling. The guiding principle behind this technique is that each element must have an equal and nonzero chance of being selected. This can be achieved by applying a table of random numbers to a numbered sampling frame. Another approach involves drawing numbers from a container. The product of this technique is a sample determined entirely by chance. It should be noted, however, that chance is "lumpy" (Abelson, 1995), meaning that random selection does not always produce a sample that is representative of the population. Imagine, for example, a sampling frame comprising 10,000 people. Furthermore, consider that race is a critical variable, and that the composition of the sampling frame is as follows: 1,500 are African American; 7,500 are white, and 1,000 are Asian. You are going to select a sample of 500 people from this sampling frame using a simple random sampling technique. Unfortunately, the simple random selection process may or may not yield a sample that has equivalent racial proportions as the sampling frame. Due to chance, disproportionate numbers of each racial category may be selected.

Systematic Random Sampling. As opposed to simple random sampling, systematic random sampling does not ensure that every element has an equal and nonzero probability of being selected. The systematic random sampling technique begins with selecting one element at random in the sampling frame as the starting point; however, from this point onward, the rest of the sample is selected systematically by applying a predetermined interval. For example, in this sampling technique, after the initial element is selected at random, every "*N*th" element will be selected (*N*th refers to the size of the interval—such as the twentieth element in the sampling frame) and becomes eligible for inclusion in the study. The "*N*th" element is selected through the end of the sampling frame and then from the beginning until a complete cycle is made back to the starting point (that is, the place where the initial random selection was made). Of note, all of the selections become predetermined as soon as the first selection is made. Thus, for example, if element 29 is the initial selection (and the interval equals 20), elements 30 through 48 have zero chance of being selected.

◆ ◆ ◆

In a Nutshell

As opposed to simple random sampling, systematic random sampling does not ensure that every element has an equal and nonzero probability of being selected.

◆ ◆ ◆

One important question is, When is systematic random sampling more appropriate than simple random sampling? The answer involves the term *periodicity*. Periodicity refers to bias caused by particular characteristics arising in the sampling frame (for example, if the list is ordered by date of birth). Sampling frames that are arranged in any meaningful fashion may possess periodicity, meaning that an inherent order exists. For example, a sampling frame of women receiving abnormal Pap test results may be arranged by date of the test (that is, women with abnormal Pap results in 1997 might be listed first, followed by those having abnormal Pap results in 1998, and so on). Systematic sampling from this sampling frame would ensure that each year of diagnosis is proportionately represented in the selected sample. Box 11.1 provides a comparison of simple random sampling to systematic random sampling with respect to this example. Note that the periodicity of the sampling frame is an advantage of systematic random sampling in comparison with simple random sampling in this instance.

Stratified Random Sampling. Stratified random sampling begins with the identification of some variable, which may be related indirectly to the research question and could act as a confound (such as geography, age, income, race or ethnicity, or gender). This variable is then used to divide the sampling frame into mutually exclusive *strata* or subgroups. Once the sampling frame is arranged by strata, the sample is selected from each stratum using random sampling or systematic sampling techniques. Imagine, for example, the following research goal: Identify key nutritional risk factors among adults living in New York State. Through conversations with people in the State Health Department, the researcher has learned that people in the southeastern part of the state (New York City and surrounding areas) are likely to be quite different than those in the northeastern part of the state and, furthermore, that people in the remaining part of the state (central and western New York) will be different from people in the east. Thus, a sample that does not fairly represent each of these three regions will have sampling error. This error can be controlled by dividing the sampling frame into three strata (southeastern, northeastern, and the remaining state). Each stratum becomes its own independent sampling frame, and a simple random sample or a systematic random sample is taken from each frame. It is important that the sample selected within each stratum reflects proportionately the population proportions; thus, you can employ *proportionate stratified sampling*. In this case, if 40 percent of the adults reside in the southeastern stratum, then 40 percent of the total sample should be selected from this stratum.

Box 11.1. A Comparison of Two Techniques to Sample Women with Abnormal Pap Test Results in the Past Five Years

Technique 1 (Simple Random Sampling)

Given a sampling frame of 650 women and a desired sample size of 100, the corresponding quantity of random numbers were drawn. This yielded 12 women diagnosed in 1997, 37 diagnosed in 1998, 7 diagnosed in 1999, 16 diagnosed in 2000, and 28 diagnosed in 2001. The proportions of women selected, by year, in comparison to those diagnosed were

1997: 105 (16.1 percent of 650) were diagnosed—11.4 percent ($n = 12$) were selected

1998: 155 (23.8 percent of 650) were diagnosed—23.8 percent ($n = 37$) were selected

1999: 73 (11.2 percent of 650) were diagnosed—9.6 percent ($n = 7$) were selected

2000: 110 (16.9 percent of 650) were diagnosed—14.5 percent ($n = 16$) were selected

2001: 207 (31.8 percent of 650) were diagnosed—13.5 percent ($n = 28$) were selected

Comment: By chance, the proportion selected in 1998 matched the proportion diagnosed in 1998. However, in 2001 the proportion selected (13.5) dramatically underrepresented the proportion diagnosed (31.8 percent).

Technique 2 (Systematic Random Sample)

Given a sampling frame of 650 women and a desired sample size of 100, a sampling interval of 6.5 was used. The first woman selected was selected at random (#456). The next woman selected was #462 (rounding down from 6.5 to 6.0) and the next woman was #469 (rounding up from 6.5 to 7.0). The sampling procedure continued until 100 women were selected (which brought the sequence back to the starting point of #456). The proportions of women selected, by year, in comparison to those diagnosed were

1997: 105 (16.1 percent of 650) were diagnosed—16.0 percent ($n = 16$) were selected

1998: 155 (23.8 percent of 650) were diagnosed—24.0 percent ($n = 24$) were selected

1999:   73 (11.2 percent of 650) were diagnosed—11.0 percent ($n = 11$) were selected

2000:   110 (16.9 percent of 650) were diagnosed—17.0 percent ($n = 17$) were selected

2001:   207 (31.8 percent of 650) were diagnosed—32.0 percent ($n = 32$) were selected

Comment: By design, the proportion selected in each of the five years matched the proportion diagnosed in each corresponding year. The periodicity of the sampling frame was used to ensure proportional representation for women in each of the five diagnostic years.

Cluster Sampling. Cluster sampling is *a* technique used when the research question is about organizational behavior or policy rather than the health behavior or disease status of individuals. Application of the technique is simple. First, a sampling frame of clusters is developed or obtained. Then, a random sample of clusters is selected (simple random sampling or systematic random sampling could be used to achieve this goal). Thus, the cluster itself is the intended unit of analysis for the research being conducted. Examples include research goals such as the following:

- To assess the established exercise programs in nursing homes
- To determine whether worksite health promotion programs provide financial incentives to employees for wellness indicators
- To assess the proportion of Nevada counties that treat their municipal water supplies with fluoride
- To identify the presence or absence of counseling protocols designed to promote proper infant hydration practices for women being discharged from maternity wards

In each case, data from individuals would not be appropriate. Instead, the unit of analysis (that is, the source of data) is the cluster. This type of research is especially applicable to health services research and to formulating policy related to health promotion.

Multistage Cluster Sampling. Multistage cluster sampling is used when an appropriate sampling frame does not exist or cannot be obtained. Rather than revert to a nonprobability sampling technique, multistage cluster sampling uses a collection of preexisting units or clusters (such as health districts, counties, voluntary health agencies) to "stand in" for a sampling frame. The first stage in the process is selecting a sample of clusters at random from the list of all known clusters. The second stage consists of selecting a random sample from each cluster. Because of this multistage process, the likelihood of sampling bias increases. This creates a lack of sampling precision known as a design effect. Of interest, specialized statistical programs are available to account for (and therefore control) design effects. One such example is SUDAAN (Shah, Barnwell, and Beiler, 1997).

An inflated design effect (see Henry, 1990, p. 108, for a computational formula) can be avoided by selecting a larger number of clusters. Clusters are likely to be homogenous (meaning that people within the clusters are relatively similar to one another) and homogeneity reduces sampling error. Given that sample size is always limited by financial or practical constraints, the question at hand is whether to select more clusters or to select more people within a smaller number of clusters. Thus, by sampling more clusters (as opposed to more people within clusters) the likelihood of sampling error can be reduced and the design effect can be minimized.

Two relatively common terms must be understood when reading or reporting research that used a multistage cluster sampling technique. The *primary sampling unit* (PSU) is the first set of clusters used in the process of obtaining a sample. For example, counties may be the PSU in a study designed to assess the prevalence of farm accidents in the state of Montana. Perhaps a second set of clusters could also be employed. For example, after randomly selecting a group of counties (that is, the PSU) from a list of all rural counties, perhaps the research team could then select zip code areas to be the second set of clusters. In this case, zip code areas would be the *secondary sampling unit* or the SSU. The final sampling unit might be cattle producers and would be selected at random from the zip code areas. The final sampling unit becomes the intended unit of analysis. At each stage, selection of sampling units (whether PSU or SSU) is made at random.

Stratified Multistage Cluster Sampling. An extension of multistage cluster sampling is stratified multistage cluster sampling. Contrary to a rather complicated sounding name, this technique is nearly identical to multistage cluster sampling. The only difference is that the clusters may be divided into strata before random selection occurs. As previously noted, stratification reduces sampling error to "zero" for variables that may otherwise introduce sampling bias into a study.

An important note: Probability sampling does not need to be overwhelming! To the contrary, the techniques used are simply variants of three basic tools. Box 11.2 illustrates the logic of probability sampling by showing that basic techniques (see step 1) can be applied in numerous ways to create a sample that best fits the needs of the research question.

Box 11.2. Probability Sampling Made Easy

Step 1. Consider three basic options:

    A. Simple random sampling
    B. Systematic sampling
    C. Cluster sampling

Use any of these options (*alone*) to meet the needs of your research question.

Step 2 (if needed). For some research questions, you may need to begin by dividing the sampling frame into strata. This creates three possibilities based on the options in step 1:

    Stratified random sample = stratification + a

    Stratified systematic sample = stratification + b

    Stratified multistage cluster sample = stratified c + a or b

Step 3 (if needed). In some cases you may need to *combine* the options listed in step 1:

    Multistage cluster sample = c + a or c + b

Common Nonprobability Sampling Techniques

Although the benefits of probability sampling are tremendous, it is nonetheless important to note that whenever the population being studied is narrowly defined, it may be difficult to employ these techniques. The term *narrow* signifies that certain distinguishing parameters are used to delineate the target population such as those highlighted in the following research questions:

- To examine associations of perceived parental monitoring with biologically confirmed tobacco cessation among *adolescents with severe mental illness*
- To identify factors that may preclude people in high-risk populations (*gay men, injection drug users,* and *low-income African American men*) from accepting an AIDS vaccine when one is approved for use
- To compare HIV-associated sexual health history, risk perceptions, and sexual risk behaviors of *unmarried rural and non-rural African American women*

As indicated, the population is narrowly defined in each of the three research goals. Because the existence of sampling frames for each of these three narrowly defined

DINCUS WORRIES ABOUT THEIR "SAMPLE"
OF NUTS FOR THE WINTER.

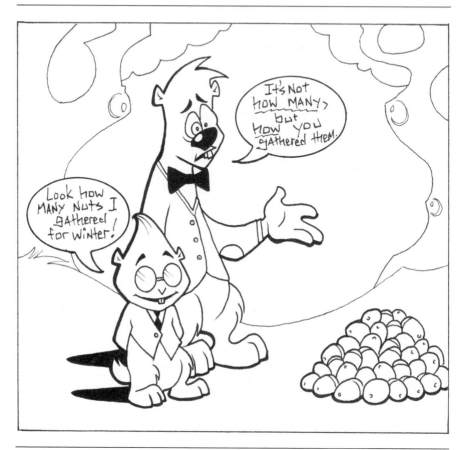

Copyright 2005 by Justin Wagner; reprinted with permission.

populations is unlikely, using a probability sampling technique is not feasible. In these instances, although a probability technique would be more rigorous, a non-probability sampling technique may be more realistic.

Convenience Sampling. Convenience sampling, perhaps the most widely used technique in health promotion research, uses preexisting groups such as a classroom of students, a support group for people with cancer, people in a waiting room of a clinic, people celebrating gay pride at a public event, and employees at work to facilitate recruitment. People in these groups can then be asked to volunteer for the study. Of course, the simplicity of this technique is attractive, but it comes with a high risk of yielding sampling bias. For example, imagine that the research question is, What are the correlates of condom use among gay men in long-term monogamous relationships? Using a convenience sample of gay men recruited from a gay bar or a gay pride event, for example, may provide a skewed view of the population in that gay male couples who attend public events may be quite different from those who stay at home.

When using a convenience sample, the key issue to consider is how well the preexisting group represents the population. Substantial and identifiable differences between the preexisting group and the population may result in study findings that misrepresent the population. Box 11.3 provides several examples of this problem. In each example it is important to note that the conclusion (despite intuitive appeal) is quite broad in scope—reaching far beyond the limitations imposed by a convenience sample.

Purposive Sampling. Purposive sampling is a technique that is targeted and specifies preestablished criteria for recruiting the sample. The need for purposive sampling is dependent on the research question. For example, "men who test positive for an STD to determine the correlates of condom use" is a research question that necessitates purposive sampling techniques. Of course, when a preexisting group is available to recruit the sample (for example, men attending an STD clinic), then

---

Box 11.3. Examples of Convenience Samples with "Large Conclusions"

Sample	*Conclusion*
952 low-income women in San Francisco	The involvement of male partners in decision making about condoms ensures greater protection against HIV infection.
789 adults recruited from a comprehensive service center in a Southeastern city	Clinicians working with adolescents should explore risk taking and prevention measures with their clients.
1,000 adolescents receiving prenatal care at one clinic	The experience of family violence is correlated with rapid repeat pregnancy among U.S. adolescents.
569 men recruited from one university	Prevention-intervention programs in high school and college reduce risk behaviors for chronic disease.

purposive sampling becomes a variant of convenience sampling. A preexisting group may not always be available, however. For example, to select a sample of delinquent youths, we may need to use a classroom as the recruitment venue and then recruit only those youths who meet the criterion for delinquency.

Quota Sampling. Quota sampling entails (1) identifying characteristics of the population to be reflected in the sample, (2) determining the distribution of these characteristics in the population ("setting the quotas"), and (3) selecting the sample based on those characteristics and their proportion in the population. These characteristics are usually sociodemographic factors such as gender, race, and age. Quota sampling can be useful if (1) the researcher determines that demographic factors such as age, gender, and race or ethnicity are critical components of representativeness, and (2) the demographic profile of the population is known. By characterizing the population and matching the sample to these characteristics sample bias is reduced.

Studies that designate college students as the target population are a good example of an opportunity to apply this technique. Suppose the research question is to identify determinants of binge drinking among undergraduates attending UCLA. Beginning with records from the registrar's office, a researcher could identify the distribution of demographics among the undergraduate population (that is, gender and race or ethnicity). Using these proportions, a matrix can be developed and would contain cells that represent the intersection between gender and race or ethnicity. One cell in the matrix is needed for each possible combination. For example, "Hispanic females" would be one cell. The quota of UCLA undergraduates, then, who are female and Hispanic would be determined based on sample size and the proportion of these characteristics in the undergraduate population (see Box 11.4). The reason for this extensive work is to have a guide for a variant of purposive sampling. The sample will be assembled to match the proportions shown in the matrix that was built from the records obtained in the registrar's office.

Box 11.4. Example of a Matrix for Quota Sampling

	Female	Male
African American/ Black	10.0 percent of enrolled students	9.0 percent of enrolled students
Asian	3.5 percent of enrolled students	1.5 percent of enrolled students
Hispanic	8.3 percent of enrolled students	6.2 percent of enrolled students
White	25.7 percent of enrolled students	35.8 percent of enrolled students

The primary problem with this technique is that the research question may or may not be one that lends itself to the assumption that demographic equivalence alone is sufficient to ensure representativeness. Perhaps, for example, binge drinking is a function of sorority and fraternity membership rather than age, gender, or race or ethnicity? Thus, representativeness is best achieved by selecting a sample that mirrors the population with respect to sorority and fraternity membership. Unfortunately, the idea that binge drinking is a function of sorority and fraternity membership may not materialize before the study is conducted; thus the researcher will not know what information should be used to build the selection matrix.

Variants of Snowball Sampling. Just as quota sampling is a specific application of purposive sampling, snowball sampling (and its variants) is also a specific application of purposive sampling. Snowball sampling is most useful in identifying and recruiting hard-to-reach populations (such as injection drug users or runaway teens). The basic technique is to begin with a "seed" (a person who qualifies to be in the study) and perform the interview (or administer any other part of a research protocol). The researcher asks the participant to identify others who meet the eligibility criteria and would possibly like to participate in the study (direct facilitation), or the researchers ask participants to contact others who meet the eligibility criteria so that they can refer them to the researcher (indirect facilitation).

Access Issues

As noted in Chapter Five, gaining access to a population is the primary starting point for health promotion research. Irrespective of the sampling technique employed, gaining access to the population may be a challenge and requires a plan to overcome obstacles and obtain the approval of certain gatekeepers that may restrict access.

The "Accounting Process"

Frequently, published reports of quantitative data will include a section that systematically accounts for the possibility of sampling bias. For nonprobability samples, such text usually begins by noting how many people were screened for eligibility and how many were found to be eligible. This first step is far less critical than the second step, which involves listing the reasons why eligible people chose not to participate and (possibly) comparing those who refused with those who agreed with respect to key demographic variables such as age, race, and sex.

FIGURE 11.2.   AN EXAMPLE OF A FIGURE USED TO REPRESENT RECRUITMENT SUCCESS.

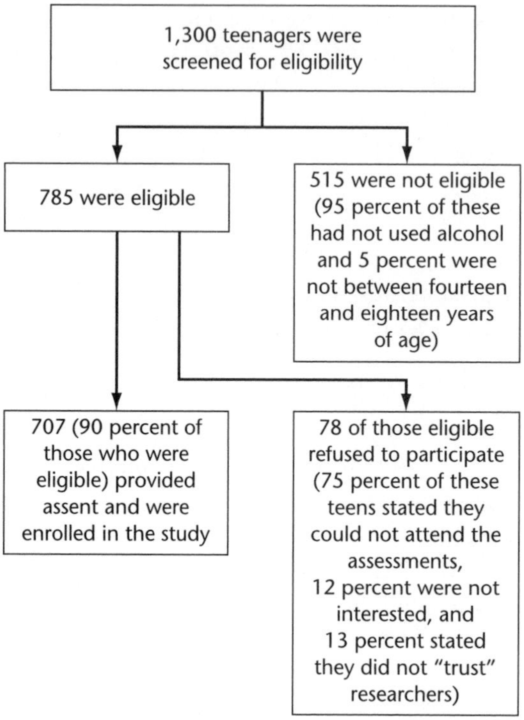

Most important, a participation rate is provided. Low participation rates suggest the possibility that *participation bias* may have occurred, while higher rates minimize participation bias. Participation bias is introduced into a sample when there may be differences between those who are eligible and participate and those who are eligible and refuse. The probability of participation bias is inversely related to the participation rate. An example of this accounting process follows and is depicted graphically in Figure 11.2.

A convenience sample of adolescent males was selected. The sample was intended to represent a broad cross-section of adolescents residing in low-income neighborhoods of Little Rock, Arkansas. Recruitment sites comprised three adolescent medicine clinics, two health department clinics, and health classes from seventeen high schools. From December 1996 through April 1999, project recruiters screened 1,300 adolescent males to assess their eligibility for participating in the study. Adolescents were eligible to participate if they were male, fourteen to eighteen years old, unmarried, and reported using alcohol at least once in the previous six months. Of those screened, 515 adolescents were not eligible to participate in the study; the majority (95 percent) did not meet the criterion of alcohol use, and 5 percent did not meet the age criterion. Of the 785 eligible adolescents, 90 percent ($n = 707$) agreed to participate and subsequently provided their assent. Of the teens who refused participation, the majority (75 percent) stated that their employment schedules would preclude them from making a time commitment (three consecutive Saturdays) to the study. Other reasons cited included lack of interest (12 percent) and a distrust of researchers (13 percent). Differences between those who refused and those who accepted the offer to participate were not found with respect to being a racial or ethnic minority ($P = .92$), age ($P = .53$), or level of education ($P = .81$).

Several points from the preceding paragraph warrant explanation. First, the participation rate of 90 percent is high and strongly suggests that participation bias is unlikely. Nonetheless, a reader who continues to suspect participation bias can be assured that refusal was mostly a function of Saturday work commitments. Three demographic comparisons between participants and "refusers" provided further assurance that participation bias was minimal. Although this process of collecting reasons for refusal and making simple demographic comparisons appears to be straightforward, an important principle of research is at odds with these practices: data cannot be collected from people who refuse study participation (see Chapter Three). Yet some researchers will argue that merely asking, "Can you please tell me why you do not want to be in the study?" is not a form of data collection. Furthermore, it can be argued that "observable" demographics (race and sex) do not qualify as collected data. Asking adolescents their age and grade level, however, is clearly a form of data collection, and engaging in this practice without their assent is a grey area with respect to ethics.

◆ ◆ ◆

In a Nutshell

Although this process of collecting reasons for refusal and making simple demographic comparisons appears to be straightforward, an important principle of research is at odds with these practices: data cannot be collected from people who refuse study participation.

◆ ◆ ◆

This accounting process is similar for probability samples except there may not be a need to determine what proportion of the people was eligible (if the sampling frame defined eligibility). Alternatively, if the sampling frame did not define eligibility, then this step in the accounting process is essential.

An Introduction to Sample Size

Before learning about the principles that guide sample size determinations, please consider the following scenario. One study ($N = 1,000$) is conducted, and the findings support the hypothesis that teens belonging to gangs will report a higher frequency of marijuana use in the past thirty days. The hypothesis was tested by performing a t-test and had a corresponding t-value of 7.5, which was significant at $P < .01$. Another study was conducted to test the same hypothesis. In this study, the sample size was much smaller ($N = 100$); however, the statistical findings were nearly identical ($t = 7.4$; $P < .01$). Knowing nothing else about the samples, determine which study had the bigger difference between means (please give this some thought before reading the next two paragraphs).

The answer to the question lies in the study's calculated effect size. Without exception, sample size and effect size are interrelated elements of any quantitative study. In the example provided, effect size can be conceptualized as "distance between group means." In the study of a thousand participants, the effect size was the difference between groups in the mean number of days that teens smoked marijuana. Teens who belonged to gangs smoked marijuana 3.7 days on average, and teens who were not in gangs smoked marijuana 1.5 days on average. In contrast, in the study of one hundred participants, the effect size was much greater. The teens who belonged to gangs smoked 9.4 days on average compared with teens not in gangs, who smoked 1.7 days on average. Figure 11.3 provides an illustration of effect size relative to this example. In this figure, effect size is portrayed as a slope. A lack of slope (a flat—horizontal—line) would represent a complete lack of effect. Conversely, an increasing slope represents an increasingly greater effect size. Note that the slope in the study of a thousand teens is quite gentle in contrast to rather dramatic slope in the study of one hundred teens.

An important (and often ignored) point is that effect size is invariant to sample size. Sample size influences the level of statistical significance only (that is, P-value). All things being equal, as sample size increases, significance is more likely to be achieved. (See Box 11.5 for an illustration of this principle.) A larger sample size (along with several other determinants) gives a study an extra "boost" to find

FIGURE 11.3.   EFFECT SIZE IN TWO SIMILAR STUDIES.

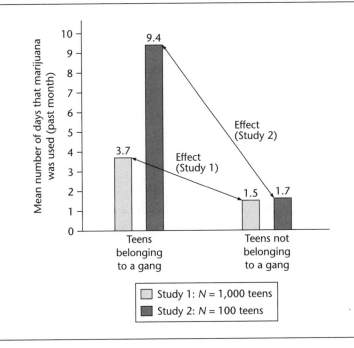

significance for modest to small effect sizes. Conversely, this boost is lacking with small samples (such as $N = 100$); thus, only large effect sizes can be detected with small samples. This point leads to a critical principle of sampling: plan for a sample size that is adequate to detect (with statistical significance) the anticipated effect size. A more thorough treatment of sample size, effect size, and statistical power is provided in Chapter Twelve.

◆ ◆ ◆

In a Nutshell

Plan for a sample size that is adequate to detect (with statistical significance) the anticipated effect size.

◆ ◆ ◆

Box 11.5. As Sample Size Goes Up, Significance Is Easier to "Find"

This principle is shown by an example. Consider an experimental program delivered to high-risk men that was designed to promote annual cholesterol testing. An index of intent to have a cholesterol test annually was constructed. The highest possible rating was 10.0 and the lowest was 0.0.

Using a pretest, posttest experimental design, with fifteen men in each of two groups, the researchers obtained posttest means as follows: Control = 6.0; Intervention = 6.9.

A significance test was conducted to determine whether the observed means were different beyond differences that could be expected by sampling error alone. The researchers used a two-tailed t-test and set their alpha at .05. The P-value achieved was .094; thus the null hypothesis was retained.

One member of the research team had a hard time accepting the finding (this person could not get over the idea that the intervention did not "change" men with respect to the measure of intent). Hence, this person suggested that the sample size "should be doubled and another study should be conducted." After the study was repeated with thirty men assigned to each of the two conditions, the same t-test was conducted (this time $N = 60$, rather than $N = 30$). This time the mean in the control group was 6.0 and the mean in the intervention group was 6.9 (exactly the same means that had been found in the study of only thirty men!). However, the obtained P-value in the test of sixty men was .001. The previously disgruntled researcher was now quite satisfied and proceeded to publish the findings.

Applied Examples

Between February and May of 1998, the Centers for Disease Control and Prevention (CDC) surveyed adolescents attending U.S. alternative schools (Grunbaum and others, 2000). Given the existence of a sampling frame, CDC used a multistage cluster sampling technique. The primary sampling unit was 121 geographical clusters of alternative high schools. Forty-eight of the PSUs were selected. For the second stage, 142 alternative schools (SSUs) were selected from the 48 PSUs. Schools with substantially greater enrollments of black and Hispanic students were purposefully oversampled. Finally, classes within the 142 selected schools were randomly chosen for study participation. Participation rates were 81.0 percent (schools) and 81.9 percent (students). A total of 8,918 students from 115 schools constituted the sample.

This preceding description illustrates the utility of a multistage cluster sample. Note that three stages were involved, thus a design effect is clearly likely. Despite this "cost" of the sampling technique, the final sample of nearly nine thousand students has a very good chance of representing the population of adolescents who attended U.S. alternative schools in 1998. The PSU is particularly important in that the CDC apparently grouped alternative schools into geographic clusters. Similar to stratification, this practice was useful in ensuring that adolescents were selected from a representative sample of geographic areas. Note that the PSUs were created by the CDC—they existed only for purposes of the sampling protocol and thus (as nonentities) they could not "refuse" or "accept" participation (hence only two participation rates were reported).

Preventive Service Utilization

A recent study investigated the effect of demographic and socioeconomic factors on elderly men's use of preventive services such as influenza vaccination, colorectal cancer screening, and testing for prostate-specific antigens (Morales and others, 2004). More than 19,000 men enrolled in Medicare health maintenance organizations and in traditional (fee for service) Medicare programs composed the sampling frame. To draw a sample that represented both high- and low-income groups, the research team used a stratified random sampling technique. In each plan (HMO and fee for service) three strata were formed: (1) men who were also Medicaid eligible and one for the remaining men, (2) remaining men who resided in a low-income zip code area, and (3) all remaining men. Men in the first and second strata were oversampled. The final sample consisted of 942 men from strata 1,700 from strata 2, and 5,354 from strata 3.

The example clearly shows the utility of stratification. Given what appears to have been a fairly detailed sampling frame (in other words, it contained much more than names), the researchers were able to ensure that three distinct groups of men were selected into the sample. This logic is an extension of the research question (that is, the research was designed to compare men in these three groups relative to their use of preventive services). Note then, that stratification was not used for its traditional purpose of eliminating sampling error for an identified variable. Instead, stratification was used to define analytic groups! This innovative use of stratification typifies the potential of using sampling techniques in a creative manner— the ultimate principle of this creativity is to serve the research question.

◆ ◆ ◆

In a Nutshell

This innovative use of stratification typifies the potential of using sampling techniques in a creative manner—the ultimate principle of this creativity is to serve the research question.

◆ ◆ ◆

Barriers to Flu Vaccination

A study reported by Armstrong and colleagues (2001) was designed to assess perceived barriers to influenza vaccination among low-income African American urban dwellers. Health system billing records served as the initial sampling frame. Selecting only people who reside in one of twelve zip code areas that defined West Philadelphia then refined this initial sampling frame. Subsequently a random sample of 825 people was drawn from this modified sampling frame.

This example is instructive on many levels. First, it illustrates that a sampling frame can be modified to suit the research question. (In this case, West Philadelphia was selected to ensure a high likelihood of selecting low-income African American urban dwellers, thus serving the research question.) Second, the example serves as a reminder that the study conclusions should never exceed the boundaries of the sample. In this case, only people receiving medical services were represented in the initial sampling frame; thus, the findings cannot be generalized to people who do not receive medical services. Furthermore, the research question was addressed only by surveying people in West Philadelphia, thereby precluding generalization to the general population of "low-income African American urban dwellers." In short, the example serves as a reminder that not all probability samples can be used as a basis for population-level conclusions. Finally, this example raises the question of why a purposive sample was not used. Given that the intent was to identify barriers to influenza vaccination among low-income African American urban dwellers, a purposive sample might have been equally effective and perhaps far less labor intensive. If recruitment for such a purposive sample occurred in nonmedical settings, then persons not receiving medical care would not have been excluded from the study. Our intent is not to "second guess" the work of this research team. Instead, this example is used here to show that probability sampling is not always an automatically superior choice to nonprobability sampling.

Integration with the Research Process

This chapter has presented basic concepts involved with step 6 of the research process (see Figure 1.2). The appropriate selection of a "parsimonious sampling technique" is indeed a critical determinant of study rigor. Although simple rules do not apply (for example, probability techniques are always better), the general principle of parsimony is very applicable. In turn, parsimony is a function of the progress in the chain of research; studies found early in the chain probably can be quite valuable based on the use of nonprobability methods. Alternatively, studies that are in advanced positions on the research chain may or may not benefit from the use of the more elaborate forms of sampling (that is, probability techniques).

◆ ◆ ◆

In a Nutshell

Although simple rules do not apply (for example, probability techniques are always better), the general principle of parsimony is very applicable.

◆ ◆ ◆

As noted previously in this chapter, formulation of the research question (step 2) may be dependent upon ability to access the sample necessitated by the question. This iterative process of asking if a research question can be fairly addressed given realistic options for sampling must occur in conjunction with step 2. Thus, sampling is very much part of the planning process rather than simply being an implementation step.

The single most important determinant of selecting a sampling technique is the selection of a priority population (step 1 in the research process) for the research. In fact, the selection of a population immediately defines and limits the sampling options. In turn, steps 8 and 9 of the research process (data analysis and interpretation followed by dissemination of the findings) are dependent on the selection of the sampling technique. For example, inferential statistics (in theory) are meant to be applied only to data collected from a probability sample. Interpretation of any study is also very much a function of the sampling—this is because the findings cannot be generalized beyond the ability of the sample to represent the population. As sampling becomes increasingly representative of a population, the ability to generalize study findings to that population also increases. Finally, it should be noted that an unfortunate reality often exists with respect to publishing (that is, disseminating) findings from research studies—probability samples are often considered "preferred" products by virtue of their ability for generalization. However tempting, this reality does not justify selecting a probability technique simply because it may facilitate publication of a manuscript.

◆ ◆ ◆

In a Nutshell

The selection of a population immediately defines and limits the sampling options.

◆ ◆ ◆

Summary

Sampling can make or break a research study. The pinnacle of success in sampling is perfect representativeness. Unfortunately, this pinnacle is rarely achieved. However, the barriers that preclude full achievement are often inevitable. One important example is the necessary compromise that must occur to protect the rights of people to refuse study participation. Another important example is extremely practical in nature: researchers are not always granted access to a potential sample of people or organizations, and they may be denied access to useful sampling frames. Once access is achieved, sampling techniques should be chosen to parsimoniously address the research question and fairly represent the selected priority population. Sampling can select elements comprising "people" or representing organized units (clusters). Again, the selection of people versus clusters is dictated by the nature of the research question. Creative use of these techniques is not only acceptable but is also encouraged—as none of the techniques has perfect utility for all research questions.

◆ ◆ ◆

In a Nutshell

The pinnacle of success in sampling is perfect representativeness.

◆ ◆ ◆

Issues to Consider

1. An important issue can be conceptualized by the following question: What constitutes a confound in the test of the research question? A confound is a measurable factor that can produce bias. For example, imagine a study that is designed to assess the protective value of condoms against the acquisition of chlamydia. The research question is largely tied to physiological processes (for example, the porosity of the latex, the size and infectivity of the pathogen, and the biology of chlamydia transmission). Thus (with the exception of sex differences, in other words, male versus female anatomy) a sample of any kind might be justifiable as the results of this study should not vary as a function of the population. In other words, if condoms "work" for one population then they should also work for another. Although this proposition is attractive, what if a factor such as "condom skill" plays a role and the sample selected has an unusually high-level of skill? Of course, the confound (skill) will create a bias

that favors condom effectiveness. Yet, if skill is measured it can be accounted for statistically; thus, the confound no longer applies. This issue then is whether a sample inherently creates confounds that cannot be controlled. When such confounds do not exist, is the use of "any sample" justifiable in studies that address largely nonbehavioral outcomes?

2. A consistently important principle in health promotion is that ethics must always take precedence over rigor. This principle, however, is often violated by even the best-intentioned researchers. For example, the "accounting process" described in this chapter suggests that knowing the reasons nonparticipants refused to be part of the study is an important aspect of gauging rigor. Yet once a person says "no," do researchers violate this principle by proceeding to ask a question and then recording the answer and treating it as data?

3. Does providing study participants with financial compensation lead to participation bias? This is perhaps one of the most contemporary issues in health promotion research. Simply stated, the use of incentives (financial or otherwise) will be a greater enticement to some people compared with others, and the reasons for this greater enticement may be a marker for a study confound. For example, offering men $20 to complete a three-hour interview about their risks of cancer may be effective at producing a high participation rate, but many of the men who say "yes" may do so simply because they cannot in good consciousness turn down this "easy money." By comparison men who say "no" may be quite different (perhaps not perceiving $20 as a substantial amount of money). Thus, the sample may have an inherent bias of low-income men. Conversely, if financial incentives are extremely low (for instance, $5) or nonexistent, it is entirely conceivable that only men with a preexisting interest in cancer risks would volunteer, thereby creating a bias sample of men who are seemingly very concerned about cancer risks. Although striking a happy median between "too much" and "too little" incentive is an apparent answer to this issue, the question becomes how much is too much and how little is too little?

For Practice and Discussion

1. After much thought and discussion, you have developed the following research question: Are immigrant Latinas in the U.S. who have not been *acculturated* (cultural modification of an individual, group, or people by adapting to or borrowing traits from another culture) less likely to receive gynecological care than their counterparts who are more acculturated? You decide that fluency in English will be a valid proxy measure for acculturation. Thus, you need a

sample of immigrant Latinas who do and do not speak English. Alone, please list your top three choices for a sampling technique and then rank these in order of desirability—be prepared to explain your thinking! Then (if possible) find another student who has also completed this exercise and compare your list with his or her list. Try to engage in discussion about the pros and cons of the selections until your lists (and your rankings) match.

2. For the articles listed below (or any other article that you may select), please answer the following questions: (1) What type of sampling technique was employed (be careful not to simply restate what the authors have said—name the technique they used based on what you learned in this chapter; (2) Are the conclusions of the article within the boundaries of the sample? Or have the authors generalized beyond the ability of the sample?; and (3) Have the authors misused the sampling technique in any way and, if so, how?

Sources for This Exercise

1. Rosenberg, S. D., and others. (2001). Prevalence of HIV, hepatitis B, and hepatitis C in people with severe mental illness. *American Journal of Public Health, 91,* 31–37.
2. Blake, S. M., and others. (2003). Condom availability programs in Massachusetts high schools: Relationships with condom use and sexual behavior. *American Journal of Public Health, 93,* 955–962.
3. Tang, H., and others. (2003). Changes of attitudes and patronage behaviors in response to a smoke-free bar law. *American Journal of Public Health, 93,* 611–617.

References

Abelson, R. P. (1995). *Statistics as principled argument.* Hillsdale, NJ: Lawrence Erlbaum Associates.

Armstrong, K., Berlin, M., Sanford-Swartz, J., Propert, K., and Ubel, P. A. (2001). Barriers to influenza immunization in a low-income urban population. *The American Journal of Preventive Medicine, 20,* 21–25.

Babbie, E. (2001). *The practice of social research* (10th ed.). Belmont, CA: Wadsworth.

Grunbaum, J. A., and others. (2000). Youth risk behavior surveillance: National Alternative High School Youth Risk Behavior Survey, United States, 1998. *Journal of School Health, 70,* 5–17.

Henry, G. T. (1990). *Practical Sampling.* Thousand Oaks, CA: Sage.

Morales, L. S., and others. (2004). Use of preventive services by men enrolled in Medicare+ choice plans. *American Journal of Public Health, 94,* 796–802.

Shah, B. V., Barnwell, B. G., and Beiler, G. S. (1997). *SUDAAN: User's manual, release 7.5.* Research Triangle Park, NC: Research Triangle Institute.

Shi, L. (1997). *Health services research methods.* Albany, NY: Delmar Publishers.

CHAPTER TWELVE

ANALYTIC TECHNIQUES FOR OBSERVATIONAL RESEARCH

Richard A. Crosby, Ralph J. DiClemente, and Laura F. Salazar

Students often experience a great deal of anxiety over the topic of data analysis. Although a modest level of anxiety may be helpful, this chapter is designed to alleviate the anxiety associated with statistics. Indeed, statistical methods applied to health promotion research do not need to be highly sophisticated (or complicated) to be effective. Although the research process is often labor-intensive and time consuming, data analysis can be a fairly short process that is straightforward by comparison. The caveat, however, is that the selection of analytic tools must be exact and the analyses must be precise. Without these two conditions, selection and precision, the entire research process is jeopardized.

As noted in Chapter One, parsimony is a critical concern with respect to data analysis. Data that tell a story worth hearing need not be "tortured" to achieve a valuable analysis. On the contrary, data analyses require the application of three basic procedures. First, the data should be described. This initial procedure is nothing more than a representation of the data in the form of frequency counts and, if applicable, means with their standard deviations. Some research questions do not require data analysis beyond this point. Second, *bivariate* associations between variables should be calculated. The term *bivariate* means that the calculated association is only between two variables. Typically, in health promotion research, the bivariate association would be between one Y variable (the outcome variable) and one X variable (the predictor variable); however, you may be interested in calculating bivariate associations between two predictor variables. Again, some research questions do not require further analysis. The problem, though, is that bivariate relationships seldom capture the complexity of health behaviors. Most health behavior is rarely, if ever, predicted by only one predictor variable. In fact, health behaviors often have complex determinants that can only be understood when a large number of X variables are taken into consideration. Studies of behaviors such as condom use (Sheeran, Abraham, and Orbell, 1999), teen pregnancy (Crosby and others, 2003), and being vaccinated against influenza (Armstrong, Berlin, Sanford-Swartz, Propert, and Ubel, 2001) involve multiple predictor variables as they relate to these single outcome variables. Thus, the third and final basic procedure is to conduct a *multivariate* analysis of the data. In this chapter, the term *multivariate* will be used to represent a statistical analysis involving multiple predictors or X variables and a single outcome or Y variable. Some scholars reserve the term *multivariate* for analyses that involve multiple Y variables, however.

◆ ◆ ◆

In a Nutshell

Data that tell a story worth hearing need not be "tortured" to achieve a valuable analysis.

◆ ◆ ◆

After presenting these three basic procedures, the chapter will also provide an overview of other related statistical issues such as power, sample size, and effect size, as these affect testing the research question. This presentation will be modest in scope. Readers who are interested in a more comprehensive treatment of these topics are encouraged to consult a text authored by Cohen (1988). The overall approach of this chapter is to provide a conceptual basis for applying analytic procedures that are commonly used in health promotion research. This chapter will serve as a springboard into statistics for observational research. Fortunately, a large number of very well-written statistics textbooks are readily available (for example, Pagano and Gauvreau, 2000; Siegel and Castellan, 1988; Tabachnick and Fidell, 1996).

Illustration of Key Concepts

Analyses generally begin with basic descriptive techniques and then proceed to employ tests for bivariate associations and, finally, for multivariate associations. When testing for bivariate and multivariate associations, it is important to understand the use of *P*-values. Last, but certainly not least, issues pertaining to statistical power and effect size must constantly be considered in the analytic process.

Descriptive Analysis

Observational data analysis seeks to describe and explain characteristics of defined groups. Ideally, these are representative samples of priority populations. (See step 1 in Chapter One.) Thus, an initial goal of descriptive analysis is to characterize the group through the use of appropriate statistics. In this section, we will use an example of an observational study of adolescents residing in detention facilities, which was conducted by the editors of this textbook, to highlight the different descriptive statistics. In this particular example, one of the research questions involved assessing the prevalence of thirty-four different health risk behaviors. After collecting the data, we produced the graphic shown in Figure 12.1. The

FIGURE 12.1.   DISTRIBUTION OF HEALTH-RISK BEHAVIORS FOR 569 DETAINED ADOLESCENTS.

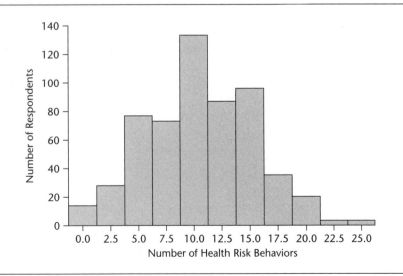

figure shows the distribution of scores and thus provides a useful overview of the data.

The Normal Curve. Scores that are distributed normally produce a distribution that, when graphed, create a specific, symmetrical curve shaped like a bell that follows a particular mathematical function. Often the normal curve is referred to as a bell-shaped curve, although, strictly speaking, not all bell-shaped curves are normal, but any distribution that is not symmetrical cannot be a normal curve. It is important to determine whether or not your data are approximately normally distributed, as this characteristic is an assumption that must be met for many statistical analyses to be performed correctly and accurately. Statistical analyses that require data to be normally distributed (for instance, linear regression) fall under the category of parametric tests. Other tests that do not require the data to be normally distributed (for example, a chi-square test) are deemed nonparametric.

A curve's deviation from normality can be judged based on two properties: *skewness* and *kurtosis*. Skewness is the degree to which scores in the distribution fall disproportionately on one side creating a curve with a long "tail." Although by graphing and visually inspecting a distribution we have a gross indicator of a distribution's skewness, it should be evaluated statistically. Most statistical software programs will determine whether or not skewness exceeds that of a normal distribution. The distribution shown in Figure 12.2 illustrates a positively skewed

**FIGURE 12.2.   NUMBER OF SEX PARTNERS (LIFETIME)
REPORTED BY DETAINED ADOLESCENTS.**

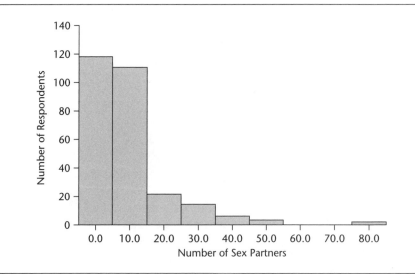

FIGURE 12.3.   NUMBER OF PAP TESTS (LIFETIME) REPORTED BY 273 WOMEN.

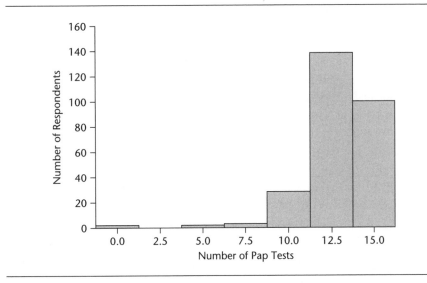

distribution in that most of the scores fall to the left side (in other words, most of the study participants reported having sex with ten or fewer partners), creating a long tail extending to the right. Whether or not a distribution is positively or negatively skewed depends on the direction of this tail. Therefore the distribution in Figure 12.2 is positively skewed. Many variables assessed in health promotion research will have a positive skew. Some examples include number of pregnancies, number of times diagnosed with a sexually transmitted disease, use of illicit substances, and frequency of driving while intoxicated.

An example of a distribution that is negatively skewed is shown in Figure 12.3. As indicated, the majority of scores are clumped together on the far right, leaving a long tail that extends to the left (the negative direction of the number line). Thus, most women in the sample reported having approximately twelve or more Pap tests in their lifetime.

Kurtosis refers to the shape of the distribution from top to bottom rather than side-to-side. A distribution with a preponderance of cases clustered in the middle—making a very tall spike-like shape—is called *leptokurtic*. Conversely, a distribution with a relatively flat shape (an absence of scores grouped around the mean) is called *platykurtic*. Again, by graphing and visually inspecting a distribution we can have a gross indicator of a distribution's kurtosis; however, it should be evaluated statistically. Most statistical software programs will also determine whether or not kurtosis exceeds that of a normal distribution.

The Mean. A mean can be calculated for any distribution assessed using ratio-level or interval-level data. *Ratio-level* data are assessed such that the distance between possible values is always equal and an absolute (rather than arbitrary) zero point exists. Age is a good example of a ratio-level measure. *Interval-level data* assume an equal distance between values but an absolute zero point is not present (see Box 12.1 for more information about levels of measurement). The obtained distribution portrays the health risk behavior profile of the entire sample of 569 adolescents (Figure 12.1). Of thirty-four possible risk behaviors, some adolescents engaged in no risk behavior, whereas others engaged in as many as twenty-five. The arithmetic average, or the *mean*, was 10.6. It is important to note

Box 12.1. Four Levels of Data

1. Nominal data represent discrete categories that are not ordered in any particular way.

Examples: sex, religion, reasons for not having a mammogram, types of illicit substances used in the past thirty days, and outcome of health promotion program (for example, improved or did not improve).

2. Ordinal data represent a value, category, or level that can be ranked or ordered in some particular way. Distances between categories are not assumed to be equal.

Examples: questionnaire responses coded as "strongly agree," "agree," "unsure," "disagree," or "strongly disagree"; decisional focus for contraceptive use (response option might be "my partner decides without my input," "I provide some input into these decisions," "I provide an equal amount of input," "I decide without my partner's input").

3. Interval data represent numerical values that are ordered, and distances between values are assumed to be equal. The value for zero is arbitrary.

Examples: psychological measures such as intelligence, special abilities, personality, and so on; temperature measured on Fahrenheit or Celsius scales.

4. Ratio data represent numerical values that are ordered, have equal distances between values, and have an absolute zero-point.

Examples: age, inches, weight, dollars, number of times a person used alcohol in the past month, number of times a person has had their blood serum cholesterol checked, number of vaccinations given by voluntary health organizations, percentage of body fat.

Note: Sometimes data can be converted from one type to another. For example, age (a ratio measure) can be converted to an ordinal measure by assigning scores that fall below 45 to a category named "young" and scores that equal or fall above 45 to a category named "old."

that the mean does not pertain to any one person; instead, it represents the average score of the group. Because it is an average score of the group, the mean is vulnerable to any extreme scores or outliers. For example, in a study of 141 high-risk men, frequency of crack (cocaine) use was assessed for the past six months. The mean number of uses was 29.1. Of interest though, one man indicated using crack a thousand times. Upon converting this score to "system missing" (as it is quite difficult to place full confidence in this extremely high value) the mean is reduced to 22.1 (a much truer representation of the group).

Spread. One important aspect of the group scores is characterized by their distribution or spread. It is important to understand two elemental indicators of spread: the *range* of the scores (in other words, the lowest score subtracted from the highest score) and the *dispersion* (that is, how much each score differs from the mean). Both the range and the dispersion are sensitive to extreme scores. For example, the initial range in the study of men who use crack was 1,000 (1,000 − 0). After excluding the extreme score of 1,000, the range decreased to 250 (250 − 0), indicating a much more narrow degree of spread.

The Standard Deviation. Because the goal is to characterize the group, it is useful to calculate an average measure of dispersion. This is called the standard deviation and can be derived by first summing each of the squared deviations (all 569) from the mean. Because negative deviations will cancel out positive deviations, the sum of all deviations will always produce a value of zero. Thus, the deviations are squared. Then, to obtain an average of the deviations, the sum of the squared deviations must be divided by the number of study participants, minus 1 (that is, 568). To return to the original metric, the square root is then calculated. The obtained value is known as the standard deviation and is always a positive value.

Like the mean, the standard deviation provides a great deal of clarity to the description of a group. It too is sensitive to influence of extreme scores. In the example of men who use crack, before excluding the score of 1,000 the standard deviation was 88.4 (this is a very large standard deviation). After excluding the extreme score, the standard deviation became much more reasonable (32.2). It is important to note that size does matter. When the standard deviation is small, this statistic indicates that the group is very similar relative to the variable being studied. This similarity is also called *homogeneity.* Conversely, when the standard deviation is large, this statistic indicates that the group is very diverse relative to the variable being studied. This level of diversity is also called *heterogeneity.*

The standard deviation can be used as a tool to characterize distributions that are relatively symmetrical. Returning to the previous example, recall that the mean is 10.6 and the standard deviation is 4.8. Moving in both positive and negative directions from the mean by one standard deviation (in other words, ± 1 SD) will account for approximately two-thirds of the scores (about 68 percent). Stated differently, slightly more than two-thirds of the sample will have scores between a low value of 5.8 (10.6 − 4.8) and a high value of 15.4 (10.6 + 4.8). Furthermore, moving in both directions from the mean by two standard deviations accounts for 95 percent of scores. Thus, 95 percent of the scores would fall between scores of 1.0 (10.6 − [4.8 × 2]) and 20.2 (10.6 + [4.8 × 2]).

The Median. The median is the score occurring at the midpoint of a ranked distribution of scores and should be used when data are skewed or when the data are measured using an *ordinal scale* (ordinal measurement means that the scores can be ranked from low to high, but that the distance between scores is not known to be equal; see Box 12.1 for more information about levels of measurement). For example, in the United States a distribution of income would have a strong positive skew, meaning that most people have low income levels whereas a small minority has extremely high income levels. Thus, the mean is not an accurate indicator of the "middle" income level for all people residing in the United States. In this instance, the median would be a better statistic to use to describe income distribution levels, as it separates the ranked order distribution at the middle. In health promotion research, many health-related variables are not always amenable to interval- or ratio-level measurement. Instead, ordinal-level measures are quite common. For example, to characterize a group with regard to satisfaction levels of physician-patient relationships when the difference between satisfaction levels are unknown and should not be assumed to be equal is conducive to the use of the median to describe the distribution of scores.

Frequency Distributions. When nominal-level data are collected, statistics are not available to characterize a distribution. *Nominal-level* measurement means that discrete categories are being assessed (such as male and female; black and white; former smoker, current smoker, never smoked); therefore, ranking from low to high or ordering in a particular way is not possible nor is it logical (again, see Box 12.1 for more information about levels of measurement). Because nominal data are not ranked, a median would be an inappropriate statistic for describing these distributions (a mean, standard deviation, or other statistic is also not applicable). Instead, simply enumerating the number of occurrences for each attribute of the nominal measure is appropriate. An example of a computer-generated frequency distribution is shown in Table 12.1. Notice that four columns appear in this table. The first provides the actual number of study participants categorized into each of the listed attributes. For example, 219 adolescents self-identified as black and

TABLE 12.1.   FREQUENCY DISTRIBUTION OF RACE OR ETHNICITY FOR A SAMPLE OF 569 DETAINED ADOLESCENTS.

Race or Ethnicity	Frequency	Percentage	Valid Percentage	Cumulative Percentage
White-not Hispanic	223	39.2	40.1	40.1
Black-not Hispanic	219	38.5	39.4	79.5
White-Hispanic	32	5.6	5.8	85.3
Black-Hispanic	42	7.4	7.6	92.8
Asian American	4	.7	.7	93.5
Native American	6	1.1	1.1	94.6
Other	30	5.3	5.4	100.0
Total	556	97.7	100.0	
Missing	13	2.3		
Total	569	100.0		

non-Hispanic. Notice in this column that data are missing for 13 adolescents. This observation is important because it suggests that converting the frequency counts into percentages could be achieved by using one of two possible denominators. The second column shows percentages based on the entire sample as the denominator (in this case 569). The third column also shows the percentages, but these are based only on the number of valid cases (meaning that the thirteen missing cases are not included in the denominator). Thus, when data are missing (which is generally unavoidable) the values in the third column will always be greater than the values in the second column. The fourth column is merely a running subtotal of the third column. This can be useful for descriptive purposes. For example, inspection of this column reveals that 92.8 percent of the sample self-identified as either white or black.

Bivariate Analysis

Before we describe a few selected types of bivariate analyses, it is important to clarify in general why statistical tests are performed. The tests yield two critical pieces of information that must be considered to answer the research question. First, the test informs us whether or not a finding may have occurred by chance. In this context, chance is determined by a probability value that when conducting statistical tests is judged against *alpha*. Alpha can be conceptualized as a cut-off point to determine the statistical significance of a test and by convention is set at .05 or less. Alpha is the probability that given the null hypothesis is true (for example, no effect) the results observed were by chance. Uppercase *P* and lowercase *p* are both used to denote the probability level associated with a particular statistical test. The second piece of critical information that statistical tests provide is a quantitative indicator of strength in relationships.

When embarking on a bivariate analysis, a key step is to select an appropriate statistical test. Three of the most basic options in health promotion research are (1) a t-test, (2) a chi-square test, and (3) the Pearson Product Moment Correlation. The t-test is used when the research question has a grouping variable that identifies only two groups (the predictor) and an outcome variable measured at an interval- or ratio-level. The chi-square test could be used with the same grouping variable (with two or more levels), but only when the outcome variable is nominal (both variables might also be ordinal, especially if only a few values are used). Finally, the Pearson Product Moment Correlation is used when both variables are represented with interval- or ratio-level measures.

T-*Test Example.* A common goal of observational research in health promotion is to compare subgroups of a sample (defined by a "grouping" variable) with respect to a second variable. Imagine, for example, that your research question involves comparing males and females on an index of health risk behavior. The grouping variable would be sex and the second variable would be the score on an index. Consider the distribution shown in Figure 12.1. Because this was assessed with a ratio-level measure, a t-test would be an appropriate method of addressing a research question involving sex differences. The test answers a basic question that is essential to all statistical tests: Are observed differences between the two groups "real" or due to chance? By convention real differences can be attributable to chance no more than five times out of one hundred tests. This corresponds to an alpha of .05. In some research studies, a more restrictive P-value may be used, such as .01. Of interest, the P-value of .05 corresponds to values of the test statistic that are greater than two standard deviations above or less than two standard deviations below the mean. This relationship is explained in Box 12.2.

The t-test will compare a mean risk score for females to the mean risk score for males. Dispersion of each distribution (one pertaining to females, the other to males) plays an important role in the calculation of t (small standard deviations will produce a larger t value). The number of study participants in each group also plays an important role in the calculation of t; larger numbers of participants will produce a larger t value. In this example, 283 females had a mean risk score of 9.9 (SD = 5.0) and 276 males had a mean of 11.3 (SD = 4.5). The obtained value for t was 3.4. This value was significant (that is, the probability associated with this test was less than .05). In fact, the obtained P-value of .001 suggests that given no sex differences, the findings would be attributable to chance only 1 out of 1,000 times! So, what can be concluded from this bivariate analysis? Given that the test was significant, it can be said that the mean for males is significantly greater

Box 12.2. Confidence Intervals

Intervals—defined by lower and upper boundaries, can be used to define a given level of confidence that a mean (or a similar estimate) is accurate. For example, a statement might read, "The mean was 19.2 (95 percent CI = 9.2 − 29.2)." The statement provides a range of confidence for the mean—implying 95 percent confidence that it is, in reality, a value that falls between 9.2 and 29.2. Values beyond this range (in either direction) would be attributable to chance—note then, that chance is set at 5 percent (corresponding to a P-value of .05). If a 99 percent confidence had been reported, then chance would be set at 1 percent (corresponding to a P-value of .01).

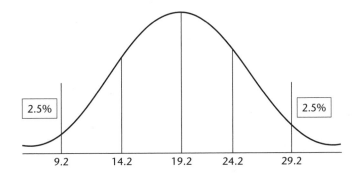

| 2.5% | | | | 2.5% |
| 9.2 | 14.2 | 19.2 | 24.2 | 29.2 |

The confidence interval is defined by standard deviations. Adding and subtracting two standard deviations from the mean defines the 95 percent confidence interval (three standard deviations defines the 99 percent CI). Given a standard deviation of 5.0, the 95 percent CI would be defined according to the picture shown here. The 2.5 percent of the cases that fall at either extreme would be "outside" of the defined interval. Wide intervals imply less precision (or confidence) in the estimate. Thus, narrow confidence intervals are a desirable standard. For example, what if the standard deviation had been 2.0 rather than 5.0 percent?

Confidence intervals can also be applied to test statistics. An odds ratio, for example, is always shown with a corresponding 95 percent CI. Again, narrow intervals are desirable. The interval can be used to compare the relative strength of two odds ratios. If the lower limit of the interval with the higher odds ratio "laps" into the higher limit of the lower odds ratio, then the two odds ratios are not significantly different from each other. However, if they do not have overlapping values between their confidence intervals, they are indeed "different," and the value of the larger odds ratio is significantly greater than that of the lower odds ratio.

DINCUS IS UNSURE OF HIS STATISTICAL PLAN.

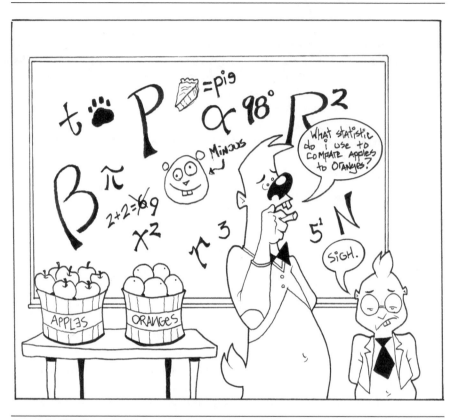

Copyright 2005 by Justin Wagner; reprinted with permission.

than the mean for females (in other words, the observed difference between 11.3 and 9.9 has a low probability of being a chance occurrence). Thus, the conclusion might read, "The average level of risk was significantly greater for males as compared to females."

Chi-Square Example. Suppose that a research study is examining whether family history of breast cancer (that is, the predictor) is related to practicing breast self-exams on a regular basis. The nature of the research question demands that women with a history be contrasted to all other women (these are two discrete categories). Those women practicing breast self-exam on a regular basis—perhaps defined as once a month—would then be compared to those engaging in the practice less frequently (again, these are two discrete categories). The public health

TABLE 12.2. CONTINGENCY TABLE OF DATA PERTAINING TO A STUDY OF BREAST SELF-EXAMINATION PRACTICES.

	Frequency of Breast Self-Examination		
	Monthly	Less Than Monthly	Total
Family history of breast cancer	79	14	93
No family history of breast cancer	66	19	85
Total	145	33	178

outcome of interest here is clearly breast self-exam; thus the predictor variable is family history of breast cancer (none vs. some). Table 12.2 displays a contingency table that contains data addressing this research question.

As shown in Table 12.2, the contingency table has four cells. These tables have an endless array of uses in health promotion research and therefore deserve extensive study by the new investigator. The outcome is shown in columns and the predictor is shown in rows. Each column and row has a total. The row totals and the column totals must, by definition, sum to the same value (in this case the value 178; this is a "grand total"). The most basic function of the table is purely descriptive. Notice, for example, that among the ninety-three women with a family history, fourteen (15.1 percent) did not practice breast self-exam on a monthly basis. Among the eighty-five women without a family history, nineteen (22.9 percent) did not practice breast self-exam on a regular basis.

Although the descriptive value of a contingency table is important, the question that arises is identical to that posed earlier in the t-test example: How likely is the difference between 15.1 percent and 22.9 percent due to chance alone? This question can be addressed by the chi-square statistic (shown as χ^2). Using the row and column totals, a value expected by chance can be calculated for each of the four cells. For example, the upper left cell has a corresponding row total of 93 and a corresponding column total of 145. To obtain the value expected by chance for this cell, multiply 93 by 145 and divide the product by the grand total of 178. Thus, the chance value for the upper left cell is 75.75. The obtained value for the upper left cell was 79. Herein lies the key to the chi-square test: the difference between the obtained value of 79 and the value expected by chance is 3.25. Across the four cells, these differences form the *conceptual* basis for the calculations needed to arrive at the χ^2 value.

After obtaining the χ^2 value, the final step is to evaluate the value for statistical significance. Again, a corresponding P-value of .05 or less would typically be counted as evidence that the difference between 15.1 percent and 22.9 percent is not readily attributable to chance. In the example shown in Table 12.2, the χ^2

value is 1.77 and the corresponding *P*-value is .18. Thus, 15.1 percent and 22.9 percent are not significantly different values. The conclusion for this study might then read: "The chi-square test revealed that the percentage of women who practiced breast self-exam and had a family history of breast cancer was not significantly different from the percentage of women who do not have a family history of breast cancer."

Before leaving this discussion of the chi-square test, it is useful to discuss the concept of a median split (as "splitting" a distribution at its median can be a useful procedure and results in the ability to apply a chi-square test). The median can be used to split a non-normal distribution of interval- or ratio-level data into two distinct parts (for example, high versus low, healthy versus unhealthy, more frequent versus less frequent). This median split can be a very useful tool for describing a group in relationship to a second variable. Consider the following research questions:

- Does a measure of attitude toward preventive practices predict ever having a colonoscopy?
- Does a measure of attitude toward preventive practices predict ever being tested for HIV?
- How do people diagnosed with depression differ from those not having this diagnosis with respect to whether they use tobacco?

In each question, the predictor variable (that is, attitude toward prevention or, in the latter question, depression level) necessitates the use of a scale measure (see Chapter Nine). However, as noted previously in this chapter, the obtained distribution for such measures may be markedly skewed (as shown in the examples displayed in Figures 12.2 and 12.3). In such cases, the lack of a normal (or nearly normal) distribution violates typical assumptions of statistical tests that might be used for these ratio-level measures. Moreover, the people represented by the skew (the long tail) are a potentially important focal point. Thus, if a median split was performed on each of these predictor variables, then the analyses could all be addressed by chi-square tests. (Note: in each test a contingency table with four cells—like that displayed in Table 12.2—could be created.)

Correlation Examples. When interval- or ratio-level data are available, the Pearson Product Moment Correlation is an efficient method of representing the strength of a linear relationship (correlation) between variables. The correlation coefficient is represented by a lower case *r*. The values of *r* range from -1.0 to $+1.0$, with a perfect correlation being found at either extreme (in other words, both -1.0 and $+1.0$ are perfect correlations). A positive and significant value of *r* means that the two variables being compared each increase together; this is known as a *direct relationship*. Consider, for example, self-efficacy for engaging in aerobic exercise (X) and the average number of aerobic workouts per week (Y). As scores on the measure of X (presumably a paper-and-pencil assessment) increase, an increase (to some corresponding degree) in Y would be expected. Because the value of r provides an indicator of how strong the correspondence is between X and Y, an r of $+1.0$ would mean they rise in perfect synchrony. However, this is only a theoretical possibility; in reality the two variables may rise together at a level of .20 or .30 or higher. Note also that r does *not* address causality; that is, X may be influencing the corresponding rise in Y, or Y may be influencing the corresponding rise in X. Sometimes, a researcher can rule out the possibility that Y could be "causing" X by knowing that X cannot be changed (age, gender, and race are good examples). However, if X and Y are related, this still does not establish that X must cause Y (as there could be unknown variables that actually cause Y—see Chapter Four).

◆ ◆ ◆

In a Nutshell

A positive and significant value of r *means that the two variables being compared each increase together; this is known as a* direct relationship.

◆ ◆ ◆

A negative and significant value of r means that an increase in one variable corresponds to a decrease in the other variable; this is known as an *inverse relationship*. Consider, for example, a relationship between age (X), ranging from fourteen to forty-five, and the average number of health risk behaviors (Y) assessed by an index. A study may have obtained an r-value of $-.35$ for this correlation. Given that this value was significant (it had an acceptably low probability of occurring by chance), the value provides an indicator of how strongly (strength) the two variables are connected inversely. The direction of this relationship (that is, negative or inverse) is not surprising, and the magnitude (that is, .35) is modest. This latter point regarding magnitude, however, warrants further consideration.

◆ ◆ ◆

In a Nutshell

A negative and significant value of r *means that an increase in one variable corresponds to a decrease in the other variable; this is known as an* inverse relationship.

◆ ◆ ◆

FIGURE 12.4.   SCATTERPLOTS ILLUSTRATING DIRECT AND INVERSE CORRELATIONS.

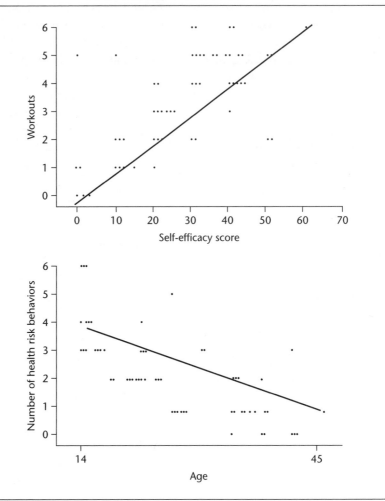

Figure 12.4 displays two scatterplots. A scatterplot is a collection of bivariate data points. A bivariate data point represents the intersection of locations on an X-axis (an abscissa) and a Y-axis (an ordinate). Through visual inspection of these data points, two observations can be made related to determining the magnitude of the linear relationship. First, a conceptual line should be "drawn" that indicates whether the two variables may be linearly related. Second, the conceptual

line may be steep or flat, indicating a perfect linear relationship or no linear relationship, respectively.

In the first scatterplot in Figure 12.4, it can be seen that a conceptual line superimposed on the data rises from left to right at a relatively sharp increase. Because the purpose of the line is to depict a linear relationship and compare how close the corresponding data points are to the line, it appears that the correlation is quite high: the closer the data points are to the line, the greater the correlation; data points that are quite distant from the conceptual line indicate a low correlation. In the second example in Figure 12.4, although the data points are close to the conceptual line, the line is not as steep as in the first example. Consequently, the correlation must be lower. Notice also that the line descends as it moves from left to right. This means that the correlation is inverse.

A caveat to each of the bivariate procedures is in order. After the two variables have been identified, it is critically important to determine which one is the outcome measure and which one is the predictor variable. (Note: the term *predictor variable* technically only applies to prospective studies; in cross-sectional studies a preferred term is *correlate*.) This determination is made based on the research question and the nature of the variables. In this example, the determination is simplified because sex cannot possibly be a logical outcome variable (that is, we could not possibly expect scores on the health risk index to be a determinant of sex, but we could fairly expect that sex would be a determinant of health risk behavior). Thus, we urge that great caution and careful logic be applied when interpreting bivariate findings; causality is often elusive and difficult to determine!

◆ ◆ ◆

In a Nutshell

After the two variables have been identified, it is critically important to determine which one is the outcome measure and which one is the predictor variable.

◆ ◆ ◆

A second caveat is in order. Imagine a graphic display of bivariate data points that takes the shape of an inverted "U." In this case, the correlation may be nonsignificant and very weak—approaching zero. This does not mean that X and Y are unrelated! This is true because not all relationships are linear. In this example, the relationship could be *quadratic*. A quadratic relationship between variables means that the two variables do not rise or decline in synchrony; rather, at some point along the X axis the relationship changes. A classic example of a quadratic relationship is anxiety (X) and performance (Y): at low levels of X, performance is low; at medium levels of X, performance is high; at high levels of X, performance is low.

Multivariate Analysis

Although several forms of multivariate analyses are available, two of the most widely selected are linear and logistic regression. Linear regression is appropriate for outcomes comprising interval-level data or ratio-level data. Conversely, logistic regression is used when the outcome is a dichotomy.

Linear Regression. The Pearson Product Moment Correlation forms the basis for simple linear regression. In simple linear regression, you are calculating an equation that determines the Y-intercept and slope of *the best fitting line.* The best fitting line refers to an actual line generated from the data and that minimizes the distance from the data points to the line. The Y-intercept and slope are termed *parameter estimates* of this equation. In turn, multiple linear regression is an extension of this test. As opposed to only one predictor variable, multiple linear regression involves several predictors.

Basically, regression serves several purposes: the first is to test the nature of the linear relationship between X variable(s) and a given outcome Y; a second purpose is to test the strength of the relationship; and a third purpose is to formulate prediction equations based on sample data that can be applied to the population. All three purposes can be achieved by generating the equation for the regression line.

One key concept in regression is the parameter estimation of the slope that reveals what the association is between X variable(s) and Y. The slope estimate, which is referred to as b, gauges how much Y would increase given a one-unit increase in X. This involves a brief understanding of *rise-to-run.* The estimate for slope is an unstandardized estimate, meaning that it is read in the original metric of the variable. Interpretation of slope estimates is as follows: "a one-unit change in X corresponds to a change in Y of b units." For example, a regression equation that was generated to examine the relationship between self-efficacy and number of days per week people exercise had a slope of 1.5. In practical terms this means that for every 1 unit increase in self-efficacy (the X variable shown on the abscissa, the run), people exercised 1.5 more days (the rise). Alternatively, if the relationship is inverse, the question becomes, How much does Y *decrease* for a one-unit increase in X?

Another function of regression is to provide standardized values of the slope estimate. Standardizing a variable places the measure on a common metric. The standardized regression coefficient is a measure of the strength of the association between X variable(s) and the outcome Y. The standardized parameter estimates are known as Beta (β) weights. Imagine three X variables: self-efficacy, age, and depression. An important question might be which of these three variables has the strongest relationship with an outcome of "attitudes toward getting a colonoscopy." Imagine further that the obtained Beta weights are .30, .21, and .15 respectively. Because they are standardized, these Beta weights can be directly compared with each other. Thus, the strongest variable in this case would be self-efficacy, followed by age, and then depression.

Another purpose of linear regression is to generate equations used for prediction. It should be noted that multiple linear regression models will generate a value for a "constant" and unstandardized parameter estimates (symbolized as b) that can be used to construct an equation that will predict Y. The assumption here is that the sample data can be applied to make inferences about the population. The equation may look familiar to anyone who can recall taking a high school math class: $Y = \text{constant} + b_1(X1) + b_2(X2) + b_3(X3)$, and so on. Using the constant and the unstandardized parameter estimates, the information from this model could then be applied to persons who were not included in the sample to make predictions of Y.

Multiple linear regression is also used to determine how well a set of variables collectively is related to Y. Specifically, multiple linear regression can be used to judge the collective strength of the X-variables in explaining *variance* in Y. Accounting for variance is an important goal of multiple regression. The statistic used to represent this value is R^2.

◆ ◆ ◆

In a Nutshell

Multiple linear regression can be used to judge the collective strength of the X*-variables in explaining* variance *in* Y.

◆ ◆ ◆

R^2 ranges from 0 to 1.0. The value of R^2 typically does not exceed the sum of the r^2-values representing the bivariate relationships between the assessed X-variables and the given Y-variable, at least when the X-variables are inter-correlated. Figure 12.5 provides an illustration of this principle, using three X-variables: level of gang involvement, level of parental monitoring, and age (the outcome of interest [Y] is number of health risk behaviors). Although the Pearson

FIGURE 12.5. THE SUM OF PEARSON *r* VALUES DOES NOT NECESSARILY EQUATE WITH R^2.

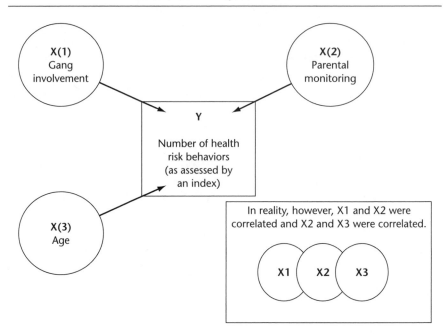

Note: Bivariate correlations: $X(1)r = .33$, $r^2 = .11$; $X(2)r = .30$, $r^2 = .09$; and $X(3)r = .10$, $r^2 = .01$ (all are significant at $P < .05$).

correlations were all significant, two were modest while the magnitude for age was very weak.

◆ ◆ ◆

In a Nutshell

The value of R^2 typically does not exceed the sum of the r^2-values representing the bivariate relationships between the assessed X-variables and the given Y-variable, at least when the X-variables are intercorrelated.

◆ ◆ ◆

While a quick glance at the *r*-values might suggest that R^2 would be about .21, the box in the lower right-hand corner of Figure 12.5 shows the common, multivariate reality. In fact, the R^2 for this model was .09. The diminished value occurs because of intercorrelation between the X-variables. Parental monitoring was significantly correlated (inverse) with the level of gang involvement. Parental monitoring was also significantly correlated with age (direct). Thus, the three X-variables exert a collective effect on Y but overlap between variables represents joint influence on Y. Of course, the overlap cannot be counted twice. Thus, the question becomes one of determining which variable (X_1 versus X_2, for example) is "credited" for explaining variance in Y relative to the region of overlap. The answer is determined by the research team and takes the form of an analytic decision relative to the order of entering X variables into the regression model. Although entry methods are beyond the scope of this introductory chapter, the curious reader should consult an excellent textbook authored by Tabachnick and Fidell (1996).

Logistic Regression. In linear regression, the Y-variable must be an interval- or ratio-level measure. Analyses that rely on outcomes that are assessed with interval- or ratio-level measures are termed *parametric*. Conversely, nonparametric analyses use outcome measures that are assessed with a categorical variable. A common form of nonparametric analysis in health promotion research is logistic regression. Logistic regression is used when the outcome variable is dichotomous. Of course, the number of research questions in health promotion that necessitate a dichotomous outcome measure is nearly infinite. Assessing the presence or absence of a disease, condition, or risk behavior, then, is clearly part of a research question that will lend itself to the use of logistic regression.

For the purposes of this introductory chapter, it can be said that the basic principles of multiple linear regression apply to multiple logistic regression. The principle behind the procedure is that an exponent (a constant value) is raised to a power of Beta (β), yielding an adjusted odds ratio. The model will then classify a given percentage of the cases correctly, based on the collective X-variables that achieve multivariate significance. Keep in mind, however, that the odds of classifying the outcome correctly are 50 percent by chance alone. Thus, for example, classifying 60 percent of the cases correctly would result in classifying only 10 percent beyond that expected by chance alone.

◆ ◆ ◆

In a Nutshell

The principle behind the procedure is that an exponent (a constant value) is raised to a power of Beta (β), yielding an adjusted odds ratio.

◆ ◆ ◆

Interpreting odds ratios is an important prerequisite to understanding research findings from logistic regression. Odds ratios are an estimate of added risk for Y based on the knowledge of an X-variable. For example, text in a manuscript might read as follows: "Adolescents identifying as members of a minority group were more than three times as likely to test positive for an STD (AOR = 3.12; 95 percent CI = 1.31 $-$ 7.43)." This adjusted odds ratio can be judged for significance based on its 95 percent confidence interval. Simply put, confidence intervals that exclude the value of 1.0 are significant. An odds ratio of one has to be nonsignificant because it means "one time as likely," which, of course, means the same as or equally likely. (Recall that 1 times anything is itself.) In prospective studies, the odds ratio can be called a relative risk ratio. In either instance, a higher value represents a greater degree of risk for Y. An exception to this occurs when an X-variable is inversely associated with Y. Consider, for example, parental monitoring (from the previous example used in Figure 12.5). A high-level of parental monitoring might be associated with a decreased risk of teen pregnancy. Therefore, the obtained odds ratio would be protective (meaning that high monitoring would equate with *lower* risk of a negative outcome). Protective odds ratios range from 0 to .99. A protective odds ratio of .50, for example, would mean that teens with high monitoring were one-half as likely as those with low monitoring to become pregnant or (if male) cause a pregnancy. As before, the significance of a protective odds ratio is judged by whether its 95 percent confidence interval excludes 1.0.

A Warning About *P*-Values

Even seasoned researchers sometimes become confused about the meaning of a significant P-value. Simply stated, a P-value less than the established alpha level means that the related finding was statistically significant, indicating that the association had a low probability of occurring by chance alone, assuming that there is in fact no association. The P-value is *not* a measure of substantive effect (that is, strength of association between X and Y).

The confusion comes from a tendency to equate diminishing P-values (those such as .01, .001, and .0001) with progressively larger associations. This is not the case. Indeed, a large (and important) association may have a high probability of occurring by chance (yielding a nonsignificant P-value). Conversely, a rather weak (and unimportant) association may have a very low probability of occurring by chance alone (thus, the P-value would be significant). How is this possible? The difference is a function of sample size. The lesson here is quite simple: P-values only speak to the question of the probability or likelihood that an association can be attributed to chance alone. To understand this concept in greater detail, it is important to have a basic understanding of statistical power and effect size.

Statistical Power and Effect Size

When considering observational research, power is the ability of a statistical test to detect true associations (effects) between variables. Power is influenced by

- Sample size (this is a "direct relationship")
- Effect size
- Dispersion or variance (this is an "inverse relationship")
- The alpha level selected for the study (a lower, more stringent *P*-level gives less power)
- The use of a one-tailed versus two-tailed test of significance (more power with one tail)

Effect size can be conceptualized as the magnitude of association between two variables. For example, suppose that 22 percent of teens who reported low parental monitoring had ever been pregnant. In comparison, only 11 percent of those reporting high parental monitoring had ever been pregnant. Teens who had low parental monitoring were two times as likely to get pregnant than teens with high parental monitoring. The "two-times" is the odds ratio and is a measure of effect size in this example.

As empirical values, effect sizes allow readers to judge whether statistically significant results are also meaningful at a practical level. Stated differently, effect size captures the "true impact" of an association, whereas significance testing merely provides a determination of whether or not the association is a chance occurrence. Unlike other determinants of power, effect size is not influenced by anything other than the observations that are collected from the research participants. Power, on the other hand, can be affected by the researcher and can be increased (for example, by using a very large sample size or a high alpha level). By the same token, power may be low due to a small sample size.

◆ ◆ ◆

In a Nutshell

Effect size captures the "true impact" of an association, whereas significance testing merely provides a determination of whether or not the association is a chance occurrence.

◆ ◆ ◆

Large effect sizes require less power than medium or small effect sizes. Conversely, small effects require a great deal of power to detect them. Thus, an important and perhaps never-ending question in health promotion research is,

When are small effects that are deemed statistically significant, substantive? The flipside to this question is, When are large effects mistakenly declared nonsignificant due to low levels of power? These questions correspond to two classic forms of error in analysis. When an effect is deemed significant but is not real (false positive), the result is termed a *Type 1 error* and is in fact represented by alpha. Recall that alpha is the probability of results occurring by chance given that there are no real effects. When large effects are mistakenly declared nonsignificant (based on problems with low power), the result is termed a *Type 2 error* (false negative). Both types of error unfortunately are common. Studies with very large sample sizes (for example, greater than a thousand participants) may be prone to Type 1 errors and, of course, studies with very small sample sizes (for example, less than two hundred participants) may be prone to Type 2 errors.

This somewhat abridged discussion of power and effect size is important for several reasons. First, a fair test of a research question implies that the power is not too high and not too low (by convention, 80 percent power is considered a "fair test" criterion). Of note, power can be adjusted before the study begins (by planning sample size) or after the study has concluded (by adjusting alpha upward). Second, power problems in small studies that have already been completed may not be resolved; thus, effect size may be an especially important value to report. Third, as previously mentioned, in studies that have high power due to a large sample size, the effect size is an important indicator of whether the findings have substantive significance. Finally, studies should be planned to detect a reasonable effect size that is not unrealistically large but substantive, and this planning should culminate in an empirical estimate of the sample size requirement. Several software packages are available (many are freely obtained over the Internet) that can calculate sample size requirements based on estimated effect sizes and the determinants of power shown in the previous bulleted list. Furthermore, after a study is done these programs can be used to calculate the available power (based on effect sizes obtained) and the determinants of power shown in the bulleted list on page 339.

Applied Examples

This chapter provides two applied examples. The first illustrates the use of linear regression and the second illustrates the use of logistic regression.

Correlates of Unprotected Vaginal Sex

A study published in the *Archives of Pediatrics and Adolescent Medicine* provides a good application of linear regression to observational research in health promotion.

Crosby and colleagues (2000) selected a priority population for the prevention of HIV, sexually transmitted infections, and pregnancy of low-income African American adolescents residing in a risky urban environment. Using social cognitive theory as a framework, the researchers investigated correlates of engaging in unprotected vaginal sex (UVS) among 522 adolescent females.

The correlates were largely composed of scale measures (each assessed using interval- or ratio-level data). The outcome variable was frequency of UVS as reported by adolescents during a six-month recall period (a ratio-level measure). Pearson correlation was used to assess the direction and magnitude of the bivariate associations between each correlate and UVS. Several correlates achieved bivariate significance. These were then entered into a multiple linear regression model. UVS was regressed on fourteen correlates in a model restricted to UVS with steady partners. Subsequently, UVS was regressed on five correlates in a model restricted to sex with casual partners. The R^2 for the first model was .235 and the R^2 for the second model was .22. The strongest predictor of UVS in the first model was the average amount of time spent with the steady boyfriend during any given week ($\beta = .26$). Several other correlates retained multivariate significance in this model (their Beta coefficients ranged from $-.10$ to $.15$). In the second model, three correlates achieved multivariate significance: (1) pleasure barriers to condom use ($\beta = .23$); (2) history of STD infection ($\beta = .28$), and (3) partner control over sexual decisions ($\beta = .23$).

Correlates of Colorectal Cancer Screening

A study published in the *American Journal of Preventive Medicine* illustrates an application of logistic regression in health promotion. Mandelson and colleagues (2000) surveyed 931 women who were fifty to eighty years of age. The study was designed to identify correlates of fecal occult blood testing (FOBT) in the past two years. Demographic, attitudinal, perceptual, and physician-based variables were examined for their relationship to recent FOBT.

First, the study reported the strength of the bivariate relationships between the assessed correlates and FOBT. The bivariate relations were based on a contingency table (like the one shown in Table 12.2) and expressed as unadjusted odds ratios. (These are odds ratios that have not been "adjusted" for the influence of variables outside of the bivariate relationship.) For example, 38.5 percent of the women in their fifties had been screened in the past two years compared with 52.5 percent of those in their sixties and 56.5 percent of those in their seventies. Women in their sixties were about 2.75 times more likely to be screened in the past two years compared with women in their fifties (OR = 2.76; 95 percent CI = 1.85 − 4.11). Women in their seventies were about 4.5 times more likely to be screened in comparison with women in their fifties (OR = 4.47; 95 percent CI = 2.91 − 6.86). Note that the odds ratios are significant (in other words, their 95 percent confidence intervals exclude 1.0), and that the range encompassed by the intervals is relatively narrow. In contrast, women who reported having a mammogram two years or less before the survey were more than nine times as likely to be screened compared with women who had never had a mammogram (OR = 9.21; 95 percent CI = 3.72 − 22.8). Notice here that the confidence interval is quite wide.

Next, a multivariate analysis was used to test variables achieving bivariate significance. Three variables achieved significance using multiple logistic regression to calculate adjusted odds ratios: (1) the extent that physicians encourage screening, (2) the degree of comfort women had in discussing FOB testing with a physician, and (3) perceptions that the unpleasant aspect of the screening is justified based on the risk of colorectal cancer.

Integration with the Research Process

Good research is brought to life by a fair analysis; the same cannot be said for poor research. Stated differently, the decision points and planning steps that lead to data analysis (step 8 in the nine-step model) are, in essence, the most important elements of an analysis. Measurement (step 5) and sampling (step 6) are particularly critical, as these steps determine, in part, the quality of the variables and the power of the analysis, respectively. Of course, the nature of the research question (step 2) is perhaps the most critical determinant of a successful analysis. A carefully crafted study will be designed to identify effect sizes that can be detected without having to sample an unduly high number of participants. More important, this careful planning will result in findings that go beyond statistical significance into the realm of practical significance.

Although a fair analysis can bring good research to life, judging what constitutes a fair analysis is problematic. Certainly, assurances that Type 1 and Type 2 errors have been avoided are important. Moreover, parsimony is important, but some research questions will demand quite complex analytic approaches. For example, data from a panel study with multiple waves of data collection cannot be fairly analyzed without controlling for the inherent correlation of responses over time within each of the study participants. These repeated-measures data sets must be analyzed using advanced tools such as Generalized Estimating Equations. Similarly, data from an observational study that is based on sampling from clusters (that is, preexisting and well-defined groups or communities of people) cannot be fairly analyzed without accounting for the unavoidable correlations found within the various clusters of participants. In such an instance, a software program called SUDAAN can be used to control for this intercorrelation effect. Although numerous other examples could be provided, the main point is that fair analyses can be complicated to a point far beyond the capacity of the few analytic tools presented in this chapter. Vigilance in analysis, then, sometimes requires the assistance of qualified statisticians. This assistance may also be needed as the findings are interpreted in the early phase of step 9 (dissemination).

Finally, it should be noted that observational research is quite distinct from experimental research. In the latter, analyses are prescribed by the study design. In observational research, however, analyses can be conceived before and after the data has been collected. Furthermore, observational research can be used to answer two distinct varieties of research questions. First (and probably most common), the research can be designed to predict Y (meaning that correlates or predictors of one given outcome are identified). Most examples provided previously in this chapter have been patterned using this approach. The hallmark here is that only one outcome variable is investigated. Second, the research can begin with only a single X-variable and then determine the relationship of this variable to multiple outcomes that are pertinent to public health. Although less common, this approach can be an effective means of addressing a broad range of health promotion outcomes as opposed to a monolithic goal. For example, a recent study found that infrequent parental monitoring of adolescent females was associated with increased risk for marijuana use, greater levels of alcohol consumption, recent arrest, having multiple sex partners, not using condoms, the acquisition of sexually transmitted diseases, and not using contraceptive methods (DiClemente and others, 2001).

Summary

Data analysis is a turning point in the research process. This chapter has presented a few of the most basic techniques that are applied to the descriptive, bivariate, and multivariate analyses of data collected in the field of health promotion. One key thread that deserves attention is that not all data are created equal. In fact, data typically follow a divide between parametric and nonparametric camps. The former involves interval- or ratio-level outcome measures and is generally based on means, standard deviations, and variance. A t-test is a common example of bivariate parametric analysis, and multiple linear regression is a common example of a multivariate parametric analysis. Alternatively, nonparametric analyses are used for data with nominal- or ordinal-level outcome measures. Frequency distributions and medians are quite useful for describing nominal and ordinal data, respectively. A common example of a bivariate nonparametric analysis is the chi square test. Logistic regression is often used to handle nonparametric multivariate analyses pertaining to health promotion research. These tools should be used with great caution to precision and with careful attention to issues relevant to power and effect size.

Issues to Consider

1. A somewhat inflammatory and certainly important issue involves Type 1 error. The essence of this issue is that effect size can be lost in the context of other factors that may ultimately have an undue influence on whether a given finding achieves statistical significance. A good example of this can be found in the analysis of a CDC study known as Project Respect (Kamb and others 1998). This study found, for example, that incidence of sexually transmitted infections (assessed six months after study enrollment) among those assigned to an enhanced counseling condition was significantly lower ($P = .0001$) than incidence among those in the control condition. Incidence was approximately 7 percent versus 10 percent. Statistically, the finding seems quite promising. However, the obtained effect size was very small, suggesting that significance may have been an artifact of an extremely large sample size (that is, greater than three thousand participants). The issue is not easily resolved. On one hand, the difference between 7 percent and 10 percent could represent a substantial number of cases averted if the enhanced counseling protocol was widely applied; yet the potential case for the operation of Type 1 error is clear. Indeed, the larger question is, "What are the ethical obligations that researchers have to disclose the liability of a study to Type 1 error?"

2. After pondering the first issue, another related issue involves the difference between statistical significance and practical significance. A case in point is the common practice of discussing significant r-values as though they represent findings in their own right. It is imperative to know that P-values do not reflect strength in a relationship; instead they merely reflect the likelihood of a chance occurrence. Significant Pearson r-values of less than .20 are commonly discussed in manuscripts as though they have great value in understanding a given outcome variable. The problem is that an r-value of .20, for example, only explains 4 percent of the variance! (This can be easily calculated by squaring r.) The ultimate value of observation research to health promotion is that it can inform practice. Investigation of X-variables, then, implies that the findings can have implications for improving practices. Yet

research that explains such a small amount of the variance can hardly be said to have value with respect to changing (or sustaining) practice. Thus, the issue becomes, How can research findings be judged for practical as opposed to statistical significance?

3. An all-too-common analytic issue is whether a skewed distribution should be transformed into a simple dichotomy. Recall that skewness implies that an interval- or ratio-level variable has a distribution that "clumps" to the right or left rather than being centered. Recall also that the "tail portion" of a skewed distribution typically represents those people who may be at greatest risk for negative health outcomes. Critics of the median split suggest that a great deal of precision is lost when an interval- or ratio-level distribution is converted to a simple dichotomy (for example, low versus high). Proponents suggest that the conversion can create a dichotomy with a great deal of utility. The utility may derive from the nature of health promotion practice. For example, the regular practice of breast self-examination (BSE) may confer a protective measure against mortality from breast cancer, whereas women who practice BSE infrequently have no more protection against breast cancer–induced mortality than do women who never practice BSE. Thus, a natural dichotomy (formed from a ratio-level measure) could be warranted. The final question may be phrased, When (if ever) is the artificial creation of a dichotomy justified?

For Practice and Discussion

1. You have been presented with a data set that addresses one research question. The question seeks to identify predictors of HIV testing in a high-risk sample of gay men. You first examine the outcome measure (frequency of having HIV tests in the past ten years) and discover that the distribution has a strong positive skew. Also, you observe that the mean is 6 and the standard deviation is 4.5. What "tools" will you use to describe the outcome measure? What tools will you use to identify the predictors of HIV testing? Most important, please justify your selection of these tools.

2. You are reading a manuscript that reports findings based on observational research of an elderly population. The research question involved determination of differences in health behaviors (nutrition, rest, exercise, and abstinence from tobacco use) between those residing and those not residing in nursing homes. Without knowing anything else about this study, what type of bivariate analysis do you suppose would be used? Again, please justify your answer.

References

Armstrong, K., Berlin, M., Sanford-Swartz, J., Propert, K., and Ubel, P. A. (2001). Barriers to influenza immunization in a low-income urban population. *The American Journal of Preventive Medicine, 20,* 21–25.

Cohen, J. (1988). *Statistical power analysis for the behavioral sciences* (2nd ed.). Hillsdale, NJ: Lawrence Erlbaum Associates.

Crosby, R. A., and others. (2000). Correlates of unprotected vaginal sex among African American female teens: The importance of relationship dynamics. *Archives of Pediatrics and Adolescent Medicine, 154,* 893–899.

Crosby, R. A., and others. (2003). Psychosocial predictors of pregnancy among low-income African American adolescent females: A prospective analysis. *Journal of Pediatric and Adolescent Gynecology, 15,* 293–299.

DiClemente, R. J., and others. (2001). Parental monitoring and its association with a spectrum of adolescent health risk behaviors. *Pediatrics, 107,* 1363–1368.

Kamb, M. L., and others (1998). Efficacy of risk-reduction counseling to prevent human immunodeficiency virus in sexually transmitted diseases: A randomized controlled trial. *Journal of the American Medical Association, 280,* 1161–1167.

Mandelson, M. T., and others. (2000). Colorectal cancer screening participation by older women. *American Journal of Preventive Medicine, 19,* 149–154.

Pagano, M., and Gauvreau, K. (2000). *Principles of biostatistics* (2nd ed.). Pacific Grove, CA: Duxbury Thompson Learning.

Sheeran, P., Abraham, C., and Orbell, S. (1999). Psychosocial correlates of heterosexual condom use: A meta-analysis. *Psychological Bulletin, 125,* 90–132.

Siegel, S., and Castellan, N. J. (1988). *Nonparametric statistics for the behavioral sciences* (2nd ed.). Boston: McGraw-Hill.

Tabachnick, B. G., and Fidell, L. S. (1996). *Using multivariate statistics* (3rd ed.). New York: HarperCollins.

CHAPTER THIRTEEN

BASIC PRINCIPLES OF STATISTICAL ANALYSIS FOR RANDOMIZED CONTROLLED TRIALS

Ralph J. DiClemente, Laura F. Salazar, and Richard A. Crosby

The aim of this chapter is to provide an overview of the main statistical principles and data analytic techniques useful in the analysis of randomized controlled trials (RCT). Many of these principles and techniques, while specifically applied to RCTs, are also applicable to the broader category of studies incorporating an experimental research design.

To begin we would like to remind you of two terms that pertain only to experimental research. These are the *independent variable* and the *dependent variable*. The independent variable is the variable manipulated by the investigator. In the context of a health promotion RCT, the independent variable is the health promotion program (HPP) and the goal is to determine its effect on the *dependent variable*. The dependent variable is the outcome of interest and is measured by the investigator, but not controlled or manipulated by the investigator.

The primary focus of the chapter is to describe the underlying purposes of statistical techniques, develop an understanding of selecting an appropriate statistical technique, and enhance understanding of the interpretation of data derived from an RCT. This chapter is deliberately written to be statistical-lite; that is to say, nonmathematical.

Illustration of Key Concepts

We will provide an overview of the data analytic process, which will entail planning for the data analysis, describing the data, assessing the comparability between groups, and understanding different types of dependent variables. Finally, and perhaps most important, we will describe a process for selecting the appropriate statistical analysis and describe those analyses as applied to an RCT.

Planning for the Data Analysis

Statistical analysis of data, while usually conducted after all data have been collected, is in reality a process that should begin much earlier in the research enterprise. The data analysis is directly related to the design of the study and how well the study has been implemented. Indeed, no matter how well designed, clever, or sophisticated a data analytic plan, it cannot compensate for a poorly designed study. A poorly conceived data analytic plan may obscure the detection of meaningful findings, obscure interpretation of the resultant findings, or both. A data analytic plan entails conducting a power analysis to determine the appropriate sample size needed to detect a statistical difference, ensuring that measurements are administered in a timely and appropriate fashion, specifying a procedure for handling participant attrition, and selecting the statistical techniques most appropriate for the design and research question. Thus, proper planning and execution of the study as well as the statistical analysis is critical to yielding reliable and valid results. Throughout this book, we have described various research designs (see Chapters Four, Five, and Six); however, without the appropriate attention on the front end of the study (the design and implementation), the data analysis on the back end will not be as useful.

◆ ◆ ◆

In a Nutshell

No matter how well designed, clever, or sophisticated a data analytic plan, it cannot compensate for a poorly designed study.

◆ ◆ ◆

Describing the Data

Once the data are obtained by following the data analytic plan, it is useful to examine the underlying characteristics of the scores for the variables collected before proceeding to more complex analyses. The first analytic activity is usually the generation of simple descriptive statistics (for example, mean, median, standard deviation, range, frequencies). These descriptive statistics are used to evaluate how scores on various variables are distributed. These variables include the dependent variables, the participants' sociodemographic characteristics, and other key predictors (in other words, hypothesized mediators of the dependent variables). Summary statistics for all of the measures should be computed separately for each arm of the trial. A visual inspection of the data, especially histograms, may reveal underlying deviations from normality of which the investigator should be aware prior to progressing to the selection of statistical techniques for the data analysis. Generation of these statistics also serves as the last quality control and quality assurance activities in data management.

Assessing the Comparability Between the Study Groups

The concept of assessing comparability between the HPP group and the control group is, at times, difficult for novice investigators to understand. An often-asked question, for example, is, Why assess comparability between groups that were created through randomization of participants in the first place? Doesn't the fact that participants were randomized, using appropriate allocation techniques, obviate the need to assess comparability? This is a common refrain. Randomization does not ensure that the study groups are equivalent, only that there is no systematic bias in the assignment of participants to the two study conditions. Indeed, for relatively small samples, it is likely that the groups will not be comparable on all variables (dependent variables, sociodemographics, and other predictors). Thus, a critical step in the data analytic plan is to assess the comparability between the study groups with respect to sociodemographics, dependent variables, and other predictors of interest. An example from our research may be illustrative.

◆ ◆ ◆

In a Nutshell

Randomization does not ensure that the study groups are equivalent, only that there is no systematic bias in the assignment of participants to the two study conditions.

◆ ◆ ◆

We conducted an RCT to test the efficacy of a behavioral intervention to increase condom use among African American female adolescents, fourteen to eighteen years of age. As participants completed their baseline assessment they were randomized to one of two study conditions using a computer-generated randomization algorithm, complying with established concealment of allocation techniques (see Chapter Six). Comparisons between the study conditions were made for a host of variables, including sociodemographic characteristics, other potential predictors of sexual behavior, psychosocial mediators of sexual behavior, and sexual behaviors. We compared the conditions using t-tests for continuous dependent variables (such as age) and chi-square tests for categorical variables (for instance, whether participants received public assistance). Results of these analyses are presented in Table 13.1.

Examination of Table 13.1 reveals that randomization was effective. The HIV risk-reduction condition and the general health education control condition were similar with respect to sociodemographic characteristics, psychosocial mediators that serve as secondary dependent variables, and sexual behaviors that serve as the primary dependent variable. In general, it is valuable to include a range of variables when assessing comparability between study conditions. If there are imbalances between the groups (for example, in this case, if there were a statistically significant mean difference for the variable "age" between conditions), then it is important to control for this age difference in the analysis. Differences between the study groups for other variables that may be potential confounders (that is, variables theoretically or empirically associated with the dependent variables) could also be controlled for in subsequent data analyses.

Understanding Different Types of Dependent Variables

In all studies there are different types of dependent variables. Two types often collected as part of an RCT are categorical and continuous variables.

Categorical Dependent Variables. Categorical dependent variables refer to the classification of participants into one of several categories according to some predefined evaluation criteria. In its most elemental form, categorical data can assume a binary format. These categories might be labeled as "has a disease or is disease-free," "changed behavior or did not change behavior," or "consistent or inconsistent condom use," and are based on a participant's responses, test scores, or medical examinations. For example, in a study of vegetable consumption, a primary dependent variable could be "heart attack" over the follow-up period. The research question is whether or not there were more heart attacks observed among participants in the control group relative to the HPP group. Thus, for any participant in the study, the range of potential values for the dependent variable "heart attack" is 1 = Yes (experienced a heart attack over the course of the follow-up) or 0 = No (did not experience a heart attack over the course of the follow-up). In

TABLE 13.1. COMPARABILITY OF THE HIV RISK REDUCTION AND GENERAL HEALTH PROMOTION CONDITIONS.

Characteristic	HIV Prevention Condition			General Health Promotion Condition			P
	Mean (sd)	Percentage	(N)	Mean (sd)	Percentage	(N)	
Sociodemographics							
Age	15.99 (1.25)			15.97 (1.21)			.87
Education (did not complete tenth grade)		45.80%	(115)		48.70%	(132)	.51
Recipients of public assistance		17.90%	(45)		18.50%	(50)	.86
Living in single-family home		74.10%	(146)		72.30%	(162)	.68
Living with someone other than a parent		21.50%	(54)		17.30%	(47)	.23
Employed		16.10%	(40)		19.70%	(53)	.28
Psychosocial Mediators							
HIV Knowledge	8.88 (3.25)		(248)	9.13 (3.03)		(267)	.38
Condom attitudes	36.02 (4.22)		(250)	35.62 (4.42)		(271)	.29
Condom barriers	42.23 (14.16)		(243)	43.13 (14.30)		(267)	.48
Communication frequency	8.61 (4.10)		(251)	8.37 (4.50)		(271)	.54
Condom use self-efficacy	30.74 (9.30)		(249)	30.52 (9.73)		(264)	.79
Condom use skills	2.91 (1.30)		(248)	3.03 (1.18)		(268)	.25
Put condom on partner	1.49 (1.01)		(232)	1.46 (0.98)		(246)	.77
Sexual Behaviors							
% Condom use, past thirty days	0.79 (0.38)		(232)	0.77 (0.38)		(246)	.68
% Condom use, past six months	0.72 (0.37)		(232)	0.70 (0.38)		(245)	.53
Unprotected vaginal sex, past thirty days	1.12 (2.84)		(226)	0.84 (2.01)		(241)	.22
Unprotected vaginal sex, past six months	4.81 (16.01)		(232)	4.23 (10.25)		(245)	.64
Consistent condom use, past thirty days		40.27%	(60)		43.35%	(75)	.58
Consistent condom use, past six months		43.53%	(101)		48.57%	(119)	.27
Condom use, last time had sex		31.90%	(74)		32.11%	(79)	.96

MINCUS USES "NO HEAD LUMP = 0" AND "HEAD LUMP = 1" FOR THE DEPENDENT VARIABLE.

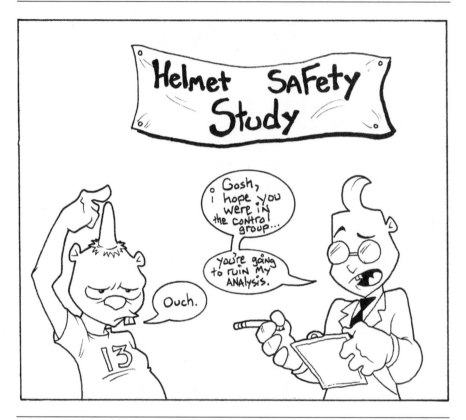

Copyright 2005 by Justin Wagner; reprinted with permission.

a study designed to test the effects of an HPP on reducing alcohol use among adolescent drivers and, as a consequence, reducing the risk of an automobile accident, we could have a categorical dependent variable of alcohol-related vehicular accidents. In this case, for any participant in the study, the range of potential values that could be obtained for the dependent variable "alcohol-related auto accident" is 1 = Yes (experienced an alcohol-related automobile accident over the course of the follow-up) or 0 = No (did not experience an alcohol-related automobile accident over the course of the follow-up).

There are circumstances when it may be desirable to have multiple levels of the categorical dependent variables. This is a logical extension of the binary categorical dependent variable described above. For example, it is possible to have an ordered categorical dependent variable—usually called an ordinal variable. This ordered categorical dependent variable would assume the form of a hierarchy or gradient. For example, in a study designed to test the effects of a stress reduction class (the HPP) on reducing headaches among college students during final exams, we could have an ordered categorical dependent variable of "headaches." In this case, for any participant in the study, the potential values for the dependent variable "headache" could range from 0 to 2 with 0 = Did not experience a headache during final exam week; 1 = Experienced a mild headache during final exam week; and 2 = Experienced a severe headache during final exam week. Oftentimes we would be tempted to treat these data as continuous when in fact the data are ordinal and should be treated as categorical.

Continuous Dependent Variables. A second type of dependent variable is a continuous variable. Continuous variables are distinct from categorical variables in that the data represent a continuous scale of measurement assessed using interval or ratio scale metrics (such as temperature, height, blood pressure, weight). Often in health promotion research, our interest is in enhancing mental health. Let's return to our study of how stress reduction may reduce headaches among college students during final exam week. RCTs, in general, have primary dependent variables; in this case, "preventing headaches." They may also have secondary dependent variables. Secondary dependent variables could include a host of other variables that the HPP is hypothesized to effect. In this study, for example, we may hypothesize that participation in a stress-reduction class (the HPP) not only would reduce headaches (the primary dependent variable) over the course of final exam week (the follow-up period) but also may have the collateral benefit of reducing depressive symptoms (a secondary dependent variable). In this example, we could collect participants' self-reports of depressive symptoms with a depression inventory at baseline, randomize them to the stress-reduction-class or no stress-reduction-class condition, then administer the same depression inventory at the scheduled follow-up assessment at the end of the final exam week. The depression inventory thus provides a continuous dependent variable, with the hypothesis that participants in the HPP will have fewer depressive symptoms during the final exam week than participants in the control condition.

Continuous dependent variables can also be transformed into categorical variables. One reason for transforming a continuous dependent variable is that the underlying distribution of the continuous variable violates assumptions of normality necessary for performing certain statistical analyses. For example, if we were also interested in hypothesizing that participation in a stress-reduction class (the HPP) would not only reduce the risk of having a headache and depressive symptoms but also result in less weight gain over the course of final examinations week, we could measure a participant's weight at baseline and at follow-up and examine changes in his or her weight as a function of his or her group assignment. While we have a continuous dependent variable, weight in pounds, this variable can be transformed into a categorical dependent variable with the following dependent variable categories: "gained weight," "lost weight," or "no change in weight." Thus, what was a continuous dependent variable is now a categorical dependent variable. However, there are some issues to consider in categorizing a continuous dependent variable. In general, use of a categorical dependent variable derived from continuous data may entail some loss of detail in describing each participant as a range of scores is reduced to only two or three categories. The issue is potential loss of statistical power. A continuous variable implies certain statistical tests that rely on variability within the data for performing those tests. When a continuous variable is transformed into a categorical dependent variable, the variability in the dependent variable is markedly reduced. Thus, when a reliable continuous dependent variable exists and it meets statistical assumptions necessary for certain statistical analyses, it is usually best *not* to transform the data.

Selection of Statistical Techniques

In health promotion research, while there are numerous statistical techniques for testing whether an **HPP** is effective relative to a control group, we will focus on those that are most readily applicable. More complex research designs, by their very nature, require the use of more complex statistical techniques. Thus, we propose a decision strategy based on the type of dependent variable (categorical or continuous) as an overarching framework to facilitate understanding, identifying, and selecting the most appropriate statistical technique.

Data analysis is a process. At each juncture in the data analytic process the investigator (that is, you) will be faced with making decisions regarding what statistical technique is most appropriate for analyzing the type of dependent variable collected. The decision-mapping approach is based on an understanding of the types of data to be analyzed and the qualities and characteristics of those data. The type of statistical approach used is directly dependent on the type of data represented by the dependent variable.

The Case of Categorical Dependent Variables. Categorical dependent variables in RCTs are often dichotomous, meaning that there is a possibility of the data assuming only two levels or categories (although dependent variables can be classified into multiple levels, in which case they are polychotomous). For example, in a long-term study (let's say it's a ten-year follow-up) of the health-promoting effects of stress-reduction classes for men, ages fifty to fifty-nine, at high-risk for a heart attack (low density lipoprotein (LDL) over 250; overweight by twenty pounds, and reporting no regular physical exercise), the primary dependent variable is a dichotomous variable representing "heart attack." Thus, for any participant in the study, the range of potential values on the variable "heart attack" is $1 = $ Yes (experienced a heart attack over the course of the follow-up) or $0 = $ No (did not experience a heart attack over the course of the follow-up).

The hypothesis is that participation in the HPP would reduce the risk of heart attacks relative to the control group. The basic approach to testing this hypothesis is to compare the proportion of participants in each condition experiencing a heart attack over the follow-up period. This can be done using a nonparametric technique (nonparametric techniques do not make distributional assumptions about the underlying normality of the distribution of dependent variables) such as a simple chi-square test of proportions. If we compare the proportion of participants in each condition experiencing a heart attack and find statistically significant differences, with the HPP group having a lower proportion of participants experiencing a heart attack, we can conclude that the HPP was effective in reducing the risk of a heart attack. Let's see Figure 13.1.

As Figure 13.1 indicates, five men in the HPP group reported having a heart attack compared with twenty men in the control group. This corresponds to 2.5 percent of the HPP participants compared with 10 percent of the control participants. The question is whether this proportional difference is statistically significant. In analyzing the study, the investigator is required to make a determination as to what statistical technique is most applicable to these data. To assist you, we have developed a simple decision map to guide the selection of a statistical test. This map is depicted in Figure 13.2.

FIGURE 13.1. NUMBER OF PARTICIPANTS EXPERIENCING A HEART ATTACK IN A STRESS-REDUCTION PROGRAM AND A CONTROL CONDITION.

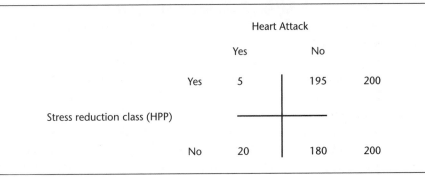

		Heart Attack		
		Yes	No	
	Yes	5	195	200
Stress reduction class (HPP)				
	No	20	180	200

FIGURE 13.2. STATISTICAL DECISION MAP.

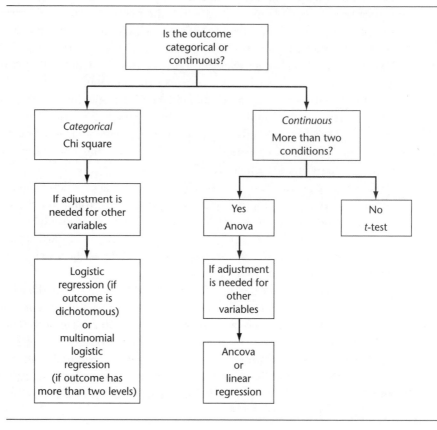

Let's use our decision map and see where it takes us. We have a categorical dependent variable (heart attack, "yes" or "no"), and there is no need for adjustment for other sociodemographic or predictor variables based on our examination of the baseline data (essentially, the groups are comparable). Thus, following our guide, a simple chi-square test would be the test statistic. The chi-square can determine whether the difference observed in the proportion of participants having a heart attack between conditions is statistically significant. Statistical significance is expressed as a probability (P), relative to chance. The customary criterion for determining statistical significance is $P < .05$.

In our example, the results are statistically significant $(P < .05)$. The findings support the hypothesis that stress-reduction classes can reduce the risk of a heart attack among high-risk men fifty to fifty-nine years of age. Please note the specificity of reporting the result. We may not be able to generalize the findings to populations with different sociodemographic characteristics, such as women, younger men, men of a particular ethnic or racial group, or men without risk indicators. External validity or generalizability is an issue related to how we select our sample and not to the type of test statistic used or the validity of the findings.

While the *P*-value is useful, it does not provide a full assessment of the effects of the HPP. Indeed, it describes the findings relative to chance. To capture more fully the effect of the HPP on the risk of a heart attack, it is useful to consider calculating a measure of effect size (ES). Effect size measures the strength of association between the HPP and the dependent variable (heart attack). In this case there are two measures that could be calculated. One is an absolute measure, the percent (or, if preferred, the proportion) difference that entails subtracting the percentage of participants with a heart attack in the HPP (2.5 percent) from the percentage with a heart attack in the control condition (10 percent), resulting in difference of 7.5 percent. A second measure of effect size is a relative measure called the relative risk (RR). The RR is defined as the risk of a heart attack in one group relative to the other group. In this example, RR = 20/200 divided by 5/200 = 4, indicating that participants in the control group had four times the risk of having a heart attack relative to the HPP. Alternatively, the RR could be expressed as .25 (5/200 divided by 20/200), indicating that participants in the HPP condition had only one-quarter the risk number of having a heart attack compared with participants in the control condition. Either calculation of RR is correct depending on how you prefer to present your findings.

The RR as a measure of intervention (or treatment) effect has a number of advantages. First and foremost, it is readily interpretable. We commonly refer to "risk" for a dependent variable. For example, dependent variables might include the risk for a heart attack, the risk of having an automobile accident while driving under the influence of alcohol, and the risk of developing cancer. Second, the RR is a "true" measure of the strength of the effect of the HPP, not a measure of chance. Third, the RR is invariant with respect to sample size. This latter advantage may require some further discussion. Thus, if the sample size was increased in each group, but the same proportions of participants in each study condition were identified with a heart attack, the RR would be exactly the same!

In addition to measuring the magnitude of the HPP effect (the RR), it is also recommended that the confidence interval around the RR be calculated. The confidence interval provides a measure of the precision of the effect. What does this mean? Well, let's illustrate. Suppose we did the exact same study one hundred times; the 95 percent confidence interval (the customary statistic) would inform us that ninety-five of those one hundred times, the RR would be between the lower and upper limits. When the confidence intervals are relatively narrow, we have more confidence that our RR calculation is precise. Conversely, relatively wider

TABLE 13.2. EFFECTS OF AN HIV RISK-REDUCTION INTERVENTION ON ADOLESCENTS' SEXUAL BEHAVIORS.

	6-Month Follow-Up Assessment		
	RR	**(95% CI)**	**P**
Consistent condom use, (past thirty days)	1.76	(1.07–3.19)	.04
Consistent condom use, (past six months)	2.46	(1.44–4.21)	.001
Condom use, last time had sex	3.94	(2.06–6.42)	.0001
Sex with new partner, (past thirty days)	0.30	(0.11–0.78)	.01

intervals detract from our confidence that our RR calculation is precise. For example, an RR of 2.1 with a confidence interval of 1.7, 2.5 suggests that the estimate is very close to its limits. An RR of 2.1 with a confidence interval of 1.2, 3.0 would not equate with the same degree of confidence.

In summary, in analyzing and interpreting data from an RCT to test the efficacy of an HPP, three statistics should be calculated: (1) the appropriate statistical test to determine if differences between conditions were statistically significant, (2) the RR as a measure of intervention effect size, and (3) the confidence interval around the RR as a measure of precision of effect. In keeping with our advice, in Table 13.2, note that we have calculated all the statistics necessary to describe the HPP effects for an HIV risk-reduction program designed to enhance consistent condom use and reduce number of sex partners. All three of these statistics should be presented when describing the results.

Interpreting the Results of an HPP with Categorical Dependent Variables. Now that we have calculated the appropriate statistics to describe the effects of the HPP, let's interpret them. The findings would be interpreted as follows: relative to participants in the control condition, participants in the HIV risk-reduction intervention were 1.76 times (95 percent CI = $1.07 - 3.19$, $P = .04$) more likely to report using condoms consistently in the thirty days prior to assessment, 2.46 times (CI = $1.44 - 4.21$, $P = .001$) more likely to report using condoms in the prior six months, 3.94 times (CI = $2.06 - 6.42$, $P = .0001$) more likely to report condom use at last sexual intercourse, and .3 times (CI = $.11 - .78$; $P = 0.1$) as likely to have a new sex partner in the prior thirty days. Thus, the use of all three statistics provides a richer description of effects of the HIV intervention (the HPP); one that includes a measure of the strength of the HPP effect that is invariant with respect to sample size (the relative risk), one that provides a measure of precision of the effect size (the confidence limits around the relative risk), and, of course, one that includes the traditional measure of statistical significance, the *P*-value.

Multivariable Models with a Categorical Dependent Variable

As we noted earlier, a key step in preparing for the analysis of any RCT is to examine the distribution of sociodemographic and other predictor variables between the HPP and the control group to assess whether the groups are comparable at baseline. In the event that differences between groups are found on sociodemographic variables or other study variables, we would want to control for them statistically. Otherwise our findings may not be valid. Including multiple variables in a model that predicts a singular dependent variable is considered to be a *multivariable* analysis. In intervention analyses, this implies the independent variable plus any identified *covariates*. Covariates are factors that vary in conjunction with the dependent variable. An analytic strategy that controls for the effects of these covariates while testing for intervention effects could be logistic regression. Logistic regression is used for categorical dependent variables that are dichotomous (Hosmer and Lemeshow, 1989); other analyses (for example, multinomial regression) would have to be employed for categorical dependent variables with more than two categories or levels (see Figure 13.2).

Logistic Regression. Logistic regression is a statistical technique that allows for the testing of an independent variable (in other words, the HPP intervention) in the presence of identified covariates. This process "controls" statistically for the effect of the covariates on the categorical dependent variable. "Controls for" in this context essentially means that the influence of intervention on the dependent variable is determined in addition to any effect the covariates may have on the dependent variable. Thus, differences between groups on the covariates are addressed.

Like linear regression, a logistic regression yields several parameter estimates. However, the primary estimate of interest is the odds ratio. The odds ratio is similar to the RR and is comparably interpreted (a 95 percent confidence interval is also derived from the analysis). For example, if a logistic regression equation that had condom use as the dependent variable, and a variable representing the HPP condition, along with several covariates, yielded an odds ratio of 3.9, it would be interpreted as "the likelihood that participants in the HPP group would report condom use at last sexual intercourse were 3.9 times the likelihood that participants in the control group would report such condom use." In addition to the odds ratio for the HPP, we would also like to calculate the 95 percent confidence interval and the corresponding *P*-value for the HPP.

Multiple Follow-Up Assessments

While the pretest-posttest RCT is the basic research design to assess change as a function of an HPP, there are, as might be expected, a number of more complex designs, and, of course, comparably more complex statistical approaches to analyze data derived from these complex designs. While it is beyond the scope of this chapter to address the range and complexity inherent in these advanced RCTs, we think it's important that students of health promotion be aware of them.

One way to extend the basic pretest-posttest design is to incorporate multiple follow-up assessments. Often investigators are curious about the sustainability of the HPP. Although we may expect that people would change their behavior, attitudes, and beliefs related to some health topic as a function of an HPP, these changes may begin to show decay over time. We might want to assess people on several occasions over a protracted time period. This design could be diagrammed as shown in Figure 13.3.

Analysis of this design with a categorical dependent variable can be accomplished through a variety of statistical techniques. One statistical approach that is gaining popularity is the use of generalized estimating equations (GEE). The GEE logistic regression model is an extension of the simple logistic regression model discussed in the previous section and can be used when the categorical dependent variable is dichotomized. With the GEE logistic model, all variables are measured on multiple occasions. Because repeated observations (measurements) collected for the same participant (for instance, measuring a participant's weight at two or more time points) are not independent of each other, a correction must be made for these within-participant correlations. This approach permits an adjustment for repeated within-participant measurement and the correlation between any one participant's measurements over time (Hardin and Hilbe, 2003).

The overall model design includes a time-independent variable, which in an RCT is the variable representing the program such as the HPP, as well as time-dependent variables (these are other predictors as well as the dependent variable that are expected to change). Additionally, a variable representing the number of time periods involved is also included in the model to differentiate the temporal order of the repeated measures. The resultant statistics are adjusted odds ratios and 95 percent confidence limits.

FIGURE 13.3.   STANDARD PRETEST-POSTTEST DESIGN.

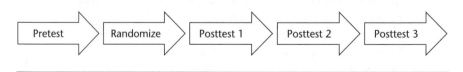

Thus, while we have simplified, for heuristic purposes, the rationale and format of a GEE logistic model, it is important to note that not all popular computer statistical packages offer this statistical routine as part of their package.

Analysis with a Continuous Dependent Variable.

Analysis with a Continuous Dependent Variable. Analysis with a continuous dependent variable is often more familiar to investigators in health promotion and health education research. In this case, the dependent variable assumes a range of scores rather than a binary response. For instance, commonly used dependent variables in health promotion research could be blood pressure (either diastolic or systolic), a person's weight, a score on an aptitude test, a score on a scale measuring depressive symptoms, number of servings of fruits and vegetables consumed, and so on. As you can see, the range of dependent variables is almost limitless.

The test statistic is one that is familiar, often learned in Introductory Statistics, the student's *t*-test. In the case of an RCT, the student's *t*-test provides a statistic that compares the means of two samples. Let's use an example to illustrate a simple analysis. In the HIV risk-reduction intervention described previously, a secondary dependent variable was to increase positive attitudes toward condom use (a continuous secondary dependent variable) among the participants in the intervention group. Attitude was assessed using a well-established scale with higher scale scores reflecting more positive attitudes toward using condoms during sexual intercourse. Participants were then randomized to either the risk-reduction group or a control group. Subsequent to completing the intervention or control group, six months later we asked all participants to return and complete a follow-up (posttest) assessment. The goal, of course, was to determine if condom attitude scores were different in the HIV risk-reduction group relative to the control group. The question is, How do we test for this important difference?

Let's assume that at follow-up (posttest), the participants in the HIV risk-reduction group had a mean condom attitude score of 32.65 (the scale range from a low of 10 to a high of 40). The control group had a mean condom attitude score of 22.40. The *t*-test assesses whether these observed means for the two study groups are statistically different from each other. It is important to note that, in the case of the RCT above, we are using an independent groups *t*-test. In our example, the results were statistically significant ($P < .05$). The findings support the motivator hypothesis that HIV risk-reduction intervention increases participants' positive attitudes toward condom use. A hypothesis may be proposed as either a *null hypothesis* (that is, there are no differences between groups) or as a *motivator* or *alternative hypothesis* (that is, differences exist between groups). However, as we noted in previous sections describing analysis of RCTs with a categorical dependent variable, while the *P*-value is useful, it does not provide a full assessment of the effects of the HPP. Indeed, it describes the findings relative to chance. To capture more fully the effect of the HIV risk-reduction intervention on condom attitude scores (continuous secondary dependent variable), it is useful to calculate a measure of effect size.

As noted earlier, but bears reiterating, an effect size provides an index of the strength of the association between the HPP and the dependent variable. In this case, a measure that could be calculated is the mean difference (D) between the group's condom attitude scores. Let's refer back to our example by examining Table 13.3.

Thus, we have calculated an absolute measure of effect on mean condom attitude scores attributable to the HIV risk-reduction intervention. On average, condom attitude scores in the HIV risk-reduction group are 10.25 units greater compared with the control group. As noted earlier, in measuring the magnitude of the HPP effect (the mean difference), and the corresponding P-value to assess its statistical significance, it is also recommended that the confidence interval around the mean difference be calculated. The confidence interval provides a measure of the *true* effect of the HPP in the population. In other words, if the study was repeated one hundred times, the 95 percent confidence interval would indicate that ninety-five of those one hundred times the mean difference would be between the lower and upper limit. In Table 13.4 we have calculated all the statistics necessary to describe the HPP effects for an HIV risk-reduction designed to enhance condom attitude scores.

Although Table 13.4 conveys a great deal of information about the effects of the HIV risk-reduction intervention on participants' condom attitude scores, it is important to understand that the statistic D is not a standardized measure of

TABLE 13.3. DIFFERENCES ON CONDOM ATTITUDE SCORES BY STUDY GROUP.

Group Assignment	Mean (at follow-up)	Mean Difference
HIV risk-reduction	32.65	+10.25
Control	22.40	

TABLE 13.4. EFFECTS OF AN HIV RISK-REDUCTION INTERVENTION ON CONDOM ATTITUDE SCORES.

Group Assignment	Mean (at follow-up)	D	95% CI	P
HIV risk-reduction	32.65	10.25	(7.38–13.86)	.03
Control	22.40			

Notes: D = mean difference (HPP – Co).
95% CI = 95 percent confidence limits around D.

TABLE 13.5. EFFECTS OF AN HIV RISK-REDUCTION INTERVENTION ON HIV KNOWLEDGE AND SELF-ESTEEM.

Dependent Variable	Mean Posttest Scores		D	95% CI	P
	Intervention	Control			
HIV knowledge	8.0	6.0	2.0	1.5–2.5	.04
Self-esteem	4.0	2.0	2.0	1.5–2.5	.04
Condom attitude	32.65	22.40	10.25	7.38–13.86	.03

Notes: D = mean difference (HPP – Co).
95% CI = 95 percent confidence limits around D.

effect size. If we wanted to compare a number of continuous dependent variables with different scale ranges, it would be problematic (similar to comparing apples to oranges). For example, the condom attitude scale used had a range from 10 to 40. Perhaps we want to examine another two scales as continuous secondary dependent variables (not an unreasonable thing to do). One scale measures HIV prevention knowledge and has a range from 1 to 10 (higher scores indicate greater knowledge) and another scale measures self-esteem and has a range from 1 to 5 (higher scores indicate greater self-esteem). Table 13.5 has information regarding these new scales.

Examining the differences between the HIV knowledge score and the self-esteem score, we note that the mean difference (D) = 2 in both instances. Hence, should we conclude that the effect of the HPP is identical for both of these dependent variables? Well, yes; if we focus only on the absolute differences. However, it is important to note that the HIV knowledge scale has a much larger range of potential scores (1 to 10) compared with the self-esteem scale (1 to 5). Thus, the same difference (D = 2) observed for each of the scales may have a markedly different magnitude of effect if we consider the relative difference. One measure that permits a relative assessment of change is called percent relative difference (RD). The RD statistic provides a common metric for measuring the magnitude of change across different scale measures. The RD is calculated by dividing the value for D by the mean posttest score for the control group. Below we demonstrate the calculation and utility of this statistic. In this example, the RD for HIV knowledge would be equal to 2/6 = .33. Likewise, for the dependent variable, mean self-esteem scores, the RD would be 2/2 = 1.00. It may be easier if the RD is then converted to the percent RD by multiplying the value by 100. Thus, as the example demonstrates, the percent RD for knowledge was 33 percent and for self-esteem, 100 percent. Thus, the HPP had a relatively greater effect on improving mean self-esteem scores compared with HIV knowledge scores. However, examining only the absolute differences in mean scores would obscure this potentially important finding. As with the other measures of HPP effects, the 95 percent confidence interval can also be calculated around the percent RD.

Interpreting the Results of an HPP with Continuous Dependent Variables. Now that we have calculated the appropriate statistics to describe the effects of the HPP, let's interpret them. The findings would be interpreted as follows: relative to participants in the control group, those in the HIV risk-reduction intervention had significantly higher scores on condom attitudes, HIV knowledge, and self-esteem. We concluded this based on the significant *t*-test. Moreover, the effect sizes indicated that the greater proportional difference was found for self-esteem, as assessed by the percent RD. Thus, the use of these statistics provides a richer description of significant effects of the HIV intervention (the HPP).

Multivariable Models with Continuous Dependent Variables

As we noted earlier, a key step in preparing for the analysis of any RCT is to examine the distribution of sociodemographic and other predictor variables between the HPP and the control group to assess whether the groups are comparable at baseline. In the event the groups are not comparable with respect to several key variables of the primary dependent variable or secondary dependent variables, we would want to control for these differences. Otherwise, our findings may not be valid. In addition to controlling for group differences revealed on baseline measures, it is important to control for the baseline measure of the dependent variable when performing analyses on the posttest data. To control for baseline measures, enter them into the analysis as covariates. This analysis strategy provides a more rigorous test of the intervention effects, such that differences between groups on posttest means are adjusted for baseline measurement. The statistical analysis used to control for both the effects of covariates and the baseline value of the dependent variable is either linear regression or its algebraic equivalent, analysis of covariance (ANCOVA).

◆ ◆ ◆

In a Nutshell

In addition to controlling for group differences revealed on baseline measures, it is important to control for the baseline measure of the dependent variable when performing analyses on the posttest data.

◆ ◆ ◆

Linear Regression and ANCOVA. Linear regression and ANCOVA are statistical techniques that allow for two or more variables to be included in a model with a continuous dependent variable. The HPP variable is included as the independent variable as well as covariates and the baseline measure of the continuous dependent variable. While the computation of the linear model is beyond the scope of this chapter, the interested reader is referred to Kleinbaum, Kupper, Muller, and Nizam (1998) for an eminently readable discussion of this approach. Linear regression and ANCOVA can adjust for the effects of group differences that would otherwise obscure intervention effects as well as adjusting for the baseline value of the continuous dependent variable. Linear regression and ANCOVA permit computation of adjusted means and mean differences (D) for continuous dependent variables similar to that discussed earlier in this section as well as constructing the 95 percent confidence interval around these effect sizes (D).

Multiple Follow-Up Assessments

As noted in earlier sections of this chapter, for categorical data with multiple assessments, the use of GEE was recommended. GEE are recommended also for continuous dependent variables, and can be used to construct a model adjusting for the correlations between the repeated measures. GEE control for autocorrelations that could distort the true effect of the HPP.

Applied Example

A study published in the *Journal of the American Medical Association* reported findings from an RCT designed to test the effects of an Internet-based behavioral intervention program. The goal of the behavioral intervention program was to promote weight loss among people with type 2 diabetes (Tate, Jackvony, and Wing, 2003). Volunteers were randomly assigned to receive an Internet-based weight loss program or the same program with the addition of an e-mail-based counseling component. Weight was assessed at baseline, three, six, and twelve months postintervention. Forty-six people were assigned to each of the two conditions ($N = 92$).

A repeated measures analysis was conducted. The continuous outcome variable suggested that a t-test or analysis of variance (ANOVA) could be used to test the study hypothesis (see Figure 13.2). The example is quite instructive because it illustrates a point that is not included in Figure 13.2. The t-test is the most parsimonious data analytic technique when the independent variable has only two levels. However, ANOVA can also be used when the independent variable has only two levels. So, why would ANOVA be a better choice? The answer involves ease of testing for the influence of covariates. Although a "controlled t-test" can be conducted, the more commonly accepted approach is to control with ANCOVA. Thus, the initial selection of ANOVA allows for an easy "switch" to ANCOVA. The authors used a repeated measures ANOVA to assess the Group (intervention or control) X Time (baseline through the multiple follow-ups) interaction. Ideally, there should be greater positive change, over time, for those randomized to the condition designated as being the treatment (in this case the Internet plus the e-mail counseling service) as opposed to the control (in this case, the receipt only of material and messages provided by Websites).

Using data collected at baseline, the authors first determined that the two groups did not differ as the study began (in other words, randomization worked). Because likely covariates were not identified, the use of ANCOVA was not necessary. The ANOVA produced the desired Group X Time interaction, showing greater weight loss among persons receiving the addition of e-mail-based counseling.

Integration with the Research Process

The analysis of an RCT is indeed an important undertaking. The amount of time and resources devoted to the RCT certainly warrant careful attention to every aspect of this analysis. However, it is critical that the analysis be constructed on a solid foundation. In particular, the RCT should have a sound design (step 4 of the nine-step model described in Chapter One), and it should include reliable and valid measurement of all variables (step 5 of the research process), including potential covariates. Of course, a great deal of attention should be devoted to measurement of the dependent variable(s); this is the primary outcome variable of interest. A well-planned analysis cannot make up for lack of planning in either of these two steps.

The quality of analysis for the RCT is highly dependent on how well the study protocol was implemented (step 7 of the research process). For example, if contamination occurred between study conditions (that is, intervention and control group participants had frequent contact) even the best statistician will not be able to rescue the analysis from this threat to internal validity. Day-to-day study procedures are also important. Consider, for example, the decline of study quality that would occur if research staff failed to collect information relative to the number of people who refused to participate in the study. Or consider the decline in quality that could occur if study participants frequently skipped large sections of the assessment questionnaires (research staff can easily help remind participants that it is important to answer all of the questions). In essence, the procedures described in Chapter Six are critical building blocks for the RCT. The subsequent analysis, then, is merely a "crowning achievement."

Fortunately, the analysis is unique in the research process because it can be reconceptualized. Consider an article published in the journal *Preventive Medicine* (Maxwell, Bastani, Vida, and Warda, 2003). The article reported findings from an RCT of a breast and cervical cancer screening program designed for Filipino American women. In a sample of 444 women, the intervention program was not significantly different from the control program in producing change in the dependent variable. However, the analysis was changed to assess intervention effects among only a sub-sample of women Filipino American women who had immigrated to the United States within the past ten years. In this subgroup analysis, intervention effects were observed.

Summary

This chapter has provided an overview of the logic and process involved in data analyses pertaining to testing whether an HPP is effective. A decision map can be used to determine the type of analytic technique appropriate for the type of dependent variable and for when other adjustments are necessary. It is critical that the decision map be followed, given the necessity to provide an accurate and valid test of the HPP, thereby avoiding biased results. In addition to choosing the appropriate statistical technique for testing of intervention effects, we also emphasized the importance of moving beyond the reporting of basic significance associated with the statistical test to include measures of effect size and confidence intervals. Including these additional statistics provides a breadth to the analysis that enhances the precision of the results while allowing for their comparability across other studies.

Issues to Consider

1. The first issue is an extension of the previous paragraph. The study was designed to test an intervention program among Filipino American women. A distinction between those residing in the United States for more versus less than ten years was not part of the a priori study hypotheses. Thus, a question that can be asked would be, Is it "fair" to conduct post-hoc analyses of an RCT when the original null hypotheses are not rejected? A skeptical position on this issue would include mention that a post-hoc analysis may be a "search" for something meaningful that can be used to vindicate the study. Alternatively, the tremendous value of the RCT to the science of health promotion could be justifiable grounds for a post-hoc analysis.

2. The issue of missing data is tremendously important to consider when analyzing an RCT. One common strategy has been to estimate the value of missing data by calculating a mean from the rest of the data. This process seems fair when the amount of missing data is small in comparison with the amount of data that is not missing. As noted in Chapter Six, the adage "once randomized always analyzed" implies that people cannot be dropped

from the analysis of an RCT on the grounds of missing follow-up data. Thus, this remedy of *imputing* data seems logical. The issue, however, becomes one of how much imputation should be consider too much?

For Practice and Discussion

1. Locate three examples of RCTs by doing an electronic search. Be sure that your examples relate to health promotion rather than medical advances. You will notice that most RCTs are indeed designed around questions in medical care such as drug effects or the effects of a new treatment procedure. Using the Decision Map shown in this chapter, determine if the authors of each study used an analytic strategy that is consistent with the map.
2. Again, using the Decision Map select an analytic approach for each scenario listed below.

   • The dependent variable is blood serum cholesterol level.
   • The dependent variable is having a Pap test in the past two years (women answered "yes" versus "no").
   • The dependent variable is an ordinal measure of cigarette use (participants answered using one of three options: "none," "less than one pack per day," "at least one pack per day."
   • The dependent variable is a scale measure of depression.
   • The dependent variable is a scale measure of depression, and several covariates are critical to the analysis.
   • The dependent variable is contraceptive use (dichotomized as "yes" versus "no"), and several covariates are critical to the analysis.

References

Hardin, J. W., and Hilbe, J. M. (2003). *Generalized estimating equations.* New York: Chapman and Hall/CRC.

Hosmer, D. W., and Lemeshow, S. L. (1989). *Applied logistic regression.* New York: John Wiley and Sons.

Kleinbaum, D. G., Kupper, L. L., Muller, K. E., and Nizam, A. (1998). *Applied regression analysis and other multivariable methods.* New York: Duxbury Press.

Maxwell, A. E., Bastani, R., Vida, P., and Warda, U. S. (2003). Results of a randomized trial to increase breast and cervical cancer screening among Filipino American women. *Preventive Medicine, 37,* 102–109.

Tate, D. F., Jackvony, E. H., and Wing, R. R. (2003). Effects of Internet behavioral counseling on weight loss in adults at risk for type 2 diabetes. *Journal of the American Medical Association, 289,* 1833–1836.

PART FOUR

CORE SKILLS RELATED TO HEALTH PROMOTION RESEARCH

CHAPTER FOURTEEN

INTRODUCTION TO SCIENTIFIC WRITING

Richard A. Crosby, Ralph J. DiClemente, and Laura F. Salazar

Students, practitioners, and researchers in the discipline of health promotion often experience a great deal of anxiety when they hear the phrase "publish or perish." The term *publish* should actually be thought of as an extension of the research enterprise, in which publishing is viewed as a necessary and logical endpoint. In reality, then, publishing is an artifact of the larger and more important process of health promotion research. Nonetheless, the published report is indeed a critical piece of dissemination (see step 9 of the nine-step model in Figure 1.2). Thus, researchers should be well versed in the "art of scientific writing." The phrase includes the word *art* because few universal standards exist with respect to the construction of manuscripts that report findings from health promotion research.

This chapter will introduce the basic structure of a manuscript and describe in detail how each section of the manuscript should be written and formatted to meet journal expectations of content and style. Moreover, we also provide guidance in how researchers can tailor their work to "fit" the intended journal to which the manuscript will be submitted. The chapter will expand on the basic themes that publishing is essentially an extension of the research enterprise and

MINCUS AND DINCUS FACE REJECTION.

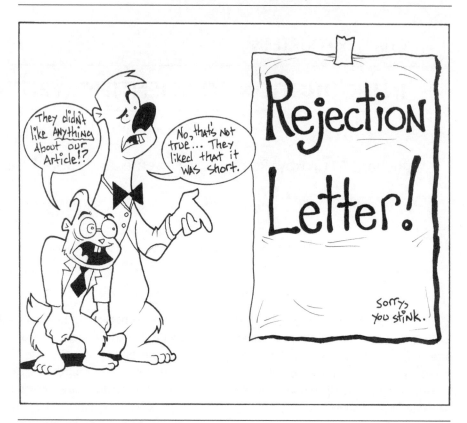

Copyright 2005 by Justin Wagner; reprinted with permission.

that producing acceptable manuscripts from rigorous research does not need to be a challenging process. Of course, no matter how well the research manuscript is prepared, publishing findings based on research severely lacking in rigor is a challenge. Thus, the chapter assumes that the "would be" authors are summarizing a rigorous research process.

◆ ◆ ◆

In a Nutshell

Of course, no matter how well the research manuscript is prepared, publishing findings based on research severely lacking in rigor is a challenge.

◆ ◆ ◆

Illustration of Key Concepts

Before the writing begins it is imperative that members of the research team carefully deliberate the question, To which journal will we submit? Once this step is complete, the remaining process is to simply begin composing the manuscript—one section at a time!

Finding the Right Fit

Three considerations are paramount when authors begin to assemble a research manuscript. First, the authors should select a journal that will provide the *maximum impact* for the topic and practical significance of the study findings. Impact ratings are frequently determined by (1) the number of journal subscribers, (2) how often journals are cited, and (3) indices related to the breadth of electronic distribution.

Second, the journal should be selected for a readership that is interested and invested in the outcomes of your study. In a discipline as diverse as health promotion, this consideration is particularly important in that the spectrum of health promotion research is vast, and, therefore, the research findings seldom appeal to a general audience. Instead, the conclusions of the manuscript may have greater impact if the manuscript is targeted to a well-defined audience. Ideally, the audience should share a common interest in the research and its findings. For example, professionals in preventive medicine may benefit tremendously from a study conclusion that has implications for clinical practice (such as "Physicians and other health professionals who counsel pregnant adolescent females should be aware that marijuana use may be common among those in their first trimester."). Professionals who have dedicated their careers to improving health practices such as fostering exercise behavior may benefit from research that supports the efficacy of a novel approach (for example, "Findings suggest that changes to the physical environment of the workplace can have a favorable impact on the exercise behavior of employees.").

Third, the nature of the study and the analyses should be understandable to the intended readership. Health promotion is multidisciplinary. Indeed, one measure of the growing strength of health promotion is the degree to which people from social sciences, behavioral sciences, law, education, nursing, and medical disciplines are mutually engaged in health promotion research. This diversity brings a welcome and critical mass of expertise to bear on a large number of disparate research questions. The drawback to this high-level of diversity is that not all researchers "speak the same language." For example, psychologists often are well versed in analysis of variance, whereas epidemiologists ply their trade with contingency table analyses. Sociologists may have a tremendous appreciation for community-level interventions, whereas physicians may be far more interested in clinic-based approaches to health promotion. One quick and efficient strategy for ensuring this fit is to know as much as possible of the professional organization sponsoring the journal (although not all journals are sponsored by a professional organization).

Once the authors have agreed upon a journal, the next task is to locate the "Instructions for Authors" (also called "Author Guidelines" or "Submission Requirements") located on the journal's Website or in a designated issue of the journal. These requirements usually change when the journal hires a new editor-in-chief; thus, authors should consult the instructions immediately prior to writing. Figure 14.1 displays a sample of journals that typically publish health promotion research.

Instructions are explicit and provide authors with a number of manuscript categories for reporting empirical findings, such as a letter, a report, a brief report, or a full-length original article. Again, the authors must strive to find an ideal fit; selecting the wrong manuscript category may severely hamper the odds of acceptance. Once the manuscript category has been identified, the authors

FIGURE 14.1. EXAMPLES OF JOURNALS THAT PUBLISH ARTICLES RELEVANT TO HEALTH PROMOTION.

Journal Name

Addiction
The American Journal of Health Behavior
The American Journal of Health Education
The American Journal of Health Promotion
American Journal of Preventive Medicine
American Journal of Public Health
Canadian Journal of Public Health
Ethnicity and Disease
Health Education and Behavior
Health Education Research
Health Promotion International
Journal of Adolescent Health
Journal of Consulting and Clinical Psychology
Journal of Health Care for the Poor and Underserved
Journal of School Health
Journal of the American Medical Association
Patient Education and Counseling
Prevention Science
Public Health Reports
Social Science and Medicine

should painstakingly adhere to the instructions that are specific to that category. Such instructions are typically broken down by section of the manuscript.

Sections of the Manuscript

The manuscript is typically divided into several discrete sections.

Abstract. The abstract is your one and only chance to make a good first impression. Often the only portion of an article that is widely available, accessible, and read in its entirety is the abstract. In fact, most journals that publish health promotion research will make article abstracts freely available through on-line search engines such as Medline®. Accessing the abstract only is often the initial goal of readers, as doing so can subsequently provide enough information to readers that they can determine whether they will benefit from reading the full article. Abstracts are also the medium for judging the quality of research that has been submitted for oral or poster presentations at professional conferences. Often the conference organizers will print the abstracts in the conference program and make them available on their Website. As is true for any first impression, a good-quality abstract can greatly enhance the odds that readers will ultimately seek (and benefit from) the full article or attend the conference presentation.

◆ ◆ ◆

In a Nutshell

Abstracts are also the medium for judging the quality of research that has been submitted for oral or poster presentations at professional conferences.

◆ ◆ ◆

Typically an abstract comprises 250 words or less. Within this limited number of words, the abstract must concisely describe the objective(s), methods, results, and conclusion(s) of the research. The abstract should convey essential information such as

- The research question(s)
- Sample size and sampling technique
- Participation rate
- Study design (retention rates if applicable)
- Key measures

- Data-collection methods
- Descriptive, bivariate, and multivariate findings (with test statistics)
- A one-sentence conclusion that addresses the research question(s)

Quick inspection of the items in this list suggests that the abstract is a "stand alone" unit within the manuscript. Indeed, the abstract should always be prepared as a digest of the complete story; it should *not* dilute the story through the use of vacuous phrases such as "implications will be discussed" or "a few examples of the findings are." Remember, space is limited so make every word count!

The important and very demanding requirements of an abstract may at first seem impossible to meet given a word limit of 250 or less. However, the judicious selection of words and the elimination of any superfluous information can greatly aid the writer in bringing the word count down within limits. Traditionally, abstracts do not have to adhere to essential rules of grammar. (See Box 14.1 for several examples.) Of course, even with a stringent selection of words and thoughts, abstracts may seem impossible to create given their strict word limits. One way to create abstracts that meet word limits is to reduce the number of findings presented. For example, it may be better to focus on the findings related to the primary research question. If space permits, then you could include the ancillary findings.

Unfortunately, universal standards for the structure of abstracts are nonexistent in the discipline of health promotion research. Some journals require that the abstract should not have specific headings, but most journals specify the headings that are mandatory and those that are optional. Knowing these requirements (based on the published "Instructions to Authors") is therefore a prerequisite to creating an acceptable abstract.

Introduction. The scope and depth of a well-written introduction is a function of journal requirements. For example, typically, journals that cater to a largely medical audience (such as the *Journal of the American Medical Association*) prefer very short introductions (two to three paragraphs), whereas journals that fall under the umbrella of behavioral and social science disciplines (for example, *Health Education & Behavior*) prefer and encourage introductions that provide a great deal of detail and allow more space. The difference between these two "camps" is not only a matter of degree but also of substance.

As described in Chapter One (steps 2 and 9), the research enterprise is focused on identifying and addressing key gaps in the existing literature. Thus, one purpose of the introduction is to describe the chain of research that led to the current

Box 14.1. Examples of Abridged Grammar in Abstracts

For the purposes of writing and submitting an abstract, the grammar used is considered correct and acceptable.

A. **Study Objectives**

This study was designed to identify factors that may preclude people from accepting an AIDS vaccine when one is developed and approved for use.

or

To identify factors that that may preclude people from accepting an AIDS vaccine when one is developed and approved for use.

B. **Study Design**

The study used a prospective design with assessments at baseline, three months, six months, and twelve months.

or

A prospective study with assessments at baseline, three months, six months, and twelve months.

C. **Study Sample**

The sample comprised 679 adult volunteers recruited from cardiac outpatient units.

or

679 adult volunteers recruited from cardiac outpatient units.

D. **Conclusion**

The study findings provide support for the hypothesis that men are less likely than women to initiate cigarette use after the age of twenty-one years.

or

Findings suggest that men are less likely than women to initiate cigarette use after the age of twenty-one years.

study—this description sets the stage for the remainder of the manuscript and clearly prepares readers for a conclusion (or conclusions) that will represent the next link in this chain. Short introductions provide this information in summary form. Consider, for example, the one paragraph hypothetical introduction that follows:

Although intensified HIV testing efforts and behavioral interventions may greatly contribute to reducing the incidence of HIV,[ref] the anticipated advent of a vaginal microbicide may represent a substantial turning point in the epidemic. Unfortunately, only two studies have investigated social and behavioral correlates pertaining to microbicide acceptance among female partners of injection-drug-using men, a population greatly at risk for HIV infection. The first study focused solely on the identification of demographic factors (such as race, ethnicity, and income),[ref] and the second investigated a large number of partner-related barriers to potential microbicide use.[ref] Related studies of other high-risk populations have found that self-efficacy for microbicide application and perceived threat of HIV infection were robustly associated with intent to use microbicides.[ref] As opposed to studies investigating intent (or actual participation) to enroll in randomized controlled trials of a microbicide,[ref] this study identified factors that may preclude women from using an HIV-preventive microbicide that was approved for use in western Kenya.

◆ ◆ ◆

In a Nutshell

One purpose of the introduction is to describe the chain of research that led to the current study.

◆ ◆ ◆

The introduction succinctly conveys the chain of research and notes the gap in the literature (in other words, no studies of women whose partners are injection-drug users and no studies of actual microbicide use). Each article is cited and described just enough to allow an interested reader to find out more by retrieving a specific article. The final sentence is the logical conclusion of the paragraph (and the entire introduction).

Alternatively, longer introductions serve the same purpose, but they provide more depth to the literature reviewed. A longer version could describe each of the cited articles in greater detail. A long introduction, however, will nonetheless take on a general form that mimics the sample shown (that is, the chain of research is reviewed, a gap is identified, and the research question is stated).

Methods: Study Sample. This subsection of the manuscript should provide details related to the generation of the study sample, such as the population from which the sample was drawn and the inclusion and exclusion criteria (as well as the number of otherwise eligible participants who were excluded based on these criteria). This section also should describe the sampling technique employed and provide the rationale for its selection. This rationale is critically important because it justifies the sampling technique (see Chapter Eleven). Consider the following hypothetical example:

> To identify differences between low-income women who have and have not ever had a mammogram, we began with a sampling frame of women receiving WIC benefits in the state of Vermont. The sampling frame was a list of all women currently receiving benefits, with women receiving benefits for the longest period of time listed first through women receiving benefits for the shortest period of time listed last. Next, every twenty-fifth name on the list was selected; this created a systematic random sample. The sample therefore comprised women who had previously been categorized as low-income and it equally represented women regardless of how long they had been receiving WIC benefits.

The text states the sampling technique used (systematic random sample) as well as the reasons the research team used this approach.

Another obligation of this section is to report the participation rate. This rate is used as a gauge to judge the potential for *participation bias* (that is, whether volunteers were systematically different from those who refused to be in the study). Although a low participation rate does not necessarily mean that the sample was biased, it nonetheless suggests that this form of bias cannot be ruled out. Consider the following example:

> From December 2000 through April 2002, project recruiters screened 1,590 men attending health department clinics to assess eligibility for participating in a cancer prevention study. Of those screened, 685 were eligible to participate. Men were eligible if they were African American, eighteen to twenty-nine years old, unmarried, and had been previously diagnosed with cancer. Of those men not eligible to participate, the majority (83 percent) were either too young or too old. The current study consisted of 605 (88.3 percent) eligible men who volunteered and provided written informed consent. The majority (91.2 percent) of eligible men who did not participate in the study were unavailable due to conflicts with their employment schedules.

Note that the paragraph provides information pertaining to eligibility requirements and shows that "age" was the primary reason why screened men were not eligible. Lack of eligibility is *not* indicative of participation bias, because this is a reason for nonparticipation that is imposed by the research question rather than a self-selection phenomenon. The important numbers are 605 (the N for the study) and 685 (the number of eligible men who were asked to volunteer). By use of these numbers as the numerator and denominator, respectively, a participation rate was obtained and reported. Although universally accepted standards do not exist, participation rates in excess of 80 percent are widely considered acceptable (that is, the potential for a strong participation bias is considered sufficiently low).

In studies that have one or more planned follow-up assessments, you should also report the *retention rate* or the *attrition rate*. The retention rate is the percentage of participants who remained in the study and completed each of the follow-up assessments. Unfortunately, in prospective studies, retaining a high percentage of participants is a challenge. Consider, for example, an article that reports only a 51 percent retention rate. This information is important to report because it suggests a possibility for *attrition bias*. (Attrition bias can be assessed analytically, and these analyses should be reported in the results section—see Chapters Five and Thirteen for analyses to assess attrition bias).

This section of the manuscript also meets several other obligations. The time period of data collection should be disclosed. This information lets readers judge whether the data represent thinking or practice that may have changed in the study population. For example, a study concerning awareness of smallpox and anthrax (among U.S. residents) conducted in 2002 would provide substantially different results than the same study conducted before the events of September 11, 2001, and the subsequent media attention to bioterrorism. Also, because this is traditionally the first section of the manuscript that reports methodology, a sentence should be included informing readers that the entire study protocol was approved by an Institutional Review Board. (Indeed, journal editors will demand that this sentence be included.)

Methods: Data Collection. This section is designed to inform readers *how* the data were collected, not *what* data were collected. A subsequent section will provide readers with specific information about the measures or instruments used in the study. As described in Chapters Nine and Ten, data-collection methods span a broad range from paper-and-pencil assessments to electronic diaries. A rationale for the selected method should be provided. Consider the following example:

> Based on studies suggesting decreased reporting bias,[ref] all self-reported measures were assessed using audio-computer-assisted self-interviewing

(A-CASI). By providing a voice track that delivered each question to adolescents through headphones, A-CASI technology may have reduced problems that otherwise would have been posed by low literacy. The A-CASI technology also created a user-friendly interview method that automatically handled skip patterns in the questionnaire and provided adolescents with an interactive experience, possibly increasing their attention to the task. The private environment created by the A-CASI may also be useful with respect to the elicitation of honest responses for questions that assessed sexual and drug-use behaviors.[ref] Adolescents' responses to the computer-delivered questions were automatically encrypted to ensure confidentiality. To help facilitate accuracy, a relatively short period of time was used when asking adolescents to recall past behaviors. Adolescents were assured that their names could not be linked to the codes used to identify documents containing their responses.

This example illustrates a good match between the research questions and the selected method of data collection. The study apparently asked adolescents to disclose information about their recent sexual behaviors and their recent drug use behaviors. Complete with references to support their position, the authors justify their selection of A-CASI with respect to these research goals.

In addition to *how* the data were collected, this section should also provide information pertaining to the physical location *where* the data were collected. This information is important because the reader must have the necessary details to potentially replicate the study and because readers may want to make judgments regarding the potential effect of the setting on participants' responses. For example, collecting data from incarcerated men in prison may inadvertently affect how they respond to certain questions (for example, Have you had sex in the past seven days) as opposed to interviewing men in a community center after their release. Finally, this section should also include a sentence that describes what compensation was provided to participants to encourage their participation.

Methods: Measures. The primary obligation of this section is to justify the constructs (for example, self-esteem) (see Chapter Nine for more details on constructs) included and describe the measures employed for assessing those constructs (such as the Rosenberg Self-Esteem Scale). If the study was guided by theory, then a sentence should be included in this section that articulates the particular theory used and that the measures chosen correspond to the theoretical constructs. This approach is mainly used in medical journals; for psychological or other social science journals, you may want to include a whole section on the theory in greater detail in the introduction. In the absence of a theoretical framework, authors should justify their selection of constructs based on previously conducted research.

Informing readers how the study constructs were measured is equally important. These constructs could be organized according to their role in the study. You could first describe the measures used to assess the X-variables (correlates in a cross-sectional study, predictors in a prospective study, or independent variables in an experimental study) followed by the measures used to assess the Y-variables (outcomes in observational research and dependent variables in experimental research). Within each category, authors may want to first describe single-item measures (such as measures of race or ethnicity, income, or geographic area) and then describe the use of scales or indexes. For each scale or index, a rationale should be provided for the choice of that particular measure. Moreover, if previous psychometric data are available, this should be provided and referenced, as well as current psychometric findings. It is also important to provide a sample question from the scale or index. The number of items constituting each scale or index should also be reported. If this information is extensive, then a table can be used. Table 14.1 provides a sample of summary information that should be reported. These measures were used to assess eight constructs among a sample of high-risk adolescents. To conserve precious journal space, the table may also provide descriptive statistics for each measure. Readers can also be referred back to this table a second time when they are reading the results section of the manuscript.

When research questions necessitate the use of directly observed or biological measures, the nature and use of these measures should be described in great detail. Two samples follow:

(1) After the interview, men were asked to demonstrate the act of applying a condom to a penile model. Trained observers scored men's performance based on six criteria: correctly opens package, squeezes air from tip, places condom right side up on model, keeps tip pinched while unrolling, unrolls to base of model, and condom remains intact. Men received one point for each of the six steps they performed correctly. Those scoring three points or less and those scoring four points or more were classified as having lower and higher demonstrated ability, respectively.

(2) Two vaginal swab specimens were evaluated for *Neisseria gonorrhoeae, Chlamydia trachomatis,* and *Trichomonas vaginalis.* The first swab was placed in a specimen transport tube (Abbott LCx Probe System for *N. gonorrhoeae* and *C. trachomatis* assays) and tested for chlamydia and gonorrhea DNA by (LCR). The second swab was used to inoculate a culture medium for *T. vaginalis* (InPouch TV test; BioMed Diagnostics, Inc., Santa Clara, California). A

TABLE 14.1. DESCRIPTION OF SCALE MEASURES AND BIVARIATE CORRELATIONS OF THESE MEASURES WITH SELF-ESTEEM AMONG AFRICAN AMERICAN ADOLESCENT FEMALES.

Scale and Sample Item	# of items	α	M	SD	Range
Body image[a] *I usually feel physically attractive.*	7	.73	27.2	4.8	12–35
Perceived family support[b] *My family really tries to help me.*	4	.86	15.2	4.3	4–20
Ethnic pride[c] *I feel good about black culture.*	13	.74	42.3	4.6	20–52
Normative beliefs favoring males[d] *Your boyfriend gets angry when you don't do what he wants.*	8	.72	15.6	5.6	8–36
Perceived support from a special person[e] *I have a special person who is a source of comfort to me.*	4	.82	17.2	3.5	4–20
Traditional sex role beliefs[f] *Boys are better leaders than girls.*	7	.64	13.2	3.9	7–28
Religiosity[g] *How often do you attend religious or spiritual services?*	4	.68	10.4	2.7	4–16
Perceived support from friends[h] *My friends really try to help me.*	4	.87	15.3	4.4	4–20

[a]Higher scores represent a more favorable body image.
[b]Higher scores represent a greater perceived family support.
[c]Higher scores represent greater ethnic pride.
[d]Higher scores represent stronger beliefs favoring male decision making in a relationship.
[e]Higher scores represent greater perceived support from special persons.
[f]Higher scores represent more traditional sex-role beliefs.
[g]Higher scores represent greater religiosity.
[h]Higher scores represent greater perceived support from friends.

number of studies have established the high sensitivity (at least 97 percent) and specificity (at least 99 percent) of these assays.[ref]

For biological measures, the authors should disclose sensitivity and specificity estimates of the test used as well as providing references. Finally, it should be noted that the name and location (city and state) of the company that produced the test should be disclosed. This practice is typically required by journals, and it also allows for replication by other researchers and possible comparison of findings across studies that use identical tests.

Methods: Data Analysis. This section should be brief yet informative. The authors have an obligation to compose a paragraph or two that informs readers about the specific statistical techniques that constituted the analytic procedures. Once described, these procedures should be followed without exception; introducing a new technique halfway through the results section creates confusion.

◆ ◆ ◆

In a Nutshell

The authors have an obligation to compose a paragraph or two that informs readers about the specific statistical techniques that constituted the analytic procedures.

◆ ◆ ◆

This section must describe the rationale and procedures used to transform any of the variables if applicable. The use of descriptive statistics does not need to be included; however, the use of each kind of statistical test employed in the analyses should be disclosed at this point. A rationale for the selection of every statistical test is *not* necessary; however, a rationale should be provided if one is not readily apparent or if the statistical test was complex. If appropriate references that support the selection of statistical tests, the rationale, or both are available, then they should be included. A manuscript may also benefit from succinct explanations of relatively novel tests or tests that are otherwise likely to be unfamiliar to readers of the journal. Finally, the authors should describe how they defined statistical significance. If statistical significance does not follow convention ($P < .05$), then a justification for choosing a different value should be provided.

When writing the methods section, it is important to note that sufficient detail should be provided to allow another research team to replicate the study. Indeed, achieving this level of descriptive detail is often considered a hallmark of well-written manuscripts.

Results: Characteristics of the Sample. This section is purely descriptive. The goal is to inform readers about the composition of the study sample. Common indices include race or ethnicity, sex, age, income-level, and marital status. However, most indices reported should be selected based on the nature of the research question. For instance, if the research question concerns associations between family structure and teen pregnancy, then basic descriptive information regarding these variables should be provided. An example of this section follows:

About one-third (34.2 percent) of the sample reported ever being pregnant, with 12.5 percent reporting a current pregnancy. The majority of participants reported residence with only their mother (59.3 percent) or with both their mother and father (32.1 percent). The remainder of the sample lived with friends (5.0 percent) or in their own apartment (3.6 percent).

When multiple sites are involved or participants are recruited from different venues, sample characteristics including number of participants can be provided for each of these different sites. Also, at this juncture, descriptive statistics for measures of key constructs should be reported. Table 14.1, for example, displays the range of scores, means, and standard deviations for each of eight assessed constructs. Referring readers to this table is therefore an important aspect of this opening part of the results section.

Results: Findings. This section is the heart of the manuscript. Describing the findings is not interpretive writing. Prose is not part of this section. The findings should be reported using technical writing, that is, using terse and precise language. Your task is to report the final output from the statistical analyses. In reporting the final output using text appropriate for this section, you should present the statistical findings in terms of the research question or study hypotheses. This context is necessary for understanding the results. As an elementary example, consider output from a logistic regression analysis that yielded an odds ratio of 3.9 and an associated P level of .001. In the text, you would say, "Women who had a regular physician were almost four times more likely to get a pap test in the past year relative to those without a regular physician."

◆ ◆ ◆

In a Nutshell

Describing the findings is not interpretive writing. Prose is not part of this section. The findings should be reported using technical writing, that is, using terse and precise language.

◆ ◆ ◆

Nearly all journals require that authors use tables and figures to extend the level of detail provided by the narrative used in the results section. The act of balancing text with these visuals, however, can be quite challenging. On one hand, the text must tell a complete story (as many readers will not inspect the visuals).

On the other hand, the visuals must also tell a complete, stand-alone story that only extends and does not replicate the story told in words. This seemingly tall order can be simplified by using a few simple guidelines:

- Tables are a good place to report test statistics, confidence intervals, and P-values.
- Figures are an efficient way of displaying associations between two or three variables (for example, linear, quadratic, and cubic trends loan themselves to the use of figures).
- Tables and figures should have footnotes when these are needed to tell a complete story.
- Text should provide a "bird's eye view" of the findings—nothing should be left out, but readers can be referred to visuals for details.

Discussion: General. Up to this point the manuscript has been guided by a blueprint that delineates the content and format of the sections. By convention, this entails a description of the research and thought processes underlying the research questions. Authors should not offer opinions or state implications of the research findings as of yet. The discussion section signals the beginning of a new set of rules and far fewer constraints with less structure. The discussion allows the authors (for the first time) to have their own voice! This voice, however, should not extend beyond the reach of the study findings. Stated differently, the study findings support the authors as they offer suggestions (albeit tempered by limitations of the study) to improve health promotion practice or policy.

Because the discussion is not driven by a rigid convention, it is much more difficult to know how to proceed with the writing process. However, several guidelines may prove quite useful.

- The opening paragraph is traditionally a place to summarize the findings. In this paragraph, avoid the use of statistics and jargon; instead strive for language that is comprehensible to the lay public.
- After the opening paragraph, it is useful to examine the findings in light of previous studies that have been reported. At this juncture authors should feel free to speculate as to why their findings may have differed from findings in other studies.
- Although the discussion should highlight findings that supported the study hypotheses, it should also offer explanations as to why any one hypothesis was not supported.
- Place the findings into a practice context. First and foremost, health promotion research should serve practitioners. Write each paragraph in a way that will put the findings to work in the field. Given that your research questions were important, this task should be relatively easy.

- Offer the findings and describe their implications in humble language. There is no such thing as a definitive study. A study that is extremely high in rigor is still just one study—it has much more meaning if it corroborates and extends evidence from previous studies.
- To help find a balance between sufficient elaboration and too much elaboration, it is helpful to read several articles that appear in recent issues of the journal you have selected. Read the discussion sections in articles that have used a study design and analytic procedures similar to the study you have conducted.

Discussion: Limitations. This section is perhaps one of the most important and most difficult sections of the entire manuscript. Virtually every research study has limitations. Study limitations are recognized weaknesses in the research that detract from rigor. Figure 14.2 provides a display of common limitations that if present, need to be addressed.

◆ ◆ ◆

In a Nutshell

Virtually every research study has limitations. Study limitations are recognized weaknesses in the research that detract from rigor.

◆ ◆ ◆

FIGURE 14.2.   COMMON STUDY LIMITATIONS.

Participation bias

Attrition bias

Social desirability bias, recall bias, and other problems inherent with self-reported measures

Limitations of the sampling technique

Limitations of the study design

Misclassification

Bias introduced by the transformation of variables

In experimental studies, bias introduced from lack of blinding and from contamination

Contrary to the instinct of some authors, limitations should be exhaustively identified. Authors should keep in mind that journal reviewers will readily spot limitations as they begin reading the manuscript. A good thing to know is that reviewers seldom expect perfection and typically anticipate that authors will disclose the study limitations and their potential impact on the findings. In keeping with this expectation then, authors need to show that they are indeed aware of each and every limitation. Thus, an exhaustive list is simply smart writing.

Discussion: Conclusions. Conclusions are the pinnacle of the manuscript. To avoid diluting the message, the conclusions should be stated in a single—preferably short—paragraph. In fact, two or three sentences can be sufficient for a well-written conclusion. Because being succinct is highly valued, authors must know exactly what to say and what not to say. The conclusions should be directly relevant to the research questions and provide a straightforward answer to each of the questions. Moreover, conclusions should not be definitive, as the research process entails ruling out alternative possibilities and providing support for hypotheses; it does not entail *proving* hypotheses. Authors should also avoid restating the findings or summarizing the research process.

One way that may be helpful when constructing your conclusion is to imagine a news story based on your study. What would the headline say? What would the thirty-second report on a local television channel be like? Indeed, few people may read the published article in its entirety, but massive numbers of people may read your three-sentence conclusion. Thus, your conclusion should be strong and striking without being overly intellectual. For all practical purposes, it should be written for a lay audience and easy to understand. Finally, high-quality manuscripts are defined by the practical value of the conclusions. Indeed, health promotion research only has value when it informs health promotion practice and policy. Thus, be absolutely sure to place the findings squarely into the context of health promotion practice. Box 14.2 displays several sample conclusions.

References. A reference list is a mandatory section of any manuscript. The list may, however, be constructed using any number of different styles. The selection of any given style is made by the journal editor and the editorial board. Although this lack of a universal system can appear overwhelming to new authors, most styles of referencing can be divided into two categories. Even within these two categories, some journals deviate from these styles; authors' instructions should always be consulted before compiling the reference list.

Numbered endnotes, of which biomedical referencing is one example, are probably the most common system used in journals that publish health promotion research. This system uses numbers in the text to denote corresponding

Box 14.2. Examples of Effective Conclusions

Research Question: The purpose of this study was test the efficacy of a structural intervention designed to increase protein intake among children residing in rural areas of Tanzania.

Conclusion: Evidence from this randomized, controlled trial suggests that a structural intervention can increase protein intake among children residing in rural villages. Widespread implementation of the intervention may contribute to substantial declines in nutrition-associated morbidity among rural Tanzanian children.

Research Question: This study identified psychosocial correlates of binge drinking among college females.

Conclusions: Binge drinking was predicted by three distinct constructs: impulsivity, loneliness, and low levels of academic motivation. Campus-based intervention programs designed to reduce binge drinking may benefit female students by addressing potential issues related to impulsive drinking decisions and drinking as a way of coping with loneliness. Such intervention programs may be especially important for female college students who are not highly motivated to achieve academic success.

Research Question: The purpose of the study was to identify barriers that may preclude low-income adults from receiving a flu vaccine.

Conclusions: Low-income adults may not receive an annual flu vaccine because they perceive the time commitment and expense as being excessive. Furthermore, African American men and women may not receive the vaccine because they lack trust in the medical system. Health departments and other organizations that provide the flu vaccine to low-income adults may need to demonstrate that receiving the vaccine involves a minimum time commitment and, simultaneously, they should seek to inspire the trust of African American adults. Findings also suggest that policies directed toward reduced price flu vaccines may promote acceptance.

---

references in a numbered reference or endnotes list. In contrast, the other style used quite often is the author-date style, of which the American Psychological Association (APA) style (American Psychological Association, 2001) is one example. This style uses the authors' last names and the publication year to denote the citation, and the reference list is alphabetized. Samples of the two styles as they would appear in the body of a manuscript follow:

Sample 1: Adolescents' lack of self-esteem has been associated with diverse health-compromising behaviors such as alcohol and cigarette use, the early onset of sexual activity, eating disorders and general emotional distress.[1-4] Conversely, high levels of self-esteem have been identified as a protective factor against adolescents' engagement in these behaviors.[5–7]

Sample 2. Adolescents' lack of self-esteem has been associated with diverse health-compromising behaviors such as alcohol and cigarette use, the early onset of sexual activity, eating disorders, and general emotional distress (Fisher, Schneider, Pegler, & Napolitana, 1991; Gordon-Rouse, Ingersoll, & Orr, 1998; Harrison & Luxenberg, 1995; Resnick, Bearman, Blum, et al., 1997). Conversely, high levels of self-esteem have been identified as a protective factor against adolescents' engagement in these behaviors (Harter, 1990; Kawabata, Cross, Nishioka, & Shimai, 1999; Vingilis, Wade, & Adlaf, 1998).

The citation style shown in Sample 2 is described in the *Publication Manual of the American Psychological Association* (2001). APA style is used by a large number of journals that publish health promotion research. Each citation gives the reader enough information to locate the reference in the alphabetized reference list—numbers (other than dates) are not used. By convention, the text citation usually comes at the end of the sentence (before the period), and multiple citations within any single set of parentheses are arranged alphabetically. For detailed instructions and other rules regarding APA style, consult the publication manual.

Before writing a manuscript, it is wise to learn the referencing style that will be required for the selected journal. Again, the endnote and author-date styles are basic categories; each has a number of variants that may be used. As a rule, a reference should have enough information that any reader could easily retrieve it from an electronic database. Rules for truncating the number of authors shown, placement of the publication year, abbreviation of journal names, and constructing other parts of the entry vary. Examples of how the reference should be written for the reference list in both endnote and author-date style follow:

1. Kawabata T, Cross D, Nishioka N, Shimai S. Relationship between self-esteem and smoking behavior among Japanese early adolescents: Initial results from a three-year study. J Sch Health 1999;69,:280–4.

Kawabata, T., Cross, D., Nishioka, N., & Shimai, S. (1999). Relationship between self esteem and smoking behavior among Japanese early adolescents: Initial results from a three-year study. *Journal of School Health, 69,* 280–284.

Applied Example

To apply the key concepts, a brief manuscript will be shown here in its entirety. Each main section will be presented separately and each will be annotated for teaching purposes.

Abstract

Background: The purpose of this study was to identify correlates of self-esteem among a sample of African American female adolescents. ← (Note that the research question is stated immediately.)

Methods: A prospective study was conducted. As part of a larger HIV prevention study, a purposive sample ($N = 522$) of sexually active, African American female adolescents, ages fourteen to eighteen years, was recruited from low-income neighborhoods characterized by high rates of unemployment, substance abuse, violence, teen pregnancy, and STDs. Adolescents completed a self-administered questionnaire that contained the Rosenberg self-esteem scale ($\alpha = .79$) and other scale measures that assessed constructs hypothesized to be associated with self-esteem. ← (Key information includes sampling technique, the sample size (N), the inclusion criteria, assessment of the primary variable, and the study design.)

Results: The regression model explained 38 percent of the variance in adolescents' self-esteem scores. Significant correlates of higher self-esteem were having a more favorable body image ($\beta = .35$), greater perceived family support ($\beta = .19$), nontraditional sex role beliefs ($\beta = .16$), greater ethnic pride ($\beta = .15$), normative beliefs not favoring male decision making in a relationship ($\beta = .12$), and greater religiosity ($\beta = .09$). ← (In a short amount of space the research question is answered using common statistical procedures.)

Conclusion: Diverse psychosocial measures were associated with self-esteem among high-risk African American female adolescents. Programs designed to enhance the self-esteem of this population may benefit by promoting more favorable body images, greater perceptions of family support, greater ethnic pride, and beliefs supporting egalitarian decision making. ← (The conclusion is suggestive and practical, not definitive and strongly related to health promotion.)

Introduction

Self-esteem, an indicator of self-worth, has been defined as a critical index of mental health[1] and is an important construct often integrated in resiliency theories, where it has been conceptualized as a protective or buffering factor.[1,2] ←(For purposes of brevity we have not included the reference list corresponding to these endnotes.) Specifically, resiliency theories posit that adolescents in high-risk social environments may be protected from adopting health-compromising behaviors because of their high self-esteem, which is reflected in their desire and commitment to overcome negative circumstances. An important aspect of enhancing adolescents' self-esteem is tailoring program content to target those psychosocial influences associated with adolescents' high self-esteem. These influences are likely to vary depending on characteristics of the adolescents.[3–12] ← (These opening sentences are based on twelve references—thus, a chain of research is now available to the reader.)

According to the U.S. Department of Health and Human Services report titled *Healthy People 2010*, minority adolescents are a priority population for health promotion interventions.[13] An especially important population is sexually active African American adolescent girls residing in communities that predispose them to risk of infection with human immunodeficiency virus (HIV), other sexually transmitted diseases (STDs), pregnancy, delinquent behaviors, substance abuse, and a range of other risk behaviors and problems that negatively affect their quality of life.[13,14] ← (This portion justifies the selected priority population.) Research identifying the correlates of high self-esteem among this population could be a valuable source of information for developing and tailoring risk-reduction programs that include the enhancement of self-esteem as one objective. ← (Here, the practical value of the research is noted.)

The purpose of this study was to identify the psychosocial correlates of high self-esteem among a sample of sexually active African American female adolescents residing in a high-risk environment. ← (The research question is concisely stated.) Previous studies have suggested that social support,[15] particularly family support,[16] may be important to the self-esteem of adolescents. Based on a literature review, we also hypothesized that several other constructs would be positively correlated with self-esteem: favorable body image, religiosity, ethnic pride, and parental monitoring.[16–19] Additionally, we hypothesized that traditional sex role beliefs and having normative beliefs that favor male decision making in a relationship would be inversely correlated with self-esteem.[20] ← (Study hypotheses and their basis are provided.)

Methods

Study Sample. From December 1999 through April 2003 project recruiters screened 1,780 female teens in adolescent medicine clinics. Of those screened, 1,609 adolescents were eligible. Adolescents were eligible if they were female, African American, fourteen to eighteen years old, unmarried, and reported sexually activity in the previous six months. Of those adolescents not eligible to participate, the majority (98 percent) were not sexually active. Of those eligible, 1,457 (82 percent) were enrolled. ← (Enough information is provided to let the reader make judgments about the potential for participation bias.) The study protocol was approved by the University Institutional Review Board prior to implementation. ← (This sentence (expressed in some form) is mandatory.)

Data Collection. Data collection consisted of a self-administered questionnaire administered in a group setting with monitors providing assistance to adolescents with limited literacy and helping to ensure confidentiality of responses. ← (The readers are now aware how the data was acquired.) Adolescents were reimbursed $20.00 for their participation.

Measures.

Criterion Variable. The Rosenberg self-esteem scale[21] was included as part of the assessment instrument. This scale has well-established psychometric properties and has been used widely with diverse populations to assess adolescents' self-esteem. The scale contained ten items, scored using a four-point Likert format, with responses ranging from "strongly agree" to "strongly disagree." Higher scores represented greater levels of self-esteem. Inter-item reliability of the scale was satisfactory ($\alpha = .79$). ← (A great deal of attention is given to this variable because it is the outcome measure (Y).)

Correlates. Two single-item measures of parental monitoring were assessed. One measure asked adolescents how often their parents or parental figure(s) knew where they were when not at home or in school. The other measure asked how often their parents or parental figure(s) knew whom they were with when not at home or in school. Eight scales were used to assess various constructs hypothesized to correlate with adolescents' self-esteem. Table 1 displays psychometric information for the eight scales as well as a sample item for each. ← (Note, the use of a table to keep the text brief.)

Data Analysis.

Pearson product-moment correlations were calculated to assess strength and direction of the bivariate relationship between self-esteem and each of the hypothesized correlates. To assess the partial contribution of each of the hypothesized correlates working as a set in explaining the observed levels of self-esteem, multiple linear regression was used. Variables representing the correlates were entered into the regression model using a stepwise procedure with the alpha criteria set at .05 for entry and .10 for exit. The *F*-statistic was computed to test the overall significance of the final model. Acceptance of statistical significance was based on an alpha of .05. ← (Enough information is provided that someone else could replicate the analysis.)

Results

Characteristics of the Sample.

The average age of the adolescents was 16.0 years ($SD = 1.2$). The majority (81.2 percent) were full-time students; 9.4 percent were part-time students, and the remainder were not enrolled in school. Nearly one-fifth of the adolescents reported that their family received welfare.

The Rosenberg self-esteem scale was completed by 98.6 percent of the adolescents ($n = 515$). Scores ranged from 16 to 40 ($Md = 34.0$, $M = 33.4$, $SD = 4.8$).

Although the distribution of scores had a slight negative skew (skewness $= -.50$), the degree of skewness was not sufficient to necessitate transforming the scores so that they more closely approximate a normal distribution. ← (Note that a great deal of descriptive attention is given to outcome measure, including a consideration to transform the measure.)

Bivariate Findings. Table 1 displays the Pearson Product Moment Correlations between each of the correlates and self-esteem. ← (For brevity, the table is not shown in this example, but it should be noted that it serves dual purposes: (1) it describes the measures psychometrically and (2) it provides bivariate correlation coefficients.)

Each of the constructs was significantly correlated, in the hypothesized direction, with adolescents' self-esteem. In addition, positive correlations between the two single-item measures assessing parental monitoring and adolescents' self-esteem were observed. ← (Text describes the table.)

Adolescents' age was not significantly correlated with self-esteem ($r = .07$, $P = .11$). ← (This text provides results that are not shown in the table.)

Multivariate Findings. Table 2 displays the standardized partial regression coefficients and the proportion of unique variance accounted for by each correlate in the final model. Overall, the model explained 38 percent of the variance in adolescents' self-esteem ($F = 49.3$, $df = 6,479$, $P = .0001$). ← (These values are rarely provided in tables.) Body image was the most important correlate of self-esteem, followed by perceived family support. Ethnic pride was an important contributor to the overall model, and religiosity played a lesser but significant role in explaining the variance observed in adolescents' self-esteem. ← (Text summarizes the values shown in Table 2.)

Discussion

Findings suggest that African American female adolescents' self-esteem may be associated with at least six relevant psychosocial constructs. The strong association between self-esteem and body image is not surprising, since some researchers have suggested that physical appearance is the most important factor in determining global self-worth for adolescents.[22] These findings also suggest that even among older adolescents, family support may be an important factor in contributing to their emotional well-being. ← (Note that the text is speculative and no longer written in the past tense.)

Influencing these six constructs may in turn promote higher levels of self-esteem, thereby providing high-risk adolescents with a valuable protective factor against health-compromising behaviors. Behavioral intervention programs may benefit African American adolescent girls with low self-esteem by helping them improve their perceptions of body image and family support while affecting their ethnic pride. Additionally, programs may benefit this population by promoting more egalitarian beliefs about sex roles and decision making in the context of adolescents' relationships with male partners. ← (The practical implications for health promotion are explored.)

Limitations. These findings are limited by the validity of the measures ← (Limitation 1) and the inherent limitations of the cross-sectional design. ← (Limitation 2) In addition, the findings can only be generalized to sexually active African American female adolescents. ← (Limitation 3) Finally, the sample was limited to economically disadvantaged African American adolescents. Therefore, the findings may not be generalized to other racial or ethnic groups, or adolescents from different socioeconomic strata. ← (Limitation 4).

Conclusions. Diverse psychosocial constructs were found to be associated with self-esteem among a sample of high-risk African American female adolescents. Several of the assessed constructs may be particularly amenable to behavioral intervention. ← (Notice that the speculative language is couched as "may.") Programs designed to increase high-risk African American adolescent females' self-esteem may benefit from promoting more favorable body images, greater perceptions of family support, greater ethnic pride, and more egalitarian sex role beliefs. ← (Again, a practical value of the research is noted.)

Integration with the Research Process

A good manuscript reflects nothing more (and nothing less) than the completion of steps 1 through 8 in the research process. Leaving out any one step of this "historical description" greatly diminishes the value of the manuscript. Indeed, a manuscript should be viewed as a historical accounting of the events that led to the conclusion. The conclusion, of course, is the penultimate product of the research. Unfortunately, this product only has value when step 9 of the research process (dissemination) occurs. The preparation of a manuscript (as outlined in this chapter), then, can be viewed as the starting point for dissemination. Indeed, once the manuscript has been completed, the researcher can also disseminate the findings by making oral presentations at conferences. Such presentations may be extremely helpful in deciding what final changes to make to a manuscript before it is submitted for review and eventual publication. Figure 14.3 displays

FIGURE 14.3. HOW A MANUSCRIPT BECOMES A PUBLISHED JOURNAL ARTICLE.

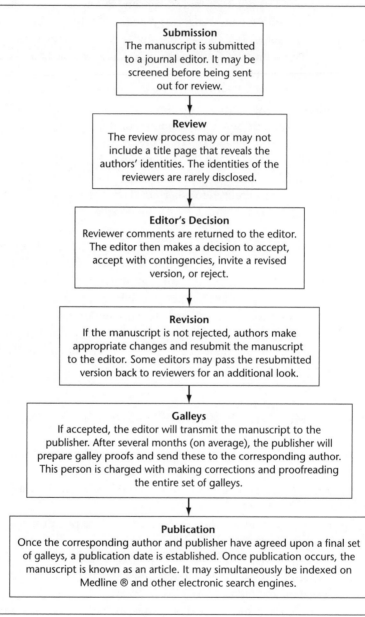

Submission
The manuscript is submitted to a journal editor. It may be screened before being sent out for review.

Review
The review process may or may not include a title page that reveals the authors' identities. The identities of the reviewers are rarely disclosed.

Editor's Decision
Reviewer comments are returned to the editor. The editor then makes a decision to accept, accept with contingencies, invite a revised version, or reject.

Revision
If the manuscript is not rejected, authors make appropriate changes and resubmit the manuscript to the editor. Some editors may pass the resubmitted version back to reviewers for an additional look.

Galleys
If accepted, the editor will transmit the manuscript to the publisher. After several months (on average), the publisher will prepare galley proofs and send these to the corresponding author. This person is charged with making corrections and proofreading the entire set of galleys.

Publication
Once the corresponding author and publisher have agreed upon a final set of galleys, a publication date is established. Once publication occurs, the manuscript is known as an article. It may simultaneously be indexed on Medline ® and other electronic search engines.

the process of taking the manuscript through the review process as it becomes a published article.

◆ ◆ ◆

In a Nutshell

Leaving out any one step of this "historical description" greatly diminishes the value of the manuscript.

◆ ◆ ◆

Summary

A manuscript is a historical accounting of the entire research process. Success in publishing is therefore a direct function of success in conducting rigorous research. The preparation of this document is not an art; indeed, the majority of journals that publish health promotion research findings will provide authors a very specific set of instructions for what should and what should not be included in the manuscript, how the manuscript should be constructed, the length of the manuscript, its citation and reference style, and a host of other considerations. Although authors should be skilled in the application of simple rules for writing (grammar, paragraphing, and so on), these skills will not "carry the day." Instead, the construction of a parsimonious and poignant manuscript—one that has an important conclusion—will ensure success. Most important is to remember that the process can be fun and exciting, especially when your manuscript is accepted for publication. Give yourself a pat on the back—you deserve it! (Go ahead.)

Issues to Consider

1. Integrity is to manuscript preparation as a roof is to a house. Without integrity, the entire process (from floor to ceiling) loses all meaning. Integrity means that the authors have purposefully avoided omitting from the manuscript any information that would otherwise help readers evaluate the strength and importance of the conclusion. It means that the authors have faithfully disclosed any conflicts of interest or any potential improprieties

in their work. It clearly implies that all statistical values are transposed verbatim from the computer output files and that "close" values are not rounded up to achieve significance. Given that science as a whole suffers when a breach of integrity is discovered, a worthwhile issue to consider is how members of a research team should ensure mutual integrity among themselves.

◆ ◆ ◆

In a Nutshell

Integrity means that the authors have purposefully avoided omitting from the manuscript any information that would otherwise help readers evaluate the strength and importance of the conclusion.

◆ ◆ ◆

2. *Publication bias* is a common problem in health promotion research. This implies that editors (and reviewers) have a preference for accepting manuscripts that confirm popular thought and may therefore shy away from (1) papers that have significant findings which support an unpopular position or (2) papers that have nonsignificant findings. Thus, an important question that peer reviewers must entertain is how to avoid, even at the subconscious level, this form of bias in science.

For Practice and Discussion

A single exercise is recommended. Working with a fellow student or colleague, select a published article that is of mutual interest and make a copy of the article for each of you. In separate locations, read and evaluate the article as though it had not been published and, instead, you have been asked to serve as a peer reviewer of the manuscript. Carefully evaluate each section of the manuscript, making detailed notations on every page. When you finish, fill out the following form and then exchange forms with your colleague. How much agreement existed between the two of you?

Please rank the quality of each section from 1 (poor) to 5 (outstanding)

| Abstract | 1 | 2 | 3 | 4 | 5 |

Main weakness: _____

| Introduction | 1 | 2 | 3 | 4 | 5 |

Main weakness: _____

| Methods | 1 | 2 | 3 | 4 | 5 |

Main weakness: _____

| Results | 1 | 2 | 3 | 4 | 5 |

Main weakness: _____

| Discussion | 1 | 2 | 3 | 4 | 5 |

Main weakness: _____

Is the title *appropriate?* Please explain. _____

_____

Is the conclusion *appropriate?* Please explain. _____

_____

Is the conclusion *important?* Please explain. _____

_____

Please write a short summary of the strong points.

Please write a short summary of the weak points.

Would you recommend this manuscript for publication?

If yes, what level of enthusiasm do you have?   1 = low, 10 = high

| | 1 | 2 | 3 | 4 | 5 | 6 | 7 | 8 | 9 | 10 |

Reference

American Psychological Association. (2001). *Publication manual of the American Psychological Association* (5th ed.). Washington, DC: American Psychological Association.

CHAPTER FIFTEEN

CRAFTING A SUCCESSFUL RESEARCH PROPOSAL

Ralph J. DiClemente, Laura F. Salazar, and Richard A. Crosby

Unlike the preceding chapters in this textbook that have each addressed an aspect of the research process, the overarching aim of this chapter is to provide guidance in how best to craft a research proposal. Rather than being an explicit part of the research process, obtaining funding to conduct research is an implicit demand that gives rise to the entire process. Because this chapter is therefore fundamentally different from the previous fourteen chapters, we have chosen to provide only an overview, the illustration of key concepts, and a summary.

First, we need to recognize that writing a research proposal is not magic. Anyone can learn the skills needed to be proficient at proposal writing. Second, proposal writing is not a one-trial learning opportunity. It is an incremental, iterative, and calibrated learning process. We need to acknowledge that proposal writing, like any other skill, whether it's surfing, gymnastics, or playing the piano, requires practice to become proficient. This is an important point that many young (and some established) investigators fail to acknowledge. Thus, to be a skilled proposal writer requires an investment of time and energy and a willingness to be receptive to constructive feedback.

While we talk of a "research proposal" as a generic product, it is useful to acknowledge that research proposals vary markedly depending on the source of funding. For example, a National Institutes of Health (NIH) proposal will have different requirements than, perhaps, a Centers for Disease Control and Prevention (CDC) or private foundation proposal. Even within an agency, NIH for example, there is an array of application types (R01, R03, R21, and so on) as well as varying research stages, purposes, and designs. For example, a research proposal that is testing the efficacy of a health promotion program (HPP) will differ in format, scope, and design from one that is proposing to conduct an observational study or a qualitative research study (that is, using focus groups, elicitation interviews, or other qualitative methods). Notwithstanding the variability inherent in these different formats, proposals do have a common core of elements. Rather than attempt to address each variation, we will provide a template of the critical elements necessary for a successful research proposal.

Illustration of Key Concepts

There is a core set of key concepts that are germane to most research proposals. These core concepts form the proverbial "backbone" of the proposal. In this section we discuss each of these concepts.

Statement of the Problem: The Specific Aims

The desire to write a research proposal is not driven by whim. Indeed, the interest in designing any study, whether it is qualitative, observational, or interventional, does not exist in a vacuum, but rather is mobilized when we identify a problem that needs to be addressed. The "problem" can range from how best to enhance vegetable consumption among adolescents, to enhance mammography-seeking behavior among women, or to promote safer sex behavior among gay men. In the discipline of health promotion, the range of problems is as limitless as our imagination. The only stipulation is that the problem should be timely and health related.

To be effective as a health promotion scientist and researcher or, for that matter, any occupation, requires an intrinsic interest in the subject matter. The first criterion in selecting a research topic is to select one that is of great interest to you. The second criterion is to select a topic that is salient to the field, something the field is wrestling with in terms of understanding how best to address the issue. The third criterion is to select a topic that has public health implications for society. This criterion suggests that the research be *applied* (in other words, research that has a practical, real-world application). Indeed, in the discipline of health promotion, our mission is *not* one of *basic* science (that is, research that may not have immediate or direct application to real-world issues).

A few ground rules may also help to weed out potential research topics. The first rule is don't select a research topic only because it is fashionable. Fashion in health promotion research, as in clothes, changes quickly. Choose something that you are passionate about studying, that needs additional research (which excludes almost nothing), and, if your study is done well, will have important implications for health promotion research and practice.

◆ ◆ ◆

In a Nutshell

Choose something that you are passionate about studying, that needs additional research (which excludes almost nothing), and, if your study is done well, will have important implications for health promotion research and practice.

◆ ◆ ◆

We will illustrate these concepts with an example from our own research. We have a strong interest and commitment to designing interventions to promote adolescents' adoption of condom use during sexual intercourse as a way to reduce their risk of becoming infected with STDs, including HIV. This interest allows us to identify potential research ideas and fuels our desire to test these ideas. Thus, criterion one (an idea driven by passion) for selecting a research topic is met. Currently, there are few HPPs that have demonstrated efficacy in enhancing adolescents' use of condoms during sexual intercourse. Thus, our second criterion (value to the discipline) is met. And, finally, there is an urgent need for the development of effective HPPs to promote safer sex behavior, as adolescents constitute a population at growing risk of HIV infection. Thus, our third criterion (value to society) has been met.

After meeting the prerequisite criteria for selecting a researchable topic, the next step is developing the research proposal. The research proposal itself has a number of sections. We'll use the Public Health Service (PHS) 398 forms as a template for heuristic purposes. As noted earlier, other proposal formats may be required, so pay careful attention to the requirements by reading the Request for Proposal (RFP), the Request for Application (RFA), or the Program Announcement (PA). Generally, the most liberal allotment for proposing a research plan is twenty-five single-spaced pages of text.

One formidable task that requires extreme attention is the preparation of an abstract (called the "Summary of the Proposed Research"). The goal of this space-limited paragraph is to provide a succinct yet comprehensive summary of the aims, significance, and proposed methodology. This will appear on a form page (see http://grants.nih.gov/grants/forms.htm for the PHS 398 forms; refer to form page 2) and does not count in the twenty-five-page limit. This paragraph will become your "first impression" to the Scientific Review Group (SRG), scientific peers who will evaluate the merits of your proposal. Thus, it is essential that the abstract be clear, articulate, and polished. This should be written only after the entire research plan has been developed, reviewed, modified, and finalized. If funded, this abstract will appear in the CRISP data file. (For a government-maintained listing of research projects, see www.http://crisp.cit.nih.gov/.)

Using the PHS 398 forms, the specific aims in a proposal are explicitly stated in Section A and labeled "Specific Aims." Typically, this section is approximately one page in length. An illustration of how to craft a specific aims section follows.

A.1 Specific Aims

1. To evaluate the efficacy of an HIV intervention relative to standard-of-care counseling in reducing HIV-associated sexual behaviors and incident STDs over a twelve-month follow-up period.
2. To evaluate the efficacy of an HIV intervention relative to standard-of-care counseling in enhancing theoretically important mediators of safer sex behavior over a twelve-month follow-up period.

The specific aims are the key research statements because they define clearly the research purpose and regulate the scope of the proposal. The aims must be parsimonious and unified. They should reflect succinctly the goals of the intended research ("less is more").

◆ ◆ ◆

In a Nutshell

The specific aims are the key research statements because they define clearly the research purpose and regulate the scope of the proposal.

◆ ◆ ◆

Corresponding hypotheses are also needed to fulfill the aims. The hypotheses must be in the form of testable statements. In this illustration, we composed the following hypotheses:

A.2 Primary Hypothesis

H1: A smaller proportion of adolescents in the HIV intervention condition compared to those receiving the standard-of-care counseling condition will engage in HIV-associated sexual behaviors and test positive for incident STDs over the twelve-month follow-up period.

H2: Adolescents in the HIV intervention condition, relative to those receiving the standard-of-care counseling condition, will demonstrate higher scores on psychosocial mediators of safer sex, including HIV prevention knowledge, self-efficacy to use condoms, communication with sex partners.

MINCUS AND DINCUS'S GRANT IS REVIEWED.

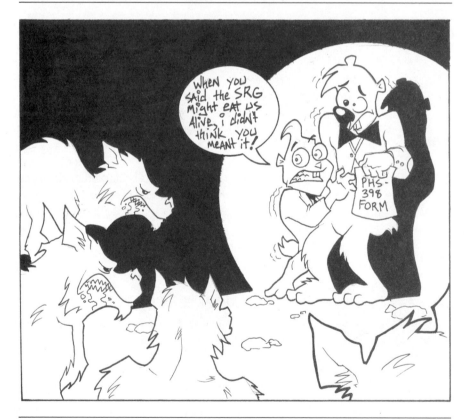

Copyright 2005 by Justin Wagner; reprinted with permission.

As shown, each specific aim has a corresponding research hypothesis, and each hypothesis is testable and directional. A hypothesis may be proposed as either a *null hypothesis* (that is, there are no differences between groups) or as a *motivator* or *alternative hypothesis*. Some people may also refer to the motivator or alternative hypothesis as a *research hypothesis*. Regardless of which one of these three terms is used, the meaning is identical (in other words, differences exist between groups). We are proposing a new intervention to enhance HIV-preventive behaviors and reduce adverse biological consequences of risky sexual behavior. Thus, in this instance, the motivator hypothesis is more meaningful than the null hypothesis because it reflects the investigators' desire to improve health conditions, practices, and programs. In proposing an intervention to enhance health behavior (or attitudes, beliefs, and so on), it is more relevant to offer a motivator hypothesis that states the direction of the HPP effects (for example, the HPP will yield positive effects). With the specific aims (Section A) clearly framed and written, the next step is Section B, "Background and Significance."

Background and Significance

The background and significance (B&S) section permits examination and framing of the existing empirical research relevant to the study. It is an opportunity to carefully consider data from diverse sources. A word of caution, however, is in order. Although the research literature may be replete with numerous studies, the B&S should be a targeted review. It is not a term paper, a master's thesis, or a dissertation. In fact, we suggest allocating only about three pages to this section. The goal of the B&S is to develop a rationale for the proposed study, for its conceptualization, and for its importance. Do not become mired in the review of the literature.

In constructing the B&S, it is important to understand the research literature—its strengths and weaknesses—so that an argument for the proposed study can be made. Indeed, if a satisfactory argument for the proposed study cannot be formulated, then the logical question arises: Why do the study? As you review the research literature, begin to make distinctions between studies. Some of these studies are well done and others are not. Some are observational and others are interventions. Not all studies are equally well designed, implemented, or analyzed. You, as a health promotion scientist, bring your unique skills to bear in analyzing the existing data. Thus, start to cull through the literature, identifying studies that may directly address your specific aims, some that may tangentially address your specific aims, and some that are unrelated to your aims but may have relevance to your intervention strategy or HPP techniques by virtue of having been used in other health promotion studies.

The B&S section for the illustration is constructed as follows, with subheadings reflecting specific sections of the B&S. Notice that topics progress from the broader to a more narrow focus.

B.1 Adolescents are at-risk for HIV infection.

B.2 Female adolescents are especially vulnerable to HIV/STD infection.

B.3 African American female adolescents are at significant risk of HIV infection.

B.4 Targeting adolescents at highest risk for HIV is a public health priority.

B.5 HIV interventions for adolescent females are needed.

B.6 Methodological limitations in assessing HIV intervention efficacy.

B.7 The importance of gender-tailored HIV interventions.

B.8 Psychosocial, gender, and relational correlates of HIV-preventive and risk behavior among adolescents and young adult women.

B.9 Peer approaches are a promising strategy for enhancing the efficacy of HIV interventions.

B.10 Significance of the proposed study for advancing the field of HIV prevention for adolescents.

This B&S section provides a brief review of the literature on adolescents and HIV, emphasizes the increased relative risk for females, and then African American adolescents. Indeed, subheadings B.1 to B.5 are crafted to make an inescapable point—this population is in urgent need of additional study to develop effective risk-reduction interventions. The B&S should firmly establish that the population is at risk, and thus there is a clear, cogent, and compelling need to address this health risk behavior among this population.

◆ ◆ ◆

In a Nutshell

The B&S should firmly establish that the population is at risk, and thus there is a clear, cogent, and compelling need to address this health risk behavior among this population.

◆ ◆ ◆

With the need to study the proposed population established, subheadings B.6 through B.9 are directly related to the proposed HPP and applicable methodological issues. These sections of the B&S provide a platform on which to build our HPP. First, however, we need to demonstrate that we are familiar with these different behavior change strategies, and that they have relevance to our proposed HPP. This is where many investigators falter. They can summarize the research literature with respect to identifying the problem (subheadings B.1 through B.5), but fail to provide an adequate discussion of the underlying theories, principles, strategies, and techniques that they will propose in their research methods. We cannot emphasize enough the importance of clearly demonstrating a thorough understanding of the underlying theories, principles, strategies, and techniques and how they are relevant to your proposed research. SRG members are often overburdened with having to read and critique many proposals in a relatively short amount of time. SRG members are not psychics or mind readers, and they may not be intimately familiar with all facets of your proposed research. When in doubt, write it out! In this instance, it is better to err on the side of redundancy than to make an error of omission by not including relevant information that is critical to building an argument to support funding your proposed study.

◆ ◆ ◆

In a Nutshell

SRG members are not psychics or mind readers, and they may not be intimately familiar with all facets of your proposed research. When in doubt, write it out!

◆ ◆ ◆

Finally, the B&S requires closure. Hopefully, you have carved a path through the morass of research literature. Now you are ready for a conclusion. How you conclude the B&S is critical. The conclusion may be what the members of the SRG remember most prominently about the B&S. We provide one more subheading that emphasizes the significance of the research to public health (B.10 Significance of the proposed study for advancing the field of HIV prevention for adolescents). Envision the information provided under each subheading as representing a piece to a puzzle. The SRG has read a number of pages, and its members are trying to put the pieces together and understand the "big picture." Thus, the last piece in the puzzle (that is, the significance to public health) is by far the most important.

What should be included in this last section? The objective is to enumerate and describe how the proposed study can significantly contribute to the field. Be brief, but be comprehensive. Also, here is an opportunity to express your passion and excitement. Research should not be a dispassionate enterprise. Quite the contrary, research is brimming with passion. Thus, you should include statements about how this study creates an exciting opportunity to interact with others from diverse scientific disciplines in a multidisciplinary approach; to develop new and innovative HP intervention strategies; and to apply HP strategies observed to be effective in other fields of health promotion research to your proposed study, population, and venue. Finally, add one statement that reiterates the clear, cogent, and compelling clinical and public health significance of your proposed study (for instance, "The proposed study of African American adolescent females will assess the efficacy of an intervention program designed to promote safer sex behaviors among a population at increasingly greater risk of STD and HIV infection").

◆ ◆ ◆

In a Nutshell

Research should not be a dispassionate enterprise. Quite the contrary, research is brimming with passion.

◆ ◆ ◆

Preliminary Studies

The next section of the PHS 398 is Section C: "Preliminary Studies" (PS). Typically, the PS section is approximately two to three pages in length and is designed to showcase previous relevant research or pilot studies conducted by the research team. This section should be tailored to the specific funding mechanism for which the proposal is written. For example, an R01 would require an extensive PS section and pilot data, whereas an R03 (a smaller developmental award) typically does not require pilot data. The team of investigators should be carefully chosen to provide a full complement of strengths to address the specific aims of the proposed research, and to develop, implement, and evaluate the research. This section is the opportunity to highlight the research team's expertise in research methods, survey design, development, implementation, and evaluation of primary prevention interventions, particularly with the proposed study population, and the use of newly developed tests or techniques. An appendix that contains relevant publications from the research team is also permitted. Describe some of the team's most relevant research; however, it is not necessary to enumerate every project or activity of the team. Although including every research experience by the team provides a cumulative index of the team's expansive array of skills and experiences, it often detracts from the focus of the skills needed to conduct the proposed study. Be judicious in selecting the research you plan to highlight. In the PS section, quality is much more important than quantity of information.

◆ ◆ ◆

In a Nutshell

This section is the opportunity to highlight the research team's expertise in research methods, survey design, development, implementation, and evaluation of primary prevention interventions, particularly with the proposed study population, and the use of newly developed tests or techniques.

◆ ◆ ◆

Most important, and this cannot be overstated, for large-scale research proposals, preliminary or *pilot research* (in other words, research that uses a small sample to inform the larger-scale research effort) is critical to convincing the SRG that the study proposed is feasible and has the potential to yield important findings that will advance the field of inquiry and benefit the population. The SRG does not expect a full-scale study; however, it does expect that you have initiated a pilot study to assess feasibility of recruiting the sample, evaluating the relevance and comprehension of the survey measures, implementing the HPP, and assessing participants' feedback about its developmental, cultural, or gender-relevance, as appropriate. Be sure to present the findings from the pilot study to justify the funding of the larger-scale proposed research. Assume that all the SRG members are from Missouri, "The Show Me State." So, show them the data! Data are critical to demonstrate that the proposed study has public health importance and significance.

Finally, the PS section requires closure. Up to this point in the section, you should have described the relevant skills, techniques, and expertise of the research team members that will enhance the probability for designing, implementing, and evaluating the proposed study. Now you need to close this section of the proposal. Again, how you "end" this section can influence strongly what the SRG remembers most about your team's skills and experience. We prefer to use a subheading titled "Significance of the Preliminary Studies for the Proposed Project." Narrative under this heading contains statements about how this study will create an "exciting opportunity" to harness the diverse array of skills and experiences of team members to conduct the proposed study.

Research Design and Methods (Overview, Site, and Eligibility)

The next section of the proposal is D: "Research Design and Methods." While all the elements of a research proposal are important, Section D is the most critical. This is where the proposed methodology and data analysis is described. This section should consume the vast majority of the twenty-five pages that are allowed when using the PHS 398 forms. There is no standard format for conceptualizing Section D. However, we provide a template that you can modify to suit your particular needs.

Step 1: Overview of the Research Design. The overview should contain the following elements: (1) the overarching aim; (2) the type of study (qualitative, cross-sectional, longitudinal, or intervention); (3) the primary outcome; (4) the sample selection; (5) the number of study participants; (6) a brief enumeration of the study's assessments procedures; (7) randomization procedures, if an intervention; (8) the theory underlying the study; (9) a brief description of the HPP, if an intervention; (10) the length of the follow-up period; and (11) data analysis.

Even with the elements articulated, it is not often intuitively comprehensible to decipher what exactly constitutes an overview. Thus, to be concrete we have provided an example of an overview.

Overview of the Research Design

The proposed study is an exciting opportunity to harness the experience and multi-disciplinary expertise of the research team to develop, implement, and evaluate the efficacy of a gender-sensitive and culturally relevant HIV intervention tailored toward high-risk African American female adolescents being treated for STDs, a vulnerable population in urgent need of intervention.

This study is a Phase III randomized, controlled trial designed to evaluate the efficacy of an HIV intervention relative to receiving the standard-of-care counseling that accompanies the treatment of STDs at the County Health Department. A random sample of 960 African American females, fifteen to nineteen years of age, will be recruited at the County Health Department STD Program following receipt of treatment and standard of care preventive counseling for STDs. At baseline, eligible adolescents will complete an audio-computer-assisted self-interview (A-CASI) and provide a urine specimen that will be analyzed using newly developed nucleic acid amplification assays to detect three prevalent STDs (chlamydia, gonorrhea, and trichomoniasis). The A-CASI interview, derived from Social Cognitive Theory and the Theory of Gender and Power, assesses sociodemographics, HIV-associated risk behaviors, cultural- and gender-relevant factors associated with risk and preventive practices, and other theoretically relevant mediators of HIV-risk and preventive behavior. After forty adolescents complete their baseline assessments, they will be recontacted and asked to return to the STD Program. When they return to the County Health Department they will be randomized to either the HIV intervention or the control condition. We expect approximately thirty-two adolescents to return for random assignment to study conditions. Adolescents randomized to the control condition will view a brief video about the importance of proper nutrition. Those randomized to the HIV intervention will participate in a group-format HIV intervention implemented over three consecutive Saturdays (four hours each day). The HIV intervention will be designed to be culturally sensitive and gender-relevant, and will be implemented by County Health Department health educators and facilitated by peer educators.

The intervention will emphasize the enhancement of (a) gender and ethnic pride; (b) HIV prevention knowledge; (c) self-efficacy for condom use skills, negotiation skills, and refusal skills; (d) norms supportive of abstaining from sex and using condoms if engaging in sexual behavior; and (e) building healthy relationships. All adolescents will be asked to return at six and twelve months postintervention to complete an A-CASI-administered psychosocial interview that is similar to the baseline interview and provide urine specimens for STD assay. An intent-to-treat analysis, controlling for baseline assessments, will determine the efficacy of the HIV intervention, relative to standard-of-care STD counseling only, in reducing HIV-associated sexual behaviors and incident STDs over a twelve-month follow-up period. Secondary analyses will evaluate the impact of the intervention condition, relative to the control condition, on hypothesized mediators of HIV-preventive behavior.

Although a succinct overview of the study provides a foundation on which to build Section D, it is usually useful to present a schematic representation of the proposed research design. A well-designed visual or figure is worth a thousand words, as it provides a snapshot of the entire project that the SRG can keep in mind as you begin to enumerate and describe, more fully, each element in the section. In Figure 15.1 we present an example of a figure outlining the research design.

◆ ◆ ◆

In a Nutshell

A well-designed visual or figure is worth a thousand words, as it provides a snapshot of the entire project that the SRG can keep in mind as you begin to enumerate and describe, more fully, each element in the section.

◆ ◆ ◆

Step 2: Description of the Study Site and Population. The next element in this section is often a description of the study site and population. This is an opportunity to demonstrate your familiarity with both the proposed study site and the

FIGURE 15.1. EXAMPLE OF A FIGURE OUTLINING THE RESEARCH DESIGN.

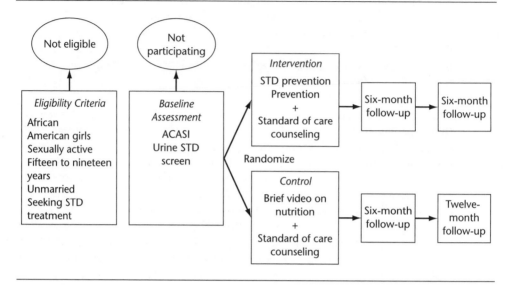

population in which you propose to conduct your study. Be succinct, but provide ample information about the site and population that is directly relevant to the proposed study. Here it is important to provide letters from site administrators that describe their support and enthusiasm for the proposed study, their willingness to commit site resources, and their willingness to provide access to the study population. Such letters are included as an appendix to the proposal. Box 15.1 provides a sample letter of support. Once the population and site(s) are adequately described, it is useful to articulate the eligibility criteria for participation in the study.

Step 3: Eligibility Criteria for Participation. In this section precisely articulate the criteria for participation in the proposed study. This typically includes the criteria such as age, race or ethnicity, gender, marital status, and presence or absence of a specific disease or risk behavior. The inclusion criteria should be tailored to correspond to the aims of the study. In addition to specifying the inclusion criteria, it is often useful to explicitly specify the exclusion criteria. An example follows:

To be eligible participants must be (a) African American females; (b) fifteen to nineteen years of age, inclusive at the time of enrollment into the project; (c) receiving STD treatment and counseling at the County Health Department STD Program; (d) unmarried; and (e) willing to provide written informed consent. Adolescents who refuse to provide written informed consent or have medical conditions that preclude participation in group-based educational programs (such as severe learning disorder) will be excluded.

Box 15.1. Sample Letter of Support

Baltimore

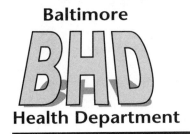

Health Department

475 South State Street, Baltimore MD 12745
555 444-8773

September 21, 2006

Gregory H. Hennington, Ph.D.
Maryland College of Public Health
1547 Baxter Road, NE
Room 542
Baltimore, MD 30322

RE: A Cancer Prevention Program for Young Women

Dear Dr. Hennington:

It was great to meet with you recently and learn about your proposal to test the feasibility of a three-session intervention designed for young women residing in Baltimore. Your idea to also test the efficacy of using support groups to promote behavior change is excellent. I fully support your proposal and will be glad to work with you to provide support for the project once you have secured funding. As you know, young women compose a large part of our clientele in our health department. Thus, we are naturally eager to assist in a research project designed to prevent them from developing both cervical and breast cancer. Clearly prevention efforts such as the one you have proposed are important to this population.

I understand that part of the project will involve hiring a health educator. I will gladly assist in the selection of this person. Good luck with your proposal for funding and please keep me posted about a possible start date for this project.

Sincerely,

Russell J. Hornby
Director
Baltimore Health Department

Research Design and Methods (Three Phases of the Research Plan)

At this juncture, let's review for a moment what we've accomplished in Section D. We have (1) provided a succinct overview of the proposed study, including a graphic representation of the proposed research design; (2) described the study site and population; and (3) specified the eligibility (inclusion and exclusion) criteria. Our next step is to begin describing the research plan.

There are countless ways in which you could present the research plan. We will show you one way to organize and present the research plan that we think provides a logical approach that the SRG can easily understand. We prefer to present the research plan in three sequential phases. Each phase represents a unique set of research activities and tasks that need to be completed to successfully develop, implement, and evaluate the proposed study. In this way we provide a logical and chronological sequence of research tasks and activities. The idea is for the research proposal to be an integrated whole, with each section of the proposal building on and informing subsequent sections. The more integrated the proposal, the easier it is to understand its flow and logic.

◆ ◆ ◆

In a Nutshell

The idea is for the research proposal to be an integrated whole, with each section of the proposal building on and informing subsequent sections. The more integrated the proposal, the easier it is to understand its flow and logic.

◆ ◆ ◆

We can categorize the research plan into three phases. Phase I describes program development, Phase II describes program implementation, and Phase III describes program evaluation. In the following sections, we review the elements commonly identified in each phase of the research plan. We describe a research plan designed to develop, implement, and evaluate an HPP. Of course, this plan is readily modifiable for observation studies (that is, for cross-sectional or longitudinal studies), as some of elements could be removed.

Phase I: Program Development

The primary Phase I activities include (1) hiring staff, (2) conducting focus groups, (3) describing the underlying theoretical framework guiding the study, (4) creating an advisory board, (5) developing the theoretically based HPP, (6) training the health educators to implement the HPP, (7) pilot testing the HPP, (8) specifying the data-collection procedures, (9) selecting measures for inclusion on the assessment instrument, (10) pilot testing the data-collection instrument, and (11) training staff to administer the data-collection instrument. In this section, we provide a brief description of each of the components included in Phase I.

Hiring Staff. In this section specify the names or position titles of staff to be hired. To facilitate the SRG's understanding of whether your staffing plan is appropriate to the research tasks and activities, it would be useful to list the project-year in which staff members are brought in (added to the project payroll). This demonstrates a degree of sophistication with respect to allocating staff time to complete project-related tasks. Unfortunately, this skill is not taught in many undergraduate or graduate courses. Experience and having conducted a feasibility study will be instrumental in guiding the assignment of staff time.

Conducting Formative Research. In many studies, *front loading* (building research activities in the beginning of the project) includes formative research to assist in tailoring the HPP. This is a sound research methodology. It's appropriate to specify the time period during which you propose to conduct formative research, for example, "During months 02 to 04 we will conduct a series of eight focus groups with adolescents recruited from the STD Program." Specify the purpose of the formative research, such as "Focus groups will be conducted to examine gender and culturally relevant causal factors potentially missing in our theoretical models that may influence African American female adolescents' sexual behavior." Next, it is useful to cite any prior experience by team members in conducting formative research; in this case, focus groups as well as those who will be designated to conduct the focus groups and analyze the resultant data. As a rule, if you propose a research activity, there should be someone specified in the research proposal that has the requisite skills and experience to conduct that activity.

◆ ◆ ◆

In a Nutshell

As a rule, if you propose a research activity, there should be someone specified in the research proposal that has the requisite skills and experience to conduct that activity.

◆ ◆ ◆

Describing the Underlying Theoretical Framework. As in the previous sections, specify the time frame when this activity or task is to be accomplished and describe the project staff dedicated to accomplishing the activity or task. Next, define the theoretical models that underlie the HPP. Briefly summarize model components and their relevance to the proposed HPP. A word of caution is called for. If more than one model or theory is specified and their conceptual components enumerated and articulated, it is important to state that you, after considerable thought, have decided that the multiple theories or models complement each other. Be sure that you fully describe how these models do so. (See DiClemente, Crosby, and Kegler, 2002, and Glanz, Lewis, and Rimer, 2003, for more information about complementary theories and models.) The obvious question from the SRG's perspective is, Why are multiple models or theories needed to guide the study? At this point, here is where it is appropriate to cite your prior research with these theories or models and their relevance and utility for explaining the phenomenon under study.

Creating a Community Advisory Board. Much of health promotion research is conducted within community settings. Thus, it is advantageous to propose a community advisory board (CAB) as part of the study. Specify the number and composition of the CAB members and how they will be identified, recruited, and compensated. Also, note the meeting schedule of the CAB and its scope of activities. One activity may be to review any project materials, such as the research survey, to ensure that they are culturally competent, comprehensive, and readable. Another activity is to ensure that the proposed HPP is culturally competent, addresses key concerns as identified by members of the target community, and is acceptable to community standards. Again, it is valuable to enclose letters of support from prospective CAB members. These letters can be attached to the proposal in an appendix.

Developing the HPP. Here is an opportunity to shine! You have read the empirical literature, you have conducted qualitative research and proposed additional research in this proposal, you have conducted a feasibility study, and you have pilot tested the HPP. Now it's time to demonstrate the culmination of this process. Begin this section by specifying the time frame in which the HPP will be developed (for example, during months 03 through 09) and the personnel who will develop the HPP. (For example, "Drs. DiClemente, Salazar, and Crosby will develop the STD prevention intervention in conjunction with the project health educators and peer educators with input from the CAB.")

Once you have described the "when" and "who," it is time to describe the HPP itself. A word of advice is to be sure to tightly integrate the HPP with the underlying models or theories. Models and theories are there to guide the development and implementation of the HPP; use them accordingly. It is critical to demonstrate a clear and obvious linkage between the underlying models or theories and your HPP activities. As an illustration, we refer to our aforementioned STD prevention study.

Social Cognitive Theory (SCT) will guide the design of the STD prevention intervention. According to SCT, behavior is the result of interactions among personal factors, environmental factors, and behavior. Personal factors include an individual's confidence in performing a certain behavior (self-efficacy), one's expectations about the outcomes associated with performing that specific behavior (outcome expectancies), and the individual's goals related to the behavior. Environmental factors include normative influences (peer norms) and the support that an individual may receive from others.

The aim of the proposed study is to enhance adolescents' confidence in their ability to self-regulate their sexual behavior. Thus, the STD prevention intervention will teach adolescents about safe and unsafe sexual practices as well as the outcomes associated with each. Given that the teens in the proposed study were treated for an STD, the intervention will teach youths about the link between having an STD and the increased risk of HIV infection. The STD prevention intervention will also teach teens skills such as (1) goal setting; (2) engaging in safer sexual behaviors (such as using condoms correctly and consistently, abstaining from sex, limiting their number of sexual partners); and (3) communicating effectively with one's sexual partner (that is, differentiating between passive, assertive, and aggressive communication styles and communicating the need to have one's partner tested for STDs). The STD prevention intervention will also be designed to create a normative atmosphere supportive of safer sex practices and self-protective communication styles. By supplying much-needed information and skills, we hope to enhance adolescents' self-efficacy to refuse risky sex and their ability to insist on condom use during sexual intercourse.

Again, the goal of this specific section is to make the connection between the underlying theory and the HPP activities transparent to the SRG. Intervention mapping, or enumerating each activity of the proposed HPP, and linking it to one of the model or theory constructs will be useful to assess how well you have used the model or theory in building your HPP.

Training the Health Educators to Administer the HPP. An important element often overlooked in research proposals by new and established investigators alike is specifying "*who*" will implement the HPP and "*how*" they will be trained. Now that you've carefully crafted your HPP, describe the personnel who will implement it. Describe their professional training (for example, M.P.H. in behavioral sciences or health education), their sociodemographic characteristics, if relevant to the effective implementation of the HPP (for example, African American health educators assisted by African American peer educators), and their background experiences (that is, prior experience in implementing an HPP with adolescents).

Once the personnel have been briefly described, it is useful to describe the training they will receive prior to implementing the HPP. This can be a brief paragraph that enumerates the training procedures used to train staff to proficiency. These could include any of the following: viewing videos, role-playing the HPP, role reversal in which the health educator may be asked to play the part of a study participant, group discussions, didactic instruction, and so on. It is useful to evaluate implementation personnel prior to their interacting with study participants. Also, have a plan available for corrective training and termination should an implementation staff member be unable or unwilling to conduct the HPP as designed. Noting that quality assurance procedures will be used to monitor implementation fidelity may be beneficial. Identifying the possibility of drift in interventions is important, as this requires remedial training of project staff.

Pilot Testing the HPP. Be sure to include language in your proposal that assures the SRG that the proposed HPP will be pilot tested. When the HPP is completed, the staff trained, and modification made to both the HPP and training protocols, a pilot test of the entire protocol is vital. In a pilot test, it is valuable to select participants from the target population who meet the eligibility criteria. The HPP will be assessed for feasibility and participant satisfaction; problems identified can be rectified, and the curriculum will be modified as necessary. Similarly, any difficulties encountered in implementing the HPP can be identified and rectified prior to actually starting the trial. A word of advice regarding this is to build in adequate time to conduct the pilot study and make modifications to the staff training protocol and HPP curriculum, and you should also specify the time frame in which the pilot study and modifications will be conducted.

Specifying the Data-Collection Procedures. This section is devoted to articulating the data-collection procedures used in the proposed study. If there are multiple procedures, it is critical to enumerate and adequately describe each procedure. For example, we used three data-collection procedures: (1) an A-CASI, (2) a urine specimen, and (3) a retrospective review of adolescents' clinic records. Describe the *first* data element with respect to time to completion. ("The A-CASI interview is approximately sixty minutes in length.") Describe where the data-collection procedure will be conducted. ("The A-CASI system will be implemented in a private room at the STD Program.") Finally, describe what type of data this procedure will yield. ("The A-CASI is designed to assess potential moderators, psychosocial beliefs, and sexual behaviors at baseline and six- and twelve-month followup.") Basically, describe each data-collection procedure in sufficient detail. Then proceed to describe the remaining data elements in a similar and systematic fashion.

Selecting Measures for Inclusion in the Assessment Instrument. A critical aspect of any study is selecting the measures (for example, scales, indexes, single-item measures) used to assess the constructs articulated in the proposal (see Chapter Nine). Furthermore, selection of constructs for assessment should be guided by a number of sources, including

- The underlying theoretical models guiding the proposed study
- A thorough review of the research literature examining potential moderators, mediators, and outcomes among the target population
- The research team's prior experience
- Input from the CAB
- Prior formative or qualitative research
- The results of the pilot study

Often, one or more of the just-enumerated factors is not available. However, the extent to which each source can contribute to the selection of constructs further strengthens the assessment component of the proposed study. Once the constructs are enumerated, select the measures to assess these constructs. Then, whenever feasible, these measures should have demonstrated reliability and validity with the target population (see Chapters Nine and Ten for a more detailed discussion of reliability and validity).

Pilot Testing the Data-Collection Instrument. As noted previously with respect to the HPP and the staff training, a pilot test can be very useful. Likewise, pilot testing the data-collection instrument(s) allows the research team to assess their utility; comprehension; and cultural, developmental, and gender relevance for the target population. This section should be brief. It should state that during a specified time period (for example, during months 08 through 10) the assessment instrument(s) will be pilot tested with a small sample selected from the target population. The pilot sample should be selected so that the individuals meet the purposed eligibility criteria. The data manager can calculate measures of internal consistency (that is, Cronbach's alpha) for all scales to determine their utility for this population. Items not well correlated with the entire scale can be deleted to improve the scale's psychometric properties. If entire scales are found to be unreliable, they should be replaced by a new measure that will undergo similar assessment procedures.

Training Staff to Administer the Data-Collection Instrument(s). Training is critical to avoid any ambiguity with respect to the study's protocol. Given the amount of time, energy, and emphasis placed on the results obtained from HPPs, training should be an integral component of any research plan. Depending on the data-collection instruments, it is useful to articulate the protocols that will be followed as well as the qualifications of the personnel involved in data collection (in other words, a trained research associate with experience in collecting similar data from the target population). Specify any training protocols that will ensure standard-ized data collection. This is increasingly important if there are multiple data collectors and the data will be collected using personal interviews, which are more susceptible to experimenter bias.

Phase II: Program Implementation

Phase II activities include

- Recruiting the study sample
- Screening and sampling procedures
- Administering the baseline assessment
- Randomizing participants to the study conditions
- Selecting and implementing the control condition
- Implementing the HPP
- Conducting quality assurance process evaluations
- Specifying follow-up procedures
- Defining strategies for enhancing retention

Recruiting the Study Sample. In this section you should propose (1) the projected sample size, (2) the time period during which it will be accrued, (3) the rate of accrual, and (4) from what population the sample will be recruited. For example, in our research the following statement was used: "We propose to enroll a sample of 960 youths over thirty months (32 adolescents per month) during months 13 through 42. Potential participants will be identified from the population of adolescents treated for STDs at the health department STD clinic."

Now that you've specified the sample, it is useful to project the participation rate. Estimating the participation rate is based on previous research, preferably by your team, or by a review of the relevant literature. For example, we noted that, "based on our previous research with African American female adolescents and young women, we projected approximately 80 percent of willing adolescents to actually return for assignment to study conditions."

A variety of recruitment strategies can be used to attract people to participate in HPP studies. Using recruitment procedures that have proven effective in other studies with the target population is invaluable. Again, experience with the target population will be useful in evaluating the type of strategies that are most effective.

To assist you we suggest that the following strategies be employed singly or in combination to enhance recruitment:

- Hire and train a recruitment-retention coordinator
- Provide a monetary allowance for completing the baseline assessment (the use of monetary incentives may significantly enhance participation in behavioral intervention trials) (DiClemente and Wingood, 1998)
- Describe the follow-up incentives to maintain interest
- Ensure confidentiality of the data and identifying information (for instance, all data will be maintained in a locked cabinet that is limited to access by key staff, only code numbers will be used on data forms and these will be kept separate from identifying information and code numbers)

Screening and Sampling Procedures. A brief section is often useful for describing the screening and sampling procedures. Again, *who* is conducting the screening? *Where* is it being conducted? *How* will it be conducted? This is important information for the SRG. Likewise, describe the sampling procedures. For example, in our research we used the following text to describe the sampling procedure: "The recruitment-retention coordinator will use a random numbers table to identify the sample of adolescents. This process will continue until the quota of forty adolescents has been recruited each month. The recruitment-retention coordinator will also collect sociodemographic information from adolescents who choose not to participate as well as their rationale for not participating in the study for later comparison with those adolescents who elect to participate." (See Chapter Five for more detail about this procedure.) If feasible, and not in violation of IRB regulations, collecting sociodemographic data from those potential participants who decline to be part of the study can provide a useful gauge of the representativeness of the final sample recruited. As in other aspects of the study, training the personnel responsible for screening and sampling is critical.

Administering the Baseline Assessment. In this section, describe the procedure for administering the baseline assessment. Again, it is vitally important to be specific in this description. The SRG is interested in knowing *who* will invite participants to complete the baseline assessment and *where* the assessment will be conducted.

Randomizing Participants to the Study Conditions. A central concern in any HPP that uses a randomized trial design (see Chapter Six) is the randomization protocol. In general, it is useful to specify *who* will determine the randomization sequence, *who* will conduct randomization, and *how* it will be implemented. Fortunately, there are a number of publications that address this important issue.

One procedure is to assign participants to the study conditions using concealment of allocation techniques (Schulz, 1995; Schulz and Grimes, 2002). These procedures have been designed to minimize bias in subject assignment to conditions in randomized trials. We have successfully used concealment of allocation procedures in our ongoing HPP interventions.

Selecting and Implementing the Control Condition. Selecting and implementing the control condition are also vital concerns when the HPP involves a between-groups design. Thus, it is useful to explain the rationale for selecting a particular control condition. A number of factors may need to be carefully weighed in selecting this control condition. First, the possibility of including a *placebo-attention condition* (structurally similar in terms of frequency, duration, and intensity, although the content should be irrelevant to the study outcomes) in the research design should be considered. This condition could reduce the likelihood that effects of the HPP could be attributed to nonspecific features (for example, group interaction and special attention should be considered). Second, consider if it is ethically feasible to include a "do nothing" control condition. For example, in testing an HPP to reduce HIV-associated risk behaviors among adolescents living in South Africa (a highly endemic area for HIV) can we ethically withhold any education related to HIV prevention? Thus, careful articulation of the rationale for selecting the control condition is imperative.

If a placebo-attention control condition is selected, implementation of the control condition, like the HPP, requires specification of *who, what, when,* and *where.* Describe the qualifications or relevant sociodemographic characteristics of the personnel responsible for implementing the control condition. Describe the control condition content. Describe when the control condition will be implemented. Finally, describe where the control condition will be implemented.

Implementing the HPP. There are two key elements that need careful clarification: (1) the personnel and logistics of implementing the HPP and (2) the content of the HPP.

First, it is important to specify *who, what, when, where,* and *how* of the HPP condition. For example, in our STD prevention intervention we noted that, "Participants randomized to the HIV intervention will receive three four-hour weekly group sessions, on consecutive Saturdays, implemented by two African American female health educators who will be assisted by two peer educators. The health educators will organize session materials, review session objectives at the beginning of every session, provide factual knowledge regarding HIV and associated risk behaviors, conduct didactic teachings, review homework, and provide reinforcement and social support. The peer educators will model social competency skills (assertive communication, refusal skills), coordinate group exercises, and provide reinforcement and social support. The health educators and peer educators will implement the HIV intervention following the guidelines in a structured implementation manual."

Describing the content of the HPP requires specifying each of the intervention elements. In a multisession HPP, specify the sessions in the sequence in which they are offered. While twenty-five pages may seem like a lot of space, you will find that being succinct is critical in preparing a coherent and comprehensive description of the HPP. A table that specifies the HPP activity and the mediator targeted by that activity can sometimes be useful as a summary mechanism.

Conducting Quality Assurance Process Evaluations. One threat to the internal validity of any HPP study is variability in delivering either the intervention or the control condition. Often health educators and program facilitators have their own style of presenting information and providing skill-based education. Even though a protocol has been developed to promote standardization of HPP delivery, there is the potential for health educators to drift (that is, to adopt a somewhat different mode of delivery). This is particularly likely when the HPP is implemented over a protracted time period. To minimize the threat of differential implementation of the intervention, it is useful to develop a detailed, structured manual that includes each session activity, the goal and objectives for the session, the person responsible for implementing the activity (the health educator or the peer educator), and the time allocated to each activity. Facilitators should be required to follow these standardized implementation procedures. At the end of the session, the facilitators will complete a session log indicating whether each activity was covered, whether the appropriate amount of time was dedicated to each activity, and any problems that may have arisen for each activity. In addition, the principal investigator or project director should schedule weekly meetings with facilitators who will review any problems and concerns arising within the sessions. All HPP sessions should, when feasible, be audiotaped (permission must first be obtained from participants) and used to evaluate the consistency of presentation and adherence to the standardized implementation protocol, to address problems within the sessions, and to suggest strategies for dealing with problems or concerns that may arise. Also useful are standardized evaluation forms that participants complete anonymously. Completed forms can be used to rate HPP fidelity. We have used these procedures in our prior research and have found them to be highly informative and helpful in monitoring implementation fidelity.

Specifying Follow-Up Procedures. The aim of this section is to clearly delineate the follow-up assessment procedures. The procedures should be well articulated, specifying *who* will conduct the follow-up assessments, *when*, and *where*. If participants are compensated for completing follow-up assessments, specify the type and amount of compensation, and when it is provided to the participant. Also of importance, specify who will contact participants, when, and if transportation will be provided to assist in accessing the data-collection venue.

Defining Strategies for Enhancing Retention. A major concern in any longitudinal study is the maintenance of the study cohort. While there are a number of tracking procedures that have proven effective, a pilot study or previous research with the target population is invaluable in determining the optimal set of tracking procedures to be used in the proposed study. (See Chapters Five and Six for a more thorough discussion of procedures used to follow a cohort.)

Phase III: Program Evaluation (Assessing Whether the HPP Was Effective)

Phase III activities include (1) conducting the last data-management and verification checks, (2) implementing the data analytic plan, (3) describing the power analysis, and (4) outlining the project timeline. Clearly conveying to the SRG that you have thoughtfully planned each of these activities is important. Also, be sure that the planned analyses exactly match the stated aims and hypotheses shown in Section A. In developing the data analytic plan it is essential to have extensive input and guidance from a biostatistician. In the following sections, we provide general guidance to writing this part of the research plan.

Conducting the Last Data-Management and Verification Checks. Data reduction, cleaning, and entry and verification of participants' responses for analysis will be performed under the direction of the data analyst, usually a statistician with expertise in the relevant statistical techniques for analyzing the data. Generally, the data-entry procedure is programmed to flag impossible values, thus providing an instant range check. Usually there are two basic data files to maintain the study operation: a sampling file, which contains information on all participants in the study, and a merged file, which contains all data. Every effort should be made to demonstrate that the study will not be plagued by missing data. If feasible, proposed use of the A-CASI system provides one additional level of quality control by reducing missing data through onscreen reminders.

Implementing the Data Analytic Plan. The primary analysis evaluates the effectiveness of the HPP: (1) in improving relevant mediators of health-promoting behavior (in other words, knowledge and relevant beliefs and attitudes), and (2) in reducing high-risk behavior. While the randomized design does not ensure that the same outcome profile (that is, distribution of behavioral risk indicators and mediators) is expected in the HPP and control group, it does avoid systematic bias as well as enhancing the likelihood of comparability between conditions on unmeasured factors. However, certain individual characteristics may be important predictors of outcome or may influence the effectiveness of the intervention. Simple analytical techniques can be used in preliminary analyses to describe the profile of participants at entry and follow-up. To evaluate the effect of the HPP together with the effect of covariates and to evaluate the interaction, a variety of statistical techniques are available, repeated measures linear (for continuous outcomes) and logistic models (for categorical outcomes) in particular.

While defining specific statistical approaches is not within the scope of this chapter, the reader should consult Chapters Twelve and Thirteen as well as a biostatistician. However, we do suggest that any intervention can benefit by conducting a general description of the study group and simple comparisons of intervention and control groups. First, propose simple descriptive statistics (mean, median, percent), scatterplots, and histograms that can be used to evaluate the distribution of participants according to study measures, such as

- Sociodemographic variables including age, education, and income
- Summary scores derived from psychosocial mediators (such as depression, self-efficacy, perceived social norms, and so on)
- Outcomes of interest

Summary statistics for all of the measures should also be proposed. Simple correlation analyses can be conducted to evaluate the association between pairs of variables. Nonparametric statistics (for example, Spearman's rank correlation coefficient, Wilcoxon's rank-sum test) are appropriate to evaluate the significance of the associations. At this juncture, the assistance of a biostatistician who will be integrally involved in the study, preferably from its inception, will be indispensable to writing a successful proposal.

Describing the Power Analysis. One other aspect integrally related to the determination of the study sample is the power analysis. (See Chapter Twelve for a more detailed description of the power analysis.) Usually, to determine a proposed study's required sample size, the investigator examines an analysis for the primary hypothesis. Using other studies or previous research by the investigative team, the principal investigator posits an estimated effect size. A thorough rationale for the estimated effect size should be provided. For example, in our STD prevention study, we estimated an incidence of 25 percent for one or more of the STDs assessed during the twelve-month follow-up in the control group. To estimate our effect size, we relied on the most recent intervention research that incorporated STDs as a measure of program efficacy. We estimated a conservative effect size of 30 percent difference for STD re-infection rates between the STD prevention condition and the control condition. We used a one-tail test, setting alpha at $P = .05$, with power of 0.80 to calculate the sample size necessary under these conditions. Always take into account attrition. Thus, if the sample size needed is eight hundred, for instance, and you assume 20 percent attrition, then be sure to recruit one thousand participants (this includes the projected 20 percent loss to follow-up), which will yield an effective sample size of eight hundred participants.

◆ ◆ ◆

In a Nutshell

Using other studies or previous research by the investigative team, the principal investigator posits an estimated effect size. A thorough rationale for the estimated effect size should be provided.

◆ ◆ ◆

Outlining the Project Timeline. The project timeline is a final and important component of any proposal. The timeline is your estimation of the start and termination of specific research activities. Again, in the absence of experience, it is difficult to construct an accurate timeline. However, pilot research and previous experience can be invaluable in developing a "realistic" timeline. Figure 15.2 provides a template using a Gnatt chart format that provides a visual overview of research activities over the five-year duration of the project.

Summary

This chapter has been devoted to providing a "blueprint" for crafting a research proposal. We have described a number of elements that are critical to a successful proposal as well as to a valid study. We are quick to remind you, however,

FIGURE 15.2. TEMPLATE FOR A FIVE-YEAR PROJECT TIMELINE.

Activities	Project Month

Activities	1	5	10	15	20	25	30	35	40	45	50	55	60
Awarded funds	X												
Hire and train staff		XXXX											
Conduct focus groups			XXXX										
Develop HIV intervention			XXXX										
Pilot HIV intervention			XXX										
Develop the interview			XXXXXX										
Pilot the interview			XXXX										
Transfer and pilot the ACASI			XXXX										
Recruit for baseline assessments				XXXXXXXXXXXXXXXXXXXXXXXXXX									
Begin four-month follow-up assessments					XXXXXXXXXXXXXXXXXXXXXXXXX								
Begin eight-month follow-up assessments						XXXXXXXXXXXXXXXXXXXXXXXX							
Begin twelve-month follow-up assessments							XXXXXXXXXXXXXXXXXXXXXXXX						
Data analysis and manuscript preparation												XXXXX	

that proposal writing is an incremental, iterative, and calibrated learning process. The suggestions presented in this chapter should be an asset to you once you begin this learning process. As you become engrossed in the process of proposal writing, we suggest that you consult a brief list of "tips" that we provide to you in Box 15.2.

We encourage readers to complement this chapter with more detailed texts. Foremost, we encourage readers to carefully consider the time, labor, and monetary needs necessary for designing, implementing, and evaluating an HPP. Given the importance of identifying effective HPPs, it is clearly worth the considerable expenditure of energy and resources to design the most rigorous study feasible. Keep in mind that writing effective grant proposals is an ongoing and iterative process. Ultimately, a prerequisite to success is dedicating ample time and effort.

Box 15.2. Tips for Successful Proposal Writing

H   Have all instructions for assembling the application been carefully followed?

O   On time (the deadline is not flexible!)

M   Make sure your budget corresponds to the personnel allocation for each project year

E   Exchange ideas with investigators of funded studies that may be similar to yours

R   Realize that a successful proposal is 99 percent perspiration and only 1 percent inspiration—there is no substitute for unwavering determination!

U   Understand the importance of carefully choosing the research team (this could be the beginning of a long and productive relationship)

N   Never, ever, give up!

Furthermore, it is often useful to involve other colleagues in the proposal process. Selecting colleagues with the requisite skills needed to develop, implement, and evaluate the proposed study is one of the most important decisions you will make. Finally, keep in mind that perseverance and fortitude will pay off in the long run.

References

DiClemente, R. J., and Wingood, G. M. (1998). Monetary incentives: A useful strategy for enhancing enrollment and promoting participation in HIV/STD risk-reduction interventions. *Sexually Transmitted Infections, 74,* 239–240.

DiClemente, R. J., Crosby, R. A., and Kegler, M. (2002). *Emerging theories in health promotion practice and research.* San Francisco: Jossey Bass.

Glanz, K., Lewis, F. M., and Rimer, B. K. (2003). *Health behavior and health education: Theory, research, and practice.* San Francisco: Jossey Bass.

Schulz, K. F. (1995). Subverting randomization in controlled trials. *Journal of the American Medical Association, 274,* 1456–1458.

Schulz, K. F., and Grimes, D. A. (2002). Blinding in randomized trials: Hiding who got what. *Lancet, 359,* 696–700.

NAME INDEX

SUBJECT INDEX

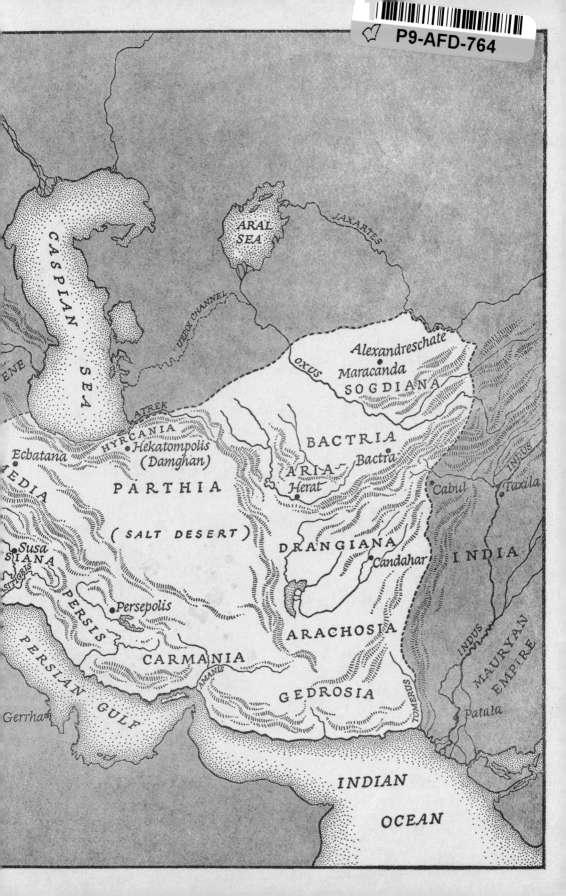

CASPIAN SEA

ARAL SEA

JAXARTES

ENE

ATREK

UZBOI CHANNEL

OXUS

Alexandreschate

Maracanda

SOGDIANA

BACTRIA

HYRCANIA

Hekatompolis
(Damghan)

ARIA

Bactra

Echatana

MEDIA

PARTHIA

Herat

INDUS

Cabul

Taxila

(SALT DESERT)

DRANGIANA

INDIA

Susa

SIANA

TIGRIS

Candahar

Persepolis

PERSIS

INDUS

ARACHOSIA

MAURYAN

EMPIRE

CARMANIA

AMANIS

GEDROSIA

PERSIAN GULF

Gerrha

TOMERUS

Patala

INDIAN

OCEAN

The World of Ancient Times

CARL ROEBUCK

NORTHWESTERN UNIVERSITY

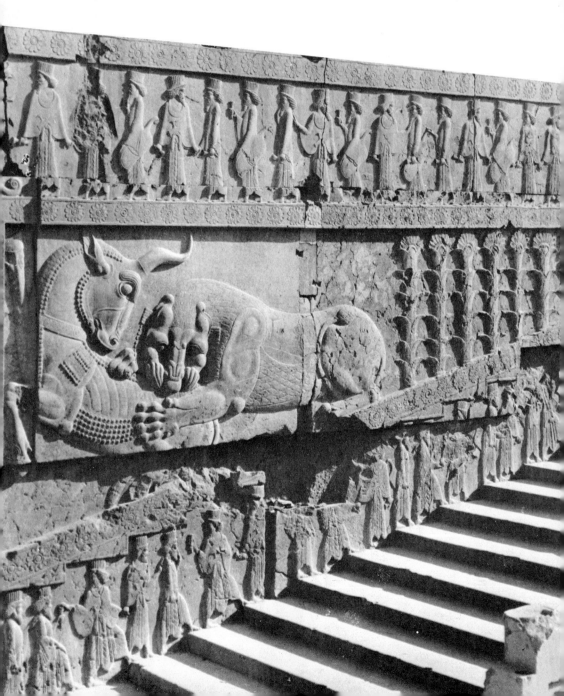

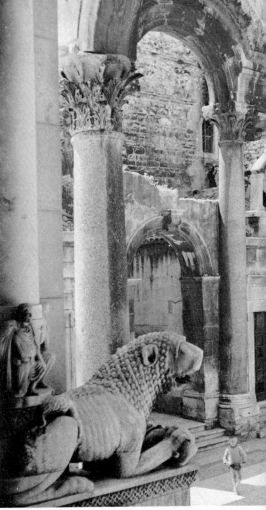

The World
of Ancient Times

CHARLES SCRIBNER'S SONS   NEW YORK

Maps by Sam'l Hanks Bryant

Title page, left: Sculptured balustrade of the monumental stairway to the Palace of Darius at Persepolis. THE ORIENTAL INSTITUTE, UNIVERSITY OF CHICAGO. *Right: Lion from the Palace of Diocletian at Split (Salonae) in Jugoslavia.* YUGOSLAV INFORMATION BUREAU.

TO My Wife

35660

Preface

THIS BOOK SURVEYS THE HISTORY OF THE NEAR EAST, OF GREECE, AND OF Rome from the New Stone Age to the fourth century after Christ. During this long period of time, almost four thousand years, many states and empires, from the cities of Sumer to the Empire of Rome, were formed, endured for a time, and then disappeared to be absorbed by their successors. The peoples and the individuals who established and tried to maintain them seem remote and sometimes their interests are hard to understand. But the events of their experience, the ideas, and the institutions which they developed not only shaped their own but subsequent history. What successive generations of men felt was useful and vital for their own lives was preserved and passed on to become, in a process of successive refinement, a part of our own civilization. The historical experience of these peoples of the Near East and of the Mediterranean forms the basis of the Western tradition.

It is on the historical experience of this "classical" ancient world that this book is focused. It has seemed important to me to understand both the individual character of these peoples and also the long process of their history. Accordingly, I have placed most emphasis on social and political institutions, tried to link cultural achievements with these in an organic fashion and to mold the whole into a balanced narrative. The approach is chronological and is designed to stress the process and continuity of history rather than to interpret its achievements broadly. The other important peoples of ancient times, of India, China, pre-Roman Europe, and the great migratory movements, whose history touched for a time that of the Near East and of the Roman Empire, have been noticed incidentally as they came within the horizon of the "classical" ancient world.

The pattern of any historical survey may seem to all but the author to be a Procustean bed, but I have tried to give a proper balance to the various parts. This purpose has resulted in more attention than usual to the ancient Near East, to the Hellenistic Period, and to the Roman Empire. Also, I have utilized so far as possible the considerable additions which archaeology has made to our knowledge of ancient history in the past several generations. Not only do major artistic monuments offer a key to understanding the minds of their makers, but the cumulative evidence of excavation has helped to amplify, and in some cases to establish, the growth and social character of communities. For example, we can see by studying the remains of Greek cities how their physical form reflected Greek social development. The Greek city of the fourth century B.C. was ready for export to the lands of the Near East following Alexander's conquest. Also, the expansive quality of civilizations in antiquity is revealed by the articles exported in trade and found in other lands as well as by political contacts. Indeed, Greece and Italy, in a very modern fashion and with somewhat the same consequences, exported their industry as well.

Acknowledgment should be made to the authors of those books which I have read. I hope that the interpretation of the past by modern scholarship is reasonably up to date, but the period covered is long and no field of ancient history is as yet embalmed. In any case, I trust that the authors will not find that violence has been done to their ideas and will accept a general statement of thanks at the outset of a book in which it is hardly possible to indicate specific indebtedness. Thanks, too, are due to the students whom I have taught. Students do exert considerable educative influence on the minds of their teachers, and the book reflects in some degree the emphases which their interest has given to my teaching. Specific thanks are owed to my colleague at Northwestern University, Mr. George Romani, who read several chapters at an early and important stage in their writing. I should also like to thank Professor William G. Sinnigen of Hunter College, Professor Donald Kagan of Cornell University, Professor Fred A. Cazel, Jr. of the University of Connecticut who read and criticized portions of the book. Professor Donald W. Bradeen of the University of Cincinnati read the entire work and made helpful comments and suggestions. And finally I should like to thank all those members of the Art Department and the College Department of Charles Scribner's Sons who worked with me in publishing *The World of Ancient Times*.

Evanston, Illinois; November 1, 1965.   CARL ROEBUCK

Acknowledgments

THE SOURCES FOR ILLUSTRATIVE MATERIAL ARE ACKNOWLEDGED SPECIFI-
cally elsewhere, but sources for quoted material are noted and acknowledged
here: from the Law Code of Hammurabi, J. B. Pritchard, *Ancient Near Eastern
Texts Relating to the Old Testament* (2d ed., Princeton, 1955); Egyptian literature,
Adolf Erman (tr. by A. M. Blackman), *The Literature of the Ancient Egyptians*
(London, 1927); from inscriptions of Cyrus and Darius, R. Ghirshman, *Iran*
(Harmondsworth, 1954); Aelius Aristides, J. H. Oliver, "The Ruling Power,"
Transactions of the American Philosophical Society, 43(1953); Andocides, N. G. L.
Hammond, *A History of Greece to 322 B.C.* (Oxford, 1959); Aristophanes' *Clouds,*
B. B. Rogers, The Loeb Classical Library (London and New York, 1927); Aris-
totle's *Constitution of Athens,* Kurt von Fritz and Ernest Kapp, *Aristotle's Con-
stitution of Athens and Related Texts* (New York, 1950); Augustus' *Res Gestae,*
W. C. McDermott and W. E. Caldwell, *Readings in the History of the Ancient
World* (New York, 1951); Euripides' *Hippolytus* and *Trojan Women,* A. S. Way,
The Loeb Classical Library (London and New York, 1912); Hadrian, Marguerite
Yourcenar, *Memoirs of Hadrian* (New York, 1963); Herodotus' *History,* A. D.
Godley, The Loeb Classical Library (London and Cambridge, Mass., 1961);
Homeric Hymn to Demeter, H. G. Evelyn-White, The Loeb Classical Library
(London and New York, 1943); Lycurgus' *Oration,* N. G. L. Hammond, *A
History of Greece to 322 B.C.* (Oxford, 1959); Marcus Aurelius, Meric Casaubon,
Everyman's Library (London and New York, 1925); Pseudo-Xenophon (The
Old Oligarch), H. Fritsch, *The Constitution of the Athenians* (Copenhagen, 1942);
Pliny the Elder's *Natural History,* H. Rackham, The Loeb Classical Library
(London and Cambridge, Mass., 1942); Pliny the Younger's *Letters,* W.
Melmuth rev. by W. M. L. Hutchinson, The Loeb Classical Library (London
and New York, 1915); Plutarch's *Lives,* The Dryden translation rev. by A. H.
Clough, Everyman's Library (London and New York, 1910); St. Augustine's
City of God, Marcus Dods D.D. (New York, 1948); Sallust, *Jugurtha,* J. C.
Rolfe, The Loeb Classical Library (London and New York, 1931); Tacitus,
A. J. Church and W. J. Brodribb (New York, 1942); Thucydides' *History,*
Benjamin Jowett (2nd. rev. ed., Clarendon Press, 1900); M. Rostovtzeff, *The
Social and Economic History of the Hellenistic World* (Clarendon Press, 1941).

Contents

Part II Greece

Part IV Rome

List of Illustrations

xvii

List of Maps

I

The Ancient Near East

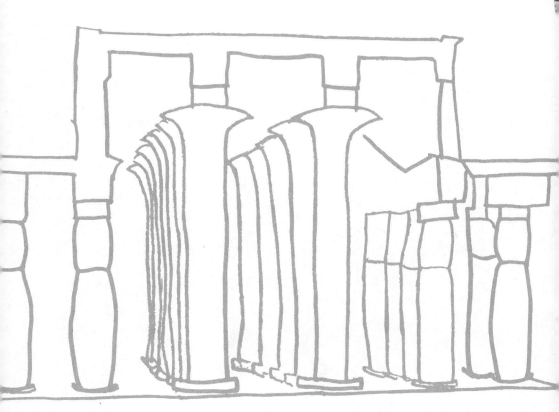

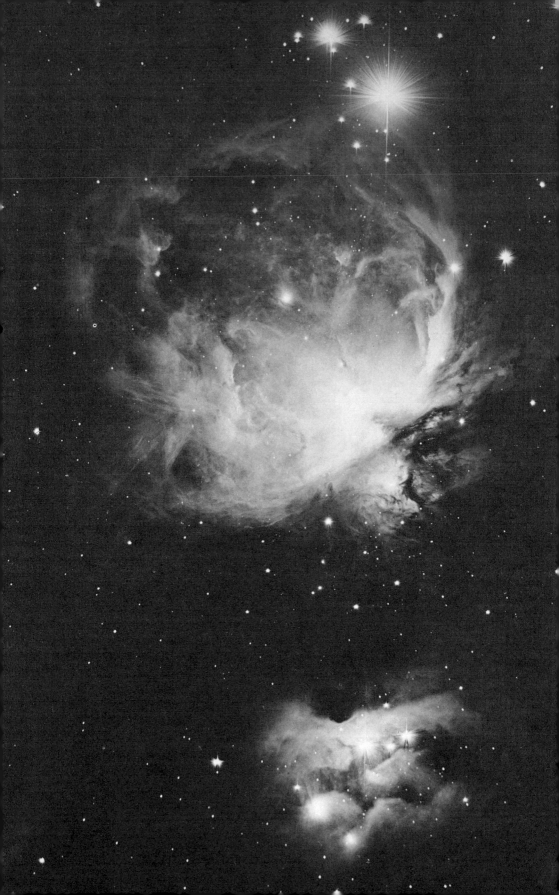

I

The Beginning

THE HISTORICAL WORLD discussed in this book is that of the ancient Near East, Greece, and Rome, where our western civilization had its origins. We can hardly speak of one ancient world from the outset, for about three thousand years elapsed from the rise of civilization in Mesopotamia and Egypt to the establishment of the Roman Empire shortly before the birth of Christ. Accordingly, we shall discuss first the countries of the Near East, where the discoveries fundamental for civilized life were made: agriculture, urbanization and writing. Then we shall pass to Greece, where the concept of a free society was born, and finally to Rome. The Roman Empire was a single world from the Atlantic Ocean to the Syrian Desert and from the North Sea to the Sahara. Rome, by applying the principles of universal law and common citizenship to the peoples of the Empire, created an organically unified society under one government. In the Roman Empire the separate strands of ancient culture were woven together and became a part of the fabric of our own civilization.

History and Prehistory

It is convenient, rather than accurate, to say that the history of western civilization began about 3000 B.C. in the river valleys of Mesopotamia and Egypt. The remark is true in the sense that writing was invented about that time, and so from then we can name some names and begin to enter more intimately into the concerns of ancient men. Yet writing was the invention of an already complex society with too much to pass along by the spoken word. Men had to keep records to carry on their business and to perpetuate the traditions of their community. Recorded history began with the use of writing, but the earliest historical societies, the city-states of Mesopotamia and the Kingdom of Egypt, had been formed in prehistory.

The span of prehistory immeasurably dwarfs the five thousand years of

The great nebula in Orion

recorded history from about 3000 B.C. to our own time, and it is impossible to fix a point in it and say, "Here is the start." A reasonable argument might be made for the era between 8000 and 6000 B.C. By that time the Recent geological era in the history of the earth had begun. Climate and environmental conditions have remained much the same to the present time. During that period, too, the most basic discovery of all for civilized life was made, the regular practice of agriculture. A continuous supply of food became available, and settled communities were formed from which the thread of growth runs unbroken to ourselves.

Yet man had survived for about three quarters of a million years before he began to sow and reap grain, to eat the seeds during the winter and keep some for the next seed time. In the course of this long period, the Age of Glaciation, our own species of man, *homo sapiens,* intelligent man, appeared. There is some recent evidence that he may have existed in Africa almost a million years ago, but he became widespread in Europe and the Near East only from about twenty thousand years B.C. In the era known as the Upper Palaeolithic, the latest phase of the Old Stone Age, *homo sapiens* replaced the other species of men. Perhaps we should start with the cultures of that time. The physical nature of man has not changed since then.

But this New Man, as he is sometimes called, shared many traits of his culture with the earlier and different species of man whom he replaced, the *hominids.* If we are to consider the problems of their physical development and cultural antecedents, we are taken still farther backwards in time. In short, our civilization is an accumulation of experience from the past. Much of it has been discarded in the course of time, and we take much for granted, so that it is hard to evaluate the significance of a discovery in its own time or the effect which an event or an idea has had on our own existence. Perhaps, living as we do in an era of rapid change, it is easier for our generation to understand that history is a process, in which men grasp for stability and happiness, and that stagnation is a quicksand. It is the historian's task to select what seems important for an understanding of the period which he discusses, for that is important, too, for the period in which he lives. In the prehistoric period we shall try to emphasize what seems most significant as a prelude to civilization.

First, it would be useful to explain the terms "civilization" and "culture," as used here and the names given to the major periods of cultural development. We have already implied that by "civilization" we mean a complex, urban society, whose records were kept in writing, and we have indicated that it began about 3000 B.C. As contrasted to prehistoric cultures, civilization has been made complex by what is sometimes called the "urban revolution," the change from farming village to urban community. An urban community had a considerable range of activities necessary for the maintenance of society, for a division of labor by specialized functions and a class structure. Men might be craftsmen, traders, priests or officials, as well as farmers. Some degree of literacy was necessary for civilization because its activity and its accumulated traditions were too complex to be transmitted orally. Through reading and writing, too, educated men could develop and continuously refine their conceptions. They were able to alter the form of their civilization.

By contrast to the civilization of history the cultures of prehistory were simple. There was probably a division of labor, but by age and sex, not by specialized function. Men hunted, tended flocks, and made war, while women gathered roots and berries, wove textiles and cooked. Prehistoric cultures are known, of course, primarily by their material remains: tools, weapons, ornaments and houses, if they had any. Much can be inferred from these artifacts about the customs and even the ideas of the people who used them. Yet the lack of writing placed a limitation both on the uncivilized, that is, primitive, society and on our understanding of it.

"Culture" may be used, too, in both a very broad and a more limited sense. The broad expression, primitive culture, refers to the whole range of material objects, institutions, and ideas of preliterate men. But within this great area we may speak of a particular culture, associated with a specific group of men who lived in a definite period of time or in a particular region. For example, we say that Mousterian culture, so named from the typical traits that appeared at the site of Le Moustier in France, was the achievement of Neanderthal man, a species of *hominid,* whose typical skeleton was found at Neanderthal in Germany. Mousterian culture is identified as the way of life for men over a wide area in Europe, North Africa, and the Near East during the fourth glaciation. Archaeologists recognize that the material remains from caves in these areas show the same traits as those from the typical site in France. Within Mousterian culture there were also regional and local variations, the result of local environment. Perhaps this rather loose usage would be clearer if we think of American culture. We might say that American culture (or civilization) is made up of elements of eighteenth-century culture (the constitution), of the twentieth century (television), and of the American south (creole cooking). The sum total of ideas, material objects, techniques, and institutions conveys the distinguishable individuality of a culture.

To work out the cultural links among different peoples and localities of prehistory is, of course, a highly technical and difficult study, and the results are often conjectural and controversial. Prehistoric men at first led a wandering existence. They were few in number and their remains are scattered, so that the record is incomplete and the gaps are many. The physical anthropologist will study the skeletal remains of men and of animals to distinguish the species and trace their evolution. The archaeologist and cultural anthropologist will study the material remains and identify their cultural characteristics and relationships by observation. He can draw inferences about the nature of the society which left the remains and about its place in the general culture of a region or period. To date the physical remains of early men and fix their cultures in time is

The reader will find Map I (page 18) useful as he reads this chapter.

equally technical. The geologist, who studies earth history, the specialist in ancient botany, who studies pollen, fossilized plants and trees, and the laboratory specialist who determines dates by measuring the rate of decay of organic materials, all play their part. The general historian can only use these results to emphasize the role of early men against the broad perspective of human history.

The conventional terms used to designate the major periods of human development were applied first by cultural anthropologists. The Palaeolithic (Old Stone) Age refers to the cultures of the Age of Glaciation, roughly from about 700,000 years ago, when man appeared as a tool-using mammal, to about ten thousand years ago, when the ice caps had reached their present line and the climate had warmed up after the fourth glaciation. Neolithic (New Stone) Age refers generally in the Near East to the period between 8000 and 3000 B.C. Formally there was a change in the technique of making stone tools in this period, but of much more significance was the discovery of agriculture and the growth of permanent communities. The latter part of the Neolithic Period, from about 4500 to 3000 B.C., was transitional to civilization and, because of the appearance of copper along with stone tools, is called Chalcolithic. The Bronze Age began soon after 3000 B.C. and ended about 1200 B.C., when the Iron Age started. These epochs were named, of course, from the chief material used in the manufacture of tools and weapons, stone, copper, bronze, and iron, but, as we have noticed in discussing the Neolithic Period, the name characterizes only one element of the culture of the period and one which is not necessarily of the greatest historical significance. The dates given above, of course, are only approximations, because in each period men continued to use the techniques and materials from the previous cultural age along with those of the new. The dates will also vary widely in different parts of the world. For example, the Bronze Age began in Italy only about 1500 B.C., and the Iron Age in America in the sixteenth century, when the white man came.

Food Gatherers of the Old Stone Age

The most important long-range factor which affected human development in the Old Stone Age was the wide fluctuation in climate and environment resulting from the successive advances and retreats of the ice caps in the Northern Hemisphere and of rainfall in the tropics. These changes created favorable or adverse conditions for human life by changing the climate and, with it, the flora and fauna on which men depended for existence. In the long run Old Stone Age men had not only to adapt themselves to their immediate environment, which might, of course, remain stable for thousands of years, but to periodic drastic changes. Groups might have been highly successful at hunting the animals of the grasslands, but die off or live miserably when the grassland changed to forest or dried up into arid desert. Presumably these long-range fluctuations were an important factor in the disappearance of some groups and species of early men who lived and then died out at different times and in various parts of the world.

Man was almost wholly dependent on nature for his livelihood, since he gathered his food from what was at hand and so was engaged in a daily struggle for survival. He hunted animals, and sometimes died by being hunted himself; he fished and collected the berries and fruits of wild trees, or grubbed out roots. The small groups of men tended to live a wandering life, sometimes moving their hunting grounds because, say, of a forest fire, sometimes, in the course of generations, shifting their habitat over thousands of miles in search of a new food supply as the result of climatic change. Under these conditions the groups were small and widely scattered. Like some animals, men lived in packs for protection and better hunting, and presumably the strongest and most experienced among them were recognized as leaders.

Yet man differed significantly from other animals in his use of tools and in his exercise of intelligence in multiplying their types and uses. Some anthropologists, in fact, would argue that man's intelligence was the result of using tools. The required dexterity and practice stimulated remembrance and imitation. Man's intelligence, however, reached farther. In the course of time he transferred fire to his own service, traded objects between regions and developed an imaginative life of the mind. Man thus created the cultures by which he tried to control and to exploit his environment for his own use. Culture, too, was progressive. For example, the simple, all-purpose implement of very early Palaeolithic times, the fist-axe, made by roughly chipping a stone to fit the hand, was replaced by the end of the Palaeolithic Age with a variety of tools for special purposes: blades, borers, scrapers, needles, fish-hooks, and arrowheads.

Old Stone Age man lived generally throughout the region with which we are concerned, southern Europe, North Africa and the Near East, although in some regions, such as Greece and Turkey, few remains have been found as yet. The earliest discoveries were made in France during the nineteenth century, and so French names from the places of discovery, the "type sites," have been applied to the cultures which they exemplify when traces of these are found elsewhere. There seems to have been a very considerable degree of similarity in culture throughout the area in Lower (Early) and Middle Palaeolithic times, from the third interglacial period to the end of the fourth ice age. After that, in Upper Palaeolithic times, beginning about twenty thousand years ago, there was much local variation. The cultures of southwestern France, with which the well-known cave paintings are associated, are the most interesting and significant.

In Lower Palaeolithic times men lived in the open, in small stations, as they are called, on the plains and the terraces of rivers. Their most important tool was the fist-axe, easily developed from a suitable stone picked up at random, and their chief preoccupations at this early stage were the daily search for food and defense against the dangerous animals of their environment. In the third interglacial era, however, the Acheulian culture used a variety of well-made flint tools, including spearheads and scrapers for cleaning hides.

In the Middle Period of the Old Stone Age culture became more complex in some respects, as illustrated by that of Neanderthal man, the Mousterian culture. This coincided with the advance of the ice in the fourth glaciation and lasted for almost eighty thousand years, until the coming of New Man and the warming up of the climate. Neanderthal man thus had to face the very adverse conditions of an ice age. He adjusted to them by moving into caves, by discovering the use of fire, with which he could roast his meat and warm himself, and by the development of new tools. Points and scrapers were common, the latter used to scrape the fat from animal skins. Presumably the group living in a cave formed a small band, consisting of several families, which from proximity must soon have become a close kinship group. The cave men showed some concern for their dead by burying them in the caves, perhaps with the idea of keeping the dead man a member of the group in order that his spirit might help to protect the living. The cave dwellers were omnivorous, their appetite even extending to their fellow men on occasion. Human bones, cracked to extract the marrow, have been found among the remains.

Mousterian culture extended beyond Europe to Egypt and to the Near East, where groups of burials have been found in caves on Mt. Carmel in Palestine, in Iraq, and Iran. When the ice retreated and the environment changed, however, Neanderthal man disappeared. Perhaps he was too specialized to adapt to new conditions; perhaps he was killed off or mingled with the New Men as they spread rapidly over his former habitat. We do not know where these New Men, our own species, had come from, but even at the time of their appearance they had subdivided into the "races" with which we are familiar in historical times.

The Upper Palaeolithic Period (*ca.* 20,000–10,000 B.C.) was short in contrast to the preceding ice age and lasted only for about ten thousand years. Yet the New Men who created its cultures made a rapid adjustment to the changing conditions of life and developed even more complex cultures. The climate was still severe in southern Europe, like that of the far north temperate zone of our own times, and the characteristic environment was that of grasslands, where such animals as deer, bison, and wild horses grazed. The best-known cultures are those of southwestern France and northern Spain, the Aurignacian and Magdalenian, established by Cro-Magnon man. The hunters pursued the animals of their habitat in organized parties and invented new weapons, the lasso and the bow and arrow, to bring them down.

There were numerous advances in technology. Men still lived in caves but also built pit houses dug into the ground. Bone, ivory and antler, as well as stone, were used for tools and were decorated with engraved ornament. Among the innovations were hafted tools and handles to give extra power, needles to sew garments of animal hide, fish hooks and harpoons. A little trade is attested by the discovery of flints on sites far from localities where flint was found, and sea shells brought inland from the coast. Evidently the desire of early man for luxuries was as strong as that for basic necessities.

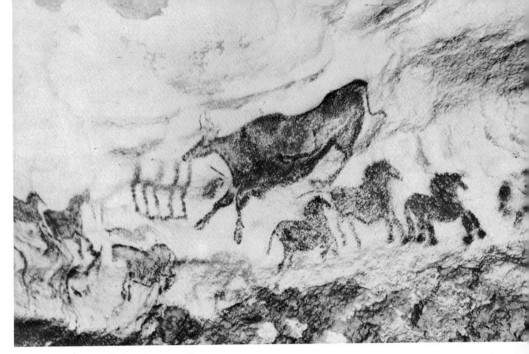

Old Stone Age cave painting. Lascaux, France

The most striking remains of these cultures, particularly of Magdalenian, are the paintings on the walls and roofs of the inner recesses of caves in the Dordogne region of southwestern France and near Altamira in northern Spain. They are artistically pleasing because of their lively, and sometimes powerful, realism and provide some clue to the imaginative life of their makers. The subjects are mainly hunting scenes and presumably had a magical significance. The mere drawing of a realistic picture of an animal being struck down was helpful, and it is likely that dances, perhaps a mimetic hunt, were performed before the pictures. Some of the paintings are chipped by blows, apparently representing hits. While most of the human figures depicted are hunters, there are a few who wear antlers on their heads and are probably to be identified as "medicine men" who made good magic for the hunt. Perhaps they received some special part of the animal killed in return for their services. In any case, some religious leaders have been distinguished. These organized hunts needed planning and direction as well as magic. Perhaps there were also recognized chieftains in the groups, men whose skill in hunting had won general recognition.

Religious life was concerned, too, with matters other than hunting. A few small statuettes have been found, carved to represent female figures with grossly exaggerated breasts and hips. Presumably these symbolized fertility in reproduction and were used in some rite to promote fruitfulness among the animals on which the group depended or within the group itself. Probably other powerful spiritual forces were associated with the natural phenomena which affected the hunters' lives, such as the weather and the heavenly bodies, but we can

9

hardly call them gods and goddesses as yet—just vaguely comprehended spirits. The importance of animals in the lives of the hunting groups probably resulted in some totemistic ideas. Men who felt some affinity of quality with a particular animal may have considered themselves its descendants; others may have eaten the flesh of specific animals to acquire their qualities. Probably this ascription of a spiritual life to the surrounding world of nature developed from an awareness by men of their own imaginative existence. In a dream or a fit of introspection, for example, a man's other self would wander freely. Thus nature, of which he felt himself to be a part, would be considered to have a similar spiritual life. Presumably, too, such conceptions explain the very considerable care taken for the dead. Weapons and tools were buried with them, and survival in an afterlife was provided for by the magic of smearing the body with red ochre to give it the appearance of life and vitality.

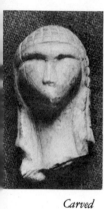

Carved ivory head. Les Landes, France

Yet the New Men who created these cultures in southwestern Europe were also too specialized to cope easily with the environmental change which came when the ice caps had receded fully. In Europe the grasslands changed to forest, and in northern Africa and Asia to desert and arid steppe land. The familiar food supply dwindled and posed the problem of survival once again. New Men did not die off like their predecessors, but a bifurcation of development took place. In the new forests of both the temperate and tropical zones, and along the edge of the arctic tundra, the traditions of food gathering and hunting were continued by cultures of the Mesolithic (Middle Stone) Age. These were of long duration and their creators became specialists in hunting the new type of game. Stone tools, called microliths from their very small size, were still used. But in the semi-arid regions of western Asia men took another direction. They began to produce their food by various attempts at agriculture and by the domestication of animals which they used for flesh and milk.

Probably there was a widespread shift in population towards the end of the Old Stone Age. In northern Africa, where there had been a phase of heavy rainfall rather than of glaciation, the Sahara Desert appeared gradually, making life difficult or impossible for both men and animals. Some of its people perhaps crossed to Europe by land bridges at Gibraltar and Sicily, while others moved east towards Libya and Egypt. A similar movement would have taken place towards the hills which rim the Arabian and Syrian deserts. From the arid steppes of inner Asia there was probably a westward movement to Europe, and southwards into the Middle East, to Iran, Armenia, and eastern Turkey. Presumably the men who made these migrations were the ancestors of those peoples who appear in historical times, but it is hazardous to make identifications. Mixing began at a very early period, and the historical peoples were formed more by environment and institutions than biology.

Food Producers of the New Stone Age

The region where men began to live by producing their food and where civilization rose is appropriately called the Fertile Crescent. The western end is the valley and delta of the Nile River in Egypt,[1] the eastern the lower courses and estuary of the Tigris and Euphrates rivers in Iraq. The crescent is made by the habitable lands of Palestine, Syria and northern Iraq, which form a great semicircle around the Syrian Desert. The first experiments in agriculture seem to have been made in the foothills and valleys of the mountains around the crescent: Lebanon and Anti-Lebanon in Palestine and Syria, Taurus and Anti-Taurus, which close off the arch of the crescent from southern Turkey, and the Zagros Mountains between Iraq and Iran. Perhaps, too, agriculture began almost as early on the central plateaus of Iran and Turkey and, by extension from the latter to Greece, in European Thrace.[2] In all these upland regions the environment was suitable. There was sufficient rainfall for plant growth, and they contained the types of grasses, wild species of wheat and barley, and of animals, sheep, goats, cattle and pigs, which could be domesticated.

The river valleys and estuaries of Egypt and lower Iraq had very rich alluvial soil, but they were not easy to cultivate. The land had to be cleared of vegetation, drained and watered by irrigation. Thus a considerable supply of labor was needed for their exploitation, and settlement does not seem to have begun until about 4000 B.C. The river valleys were to be the scene of the rise of civilization, but first the cycle of agriculture had to be established.

THE TRANSITION TO AGRICULTURE

Just how and where the transition from food gathering to food producing took place is obscure and, judging from the nature of early agriculture, probably will remain so. It is likely that at first wild grains were reaped regularly but that no sowing was done. An example of this practice is found in the culture of a group called Natufians who lived in the caves on Mt. Carmel in Palestine[3] between 8000 and 6000 B.C. The people were primarily food gatherers, who hunted and fished for most of their livelihood, but in their caves stone sickles and the seeds of wild grains were found. Apparently these Natufians had not domesticated animals because only the bones of wild species were discovered. The people themselves were New Men, whose habitation levels overlay those of the Old Stone Age men of Mousterian culture, who had lived in the caves during the last ice age.

The important step, of course, was to plant seeds, reap a harvest and re-plant from the stored grain, thus establishing a cycle of production. We can only conjecture how this might have been done. Perhaps the women of a group of food gatherers, who collected berries and fruit, protected young plants for future use and observed their process of growth. Whether the women tried to reproduce a plant by pushing a branch into the ground or covering up a seed with earth we cannot tell. In any case, such wandering groups seem to have

[1]See Map II, page 48.
[2]See Map VII, pages 172–173.
[3]See Map V, page 126.

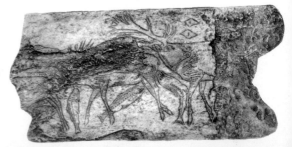

Reindeer carved on ivory

made temporary settlements of huts in the open and to have cultivated the ground nearby by scratching its surface with a branch or a crude hoe. Such cultivation was not very productive and could hardly be carried on in the same area over many seasons. Probably, then, the first agriculturalists moved about frequently and still obtained most of their food by hunting and gathering. They do seem, however, to have domesticated sheep and to have invented the mortar and pestle for preparing their grain.

Between 7000 and 6000 B.C. a cycle of agriculture carried on by stable communities seems to have been established. Used thus, *stable* is a very relative term, for the settlements were very small and their remains, apart from the stone tools, flimsy. Perhaps a brief discussion of two typical sites will illustrate the problems involved. They are Jarmo, located in northeastern Iraq near modern Kirkuk, and Jericho in the Dead Sea valley of Palestine. Jarmo was a village of about 150 people living in a group of some twenty huts. It was an open community, unfortified, and the huts were built of sun-dried brick. The huts did, however, contain several rooms and were rectangular in shape. The inhabitants grew wheat and barley and, perhaps, peas and had domesticated goats, sheep, and pigs. The evidence indicates that the regular practice of agriculture and the domestication of animals went hand in hand. Perhaps the latter was accomplished in the first instance by raising the young of wild animals until they reproduced in captivity and became partially dependent on man. For about two thirds of its existence, Jarmo was what is called a "pre-ceramic" site. That is, pottery was not in use. By the latter part of the village's existence, however, knowledge of it had come to Jarmo. Again we can only conjecture about the invention. Man's first containers were baskets made of pliable boughs and lined with clay to seal the gaps. One may have been left near a fire which baked the clay lining, and thus the owner was presented with a new type of vessel. The "invention" became established rapidly, and pottery-making was a regular practice of the cultures of the New Stone Age after 6000 B.C.

The first village settlement at Jericho may have lived by food production, and it is dated by some archaeologists earlier than that at Jarmo. Since Jericho is in an oasis, this presumed earlier date has been used to support another theory of the development of agriculture. It may be called the "oasis theory." The hypothesis is that, because of the transformation of the grasslands to desert, the river valleys and oases became havens of refuge and the start of the new life. Since many animals had perished or wandered off to find a more satisfactory habitat, man depended more on a diet of plants and learned to cultivate those species most suitable for food. Those animals which took refuge in the oases and lived close to men were domesticated. Aside from the very technical question of assigning priority to Jarmo or to Jericho, there are other more general objections to the oasis theory. Other very early pre-ceramic settlements, which practiced agriculture and had domesticated animals, have been found in northeastern Iraq and elsewhere in the upland region. This general area seems to have been a center from which knowledge of the new practices was rapidly diffused.

The problems are difficult and technical, however, and enlarged almost annually by new discoveries.

By about 6000 B.C. agriculture and village communities were establishing a new pattern of life over a wide area in the Near East. Presumably the highlands could not support the growing population brought into existence by the increased food supply, and so men had moved down into the plains when they spread along the natural routes of communication. Recent archaeological work has added much to our knowledge of the regional cultures which were established and to their interrelationships. There were two areas of intensive development. One, which has been long known, was in northern Mesopotamia and across the Fertile Crescent through northern Syria to the Mediterranean. An example of the early culture of this region is offered by the site of Hassuna, near modern Mosul, and the developed stage by Halaf (Halafian culture). The other region, currently being explored, was in southwestern Turkey, in the Konya plain,[1] where there was very intensive settlement in the New Stone Age. At present the culture of this region is known mainly by the excavation of sites at Haçilar and Çatal Hüyük. At the latter have beeen found the earliest paintings on man-made walls. They date from about 6000 B.C.

Farther from these regions the development of village communities was delayed. Perhaps those in Greece were almost as early as in Turkey, judging from the evidence of incipient agriculture in Thrace and recent study of communities in Thessaly and Central Greece. In Egypt, however, the new techniques of food production do not seem to have been established until about 4500 B.C. Perhaps the knowledge of farming was introduced by migrants from the coast of Syria or Palestine, but Egyptian prehistoric culture was African, rather than Asiatic, in character. It remained remarkably homogeneous and isolated until the rise of civilization (pp. 51–54). In the valley of the Indus River in northwestern India, the third of the great river valley civilizations, village communities do not appear before 3000 B.C. and civilization not before 2500 B.C. (pp. 40–41). While each region had its individual techniques of making pottery and tools, they all shared the agricultural manner of life which characterized the New Stone Age. We will leave the difficult problems of interconnection, of priority, and description of the regional cultures to the experts and simply summarize the general character of Neolithic culture.

NEOLITHIC CULTURE

In the New Stone Age there was a marked development in the technique of making stone implements and in their size and variety. It is from these, of course, that the age takes its name. The old practice of chipping and flaking stone was still used, but grinding and polishing were introduced. Large tools, a true axe, stone bowls, mortars and pestles were skillfully made. In addition, in some regions a considerable use was made of wood, which was preferred even to pottery after the latter had come into use.

[1]See Map III, page 74.

The regular practice of agriculture which, as one prehistorian has remarked, made men partners of nature instead of parasites on it, resulted in extensive changes in society. Men settled down in stable, permanent communities to raise their food on the adjacent land. They still hunted, fished, and gathered berries and nuts, but a precious margin of security had been obtained. The grain could be stored over the nonproductive season, while the flocks of animals provided a steady supply of milk and meat. Apparently the weaving of textiles was invented early in the period, perhaps by the transfer of the methods of basketry to the long fleece of sheep. Men began to clothe themselves in garments of cloth rather than the skins of animals. Diet, of course, was improved both by cereals and meat and by the practice of boiling food in pottery containers.

The village communities were small, with a population of about five hundred to a thousand people, but families lived in separate houses of a permanent type. They were built of mud bricks, dried in the sun, usually laid on a foundation of field stones, and consisted of several rooms. Domestic architecture thus had its origin in this period. Perhaps we can also say that religious architecture had a start, because one structure at Çatal Hüyük appears to have been a shrine. For the most part the villages remained open and unfortified, but in the latter part of the period defense walls were built.

Community life, of course, resulted in the growth of new social institutions. Land itself became valuable, thus giving rise to ideas about property. We can only conjecture about the system of ownership, and there is controversy as to whether the land was regarded as communal property and its yield divided among the villagers, or whether separate lots were worked as the property of a family. Perhaps grazing land was used in common, while the more valuable cultivated land was held partly in common, partly in family hands. Feeling for the welfare of the group would have been strong, and it is improbable that any one individual would have owned more than personal items. Certainly there are no indications of great wealth in the possession of any one individual or household, and probably a rough equality prevailed.

The community needed leadership for defense in war and for settlement of disputes among its members. There was need, too, to be on good terms with the spirits who controlled the weather and the new activities of agriculture and those who were thought to live in the locality of the village. The village headsman, then, was probably a combination of king, to lead in war, judge, to settle disputes, and priest, to mediate with the gods. Perhaps, however, religious activity was so important and complicated that a special class of priests, who knew how to address the spirits and how to use the proper rituals in worship, began to crystallize. The elders of the village would have been revered and their opinions given weight simply because they had contrived to live to the ripe age of twenty-five or thirty. Life expectancy was very short. Thus, law, in the sense of traditional custom, and government, however rudimentary, had its beginning.

While virtually every member of the village was a farmer, it is probable that there was a division of labor by age and sex. Women would perform the household work and much agricultural labor, while men looked after the animals, hunted and fought for the community. Since the households were self-sufficient, the share of labor performed by the women was great; they were responsible for cooking, weaving, and making the family's pottery. The village itself was virtually self-sufficient, and few articles were imported from other localities. In the latter part of the period, when copper came into use, that metal would have been brought by wandering traders, and at all times flint and obsidian were traded. Obsidian, for example, was brought to Jarmo from some producing area. Yet the quantities involved were very small, and in the farming village only the germ of a division of labor by special function existed.

Not all men, however, settled down to farm. The establishment of new communities was probably made by wandering groups who found a favorable location, but a new type of nomadic life, based on the domestication of animals, developed. It was to remain characteristic of the Near and Middle East and North Africa to the present day. The pasturage over much of this area is seasonal, appearing in the lower hills and at the edge of the desert in the wet season but lasting in the high hills and mountain valleys throughout the summer. The environment was conducive to a seminomadic life, in which men moved their flocks seasonally to find new pasture. Frequently, of course, the nomads raided the settled villages and sometimes were tempted to settle down and change their mode of life. Then tension thus established between semi-nomad and agriculturist was to become one of the formative factors in Near Eastern history.

The characteristic form of social organization in historical times throughout the Near East, both for nomad and agriculturist, was the patriarchal family, in which the father was the head of the household and exercised unquestioned authority over its members and property. It is easy to understand why this should be so in the nomadic groups, because care of the animals, man's work, was all important, but in the farming villages women did the essential work of agriculture. Perhaps, as frequently suggested, agricultural groups were originally matriarchal but changed in the latter part of the Neolithic Age when new activities were introduced. Metallurgy was practiced, the plough, pulled by animals, replaced the earlier hoe culture, and, as population grew and land became more precious, war became an important method of adding to the community's wealth. All these new activities were the work of men.

Religious concepts and practices changed in accordance with the establishment of new traditions and institutions. As in the past the new activities were associated with ritual and magic to ensure their success, while new spirits were conceived to preside over them. When man lived in a fixed locality, certain features of the landscape, like a spring vital to the life of the group or a spot with some traditional association in its history, were considered to be the residence of a spirit. The times of sowing and reaping and of the growing crop were thought to need divine protection. The forces of nature were of as much importance to the agricultural villages as to the nomads and hunters. In short, the practice of animism, the endowment of nature with a spiritual life, was extended. Probably, too, the more important spirits became personal and were made into gods. The number of spirits was almost inexhaustible, and so, when man made gods in his own pattern, he made many of them. Religion was polytheistic.

The most widespread conception seems to have been that of a mother-goddess, a divine force to provide fertility. She was represented by statuettes essentially similar to those of the Upper Paleolithic Period as a big-breasted, wide-hipped woman. Whether she had a name as yet in the different regions where she was worshipped we do not know, but the conception is obviously akin to those of many later goddesses, like Ishtar of Babylonia and Aphrodite of Greece. The new religious festivals celebrated by the whole community and geared to the cycle of agriculture similarly became and remained a part of ancient life, for agriculture was to continue as the basic activity of men.

In the earlier Neolithic Age, however, the older activity of hunting was still important, as the murals from Çatal Hüyük reveal. They were painted in earth colors on the mud walls of houses and of one structure which has been identified as a shrine. If so, its construction would mark an important step in religious development—a place of worship for the chief deity of the whole community. The scenes represent animals and men, lively vigorous figures, in the hunt and in a ritual, hunting dance. One, of a more macabre nature, depicts a flock of vultures attacking men. In this region of southwestern Turkey the bull had religious significance, perhaps as an embodiment of strength and vitality. Bulls were represented in the paintings and, in a new artistic technique, their skulls were modelled in relief as part of the wall decoration.

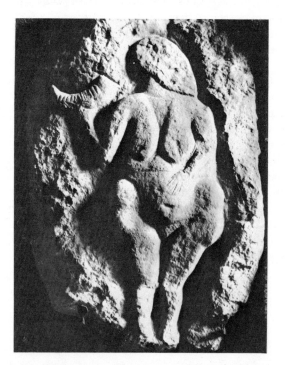

Figurine of the mother-goddess used in fertility rites. Çatal Hüyük, Turkey

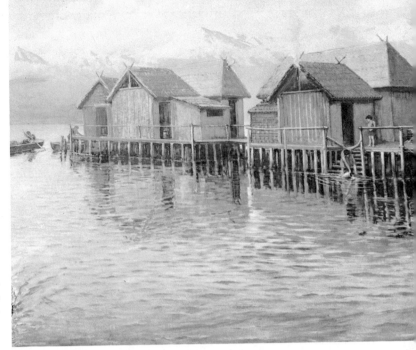

Reconstruction of Swiss lake dwellings of the New Stone Age. These settlements were built along the shores of the large lakes in Switzerland by driving piles into the lake bottoms to support the beams on which the houses rest. The inhabitants practiced agriculture on the shores, as well as fishing and hunting. Investigated in the nineteenth century, they were among the first Stone Age settlements known to modern archeology.

Myth, too, must have been greatly elaborated in this period when a new relationship to nature was being worked out. We do not, of course, know the myths of early man until the techniques of art and literature were able to record them in permanent form. Yet early men thought of themselves as a part of nature, or, to put it another way, of nature being of the same stuff as themselves. Their consciousness of a spiritual life within themselves was transferred to nature, and they explained its phenomena as they would their own. Thus stories, expressed in terms of vivid human experience, were invented. When the story was told the listener would have the vicarious experience of living through its action and feeling its truth as an emotional experience. The coming of a storm could be explained as the darkening of the sun by the wings of a great bird, or the creation of the world recounted as a union between heaven and earth, like that between man and woman.

By about 4500 B.C. neolithic farming villages were numerous and widely spread across northern Mesopotamia and Syria to the Mediterranean coast. Many had reached a state of balance, in which their population was nicely adjusted to the production from the adjacent land. They were largely self-sufficient and static, and perhaps we may assume that their inhabitants were also self-satisfied and content. In some, of course, this balance could not be retained because of natural disasters, exhaustion of the land, or the pressure of nomads crowding in to settle. To advance, an "escape" was needed. Men moved to the areas of the river valleys and their estuaries where agriculture had previously seemed too difficult. Towards 4000 B.C. settlement began in the alluvial regions of lower Mesopotamia and of the Nile. The transition to an urban, civilized society was made earliest in Mesopotamia, the subject of the next chapter.

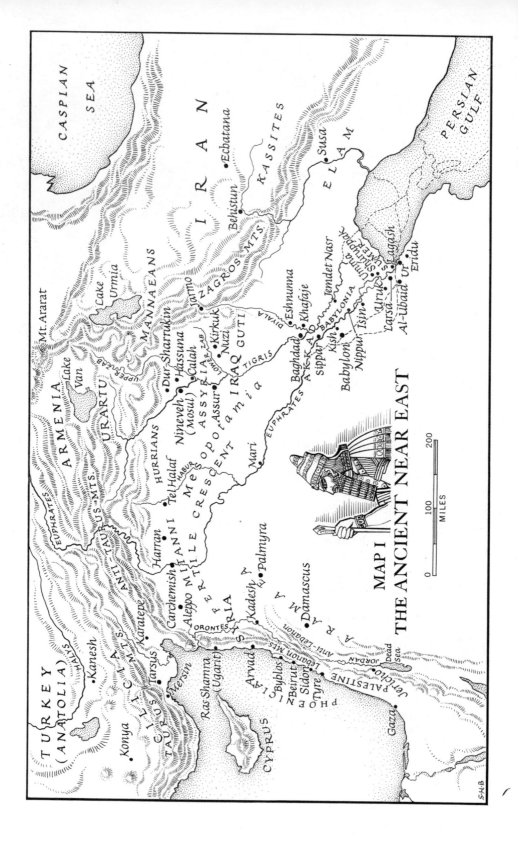

MAP I
THE ANCIENT NEAR EAST

0   100   200
MILES

TURKEY (ANATOLIA)

Konya
•Kanesh
Karatepe
HALYS
TARSUS
Tarsus
CILICIA
ANTI-TAURUS MTS.
TAURUS MTS.
Mersin
Ras Shamra (Ugarit)
CYPRUS
Arvad
Byblos
Beirut
Sidon
Tyre
Gaza
PALESTINE
Jericho
Dead Sea
JORDAN
Lebanon Mts.
Anti-Lebanon
PHOENICIA
Damascus
ARAM
Palmyra
Kadesh
ORONTES
SYRIA
Aleppo
Carchemish
MITANNI
Harran
HURRIANS
Tel-Halaf
HABUR
UPPER ZAB
FERTILE CRESCENT
Mesopotamia
Mari
EUPHRATES
Baghdad
AK-KAD
Babylon
Sippar
Kish
Nippur
Babylonia
Jemdet Nasr
Isin
Shuruppak
Umma
Uruk
Larsa
Lagash
Al-'Ubaid
Ur
Eridu
SUMER
Nippur
TIGRIS
DIYALA
Eshnunna
Khafaje
Baghdad
IRAQ
GUTI
Nuzi
Kirkuk
LOWER ZAB
ASSYRIA
Assur
Nineveh
(Mosul)
Calah
Hassuna
Dur-Sharrukin
Jarmo
MANNAEANS
Urmia
Lake Urmia
ZAGROS MTS.
KASSITES
Behistun
•Ecbatana
IRAN
Susa
ELAM
PERSIAN GULF
URARTU
Lake Van
ARMENIA
•Mt. Ararat
CASPIAN SEA
EUPHRATES

S-H-B

Mesopotamian Civilization

(*ca.* 3500–1500 B.C.)

THE EARLIEST AND MOST INFLUENTIAL civilization of the ancient Near East rose in Mesopotamia, the region between the Tigris and Euphrates rivers from the Persian Gulf to the district of Mosul, near the modern frontier between Iraq and Turkey. The northern part of the region, the land around the middle Tigris and the Upper and Lower Zab rivers, was called Assyria. Below Baghdad, where the Tigris and Euphrates draw close together, was Babylonia, divided into a northern region, Akkad, and the delta land of Sumer. Here, on the low alluvial islands and the river banks of the delta the Sumerian people made the discoveries upon which Mesopotamian civilization was based. The rich alluvial soil, reclaimed by cooperative works of clearing and irrigation, produced a surplus of food by which the growing population and increasingly diversified social organization could be maintained. The Sumerians invented a system of writing, cuneiform, to serve the needs and to preserve the records of their civilization. Their communities grew rapidly into city-states, and from them the elements of Sumerian civilization spread northwards along the rivers into Babylonia and Assyria. Communication was easy by boat on the rivers and by cart and donkey across the flat river plains. From Mesopotamia the civilization was widely diffused, west to the Mediterranean coast, north into Anatolia and east to Iran and Elam. Elements of Sumerian culture, too, were carried by the sea routes through the Persian Gulf to Bahrein Island, to the Oman coast of Arabia, and to northwestern India, where the cities of the Indus River civilization were affected.

The Physical Character of Mesopotamia

Widespread cultural diffusion was possible because Mesopotamia was accessible to neighboring lands. The chief route to the west lay along the river valley of the Euphrates. In the middle stretch of the river the city of Mari devel-

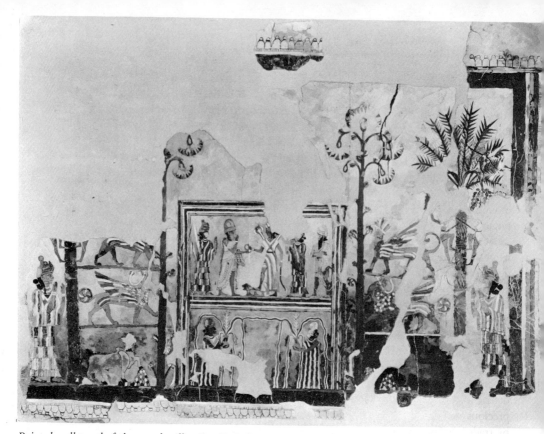

Painted wall panel of the second millennium B.C. from Mari on the Euphrates River. Religious scene (center) framed by mythological creatures and palm trees in a landscape. The fish are a symbol of life.

oped early as an important crossing point on the river. (Excavations by French archaeologists have revealed the palace and archives of Mari's rulers and the important part which they sometimes played in Mesopotamian history.) Beyond Mari the river bends west into northern Syria, where there was another crossing at Carchemish, which became important at a later date. From Carchemish the Syrian coast might be reached by way of Aleppo and the Amuq plain. From this area and from Assyria, too, passes led into Anatolia, but generally speaking, the mountain ranges of Taurus and Anti-Taurus formed a barrier between the Anatolian plateau and northern Mesopotamia and Syria.

Along the natural routes came foreign peoples, attracted by the rich fields and the growing cities of the river valleys. Sumerian and Babylonian rulers led raids and sent their traders along these same routes. To the west of Mesopotamia were the Arabian and Syrian deserts, inhabited by nomadic Semitic tribes. Some of these Semites infiltrated into the territory of the cities as individuals or family groups and were soon assimilated. Others came on raiding parties for plunder, while larger invasions sometimes resulted in permanent settlement and the establishment of Semite rulers. From the outset the population of Sumer was infiltrated by Semites, and in Akkad and Assyria they formed the bulk of the population as these regions developed.

The fields and cities of Mesopotamia were also a magnet to the hill peoples living in the Zagros Mountains between Mesopotamia and Iran. The mountaineers raided into the river valleys and, in turn, their lands were ravaged and sometimes controlled by the rulers of Mesopotamia. The main route into Iran from the middle Tigris lay up the Diyala River to the sources, from which it crossed to Ecbatana (Hamadan) by a lengthy caravan track. Farther to the south the people of Elam exerted continuous pressure on Babylonia. While we read much in Mesopotamian documents of hostilities between the peoples of the mountains and of the river valleys, the former were strongly affected by Mesopotamian culture and formed a part of its domain.

Although the soil of Babylonia was fertile, the yield depended entirely on irrigation from the rivers, for the rainfall was scanty and in summer the climate desperately hot. A choice could be made only between the scorching heat of the desert and the stifling humidity of the delta. With proper irrigation, however, the food supply was ample for a large population. Grain, vegetables, fruit and dates were grown near the rivers, while there was seasonal pasture on the adjacent steppes of the desert for sheep, goats and cattle. No stone and little timber for building existed in Mesopotamia, but a ready substitute was found for these in the clay and reeds along the rivers, so that sun-dried and kiln-dried bricks became the standard material of Mesopotamian architecture. A more serious deficiency was the lack of metals, copper and tin for weapons and tools and the precious metals for jewelry and a medium of exchange. These were sought out by trade and by raids on the sources of supply in an ever widening circle beyond Mesopotamia. Copper came from Oman, Sinai, the Zagros Mountains, and Anatolia. The sources of tin are obscure, but perhaps fields in Syria and Armenia, exhausted in antiquity itself, supplied that commodity. There were deposits of silver in the Taurus Mountains, but gold was brought from farther afield, from Armenia and perhaps from Nubia and the eastern desert of Egypt. Some timber came by sea to the delta at an early date and from the Zagros Mountains, but most highly prized were the famous cedars of Lebanon. Building stone, too, could be procured from the mountains with great labor, and semiprecious stones, like lapis lazuli and carnelian were traded from Iran and Baluchistan. Sources of supply were sought out continuously, and many of the military expeditions recorded in the documents were designed to procure goods lacking in Mesopotamia rather than to acquire territory. The commodities which came in trade were paid for by the craft products and textiles of Mesopotamian workshops.

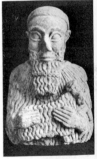

Man carrying a lamb for sacrifice. (From Mari on the Euphrates River.) Early second millennium B.C.

Conditions of life in Mesopotamia were never easy and at times very difficult and dangerous. The price paid for an ample food supply was hard work on the irrigation channels and the land. The rivers might rise in sudden flood, or destructive tides and gales roar into the delta from the Persian Gulf. The cities fought aggressively to control the precious land within reach of the water from the rivers and the canals. Threats of raids from the desert and the hills were constant. Nevertheless, the transition from barbarism to civilization was made by the people of Sumer in the course of the fourth millennium before Christ.

The Formation of Sumerian Civilization (ca. 3500–2800 B.C.)

Although agricultural villages had become well established in northern Mesopotamia in the course of the fifth and fourth millenniums before Christ (pp. 13, 17), it was in the southern delta region that the transition to urban culture and to civilization was made. The earliest remains of habitation in the delta date from about 4000 B.C., by which time the swamps had begun to dry out and settlers had begun to realize the potentiality of the alluvial soil for growing food. With proper irrigation and care a surplus of food could be obtained, but in the north the self-sufficient farming villages lacked this stimulus to develop. The change from village to city seems to have been rapid. It took no more than a few generations and was evidently stimulated, if not initiated, by the arrival of the Sumerians, the "blackheads," as they called themselves.

Although not the first people to settle in the delta, the Sumerians began to arrive about 3500 B.C. Their place of origin is obscure, but most scholars regard them as migrants from the hill country to the northeast, probably entering Mesopotamia from Iran by the Diyala River valley. The Sumerians were evidently of a different racial stock from the earlier settlers, because the names of the cities, which grew out of the original farming villages, were not Sumerian. The Sumerians, too, were different from the Semites of the desert, for the Sumerian language is isolated, agglutinative in character and thus non-Semitic. Perhaps the earliest settlers of the delta had come from northern Mesopotamia and from the outset their numbers were increased by Semites from the desert.

Before the arrival of the Sumerians these earlier settlers had already made important steps toward urbanization. These are revealed by the lowest levels of the cities of Eridu, of Uruk and of a site at Al Ubaid, to the northwest of Ur. A distinctive culture, Ubaid, which spread northwards into Babylonia in its latest stages, was so named from the remains found there. The people based their farming on irrigation, used molded bricks for building, and had developed distinctive structures for the gods who protected their community. A few of their tools were made from copper brought by wandering traders. At Uruk a temple set on a raised platform, foreshadowing the form of the later ziggurats, Mesopotamia's characteristic temples, was discovered. Carts were used there, and at Eridu the earliest representation of a sailing ship, dating about 3000 B.C., was found.

The Sumerians, however, seem to have been the inventors of cuneiform writing, which was to serve Mesopotamian civilization for almost three thousand years. The earliest examples have been found at Uruk, at Jemdet Nasr, about 15 miles northeast of Kish, at Ur and Shuruppak, but by 2800 B.C. the practice of writing, along with the other elements of Sumerian civilization, was widely spread throughout the delta. The name given to this formative period between 3500 B.C., when the Sumerians began to appear, and 2800 B.C., when the city-states emerged into the light of history, is Proto-Literate Period.

While the invention of writing was only one of the phenomena which accompanied the emergence of civilization, it is the most significant for the historian. The invention itself was a response to the needs of a complex society, which could not function without keeping a record of activities.[1] Their detail had grown beyond the ability of human memory. The earliest documents were lists of commodities, recorded in the temples, and of the signs used in writing, to be learned by would-be scribes. As writing developed, however, other activities were recorded: the official acts and exploits of rulers, laws and regulations, the business transactions of private citizens and, in time, the thought and traditions of individuals and societies. In short, not only was a complex civilization facilitated by the keeping of records, but detailed reconstruction of history became possible, so that men began to live consciously with their past, as well as in their present.

In a sense writing had already been invented in the latter part of the Old Stone Age, when pictures of the hunt had been drawn on the walls of caves. The imagination of the artist had given a coherent organization to his work, a composition to tell a story, but pictorial writing was limited to the representation of objects. Its effect was to produce an aesthetic or emotional reaction to

[1] Although the invention of writing made it possible for men to keep detailed records, it is a difficult and highly technical task to fix the time of the events which they recorded in terms of our own Christian era. Not only are the gaps in our information numerous and large, but each people of antiquity had its own methods of reckoning time and dating events. The Christian era itself came into use only in the sixth century after Christ. About A.D. 540 a monk, Dionysius Exiguus, calculated by historical methods that the 248th year of the era of the Roman Emperor Diocletian, in which Dionysius lived, was the 532nd year from the birth of Christ. Even so, it was not until the eighteenth century that the practice of expressing events as occurring before the birth of Christ (B.C.) became regular in the western world. While Diocletian's era (beginning in A.D. 284) helped to serve the Late Roman Empire, the usual Roman practice was to refer events to the years which had elapsed from the traditional founding of Rome (ab urbe condita, a.u.c.; from 753 B.C. in our own terms). Greek historians after the time of Alexander the Great usually referred events to an Olympic era, dating by Olympiads, the four-year periods of the Olympic Games (their start was traditionally in 776 B.C.). The Egyptians kept lists of their kings, ultimately dividing them into periods of rule of a single family, a dynasty (pages 53–54). The Assyrians in the first millennium B.C. made very detailed annual chronicles by listing their kings and indicating the year by reference to the name of an annual magistrate (the limmu lists; this practice was also followed by certain Greek states, like Athens, and by Rome). From such records as these it is possible for historians to establish a relative chronology, to arrange events in the order of their occurrence in the history of a single people. But how do we transfer such relative schemes to the Christian era? In general, ancient peoples reckoned the passage of time as we do, if not quite as accurately, by the passage of days, months (lunar) and years (solar). Accordingly, the notice in ancient sources of astronomical phenomena of a recurring nature, such as eclipses of the sun and moon or the rising of certain stars are very helpful. These may be fixed in the absolute terms of our era by the use of modern astronomical tables. For example, an Egyptian record mentioned the heliacal rising of the star Sirius (Egyptian New Year's Day) in the seventh year of the reign of a king of the Twelfth Dynasty. This was apparently the seventh year of King Sesostris III and is equivalent to 1872 B.C. Calculations may be made forwards and backwards from this, and other such absolute dates, by the relative data. Ancient sources, too, mention synchronizations of events which occurred in different places. Sometimes these are false and represent a wish to correlate two great happenings; frequently, however, they are incidental and may be accepted as valid. For example, clay tablets found at Mari on the Euphrates River linked the great King Hammurabi of Babylon with an Assyrian king known from the king lists. The result of this discovery was to set Hammurabi's dates about 1700 B.C. Previously he had been placed in the twentieth century B.C., so that a far-reaching revision of the chronology of Mesopotamian history in the second millennium had to be made as the relative data was brought into line. In general, of course, the earlier the date in the historical period (in the third millennium, in particular), the more uncertain it is because of our lack of information. The ancient peoples themselves knew little of their early history and frequently remedied the lack of knowledge by giving their legends and myths a setting in the obscure early periods.

the narrative depicted rather than to convey an idea. Sumerian writing presumably grew from such a pictographic stage, but the earliest known examples had already advanced to the use of some abstract symbols, ideographs, which represented an idea. For example, while a picture of a man standing with legs closed might represent a man, a picture of him with legs astride could suggest the idea of running, "to run," rather than a particular man running. An important step from the stage of ideographic writing was that to phonetic symbols, where a sign represented a sound. This was soon taken by Sumerian scribes, but at the same time the writing remained composite, using a mixture of simplified pictures to represent objects, ideographs for simple ideas and phonetic symbols for the sounds of speech. The script permitted considerable expression but the method was very awkward. The Sumerians used several hundred word symbols and about one hundred sound symbols, but neither they nor their Babylonian successors developed the writing to an alphabetical stage. That important development occurred in the Late Bronze Age, about 1600–1400 B.C., in the busy commercial cities of the Syrian coast (pp. 99–100).

The initially rapid development of writing in Sumer was facilitated perhaps by the method used to make the symbols, although this, too, imposed some limitations. The signs were made at first by pressing the cut end of a stiff reed on soft clay, later by a bone stylus formed to essentially the same wedgelike shape. Marks of this shape could not make a continuous line, so that the pictures made by them soon passed into an almost unrecognizable shorthand representation. It is from the wedge-shaped symbols that the name *cuneiform* was given to the writing (Latin: *cuneus,* a wedge). Tablets of clay, baked to preserve them after the symbols were marked, remained the standard material for writing, although important documents were also chiseled on stone and set up in a public place. The use of such materials, of course, required that documents be relatively short and that expression be mainly in stereotyped formulas. The very difficulty of learning to read and write hundreds of symbols restricted the use of writing to a small class. Mesopotamian society did not become generally literate, however valuable the writing proved for its growth.

Another hallmark of Mesopotamian civilization was the cylinder seal. These were small, cylindrical objects made of stone, usually of some semi-precious variety, about the size of a man's thumb and engraved with designs. The latter were frequently of religious significance, and the object presumably was thought to have a magic potency. The seal was rolled on a blob of soft clay to impress the design, and the resultant "tag" was affixed to an object to protect it from harm by the power of the owner's seal. The designs were very carefully

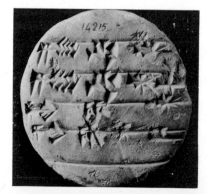

A school practice tablet for cuneiform writing. Sippar, Iraq. Most tablets are roughly rectangular in shape, small enough to be held in the hand

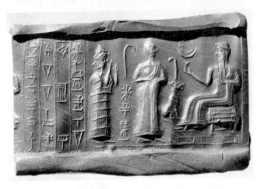

Design cut on a cylinder

cut, so that in addition to their being considered magic amulets the seals are minor works of art as well.

Writing was one of the later inventions of this urban revolution, as it is sometimes called, and there were many others. We can scarcely reconstruct the process of growth in detail, for it was complex and is visible to us only in the material remains from the communities. Technological discoveries were numerous: the plough, by which land was made much more productive than by working the surface of the soil with hoes; the wheel, which led to transportation by cart on land; the sailing boat, which opened up navigation by sea, as well as by rafts and logs on rivers. Metalworking was a primary discovery. At first only copper was used, and copper tools began to replace some of the stone implements of the previous era, but the use of bronze, a harder and more useful metal, was generally established by 2500 B.C. Gold and silver were employed at first only for precious objects, but, as trade developed, they were used as a medium of exchange, not in the form of coins, but by standard weights.

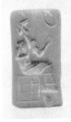

A cylinder seal

The emergence of the urban community itself, which had a centralized structure of government and a class society, was the end product of the revolution. The germ of such a community had been planted in the farming villages of the New Stone Age when a few members of the group began to make tools for the farmers and when traders appeared to exchange flint and obsidian or some small luxury object for the products of agriculture. Yet these simple exchanges could not become more complex without the considerable surplus of food which rich, irrigated land and better agricultural techniques provided. The surplus was obtained by the direction and organization of labor in the community, and a chain reaction was started. The surplus of food provided support for artisans and traders, for directors of the community, the rulers and priests, and as these multiplied a greater surplus was obtained. In the lower river valleys of Mesopotamia the circumstances were very favorable for this development. The soil was rich, there was a reservoir of manpower in the desert to enlarge the population, and needed metals could be obtained by trade with the sources of supply.

Yet the primary activity of agriculture tended to shape the political and social structure of the growing cities. In the minds of the people the production of the soil depended not so much on their own labor, which was taken for granted, as on the goodwill of the gods who controlled the flooding of the rivers, the weather and the processes of growth and harvest. The headman of the former agricultural village, who had acted as the mediator of his community with the gods, quite naturally continued this function and added to it the direction of the works of irrigation and of agriculture. As an effective representative of the gods he exercised the functions of government. Accordingly, the political structure which resulted tended to be a theocracy, and the earliest monumental type of building to develop was the temple of the god. As the towns became larger, the apparatus needed to organize the work of the people also grew. The headman required assistants, so the officials of government came into existence. As a priest he had to have lesser priests and temple attendants. Apparently in some towns chief priest and ruler were identical, as we have theorized, while in others a separation of function occurred early. Perhaps in the latter the need of a strong political ruler for defense was paramount. In all, however, rulers and priests were supported by the production of the community in return for their services. This, of course, involved the subordination of the laborers, farmers, and craftsmen to the governors and ultimately to the gods who protected the community.

The social stratification which resulted was apparently very rigid. The rulers and officials of the state formed a noble class distinguished from the lower groups of society by the wealth which they obtained as pay for their services. The nobility, too, maintained its position by leadership and effective fighting in war. There was a limit, of course, to the amount of land which could be successfully irrigated; therefore, when the food supply was insufficient to maintain the population, additional territory could be obtained only by conquest or by unprofitable reclamation of marginal land. War seemed the easiest remedy, and we find conflict among the Sumerian cities from the beginning of recorded history. As the towns grew in size, a middle class developed from the increase in number of craftsmen and traders. They occupied a position midway between the noble and the farmer. While all the citizens were freemen, the farmer, from the very nature of his occupation, with its fixed routine and directed activity, tended to be subordinated to a serflike position. In this early period there were apparently very few slaves. Those who were slaves had been taken as prisoners of war and seem to have served in the temples as menials, rather than as the property of private owners.

During the Proto-Literate Period the transition from farming village to city-state was made throughout Sumer, and a similar process began in central and northern Babylonia. For the time being Assyria, less fertile and more arid, did not share in urbanization. Yet some of the elements of Sumerian civilization spread surprisingly far. In Egypt, where a similar transition to civilization was under way, unmistakable Sumerian cultural traits appeared: cylinder seals, certain art motifs, the practice of burial in brick-lined tombs, and the principle, if not the method, of writing. These may have been the result of trade from Sumer by way of Syria and Palestine or across Arabia and the Red Sea, but it seems more likely that they were brought by Asiatic migrants. The traits seem too deep-rooted in social habits to be the result of casual trade. Yet the African character of Egyptian culture overpowered the Mesopotamian influences, and each of the two great early civilizations, Sumerian and Egyptian, developed in relative isolation from the other throughout the third millennium.

The Sumerian Cities: Early Dynastic Period
(ca. 2800–2340 B.C.)

In the Early Dynastic Period the Sumerian cities emerged into the light of history. While the documents are at first few in number and their interpretation difficult, it is apparent that in Sumer there were a dozen or more separate city-states, each of which tried to retain its independence and, when opportunity offered, to extend control over its neighbor's lands and irrigation canals. If a city were to survive, a strong centralized administration was necessary, so that new institutions developed. Kings were chosen to lead the cities in war. Some extended the territory of their cities and formed ephemeral coalitions on the strength of which they claimed to be overlords of the whole land. Within the cities the temples continued to direct much of the labor of the community in the service of the gods, but, along with the great temple estates, a system of private ownership seems to have grown as well.

Among the important cities of this period there was Kish, the temporary supremacy of which was indicated by the title, "King of Kish," used in later times by kings who claimed to rule over all of Babylonia. Uruk, too, was important under its King Gilgamesh. He was worshipped as a god after his death and became a hero of legend, whose exploits were recorded in the best known of Sumerian-Babylonian literary works, the *Epic of Gilgamesh*. This early period of Sumerian history was the heroic age of Sumer when traditions were formed and crystallized into the myth and legend embodied in the later religious literature. The exploits of the early kings were glorified, and the gods of the cities were pictured in stories which reflected the vicissitudes and triumphs of their worshippers.

The City of Ur is known, in particular, through the excavation of a group of richly furnished tombs, dating from about 2750 to 2650 B.C. They contained jewelry and ceremonial objects, which mark them as royal burials, although it is surprising that the names of their dead were not written in the traditional lists of kings of Sumerian history. A survival of savage custom was the practice of killing the attendants of the ruler and burying them with their lord. The wealth of the royal family at Ur was apparently obtained in part from a territory extending over the lands of its neighbors, Kish and Nippur.

While overall unity was never obtained in this early period of Sumerian history, we find perhaps a hint of occasional coalition against Semitic invaders in the great importance which Enlil attained, the local god of Nippur. In later times the rulers of the whole land found support for their rule in the approval of Enlil, while Nippur became the most important religious center of the land. The characteristic unit of early Sumer, however, remained the small independent city-state.

It has been argued that the earliest form of government in the cities was a

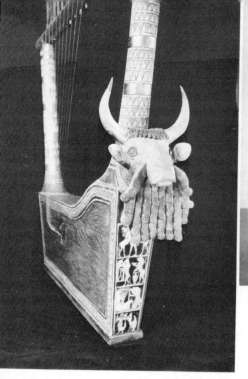

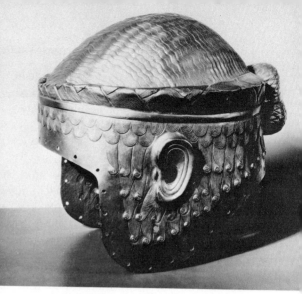

Gold wig-helmet. Royal Tombs of Ur

Lyre with gold bull's head.
Royal Tombs of Ur (2750–2650 B.C.)

sort of primitive democracy in which a council of elders and an assembly of the citizens were sovereign. While no direct evidence to that effect exists, such an arrangement has been conjectured from the action of the gods depicted in myth and epic. It is assumed that this is a reflection of the political organization of the earthly city-states. In the myths a supreme god presided over a general assembly of the gods which met at times of emergency and, in addition, was advised by a special council of seven important gods. The latter might correspond to a council of elders, and the heavenly assembly might be the divine counterpart of a town meeting of the citizens of a Sumerian community. The advice of the elders, of course, would carry special weight, and the aim of the whole assembly was to reach a consensus of opinion by debate rather than by voting to express the will of the majority. This unanimous decision would be announced as a decree of the city-state.

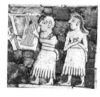

Lyre player from the "Standard" of Ur

Kingship may have developed out of this town meeting in response to the need for a single competent leader in war. At first the citizens would select a known and experienced commander for the duration of a military emergency to lead them into battle. In Sumer military emergencies were frequent, and so the opportunity for a consolidation of power by the king was favorable. Under pressure of war the kingship would tend to become permanent and hereditary in character. Provision for military action, too, would become a normal part of the city's business. The kings established armies, in which a chariot force and heavy

28

armed infantry, fighting in close order of battle, were the most effective branches. The palace of the king took its place alongside the temple of the city's god to become a second center of wealth and power. Presumably the early kings were not absolute in their rule but consulted the elders of the community and, of course, sought a sanction for their authority by representing themselves as servants of the gods. Thus two centers of authority developed in the Sumerian state, the temple establishment of the god of the city and the palace establishment of the king. There was a clash of power implicit in the situation, but, generally speaking, the feeling of the citizens was to support their gods, that is, the temple and the priests, and in Mesopotamia the role of the king was primarily that of a servant of the gods. He worked with the priests and at times had to account to them for his conduct of the state's affairs. Rarely did a king feel strong enough to claim divinity and worship for himself.

The titles born by the officials of the state in this early period are obscure. At a later date the title *lugal* was used by a king who ruled over a wider territory than that of his own city. *Ensi* seems originally to have designated the ruler of a city who organized its economic, that is, agricultural, life, but later the *ensi* was a city governor, administering it as the subordinate of a "great" king who held sway over several cities. Presumably originally independent *ensis* had been subordinated to the rule of the *lugals* as the latter extended their control.

The term, city-state, should be thought of as including both the urban agglomeration of the city and its rural territory, a few hundred square miles at most. We can only conjecture about population, but sixty thousand seems a fair estimate for the city of Lagash in the latter part of the Early Dynastic Period. The cities were protected by a wall of brick, and in them the most conspicuous structures were the temples of the main god of the city and of the less important gods. These were raised on a high terrace but did not develop the typical ziggurat form, a sort of stepped tower, until about 2000 B.C., towards the end of the Sumerian Period. The temple itself consisted of a rectangular central room in which there was a statue of the god visible from the doorway. In front of this chamber was a forecourt, surrounded by rooms for storage and for the attendants and officials. The whole complex was walled. The drab brick construction was enlivened by colorful mosaics formed from cones of clay painted on their butts and pushed into the columns and wall buttresses. Sumerian cities grew without planning along narrow twisting streets where houses of various shapes were set close together to fit the available space. The homes of the wealthier citizens might have courtyards, but all were built of brick with thick, windowless walls to afford some comfort in the merciless heat of summer. Apart from the temples and the palaces the cities were undistinguished in appearance, and their brick buildings have collapsed into mounds of earth, formed from the dissolved brick.

Beyond the city the fields of its territory, stretching across the flat river plain, were broken by clumps of trees, such as date palms, by the checkerboard pattern of irrigation canals and, near the city, by small suburban villages. In the fields were grown the staples of Sumerian diet: barley and emmer (a coarse wheat), vegetables, among which the onion was a favorite, peas, beans and lentils. Beyond the cultivated land was desert steppe which provided seasonal pasture. Meat, however, was only a treat at festivals, and protein was furnished by the fish in the rivers and canals.

The system of landholding in the Sumerian cities was apparently a mixture of temple estates and private property. Most of the documentary evidence for economic organization was found in one city, Lagash, and most of the documents were from one of its temples, that of the goddess Baba. When these tablets were first studied, scholars had the impression that the whole land of the city belonged to the temple and extended this pattern of ownership to other Sumerian cities for which evidence was lacking. A thesis was developed which pictured the economic life of the city as organized and directed by the temple officials of the main god of the city, the owner of the cultivated land. Recently, however, this view has been revised, although the degree to which the revision is to be accepted is controversial.

Presumably a large part of the cultivated land in the city's territory was owned and administered by the temple organizations, both those of the main god and of the less important gods. Yet some documents indicate that the king and nobles had large holdings of their own, while others show that private citizens could buy and sell land as well as personal property. In Lagash the temple of the chief god seems to have administered about one-sixth of the arable land. Perhaps at the outset the chief god of the community had been thought of as the actual owner of the whole city, which was administered for him by the governor who combined political and sacred functions. The kings who defended the community, however, and established their families as rulers would have needed land for their own support. Such land seems to have been obtained partly by purchase and partly by seizure of temple holdings. The kings, of course, might grant land as gifts to loyal officials, thus establishing the nobility as landholders. Small private holdings perhaps became the property of a single family by continuous usage. It is suspected that these holdings were mainly garden plots, and they seem to have been held by the family as a group, not by individuals.

The method of administration for the temple lands is well known through the documents found at Baba's temple in Lagash. Some fields and pasture land were used to support the temple directly, that is, their production provided offerings for the god's cult and goods for exchange. These lands were administered by the priesthood and worked by temple personnel in exchange for rations and clothing. Other fields were granted to the officials of the temple as pay for service, while still another category of land was rented to citizens, unaffiliated with the temple, on a share-cropping basis. This latter arrangement, of course, might permit an increase in private wealth if the tenant managed well and had a series of good crops. While the system did place very great power in the hands of the priests, who sometimes abused it by exploiting the workers, it also placed responsibility of supplying grain for seed and food and clothing on the temples.

The great bulk of the population of a Sumerian city consisted of farmers, boatmen, craftsmen, merchants, traders and scribes. The poor lived on small lots of land or served on big estates as clients of the wealthy and of the temples. Craft labor consisted in working for the temple to produce the goods needed for its services or for private sale on a free market. Women, for example, did the spinning and weaving for the temple. Trade, too, was divided between traders for the temples and the palace and private traders working for their own profit.

The patriarchal family was the basis of society. Marriage alliances were a matter of contract between families, and the bride so obtained became the principal wife in the household of her husband. Since concubinage, however, was a regular practice, divorce was easy to obtain in the event of sterility because of the strong feeling that the family line must be maintained. The number of slaves apparently continued to be small, with most serving in the temple or palace.

In one sense, however, all the people of a Sumerian city were servants, for the main god of the community was considered to have a claim on their labor, priest and king, rich and poor alike. Yet man had also created a complex urban society for himself. Soon, he was to work out conceptions of unity among the cities and to devise methods of administering a large territorial state.

The transition to a large state is exemplified by the history of Lagash in the latter part of the Early Dynastic Period. At that time its kings established a fairly extensive rule over central and southern Babylonia. About 2500 B.C. Messalim, the king of Lagash, took the old title, "King of Kish," to indicate his suzerainty, and he established a dynasty of rulers which lasted for five generations. Lagash was in a favorable position to profit from land and river trade, and it increased its territory by taking over a frontier strip from the nearby city of Umma, long in dispute between the two cities. The third king of Lagash, Eannatum, not only raided Umma successfully but ventured as far as the hills of Elam to the east and to Mari on the middle Euphrates. His exploits were commemorated on one of the famous works of Sumerian art, his victory monument, called the Stele of the Vultures. Eannatum is represented at the head of his phalanx of warriors, while the chief god of Lagash, Ningirsu, holds the prisoners of Eannatum in a great net, and vultures tear at the dead.

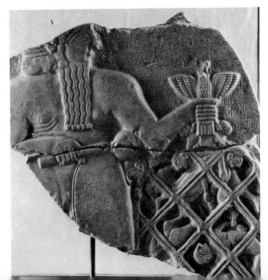

The victory monument of Eannatum of Lagash. The god Ningirsu holds King Eannatum's enemies in a net.

Towards the end of the Early Dynastic Period the city of Lagash was torn by internal social conflict. We know something of this struggle from the record of a reformer, Urukagina, who restored to the temple lands seized by the kings of Lagash and rescued the ordinary citizens from the extortion and abuse of wealthy officials. Presumably Urukagina's reform was the climax of a struggle between temple and palace. The kings had supported their wars and military establishment by high taxation and by setting up a bureaucracy. Urukagina claimed that his reforms restored divine law, that is, the ascendancy of the temple, and protected the poor from arbitrary seizure. Yet Lagash was defeated by the ruler of Umma, Lugalzaggisi, and the city fell into temporary eclipse. The first really effective unity in Babylonia was accomplished by Semitic rulers from the northern part, Sargon of Akkad and his descendants.

Sargon of Akkad and the Akkadian Empire (ca. 2340–2150 B.C.)

Sargon, the founder of the first large territorial state in Babylonia, became a hero of legend after his death, so that it is difficult to separate his historical accomplishments from those with which posterity fictitiously credited him. For example, one story recorded that Sargon, like the Hebrew Moses, was a foundling, picked from the rushes of the river, and another made him out to have been the cupbearer of the King of Kish. Perhaps the latter was true since such a position was an important, confidential office and could have served as a start for Sargon's rise to power. He is said to have ruled from the Lower to the Upper Sea, that is, from the Persian Gulf to the Mediterranean, but presumably his expeditions beyond Babylonia were raids for plunder rather than firm conquests. He did, however, defeat Lugalzaggisi, the king of Umma, who had destroyed the power of Lagash and had taken over most of the cities of Sumer. Sargon's actual control seems to have extended as far as Mari, and his raids perhaps reached the Lebanon Mountains and the borders of Anatolia. Many campaigns were also made against Elam to the east, and thus Sargon was able to provide protection for his kingdom against both those mountaineers and the Semites of the Syrian Desert.

Sargon's consolidation of rule is a sign of the growth of the northern, (Semitic) area of Babylonia, and he established a new pattern of organization throughout the whole land. He and his descendants ruled from the city of Akkad, as yet undiscovered, which gave its name to the northern part of Babylonia and to the Semitic language used by its inhabitants. While the population had long been Semitic, the people had thoroughly assimilated Sumerian culture, and their scribes wrote the Akkadian language in cuneiform symbols. The kings established a centralized administration, using Semitic officials from Akkad as governors in the subject cities and putting in garrisons which were probably drawn from a standing army. Sargon's grandson, Naram-Sin, further strengthened the kingship by claiming worship as a living god and by taking the title,

"King of the Four Quarters of the Universe," to describe the extent of his rule. Naram-Sin also treated severely those Sumerian cities which tried to break away from his domination. Even the temple of Enlil in the holy city of Nippur was looted. While Naram-Sin was able to exalt his position as king of a unified Babylonia, his successors were less fortunate. The Empire crumbled away under attacks from the Semites in the northwest, revolts in Elam and, in particular, through the heavy raids of a new people, the Gutians, from the mountains to the east in Iran.

The Gutians acquired control of much of Babylonia for about two generations after the fall of the Akkadian Empire. They raided the fields, harassed the cities, and destroyed the unity of administration which had been established. Many cities acknowledged their authority and paid tribute, but a few remained independent. Among the Gutian dependents Lagash seems to have been especially favored, probably because of its important trading activity. This latter is revealed by the records of the *ensi,* Gudea, who described his work as a temple builder. He organized the people of Lagash for this task and imported gold from Egypt and Anatolia, silver from the Taurus Mountains, cedar from Mt. Amanus in Syria, and copper from the Zagros range. Evidently, despite Gutian and Semitic raids, the far-flung trading activity of the Akkadian Empire still survived, and the routes remained secure. In fact, the cities of Sumer were fundamentally stable and prosperous. They might have been harassed by raids and resented paying tribute to the Gutians but probably preferred the loose control of the latter to the stricter authority of the Akkadian kings. About 2135 B.C., however, the king of Uruk, Uterhegal, defeated the Gutians decisively but did not live long to enjoy his success. His governor, Ur-Nammu, who administered Ur, revolted against Uterhegal and established Ur as the dominant city of Sumer. Under Ur-Nammu's rule and that of his family, the Third Dynasty of Ur, the Sumerian states reached their highest point of prosperity and development.

The Third Dynasty of Ur (ca. 2135–2027 B.C.)

The kings of Ur re-established political unity in Babylonia and built on the practices of the Akkadian Empire to create an even more centralized system of administration. Their period of rule is better known than any other of Sumerian history from the very large number of documents which have been found. The tablets provide evidence for the details of administration both of the palace and of the temples. The latter were made a part of a planned state economy, while the kingship was exalted in a manner similar to that of Naram Sin. Ur-Nammu, the first king of the Third Dynasty, added the title "King of Sumer and Akkad" and was deified after his death, while his successor, Shulgi, through the prestige of a successful reign which lasted almost half a century, became "King of the Four Quarters of the Universe" and was worshipped as a god during his lifetime. Both Ur-Nammu and Shulgi were highly successful military rulers. The former

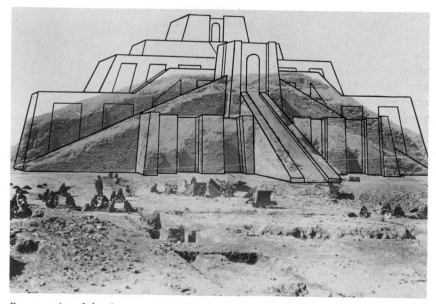

Reconstruction of the ziggurat at Ur. The "high temple" at the top perhaps was considered to be a resting place for the god on his way between heaven and earth.

took over many of the cities of Sumer, and Shulgi completed the acquisition of all Babylonia and led expeditions into Elam and northwards to Assyria. They and their successors were able to provide a general condition of freedom from foreign invasion and of internal peace, thus winning the opportunity to set up the elaborate, planned economy about which we know from the documentary material.

The kings of Ur ruled their subject cities through local governors, the *ensis,* who might be transferred to new districts from time to time to forestall the growth of local loyalties and ambitions. The power of the *ensi* was also limited by the appointment of a separate military official, responsible to the king, and by the installation of garrisons of the king's troops. Ur-Nammu collected the local laws of his cities and published them in a code designed for general use, thus giving his Empire a single legal system enforced by the king's authority. Unfortunately the code survives only in fragmentary form, but it is evidently the first of a series which led ultimately to the great code of Hammurabi of Babylon several hundred years later. While external security was obtained mainly by raids beyond Babylonia, the kings of Ur also showed some appreciation of statecraft by making interdynastic marriages with the daughters of kings in Elam. Ur, as the political capital of the kingdom, was glorified by the construction of the first great ziggurat in Mesopotamia. Nippur, however, was developed as the most important religious center. The temple of its great god Enlil, who was regarded as the sponsor of the kings, was enriched by offerings sent from other cities of the Empire.

This political and religious centralization was accompanied by elaborate economic planning to organize agriculture, trade and communications from the palace of the kings. Presumably the existing practice of the temples furnished the model, but the kings of Ur worked out a state-wide system administered by an elaborate bureaucracy. Agriculture was regulated by recording the amount of seed sown, the labor in the fields, and the yield of the harvest. The number of animals and the time of delivery to designated state centers was all carefully recorded. The produce so obtained by the government was used for various expenditures and sacrifices to the gods, while the surplus was stored. Metals, obtained by raids and through trade, were allocated to forges to be made into tools and weapons for the state. Similarly, transport and communication services, mainly on the rivers, were systematized. Temple and palace each had its own craftsmen and workers to whom rations were issued, while the products of their labor were stored for later use. An elaborate system of account-keeping was required for the recording and for the planning based on it. Income and expenditures were scrupulously drawn up with summary balance statements by the officials of the separate districts. These were forwarded to the king's officials in Ur, and so each year the agricultural yield could be planned. The fields were surveyed and allocated, seed provided, maintenance work was done on the canals, and the projected amount of crop set.

The well-being of the kingdom, however, depended on continued security from invasion. By the reign of Ibbi-Sin, the fifth king of the dynasty, pressure had become intense on the northwest from the Semites of the desert, and on the east from Elam. The desert tribes, known collectively as Amorites, were moving down the Euphrates, while in Elam Sumerian pressure and cultural influence had promoted coalescence into a strong state. The ability of Ibbi-Sin to defend his kingdom was weakened by the disloyalty of local governors and by officials who sought their own advantage in the military crisis. Akkad was lost when an official in the city of Isin, Isbi-Erra, blackmailed his superior and set himself up as king of Isin. The Amorite raiders poured into Akkad, preventing the shipment of grain down river to Sumer, where the cities were suffering famine as the result of a bad season. The Amorites took over some cities of Akkad, while others declared their independence of Ur. The Elamites attacked Ur, pillaged the city and carried off Ibbi-Sin as a prisoner of war. Disintegration followed rapidly in Sumer as the land was thrown open to Amorite raids and the cities were left to their own resources.

In the following period of anarchy, civilization was not lost in Babylonia, but the Sumerian people were submerged by the great influx of Semites. The civilization which they had created was carried on and modified by their Semitic successors. Before discussing the rise of Babylon and of Hammurabi's Empire, however, it would be useful to survey Sumerian culture.

Sumerian Culture

As we have noticed, the political institutions and economic life of Sumer were very closely associated with religious conceptions and practice. The kings were regarded usually as representatives of the gods, and some of the more powerful rulers established worship of themselves as living gods, divine kings who ruled directly. The priests administered the lands and workshops of their temple as stewards of its god. This pervasive influence of religious conceptions seems to have affected almost every activity in Sumer. Imaginative literature was primarily religious, part of the ritual of worship or poetry which embodied theology and myth. Art was largely religious in inspiration and use, and the most characteristic building of Sumerian architecture, the ziggurat, was a religious monument. The beginnings of science and of mathematics are to be sought in connection with religious practice, and their advance was hampered by taboos and magic. With our own very different frame of reference it is difficult to attain an imaginative understanding of such modes of thought. We can perhaps see how the priests looked at the world because they wrote the literature and prescribed the system of education, but is it hard to know to what extent the ordinary Sumerian shared in these religious preoccupations. Presumably, like men at every period of history, he was concerned mainly with the problems and work of his daily existence and was jolted from them only by some unusual personal experience. But on the whole the Sumerian seems to have regarded his life as set in a world governed by the will or caprice of the gods. He felt that they preferred justice and truth, but found their actions obscure and was moved to complain but not to question. This passivity of mind seems to have bred a fundamentally pessimistic attitude to life. The Sumerian was concerned above all with his life on earth and speculated little about a life after death or about betterment of his condition.

EDUCATION

Formal education in Sumer was neither universal nor compulsory but a privilege of the sons of the wealthy families who had the means and the leisure to attend the scribal schools. On completion of their work they were rewarded by appointments to the upper class of officials and priests and thus perpetuated their own kind. While the schools were at first an institution of the temple, they eventually became secular, and the teachers were paid from tuition fees. The curriculum, however, remained traditional in content and method. Above all the students had to learn to read and write cuneiform, since the aim of the schools was to turn out trained scribes. In addition to memorizing and copying examples, the students learned mathematical tables, wrote essays, and worked at practical problems of accounting and land measurement of the type which would confront a future official. The textbooks were the religious literature composed by the priesthood: hymns, proverbs, theological poetry, laments of the fall of cities, and the epics of legendary kings.

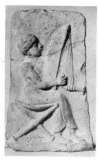

Harpist. Ischali, Iraq

RELIGION AND LITERATURE

The Sumerian universe was operated by a great pantheon of gods of various origins and functions who, in the course of time, had been arranged in a hierarchy of rank. The gods were thought of as human in form and behavior, but were immortal and had the power to direct action in the universe. The great gods of the elemental forces of nature, heaven, earth, the sea, and the air were creative gods, and by their word alone could create the forms of existence. All gods and spirits, however, might affect the welfare of human beings. Many gods were local in origin and, as we have noticed, each city had its own particular god about whose figure there grew a web of myth and specific rituals of worship. The agricultural gods were more universal in type, inasmuch as they presided over the planting and growth of crops and raising animals. They were the central figures of the great festivals associated with the activities of agriculture, particularly at the time of planting and harvesting. The relations of the separate cities to one another during wars and raids were mirrored in stories of the gods of each city and of their dealings with people and rulers. The god of a conquering city was obviously a more powerful deity than that of his defeated rival, and so might be in the process of becoming a great god. Accordingly, the hierarchy of gods was formed from the great gods of powerful cities to the agricultural gods and the creative gods of nature. All these had their favorite cities and might be identified with lesser gods of local importance as the latter rose in the scale.

The most important god of the developed hierarchy was An, the sky-god, who was considered to be the father and ruler of the gods. An was remote and concerned with the great matters of the universe. He was not in as direct touch with the other gods and with human beings as Enlil, whose chief seat of worship was at Nippur. Enlil was god of the air and had brought order out of a primeval chaos. He presided over the assembly of the gods. Enki, the water-god, was third in the series and was considered to have brought civilization to men, teaching them wisdom, medicine, and writing. Most important among the goddesses was Inanna (the Semitic Ishtar), in origin a fertility and mother-goddess. She had as consort a youthful god, Dummuzi (the Semitic Tammuz), perhaps in origin a deified king. Dummuzi was believed to die each winter with the vegetation and to rise again in the spring. Some of the deities were also identified with planets, as Inanna with Venus, and each god had a number from the Sumerian notation to indicate his relative importance: An was sixty, the basic number, Enlil fifty, Enki forty, and Inanna fifteen.

The worship of the gods was carried out in highly developed rituals at which the priests officiated, sacrificing victims, making offerings of produce, conducting the prayers and hymns, and leading religious processions. The most important festival was that of the New Year in April, when a feast was held and a holy marriage performed between the king of the city and the priestess of Inanna and Dummuzi. Its purpose was to ensure an ample harvest when the crops were reaped in May and June.

The myths of the gods, which depicted their mutual relationships and dealings with men, were told in many vivid stories. Some myths accounted for the origin of nature in terms of human procreation. The primeval sea had born heaven and earth, and out of their union and the marriages of their descendants were born the moon and the sun and the other forces of nature. Stories were told about the creation of man and about a great flood which covered the earth, but men and animals were saved by a Sumerian Noah. Like his Hebraic counterpart he built an ark, in which he, his family and their animals floated until the water receded. The story of the flood, along with other tales, became a part of the general mythology of the Mesopotamian region in which the Hebrews shared. Thus the Sumerians, like other early peoples, accounted for their world by myths based on familiar experience which had an immediate emotional impact. They regarded themselves as a part of nature, together with the gods and the animals and a host of malevolent spirits. The latter were pictured in Sumerian art as demons, some human and some bestial, who surrounded men and did them harm.

The epic poems about early kings were also set in a world where men and gods moved on the same plane of existence. The material for the Sumerian epics was drawn from the Proto-Literate Period, the heroic age of settlement, and of the foundation of cities. The heroes were the kings of the early city-states who held control by their military valor and led bands of soldiers in war and adventure. The poems were short and simply organized, concentrating on a single episode rather than woven together in intricate and sophisticated fashion like the Homeric epics of Greece. Seven epics are known, the most famous of which is the story of King Gilgamesh of Uruk. In Sumerian times a number of short poems were current about Gilgamesh, but we know of his exploits from the Akkadian versions in which the Sumerian ballads were pieced together to form an epic of about three thousand lines.

The poem began with an account of the wanderings of Gilgamesh with his friend Engidu, a "natural" man of the wild countryside. The pair met the goddess Inanna, who fell in love with Gilgamesh. When the hero repulsed her love, the goddess sent a wild bull to kill him, but Engidu, not Gilgamesh, was slain. Gilgamesh, confronted with death and stricken with grief, set out to find some means by which his friend might be restored to life. In the course of his search Gilgamesh obtained a plant from the bottom of the sea which would bring immortality. It was snatched from his hand by a serpent. Then Gilgamesh went to the underworld to recover his friend but could not restore him to life. The profoundly simple experiences of man's existence, love, death, grief and

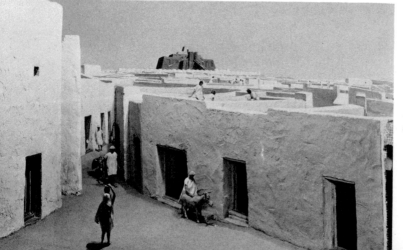

Diorama of the city of Ur about 2000 B.C.

the desire for immortality are embodied in story form set in a world of magic and the supernatural.

ART

The development of monumental sculpture and architecture in Sumer was handicapped by the lack of stone, but craftsmen were particularly skillful at metalwork and engraving. Many fine examples of work in gold and jewelry were found in the royal tombs of Ur, among which are the harp, decorated with a bearded bull's head, and the golden wig-helmet. In the engraving of cylinder seals Sumerian and Babylonian craftsmen used a wide range of subject matter from scenes of everyday rural and religious life to the mythical world of beasts and demons. Many seals were painstakingly and delicately cut, despite the awkward field which the cylindrical form of the seal offered.

Sumerian builders knew the principle of the true arch in their brick construction, and in the ziggurat produced a notable theological concept. The structure seems to express the ascent of man to heaven in its stepped construction reaching toward the sky. The more elaborate buildings were decorated with mosaics, reproducing colorful and intricate textile patterns by the use of pointed clay cones. Apparently walls were painted with frescoes, but we have little knowledge of Mesopotamian painting before the examples preserved on the palace at Mari in the Babylonian period. There, human figures, mythological conceptions, and landscape elements were blended in an irrational but colorful and pleasing composition.

Life-size figures in sculpture were few in Sumer, but one of the earliest, a marble mask from Warka, designed apparently to be fitted to a wooden figure, shows severe but sensitive modeling. The most appealing figures of Sumerian sculpture are the statuettes of worshippers placed in shrines, like the group found at Tell Asmar. The figures stand with hands clasped across the breast in an attitude of devotion, and, despite the formalistic expression and awkward stance, are intensively alive and alert. The statuettes seem to have been substitutes for the worshippers themselves, to assure the god in whose shrine they were placed

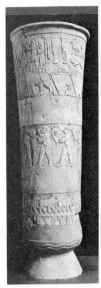

Alabaster vase. Uruk, Iraq

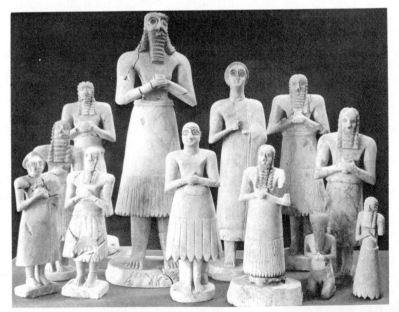

A group of worshippers from a shrine at Tell Asmar, Iraq

of continuous loyalty. Some of the sculpture, too, is vigorous and powerful, like the relentless advance of Eannatum of Lagash at the head of his phalanx on the Stele of the Vultures. The masterpiece of Sumerian art, however, is the bronze head of an Akkadian king. The head combines a monumental majesty of conception with a delicate pattern of hair and ripely smooth flesh surface.

SCIENCE

The origin of astronomy and of mathematics in Sumer and their development in Babylonia are difficult and technical subjects, but we should notice that mathematics probably had its beginning in the accounting practices of the Sumerian temples and astronomy in reckonings for the calendar. The Sumerians used a sexagesimal system of counting, in which sixty was the basic unit, and they combined it with the decimal system. This form of reckoning has, of course, left a mark on our own reckonings of time and measurement. A careful system of dating was employed for documents in which the year, month, and sometimes the day were listed. The year was named for some notable event, like the accession of a king or a decisive battle, and was divided into twelve lunar months of twenty-nine to thirty days. The discrepancy between this and the solar year of 365 days was made up by intercalating a thirteenth month into the calendar every three years. It was natural, of course, that close observations would be made of celestial phenomena, the movements of the sun, moon and stars, in a desert land, and perhaps equally natural that they should be correlated to human experience. Along with the sciences of astronomy and mathematics were born astrology and numerology.

The Diffusion of Sumerian Culture

By the end of the third millennium, when the Sumerians lost their identity as a people in the influx of Semites into Sumer, elements of their culture had been widely disseminated along the trade routes from Mesopotamia. Traders moved up the Euphrates beyond Mari, along the Tigris into Assyria and through the Zagros Mountains to Iran and Elam. Voyages were made into the Persian Gulf to Magan (the Oman coast of Arabia), where the Sumerians exchanged textiles, vegetable oils, wool, and leather for copper, ivory, and semiprecious stones. Tilmun (probably Bahrein Island) was becoming a clearing port for these goods and for the incense and spices of southern Arabia. There was also trade by sea with Melukkha, the identity of which is obscure. Some scholars identify it as African Somaliland, others as Baluchistan or northwestern India with which the Sumerians had trading and perhaps even closer cultural relations.

In the river valley of the Indus an urban civilization had developed in the course of the third millennium. Its history is more obscure than those of Sumer and Egypt, for it is known only through archaeological excavations made since the 1920's. The people of the Indus valley had invented a script for writing, but the language is unknown and the texts still untranslated. Apparently urbanization originated in environmental conditions essentially similar to those of Mesopotamia, and the economy depended on intensive cereal production based on irrigation from the Indus River.[1] Cities developed by 2500 B.C., among which the best-known centers were at Harappa and Mohenjo-daro. These two are about four hundred miles apart, but their remains show a remarkable similarity of culture. The cities were regularly planned on a checkerboard layout, using blocks of uniform size, and the chief architectural feature was a citadel enclosing palaces and temples. Apparently a theocratic type of organization prevailed in them as in the Mesopotamian cities. This civilization flourished until about 1700 B.C., when a period of stagnation set in, which was followed by destruction about 1500 B.C.

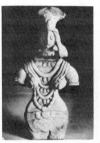

A mother-goddess of the Indus River civilization. Mohenjo-daro

The relationship between the cities of Sumer and those of the Indus River valley is difficult to define, because they seem to have shared cultural traits as well as trade. The evidence of the latter is quite clear: Sumerian cylinder seals have been found at Mohenjo-daro, and a type of seal made at Harappa, perhaps in imitation of Sumerian types, has been found in Mesopotamia. The presence of a group of Indian traders in Mesopotamia may be indicated by reliefs carved on a vase from Khafaje in the Diyala River valley. On it a humped bull of Indian type is represented, so that it is suggested that the vase was used by Indians in a religious ceremony of their own. Probably the trade between Mesopotamia and India moved both overland across Iran and by sea through the Persian Gulf and the Indian Ocean to the delta of the Indus. Some scholars have suggested that the Sumerians themselves came by sea from India to the shores of the Persian Gulf. There is some affinity in the early remains of each civilization, and one Sumerian tradition points to arrival in their land by sea rather than overland from the mountains. Yet it is more probable that both Sumerians and the people of the Indus River valley had a common origin in migrations into Iran at the close of the New Stone Age, which sent some groups westward to Mesopotamia and others east towards India. In any case, when the center of gravity in Mesopotamia shifted north to Babylonia after the fall of the Third Dynasty of Ur, trade with India diminished.

The Babylonian Empire of Hammurabi

When Amorite invaders moved into Mesopotamia from the west and Elamites pressed on the Sumerian cities from the east, the land fell into anarchy.

[1]See Map VI, page 156.

Panoramic view of Mohenjo-daro

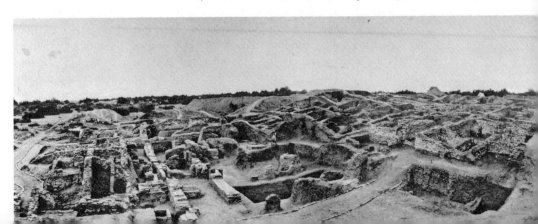

For a time the city of Isin, where Ishbi-Erra had established himself as king, ruled over a remnant of Ur's Empire, but about 1900 B.C. Isin's authority was challenged by Larsa, situated near Ur, and soon both cities fell to the Elamites. The latter took over control of most of Sumer, but in the land of Akkad new Semitic dynasties began to rise, chief among which was that of Babylon. This shift of importance to the north probably resulted in large part from the arrival of a new and vigorous people, but other factors, too, were at work. Apparently the land of the Sumerian cities in the delta was being gradually silted in or invaded by the salt water of the Gulf. Also, the lines of trade had shifted north as urbanization spread to Syria on the northwest and to Assyria in the north. Babylon was better situated to serve as a center for traffic up the Euphrates to Mari and Syria and along the Tigris into Assyria.

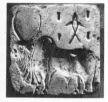

Indian humped bull. Seal from Mohenjo-daro

While little is known of Assyria during this period of history, it is evident that small kingdoms were forming under the leadership of Semitic chieftains and their followers, the "tent-dwellers," as they were called. The chief town of Assyria, Assur, played an important role in the metal trade with eastern Anatolia. Assyrian merchants crossed to the Anatolian plateau through the mountains north of their land and established colonies in the towns of local rulers. One such settlement has been excavated at Kanesh (Kultepe), near modern Konya. The Assyrian merchants and their families lived in a separate quarter of the native city, where they were allowed their own jurisdiction but were under the general authority of the local king. The goods of trade were carried by donkey caravans, which seasonally brought Assyrian textiles to exchange for copper. The tablets found at Kanesh, written in Old Assyrian, indicate that up to two hundred animals were used in a caravan and that loads of five tons of copper were carried back to Assyria. The colony at Kanesh was founded about 1900 B.C. and destroyed about the end of the following century in the disturbances preliminary to the rise of the Old Hittite Kingdom in central Anatolia (pp. 91–93.)

While the new kingdoms of Assyria had begun to play some part in history, the city of Babylon became the dominant power of Mesopotamia under King Hammurabi, who ruled for over forty years from about 1792 to 1750 B.C. He was able to re-establish political unity and to leave a large territorial empire to his descendants. Hammurabi gained his Empire by a mixture of diplomacy and hard fighting, some of the details of which we know from the royal archives of Mari. At the outset of Hammurabi's reign Mari was subject to Assyria but switched its alliance to Hammurabi, thus giving the king an opportunity to concentrate his attention against his enemies to the south. Rim-Sin, the king of Elam, who had occupied most of Sumer was defeated, and Hammurabi added the Sumerian cities to his own kingdom. Later Mari turned against Hammurabi and was destroyed by the king. Free to act in the north, Hammurabi defeated his greatest enemy, the city of Eshnunna and held Assyria at bay. The king ruled all of Babylonia and controlled the important trade routes and outlying districts.

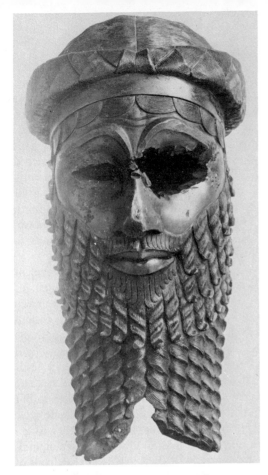

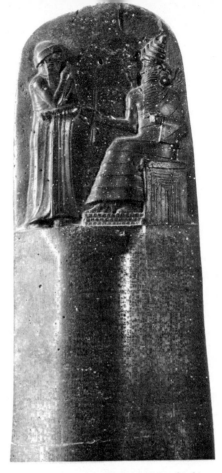

Bronze head of an Akkadian king. The eyes were probably of precious stones. Nineveh, Iraq

Hammurabi (standing) receiving his law code from the god Shamash

Hammurabi and his successors made Babylon into one of the great cities of the Near East, a position which it held throughout the remainder of antiquity. Canals were dug to provide water for the nearby fields, and temples and palaces were erected. The local god of Babylon, Marduk, was deliberately promoted to a prominent position in the Sumerian-Babylonian pantheon and represented as the sponsor of his earthly representative, Hammurabi: "When lofty An . . . and Enlil . . . determined for Marduk . . . (dominion) over all mankind . . . at that time An and Enlil named me, Hammurabi, . . . to cause justice to prevail in the land, to destroy the wicked." The Babylonian priests even rewrote old myths to picture Marduk as a creator god, who slew the dragon, Tiamat, and brought order out of chaos.

Hammurabi's administration was thoroughly centralized. Local governors and officials in the subject cities were made responsible to the king, and Akkadian became the official language. Sumerian passed entirely into the role of a dead language when the religious literature was rewritten in Akkadian. Acting

43

in the name of Marduk, Hammurabi presented himself as the source of justice for his subjects and established a single legal system for the Empire by his famous Code of Law. Yet some measure of independence was left to the cities by allowing their assemblies to act as courts for local cases referred to them by the king's representative.

Hammurabi's Code, much of which is extant, is one of the most important documents of Mesopotamian civilization. It not only illuminates the society and concepts of justice in Hammurabi's reign, but is the culmination of a long history of the reign of law in the Sumerian and Babylonian cities. From the outset, of course, the extreme regimentation of activity in them had encouraged the rule of law. Probably the cities of Sumer had codified their laws at an early date and gradually a generally recognized body of practice and precepts had come into existence. We know of four earlier codes, beginning with that of Ur-Nammu of the Third Dynasty of Ur, by which rulers had attempted to establish a common legal system for the cities under their control. Hammurabi's Code both summed up what was currently useful from the previous codes and modified practice to bring it into line with conditions in his own period. Copies were set up in the cities of the Empire for reference, and it is one of these which has survived. The stele on which the laws were recorded came originally from the Sumerian city of Sippur, from where it was carried off to Susa as a prize of war by the Elamites. It was found there in excavations in 1901. The document, although not complete, is one of the longest of cuneiform inscriptions, consisting of about eight thousand words.

Hammurabi's Code was represented as being given to him by Shamash, the sun-god, and thus had a divine sanction. A prologue recounted the king's exploits, and an epilogue promised rewards for those who obeyed the law and punishment for those who transgressed. The laws themselves were set out in 260 sections in the form of cases which embodied a legal principle. Here are typical sections: "If a seignior has destroyed the eye of a member of the aristocracy, they shall destroy his eye. If he has broken another seignior's bone, they shall break his bone. If he has destroyed the eye of a commoner or broken the bone of a commoner, he shall pay one mina of silver." The Code is not a complete system of law, but its sections cover a very wide range of subject matter, and in them we can see the structure of society and the principles of justice which were observed.

Babylonian society consisted of three classes: a nobility, a middle and lower class of free commoners, and slaves. The nobles were the high officials of the palace and the priests of the temples, who lived partly on their salaries and gifts from the king, partly on the revenue from large estates. The latter were frequently divided into small plots of land leased to tenant farmers. The commoners were made up of the tenant farmers, craftsmen, merchants, small-scale landowners and hired laborers. The slave class was apparently much larger than it had been in Sumerian cities of the third millennium and was recruited both from prisoners of war and by purchase and breeding. Slaves, however, might buy their own freedom by accumulating property or borrowing the amount necessary for that purpose—the temples made such loans. Also, marriage to a free woman brought freedom to the children of the pair.

The types of penalties stipulated in the Code reveal that each individual was not on an equal footing before the law. Generally speaking, the nobility seem to have borne a more serious social responsibility than the free commoners, for the penalties for their offenses were of a primitive type: an eye for an eye and a tooth for a tooth. This may be a reflection of the code of behavior observed by the Semites of the desert and retained by them after settlement. For the commoners penalties were usually monetary, that is, a fine payable in a weight of precious metal. Penalties for violence against another man's slave entailed payment of a sum in compensation, but offenses of physical violence committed by slaves themselves were punishable by mutilation.

There is much that is primitive in the Code. The death penalty was frequent, used not only for such crimes as murder, rape and desertion in military service, but also for the flagrant extravagance of a wife and the adulteration of beer. Trial by ordeal, ducking in the water, was used, but apparently in most cases as a last resort, when both parties seemed to be falsifying their oaths. The trial by ordeal left the decision to God. A summary of the subject matter of the Code gives some idea of its minute regulation: administration of justice, offenses against persons and property, assault and injury, the family and inheritance, contracts, prices and fees. The amount of privilege enjoyed by women is interesting. They could, as we have noticed, marry slaves, carry on business in their own right and own property.

In addition to the changes in practice perceptible in Hammurabi's Code, which seem to have resulted from the Amorite invasion, others are revealed by the business documents of the period. The temple estates and the former ruling families lost a considerable amount of land. This was taken by the new rulers and parcelled out among their own followers. As the new estates were split up in inheritances or sold for various reasons many transfers were made, and owners frequently preferred to lease their holdings rather than to work them directly. Thus the Babylonian period saw a considerable development of private enterprise and the organization of trade. Exchange was facilitated by the use of fixed weights of precious metals, usually of silver, as a medium. A typical entrepreneur was the *tamkarum,* a combination of merchant and moneylender. He employed agents to carry on his business over a wide area, supplying them with goods and credit. Trade extended more widely to the west, to the coast of Syria, where cities of a predominantly commercial character arose. There was some intercourse, too, with Egypt as the rulers of the Middle Kingdom extended their interest northwards to Palestine, Syria, and the Aegean. This activity was a prelude to the knitting together of the lands of the Near East into something like a common international life in the Late Bronze Age. Before such a life was achieved, however, new peoples, mainly Indo-European invaders, who had entered the region, had to be assimilated.

Hammurabi's Empire was of relatively short duration. In the seventeenth century the rulers relaxed their hold on the cities of Sumer. Some revolted successfully, others were again attacked and made subject by the Elamites. The chief blow, however, came from the new Indo-European peoples. About 1595 B.C. the Hittites[1] made a great raid from the Anatolian plateau into North Syria and swept down the Euphrates. Aleppo was taken and sacked, Mari plundered, and Babylon captured. The Hittite king, preoccupied with internal difficulties in his own homeland, gave up his conquests and withdrew to the north behind the mountains. In the following generations, however, other Indo-Europeans, Kassites from the Zagros Mountains, who had perhaps collaborated with the Hittites, began to attack the cities of Babylonia, and by 1500 B.C. their chieftains had replaced the Babylonian kings and governors. The Kassites were to rule in Babylon for about five hundred years. Yet the cities were not destroyed, and, like the desert Semites before them, the Kassites were assimilated into Mesopotamian civilization. The same was true of other new peoples who entered the region. Hurrians, who had moved into Assyria and northern Babylonia, began to spread westwards after 1500 B.C. to northern Syria. They carried with them the techniques and traditions of Mesopotamian culture, which they had adopted, and strengthened the impact already made through trade in Syria and Palestine.

The first great era of Mesopotamian civilization drew to an end with the entry of these new peoples into the land. Their appearance was but one phase of movements which had already brought the Hittites into Asia Minor, the first Greeks into the lands around the Aegean, and the Aryans into northwest India, where they destroyed the cities of the Indus River valley. Before discussing the nature and the impact of these migrations, it is necessary to turn to Egypt and trace the growth of its highly individual civilization in the valley of the Nile River. The Egyptians were to dominate the international life of the east in the new epoch which began in the sixteenth century B.C.

[1]See Map III, page 74.

Bronze stags from the royal tombs of Alaja Hüyük, Turkey. This animal-style of art was used by the nomadic invaders of the Near East.

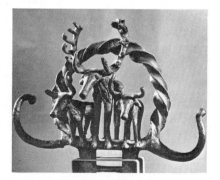

The Kingdom of Egypt

(*ca.* 3100–1600 B.C.)

DURING THE THIRD MILLENNIUM before Christ, while the city-states of Sumer were growing in size and prosperity, the Egyptian people developed their own civilization in the valley of the Nile River. Environmental conditions there were very similar to those in Sumer. In an annual flood the Nile carried along rich alluvial soil, the deposit of which had made its banks and delta a great swamp choked with reeds and other plant growth. If the land could be cleared and drained, protected by dikes, and watered by controlled irrigation, there would be an ample surplus of food for a growing and diversified population. In the course of the fourth millennium as the land was exploited by applying the necessary direction and cooperative labor, peasant villages formed along the river valley and in the delta and gradually coalesced into local territorial units, later called nomes. These achievements were made by the Egyptians themselves, but towards 3000 B.C. cultural influences from Sumer seem to have stimulated the arts of civilization, in particular, architecture and writing. Yet in Egypt the resulting civilization was very different from that of Mesopotamia.

Egypt was protected from large-scale immigration and invasion by the deserts which enclosed the valley of the Nile, and so Egyptian institutions acquired a unique character, adapted to Egypt itself. The Egyptians, comfortable in the prosperity of their land and convinced of the superiority of their own way of life, resisted change and were reluctant to accept new ideas. Egyptian civilization clung to its traditions through the vicissitudes of history and seemed to the Greeks, when they first visited Egypt, immensely old and changeless. Such an impression was strengthened by the architectural monuments, the great pyramids and temples, and by the unchanging statues of the long series of Egyptian kings, whose rule extended over almost three thousand years of recorded history before Alexander the Great entered the land in 332 B.C.

The character of Egyptian civilization resulted in large part from the focus of life on the divine ruler, the Pharaoh. When Egyptian records began towards

47

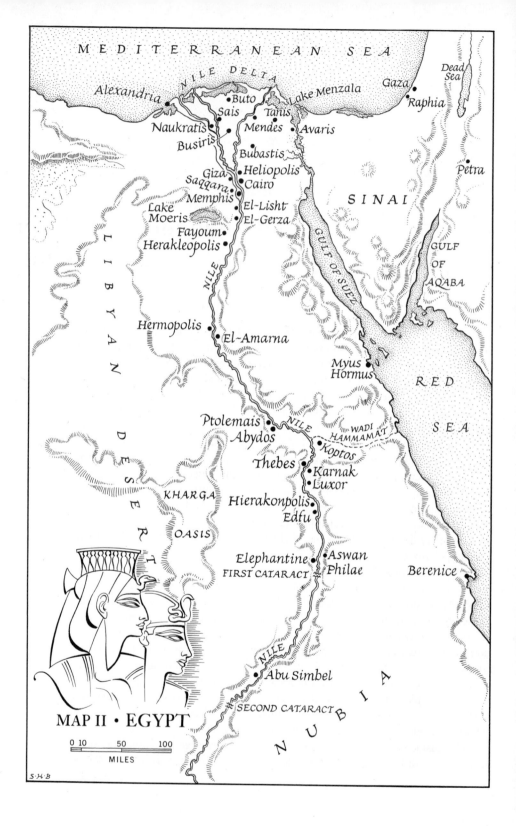

MEDITERRANEAN SEA

Dead Sea

NILE DELTA

Alexandria

Buto
Sais
Lake Menzala
Gaza
Raphia

Naukratis
Tanis
Mendes
Busiris
Avaris

Bubastis

Heliopolis
Giza
Saqqara
Cairo
Memphis

El-Lisht
El-Gerza

S I N A I

Petra

Lake Moeris

Fayoum
Herakleopolis

L I B Y A N   D E S E R T

NILE

GULF OF SUEZ

GULF OF AQABA

Hermopolis
El-Amarna

Myus
Hormus

R E D

S E A

Ptolemais
Abydos
NILE
WADI HAMMAMAT
Koptos

Thebes
Karnak
Luxor

KHARGA

Hierakonpolis
Edfu

OASIS

Elephantine
Aswan
Philae
FIRST CATARACT

Berenice

NILE

Abu Simbel

SECOND CATARACT

N U B I A

MAP II · EGYPT

0 10   50   100
MILES

S·H·B

3000 B.C., the country had already become a unified state under the rule of a sacred king. Soon he was regarded by his subjects as a living god, responsible for their welfare. Around his figure the institutions of Egypt came into being during the period of the Old Kingdom from about 2686 to 2180 B.C. The most characteristic monument of that age, the pyramid, was the tomb of the king and symbolized the magnitude of his position in the eyes of his subjects. The people of Old Kingdom Egypt were satisfied with their mode of existence and concerned to ensure its continuance under the king's direction. Egyptian art and literature reflected this focus of thought, and the institutions of government and society were formed to express it.

The Physical Character of Egypt

The Egyptians called their country the "Black Land" because of the black soil made by the annual Nile flood which was in contrast to the "Red Land," the sand and rock of the surrounding desert. Egypt, in fact, was the valley and the delta of the Nile, stretching from the Mediterranean Sea for about 750 miles to the First Cataract near Aswan, where masses of granite block the river and form a natural frontier on the south. To the east and west of the river was the desert, rising in gradual steppes to the west and to high, steep cliffs on the east. The floor of the valley was a narrow strip, seldom more than seven miles in width and frequently much less. The valley of the Nile, about six hundred miles in length from Aswan to Cairo, at the apex of the delta, is known as Upper Egypt. The delta, Lower Egypt, was a great triangle of marsh, and some of it near the sea coast was salt marsh and unfit for reclamation. In antiquity the delta was cut by about a dozen channels of the river, making their way to the sea and dividing the land into small units. On either side of the marsh was good pasture land. River valley and delta were in natural contrast, and in the course of settlement each acquired an individual quality. Although political unity was achieved early in Egypt, as soon as central authority was relaxed, Upper and Lower Egypt fell back into their old division.

The Nile flood, which reached the area of Cairo in late September, was vital to Egyptian welfare, and the lives of the people were geared to its progress. A low Nile meant temporary famine for rainfall was very scanty. Cairo receives about one and one-half inches annually, while the amount decreases farther up the valley. The flood which of course set the rhythm of agricultural work is reflected in the names which the Egyptians gave to the seasons of the year: Flood Time, Seed Time and Harvest Time. As soon as the waters receded, dikes and irrigation channels were put in order, ploughing and seeding began, and, when the harvest was gathered, the workers tried to grow another where that was possible. The Greeks aptly called Egypt "the gift of the Nile" for the river not only made its annual donation of new land, but it was the source of Egypt's wealth and unity. The stream provided a road of communication through the whole land, helping to bind it together. It provided the soil and water for the chief crops: barley, emmer, fruits, vegetables and flowers. Flowers made honey possible for the Egyptian diet, and they were also the source of considerable aesthetic pleasure. Flax and papyrus reeds were abundant, from which came linen for clothing and cordage, and paper for writing. Fish were taken from the river, and of the wildfowl attracted to it, geese and ducks were soon domesticated, while on the fringe of the desert there was game in plenty. The very abundance of such food perhaps slowed the advance of agriculture in its initial stages. In all, there were about twelve thousand square miles of cultivable land in Egypt, a relatively small but very fertile area. At all periods Egypt was able to feed its population, and in Greek and Roman times produced a surplus of grain for export by means of intense cultivation.

The desert, too, furnished much of use for Egyptian civilization. In contrast to Mesopotamia there was ample stone for monumental architecture and sculpture: limestone and sandstone, easily cut and trimmed for ordinary building material, granite, diorite, and other hard stones for fine lapidary work. Although gold was plentiful in the eastern desert, when that supply was depleted, more was procured in Nubia to the south of Aswan. Copper and turquoise were discovered at an early date in the Sinai peninsula. The Egyptians sought out and exploited the considerable mineral resources of the desert and were able to carry them down the Nile for use throughout the whole land. Egypt's most serious deficiency was suitable wood for shipbuilding and fine furniture. This was supplied, however, at an early date by trade with inhabitants of the Syrian coast, where the cedar of Lebanon was obtained, and of eastern Africa, by way of the Nile or the Red Sea, where hard tropical woods, like ebony, could be procured. On the whole, Egypt did not need to develop an extensive trade to supply deficiencies and tended to be content with what it could get relatively close at hand. For example, the use of bronze and iron was delayed in Egypt long after those metals had been introduced elsewhere in the Near East. Trading, too, tended to remain a project of the king, who sent out expeditions and his own traders, so that the rise of a middle group in society was slower than in Mesopotamia.

The most important approaches to Egypt were along the valley of the Nile from the south and across the Isthmus of Suez on the northeast, where a short strip of desert connects the Nile delta to Palestine. The latter has always been the historic avenue of invasion into Egypt, by which desert nomads, then Assyrians, Persians, Greeks, and Arabs have successively entered and taken over the land. No organized power, however, threatened Egypt from the north until late in its history, so that it was the lands to the south, Nubia and Kush (called Ethiopia by the Greeks), which were of great concern to the early Egyptians.

Beyond the First Cataract the valley of the Nile offered no invitation to agricultural settlement. Lower Nubia, stretching south from Aswan, has been described as a land five yards wide and two hundred miles long. Its rocky desert, however, had valuable building stone and gold, and was a vital link for trade in African exotics: ebony, ostrich feathers, and certain vegetable oils. To control the desert tribes the Egyptian kings established forts along the Nile and ultimately made Nubia, the region up to the Second Cataract at Elephantine, a regularly administered province. Beyond this point the Egyptians eventually penetrated into the land of Kush, the Sudan, to the Fourth Cataract, about 350 miles short of modern Khartoum.

To the east and west of Egypt, however, the deserts were more easily controlled, because neither was a reservoir of manpower like the Arabian and Syrian deserts. The Libyan Desert west of the Nile was probably not as arid as it is at present and had centers of habitation in the string of oases along the river. Control of the desert people, with whom Egypt continuously carried on trade, could be secured by raids or by holding the oases. In fact, one oasis, the Fayoum, near the apex of the delta, became a part of Egypt when Lake Moeris was connected to the Nile to serve as a sort of reservoir for water control. The eastern desert rose into high, rugged mountains between Egypt and the Red Sea, and these, along with the Red Sea itself and the Gulf of Suez, formed a formidable barrier. A track was developed from Koptos on the Nile by way of the Wadi Hammamat to the Red Sea to serve as the land leg of a trading route to the Land of Punt, the Somali coast of east Africa.

Although the Isthmus of Suez was ninety miles of very dry desert, which separated the Egyptian delta from Palestine, it tended to be a corridor of passage rather than a barrier. While it was the historic invasion route into Egypt, it was also the path which Egyptian raiding parties and armies took into Palestine and Syria after 1600 B.C., when Egypt became a powerful, militant state. The coast of the Mediterranean offered access to the sea, but long voyaging was not attractive to the Egyptians. Most of their sea traffic was to the coast of Syria, although in the second millennium some ships traveled to Cyprus, Cilicia, Crete, and perhaps occasionally into the Aegean Sea. The Nile delta was open to sea raids, but raiders did not appear until the thirteenth century B.C., when the era of the first great civilizations of the Near East was drawing to an end.

Prehistoric Egypt (ca. 4500–3100 B.C.)

The successive steps by which Egypt achieved the unity of culture and government, in which its recorded history began about the end of the fourth millennium, are very obscure and difficult to trace. In general, the start and the pace of development were slower than in Mesopotamia. The transition to a food-producing economy seems to have started about 4500 B.C. on the fringes of the Nile valley. At that time the practice of growing grain and storing it over the nonproductive season was perhaps introduced by migrants from Palestine, where it had been known for some time. Egyptian culture, however, was African in character and remained so, with its affinities in Libya and Nubia rather than in western Asia. The valley of the Nile was unfit for habitation until the tasks of clearing and irrigation were started. But by 3600 B.C. neolithic cultures based on agriculture and the domestication of animals had been established in the valley of the river and in the delta. The people were almost self-sufficient: they grew barley and emmer and stored it in pits lined with reed mats; they raised cattle, goats, and pigs; and they wove linen and baskets. While tools and weapons were of bone or local stone, some copper pins and obsidian beads indicate that trade was carried on beyond the limits of Egypt.

We can only conjecture about the process of social development. Probably family groups moved down from the tops of the cliffs along the river to form little village communities on the low mounds projecting above the level of the swamp which choked the valley floor. Cohesion was strengthened in the villages by the common labor of clearing and protecting the land so won by dikes. Probably the villages in a single, naturally defined locality were gradually united into the territorial units, later called nomes by the Greeks. In later Egypt these nomes became basic administrative districts, but each retained old traditions of its own, mainly of a religious nature. Each nome had a town or group of villages as its center. Their local gods were the totemistic animal gods of Egypt and evidently originated at a time when men lived on very close terms with the animals of their environment. The rulers of these early communities were probably like medicine men who ensured the growth of crops and the welfare of their communities by magic. Like their counterparts in African societies of the region in more recent times, the leaders seem to have been killed when their powers failed. In historical Egypt the tradition persisted that the king should die to save the land and that it was his primary function to nourish and to safeguard Egypt by his divine power.

The early settlers of Egypt were short, slender people, fine-boned and delicate-featured, who are identified as native to Africa and who are called Hamites. Their physical characteristics appear still among the Berbers and in southern Egypt. About 3600 B.C. people of a different physical type appeared in Egypt, stockier, broad-faced and heavy in appearance. These were probably Armenoids who came in small groups from Syria and Palestine. Possibly they brought the knowledge of metalworking with them, for after 3600 B.C. the static agricultural communities began to grow and Egypt moved towards civilization.

Predynastic Egyptian pot

This latest phase of prehistoric Egyptian culture is known as Gerzean from excavation at the modern town of El-Gerza. Here we find not only the more extensive use of copper, but also new and distinctive pottery types related to those of Palestine. The Mesopotamian influences, noticed before (p. 26), appeared now and helped to develop the arts of civilization. These were the use of sun-dried bricks and certain architectural principles in building, the arch and the recessing of walls for decorative effect. Cylinder seals were used for a few centuries, and some artistic motifs, which originated in Proto-Literate Sumer, were introduced. But above all, there was writing. Egyptian hieroglyphic writing, like Sumerian cuneiform, originated in pictographs, but from the outset it was more truly pictorial.

Political unification seems to have accompanied these advances in culture, but we have only hints of the process in archaeological evidence and later tradi-

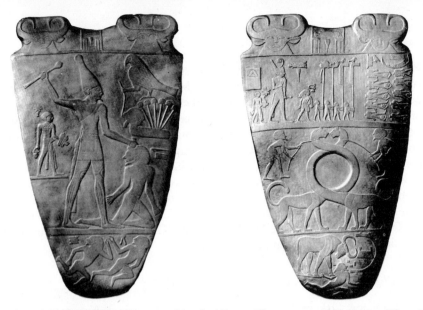

The votive palette of King Narmer who united Egypt. The scenes record his victory. The animals with entwined necks are found also in Mesopotamian art.

tions. In Upper Egypt a general uniformity of culture was established along the valley of the river and presumably the nomes were consolidated into a kingdom under central authority. A similar process of unification took place in the delta, but about that we have little information because of the difficulty of excavation in its watery soil. Warfare flared between the two kingdoms. It has left a record in pictorial representations of battles cut on slate palettes, used to grind malachite for eye paint, and on stone mace heads. Myth told of a conquest by Horus, the falcon-god of Lower Egypt, of Seth, the god of Upper Egypt. In this period the tradition of two separate kingdoms was stamped on Egyptian history, whose records begin with their unification under a single ruler. Such a merging is portrayed on the palette of Narmer, the king of Upper Egypt, who defeated his enemies of the delta, and later in the written chronicles of Egypt where Menes is named as the first king of the First Dynasty. Narmer and Menes are considered to be one and the same person, with whose reign recorded history, the Dynastic Period, began. The palette of Narmer shows the king wearing a double crown, the white crown of Upper Egypt and the red crown of Lower Egypt. On one side the king is represented towering over a defeated foe whom he is about to brain with a mace. Above the latter an embryonic hieroglyph explains the action in symbolic language: a falcon, representing Narmer, is leading a human-headed figure above whose back papyrus reeds grow—the symbol of the delta.

The reigns of the Egyptian kings known to history are conventionally divided among thirty-one dynasties, periods of rule by successive members of the same royal family. The series begins with Menes, conjecturally placed about 3100 B.C., and ends at the conquest of Egypt by Alexander the Great in 332 B.C. This division of the reigns was made by an Egyptian priest, Manetho, who wrote the history of his country in Greek for its first Macedonian rulers,

Ptolemy I and II (p. 405). His work has survived only in summary form in later Greek writers, but the designation of Menes as the first king agrees with other fragmentary lists of earlier date. All the lists have gaps and include names of dubious authenticity, so that reconstruction of the king lists is difficult, particularly for the earlier period of Egyptian history. In addition to this dynastic division, modern scholars also refer to the important phases of Egyptian development by the terms, Archaic (*ca.* 3100 to 2686 B.C.), Old Kingdom (*ca.* 2686 to 2180 B.C.), Middle Kingdom (*ca.* 2080 to 1640 B.C.), and New Kingdom or Empire (1570 to 1075 B.C.). These represent the periods of prosperity and of firm central authority, while the First and Second Intermediate Periods between the Old and Middle and the Middle and New Kingdoms respectively, indicate a weak central authority and political anarchy.

The Archaic Period (ca. 3100–2686 B.C.)

We know little of the kings of the first two dynasties, whose reigns fall in the Archaic Period, for written records were few and the royal tombs have been damaged and plundered. The tombs of the rulers of the Second Dynasty, in fact, have not yet been discovered. The kings came from Abydos in central Egypt, but Menes is said to have established his capital near the apex of the delta by founding the city of Memphis, "White-Walls," from which control could be more easily exercised over both parts of the kingdom. The tombs were built at Saqqara, near Memphis, but apparently in recognition of the origin of the kings in Upper Egypt it was considered necessary to have funeral monuments at Abydos also. There cenotaphs were constructed on as lavish a scale as the tombs at Saqqara. Some hint of continuing political strife is given by the fact that the tombs of the rulers of the First Dynasty were plundered and deliberately set on fire by their successors, but we have no detailed knowledge of the steps by which rule was consolidated.

A noble's tomb (mastaba) *of the Sixth Dynasty. Saqqara, Egypt*

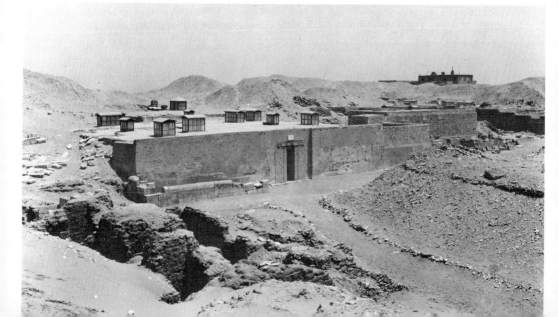

The remains of the royal tombs, despite their damaged and plundered condition, indicate that Egypt became a highly organized and civilized state during the Archaic Period. The tombs, called *mastabas,* were developed from simpler forms of burial used in prehistoric times. In that epoch the earliest graves were pits dug in the desert sand and lined with reed mats, in which the dead man was laid in a contracted position with a few pottery vessels and tools for use in the hereafter. Then the pit was converted into a more permanent tomb by lining the sides with stone or bricks to form a chamber. The royal *mastabas* of the Archaic Period were greatly enlarged by building double rows of graves on each side and at the ends of a great central chamber and by covering the whole complex with a benchlike superstructure of brick. The walls of the bench were decorated by recessed panels as in Mesopotamian architecture and the roof was spanned by large beams of cedar. The central chamber was destined for the body of the king, while around him were buried servants and attendants, apparently sacrificed to accompany their master in death, as they were in the royal burials at Ur in Mesopotamia. The objects left in the tombs, even after the plundering, indicate that the kings were already obtaining luxuries from far afield and that Egyptian craft work had reached a high level of skill. The cedar beams would have been imported from Syria, while objects of ebony and ivory show that trade with east Africa had begun. In fact, a king of the First Dynasty has left an inscription in the Sudan, the memento of an expedition far up the Nile. Copper tools, utensils, and vessels cut from hard stone show advances in metallurgy and lapidary work over the preceding period. The monumental tombs themselves, of course, indicate that the king was able to command and to organize the labor of his kingdom for their construction.

The development of writing facilitated the establishment of an administrative system for the whole of Egypt and probably, too, prompted the development of methods of calculation and of reckoning time. There was need after the havoc of every flood to survey the land, and so mensuration and practical geometry developed rapidly. Towards the end of the Archaic Period a new system of reckoning time seems to have been introduced. The year was divided into twelve months of thirty days each, with a total of three hundred and sixty-five days obtained by the intercalation of five extra days. In this period, too, the practice of dating events by the regnal years of the king was established, and so a body of record gradually accumulated which, at a later date, could be molded into a chronicle of history. By the end of the period Egypt had the wealth and skill necessary to construct the great pyramids which are the characteristic monuments of the Old Kingdom.

The Old Kingdom (ca. 2686–2180 B.C.)

Throughout the period of the Old Kingdom, for about five hundred years, Egypt enjoyed internal stability and prosperity during which the essential elements of its civilization were thoroughly established. The Pharaoh became a living god, ruling absolutely and able to command the services and wealth of the people. The center of the kingdom was the Pharaoh's court at Memphis, where he lived surrounded by his family and nobles. After death his pyramid tomb became a sacred center, the chief monument of a burial complex in which his former associates had their own tombs so that they could be as near him in death as in life. The kings exploited the copper and turquoise mines of Sinai and sent expeditions to Nubia and to Punt for the luxuries which they desired. At Byblos in Phoenicia it is likely that a colony of Egyptians was established to procure the cedar of Lebanon because an Egyptian temple and inscriptions bearing royal names have been discovered there. The local ruling family in Byblos was strongly affected, too, by Egyptian culture. Otherwise Egypt's influence abroad was extended by occasional punitive raids into the Libyan Desert and into southern Palestine. Since no territory seems to have been annexed, the immense wealth of Egypt, apparent in the construction and furnishings of the pyramids and tombs, must have been drawn from the land itself, the private estate of the Pharaoh.

The advent of a new era was marked by the building at Saqqara of the Step Pyramid of King Djoser, the second king of the Third Dynasty. His architect, Imhotep, who became one of Egypt's legendary wise men, is credited with the conception of this new architectural form and with the development of the technique of building in stone. The Step Pyramid is, in fact, the first great stone building of the world. The king's tomb lay under six steps of stone, rising like a stairway to a height of 204 feet. The structure was a logical development of the *mastaba,* made by superimposing one such "bench" upon another, but the form seems to symbolize a new conception of the Pharaoh. Djoser's tomb was not so much a house, in which he lived after death, as an ascent to heaven, by which he joined the other gods. The pyramid was the center of a complex of buildings,

The Step Pyramid of King Djoser of the Third Dynasty (Saqqara, Egypt). On each side of the pyramid are funerary buildings and the mastabas of his nobles.

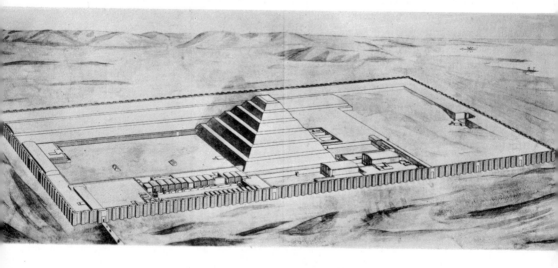

some for the dead associates of the king and some for the celebration of his worship. As a god among the gods, a dead Pharaoh could help his people almost as effectively as he did on earth. The complex was surrounded by a wall thirty feet in height and more than a mile in circumference, a veritable capital city for the dead.

Djoser's was the first pyramid, but the fully developed form of the pyramid was not attained until the Fourth Dynasty, when the Great Pyramids were built at Giza between 2600 and 2500 B.C. for Khufu (Cheops), Chephren (Khafre), and Mycerinus (Menkaure). These, too, were centers of cities of the dead and even more grandiosely conceived. At the edge of the cultivated area along the Nile, a temple was built for the Pharaoh's worship, from which a processional roadway led up to each pyramid and its complex of buildings. Adjacent to the pyramid there was a special building for the cedar boat of the Pharaoh to carry him on his voyages after death. Around the pyramid of the king smaller ones were built for his wives and daughters. The nobles were buried, however, in *mastabas,* as befitted their less important position. All these structures were laid out on an ordered plan like the streets of a city.

The largest pyramid, that of Khufu, combines a remarkable skill in planning and construction with an impressive monumentality. The structure was laid out almost exactly on the cardinal points of the compass, and its corners form almost perfect right angles. This was a remarkable achievement in mensuration for a building which covers thirteen acres of ground and measured 786 feet on each side of its base. The height of the pyramid was 481 feet, and it is calculated that over two million blocks of limestone were used for its construction, some weighing as much as fifteen tons. Granite was used only sparingly in Khufu's pyramid for door jambs and some beams, but the lower part of Mycerinus' pyramid was encased with red granite blocks, and it became the usual practice to use this hard stone for lining the interior walls of corridors and chambers. The working of the stone and its final polishing had to be done with stone tools. Much of the stone was ferried to the building site at high water and the blocks pulled and levered into position up long earth ramps. For a project of this kind, almost all the years of a king's reign and the labor of a very large proportion of his subjects were required. In the buildings of the pyramid complex, as well as in the burial chamber of the Pharaoh, were immense stores of wealth, furniture, weapons, tools, jewelry, and precious objects. To maintain the buildings and the worship of the dead Pharaoh, endowments were created by setting aside revenues from the king's lands. Although the building of pyramids continued throughout the Old Kingdom, those of the kings of the Fifth and Sixth Dynasties were on a smaller scale, and some were of hasty, cheap construction. Evidently the position of the Pharaoh, who could command the wealth and labor of his subjects on such a great scale in the Third and Fourth Dynasties, had begun to decline.

The earlier Pharaohs of the Old Kingdom ruled directly and personally, leading the army and conducting civil and religious duties themselves. Their subjects regarded them as gods, able to provide a good flood on the Nile, protect them from raiders out of the desert, and see to it that justice was done. The Pharaoh was the source of all favors to noble and peasant alike, both of whom were on the same low human level. His exalted position was indicated by an elaborate set of titles to express different facets of his power and divinity. Pharaoh, the word commonly used of the ruler, did not come into use until the New Kingdom. It means "Great House," and refers to the elaborate administration centered in the king's palace which had grown up by that time. The majesty of the kings of the first four dynasties is strikingly represented on their sculptured monuments in which the king, larger than life, towers over subjects and enemies alike. The older hereditary nobility of the Predynastic and Archaic Periods probably still held some place in the Third Dynasty, but they were replaced by members of the king's family and by individuals on whom his favor fell. These latter might in some cases be men of humble birth who had caught the king's eye and were rewarded by gifts of land, titles of office and special assignments. A signal mark of his favor was assistance in the building or furnishing of a tomb. The king would make use of these associates as he desired, and only gradually did a fixed system of administration come into existence.

The great pyramids of Khufu and Chephren at Giza, seen from the Nile

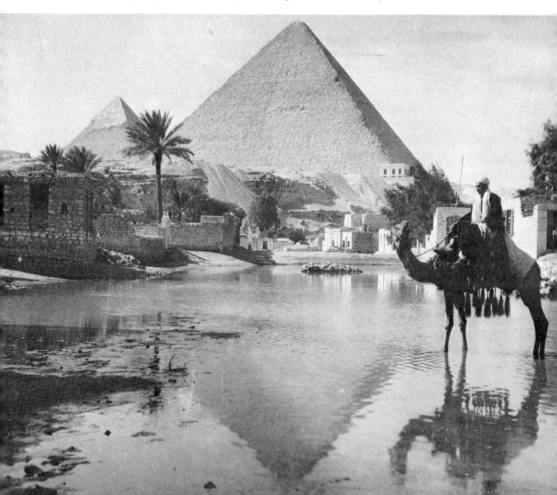

The ordinary people of Egypt were all subject to the king's service, be it military assignments, labor on the irrigation works or on the pyramids and other building projects. There was no regular army, but simply a system of levying men as needed, and the soldiers might find themselves assigned to protect frontiers, to make raids into the desert against the nomads, or to get building stone. Peasants and workmen paid a part of their production to support the divine establishment. Yet the general tone of the regime was patriarchal. Men felt that authority resided where it should, with their chief god. He might be so remote that men feared to touch him, even accidentally, but his personal care and responsibility for his subjects pervaded the whole land.

In the Fifth and Sixth Dynasties, however, other gods, who overshadowed the Pharaoh, rose to prominence so that his office lost its compulsive authority. At the time of the Fifth Dynasty Re, the sun-god of the city of Heliopolis, was honored especially, and the Pharaohs began to call themselves sons of Re. Similarly in the Sixth Dynasty Osiris, a hero-god and ruler of the hereafter, emerged as a great god, and in myth the Pharaoh became Osiris' son, of less importance than his father. Perhaps some discontent had entered men's minds as king after king sought to build a greater pyramid than his predecessor, and the labor and wealth of the kingdom were tied up in such projects for generation after generation. More probably, the growth of an administration to supervise the working of this highly centralized system encroached on the king's authority, and his nobles and officials rose to a status comparable in dignity to that of the Pharaoh himself. In the Fifth and Sixth Dynasties the tombs of the great nobles rivaled those of the kings in size and wealth of furnishings. Moreover, they were built in the nobles' own family districts, instead of around the pyramid of the king. The economic power of the kings had declined, too. A considerable part of their wealth had gone into the creation of endowments for the maintenance of the pyramid cults and much had been lavished on gifts to officials.

A great official, the vizier (or superintendent), had appeared, who stood next in importance to the king, and if the ruler were not a man of strong personality, the vizier might overshadow him. At first the vizier was a royal prince, a member of the king's family, but in the Fifth Dynasty prominent officials were raised to the office and it came to be regarded as hereditary in the holder's family. The vizier executed the king's orders through a hierarchy of officials and scribes, procured building materials and labor, and acted as a judge. Other nobles were placed in charge of the nomes, where they consolidated their family's position and came to look on their posts as hereditary. The new nobles had a following of tenants and workmen on their lands and vied among themselves for favor.

In fact, we know more about some of the nobles of the Fifth and Sixth Dynasties than about their rulers. The nobles inscribed their autobiographies on the walls of their tombs and had reliefs cut depicting the daily life on their estates. The career of one such man, Weni, is illuminating. Weni served the first three kings of the Sixth Dynasty and rose from humble status to the governorship of Upper Egypt. At the outset of his career he was a minor court officer and pyramid priest, then a judge, in which capacity he heard cases of conspiracy in the royal harem. His discretion in this last was rewarded by the king's help in decorating his tomb. Then Weni led five military raids into southern Palestine to chastise the nomads, the "sand-dwellers," and ultimately became governor of Upper Egypt. In this capacity he collected revenues, levied labor, obtained granite and alabaster by expeditions into the desert, cut channels in the river, and built ships for the transport of stone down the Nile.

Although Weni was a loyal official, who ascribed his successful career to the favor of his successive masters, the Pharaoh's authority was gradually undermined by the rise of such figures and by the consolidation of local power in the hands of their families. The last ruler of the Sixth Dynasty, Pheops II, had a very long reign of about ninety years. Evidently his hold on the government was something of a token in his last years, for, upon his death, a tide of anarchy suddenly swept over Egypt. In this First Intermediate Period the nomarchs asserted their independence and the nomes once again became small independent states. The local rulers thought only of their own interests and some claimed the titles and attributes of the Pharaoh. Civil war and disorder became widespread, much of the wealth of the Old Kingdom was destroyed, temples were damaged, and the tombs of the kings looted. Some great families were broken, while others rose to take their place by force of arms. Egypt's foreign trade vanished, and the land suffered to some extent from raids and the infiltration of new settlers from Nubia or from the desert on the northeast. The chief cause of distress, however, was the breakdown of central authority, and for well over a century the stability and ordered regimen of existence which had characterized Old Kingdom Egypt vanished.

It is scarcely possible to trace the political history of this period, in which tradition placed the rulers of Dynasties VII through X because these so-called Pharaohs had very transitory and local reigns. Reconsolidation began from Thebes, far up the Nile from the old capital at Memphis, where an energetic line of local rulers began to extend their power north and south along the river to pull Egypt together again.

A scribe

The Middle Kingdom (ca. 2080–1640 B.C.)

The city of Thebes, on the east bank of the Nile near modern Luxor, had been an insignificant town in the Old Kingdom. During the disorders of the First Intermediate Period, however, the ruling family of nomarchs not only held on to their own nome but also extended their authority along the river valley from Abydos to Aswan. In the southern part of Upper Egypt there had been a considerable infiltration of Nubians, while north of Abydos the land was held by the rulers of Herakleopolis, whose authority as Pharaoh the Theban kings nominally acknowledged. About 2080 B.C. a vigorous king, Menthu-Hotep I, came to power in Thebes and in the course of a reign of fifty-one years reunited the whole land under his rule. By 2040 B.C. the rulers of Herakleopolis had been defeated and the Nubians cowed, so that Menthu-Hotep was recognized as the founder of the new, Eleventh Dynasty. He himself ruled from Thebes and was buried at Deir-el-Bahri in the vicinity. His successor, however, was deposed with some violence by his own vizier, Ammenemes, who established the line of rulers known as the Twelfth Dynasty. They ruled until about 1785 B.C. and in the course of long reigns brought Egypt to a new peak of prosperity in the period of the Middle Kingdom. Under their stable, centralized authority the state made a rapid recovery. Trade was revived and Egyptian influence extended to the Sudan, into western Asia, and the Aegean. The patronage of the kings brought Egyptian art and literature to their classical forms and established Amon, the god of Thebes, as the national god of Egypt under the name of Amon-Re.

While Ammenemes and his successors adorned Thebes and Abydos with monumental buildings and promoted the worship of their respective gods, Amon and Osiris, they preferred to rule from a new capital founded near modern El-Lisht, about twenty miles south of Memphis. Even though the whole kingdom could be more easily controlled from El-Lisht, at first it was necessary for the new Pharaohs to keep a watchful eye on the nomarchs. Since some of them had supported Ammenemes' coup, Ammenemes had to continue their privileges and powers of local government. Yet the boundaries of the nomes were carefully defined and the nomarchs were brought into the king's service by making them responsible for the levying and command of troops from their own nomes. At the same time an administration responsible to the Pharaoh was formed, and by the reign of Sesostris III, the great Sesostris of legend, the power of the nomarchs could be drastically reduced. Sesostris formed three territorial departments to administer Egypt, each headed by an official called the "reporter," aided by an extensive bureaucracy of lower officials and scribes and under the supervision of a vizier.

Because the social structure of Egypt was affected by the suppression of the great landowners, a middle class began to rise, composed of the lesser officials, traders, craftsmen and small-scale farmers. While the power of the Pharaohs thus became absolute once more, the shock which the office had suffered by the breakdown of the Old Kingdom impaired the ruler's divinity. The Pharaohs of the Middle Kingdom dominated by their own personal abilities as rulers and by political means rather than by virtue of being gods. They were, of course, called the sons of Amon-Re, as the new national god was designated, and their patronage of his great temple at Karnak, near Thebes, closely identified them with the national worship. Yet the exalted position of the kings was owed in large part to the vigorous and expansive policies which they pursued.

To the south, Ammenemes I made Nubia a province, and his successors, notably Sesostris III, extended Egyptian control to the Third Cataract of the Nile, into the land of Kush. Forts were built along the river to control the desert tribes and to protect the quarries and trade routes into the Sudan. In this period Nubia became the chief source of gold for Egypt; the deserts were explored widely for building stone, such as basalt and diorite. The route from Koptos on the Nile to the Red Sea via the Wadi Hammamat, opened during the Eleventh Dynasty, was made easier by digging wells to provide a water supply and by regular patrols. The corridor across Suez was protected by a line of forts known as the "Walls of the Prince," and diplomatic relations were established with the petty chieftains of the desert and hills in Palestine. As a result there was an appreciable development of trade and exchange of gifts between the Pharaohs and these Semitic princes. Trade by sea to Byblos was intensified and extended into the Aegean to the island of Crete. Its Minoan civilization (pp. 109-11) developed under strong influence from Egypt and Syria, as Minoan traders brought their fine pottery and textiles to the older lands and became familiar with their cultures.

Egypt, however, made no territorial acquisitions, except for Nubia; therefore, the prosperity and luxury of the Middle Kingdom were founded essentially on Egyptian agriculture and the trading ventures of the Pharaohs. The last great ruler of the Twelfth Dynasty, Ammenemes III, being able to concentrate his long reign of fifty years on internal development, brought Egypt to a peak of prosperity. The desert quarries and the mines of Sinai were intensively worked, and a considerable amount of land reclaimed and diked in the region of Lake Moeris. During his reign, too, new influences had come to Egypt through its widened contacts. Nubians and Semites were absorbed into the population, most as anonymous serfs and slaves, but some became figures of importance in the administration. Conversely, of course, Egypt became known to the peoples of Palestine and the desert as a great center of wealth and luxury.

Upon the death of Ammenemes III about 1785 B.C., a decline in the position of the Pharaoh began. Possibly Ammenemes' reign had been too long to maintain the vigilance necessary to keep the high officials in hand, possibly his successor was a weakling. In any case, a weakening of central authority is indicated throughout the remainder of the eighteenth century by a series of short reigns and weak kings who were the tools of their viziers. Egypt's prestige abroad was maintained for several generations, but by the end of the century Nubia had broken away to become an independent kingdom, while a foreign people, the Hyksos from Palestine and Syria, were established in the eastern part of the Nile delta. The Middle Kingdom had begun to crumble away; by 1640 B.C. Lower Egypt was ruled by Hyksos kings, and a new line of rulers in Thebes seem to have acknowledged the Hyksos as their masters and to have held their own land with difficulty against Nubian encroachment. The Egyptian forts were taken and Egypt pushed back to the old frontier at the First Cataract of the Nile.

The coming of the Hyksos was a turning point in the history of Egypt. During the Old and Middle Kingdoms the Egyptians had been generally secure from foreign invasion, if not isolated. They had acquired a feeling of self-complacency, which was lost in the period of Hyksos rule. From it a new Egypt emerged, aggressive and nationalistic, bent on punishing the Asiatics who had entered the land and pushing Egyptian frontiers to the limit of power. Egyptian tradition of this imperialistic period represented the coming of the Hyksos as a great invasion. The Asiatics swept into Egypt from Palestine, took over the cities of the delta, and pushed up the valley of the Nile beyond Memphis. The invaders were pictured as merciless barbarians, who looted temples, killed Egyptians, and oppressed the land by cruelty and a heavy tribute.

There is, however, little archaeological evidence for such a large-scale invasion and devastation. Relaxation of vigilance in the Isthmus of Suez in the eighteenth century probably allowed some initial infiltration by the people of the desert and then a fairly large-scale migration from Palestine. Since the term, Hyksos, meant something like, "Rulers of the Uplands," the leaders of the migrants were probably the petty princes from the hill country of Syria and Palestine. Their followers seem to have been a composite group, preponderantly Semitic, who had moved into Syria and then made their way south establishing fortress cities. Presumably the movement is to be connected with the general disturbances which were attendant on the breakdown of the Babylonian Empire in Mesopotamia. As we have already noticed, Hittites were pushing into Syria from Anatolia and Hurrians moving westwards across the arch of the Fertile Crescent. These pressures propelled the desert and hill peoples south to the magnet of Egypt. About 1720 B.C. the Hyksos seized a fortress city, Avaris, in the eastern delta. From that center, rule was extended throughout the delta until Memphis was taken about 1674 B.C. Although Memphis seems to have been the effective limit of Hyksos control, the shock was sufficient to break the continuity of rule in the Middle Kingdom and to throw Upper Egypt into some confusion. No doubt the Hyksos expansion was accompanied by some destruction and warfare, but the people of the delta seem to have accepted foreign rule without much opposition. The Hyksos kings were attracted by Egyptian civilization; consequently their names were Egyptianized and they adopted Egyptian customs and religious worships. They were in a sense recognized as Egyptian kings, being grouped into Dynasties XV and XVI by later chroniclers.

The Egyptians, too, learned much of value from the Hyksos. Bronze became established as the usual material for weapons and utensils, replacing copper. The Egyptians adopted a new weaponry: horse-drawn war chariots, the Asiatic composite bow, and various striking weapons. Even the craft of weaving was improved by the introduction of the standing loom. Above all, the Egyptians were shaken from their complacency by the pressure of the Hyksos who provided a stimulus to reorganization. Consolidation of Upper Egypt started once more from Thebes and rapidly grew into a national movement to throw the Hyksos from the land. Beginning with the reign of King Kamose of Thebes in the latter part of the seventeenth century, a new line of rulers drove the Hyksos back into Palestine, recovered Nubia and Kush, and led Egypt to empire in western Asia. Egypt entered the period of the New Kingdom as a strong nationalistic state, able to rule Palestine and to contend for Syria with Mitanni and the Hittites. Since Egyptian civilization had been formed in the

Old and Middle Kingdoms, it would be useful to review its characteristics before discussing the Empire.

Egyptian Civilization

The character of Egyptian civilization seems to have changed very little in the thousand years of history through the Old and Middle Kingdoms. Most Egyptians, of course, were farmers engaged in a continuous routine of agricultural work, set by the annual rhythm of the Nile flood. Because their occupation was unchanging, they tended to accept the traditions of their life as equally stable and fixed. There was a great burst of creative energy in the early years of the Old Kingdom and again in the Twelfth Dynasty, but in general change came slowly in Egypt and worked within the limits imposed by tradition. On the whole, the Egyptians seem to have had a decided bent toward the practical and material side of life, whether in their daily work or in providing for existence in the hereafter, which they conceived of as taking place under conditions similar to those on earth. Yet, of course, ideas did deepen in response to historical experience. As the position of the Pharaoh weakened and his divinity was impaired, the nobles, and ultimately the ordinary people of Egypt, acquired individuality and lived in their own right rather than through their king. We are more conscious of this among the upper classes, but we can get some glimpse of the lives of ordinary people in the paintings in the tombs of the nobles.

The life of the Egyptian nobles and of the upper class of high officials, administrators, and priests was comfortable and luxurious. They might, of course, be very busy with the routine of administration, but had time to enjoy their estates and leisure activities. They lived in great houses with elaborate gardens, orchards, and pools and a variety of buildings for the varied activities on their estates. Leisure might be strenuous; for example, they hunted dangerous game of the desert and river such as the lion and hippopotamus, or they fished and snared the wildfowl of the rivers and marshes. Private life was comfortable and sensibly adapted to the excessive heat. The Egyptian shaved his head to the skull and wore elaborate wigs for ceremonial purposes; he protected his eyes with paint of black or green, and used a wooden headrest as a pillow to allow free circulation of air around the head. His house was of brick, thick-walled and rambling, with dark rooms and courtyards. The lives of the officials were ordered and ceremonious, and they speak of themselves in highly laudatory terms as dutiful, discreet, and prudent. In the Old Kingdom their lives were spent in patient and unquestioning service of the Pharaoh, a testimonial of the stable and conservative society that was Egypt.

Craftsmen and traders worked mainly for the kings and the nobles on commissions rather than for a free market or for trade. Accordingly, a middle class was slow to develop and scarcely appeared before the Middle Kingdom. Because craftwork tended to be hereditary, the craftsmen attained a very high degree of skill, not only in fine works of art but in the objects made for everyday use.

Perhaps the quality of production was higher than among any other people of antiquity, except the Chinese.

The bulk of the people, of course, were farmers who lived in rural villages and worked the lands of the king, of the nobles, and of the temples. In addition, their labor was subject to the king's call for any purpose: work on the building projects, in the quarries, in repairing and extending the irrigation system, and in service on the king's expeditions. To organize this labor and to collect the taxes fixed in agricultural produce, there was an elaborate bureaucracy, whose petty officials seem to have bullied and harassed the peasants. Yet, to judge from the wall paintings in the tombs, the Egyptian peasant was a cheerful, happy worker, satisfied with his lot and accepting it as part of the normal order of life. Herdsmen and farmers were represented joking with one another; women brought out lunches to their menfolk; children squabbled happily, and shepherds went to sleep under a tree, with a dog or a bottle of beer beside them. When the Nile flood failed or the landlords became unduly oppressive, however, the peasant might run away or go on strike. At all times he enjoyed hiding his assets from the bureaucrats and owners, but between laborer and landlord a patriarchal tie existed. Masters were naturally arbitrary and unreasonable, but the farmer expected, and usually got, responsible care. Above all, the farmer felt that ultimate authority rested where it should, with the Pharaoh at the apex of the Egyptian social pyramid.

RELIGION

Egyptian religion, like that of Mesopotamia, was an accumulation of beliefs and practices which had grown through the centuries and were organized and refined sporadically by the development of a theological system or the application of new concepts. In origin Egyptian religion seems to have been associated with the worship of local gods of the villages and nomes, but, when Egypt was united, the Pharaoh became a focus of national worship and the gods important to him were promoted to prominence. Accordingly, at any given time, the religion was very complex and grew steadily more so, for the Egyptians applied their conservatism to religion and added rather than replaced gods.

Deities of animal form predominated among the local gods, although certain trees and plants were endowed with spiritual life, and the universal forces of nature, like the sun, were revered. In the early years of settlement the people of Egypt had lived very close to the animals and birds of the river valley and of the desert steppes. Some were domesticated and put to use, while others were feared and respected, but all were endowed with supernatural qualities. In time these animal gods were partially humanized, perhaps because men observed that animals did act to some degree like human beings. Then they were represented as a composite of man and beast. Anubis, for example, was depicted with the body of a man and the head of a jackal. Representations of the gods were shown on the battle standards of the nomes, and the gods shared the vicissitudes and triumphs of their worshippers, so that in time a loose and shifting divine hierarchy was established. Presumably in this manner Horus, the falcon-god, who was associated with the early Pharaohs, was depicted as hovering behind their heads in a protective manner. Other local gods became patrons of the new arts of civilization, like Thoth, the ibis-god, who was the patron of writing. The Pharaoh officiated as priest of his own god, and when he visited other localities he acted as priest also of their gods. He could scarcely be everywhere, and we may assume that from the outset there were local priests in Egypt. Unlike Mesopotamia, however, there was no implicit conflict between king and priesthood. The Pharaoh, as a god and high priest himself, towered far above them.

The kings of the Fifth Dynasty sponsored the worship of the sun-god, Re, for whom a special liturgy and system of theology was worked out by the priests of Heliopolis. As we have noticed, Re, a universal god, tended to overshadow the Pharaoh himself, and so the latter was spoken of as the son of Re. This worship, more than any other, became a national religion in Egypt which was supported by the kings and adjusted to older traditions. Some of its concepts are revealed in the Pyramid Texts, as they are called, inscribed on the interior walls of the pyramids from the end of the Fifth Dynasty. The texts were religious formulas and spells, designed to help the Pharaoh's entry into the hereafter by their magical efficiency. Some were evidently revised by the priests of Heliopolis to show Re playing a decisive part in the creation of the world and to set him in prominent relationship to other gods. Re, however, suffered some eclipse when the rulers of the Middle Kingdom brought forward their local god of Thebes, Amon. The priests obligingly identified the two as Amon-Re and, under this name, Amon became the national god of Egypt. The Theban rulers of the New Kingdom, who expelled the Hyksos and founded the Empire, continued to glorify Amon-Re and rewarded his priesthood and temple at Karnak with gifts of land and plunder from their wars. Amon-Re, however, as a god of war and conquest, represented the fierce heat of the sun, as well as its universality and gentle, life-giving warmth. This latter idea was closely linked to the older conceptions of Re, and in the New Kingdom its revival was to provoke a religious revolution in Egypt.

A very important part of Egyptian religion was the provision for existence in the hereafter. This firm belief in immortality is usually explained as having originated in the obvious fact that decay was very slow in Egypt because of the extremely dry climate. Thus death might seem a prolongation of life because little change in physical form was apparent. Life after death was pictured in essentially the same conditions as on earth. The dead needed food and drink, a house, tools and furniture and, in the case of the wealthy, servants and animals. Apparently the dead man was thought to center his life in the vicinity of the tomb, and so it was important to preserve his physical identity. This might be done by placing statues in the burial chamber to perpetuate both his memory and his existence as an individual personality. At a later date mummification served the same purpose. The Egyptians seem to have made no very clear differentiation between the soul and the body. Sometimes the soul seems to be

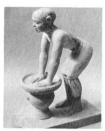

A beer maker

regarded as living a phantom-like existence near the tomb as a double of the personality, *ka,* and sometimes able to leave the body in the form of a bird, *ba.* Several beliefs, essentially contradictory but not felt by the Egyptians to be so, existed about the hereafter. At first, as noticed above, life after death was supposed to go on in the tomb itself, but a more sophisticated age removed the next world more completely from this one. In popular thought it was an underworld like Egypt in that it had a Nile which never failed and a benevolent king. Another more priestly view pictured the next world as lying far to the west of Egypt, the Land of Reeds, a world of the blessed.

At first only the kings could enjoy a proper immortality in their great tombs, but they took care to provide themselves with servants. Apparently the attendants of the rulers of the First Dynasty were killed at the funeral and buried in the *mastaba* to serve their masters after death as they had in life. Later, the practice of building smaller pyramids for members of the king's family and of granting permission to favored nobles to build their own *mastabas* near the royal pyramid extended the privileges of immortality to the king's associates. Sculptured replicas of daily life on the walls of the tombs provided for its continuance without actually killing servants and slaves. In the Fifth and Sixth Dynasties the nobles began to build their tombs in cemeteries near their seats of administration in the nomes, thus usurping the king's privilege of providing immortality, as well as encroaching on his earthly administration. Full democratization of the hereafter came with the rise of Osiris as a god of the dead in the First Intermediate Period and in the Middle Kingdom.

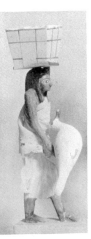

Wooden funerary statuettes of the Eleventh Dynasty. Thebes

In origin Osiris seems to have been a god of vegetation brought by Asiatic migrants to the delta in the prehistoric period and identified there with a deified local king, a hero-god. According to legend Osiris ruled with his step-brother, Set, who killed Osiris, dismembered his body and scattered its parts over the land. Isis, the wife of Osiris, searched out and reassembled them, restoring him to life and to corporeality by a knowledge of embalming. Their son, Horus, avenged his father's death, while Osiris himself became a symbol of resurrection and a god of the dead who could help men to achieve immortality. By the end of the Fifth Dynasty Osiris had risen to some prominence because in the Pyramid Texts he is identified with the dead Pharaoh. In the period of anarchy which followed the Old Kingdom he took over the function of the Pharaoh as a giver of immortality and that of Re as a judge.

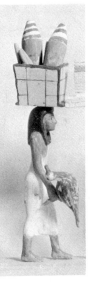

Ordinary men might gain immortality by meeting the requirements of Osiris for admission to the hereafter and by identification with him. While the requirements could be partly met by embalming, an act of magical potency, and by the use of magical spells and formulas, ethical ideas were also involved. To gain the blessings of the hereafter the dead man had to have lived a just life, like that of Osiris, the just king. This extension of immortality was marked also by the use of symbols and formulas, previously reserved for the Pharaoh, on the wooden coffins of ordinary men. These texts, written inside the coffins, are known as the Coffin Texts. By the end of the Middle Kingdom it had become customary to shape the coffins in anthropomorphic form and to paint the picture of Osiris on them to represent the dead man. Texts, known as the Book of the Dead, were written on the linen mummy wrappings or papyrus rolls and placed inside the coffin. These were obtainable at a price from the priests, who in fact conducted the whole funerary ritual. Ethical ideas, however, continued to be associated with entry into the next world, and even the Pharaohs had to pass an examination on their conduct before they crossed a sacred lake to join the sun-god. In this period, too, the practice of placing wooden statuettes in the tombs developed. They are called *ushtabi* figures and reproduce in miniature the houses, stables, workshops, animals, boats and the like which the dead used in the afterworld. Such replicas of the dead man himself were designed to perform the labor which might be required of him in the hereafter.

ART

The art in Egypt was associated almost exclusively with religious ideas. Many art works were sealed in the tombs, thus cloaking the artists with anonymity and to our mind depriving the living of much aesthetic enjoyment. The great stone buildings of Egyptian architecture were mainly tombs and temples, while brick served for the public buildings and houses of the living. During the Old Kingdom the important works of sculpture commissioned by the king and nobles had a magic significance in the tomb, and much jewelry and furniture was made to be buried with the dead. Perhaps because of this predominantly religious purpose, Egyptian artists tended to follow strict artistic conventions which were fixed in the Old Kingdom. Nevertheless, the artists worked with extreme skill and virtuosity within them and made Egyptian architecture, sculpture, and painting one of the treasured heritages of antiquity.

The techniques of building in stone, as we have noticed, were attributed to the architect, Imhotep, who built for Djoser in the Third Dynasty. While these techniques were not his invention (earlier essays had been made and much remained to be learned), he did produce the first great stone building of Egypt and of the world, the Step Pyramid. This gave an impetus to the rapid development of monumental architecture under the patronage of the Pharaohs. They had unlimited supplies of stone with which to work and commanded huge resources of labor. Although the chief impression of Egyptian architecture is its monumentality and grandeur, represented in the pyramids and the temples, the early builders translated the older forms of mud-brick and wood into delicate, crisply cut stone forms. Plant shapes of the lotus and papyrus in particular were used for ornament and for the capitals of columns, while the cutting and finishing of hard stones were exquisitely done.

The principles of building were simple, consisting essentially of a structural system of post and lintel. Stone columns divided areas into small units which could be spanned easily by stone lintels and covered by a ceiling of slabs. The problem of lighting was solved by the development of the hypostyle hall. Two rows of columns along the central axis of the building projected above the others to make a clerestory in which windows were set. Monumentality was achieved partly by mere size, partly by axial planning on the grand scale to lead the eye to the central structure. In the large temple complexes a roadway lined on either side with sculptured figures led to a forecourt, across which a pair of great pylons gave access to the temple area. The temple itself was a hypostyle hall, a literal forest of columns, engraved with hieroglyphs and relief sculpture, behind which were dark inner chambers for the cult ceremonies. Egyptian architects, too, made skillful use of natural features of the landscape, as at Deir-el-Bahri, where great terraces and temples were built at the base of the cliffs, towering above them to form a huge backdrop (pp. 79–80).

The sculpture of the Old Kingdom, both in wood and stone, is also an impressive witness to the confidence and vitality of Egypt at that time. At first only portrait statues of the kings were made to be placed in their tombs, but in time this privilege was extended to the nobility and ultimately to all who could afford it. Since the purpose of the statue was to perpetuate its subject's identity, the figures were reduplicated for insurance. As many as fifty identical statues might be placed in the tomb. The artists achieved a remarkable combination of a realistic portrayal of the individual's personality and, through the conventions which they used, at the same time a portrayal of an enduring type. The figures

Columns in the hypostyle hall of the Temple of Amon at Karnak

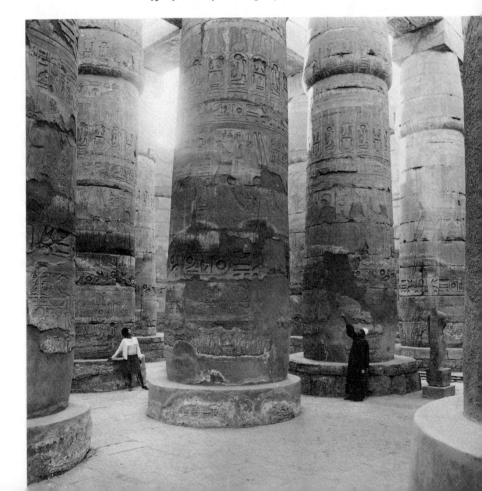

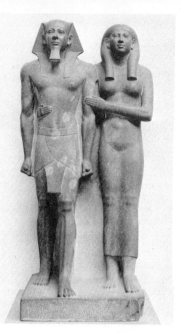

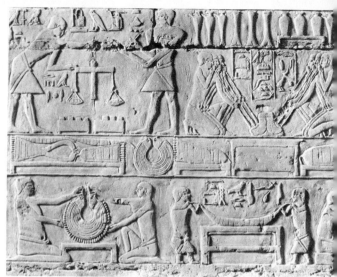

Goldsmiths at work. Relief from a noble's tomb of the Sixth Dynasty

King Mycerinus and his Queen. Fourth Dynasty. Boston Museum

of the kings were strong and vital, whether represented as erect and striding or seated in massive, fixed dignity on a throne. The canons of proportion and the types of representation were set in the Third and Fourth Dynasties and remained fixed. No perspective was used in representation, but the artist combined the most characteristic aspects of his subject—memory pictures—from different points of view. In the relief work, for example, profile-head and legs were combined with a frontal torso. This law of frontality was observed, too, in the portraits, which were cut from a massive cube of stone to be viewed squarely.

Many of the reliefs carved on the walls of the tombs have great historical, as well as artistic value. They depicted scenes of life familiar to the occupant of the tomb, agricultural work on his estate, hunting, boating, and festivals, in which he could share with a nostalgic interest. The reliefs were very shallowly cut and painted in high colors. While depth and imaginative composition were lacking, their subtle linear patterns and color contrasts mirrored a happy and lively world.

There was a decided change of tone in the art of the Middle Kingdom. The royal portraits were equally strong, but the heads were introspective and severe. Evidently the artists had absorbed the loss of confidence produced by the suffering of the First Intermediate Period, and they represented the king as brooding like a statesman on the cares of office, not with the serenity of a god. The subject matter of the tomb paintings changed too, and scenes of warfare replaced those of country life. A new technique came into use, painting in tempera, which imitated the conventions of the preceding relief sculpture. In this period the style of Egyptian painting was set for the future: decorative, lively, and linear in character. In general, the conventions and style of Egyptian art were fixed in the Old and Middle Kingdoms and were to endure, with one significant exception, to the end of Egyptian greatness. In the New Kingdom, in the four-

70

teenth century B.C., a revolution in art accompanied a revolution in religion (p. 85).

WRITING AND LITERATURE

The hieroglyphic writing used by the Egyptians developed from pictorial representations and, like cuneiform, grew into a mixed system of pictographs, ideographs, and sound symbols. Unlike cuneiform, however, the hieroglyphic symbols retained a pictorial appearance and were highly decorative when carved or painted on the walls and columns of buildings. Fairly early a potential alphabet was invented, in that each of the twenty-four consonantal roots had at least one sign to represent it in combination with certain vowel sounds. These signs were never refined into a proper alphabet, and hieroglyphic writing remained quite ambiguous throughout the period of the Old Kingdom. No logical system was devised for spelling, although ultimately usage brought about considerable consistency. Since normally vowel sounds were not indicated, pronunciation of Egyptian words and their transliteration into modern languages are obscure and controversial. The Egyptian scribes, to avoid ambiguities, added determinatives to pictorial signs and phonetic complements to sound symbols. Yet the hieroglyphs remained an esoteric means of communication, only used in later times for inscriptions on temples and walls for formal official purposes.

Two simplified scripts were developed in the course of time, hieratic and demotic. Hieratic writing was a sort of abbreviated hieroglyphic, written in cursive form rather than carefully drawn. It was used for literary and business writing and for ordinary religious purposes. Demotic, a still more cursive form, used for the purposes of daily life, grew from hieratic only about 700 B.C. and continued in use throughout the Greek and Roman periods. Some demotic characters were ultimately used for Coptic, the language of Egypt in late antiquity. Coptic was written mainly in Greek alphabetic signs and was full of Greek words. The last records of hieroglyphic writing were made by a group of priests in the temple of Isis on the island of Philae, far up the Nile near the First Cataract, in A.D. 394.

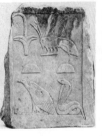

Hieroglyphs

Egyptian writing served a variety of purposes in addition to the religious uses to which it was put, as in the Pyramid and Coffin Texts. There were historical and commemorative records, technical treatises, business and archival records, and an interesting and extensive literature of an imaginative, secular type. The historical records are somewhat disappointing as sources of information. In the Old Kingdom no official records were made of the king's achievements, presumably because he was a god, and so did not need to be commemorated in this fashion. At a later date the reigns were usually described in conventional and stereotyped form, with a great amount of self-glorification. Each king spoke of himself as a great warrior and builder, but in many cases he became so only by using the same descriptions of his exploits as his predecessors. Biographies of the nobles are more illuminating, but because they too were anxious to put themselves in the best possible light they were often more concerned with listing their titles than giving the details of their careers.

The First Intermediate Period had as formative an effect on Egyptian literature as it had on art. The impact made by disorder and suffering on the minds of the scribes resulted in imaginative and psychologically interesting writing. *The Admonitions of the Prophet Ipuwer* described the social upheaval which accompanied the collapse of the Old Kingdom:

> Nay, but the son of the high-born man is no longer to be recognized(?). The child of his lady is become the son of his handmaid. . . . Men do not sail to Byblos today. What can we do to get cedars for our mummies? . . . Gold is diminished. . . . To what purpose is a treasury without its revenues? . . . Nay, but laughter hath perished and is no longer made. It is grief that walketh through the land, mingled with lamentation.

This type of lament became a prototype for those of later times during similar periods of disaster, but many of them appear to have been exaggerated to glorify the Pharaohs who restored order. Another interesting document is an *Argument Between a Man Contemplating Suicide and His Soul.* His soul, which held out for life, won the debate. In the same pessimistic vein are the instructions purported to have been given by Ammenemes I, the founder of the Twelfth Dynasty, to his successor: "Be on thy guard against subordinates . . . Trust not a brother, know not a friend and make not for thyself intimates." The advice loses none of its poignancy by the fact that it was written after Ammenemes' assassination.

During the Middle Kingdom romantic tales became a popular form of writing, the best known of which is the *Story of Sinuhe,* set in the reign of

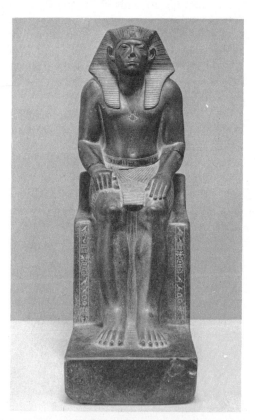

King Sesostris III. Twelfth Dynasty

Ammenemes' successor, Sesostris I. Sinuhe, a minor official at the court, became aware of an important court secret concerning the assassination of Ammenemes and, to ensure his own survival, fled from Egypt to Lebanon. There Sinuhe married the daughter of a king and was given lands and high office as a commander of the king's army. He fought his father-in-law's battles successfully and entertained Egyptian officials who called at his court. Through them he petitioned Sesostris successfully to allow him to return to Egypt, where he wished to end his days. The story closes with an account of Sinuhe's warm reception by the king and the royal family. While the story is skillfully and realistically written, it had, of course, the purpose of glorifying Sesostris as a benevolent ruler. In addition to imaginative literature the scribes of the Middle Kingdom produced many technical treatises; some were on mathematics, which contained practical problems of arithmetic; some were on medicine, which described the practice of embalming. Because the style in which the literature of the Middle Kingdom was written made many of its works classics, they continued to be read and used as models in the scribal schools.

Egyptian and Mesopotamian civilization had much in common: discovery of the techniques of writing, metalworking, intensive agriculture based on irrigation, and institutions with basically religious sanctions. Yet the individual character of each was markedly different. In Egypt unity had been early achieved and remained the normal condition, while in Mesopotamia disunity was the rule, and a single government of the land was attained and kept with difficulty. Each civilization had grown largely in isolation from the other and thus had produced its own very distinctive patterns of thought and life. In the early part of the second millennium, however, the two were drawn together to some degree as the Babylonian Empire reached out along the Euphrates into North Syria and as Egyptian interest in Palestine and Lebanon grew. The great migrations, first of the Amorites from the Syrian Desert into Mesopotamia and Syria, then of the Indo-European peoples into the lands of the Near East, accelerated this process. Both Egypt and Mesopotamia suffered from these movements. Egypt fell under the rule of the Hyksos kings, and the Babylonian cities under the Kassites. Yet the invasions also acted as a stimulus, so that after 1600 B.C. the whole of the Near East, from the Aegean region and Anatolia to Egypt and Babylonia began to coalesce in a common international life.

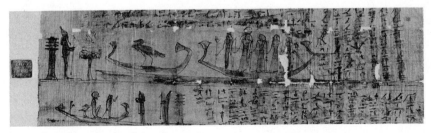

Magical papyrus, showing late script

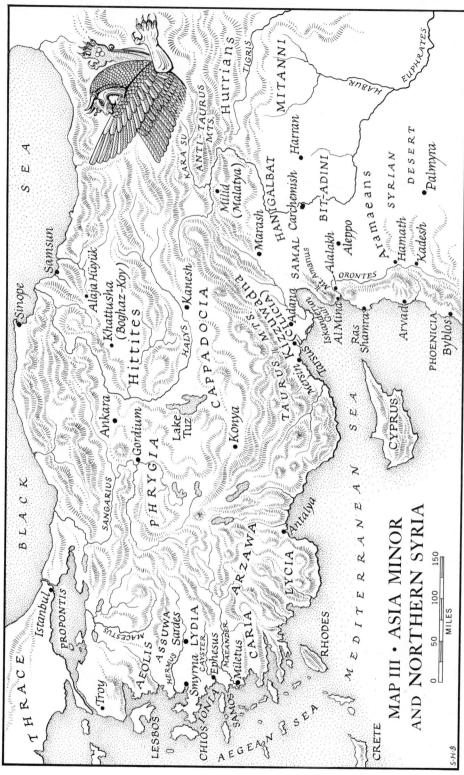

MAP III · ASIA MINOR
AND NORTHERN SYRIA

MILES

0   50   100   150

S·H·B

BLACK   SEA

THRACE

Istanbul

PROPONTIS

Troy

AEOLIS

ASSUWA

LESBOS

Smyrna

LYDIA

Sardes

CAYSTER

HERMUS

Ephesus

CHIOS·IONIA

Miletus

MAEANDER

CARIA

SAMOS

RHODES

CRETE

AEGEAN SEA

MEDITERRANEAN SEA

Antalya

LYCIA

ARZAWA

SANGARIUS

PHRYGIA

Gordium

Ankara

Lake
Tuz

Konya

HALYS

CAPPADOCIA

Kanesh

Khattusha
(Boghaz-Köy)

Alaja Hüyük

Hittites

Samsun

Sinope

KARA SU

ANTI-TAURUS MTS.

Marash

Milid
(Malatya)

HANIGALBAT

Hurrians

TIGRIS

MITANNI

Harran

Carchemish

SAMAL

BIT-ADINI

Aleppo

Mt. Amanus

Alalakh

Al Mina

Iskenderun

ORONTES

Ras
Shamra

Aramaeans

Hamath

Kadesh

Arvad

PHOENICIA

Byblos

SYRIAN DESERT

Palmyra

HABUR

EUPHRATES

CYPRUS

Adana

CILICIA
(ADANA)

TAURUS MTS.

KIZZUWADNA

Tarsus

Mersin

AMANUS MTS.

The Egyptian and Hittite Empires

(*ca.* 1600–1100 B.C.)

A STRONG REACTION began in Egypt against the Hyksos about 1600 B.C., while in Mesopotamia the Babylonian Empire started to crumble under the attacks of new peoples, the Hittites and Kassites. These changes were symptomatic of the effects of the arrival of the Indo-European peoples into the Near East. The impact of the newcomers varied considerably because in some areas they settled and ruled the former populations while in others their influence worked only indirectly. In the less advanced regions to the north, such as Asia Minor and the Aegean area of Greece, the Indo-Europeans were able to impose their languages and social organization and to establish the first large states. In Mesopotamia and across the arch of the Fertile Crescent, although they were able to establish themselves as ruling aristocracies, the invaders were assimilated rapidly to the patterns of a higher culture. In Egypt the effect was entirely indirect. Probably disturbances in Syria had propelled the Hyksos towards the delta of the Nile, but the Hyksos themselves were preponderantly Semitic. Yet they had learned from the newcomers to use horse-drawn chariots and a new weaponry, both of which were adopted by the Egyptians. In general, the Indo-Europeans introduced the use of the horse and new methods and weapons of war and stimulated energy in the older lands, while in Greece and Asia Minor they established new patterns of social organization. We will review first the course of Indo-European settlement and the establishment of new states and then turn to the growth of Egypt as the dominant power of the Late Bronze Age.

The Indo-Europeans

The words common to the various Indo-European languages for animals, trees, and cereals seem to indicate that Indo-Europeans came originally from the temperate zone of Eastern Europe. It is plausibly suggested because of their domestication of the horse that they came from the grassy plains and steppe

In addition to Map III on the facing page, the reader will also find useful for this chapter, Map II on page 48.

lands between the lower Danube and the Volga rivers. By the time the migrants began to move to the east and south they had some skill in agriculture and herding, worked copper and bronze, and were organized in a strongly patriarchal society. With regard to such great mass movements in early history, we can only conjecture about the causes of migration. Climatic change, overpopulation, local food shortages, and a desire to satisfy needs by roving and plundering, congenial to a seminomadic society—all contributed to the causes of migration at different stages. Fairly early, however, the Indo-Europeans evidently split into an eastern and western group because the basic language, by which the people is identified, divided into two main branches. The eastern group of peoples, the Aryans, used what is called the *satam* group of languages, and the western, the *centum* group. They differed in the pronunciation of the gutturals, as these Sanskrit and Latin words for "hundred" indicate. The western languages retained the hard sounds of *k* and *g*, while the eastern converted them into some form of sibilant. The main languages of the eastern group were Sanskrit and Iranian, while those of the western group were Latin, Greek, Celtic, and the Germanic languages.

The Aryan migrants who entered the Middle East settled in Iran and eventually in northwestern India, where they seem to have destroyed the cities of the Indus River civilization about 1500 B.C., and imposed their Sanskrit language and customs on the region. Of those who settled in Iran one group, the Kassites, moved into the western mountains, and from about 1550 B.C. began to take over the cities of Babylonia. We can recognize their kings and gods by the Aryan names, but on the whole the Kassites were assimilated to Babylonian culture and brought little fundamental change to Mesopotamia.

Another group of Indo-European conquerors, the rulers of Mitanni, entered northern Mesopotamia soon after 1600 B.C. They ruled over the population, Semitic and Hurrian, from Assyria to the Euphrates River and into northern Syria, establishing a feudal type of regime in which vassal kings acknowledged the authority of a great king. The capital city of Mitanni, Wassukkanni, lay in the land called Hanigalbat to the northwest of Assyria. The city is still undiscovered. As in the case of the Kassites, the rulers of Mitanni are identified as Aryans by their own names and those of their gods, and something of their history is known from Egyptian and Hittite records. The culture of their land, however, remained essentially Mesopotamian.

The rulers of Mitanni found a non-Semitic and non-Indo-European people, the Hurrians, living across the arch of the Fertile Crescent. They had appeared in northern Mesopotamia as early as the seventeenth century and had subsequently spread westward into Syria and Palestine. The Hurrians were originally from the region of Armenia. Their culture is known, however, particularly from the excavations at Nuzi, near modern Kirkuk, where they had penetrated in the seventeenth century. From their language, which has been recognized and read comparatively recently, it is evident that their culture was greatly affected by that of Mesopotamia. Those Hurrians who remained in Armenia coalesced into a kingdom in the fifteenth century and exerted considerable influence on the Hittites with whose rulers dynastic marriages were made.

Indo-European movement into Asia Minor seems to have begun from the northwest by 2500 B.C., and at the end of the third millennium the western and southwestern parts of the peninsula were occupied by the Indo-European Luwians. Their language is known mainly from documents found in the later Hittite archives. In southwestern Asia Minor the Luwians eventually established the kingdom of Arzawa, for a time a rival and later a subject state of the Hittite Empire. The Hittites themselves entered the region of central and southcentral Anatolia, which was to be the heart of their Empire, from the northeast, probably before the end of the second millennium. They settled and mixed with the original inhabitants, the Khattians, but did not establish a kingdom until the seventeenth century. In the fourteenth century the Hittite Empire was formed, when the Hittites advanced to the west to take Arzawa, crossed the Taurus Mountains to crush the Kingdom of Mitanni, and became the rivals of Egypt for control of Syria.

Greece seems to have received its first Indo-European, Greek-speaking settlers about 1900 B.C. They are usually regarded as having entered the land from the north and having made their way down through the peninsula, although a more recent theory holds that they crossed the Aegean from northwestern Asia Minor. In any case, by about 1600 B.C. the first "Greeks" had absorbed much of the higher civilization of Minoan Crete and were establishing small kingdoms in central and southern Greece (pp. 113–14). From Greece they took to the sea, overwhelmed the centers of Minoan civilization on Crete and followed the sea routes to the southeast where colonies were founded on Rhodes, Cyprus, and along the shore of southern Asia Minor. An intensive trade was established with the coastal cities of Syria, and towards the close of the Late Bronze Age (in the thirteenth century) the Greeks had begun to play some part in the political life of the large states, Egypt and the Hittite Empire.

Thus, from about 1600 B.C. a new order was being established in the Near East. The most important state was Egypt, which reached a new peak of wealth and power in the fifteenth century and became the focal point of Near Eastern history. As the great states extended their influence and came into mutual contact, the lands of the Near East were drawn together. The rulers conducted their relations by diplomacy as well as by war, and traders and officials traveled regularly over the routes of communication from Egypt to the Tigris and into Anatolia to the Hittite cities. Yet, despite this growth, by 1200 B.C., the big states were on the defensive and had begun to fight for their existence. A second and more destructive round of invasions by new Indo-European peoples was beginning. The Greek kingdoms of the Aegean and the Hittite Empire were to be destroyed and Egypt reduced to isolation. But in the Late Bronze Age, between 1600 and 1200 B.C., the early civilizations of the Near East reached their climax.

The New Kingdom of Egypt (ca. 1600–1075 B.C.)

THE ESTABLISHMENT OF THE EMPIRE

Early in the sixteenth century much of Egypt was under foreign rule. The Hyksos kings were in control of the Nile delta and the city of Memphis at its apex, while a Nubian king occupied the southern part of Upper Egypt and encroached on the territory of Thebes. Thebes itself was ruled by a native Egyptian dynasty, the Seventeenth; but as a result of the collapse of the Middle Kingdom the prestige of the kings was low, and challenges to their authority by local nobles and pretenders to the throne were frequent. Yet in the Egyptian people bitter resentment was growing toward the Hyksos, and a militant, nationalistic state was in the making. Recovery began in the sixteenth century under the last two kings of the Seventeenth Dynasty. Sekenenre was killed in violent battle, but his successor, Kamose, won a decisive victory over the Hyksos king, Apophis. Kamose ignored, or temporarily quelled, the Nubian threat to his rear and sailed his fleet down the Nile to challenge the Hyksos king. Victory enabled him to extend Theban territory almost to the Fayoum, but the expulsion of the Hyksos from Egypt was completed by his younger brother and successor, Ahmose, the founder of the Eighteenth Dynasty, who came to the throne about 1570 B.C. The period of the Eighteenth Dynasty, from 1570 to 1365 B.C., was to be the most glorious of Egypt's history. The kings made Thebes into a great imperial capital, and the temple of its god, Amon-Re, at Karnak into the greatest of Egyptian religious establishments. The rulers were buried in the Valley of the Kings to the west of Thebes, while their important officials were entombed in the hills nearby.

Ahmose (1570–46 B.C.) was an able and experienced general who, like his brother, was devoted to the reconsolidation of Egypt. He drove the Hyksos from the delta by taking the fortified city of Avaris and pursued them deep into Palestine, while in Upper Egypt the Nubian king was killed and the frontier restored at the First Cataract. Those Egyptian nobles who opposed Ahmose were crushed, but his allies were rewarded with gifts and titles. Since the restoration of central authority had begun by the expulsion of the Hyksos, Ahmose won general support from the people for his new regime and was able to turn Egypt again into a powerful, ordered state. The Egyptians were proud to serve in the new army, recruited mainly from the middle groups of society and officered by the nobles. The latter could satisfy their ambitions under the warlike and energetic Pharaoh. The army became a professional, standing force, brigaded into chariot squadrons and companies of archers and infantry. They were well trained in the use of the new bronze weapons, chariot tactics, and the deadly composite bow, all of which had been learned from the Hyksos. Ahmose reconsolidated the power of the Pharaoh in Egypt and prepared the tools for Egyptian expansion, but the building of the Empire was done by his successors.

Egyptian expansion abroad began under Amenophis I (1546–26 B.C.) and Thothmes I (1526–12 B.C.). Amenophis I recovered Nubia and made it into a province by a policy of colonization and the appointment of a viceroy called the "King's Son of Kush." The war against the Hyksos was enlarged into a crusade against all Asiatics when Amenophis thrust into Palestine and Syria as far as the Euphrates River, bringing back booty and prisoners of war to impress Egypt with his might. Thothmes I advanced even farther by crossing the Euphrates into the kingdom of Mitanni and pushing up the Nile to the Third Cataract. The ventures into Palestine and Syria, however, were essentially raids for plunder despite Thothmes' boast of extending the boundaries of Egypt.

Palestine and Syria were divided among many petty kings and city-states, whose reduction by a foreign power was very difficult. Because they were constantly fighting or conspiring among themselves, they were ready to join an outsider for their temporary advantage, or were just as willing to turn against him. In this fertile field for intrigue the rulers of Mitanni began to work against Egypt, and consequently large-scale and prolonged campaigns were needed to secure Egyptian control. Projects of conquest, however, were given up for a generation after the death of Thothmes I in 1512 B.C. His successor, Thothmes II (1512–04 B.C.), was a weaker king than his father and had to deal with revolt in Nubia, while his successor, Queen Hatshepsut, preferred to rule in luxurious splendor in Egypt and to make herself a Pharaoh in fact and name.

Hatshepsut (1504–1482 B.C.) was not the first queen of Egypt to rule directly, but the first to represent herself as Pharaoh by wearing the double crown of Egypt and describing herself officially as "His Majesty." According to Egyptian thought, she did have a legitimate claim to the throne, for, as a daughter of Thothmes I and the sister and wife of Thothmes II, she had more divinity than her stepson, Thothmes III, who was the younger son of her husband by a concubine. In Egypt descent was traced through the mother; consequently both the eldest son and the eldest daughter of a Pharaoh by his principal queen were of significance in the succession. In fact the brother normally married his sister as a principal queen in order to preserve the purity of divine descent. However, under the circumstances it was probably more important that Hatshepsut had the backing of a group of powerful officials at the court and that Thothmes III was still a child. He was named king and she regent, but within a year Hatshepsut, adopting the titles of the Pharaoh, kept the young king well in the background.

Hatshepsut's favorite and chief aide was Senemut, a very able administrator, who became the "Steward of Amon" and probably brought the useful support of Amon's priesthood to his mistress. The "king" dutifully rebuilt many temples in Middle Egypt, celebrated festivals, and concentrated her attention on the pomp and circumstance of rule. Her greatest building project was the magnificent funerary temple at Deir-el-Bahri near Thebes at the foot of the cliffs on the east bank of the Nile. One sculptured relief in the temple affirmed Hatshepsut's claim to rule by representing her conception by the great god

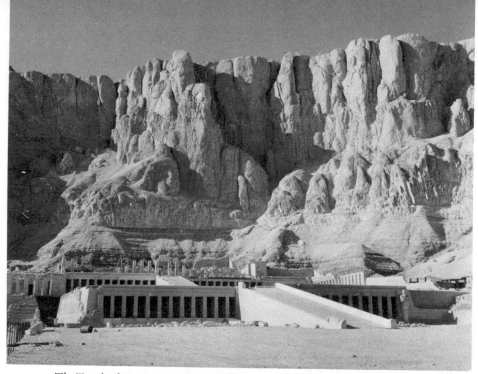

The Temple of Queen Hatshepsut (1504–1482 B.C.) at Deir-el-Bahri

Amon, as well as by her mortal father, Thothmes I, while another depicted a famous expedition to the land of Punt. Hatshepsut's officials were shown among the grass huts of the people of Punt getting myrrh or frankincense (a tree gum), ebony, ivory, gold, apes, and leopard skins in exchange for Egyptian weapons and jewelry. Although Hatshepsut maintained the Egyptian army, no military action was taken in Palestine or Syria, and by the end of her reign a reaction in favor of conquest and war had set in. This desire for war was presumably fostered by Thothmes III, for he seems to have taken over the throne in 1482 with the support of the army. Like an angry lion, he emerged from the obscurity of the military camps to obliterate the records of Hatshepsut's rule and to chasten the Asiatics.

Thothmes III (1482–50 B.C.), the greatest military figure in Egyptian history, established Egyptian power for a century in Palestine and Syria. His bitterness toward Hatshepsut was vented by erasing the queen's name from her monuments and substituting those of Thothmes I and II, as if she had never reigned. His own campaigns were recorded in many inscriptions in the great temple of Amon at Karnak and by the erection of an obelisk, a monolithic needle of stone, 165 feet in height, weighing 445 tons. His campaigns, unlike those of many Pharaohs, were worthy of record.

Thothmes III marched into Palestine and Syria seventeen times in over twenty years, devoting his summers to fighting and his winters to inspection tours and administrative problems in Egypt. His first important victory was at Megiddo, the fortress town which commanded the coastal passage from Palestine into Syria. There he defeated a coalition of the kings of Palestine and Syria, led by the king of Kadesh, an important city on the Orontes River and the key to North Syria. Many prisoners were taken on the field of battle, but Thothmes had to lay siege to Megiddo for several months before the fortress was taken. When the king of Kadesh escaped, Thothmes launched campaign after campaign to win North Syria. He built a fleet and made skillful use of the Syrian coastal cities as bases for thrusts into the interior, in which the land was laid waste and tribute imposed on the local kings. Finally Thothmes took Kadesh itself and was able to push across the Euphrates into the Kingdom of Mitanni. Although the Mitannian king was defeated, Thothmes was too far from his bases to occupy the land successfully. Mitanni remained hostile to Egypt, fomenting revolt among the latter's vassal kings until an alliance was made in the reign of Thothmes IV (1424–17 B.C.) and a Mitannian princess entered the Pharaoh's harem to seal the bargain.

The Empire which Thothmes III had formed was held by putting garrisons into key fortress cities, installing new rulers in the place of former enemies, and taking hostages to Egypt. The sons of royal families were educated there and sent back to their lands in the expectation that they would remain pro-Egyptian. Yet Syria and Palestine never became provinces of Egypt after the fashion of Nubia. Tribute was collected, and many Semites came to Egypt as prisoners of war or as voluntary immigrants, but Egyptian cultural influence was limited to the localities where Egyptian troops were quartered. Egypt's interest was essentially in the tribute and in the goods of trade which the land provided. Thus the Egyptians remained contemptuous of Asiatics, while the Semite rulers grasped any opportunity to renounce their ties with Egypt and to make the Pharaoh pay for their continued loyalty.

The profits of empire, of course, contributed much to Egyptian wealth and pride. The great vizier of Thothmes III, Rekhmire, decorated the walls of his tomb near Thebes with pictures of foreigners bringing tribute to the Pharaoh's palace. Even diplomatic gifts from the rulers of the Hittites, of Crete and Assyria, sent to acknowledge the power of Egypt, were represented as tribute. Thothmes

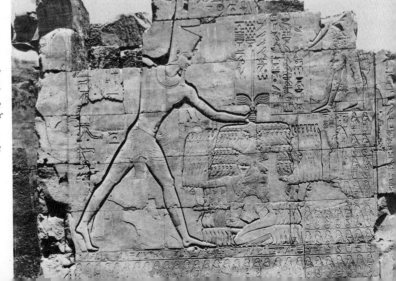

King Thothmes III (1482–50 B.C.) punishing his captives. The pose of the king is similar to that of Narmer on his palette. Karnak

III rewarded the Egyptian gods, the patrons of his Empire, with gifts of land and plunder, founded new temples and festivals, and made Thebes into a metropolitan imperial capital.

Thothmes' successors, Amenophis II (1450–25 B.C.), Thothmes IV (1425–17 B.C.), and Amenophis III (1417–1379 B.C.), were able to enjoy the Empire in relative peace. Their reigns were marked by occasional revolt in Nubia and Syria, but the kings had the power to quell the revolts without difficulty and embarked on no large-scale conquests. As yet the Hittites were too weak to strike southwards across the Taurus Mountains into Syria. The Egyptian kings continued to lead strenuous lives, taking part in military exercises, hunting big game from chariots, and taking care of their administrative duties. Amenophis II, for example, passed into Egyptian legend as a great archer, and Thothmes III set a record of 120 elephants killed in a single hunt at Niy in Syria. During the reign of Amenophis III Egypt reached the peak of power and prosperity. He lavished the vast tribute from the Empire on building and, after the first ten years of his reign, on an unusually ostentatious and luxurious palace life. He built a new palace at Medinet Habu and set a new fashion in sculpture by the erection of colossal statues of himself. One of these, the Colossus of Memnon, was fifty feet in height. Under the patronage of the Pharaoh, Egyptian craftsmanship reached a new level of technical skill and sophistication. Yet in the latter part of Amenophis' reign a turning point in the fortunes of Egypt was reached. The Pharaoh, presumably from the indolence of his advancing age, began to neglect the tasks of administration.

We know a considerable amount about the latter part of Amenophis' reign from the royal archives, found in the palace of his son, Akhnaton, at El-Amarna. The El-Amarna Letters, as they are called, were discovered in 1887 by Egyptian peasants and were widely scattered through private purchase before excavation began on the site. Despite their incompleteness, the documents contain much information about the diplomacy and administration of the Egyptian Empire on the eve of its decline. The letters, written in Babylonian cuneiform, the language used for international correspondence, were addressed to the Pharaoh by rulers of the Near East from Syria to Babylon. Relations were cordial between Amenophis III and Tushratta, the king of Mitanni, and apparently no more than usually irritating to the minor subject kings and allies. It is apparent that Egyptian influence was maintained as much by gifts and subsidies as by garrisons and officials, because the subject kings were unanimous in extolling their own importance and in asking for Egyptian gold. Amenophis' most serious problems seem to have been in curbing this almost whining greed and in keeping his marital alliances in order. His stewardship of both was rather haphazard. For example, the Kassite king of Babylon, in reply to a request of the Pharaoh to add a Kassite princess to his harem, plaintively inquired what had become of his sister, married to Amenophis some years before. Nevertheless, the power of Egypt, as well as its gold, was still real, and the court at Thebes the center of adulation in the Near East.

The Pharaohs, to the end of Amenophis' reign, enjoyed the prestige of military success. The greatest of them had led their armies in person, and they all cultivated a military aspect which strengthened the traditional sanctions of divinity. They were strong absolute rulers in a very personal fashion. The complexity of government had grown since the days of the Middle Kingdom, and under the supervision of the Pharaoh a chain of officialdom led down to the peasants of Egypt and to the subjects in the Empire. There were two viziers, one for Upper Egypt and one for Lower Egypt, who were responsible for the whole conduct of administration and acted as financial comptrollers, judges, and personal agents of the Pharaoh, to whom they reported daily when they were in residence in the palace. Two overseers of the treasury kept account of the taxes from Egypt and of the tribute and booty from the Empire, while the "King's Son of Kush" governed Nubia and another viceroy supervised Palestine and Syria. The number of nomes in Egypt was increased to fifty-five, each governed by a nomarch under whom town mayors and various petty officials acted at the local level. The lands and the population of Egypt were carefully registered and the economy planned to exploit the agricultural production.

While the Pharaoh was still regarded as the nominal owner of Egypt, the amount of land assigned to support the temples and given to favored individuals increased greatly. The temple of Amon, of course, was particularly privileged and drew its support from an estate second only to the Pharaoh's. The Steward of Amon controlled land, serfs, artisans and workmen, herds of animals, and a fleet of ships. The high priest of the god was a great dignitary, appointed by the Pharaoh and high in his councils. Exemptions from taxation were granted to many temples, but this did not affect the revenues seriously, as long as the tribute came from the Empire.

Nubia and Kush became culturally and economically a part of Egypt. Nubians were used as soldiers in the Egyptian army, as police, and as servants in Egyptian families. Some rose to high office and most were thoroughly Egyptianized. On the one hand, as a province of Egypt, Nubian agriculture was improved by irrigation and the population increased; on the other, however, Egypt gained the most by the supply of gold it obtained from Nubia. The mines were a government monopoly, worked by gangs of slaves and criminals. Egyptian influence extended beyond Nubia to the Fourth Cataract of the Nile in the Sudan, where the Egyptians came into contact with Negroes. Some were brought to Egypt and perhaps even sent as gifts to foreign rulers, as a painting on the walls of a palace in Crete reveals. It shows a Minoan officer leading a file of Negro soldiers.

As the Empire developed and as the governing bureaucracy tended to grow into a closed and hereditary class, many officials boasted of their rise from humble birth to high position. For a successful career in the army, the administration, or the priesthood, an exacting scribal education was needed. In the scribal schools, years of training were devoted to memorizing the glyphs, copying excerpts from the Egyptian classics, and acquiring general information. Graduates formed a new nobility of office which took the place of the hereditary nomarchs and local dignitaries. In this society the generals of the army, the high priests, and the great state officials were the leaders and had the ear of the king. The Pharaoh, however, always represented himself as personally making the important decisions of state. The middle groups in Egypt increased in number, drawing their membership from the lower ranks of officials as well as from traders and merchants. While foreign trade remained largely in the Pharaoh's hands, the great increase of wealth resulted in the development of local trade and craftwork. The life of the peasants, however, followed its age-old course, geared to the flooding of the Nile. In the New Kingdom the Pharaohs continued to be dependent on the real elements of power rather than their divinity, and so personal ability in war and government were necessary to preserve their authority. Amenophis III became careless, and his successor, Akhnaton, completely neglectful.

THE REIGN OF AKHNATON (1379–65 B.C.)

Amenophis III died in 1379 B.C., an aging man who had enjoyed the luxuries of his palace too much and who had ignored the tasks of imperial administration. Although Egyptian garrisons and vassal kings still controlled Palestine and Syria, and an equilibrium had been established there by peace and alliance with Mitanni, both the Hittites to the north in Anatolia and the Assyrians to the east were on the move. About the time of Amenophis' death, Shuppiluliumash, the greatest king of Hittite history, came to the throne. He wrote a letter of condolence to the Egyptian court but, when it was neglected, speedily initiated attacks on Mitanni and intrigued against Egypt in Syria. The Assyrians pressed against Mitanni from the east, and the vassals of King Tushratta were split into pro-Assyrian, pro-Egyptian and, ultimately, pro-Hittite groups. At a time when Egypt needed a resolute and energetic king, a youthful, religious fanatic came to the throne, bred in a cloistered palace life and indifferent to the Empire.

The first four years of Akhnaton's reign were conducted in orthodox fashion, probably under the influence of his mother, Queen Ty, the indomitable and powerful principal wife of Amenophis III. Akhnaton retained his alliance with Tushratta by marrying a Mitannian princess. In Egypt he was depicted on the monuments as one who conducted himself in traditional fashion. Then came an abrupt change. When the king's Mitannian wife died, he married his sister, the remarkably beautiful Nefertiti. The royal couple broke with the traditional religion of Egypt and threw themselves into the promotion of a new god, Aton, symbolized by the disk of the sun. Akhnaton, who had reigned up to this time as Amenophis IV, changed his name to Akhnaton, "Serviceable to Aton," while Nefertiti became Nefer-nefru-aton, "Beautiful is the beauty of Aton."

The worship of Aton had begun in the preceding generation and had, in fact, deep roots in Egypt's past, in the worship of the sun-god, Re, at Heliopolis. Yet it contained much that was novel and even revolutionary. Aton was represented in art as the disk of the sun whose rays terminated in hands as if to bestow warmth and life on all living things. Perhaps this conception had been present in the worship of Re. Certainly universalism was shared with Amon, the god of empire, but this representation of Aton remained unique. The new god was almost entirely divorced from the zoomorphic and anthropomorphic associations of other Egyptian gods. Novel, too, in the conception of Aton, was the stress laid on his role as the creator and nourisher of the universe. Apart from Aton, there was only Akhnaton. The king shared the divinity of Aton and spoke of himself as Aton's son and co-regent, but the other gods of Egypt were laid aside.

Akhnaton, as the royal patron of art, was in a position to foster an artistic revolution. The art of the Amarna Age broke with the conventions and formalism of the past to represent its subjects in a frankly realistic fashion. Akhnaton was depicted as a sickly, almost deformed man—pot-bellied and spindly legged—but with a strong, intense face. Nefertiti's portrait, now in the Berlin Museum, has become almost as much a symbol of Egypt for its sophisticated beauty as the pyramids are for the massive authority of the Pharaoh. The royal couple were shown by Akhnaton's artists in intimate scenes of domestic life, eating, playing with their children and talking affectionately in a complete reversal of the stereotype of the Pharaoh which had characterized Egyptian art for centuries.

Akhnaton established a new capital city to symbolize his new regime. It was dedicated to Aton and called Akhetaton (El-Amarna), the "Horizon of Aton." The city was complete, containing palaces, official buildings, a great temple complex for Aton, and houses for officials and workmen, but construction was hurried and flimsy, of brick and stucco and not in the traditional stone. The court and administration moved to Akhetaton from Thebes, bringing with

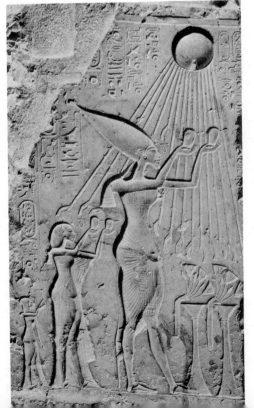

King Akhnaton and Queen Nefertiti worshipping Aton, symbolized as the sun's disk. The rays end in hands to bestow life by their touch. El-Amarna

them the royal archives of Amenophis III, to which those of Akhnaton's own reign were added. Those dignitaries who followed Akhnaton and accepted the new religion were handsomely rewarded with gifts and titles while the traditionalists descended into oblivion.

Akhnaton attempted to discourage the worship of Amon by erasing the god's name from monuments and by cutting off the revenues to his and other temples, but the new faith received little popular following. Aton had a temple in Memphis and apparently one in Thebes itself, dating from the time of Amenophis III, but, in general, the Egyptian people were not affected. The concepts associated with Aton were too difficult and too strange for ordinary men to understand; and, while they might easily assent to the emergence of a new god, they could not forget Amon and their old local gods. Amon, in fact, might seem much more powerful than Aton, under whose patronage the Empire was dissolving. In the Amarna Letters we can read the pleas for help which came from Egypt's allies. The city of Byblos, in particular, was hard pressed by the anti-Egyptian king of Amurru. Akhnaton, if he read his correspondence, paid no attention. Tushratta was assassinated in Mitanni, and his kingdom became a vassal state of the Hittites. Byblos was taken by the king of Amurru, and Shuppiluliumash intrigued and advanced his power southwards toward Palestine. Parts of that land, too, broke away from Egypt. The damage, if not fatal to Egypt, was irreparable. The Hittites became firmly established in Syria, and so the booty and tribute from that land were lost to Egypt.

Toward the end of Akhnaton's reign palace intrigue against the Pharaoh brought about the dissolution of the Eighteenth Dynasty. Nefertiti either died or fell into disgrace, and apparently Akhnaton had to associate himself with

Nefertiti. Idealized portrait *Akhnaton. Idealized portrait*

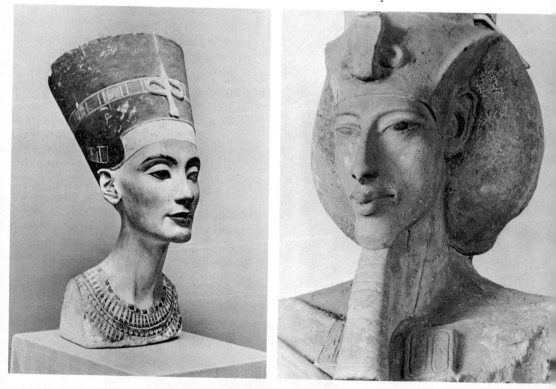

his half-brother, Smenkhare, as co-ruler. Smenkhare returned to Thebes to make peace with the priests of Amon and to propitiate the outraged god. To judge from the sequel, the moving spirit behind the intrigue was a priest, Ay, who later emerged as the ruler of Egypt. But Akhnaton's mother, Queen Ty, although not a convert to his new faith, seems to have been loyal to her son to the end. Akhnaton himself died in 1365 B.C. and Smenkhare shortly afterwards. The new Pharaoh was the well-known Tutankhamon, at this time a boy of eleven, married to one of Akhnaton's six daughters.

Tutankhamon's reign of seven years was spent under the influence of the priest Ay, who became his vizier, and was devoted to reconciliation with Amon. Evidently there was considerable disorder within Egypt itself as well as in the Empire because Tutankhamon's records speak of neglected temples, and the king's own burial, despite its costliness, was very hastily performed. Upon Tutankhamon's death his young wife tried desperately to assert her power against Ay. She wrote to Shuppiluliumash asking him to send her one of his sons as a husband, evidently intending to found her rule on a Hittite alliance. Shuppiluliumash, disbelieving at first, verified that her request was genuine and sent a young Hittite prince to marry the queen. The prince disappeared en route, probably killed by agents of Ay, and the queen was forced into marriage with Ay. Ay's reign was brief, lasting about three years, and in 1352 B.C. the generals of the army with the approval of the priesthood of Amon took the situation in hand. The descendants of Amenophis III and of Akhnaton were thrust aside, and an able general, Harmhab, was put on the throne by a military coup.

Harmhab (1352–19 B.C.) was an experienced soldier and administrator who had served under Akhnaton and Tutankhamon but had not been associated with the religious reform. Under his direction strong government was restored in Egypt. Temples were repaired and supported by new endowments. The epidemic of tomb robbery, which always accompanied a breakdown in Egypt, was checked and corrupt officials severely punished. The memory of Akhnaton's reign was obliterated by erasing his name from the monuments, but the damage which he had done to the state was too great to be repaired. The primacy of Egypt in the Near East perished with the Eighteenth Dynasty.

RECOVERY AND BREAKDOWN

Even though Harmhab restored administrative efficiency to Egypt and his successors did succeed in recovering Palestine and southern Syria, Egypt faced a rapidly changing world in the thirteenth and twelfth centuries B.C. The Hittites had acquired control of northern Syria, and Semites from the desert were again pressing into southern Syria and Palestine, among them the ancestors of the Hebrews. Greeks were sailing out of the Aegean to raid and trade in the southeastern Mediterranean. In western Asia Minor restlessness among its peoples heralded new migratory movements.

In Egypt there was an evident failure in vitality following the religious experiment of Akhnaton. The return to orthodoxy checked the development of the new artistic expression of the Amarna Age and hastened Egypt's decline into sterile sacerdotalism. There was much building, particularly in the reign of Rameses II (1298–32 B.C.), but workmanship was crude and originality was lacking. The temper of the age is revealed in the subject matter of the tomb paintings, where the lively scenes of everyday life were replaced by the Judgement of Osiris in the afterworld. This religious preoccupation was accompanied by an increase in the power and wealth of the priesthood. Temple estates grew in size and their administration almost rivaled that of the nomes in complexity. Spiritually and temporally Egypt was changing into a theocratic state for the service of the gods, and the palace of the Pharaoh giving way to the cloisters, of the high priests. The energetic kings of the Nineteenth Dynasty, however, provided one last century of grandeur before Egypt was eclipsed.

The founder of the Nineteenth Dynasty was Rameses I, a soldier who had served Harmhab as vizier and general. His reign was short but he did establish the succession for his son, Seti I (1319–1298 B.C.). Seti began the restoration of the Empire by a skillfully executed campaign which carried him through Palestine to Lebanon. Egyptian garrisons were put into the fortress towns and local rulers reduced to tributary status. Another thrust resulted in the capture of Kadesh in northern Syria, but Seti was forced to conclude an agreement with the Hittites and to concentrate his attention on other projects. He was able to consolidate his rule in Palestine and found time to start a great temple at Abydos for Osiris, Isis, and Horus. Seti, however, had restored the prestige of Egypt in the north and prepared the way for the grandiose schemes of Rameses II, the last great king of Egypt.

Coming to the throne in 1298 B.C., Rameses held it for sixty-six years until 1232 B.C. in a reign remarkable for its building projects and for the Pharaoh's vainglory. The great military project of his career was the reconquest of North Syria from the Hittites. In 1287 B.C. Rameses prepared a full-scale campaign, leading an army of about twenty thousand Egyptians, Libyans, Nubians, and Semites against Kadesh, which was again in Hittite hands. The force arrived safely in the neighborhood of Kadesh, but Rameses pressed on incautiously with only a part of his army to seek out the enemy, who were lying in wait and ambushed the Pharaoh. Rameses managed to extricate himself, partly by great personal bravery and partly by the timely arrival of the rest of his army, but the campaign was lost. The battle, however, was represented as an Egyptian victory, and its account furnished material for inscriptions and monuments throughout the remainder of Rameses' reign. Since the Hittites held on to North Syria, Rameses had to satisfy his thirst for military exploits by organizing Palestine and raiding into south Syria. He did prevent the Hittites from advancing southwards; consequently in 1268 B.C. the two powers recognized this stalemate by concluding a treaty of peace and alliance.

Both the Hittite and the Egyptian copies of the treaty have survived and give a good idea of the international diplomacy of the period. The pact was made in the name of the two kings, Rameses and Khattushilish, and is rep-

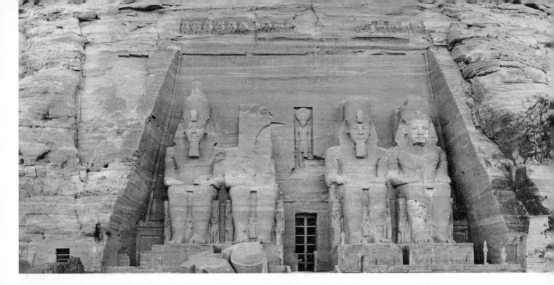

Colossal statues of Rameses II (1298–32 B.C.) before his funerary temple at Abu Simbel. They are over sixty feet in height.

resented as restoring the permanent state of peace which the gods had created. Each king pledged not to invade the lands of the other and to give assistance in the event of an attack by a third party. Provision was made for extraditing deserters, with the proviso that no punishment would be inflicted. The queens of Egypt and of the Hittites wrote to each other as sisters after the treaty was sealed by oaths taken in the names of the thousand gods of Egypt and of the Hittites. A few years later Rameses married Khattushilish's daughter in a ceremony attended by the Hittite king and the soldiers of each army.

The establishment of peace enabled Rameses to devote his full energy to building projects. He had begun his reign in proper filial fashion by completing his father's temple at Abydos and then proceded to glorify Amon and himself. The great hypostyle hall at Karnak was built for Amon and a funerary temple, the Rameseum, at Thebes for himself. At Abu Simbel, above the First Cataract, colossal statues of Rameses were cut high on the cliffs overhanging the river to serve as portals for a funerary chapel tunneled into the rock. Its entrance hall was lined with another set of twelve colossal statues of the king. Rameses found much of his building stone by pulling down the monuments of his predecessors, an easier method than quarrying blocks in the desert and floating them down the river, as earlier kings had done.

The reign of Rameses was the autumn glow of Egypt's Empire. In the reign of his successor, Merneptah (1232–14 B.C.), who came to the throne a tired old man, the first of a series of blows fell on Egypt. Libyans from the western desert, perhaps lured toward Egypt by the increasing aridity of their own land, attacked the northwestern delta with the aim of settlement. They were accompanied by their wives and children and were helped by the Peoples of the Sea. The latter were sea raiders from the Aegean and southern Asia Minor, some of whose names appeared later in Greek traditions as well as in the records of Merneptah's reign: the Akaiwasha (Achaeans), Luka (Lycians),

Turchi (Tyrrhenians ?) and Sherdani (Sardinians). Their object was to plunder rather than to settle. Merneptah defeated this invasion, but a generation later, in the reign of Rameses III (1198–67 B.C.), a second formidable attack was made by the Peoples of the Sea from the northeast. They struck down to Egypt through Syria and Palestine by land and sea. Among them were new peoples, the Danuna (Danaans) and the Peleset (Philistines). The Danuna, perhaps originally Greeks from the Aegean, came from southern Asia Minor, for they are referred to as inhabiting the plain of Adana in an inscription of the eighth century B.C. found at Karatepe in Cilicia (p. 97). Presumably the Peleset were from the same general area, but we cannot locate their homeland definitely. Although Rameses was able to repulse them from the delta, they settled on the coastal plain of Palestine.

In the twelfth century B.C. the pressure of Libyans and of sea raiders on the delta increased. Palestine had to be abandoned to the Philistines and to Semitic invaders, among them the Hebrews, coming in from the desert. The Libyans infiltrated into the western delta and the valley of the Nile. Egypt shrank back to its ancient limits, and once again the natural division in the land asserted itself. The Pharaohs after Rameses III seem to have resided mainly in the delta, at Tanis, while at Thebes, far up the river valley, the high priests of Amon took over. Their succession became hereditary, and in 1075 B.C. the priests became Pharaohs. Egypt's government was thus split between Tanis and Thebes. For the next four hundred years the state was weak and small, maintaining independence precariously and living on the traditions of the past.

The blows which had fallen on Egypt were only local repercussions from another cycle of Indo-European migration and invasion. Before noticing its effects, however, we should discuss the growth of the earlier Indo-European states, the Hittite Empire and Mycenaean Greece.

Anatolia and the Hittites

THE HITTITES

The Hittite Empire, which had defeated Rameses II in Syria and later made an alliance with him, was the first great state to rise in Asia Minor. Its history and organization are known chiefly from the archives discovered in the excavation of the capital city, Khattusha (Boghaz-Koy), about 110 miles east of modern Ankara. The archives are in several languages, in addition to Hittite, and reveal the variety of peoples with whom the Hittites had dealings. Unlike the Kassites, however, the Hittites retained in some degree their Indo-European social and political institutions, although Hittite culture was strongly influenced by that of their predecessors on the Anatolian plateau and by the civilizations of the Hurrians and of Mesopotamia. For example, the Hittites used cuneiform writing and took much of their religious practice from their subjects and neighbors, but their kingship tended to remain Indo-European in character rather than oriental.

The chief centers of the Hittite Empire lay in the Anatolian plateau, the central tableland and dominant physical feature of Asia Minor. The plateau, rimmed with mountains and studded with salt lakes, rises steadily eastwards to the mountains of Armenia. It is cut off from easy access to the Black Sea, the Aegean, and the southeastern Mediterranean which lap the coasts of Turkey. On the north, heavily forested ridges sink to the Black Sea, while on the south and southeast the mountain ranges of Taurus and Anti-Taurus form a barrier toward Cilicia and northern Syria, traversable only by mountain passes. The western edge of the plateau, toward the Aegean, was cut by the valleys of the Hermus, Cayster and Maeander rivers, offering routes to the coast, but these were lengthy and seasonally difficult. The eastern part of the plateau is drained by the Halys River, which makes a big bend to the west before cutting its way through the ridges to the Black Sea, and the western part, later the land of Phrygia, is crossed by the Sangarius.

The plateau was not an easy land in which to live. The climate is continental with hot summers and severely cold winters, but there were adequate resources for agriculture and herding in the sheltered river valleys, while the mountains had deposits of copper, silver, and iron. In antiquity there was also much more timber than at present, and probably the rainfall was greater; so the landscape did not present the same bleak, eroded appearance as it does today. Generally speaking, inner Anatolia was oriented towards Cilicia, Syria and Mesopotamia and its life connected with theirs, while that of the western coast was bound more closely with the Aegean. Far to the east, of course, through modern Kurdistan and Armenia, Asia Minor was connected with the Caucasus and the lands of the Middle East, Assyria, Media, and Iran (Map VI, p. 156). Thus it is difficult to discuss Asia Minor as a unit, for the peninsula was a bridge with avenues to the Aegean and to southeastern Europe, as well as to the lands of the Near and Middle East. Its separate regions might have different cultural and political connections and one area might be little affected by events in another until a considerable lapse of time. Generally speaking, the eastern part of the plateau seems to have remained pastoral for a long period, but in the south and western regions there was an early transition to the metalworking and urban culture of the Bronze Age.

PREHISTORIC ASIA MINOR

Historians know little as yet of early Asia Minor in comparison to Mesopotamia or Egypt because archaeological investigation over its vast area and widely differing regions has become intensive only in the present generation. There are still great gaps in the record and the interpretation of important discoveries is conjectural. To judge from recent excavations in the plain of Konya in southwestern Anatolia, agriculture had been practiced there, and settled communities had formed in the seventh millennium before Christ (above, pp. 13, 17). Yet recorded history began in Asia Minor in the colonies of Assyrian merchants in the nineteenth century (p. 42). Their records contain Hittite names, which indicate that Hittites had entered the land before that time. The Hittites were not then rulers of the land, but Anatolia was organized in local kingdoms, whose kings lived in fortified strongholds and whose people practiced their traditional agricultural and pastoral economy. As the presence of the merchants shows, however, the mineral resources of Asia Minor had become known to Mesopotamia and Syria. Asia Minor supplied those areas with copper. The Anatolian Bronze Age had, in fact, begun about the same time as in Sumer, towards 3000 B.C. Archaeology has recovered something of its early history.

In the Konya plain the transition from Stone to Bronze Age, gradual and continuous, was made by the indigenous population itself. Immigrants into Cilicia from the Konya region probably carried the new metallurgical techniques to the southwestern part of Asia Minor, from where they were transmitted across the Aegean to the island of Crete and to the mainland of Greece (p. 106). The knowledge of metalworking spread also to northwestern Asia Minor and was carried from there into Europe. As wealth increased, urban communities arose, and small kingdoms were formed. The kings lived in heavily fortified citadels. As the objects in their tombs indicate, they had considerable wealth, and in some cases a wide range of trade was carried on. One surprising object, perhaps a royal gift, was a gold chair casing found at Dorak near Troy in northwestern Asia Minor, inscribed with the name of Sahure, an Egyptian king of the Fifth Dynasty. Northwestern Asia Minor, however, formed a distinct cultural region, linked more closely to the Aegean than with the central plateau, as the history of its most important site, Troy, indicates (pp. 117-18).

The arrival of the Indo-Europeans into Asia Minor resulted in the destruction of many of the cities and started a new process of growth in which both the migrants and indigenous population shared. A recent theory develops the view that the first Indo-Europeans entered the peninsula across the Dardanelles about 2500 B.C. Their numbers were small, but about 2300 B.C. the first arrivals were caught up in a massive new invasion which swept from the northwestern corner of the peninsula to the south and east into Anatolia. The cities of western and southwestern Anatolia were destroyed in a wholesale manner. In the Konya plain, for example, every town was burnt, deserted by its population, and the land converted to grazing for the herds of the nomadic invaders. The newcomers are identified as the Luwians, known from the records of the Hittite Empire at a much later date. By that time they seem to have formed the Kingdom of Arzawa in southwestern Asia Minor, against whose rulers the Hittite kings made war.

Little is known about the arrival of the Hittites, the other main Indo-European people of Anatolia. As noted above, some Hittite names are found in the documents of the Assyrian merchant colonies, which proves that they were mingling with the native population in the nineteenth century. It is suggested that the Hittites entered the land from the northeast, coming through the Caucasus and spreading westwards to the Halys River, probably in the twenty-first century B.C. In any case, the main Hittite cities were in the bend of the

Halys, the district which remained the center of their state. The older inhabitants of the Hittite land were known as the Khattians. By the time that Hittite records begin, in the seventeenth century, the two peoples were thoroughly mingled. As might be expected of newcomers in a strange land, the Hittites took over much of the vocabulary of their predecessors and were also concerned with propitiating the native gods whose anger they feared. They borrowed heavily, too, from the Hurrians to the east, adopting many Hurrian gods and myths.

THE OLD HITTITE KINGDOM

A unified Hittite state did not emerge until about the middle of the seventeenth century. Because the Hittites entered the plateau as nomadic invaders, they presumably had to subdue the small kingdoms which were in existence there. At first each Hittite chieftain was intent on carving out a principality for himself. Temporary coalitions were formed, but not until about 1650 B.C. did a king, Labarnash, form a more solid union. He ruled from a capital city, Kushshar, still unlocated, and was able to leave his small kingdom to his son, Khattushilish I. Khattushilish moved the capital to Khattusha (Boghaz-Koy), which was rather far to the north for a center of the kingdom but controlled a broad fertile plain and the communications from the northeast. It was a natural fortress surrounded by deep gorges, which later Hittite kings further protected by an elaborate wall system. These early kings raided down into Cilicia and northern Syria through the mountains, probably bringing back scribes who began the practice of writing Hittite in cuneiform. The farthest thrust to the south was made in 1595 B.C. by Murshilish. He marched across the Taurus Mountains and took Aleppo; then, in a great raid down the Euphrates, captured Mari and Babylon. Internal dissension, however, forced a withdrawal, and throughout the remainder of the sixteenth century the Hittite kings were held to their homeland by dynastic quarrels and by warfare with the Hurrians to the east. About 1525 B.C., however, a usurper, Telepinush, seizing the throne, managed to consolidate the kingship. He issued an edict which set the rules of succession and regulated the behavior of king and nobles. While these were generally followed by his successors, circumstances were not propitious for Hittite expansion in the fifteenth century. Mitanni blocked the way to the south, and although a nominal alliance was made with Thothmes III of Egypt, this advantage was lost when the Egyptians and the Mitannians came to terms. As Egypt weakened under Amenophis III and Akhnaton, however, the Hittites acted.

THE HITTITE EMPIRE (*ca.* 1400–1200 B.C.)

About 1380 B.C., at the time of Amenophis III's death, the greatest of Hittite kings and the builder of the Empire, Shuppiluliumash (1380–35 B.C.), came to the throne. As we have noticed, he wrote a letter of condolence to the Egyptian court, but evidently Akhnaton's behavior convinced Shuppiluliumash

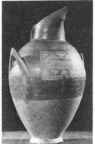

An early Hittite vase

that no attention need be paid to Egypt, and so he set about the reduction of Mitanni. A raid made directly across the Taurus Mountains failed, but about 1370 B.C. Shuppiluliumash crossed the Euphrates River near modern Malatya and attacked Mitanni from the rear. The capital city, Wassukkanni, was sacked and the Hittites advanced into Syria, where the defeat of the king of Kadesh opened the way to Damascus. The Hittites replaced Egypt as the arbiter of northern Syria. Although Mitanni was later lost to Assyria, Hittite control remained firm in Syria. The important cities of Kadesh and Carchemish were held, and the various attempts of the Pharaohs of Egypt to regain Syria were defeated. In Asia Minor the Hittites ringed their homeland with vassal states, ruled by native kings in subject alliance or by princes of the Hittite royal family.

Although the names of these vassal states survive in the Hittite archives, there is considerable difficulty in identifying their locality. Among them was Assuwa which seems to have been in western Asia Minor, between the Maeander River and the Propontis (Sea of Marmora) on the north. Troy, however, was not included in Assuwa, judging from the fact that no Hittite objects have been found there nor have Trojan objects been found on Hittite sites. The name Assuwa seems to have survived into Greek times, when, as Asia, it was applied to the same general region and gradually extended to include the whole continent. In the southwest were Luwian Arzawa, as we have noticed, and in Cilicia, Kizzuwadna, which also had a preponderantly Luwian population. The records mention difficulties with the king of Ahhiyawa, perhaps a Greek kingdom on Rhodes, which held some territory on the south coast of Asia Minor, perhaps Mycenae itself. Yet, as their history indicates, the Hittites were drawn primarily to the older lands to the south of Anatolia rather than to the Aegean. Hittite control over the hill people to the north and east of their land was troubled by sporadic revolts in the thirteenth century, but the only organized state in the latter direction was the Hurrian Kingdom with which they came to terms.

HITTITE CIVILIZATION

The political instability which characterized the Old Hittite Kingdom is to be explained partly by the nature of the Hittite kingship, as well as by the difficulties of settlement. As in other early Indo-European societies, the king was essentially a first among equals, a military leader elected by an assembly of warriors called the *pankush*. He also acted as a priest, sacrificing to the gods in behalf of his people and as a judge in settling their disputes. The *pankush*, however, being an assembly of the warriors, also had some judicial functions. As the Hittites settled down and formed contacts with other peoples, the kingship became hereditary and was bolstered with more sophisticated sanctions of authority. During the Empire the king had an aura of superhuman power and might be called "My Sun." He also acted as a high priest for the whole kingdom, making an annual tour of the Hittite holy cities, conducting festivals and supervising the upkeep of the sanctuaries. Until the end the Hittite kings ruled directly and personally, leading the armies in war and delegating power mainly to the members of their own family. It is noteworthy too that the Hittite queens were personages of importance and dignity, as in Homeric Greek society and in the great households of early Rome.

The kinsmen of the king, his Great Family, held high administrative posts in the palace and acted as generals in the army and governors of key provinces and cities. Their wealth was drawn from large estates and the possession of great herds of animals. Yet it is interesting to find that local government continued to be strong. While the king was regarded as the ultimate source of justice, district elders acted as a court and in the holy cities priests might serve in the same capacity. The Hittite rule was, in fact, like that of Sumer and Babylonia, essentially a rule of law, although the king's will might override the law on occasion. Several fragmentary law codes which follow the model of that of Hammurabi have been preserved. Their articles cover a very wide range of activities and are expressed in the familiar form of cases involving principles. The Hittites also followed the international usage of the older civilizations, as indicated by the treaty made with Rameses II, and used Akkadian for their diplomacy.

Despite the considerable amount of intermingling with the older population, the Hittites were a ruling class, and, as the government of the Empire became more centralized, old privileges, perhaps given at first to win allegiance, were withdrawn. The local courts, for example, were curtailed in jurisdiction and a bureaucracy developed. Yet the indigenous Khattians were not converted into serfs. There were some serfs on the great estates, but the majority of the population remained free, living by farming and herding, which continued to be the basic occupations of Anatolia. Hittite life never became urbanized and sophisticated to the same degree as that in the great cities of Babylonia and Egypt, but retained a military character as a result of the turbulent conditions of settlement and expansion.

Hittite cities were strongly fortified, dominated by a citadel in which the rulers lived, and were enclosed by massive walls and monumental gates. The Hittite nobles formed a very formidable chariot force, fighting in heavier and faster chariots than those used by the Egyptians. A battle axe and short curved sword were the principal weapons of the foot soldiers. But in full levy, as at the battle of Kadesh against Rameses II, the Hittite army presented a variety of weapons and dress, for the king conscripted men from his vassal states as needed: spearmen, bowmen, cavalry, labor troops, and slingers.

The grim massiveness of Hittite art is expressed above all in the fortress architecture. At Khattusha the circuit of the fortification wall enclosed an area of over three hundred acres, and the more open areas were protected by a double line of walls. The inner (and stronger) line was built of rubble masonry packed between two faces constructed of great blocks. The stones of the outer face, in particular, were huge and roughly dressed, giving an impression of crude strength, rather like the Cyclopean masonry of Mycenaean Greek walls (p. 114). Hittite military architecture, however, was quite sophisticated, making use of projecting towers and elaborate entrance systems to bring attackers under cross fire. The gates, protected by flanking towers, were constructed in the form of a corbeled arch resting on great monolithic blocks. These were usually decorated with sculptured reliefs, depicting lions, sphinxes, or warriors.

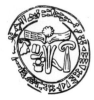

Hittite sculpture was mainly relief work, cut on the gate blocks, or the lowest course of palace and temple walls, or high up on rocky cliffs to form a feature of the landscape. The range of subject matter was small: the king presiding over religious functions, representations of the gods and of religious ceremonies. The chief monument of this type is the gallery of deities and dignitaries at the shrine of Yazilkaya, about two miles from Khattusha, evidently a holy place of the highest importance. The pantheon represented there is that of the Hurrians, rather than of the Hittites, and it is suggested that this assemblage of foreign gods was introduced by Queen Puduhepa, a Hurrian princess, who became the wife of Khattushilish III. It was she who wrote to the Queen of Egypt as "sister," after her husband made his treaty with Rameses II.

Royal Hittite seals

The "thousand gods of the Hittites," by whom the king swore to observe the treaty, were mainly local to Asia Minor rather than Indo-European in origin. Important among them were Teshub, a weather-god, his wife, Hebad, both of whom presided over clouds and storms, and Sharsha, a fertility-goddess, the Hurrian counterpart of Ishtar. The particular patroness of the kingdom, a sun-goddess, was Hittite. Among the hundreds of less important deities one goddess, Kubaba, was to have a very long history. She became the great goddess of the Phrygians under the name of Kubebe and entered the Greco-Roman world as Cybele. Her worship, spread widely through the Roman Empire, was one of those oriental religions which competed with Christianity in the third and fourth centuries after Christ. The Hittite gods were conceived of as human in form, immortal and powerful, and were worshipped in temples. The temple plan had considerable resemblance to the palaces of Minoan Crete (pp. 110–11), in that the structures consisted of a series of rooms and porticoes built around a central open court.

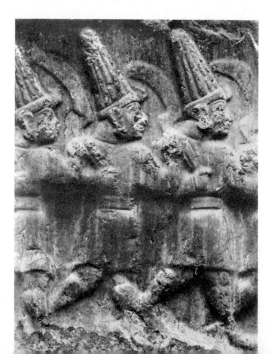

Running Hittite warriors from the rock-cut relief in the royal shrine at Yazilkaya, Turkey

The Hittites seem to have taken over most of their mythology from the Hurrians, and perhaps transmitted some stories to Greece. For example, a cycle of stories was told about Kumarbi, the father of the gods, who won divine kingship against his rivals. There is a similar story told about Zeus in the *Theogony* of the Greek poet Hesiod, who lived in the seventh century B.C. Another story about Kumarbi's wars, the *Story of Ullikumma,* contains elements similar to those in the myth of the Greek Typhon, who warred on Zeus. Probably these Hittite myths came to the Greeks through North Syria where the traditions of the Empire were preserved after the destruction of its centers in Anatolia.

We do not know how the Empire fell, for the Hittite records end abruptly soon after 1200 B.C., when Khattusha and the other cities of Anatolia were destroyed. The invaders are usually identified as Indo-European peoples, Thracians and Phrygians, who entered Asia Minor from the northwest and, like their Luwian predecessors, fanned out into the plateau. Probably the strongly fortified Hittite citadels were attacked continuously and cut off from supplies of food, rather than taken by direct assault. With the centers of the Empire under attack the vassal states had to look to their own safety. Some of their inhabitants were probably among those Peoples of the Sea who pushed down the coast of Syria and Palestine with the aim of attacking Egypt.

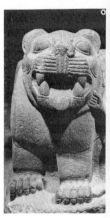

Syro-Hittite sculpture. Supports for the enthroned statue of a god-king of Carchemish

The traditions of Hittite culture were preserved in the southern provinces of the Empire, in Cilicia and northern Syria, where a group of small kingdoms, the Syro-Hittite states, rose to local prominence in the tenth and ninth centuries. These Syro-Hittites (pp. 135–36) were the Hittites of the Old Testament, contemporary with the Hebrew Kingdom. A recently discovered inscription has established a new link between their epoch and that of the Hittite Empire. The inscription was bilingual, written in a Phoenician and a Hittite hieroglyphic version, and was found at Karatepe, a Syro-Hittite fortress city located in Cilicia in the foothills of the Taurus Mountains. The Hittites of the Empire had used hieroglyphic writing for their monuments, in addition to cuneiform, but it had been imperfectly understood. The new inscription added much to the knowledge of vocabulary; its content referred to traditions of the Late Bronze Age, thus attesting the filiation between the two epochs in this provincial region of the Empire. Farther south in Syria and Palestine, however, the Canaanite culture, established there in the Bronze Age, was relatively unaffected by the Hittite rule.

Syria and Palestine

During the period of the Egyptian and Hittite Empires the small states of Syria and Palestine (Map V, page 126) occupied an unenviable position at the political cross-roads of the Near East. Palestine remained for the most part in Egyptian possession, but Syria was caught first in the rivalry between Egypt and Mitanni and then between Egypt and the Hittites. While political independence was extremely precarious under the pressures of the big powers, the cities flourished materially. Their rulers were subsidized, and the cities of Syria, in particular, became the middlemen of international trade. The main land route from Egypt to Mesopotamia and to Asia Minor passed through Palestine and Syria, and the coastal cities were the ports of call for the developing trade with the Aegean, as well as with Egypt.

Palestine and Syria were limited by the Taurus Mountains and the upper Euphrates River on the north, by the Syrian and Arabian deserts to the east, and by the strip of desert between Gaza and the Nile delta on the south. For the most part the land is rough and mountainous, with the coastal strip along the Mediterranean cut off from the interior by high hill country in Palestine and by the Lebanon Mountains in Syria. Although the coastal strip is relatively level in southern Palestine, the mountains reach to the coast beyond Mt. Carmel. Phoenicia, roughly coterminous with modern Lebanon, is divided into small enclaves of territory by the deep gorges which carry mountain torrents to the sea. Since natural harbors are plentiful, the coastal cities of Phoenicia very early began to play the maritime role for which they are known in history. The mountain region is also cut into small valleys and natural enclaves, so that political unity was difficult to establish over an extensive area. The natural pattern of organization, as in Greece, was that of small city-states, each controlling its adjacent territory and striving to maintain its independence. It was both difficult for a large power to control them and likewise for the cities to achieve complete freedom of action.

From the beginning of the third millennium B.C., Syria and Palestine shared in the rapid growth which had characterized Mesopotamia and Egypt. There was a marked increase of population, with the agricultural towns being urbanized and developed into city-states. In this early period Byblos became the chief center for the timber trade to Egypt, and, as we have noticed, probably housed a group of Egyptian traders for the Pharaohs of the Old Kingdom. Many of the cities were heavily fortified, like Jericho in Palestine, both for protection against their neighbors and against raids and invasion from the desert. Semites had entered the land as early as 3500 B.C., but the main influx, which made the population permanently Semitic, was about 2000 B.C. At that time Amorites from the Syrian Desert moved westwards into Syria and Palestine, while their kindred were entering Mesopotamia. Despite the infiltration of Hurrians, Egyptian officials and soldiers, and Luwians and Hittites in the second millennium, the population continued to be preponderantly Semitic and was reinforced towards the end of the Bronze Age by new Semitic peoples, the Aramaeans and the Hebrews. The Semitic population west of the mountains is conveniently, if not entirely correctly, called Canaanite, while that in the interior and on the desert fringe is Amorite. More specifically, Canaanite is used of the northwest Semitic language group, including Hebrew and Phoenician.

From about 1900 to 1200 B.C. the small states in Palestine and Syria experienced a renewed phase of material prosperity and cultural growth, paralleling that of Egypt and of the Babylonian Empire. They experienced also the vicissitudes of the Hyksos invasion, an obscure period in the eighteenth and seventeenth centuries, but in the main their Canaanite culture became firmly established. There was a general uniformity of civilization throughout the whole area, although, as might be expected, Egyptian influence was strong in the south and in Palestine, while the influence of Babylonia was felt in Syria to the north. The practice of writing in cuneiform was adopted, and here too Akkadian was the international language of communication. But alphabetic scripts were developed in the cities to express the Semitic dialects. Perhaps alphabetic writing was used first in Palestine where scripts, dating between 1600 and 1500 B.C., have been found at Gezer, Shechem, and Lachish.

The political structure of the city-states was uniform in this period, in that all were ruled by local kings. Each city intrigued to make the best bargain possible with the great powers or it fought, when that seemed appropriate, to hold its independence and to increase its territory. Yet, because of the diverse nature of the country, there was considerable variety in the cities. Some were hill fortresses, holding strategic passes and valleys in the mountains, some on the fringe of the desert ultimately grew into centers for the caravan trade, while others, such as Byblos and Arvad in Phoenicia, were seaports. Kadesh and Carchemish, as we have noticed, were key centers for communication, on the Orontes and Euphrates rivers respectively. Byblos enjoyed primacy among the Phoenician cities because of its trade with Egypt. A remarkable testimony of its rulers' wealth is furnished by the gold jewelry of Egyptian manufacture found in the royal tombs of the eighteenth century B.C.

Perhaps the best-known example of Canaanite civilization in Syria is furnished by Ugarit (Ras Shamra). The city was situated close to the sea in northern

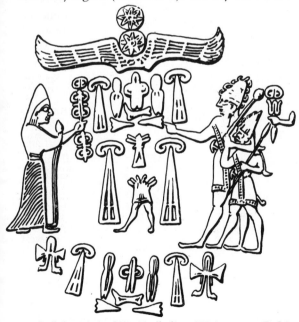

Seal of the Hittite king Tudhaliyas IV (1250–20 B.C.).
The king is the small figure on the right, protected by a god
and goddess, between whom are Hittite hieroglyphs

Statuette of a goddess from Ugarit (Ras Shamra)

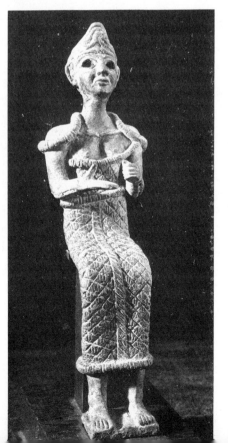

Syria in an advantageous position for trade with Cyprus, the Aegean, with Aleppo and the big cities of Carchemish and Mari on the Euphrates. This position, of course, not only exposed Ugarit to the tides of political change, but also offered commercial advantage. The city, founded about 4000 B.C., had been destroyed in the Amorite invasion at the end of the second millennium but was rebuilt by the new Semitic population. Before 1500 B.C., while independent, it had diplomatic relations with Aleppo and Mari, then came under Egyptian control at the time of the conquests of Thothmes III. About a century later, coming under Hittite rule, it continued to flourish until its destruction by the Peoples of the Sea.

The population was polyglot as a result of the presence of foreign officials, soldiers and traders, among whom were Cypriotes and Mycenaean Greeks from the Aegean. In this period Cyprus became important as an exporter of copper, shipping the metal in the form of ingots shaped like an outstretched oxhide. The Greeks obtained costly articles at Ugarit such as ivory, jewelry and textiles, for which they exchanged their own agricultural surplus of hides, wine and olive oil. Local crafts developed there, for which the copper from Cyprus, silver from the Taurus Mountains, and purple dye from the local beds of the shellfish *murex* provided some of the raw material.

The variety of languages used is revealed in the archives of the main temple and the palace of the local ruler. In addition to the Ugaritic variety of Canaanite, six other languages were written; therefore it is not surprising that among the documents from the temple schools were dictionaries of the various cuneiform scripts. The Ugaritic dialect was written in an alphabet of thirty-one cuneiform symbols, presumably selected and simplified to serve the needs of trade. The temple archives also contained religious texts which throw a light on Canaanite mythology and beliefs. The texts reveal the matrix of thought and practice in which the Hebrew religion developed and offer parallels, too, with Greek mythology.

About 1200 B.C. Ugarit and other coastal cities were destroyed in the second raid of the Peoples of the Sea which swept on to the delta of the Nile, where it was turned back by Rameses III. Probably some of the raiders, as well as the Philistines, settled along the coast and mingled with the Phoenicians. During the same period the desert fringe of Syria and Palestine was assaulted. The Hebrews had begun to enter the central hills of Palestine already in the thirteenth century, and to the north, along the Euphrates, a kindred Semitic people, the Aramaeans, were moving in from the desert. Unlike the Hittite Empire and Mycenaean Greece, however, Syria and Palestine were not overwhelmed. The newcomers absorbed Canaanite culture, and their cities, free from domination by a great power, were able to play a significant part in the history of the Early Iron Age. Before discussing their history we should turn to the Aegean area and to the first civilization of Greece. Greek history, too, was following a similar rhythm to that of the Near East.

V

Early Greece: Minoans and Mycenaean Greeks

(*ca.* 3000–1100 B.C.)

THE LAND OF GREECE was the scene of the first great Mediterranean civilization. In the New Stone Age its inhabitants apparently made their way to the islands of the Aegean Sea and to the Greek peninsula from western Asia Minor. At first the development of Greece was spurred by contacts with the older civilizations of western Asia. The techniques of metalworking and the other crafts, some architectural forms, the principle of writing, some religious concepts, and artistic motifs were owed to migrants and to imitation. Yet the people of early Greece, despite the derivative character of much of their material culture, adapted and transformed their borrowings to express their own needs and individual character. The history of Greece in the Bronze Age is a link from the Asiatic Near East to the first high civilization of Europe.

The island of Crete was the most important center of early Greece. Its civilization is called Minoan, from the legendary King Minos, who ruled at Cnossus, the chief city of the island. But about 1900 B.C., as we have noticed (p. 77), Indo-Europeans entered Greece and introduced the Greek language. These first "Greeks" overran the peninsula and by 1600 B.C. began to take to the sea in order to raid and to trade. They adopted much of the sophisticated culture of Crete, but remained warlike and predatory. The Greek chieftains established small kingdoms, each with a strongly fortified citadel as its center. The best known of these is Mycenae, the seat of King Agamemnon, traditional leader of the Greek forces in the Trojan War. Although later Greek tradition preserved few recollections of Mycenaean relations with Egypt and the Hittite Empire, in the Late Bronze Age the Greeks did share in the life of the Near East in a very real sense. Trade with Syria and Egypt, established originally by the Minoans, was intensified, and about 1200 B.C. some peoples of Mycenaean culture took part in the raids by the Peoples of the Sea on Egypt. Others were

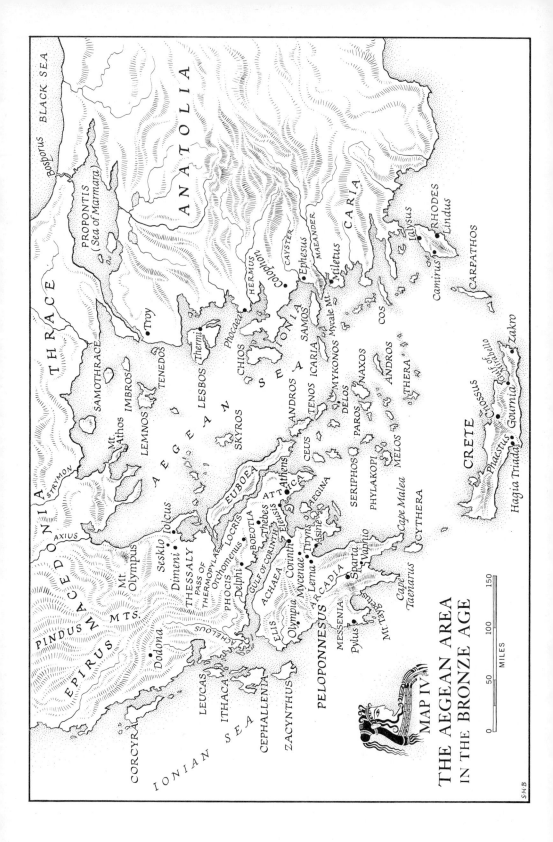

THE AEGEAN AREA
IN THE BRONZE AGE

MAP IV

MILES

0   50   100   150

BLACK SEA

Bosporus

PROPONTIS
(Sea of Marmara)

THRACE

ANATOLIA

MACEDONIA

EPIRUS

PINDUS MTS.

Strymon

Axius

Mt. Athos

SAMOTHRACE

IMBROS

LEMNOS

Troy

TENEDOS

Thermi

LESBOS

Phocaea

CHIOS

AEGEAN SEA

SKYROS

EUBOEA

Mt. Olympus

Sesklo

Iolcus

Dimeni

THESSALY

PASS OF
THERMOPYLAE

Orchomenus

LOCRIS

PHOCIS

Delphi

BOEOTIA

Thebes

ATTICA

Athens

Eleusis

GULF OF CORINTH

ACHAEA

Corinth

Mycenae

Tiryns

Asine

Lerna

ELIS

ARCADIA

Olympia

AEGINA

Vaphio

Sparta

MESSENIA

Pylus

Mt. Taygetus

PELOPONNESUS

Cape
Taenarus

CYTHERA

Cape Malea

DODONA

CORCYRA

LEUCAS

ITHACA

CEPHALLENIA

ZACYNTHUS

IONIAN SEA

ACHELOUS

HERMUS

Colophon

CAYSTER

Ephesus

MAEANDER

IONIA

SAMOS

Mycale Mt.

Miletus

CARIA

ICARIA

TENOS

MYKONOS

DELOS

ANDROS

CEUS

SERIPHOS

PAROS

NAXOS

ANDROS

THERA

MELOS

PHYLAKOPI

COS

CARPATHOS

RHODES

Ialysus

Lindus

Camirus

CRETE

Cnossus

Gulf of Mirabello

Zakro

Gournia

Phaestus

Hagia Triada

S-H-B

apparently in direct military and diplomatic contact with the Hittites. Further development of these relationships, however, was broken by the destruction of the centers of Mycenaean civilization about 1200 B.C. Along with Anatolia, Greece suffered the brunt of the Indo-European invasions at the outset of the Iron Age with the result that its first start was abruptly ended.

The Aegean Area

The Aegean area was oriented by nature to play the historical role of intermediary between western Asia and Europe. Its center was not so much the whole peninsula of Greece as the Aegean Sea itself, with its islands and coastlines in both Europe and Asia. The Aegean opens to the southeast, where chains of small islands draw the lines of travel to Crete, Rhodes and Cyprus, the stepping stones to Syria and Egypt. Along the west coast of Asia Minor are gulfs where large rivers—the Hermus, Cayster, and Maeander—drain from the central Anatolian plateau. But the routes to the plateau were long and seasonally almost impassable, limiting the use of the river valleys into the interior of Asia Minor. Throughout antiquity the seaway to the southeast remained the main line of connection between the Aegean area and the Near East.

Communications from the Aegean to the western Mediterranean and to Europe were not as easy as those to the Near East because of the terrain of Greece. Since the mountains march close to the sea on the west coast Greece naturally turned its back to the Adriatic and to Italy. The Mycenaean Greeks did cross the lower Adriatic to South Italy to establish some trading posts, but their main line of expansion followed that of Minoan Crete from the Aegean to the southeast. Later, from the eighth century B.C., intensive colonization from Greece made South Italy and Sicily a part of Greek civilization. Access to the Danube River valley and to Central Europe from northern Greece was impeded by the mountain barriers of the Pindus and Rhodope ranges. The mountain passes were used by invaders from Europe, but normal communication was intermittent. In fact, the mountainous northern and western regions of Greece, like Central Europe itself, remained a hinterland until the Macedonian and Roman eras. Such trade as existed with Central Europe went from the head of the Adriatic Sea or into the estuary of the Danube by way of the Bosporus and the Black Sea.

The terrain and resources of Greece differ greatly from those of the river lands of Egypt and lower Mesopotamia which are enriched by regular alluviation and irrigation. The streams of Greece are short and unnavigable, and only the largest carry water throughout the summer. Melting mountain snows and heavy rain cause the rivers to become brawling torrents whose fast runoff damages the land by erosion. Greece is a mountainous country whose steep, bare ridges cut the land into narrow valleys and small plains that make travel by land toilsome and difficult. The lower hillslopes are terraced and exploited to the last inch of cultivable soil. Above these shelves flocks of sheep and goats

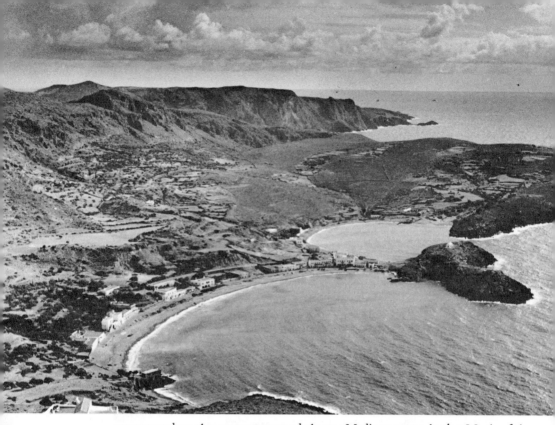

are pastured on the sparse grass and thorny Mediterranean shrubs. Much of the forest growth on the mountains was cut or browsed off at an early date, and in antiquity only the more undeveloped areas in the northwest and in Macedonia were still able to provide timber for shipbuilding. In general, about 80 per cent of the land area of Greece is too mountainous or eroded for cultivation. The proportion does not seem to have been very different in antiquity, so that the balance between production of food and population was easily reached.

The mountains, composed mainly of limestone, contain few useful minerals, and the basic metals needed for ancient economy were absent or in very short supply. There was no tin for the making of bronze; copper and iron deposits were small and scattered. Some regions, notably Attica and Macedonia, did have silver mines which contributed greatly to the prosperity and strength at certain periods, but the lodes were soon exhausted. Throughout Greek history the spurs of want and hunger drove the Greeks to work out very different solutions to the problem of existence than the people of Egypt and Mesopotamia.

Greece also had valuable physical assets. Since the soil and climate were well suited to the cultivation of olives and grapes, olive oil and wine could be traded for metals and grain. The mountains provided a plentiful supply of limestone and marble of high quality for architecture and sculpture. In many places there was also excellent clay for the manufacture of pottery for local use and export. The gregarious outdoor life which was characteristic of ancient Greece was encouraged by a stimulating climate. In the islands and the coastal districts the clear fresh air from the sea offers relief in the hot, dry summers and only in northern Greece and the higher mountain slopes does the winter temperature fall steadily below freezing.

The sea offered means of communication and trade which the mountainous character of the land denied. Along the coast are many little harbors and shelving beaches on which ships could be drawn, while the chains of islands furnished convenient landfalls and lee shores along which boats could run and lay up at nightfall. Navigation in the Aegean, however, had to be seasonal from April to October. In winter strong northeast winds, which were very dangerous for the small ships of ancient Greece, blow from Thrace and the Black Sea. Despite this unifying influence of the sea, the physical barriers to communication were too great for Greece to become a politically unified state. Throughout ancient history, except under extreme political pressure, the land remained divided into hundreds of small states, each cherishing its local traditions and striving to remain independent behind its mountain frontiers. Part of the interest in studying Greek history lies in the variety of response made by individual city-states to the limitations of their environment.

Settlement

The rhythm of growth was slower in early Greece than in the lands of the Near East because Greece seems to have been settled rather later and was re-

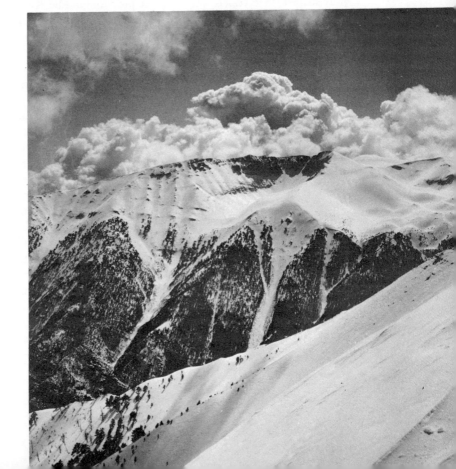

Above, left: Greek coastal landscape. The Island of Cythera

Mt. Olympus in Thessaly

mote from their important early centers. We know very little as yet about the Old Stone Age in Greece, and the traces of the earliest agricultural communities of the New Stone Age are just being revealed. While incipient agriculture seems to have started almost as early as in southwestern Anatolia (p. 11), developed communities formed more slowly. They are known from about 5500 B.C. in the fertile plains of Thessaly, Central Greece, the northeastern Peloponnesus, and at Cnossus in Crete. The pottery found in the villages gives us a clue to the origin of the population, for influences from western Asia Minor are apparent in the shapes and decoration. Probably settlers had spread across the islands of the Aegean and around its northern shore. Since conditions of life in Greece were generally peaceful, the typical form of community was the small unfortified village. The settlers began clearing and cultivating the land, but increase of population and extension of the settlements was gradual. Even the introduction of metalworking early in the third millennium did little to accelerate the process of urbanization.

Metalworking in Greece began about a thousand years after it did in Sumer after another wave of migration from southwestern Asia Minor. There is more tangible evidence of these connections in the Early Bronze Age than the influences revealed by pottery. At Lerna in the northeastern Peloponnesus the massive foundations of a large building reminiscent in plan of structures in southwestern Anatolia have been found. It is probably to be identified as the palace of the rulers. On the little offshore island of Mochlos near Crete beautifully shaped stone vessels, akin to those produced in Old Kingdom Egypt, were made. Crete had begun to enter the cultural circle of the East and its rate of growth was accelerated. The island had an area of about 3400 square miles; its central part contained relatively large, fertile plains and good harbors. The central and eastern half of the island soon became studded with growing settlements, which from 2000 B.C. developed rapidly, outdistancing the Greek peninsula where a new beginning had to be made.

About 1900 B.C., Indo-Europeans, probably the first people to speak Greek, began to enter and spread through the peninsula. The newcomers are usually regarded as entering Greece directly from the north, but recently it has been suggested that this movement into Greece was an offshoot of the Indo-European migration into Asia Minor (p. 92). The invaders were nomadic and warlike, intent at first on plunder and destruction rather than settlement. In Thessaly, where the stagnant neolithic culture was lingering on, their impress is probably to be seen in the rough fortification walls thrown around older towns at Sesklo and Dimeni and in the introduction of a type of house called the megaron. It consisted of a narrow rectangular room with a hearth in the center and the side walls extended to make a protective porch. The invaders burnt and plundered the towns of the Early Bronze Age, sometimes settling on the ashes, if the site pleased them, but frequently founding new settlements chosen with an eye to communication and defense. Several hundred years of adjustment and reorganization were necessary, but by 1600 B.C. the Greeks of the peninsula had formed stable communities and had begun to adopt elements of the Minoan culture. The fusion of these elements, Minoan and Greek, produced the widespread Mycenaean culture of Greece in the Late Bronze Age, which is known to us through later Greek tradition and modern archaeological excavation.

The Discovery of Prehistoric Greece

The civilization of Crete (Minoan) and its adaptation by the invading Greeks (Mycenaean) were known to the later Greeks themselves only through legends, such as the story of Theseus and the Minotaur or the Trojan War, which Homer used in the *Iliad*. These stories pictured Crete as the center of a sea empire ruled by King Minos and the peninsula of Greece as divided into kingdoms whose rulers were the heroes of the war against Troy. The rational skepticism of historical scholarship in the nineteenth century firmly dismissed these traditions as the fiction of legend and saga. Probably the narrative detail is fictitious, but archaeological investigation, beginning with the site of Troy in the 1870's, has established the reality of the historical setting of the tales. We can understand something, too, of the religious and artistic concepts of Minoan and Mycenaean Greece from the material environment revealed by excavation. A more detailed knowledge of social institutions and organization, which written documents can give, has been made increasingly available since 1953. In that year decipherment of the writing on clay tablets (Linear B script), discovered at Pylus in Messenia and at Cnossus in Crete, was made by Michael Ventris, a gifted young linguist and cryptanalyst. Interpretation of the documents remains controversial and uncertain, but they reveal a highly organized economy centered in the king's palace, similar in character to that of the contemporary kingdoms of the Near East. The documents from Pylus, however, are from the administrative archives of a brief period of time at the end of the Mycenaean civilization. They do not give even a chronological skeleton of Mycenaean history, let alone the information needed for a full reconstruction. Knowledge of prehistoric Greece still relies largely on the results of excavation.

The founder of prehistoric archaeology in Greece was Heinrich Schliemann, a retired German businessman whose profitable grain exporting business in Russia provided the means to test his idea that the Greece of Homer's heroes had actually existed. In 1870 he began the excavation of Troy (Hissarlik) and had the good fortune to find the impressive remains, including a royal treasure of gold, of a city which he identified as Homeric Troy. Subsequent excavation and checking have established that Schliemann's "Homeric" city (pp. 117–18) should be dated about 2000 B.C. and that he had cut through the levels of the Troy of the traditional period of the Trojan War in the thirteenth century. Yet Schliemann's excavations at Troy demonstrated the possibility of reconstructing the prehistory of Greece. He went on to excavate at Mycenae, Agamemnon's city, where he again found gold treasure in the royal burials. He planned to excavate also at Cnossus in Crete, the city of King Minos, but was prevented by political disturbances on the island which was then under Turkish control. The Minoan civilization, which had preceded the Mycenaean, was later revealed by Sir Arthur Evans who began in 1900 a lengthy excavation at Cnossus. The well-preserved palace and striking remains of its art tended to overshadow and obscure the significance of the Mycenaean development on the Greek peninsula until the balance was corrected by further excavation and study, notably at Mycenae and Pylus, and by the decipherment of the Mycenaean inscriptions.[1]

Minoan Civilization

The promise apparent in the growth of Crete in the Early Bronze Age was fulfilled in the Middle Minoan Period (2100–1600 B.C.), during which the island reached its peak of prosperity. More land was brought under cultivation, sea trade was intensified, especially with Syria and Egypt, and colonies were established on some Aegean islands. Although all the Minoan towns grew in size and population, two in the central part of Crete forged ahead of the others— Cnossus, near the north coast, and across the island, Phaestus. Both were wealthy and evidently had established political control of their adjacent districts, from which they drew revenues. We do not know in what relationship each stood to the other, but we do know that intercourse between the cities was continuous, for a good road through the mountains had been built to connect them. This centralization was accompanied by a greater uniformity of culture as the small towns on Crete followed the fashion of the large centers. All seemed

---

[1] The archaeological work has provided a chronological framework for prehistoric Greece by which we can study its development. The name, Minoan, is applied to Cretan culture, and Helladic (since the Greeks' name for their land was, and still is, Hellas) to that of the Greek peninsula. Mycenaean is used for the Greek culture of the period from 1400–1100 B.C., when its most important center seems to have been Mycenae. The dates are obtained by cross-connections, mainly with Egypt, and by study of the stratification and cross-connections of the Aegean sites. Such dates are, of course, approximations and are still provisional. A third cultural region, the Cycladic, so-called because it comprised the Cyclades islands of the Aegean, is still very imperfectly known.

AEGEAN AREA

New Stone Age: 6500(?)–2900 B.C.

Crete		Greek Peninsula	
Early Bronze Age: 2900–2100 B.C.			
Early Minoan I		Early Helladic I	
Early Minoan II	2900–2100	Early Helladic II	2800–1900
Early Minoan III		Early Helladic III	
Middle Bronze Age: 2100–1600 B.C.			
Middle Minoan I	2100–1900	Middle Helladic I	
Middle Minoan II	1900–1750	Middle Helladic II	1900–1580
Middle Minoan III	1750–1600	Middle Helladic III	
Late Bronze Age: 1600–1150 B.C.			
Late Minoan I	1600–1500	Late Helladic I	1580–1500
Late Minoan II	1500–1400	Late Helladic II	1500–1425
Late Minoan III	1400–1150	Late Helladic III	1425–1150

to live in peace, because the towns were unwalled and their wealth was evidently spent on the cultivation of an increasingly sophisticated and comfortable life.

This peaceful growth enabled the Cretans to expand and diversify their exports by sea and to establish that maritime activity in the Aegean, which was remembered in Greek tradition. Their pottery, which good craftsmanship and the fine clays of Crete brought to perfection, has beeen found in Egypt, Syria, and the southern islands of the Aegean. The export, which reached its greatest range and volume towards 1600 B.C., probably included olive oil, textiles, and metalware in addition to pottery. The Minoans imported exotic luxuries from Egypt and Syria and were introduced to new techniques of craftwork, painting, and architecture which the rulers could afford to utilize in their palaces. The existence of a small palace at Phylakopi on Melos, decorated in the Minoan style, suggests that there was Cretan control of at least one of the Aegean islands. It was probably that of a Minoan governor of the island. Some harbor towns were called Minoa in later Greece, and traces of a Minoan settlement of about 1600 B.C. have been found at Miletus on the west coast of Asia Minor. The invasion and settling of the Greek peninsula by the Greeks retarded Minoan trade in that direction until about 1600 B.C. In Crete the need to organize production and trade fostered the development of writing. From a pictographic representation, called Minoan hieroglyphic, scribes developed a linear script (Linear A) in the Middle Minoan Period. This script is still not deciphered satisfactorily, but because of Crete's contacts with the coastal cities of Syria, the script writers seem to have borrowed some Semitic words and also the practice of inscribing their symbols on clay tablets.

There are indications that Minoan prosperity was waning in the first century of the Late Minoan Period (1600–1500 B.C.), as the more warlike Greeks from the peninsula took to the sea. The markets in Egypt and Syria were gradually lost, for in them Mycenaean Greek pottery replaced Minoan. Probably in the following century Mycenaean Greeks raided the Cretan palaces and ruled over parts of the island, but our knowledge of the decline of Minoan civilization is based on inference from controversial archaeological evidence. A plausible theory is that Greeks took over Cnossus about 1450 B.C. and established their chieftains as rulers. Their control is most clearly indicated by the tablets written in Greek in the Linear B script in place of the earlier Linear A. The taste of the new rulers may be indicated by the introduction of new architectural elements in the palace and by a change of style in its wall paintings. The drawing is stiffer and the composition more symmetrical, like the paintings in the palaces of the Greek peninsula. However, this new regime at Cnossus itself came to an end by 1400 B.C. The palace was burnt and looted, probably by other Greeks from across the Aegean. The other palaces on Crete had already been damaged by attack or by earthquake; consequently with the destruction of its main centers Minoan civilization lost its driving force. The towns dwindled and reverted to isolation and to their originally agrarian character. By 1150 B.C. the brilliant civilization of Minoan Crete had virtually disappeared.

Libation bearer on a wall painting. Cnossus

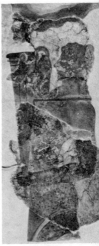

Yet many of its elements had been adopted by the Mycenaean Greeks and had become a strand in the complex growth of Greece.

The character of Minoan civilization is best revealed by the remains of the royal palaces, particularly the one at Cnossus. Although the city was located about three miles from the sea, it was connected by a road to a harbor town. A low hill in the central part of the city furnished a dominating site for the palace and for several large houses, probably those of important officials or other members of the royal family. Cnossus was evidently the chief center of Crete. The population of the city is estimated, rather generously, at about fifty thousand.

Building of the palace started about 2000 B.C. and extended over several centuries, as various units were built around a great central courtyard. In its final form the structure covered an area of about three acres, with some sections four stories in height. Providing for all the activities of the royal family and the administration, it was a composite dwelling, royal court, workshop, and storehouse. The roads which led to Cnossus from Phaestus on the south and from the harbor town on the north terminated in entrances on those respective sides, but the ceremonial entrance was from the west. It gave access to the principal, or west, wing of the palace in which there were ceremonial halls, galleries, and shrines on the upper floors, and in the basement a labyrinthine complex of corridors and storage chambers. Here were set huge jars to hold the grain and olive oil collected by the king as taxes from his subjects. Across the central courtyard the northeast corner provided rooms for the manufacture of pottery, jewelry, and other fine objects that were used in the palace or were sent abroad for trade and as gifts from the king of Cnossus. Most of the east wing was taken up by the domestic rooms in which the residents lived in considerable comfort, enjoying sitting rooms and even bathrooms, for which water was piped into the palace. This quarter, rising to four stories, was served by a skillfully built staircase and light shaft. Throughout the palace the walls were

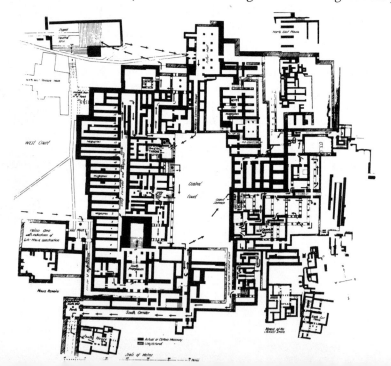

Plan of the Palace of Minos at Cnossus

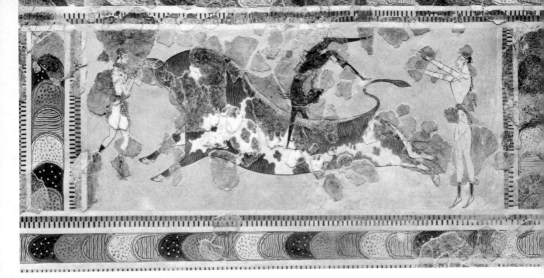

Bull-leapers on a wall painting. Cnossus

decorated with paintings depicting scenes of the countryside and of the sea, religious and court festivals, sports and games. The arrangement of the building recalls the contemporary palaces of Syria and Asia Minor, while the paintings owe much in technique to Egypt. Yet, they have a freshness of treatment, vitality, and selection of scene which were peculiarly Minoan; thus the palace itself was designed to serve the needs of Minoan life.

The paintings themselves are most informative, despite the primitive conventions which Minoan artists shared with their contemporaries in Egypt. In the paintings, for example, there is no representation of old age or death. The men and women pictured are all young, lithe, and vigorous, engaged in procession, dance, or festival. In contrast to the hectic life of the court are the scenes from nature, of plants, birds, and the sea. The Minoan artists mirrored their own familiar world with little thought or serious purpose, but they caught its action and lively joy. The king and young noblemen are red-brown, striding figures, clad in the typical Minoan male costume—a kilt held by a tight rolled belt around an abnormally slim waist. The ladies of the court are sitting to watch a festival or are taking part in dances and religious ceremonies.

Some scenes hint, underneath the enjoyment and pageantry, of a thread of cruelty which may have involved virtual human sacrifice. In the dangerous sport of bull-leaping, a bull was released among athletes, both young men and women. The leaper, who waited the bull's charge, would grasp the lowered horns and vault over the bull's back in a somersault to land in temporary safety; or he might slip, and be gored on the horns. The victims were perhaps regarded as a sacrifice to the bull-god, not merely as casualties of the arena. The dangerous sport was recalled in Greek tradition by the story of Theseus of Athens, who killed the Minotaur, the half-bull, half-man of the Labyrinth who demanded young men and maidens as tribute.

Minoan religion retained many primitive traits of an animistic character in which each object in nature was endowed with a spiritual power of its own.

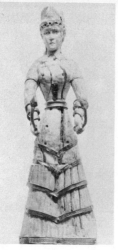

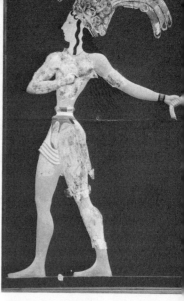

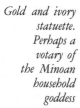

Gold and ivory statuette. Perhaps a votary of the Minoan household goddess

The priest-king. Painted relief from Cnossus

The kings did not build great temples like the Pharaohs of Egypt, but, like their people, worshipped in simple household and rustic shrines. Caves, groves of trees, springs, and hilltops were revered as sacred places. Some of these were transferred and given architectural form in the palace. There, the sacred cave was recalled in a pillared basement. The supporting pillars were fetishes, worshipped for their strength in a land of earthquakes and decorated with another symbol of strength, the *labrys* or double axe.

There are also indications of more sophisticated, anthropomorphic conceptions, stemming from the worship of the mother-goddess who ruled over all of nature. By the Late Minoan Period her functions had been distributed, and various minor goddesses were thought to preside over the activities of hunting, seafaring, the harvest, and the household. Some of these deities were probably the prototypes of later Greek goddesses, Artemis, Demeter, Athena, and Aphrodite. One striking representation, perhaps a worshipper of the household goddess, shows a woman holding snakes entwined about her body and arms. The snake was an attribute of the later Greek Athena. The important position held by women in society parallels this feminine predominance in religion. Women were not secluded in a harem or in the household, but, as shown in the paintings, sat with men and took an equal part in public festivals. Perhaps Cretan society was originally matriarchal, but in the paintings a male is represented in kingly costume, and the worship of a bull-god is indicated by the ceremony of bull-leaping. The names of Minoan rulers, too, as preserved in Greek tradition, are those of men.

The character of the palace gives some hints of administration and government. There was evidently a highly centralized organization headed by a king. Perhaps Minos was his title. The ruler has been called a "priest-king" by Sir Arthur Evans and certainly the palace resembled the temples and palaces of western Asia, which administered the economic life of their community. The produce of the farmers on the royal lands was collected, recorded, and stored in the palace; goods were manufactured there, and we can assume that a hierarchy of officials was set up to administer these processes. It is likely, too, that the overseas trade was organized by the palace officials and the goods provided from the king's storehouses. The building of seagoing ships for the long voyages to Syria and Egypt would have been very costly for an ordinary merchant. Possibly, too, the various localities of Crete had become subject in some manner to the king of Cnossus, for the size and wealth of the city and of the palace seem too great for local resources.

Along the coasts and in the mountain valleys of Crete there was a vigorous local life. We can get a glimpse of it in one community, the little town of Gournia, which lies east of Cnossus in the Gulf of Mirabello. The town's buildings cover the slopes of a hill overlooking the gulf and commanding a small coastal plain. Narrow cobbled streets and alleys wander irregularly up the hillside to the palace of its ruler. The houses along them were small and irregularly planned, often containing a workroom or shop. Gournia was a market for the surrounding countryside and coastal area. The excavation of its palace yielded some luxuries like those found at Cnossus. In both towns there was evidently a great gulf between ruler and ruled, and in Gournia itself, little distinction among the ordinary people. Perhaps a middle class of officials and merchants existed in the big city of Cnossus, but the prosperity of Crete does not seem to have resulted in a middle class in the small towns which might have transformed its society in the course of time. Government and economic organization remained centered in the palaces.

Mycenaean Civilization

During the rise of Minoan civilization, the Greeks, who had invaded the peninsula, were involved in the turbulent process of settlement. By 1600 B.C. they were established from Thessaly to the southern Peloponnesus. By that time they had taken to the sea themselves and had begun to adopt the more civilized customs of Crete. Military needs are apparent in their selection of town sites, and that of Mycenae, which has given its name to the civilization, is typical. The royal citadel crowned an easily defensible hill, lying well inland from the sea, at the end of the pass through which led the main road from the Isthmus of Corinth into the Peloponnesus. As Mycenae's power extended over the adjacent countryside, guard towers were built on the hills to control the lesser roads and paths, and a harbor town came into being. Mycenae became the center of a thickly populated area, the Argolid, in which smaller citadels and towns developed, like Tiryns, Asine and Corinth, all probably subordinate to the king of Mycenae. Other great centers in the Peloponnesus were Pylus, the traditional seat of King Nestor, and Sparta, where Agamemnon's brother, Menelaus, ruled. The Peloponnesus was the most important Mycenaean area, developing earliest, for it was closest to Crete. Central Greece, however, also became an important Mycenaean region with citadels and royal tombs at

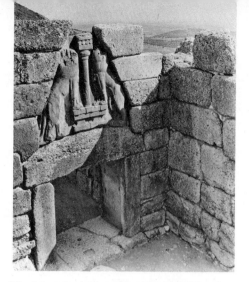

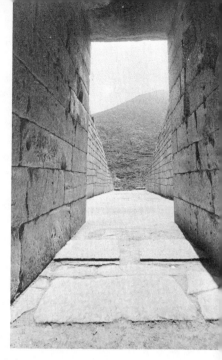

The Lion Gate at Mycenae, the principal entrance to the citadel. The lions are perhaps a heraldic symbol of the royal family. Right: The entrance corridor of the Tomb of Atreus, the best preserved of the beehive tombs at Mycenae

Athens, Thebes and Orchomenus, and, at Iolcus in southern Thessaly, a large palace has been excavated.

In contrast to the peaceful conditions of life in Minoan Crete, Mycenaean Greece remained restless and warlike, judging from the development of the fortifications surrounding its citadels. These strongholds, like medieval castles, were occupied by the ruling family and its establishment. The palace of the king was set on the hilltop and, surrounding the palace, were quarters for servants, soldiers and officials, storerooms for grain, pottery, weapons, and other possessions. Around the citadel well-engineered and immensely strong fortification walls were built, skillfully following the contours of the hillside to take advantage of the most defensible slopes. Jogs were made in the wall to control accessible slopes. The gates were constructed to expose the undefended side of attackers to fire from the walls, which, as indicated by well-preserved stretches at Tiryns, were built with inner corridors and storerooms for food and arms. Huge, roughly cut blocks were used in their construction with some stretches of wall as much as fifty feet in thickness. Such strength was unnecessary, for siege machinery had not yet come into use in Greece. Apparently the construction was intended to express the might of the king and designed to impress, as well as to defend. The weak point of the citadels was, of course, the need to store food and water, and their ultimate fall to invaders is probably to be explained by the cutting off of supplies rather than by direct assault.

The same quality of rather barbaric ostentation is apparent, too, in the rich burials and tombs, particularly at Mycenae. There, the royal families, from 1650 to about 1500 B.C., were buried in rectangular pits—shaft graves as they are called—arranged in two circular areas marked off by a curb of stone slabs. The earlier graves reveal a very warlike society which had just begun to lead a settled

life and acquire luxuries. Many bronze weapons and pottery jars of local manufacture and style had been placed in the tombs, but there was little gold and
jewelry. The head of one body had been covered with a death mask of thin
gold, and in another grave was a gem carved with a striking portrait of a
bearded man, the earliest Greek portrait. In contrast, the later shaft graves
(1550–1500 B.C.) show the full adoption of Minoan luxuries and a very great
wealth of gold. There was much fine pottery, gold and silver vessels, and beautifully inlaid daggers. The bodies, twenty-three in all, had been clothed in robes,
sewn with gold disks, and the faces of the kings were covered with gold death
masks. This wealth was evidently the fruit of piracy and raiding, for Greece
produced no gold in this period.

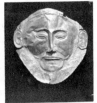

*Gold death mask
from the
shaft graves
at Mycenae*

Unfortunately the burial places of Mycenae's kings during the period of
its greatest power from 1500 to 1200 B.C. were plundered, probably at the time
of the city's destruction. The burial chambers, however, have survived and are
among the most impressive of Greek structures. They are large stone chambers,
shaped like a beehive and are called *tholos* tombs. The tombs were constructed
by cutting a horizontal shaft into the base of a hillside and lining the entrance
corridor and the burial chamber with regular courses of well-cut stone blocks.

The Mycenaean palace owed much to Crete in its decoration, but a typical
and most important room was developed from the megaron type of house. In
the palaces the megaron element had a separate entrance portico and a great
hearth in the center, surrounded by four tall columns to help support the roof
and to form a clerestory for the exit of the smoke. In it the king presumably
held council, banqueted with his nobles, and gave audience to visitors. While
the wall paintings from the Greek palaces are not so well preserved as those
from Cnossus, the fragments reveal a different style, more symmetrical and
balanced, and show that the Greek kings had a taste for hunting and battle
scenes.

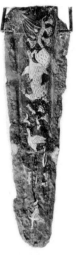

In Mycenaean society, as in Crete, the wealth of the community was largely
concentrated in the king's establishment, both during his life and even after
death by the treasure placed in his tomb. We know relatively little of the manner of life of the ordinary Mycenaeans. Their houses were built outside the
citadel, but in time of war the people took refuge within its walls. In the
countryside were small towns and villages, the seats of the king's nobles, and
centers for the agricultural life of the kingdom. From the inscribed tablets,
however, we can get some idea of the organization of Mycenaean society.

*Inlaid bronze
dagger from
the shaft
graves at
Mycenae*

Clay tablet (No. 731) with Linear B writing from Pylus, Messenia

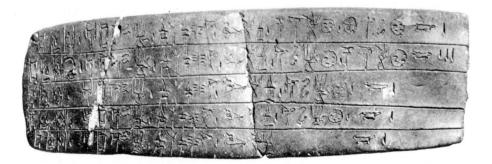

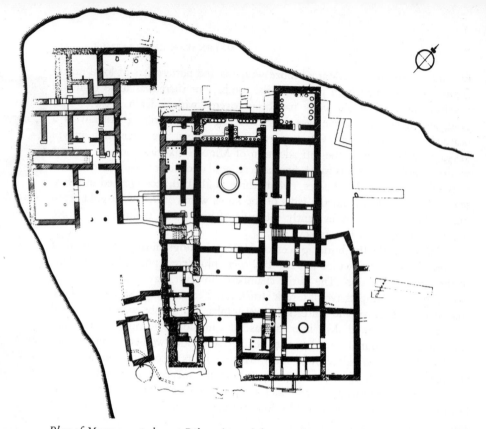

Plan of Mycenaean palace at Pylus. Around the central megaron, with its round hearth, are service corridors and storerooms.

The title of the king was *wanax*. His court was composed of a group of nobles, the king's companions, who lived close to him and served as officials. The king's duties were mainly administrative and religious, since his position probably rested in part on a belief that he was divine. There was a war leader, a *lawagetas*, whose ambition must at times have challenged the king's authority. The settled character of the Mycenaean centers and the example of the Near Eastern courts, which they came to know, probably kept the thrones secure in a hereditary descent. Below the king was a nobility, the *basileis,* who lived in towns on their estates and were responsible to the king for part of their produce and for service in war. Below them in the social scale were numerous craftsmen, peasants, and shepherds. Despite the detailed information on the tablets, they are disappointing in some respects. They give lists of names, record the payment of produce for taxes and contributions of material for war, but do not preserve decisions of government or chronicled history. While the names of some gods are recorded, there are no hymns, prayers, or imaginative literature. Apparently writing was a possession of the palace scribes and served only the purpose of administration.

The Mycenaean expansion abroad was as vigorous as it was in their own centers. Trade was started across the Adriatic Sea to South Italy before 1600 B.C., even earlier than across the Aegean, but trade to the west was of secondary interest. The main line of expansion, by trade, raiding expeditions, and the founding of colonies, followed that of Crete to Syria and Egypt, where Mycenaean goods replaced those of Crete. Pottery, olive oil, and hides were exported in exchange for luxuries such as spices, ivory, and jewelry. A skillful craft of ivory carving was developed with Syrian ivory. In fact, a considerable trade was developed with Syria, where some Greeks found it profitable to settle in the cities of Tarsus and Ugarit. Small colonies were founded to serve as trading posts or bases for piracy rather than for the relief of population pressure. The most important colonies were on the islands of Rhodes and, near the end of the Mycenaean era, on Cyprus, but a few smaller settlements were established on the west coast of Asia Minor, notably at Miletus, and along the south shore. As the Greeks were thus being drawn into the circle of Near Eastern powers, the Hittite kings began to deal directly with them in the thirteenth century. Unfortunately the Linear B tablets do not contain any letters of negotiation like the documents from El-Amarna in Egypt, but Hittite inscriptions do mention the Ahhiyawa. It is likely that these were the Achaeans, a Homeric name for Greeks, and scholars identify them with the settlers on Rhodes or, less probably, with the peoples of the great centers in the Argolid, the heart of Mycenaean civilization. This closer connection, however, was cut short by the invasions which destroyed or weakened the states of the Bronze Age.

The Trojan War and the Destruction of Mycenaean Greece

Perhaps one of the last Mycenaean ventures overseas was the expedition against Troy, which survived in Greek tradition as the Trojan War. The war was pictured by Homer as a full-scale effort of the Greek kingdoms under the leadership of King Agamemnon of Mycenae. Despite the size of their force, the Greeks besieged Troy for ten years before taking the city by deceit. There are difficulties, of course, in accepting both the reality of the war and Homer's picture of it as the effort of a united Greece. Part of this difficulty lies in the history of Troy as revealed by excavation.

Troy (Hissarlik) was founded at the beginning of the Bronze Age, about 3000 B.C., on a low ridge several miles from the sea in the northwestern corner of Asia Minor. The town controlled its own fertile coastal plain and lived mainly from this resource and by commerce with other towns in the northwestern corner of the Aegean. From the outset, however, Troy was heavily fortified and became the most important community of the region. In the Early Bronze Age the second level of habitation, Troy II, was a relatively wealthy community, judging from the large buildings on its citadel and the considerable treasure of gold jewelry found by Schliemann. Troy II was destroyed about 1900 B.C., but the new population rebuilt it on a substantial scale. Troy VI of the Middle and Late Bronze Ages was also large and prosperous, rivaling the Mycenaean centers of the Greek peninsula. Its heavily fortified citadel was enlarged to a total length of about 225 yards, and a palace crowned the ridge on which the town was built. Troy's chief connections during this period continued to be with the northern islands of the Aegean and the Greek mainland, but Crete lay beyond its horizon. There seems, too, to have beeen no connection with the Hittite Empire (p. 94).

Troy VI, which seems to be an ideal candidate for the Troy of the Trojan War, was, however, destroyed by earthquake about 1300 B.C. It was replaced by a much smaller town, Troy VIIa, and it is this town which is proposed as the Troy of the Homeric poems. Troy VIIa was destroyed about 1250 B.C., a possible date for the war according to later Greek tradition, and the destruction seems to have been by the violence of men. The town was a moderately prosperous little place, but certainly its capture should not have required the mobilization of all Mycenaean Greece and ten years of siege. It is difficult, too, to imagine that a single king of Bronze Age Greece could recruit its many rulers in his family's interest. Presumably, then, we should assign the scale of the war to the poetic imagination of Homer, but admit that the germ of the tradition may have lain in a small-scale raid made by a transitory coalition of some Mycenaean kings and their followers. Even more prosaically, it has been suggested that Troy fell to the Indo-European invaders from Europe who ultimately destroyed the Hittite Empire. Its destruction, in any case, was closely contemporary with that of the invasions which heralded the Early Iron Age.

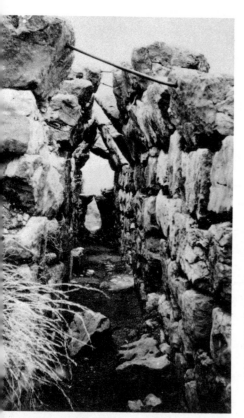

Corridor with corbeled vaulting inside the fortification wall at Tiryns. The style of masonry, constructed of large, roughly dressed stones, is called Cyclopean.

Troy. Tower and fortification wall of Troy VI. The inward slope of the wall was designed to make its scaling more difficult.

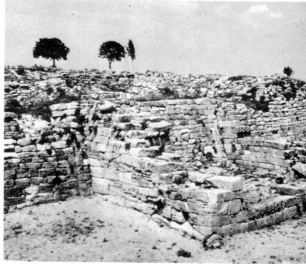

By 1200 B.C. the tide of destruction was sweeping over Greece. The end of the widespread civilization which the Minoans and Mycenaean Greeks had established was of course a complex process which we can only understand imperfectly by the evidence of archaeology and the survival of institutions and traditions into the better known age of historical Greece. Apparently the main centers of Mycenaean Greece were under attack in the latter part of the thirteenth century and most had perished by 1200 B.C. For example, the town of Mycenae outside the citadel was destroyed about a generation before the palace on the citadel was looted and burnt. Presumably invaders were attacking in groups, and, if the first attack failed, they might veer off elsewhere to return again later. An indication of the efforts made to protect the Peloponnesus is furnished by the discovery of a fortification wall thrown across the Isthmus of Corinth. The wall was ineffective, for, although Mycenae survived for a brief time, the palace at Tiryns was burnt about 1200. Pylus, too, perished about the same time. Athens, however, seems to have beaten the invaders off or was by-passed and according to tradition became a haven for fugitives from other kingdoms. When the citadels fell and the administrative systems collapsed, the small towns in the countryside were abandoned and the populations scattered or were enslaved by the newcomers. Mycenaean traditions were preserved for a few generations in the more remote sections of the Peloponnesus, in Achaea and Arcadia, and in the Mycenaean colonial regions—in the Ionian islands to the west, in the islands of the Aegean, as well as in Rhodes and Cyprus, to the east—but the collapse of the great centers meant destruction for the civilization.

The skilled techniques of writing, fine craftwork, and monumental architecture, which had depended on the patronage of the palaces, were forgotten. The ties of trade were almost completely cut and Greece reverted to an agrarian and pastoral economy. Those institutions embedded in religious practice and folk memory lasted longer. The gods lived on to become the well-known deities of classical Greece. The great cycles of myth and legend which we know from Greek literature were derived from memories of the Mycenaean kings and of their seats of power.

Greek tradition and some modern scholars have identified the destroyers of Mycenaean civilization as the Dorian branch of the Greek people, who were said to have entered Greece about 1100 B.C. and to have founded the Dorian states of Corinth, Argos, Crete, and Sparta. Perhaps the actual destroyers were forerunners of the main Dorian groups, known from historical Greece, who began to settle only after 1100 B.C. In any case, from that time a Dark Age obscured Greece until the rise of the historical city-states in the eighth century.

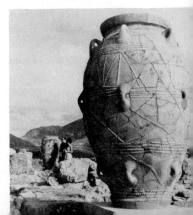

A storage jar from Cnossus

V I

New States of the Near East

(*ca.* 1200–700 B.C.)

IN THE AEGEAN REGION and in the Near East the Bronze Age came to an end about 1200 B.C. in a series of raids and migratory invasions which pushed the Egyptians back into the valley of the Nile and which destroyed the Mycenaean and Hittite kingdoms. As we have noticed, new elements were introduced into the populations of Syria and Palestine by the Peoples of the Sea, who raided the coasts, and by the seminomads from the desert, who entered the cultivated regions to settle. These movements, however, were only a part of the great migrations. Far to the east, Aryan peoples, the forefathers of the Medes and Persians, came into Iran from the steppes of Asia by the land corridors east and west of the Caspian Sea. They gradually worked their way into the fertile valleys of the Zagros Mountains, settling and forming local kingdoms. In the west, repercussions from the invasions of Greece brought other Indo-European peoples from the Balkans to Italy. Among them were the Latin people, who settled in Latium and the hills of Rome. Thus a new phase, called the Early Iron Age, began in the history of the ancient world between 1200 and 1000 B.C.

This second round of migrations was on a larger scale and more destructive than that of the early second millennium before Christ. In the Aegean region and in much of Anatolia where the brunt of the impact was felt the invasions were followed by a period of wandering and fresh settlement. A new start had to be made from a pastoral and seminomadic way of life, villages formed, and new systems of social and political union worked out. Few traditions endured from the civilizations of the past, and until the ninth century the Greeks and the Anatolian peoples were almost completely isolated from the older and still largely intact centers of the Fertile Crescent. By that time, however, the city-states of Greece and the fortress cities of Phrygia in central Anatolia had begun to coalesce. In contrast to this Dark Age of Greece and Asia Minor the new

The reader will find Maps III and V (pages 74 and 126) useful as he reads this chapter.

peoples in Syria and Palestine brought vigor to the surviving traditions. Small states developed quickly and were able to maintain their independence in the political vacuum left by the destruction of the great powers of Egypt and the Hittites. In the Early Iron Age the focus of history is first on the cities of Phoenicia, on the Hebrew Kingdom of David and Solomon, and on the Aramaean and Syro-Hittite cities of North Syria. While the Assyrian Kingdom was maintained in northern Mesopotamia, it was not until the ninth century that the Assyrians began to raid to the west and not until the late eighth century that they brought all the small states from the Mediterranean to western Iran into a new empire.

Despite the damage done by the migrations, recovery and renewed growth were relatively quick because communications were extended and the new metal, iron, came into general use. In the tenth and ninth centuries the Phoenicians began long-range seafaring in the Mediterranean. They founded trading colonies on Cyprus, sailed into the Aegean, then to the big islands of the western Mediterranean, to the north coast of Africa, and to Spain. The Aramaeans used camels domesticated in the Arabian Desert during the Late Bronze Age on the caravan routes of the Fertile Crescent. This long-range trade was mainly in metals and small luxury goods, but their distribution had an important civilizing effect. In the ninth century the Aegean and Anatolia were drawn again into contact with the older centers. By the eighth century the first important ties between the western and eastern basins of the Mediterranean were being forged and in the Near East renewed prosperity was apparent.

By that time, too, iron had come into general use for weapons and tools. It had been known to the Egyptians and Hittites of the Late Bronze Age, but only as a rare metal, a gift between kings. The Indo-European invaders from Europe had been armed with iron weapons, giving them an edge of superiority over their enemies, and from about 1100 B.C. the use of iron was gradually disseminated. Sources of supply were sought out, particularly in Asia Minor, and the techniques of smelting and working were developed. Iron was cheaper and easier to work than bronze and was more efficiently used in war and agriculture. While the Assyrians in particular were to profit from the new iron weapons of war, iron ploughshares increased the yield of food everywhere. Population increased and the standard of living for ordinary men improved. The second great era of ancient history had begun in which the lands from the Atlantic Ocean to the steppes of central Asia were to be drawn together. First, however, our focus must be on the Fertile Crescent where the ties with the past were strong.

The Phoenicians

From about 1100 B.C. until the late eighth century the sailors and merchants of Phoenicia carried on most of the sea trade of the Mediterranean. Phoenician culture remained Canaanite, however, despite the fact that some of the Peoples of the Sea mingled with the Semitic population. Perhaps this fusion gave additional stimulus to maritime activity. By 700 B.C. Assyrian domination of Phoenicia was draining the profits of trade in tribute; competition from the maritime cities of Greece had largely excluded the Phoenicians from the waters of the Aegean and was disturbing their trade elsewhere in the Mediterranean. Yet the Phoenicians remained an important maritime people throughout the rest of antiquity. They provided the ships and sailors for the Persian Empire, and in the Hellenistic and Roman periods their big port cities continued to play an important role in eastern Mediterranean commerce.

During its period of independence, Phoenicia, as in the past, was divided into separate city-states. The territory of each was predetermined by the deep gorges which carried the torrents from the Lebanon Mountains to the sea and cut the land into natural enclaves. In the Early Iron Age, however, there was a shift in importance among the cities. Byblos, which had risen to prosperity by its early trade with Egypt, took second place to Tyre and Sidon. King Hiram of Tyre, known from the Old Testament stories of his dealings with Solomon, built Tyre into an almost impregnable port in the tenth century by shifting its main harbor facilities to the off-shore islands and fortifying them with great sea walls. We possess a plaintive commentary on the decline of Egyptian trade with Phoenicia in the account of an envoy, Wenamon, who had come from Egypt to purchase timber. The Phoenician authorities kept him waiting while they attended to more important business. They were beginning to forge new trading connections by a foreign policy of diplomacy and alliance with their neighbors, the Aramaean and Syro-Hittite cities beyond the mountains in Syria, and the Philistines and Hebrews to the south in Palestine. The Phoenicians' role in trade was primarily that of middlemen. Their front door opened to the Mediterranean and their back door to the developing caravan trade beyond the mountains from Syria, Mesopotamia, and Arabia. Kingship remained the normal form of government in the Phoenician cities, but the rise of a wealthy merchant class is perhaps to be seen in the existence of a council of elders to advise the ruler.

Since Phoenicia itself had few resources to provide the goods of trade, the merchants were essentially carriers, buying and selling in double transactions for their own greater profit. The Phoenicians did have one valuable native product, the purple dye obtained from the shell-fish, *murex,* found in large beds along the coast. This dye and the wool from their own flocks of sheep pastured in the mountains, provided the materials for a famous textile industry. Phoenician craftsmen also manufactured fine furniture, jewelry, ivories, and metalware for export. Cedar for the furniture came from the Lebanon Mountains, copper and iron from Cyprus, silver from the Taurus Mountains and ivory from the elephant herds which still survived in Syria. Many articles were also brought by the carrying trade. The products of Mesopotamian and North Syrian craftsmanship were available in the Aramaean caravan cities, particularly in Damascus. The exotics of Arabia, myrrh and spices, were brought by desert routes from the south. Some idea of the nature of trade and the wealth of Tyre is given by the chapters in Ezekiel (26–27) which tell of the fall of Tyre at the hands of Nebuchadrezzar of

Babylonia in 571 B.C. The Hebrews considered Tyre the world's great trading city because of its commerce with Cilicia, Syria, Palestine, Egypt, Arabia, and the lands to the East.

The most striking achievement of the Phoenicians, however, was the establishment of long sea routes to the western Mediterranean. In the eleventh century they resumed trade with Cyprus and established an important colony at Kition. Phoenician and Cypriot traders then penetrated into the Aegean and worked along the coast of Asia Minor. Probably a few ports of call were set up, but these ventures into Greek waters were primarily to exchange metals and small luxury articles for hides, grain, olive oil, and slaves. Phoenician captains were not above piracy and kidnapping and, judging from the stories told in the Homeric poems, they were slippery, unscrupulous dealers who might sail away with their customers on board. Evidently the Phoenicians got the better of the Greeks. Probably by the end of the ninth century the Phoenicians had entered the western Mediterranean, where colonies were founded on Sardinia, and at Utica and Carthage on the coast of North Africa. Carthage, according to tradition, was founded in 814 B.C. by the sister of the king of Tyre, Dido, whose husband the king had put to death. This tradition, of course, scarcely accords in its timing with that told by the Roman poet Vergil in the *Aeneid*. His hero, Aeneas, found Dido building Carthage when he came from the fall of Troy four centuries earlier. Neither story seems to agree with the scanty and disputed archaeological evidence of early Phoenician activity in the western Mediterranean, but the important fact is that the western Mediterranean was brought into connection with the older centers of the East in the eighth and seventh centuries. Phoenician trading posts were set up in western Sicily, Malta, the Balearic Islands, along the north coast of Africa west of Carthage and in southern Spain.[1] Carthage ultimately welded them together in a great trading empire, which became the chief rival of Rome in the third century B.C. (p. 312). The primary goal of this early trade in the far west was the metals of southern Spain, copper and silver, and the tin brought there from as far afield as Cornwall in England. The point of exchange seems to have been at Gades (Cadiz), where a Phoenician colony was established.

As might be expected, the Phoenicians were renowned as shipbuilders and navigators. They developed a type of ship rowed by tiers of oarsmen, fast and seaworthy for long voyages. It was probably the prototype of the famous Greek triremes, which came into use in the late sixth century. Apparently, too, the Phoenicians wrote navigation guides in which information about the islands and coasts of the Mediterranean was collected. Phoenicia seems to have transmitted the alphabet to the Greeks in the mid-eighth century (pp. 230–31). By that time Greek traders from the islands of the Aegean had been attracted in their turn to the Syrian and Phoenician coasts and had established small trading posts. Perhaps the actual transmission of the alphabet took place in the Greek settlement of Al Mina near the mouth of the Orontes River. Through these

[1]See Map VIII, page 184.

small Greek ports, as well as through direct Phoenician trade, many of the orientalizing influences apparent in early Greek art, from Phoenicia, North Syria and Mesopotamia, were derived (p. 222).

In the ninth century the Assyrians, seeking an outlet to the Mediterranean, began to attack the Phoenician cities. Much plunder was carried off and tribute was imposed. Despite stout resistance by the Phoenicians and desperate attempts to form coalitions with their neighbors against the new enemy, the Assyrians were victorious. From about 850 B.C. tribute was paid fairly regularly, and in the latter part of the eighth century Phoenicia became a province of the Assyrian Empire.

The Aramaeans

To the east of the Lebanon Mountains, the Aramaeans had taken a position in land trade similar to the Phoenicians' sea trade. They were Semites who had lived a seminomadic life on the edge of the desert in the Late Bronze Age and settled in the region of the Upper Euphrates, mainly north of Damascus, in the course of the twelfth and eleventh centuries. Here they took over or founded new city-states, each ruled by its own king and frequently at war with its neighbors. Despite the fact that no large, centralized state was organized by the Aramaeans, their influence in Syria and Mesopotamia was great. Their settlement cut the routes to the Mediterranean coast from Mesopotamia and enabled them to press hard on the western cities of Assyria and Babylonia. Some of the latter cities were forced to accept Aramaean rulers and the population of central and northwestern Mesopotamia was heavily infiltrated by Aramaean settlers. Despite their mutual political friction, the Aramaeans developed the caravan trade of the region and prospered on both the tolls imposed and on the conduct of trade. Although the Aramaean cities were absorbed into the Assyrian Empire in the latter's westward expansion, the Aramaean language by that time had been thoroughly and widely disseminated as a sort of *lingua franca*. The Persians, for example, used it for official purposes in their Empire. Aramaeans used an alphabet of twenty-two symbols, with which the old cuneiform scripts could not compete, and by the time of the birth of Christ, cuneiform had gone out of use even in Babylonia. Thus Aramaic became the chief rival of Hellenistic Greek, the *koine,* in the Near East and was used by early Christian writers almost as freely as the latter.

The Philistines

The Philistines, who are known to history chiefly from the tales of their conflicts with the Hebrews, had been among those Peoples of the Sea repulsed from the delta of the Nile by Rameses III in the early twelfth century. When the raiders were turned back, the Philistines seized control of the southern part of the coastal plain of Palestine. Their origin is obscure, but, judging from their costume and weapons, they seem to have come from the colonial area of Mycenaean influence in southern Asia Minor. Although the Philistines settled in a group of five separate city-states, Gaza, Askalon, Ashdod, Ekron, and Gath, each ruled by its own king, they combined into a confederacy for war. Their fighting ability and a temporary monopoly of the supply of iron in Palestine enabled them to rule over the Canaanite cities on the coastal plain and for a brief time to dominate the whole land west of the Jordan River. This supremacy during the twelfth and eleventh centuries resulted in the designation of the land as Palestine, the land of the Philistines.

A bowl from Gath

The pressure by the Philistines on the Hebrews who had settled in the hill country behind the coastal plain was one of the main factors in the rise of the Hebrew Kingdom. The early years of struggle which was remembered in the stories of Samson and Delilah, of David and Goliath, and of the exploits of Saul became a heroic age to the Hebrews. At first the Philistines were successful. They defeated the Hebrew tribes at the battle of Aphek about 1050 B.C. and seized the Sacred Ark of the Covenant. Garrisons were placed at strategic points in the hills, but their hold on the land was obviously incomplete. Saul was able to rally the Hebrew tribes to fight against the invaders, and finally David succeeded in defeating them decisively and penning them into the southern corner of the plain where their chief cities lay. Despite this defeat and considerable Canaanite influence on their culture, the Philistines seem to have retained their identity as a people at least until the eighth century B.C. At that time Philistine names appeared in the annals of the Assyrian conquest. Soon, however, the Philistines had merged indistinguishably with the native people of the region, leaving little trace in history except for the record of the Old Testament and the archaeological remains of their settlements.

The Hebrews

In our own historical perspective the Hebrews loom far larger than they did to their contemporaries in the ancient Near East. The Kingdom of David and Solomon, to which Hebrews later looked back as their period of greatness, did play a significant role in the history of the tenth century B.C. After the death of Solomon, however, in 922 B.C., his kingdom split into the separate states of Judah and Israel. Each was a weak, small kingdom and except for a few brief spells of relative peace, led a harassed existence until it was taken over by larger powers, Israel by Assyria in 721 B.C. and Judah by the New Babylonian Kingdom in 586 B.C. Thereafter the Hebrews were subject to the great states which ruled the Near East, to the Persian Empire, to the Greek Ptolemies and Seleucids, and to Rome. Yet, in their short spell of independence the Hebrews established their lasting identity as a people and worked out the fundamental tenets of their religion. The Bible, too, began to take form in this period. The subsequent influence of Hebrew religion, of course, seems more significant to us

The holy place in a Canaanite sanctuary

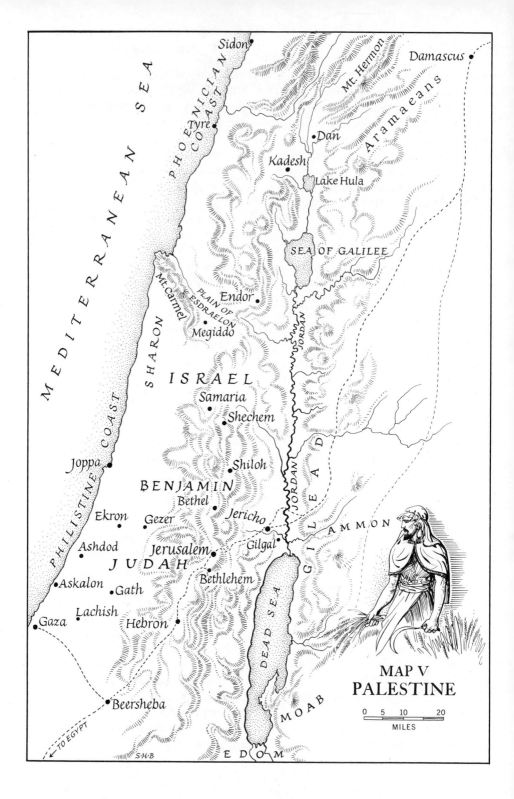

MEDITERRANEAN SEA

PHOENICIAN COAST

Sidon

Tyre

Damascus

Mt. Hermon

Aramaeans

Dan

Kadesh

Lake Hula

SEA OF GALILEE

SHARON

Mt. Carmel

PLAIN OF ESDRAELON

Endor

Megiddo

JORDAN

ISRAEL

Samaria

Shechem

Shiloh

GILEAD

Joppa

BENJAMIN

Bethel

Jericho

Ekron

Gezer

JORDAN

AMMON

Ashdod

Gilgal

Jerusalem

JUDAH

Askalon

Gath

Bethlehem

DEAD SEA

Lachish

Gaza

Hebron

PHILISTINE COAST

Beersheba

TO EGYPT

MOAB

EDOM

S·H·B

MAP V
PALESTINE

0   5   10   20
MILES

than their early history, but that is a lengthy and complicated subject. Here we are concerned only to sketch the circumstances in which the Hebrew people emerged into history.

The Hebrews were to find Palestine a land of few resources and very difficult to unify. The area of Israel proper, west of the Jordan River, was only about six thousand square miles and much of that was rocky hill country, offering pasture but little good land for agriculture. The Jordan, flowing in a deep rift from the Anti-Lebanon Mountains to the Dead Sea splits Palestine in two. While the valley of the river is hot and desert-like with oases, beyond it to the east in Transjordania were fertile plains, reasonably well-watered and productive until they petered out into the desert. But Israel, the chosen land of the Hebrews, was the rugged hill country which lay between the Jordan and the coastal plain. It fell into three main subdivisions: Judah in the south, from Jerusalem to the desert, Israel in the center, and Galilee to the north near the Sea of Galilee. Because it was a land of mountain shrubbery, a land well suited to herding sheep and goats and to a small-scale cereal production, it was quite literally a land of milk and honey. Water was scarce and had to be stored in cisterns for use during the hot summer season. Although the coastal plain was productive, it was bordered by sand dunes and had no good harbors for sea trade. Yet Palestine, because it was situated between Egypt and Syria, was a vital link in the communications of the Fertile Crescent, and is usually described as a "land of passage." The road from Egypt ran through the coastal plain to Mt. Carmel on the north. From Megiddo, an important control point, it turned along the north side of Carmel into the large plain of Esdraelon, then crossed the Jordan River and bent northeast to Damascus. Except for this gap to the northeast, northern Palestine was closed by mountains. The hill country itself was isolated, and the Hebrews living there tended to maintain an ingrown and provincial life.

THE SETTLEMENT

The Hebrews learned to write from their Canaanite neighbors only after settling in Palestine, and their recorded history began at the time of the kingdom in the tenth century. The vivid Biblical stories of presettlement days, of the wanderings of the patriarchs and of the Exodus from Egypt, are legendary and, like the early legends of other peoples, were subject to the variations and embroidery of oral transmission. They can scarcely be checked from the records of other contemporary peoples, yet legends contain some truth. Scholars have pointed out that the stories of the wandering of the patriarchs, Abraham and his descendants, from Harran in northern Mesopotamia to Palestine could fit the historical conditions of the early part of the second millennium. They suggest, too, that this early contact with Mesopotamia may account for the parallels between the patriarchal law of the Hebrews and that of Babylonia and that stories, like that of the Flood, may have become a part of Hebrew tradition at that time. Both law and stories, however, could have been learned from the Hurrian element of the population of Palestine after the Hebrew settlement.

Sometimes the Hebrews are identified as the Habiru, mentioned in Egyptian sources as a desert people. Habiru, however, seems to have been used to describe any wanderers who had no homeland, rather than a specific people. The Habiru sometimes served as hired soldiers and laborers in the settled countries. Rameses II, for example, employed them on building projects in Egypt. Perhaps the Exodus from Egypt was made partly by these Habiru of Rameses II and partly by Israelites, to use their later name, who were wandering in the desert of Sinai in the thirteenth century. This group of migrants does seem to have been the nucleus of the later Hebrew community, judging from the strong tradition of the Covenant made between their leader Moses and their god Yahweh.

In any case, the most intensive period of Hebrew settlement seems to have been the latter part of the thirteenth century. At that time the more fertile parts of Palestine were dominated by fortified Canaanite towns situated in the coastal plain and along the main roads in the hill country. In the early twelfth century, as we have noticed, the Philistines settled in the southern part of the coastal plain, taking over the Canaanite towns there by force. Both Canaanites and Philistines were obstacles to occupation by the Hebrews and the kindred desert tribes who entered the land from the south and east. Like the Aramaeans, to whom the Hebrews were closely related, the Hebrews had been living a semi-nomadic life, moving along the edge of the desert in search of seasonal pasturage. Since the Hebrews apparently found the good land east of the Jordan River already occupied by recent arrivals, the Edomites, Moabites, and Ammonites, they therefore settled in the hill country west of the Jordan. Some Canaanite communities were attacked and taken over by bands of Hebrews, but the Hebrew settlement should not be regarded as a conquest by a united people. In fact, the Hebrew tribes themselves were in the process of formation and did not unite under a king until about 1000 B.C. At first the Hebrews settled down beside the Canaanites from whom they learned much that was useful in the transformation from a nomadic to an agricultural life.

The tribal structure of Israelite society which had existed in embryo before the entry into Palestine was completed and strengthened. Because the hill country in which the Hebrews settled was split by nature into separate cantons, the settlers in each were confronted with local problems of defense and co-existence. Local tribes developed as strong, compact groups, made up of the new settlers as well as elements of the local population which had been assimilated. Each tribe chose its own leader as described in the Book of Judges in the Bible, men like Gideon, Jephthah and Samson, who exerted a vigorous personal leadership in war. Only on rare occasions did some of the tribes band together. The economic difficulties of settlement also slowed coalescence. Land had to be reclaimed for agriculture, and because pasturage was seasonal, nomadic habits were prolonged. Towns were slow to form and remained small and crudely built.

Working for unity at this time was the moving force of religion. The twelve tribes formed a loose association to worship Yahweh which we call an amphictyony, by analogy with similar associations formed by the Greeks (p. 176). The tribes had a common shrine, apparently a tentlike structure reminiscent of their nomadic days, at Shiloh, in which the Ark of the Covenant was kept. A priesthood was chosen to conduct the ceremonies of worship and, presumably, to settle disputes left unresolved by the village elders, through oracles from Yahweh or by their knowledge of the sacred law. Despite this general recognition of Yahweh as a national god, local religious attachments were strong; thus the Canaanite religious practices were freely adopted. The Israelites had entered an alien land, whose gods had to be propitiated; they were learning new ways of life, agriculture, for example, which were governed by age-old rituals. Accordingly, the local Baals of the Canaanite population were recognized and rituals associated with sowing and the harvest were practiced along with their own rites which were more appropriate to a seminomadic people from the desert.

The first two centuries of Israelite history were turbulent with warfare and, indeed, ended in the occupation of Israel by the Philistines. The Canaanites proved difficult to dislodge from the plains because they fought in chariots. Other desert peoples, like the Midianites, attacked the Hebrew lands in swift camel raids. The Philistines pressed into the hills from the coastal plain. This era of fighting became the heroic age of Hebrew tradition, made illustrious by warriors like Gideon, who triumphed over the Midianites; by Samson, who raided and tricked the Philistines; and by Deborah, whose victory over the Canaanite chariot forces in the plain of Esdraelon was sung in one of the earliest ballads of Hebrew literature. The Philistines, however, proved too formidable. They were soldiers by avocation who possessed the advantages of iron weapons and a disciplined organization. As we have noticed, the Philistines defeated the Hebrews at the battle of Aphek about 1050 B.C., carried off the Ark of the Covenant as a trophy, and established a limited control over Israel by placing garrisons in the hills. Yet the battle of Aphek was also a landmark in the growth of Hebrew unity. For the first time the separate tribes offered a concerted resistance. The tribal leaders were becoming conscious of the need for some centralized authority, and in the latter part of the century they gave their support to Saul, the first king of a united Israel.

THE KINGDOM OF ISRAEL: SAUL

The kingship to which Saul was elected by the tribes of Israel was formed in response to the needs of war. Because he defended his own tribe of Benjamin from Ammonite raids, Saul was hailed by other tribal leaders when proposed as king by the Judge, Samuel. Resistance to the Philistines had been kept alive after the defeat at Aphek by the wandering prophets of Israel, among whom Samuel was trusted and influential. The Hebrew kingship thus came into existence with religious and political approval. Saul's reign began in victory. An army formed under his over-all command drove the Philistines from their garrison posts. It soon proved difficult, however, for the tribal leaders to acknowledge the demands of a central authority. Saul himself was ill-fitted for the compromise necessary to leadership because he seems to have been violent and unstable, jealous of distinction among his followers, and, worst of all, ultimately unable to defeat the Philistines decisively.

Samuel was estranged, perhaps because of Saul's failure to reconcile the older traditions of religious authority and the new political needs of kingship. Then Saul quarreled with his young favorite, the hero David. When Samuel withdrew his support, David fled for his life to the hills of Judah. There he gathered a band of followers and became identified as a potential leader of the people of Judah. Soon, however, he took refuge among the Philistines to escape the vengeance of Saul. Saul's reign ended in tragedy about 1000 B.C., when the Israelite army was defeated in battle on the plain of Esdraelon. Saul, in despair at the defeat and the death of a son who was killed in the battle, committed suicide, leaving Israel leaderless. The Philistines reoccupied the land and recognized David as a vassal king in his native Judah.

DAVID (*ca.* 1000–961 B.C.)

The real founder of the Kingdom of Israel was David, who consolidated all of Palestine and much of Syria under his rule and established his descendants as kings in Jerusalem for four centuries. David seems to have played a skillful double game while in the service of the Philistines, both contriving to hold their confidence and to establish himself as leader of the southern tribes in Judah. He took no part in the battle in which Saul was defeated, and shortly afterwards was elected king of Judah. Saul's posterity, who attempted to carry on the kingship among the northern tribes in Israel, failed to assert their position and were removed by David. The northern tribes then elected him king and thus the united kingship of Judah and Israel was combined in his person.

The new state, unified under a young and vigorous ruler, offered a threat to the Philistines. Their attempt to oust David failed and, instead, he penned them into the southern part of the coastal plain. In the following years the Canaanite cities of Palestine were peacefully taken over and made tributary to Israel. In a series of difficult and bloody wars David conquered the lands beyond the Jordan—Ammon, Moab and Edom—and extended his power northeast to include Damascus. An alliance was made with Tyre and friendly relations established with the other cities of Phoenicia. David had built his kingdom into the strongest power of the region in the course of a generation; from the revenues he was able to form an administration and to make Jerusalem his capital city.

Jerusalem was not a Hebrew foundation, but had first appeared in history about 2000 B.C. in the records of Middle Kingdom Egypt. David, at the outset of his reign, had taken it over from the native Jebusite population. The city was a natural fortress, built on a great bastion of rock surrounded by ravines on three sides which could be heavily fortified. Probably, however, political as well as military considerations prompted David's choice. His regime was new, and the union between the northern tribes of Israel and the southern tribes of Judah was shaky. Jerusalem was, in a sense, neutral ground, the choice of which would offend neither group. Yet it was in the northern part of Judah on whose tribesmen David principally relied. The city became the political and religious center of the kingdom. David built a palace there and housed his court and harem in it. The Ark of the Covenant, recovered from the Philistines, was brought to Jerusalem, and a priesthood appointed to preside over religious worship. In this manner the religious life of the Hebrews was focused on the new capital, where the kingship and the formal worship of Yahweh were closely associated.

While the rule of David was personal and direct, the large size of his kingdom required that he begin to form a bureaucracy. Generals were selected to lead the army in some operations, governors were appointed to the tributary districts, and scribes and minor officials were assigned to keep records and to relay orders. A census was taken on which taxes and levies for work on building projects and for military service could be based. While these innovations were not popular, they were necessary for the transformation from tribal to centralized government and were generally accepted. The last years of David's reign, however, were marred by revolts caused partly by resentment at the demands of the new state and partly by his own indecision in arranging for the succession. In Israel a revolt of the northern tribes, who acclaimed David's son Absalom as king, had to be suppressed. Finally David, swayed by his favorite wife, Bathsheba, selected her son Solomon as co-ruler and successor. Solomon presumably had the backing of a powerful faction at court, but David's vacillation and the indications of hostility to him among the northern tribes boded ill for the stability of the kingdom.

SOLOMON (961–22 B.C.)

Because Solomon came to the throne through palace intrigue, he had to make a show of force at the outset to consolidate his position. He removed potential rivals and devoted his reign to exalting the kingship and to organizing Israel on the pattern of other oriental monarchies. These aims were achieved by intensive economic development within Israel itself and through a policy of foreign alliances to facilitate trade. Solomon gave up, perhaps unwisely, David's aggressive warfare, but established a large army to defend his kingdom. The soldiers were enlisted by conscription and quartered in fortified bases throughout the country. An expensive but necessary chariot force was organized, part of which was placed in the key fortress of Megiddo. Excavation there has uncovered the stables for about 450 horses. Despite these measures, Solomon had to give up some of the territory which David had conquered. Edom revolted but was only partially recovered, and Damascus was lost to the Aramaeans.

Yet Israel was counted a strong state among the kingdoms of the Fertile Crescent; consequently Solomon was able to work out advantageous alliances with his neighbors and to exploit Palestine's strategic position for trade. The alliance made by David with Hiram of Tyre was renewed, and Phoenicia was brought into a close economic relationship with Israel. The agricultural products of Palestine, wheat, olive oil, and wool were exchanged for the timber of Lebanon and Phoenician craft products. Phoenician craftsmen, shipbuilders, and sailors were used by Solomon for his building projects and trading ventures. Solomon, like other oriental rulers, by holding a monopoly on the production and labor of his kingdom, channeled the revenues from its development into his treasury.

Particularly noteworthy was Solomon's expansion of trade in the Red Sea, to which Israel had access by desert routes across Sinai to the Gulf of Aqaba. There a port was built at Ezion-Geber to serve a merchant fleet, probably constructed by Phoenician shipbuilders and manned by Phoenician sailors. It operated along the Arabian coast and carried on trade with Ophir (the Somali coast of Africa?). Solomon also encouraged the caravan trade by land routes in western Arabia to obtain the spices, incense, and other exotics of the south for Palestine and Phoenicia. The famed visit of the Queen of Sheba may well have had a basis in fact, for Sheba was the Sabaean land of South Arabia. More prosaically, but perhaps more usefully, Solomon exploited the copper mines of Sinai and built smelting works at Ezion-Geber. Also, he seems to have been a horse trader on the grand scale, importing horses from Cilicia and chariots from Egypt and selling both to the Syro-Hittite kingdoms in North Syria.

The revenues from Solomon's intensive development of agriculture in Palestine and from foreign trade brought a general rise in prosperity. Large-scale building projects were undertaken, urbanization was accelerated, and craftwork was encouraged by royal patronage. Much of this was evident in Jerusalem, where Solomon fostered a luxurious court life and rebuilt the simple structures of his father on a grand scale. Workmen and building materials, like the cedar of Lebanon, were imported from Phoenicia. Solomon's new palace was a great complex of buildings, presumably constructed on the Canaanite model and providing ample room for his varied harem, officials, and servants. The harem, seven hundred wives and three hundred concubines, was a testimonial to the success of Solomon's political and business ventures. In this group were girls given by their fathers to seal bargains. There was even a daughter of the Pharaoh of Egypt. Like David, Solomon maintained a close association between religious and political leadership. A new temple was constructed within the palace complex and a high priest appointed, thus making the center of Hebrew religion almost a dynastic shrine of the king. David's rudimentary bureaucracy was enlarged, and Jerusalem, or rather the court, became the scene of the first flowering of Hebrew intellectual culture.

The proverbial wisdom of Solomon himself was a reflection of the growth of this intellectual life at his court, where an educated class of administrators and priests both wrote and formed an audience. In addition to the work of the official scribes, who compiled records and attended to correspondence, Hebrews wrote their first imaginative literature. Pride in the traditions of settlement had been stimulated by the achievements of David and Solomon, and so the old legends and heroic exploits of early Hebrew leaders were written down. Historical chronicles, composed with skill and imagination, replaced legend. We can see the results in the Bible, where accounts of the rise of David and of

Solomon's reign exhibit a new reflective attitude on the significance of Hebrew history. In it Yahweh was presented as the arbiter of men's actions, shaping events in accordance with his plans for the chosen people.

Yet this brilliant court life rested on an insecure basis. Solomon's grandiose building projects, extensive diplomacy and the upkeep of the court and the army cost more than the revenues provided. Despite his efficient new bureaucracy, the burden was heavy and the people grumbled. Solomon's tax system seemed particularly onerous. Israel was divided into twelve administrative districts which obliterated the old tribal frontiers. Each district was headed by a governor who was called on to provide the court with food for one month in addition to other services and taxes. The Hebrews were liable to military service, but not work levies, while the Canaanites provided labor. The new urban structure which Solomon's economy was imposing on agricultural life began to produce a well-marked upper class of officials, merchants, and large-scale landowners, whose interests diverged from those of the farmers and shepherds. The upper class profited, while the farmers remained at a subsistence level, and division grew between rich and poor and between town and country.

The monarchy itself tended to become a bone of contention, for centralized kingship was destroying the older traditions of tribal society and of religious leadership by the prophets. While the Hebrew king was not himself divine, like the Pharaoh of Egypt, he was regarded as a servant of Yahweh, and so was not above criticism as an interpreter of Yahweh's intentions. The prophets might consider that they were better able to understand God's will than the king or the high priest. Thus the new monarchy rested somewhat uneasily in the structure of Hebrew society. These reflections, however, were more a product of the future than of Solomon's own reign. His taxation bore very heavily on the northern tribes in Israel whose people grumbled that they carried an unfair share of the cost for the court in Jerusalem. Solomon himself was able to hold the kingdom together, but after his death Judah and Israel divided into separate kingdoms.

THE DIVIDED KINGDOM

After Solomon's death Hebrew power disintegrated rapidly. His son, Rehoboam (922-15 B.C.), was accepted without difficulty as king by the people of Judah, but the northern tribes in Israel demanded that their tax burden be relieved. When Rehoboam refused, revolt flared, and a separate kingdom was set up under the rule of the Israelite Jeroboam (922-01 B.C.). Neither Judah nor Israel could hold the outlying territories of the kingdom. Israel held or fought for Moab for about a century, and Judah retained a small part of Edom, but southeastern Syria and nearly all the land east of Jordan was lost. The new kingdoms had to live on their own scanty resources and from them maintain their own courts and armies.

Israel, which was larger and more fertile than Judah, was better able to support itself, but the new ruling family of Jeroboam failed to establish stable rule. The people of Israel were more divided by tribal rivalries and religious traditions than those of Judah. The population contained a large Canaanite element, to whom some religious concessions had to be made, while the Hebrews were pulled towards Jerusalem which was then established as the traditional religious center of the Hebrew people. Jeroboam made a vigorous effort to create new religious sanctions for his kingship, but failed. The government was located at Shechem, a venerable place in Hebrew tradition, and royal shrines were founded at Dan in the north and at Bethel in the southern part of the kingdom. Apparently the king permitted Canaanite practices of worship in the new shrines, and was therefore criticized by the religious leaders. The kingship remained unstable, and in the course of Israel's brief history seven dynasties occupied the throne.

Israel, however, did have a renaissance of material prosperity under the rule of Omri and of his son Ahab (876–49 B.C.). These kings modeled their government on that of Solomon and cultivated close commercial relations with the Phoenician and Aramaean cities to the north. Ahab married the famous Jezebel, daughter of the king of Tyre, to seal the alliance and moved his capital to Samaria, where the royal couple sponsored a brilliant court life. As in Solomon's reign, the brilliance of the court was supported by heavy taxation and exploitation of the farmers to provide the goods for trade with Phoenicia. Hebrew discontent was enflamed by Jezebel's injudicious attempt to establish the worship of her Phoenician Baal as an official cult. The king built a temple for Baal in Samaria and staffed it with a retinue of Phoenician priests. While this may have encouraged the loyalty of the Canaanite element of the population and strengthened the alliance with Tyre, the Hebrews reacted strongly, and the prophets Elija and Elisha preached a holy war against the monarchy. In 842 B.C. a general of the army, Jehu, took over command in a military revolt during war against the Moabites and was anointed king by Elisha. Jehu took a bloody revenge, throwing Jezebel to the dogs in the palace courtyard and killing the priests of Baal and the Phoenician faction in the palace. Perhaps Israel was saved from becoming a satellite of Tyre, but the damage done to its alliances and economic life was heavy. The state remained weak and its government anarchic. In 734 B.C. Tiglath-Pileser III made Israel subject to Assyria and in 721 B.C. his successor, Sargon II, reduced it to provincial status. Many of the governing class and the wealthy merchants, traditionally remembered as 27,290, were carried off to northern Mesopotamia. The Hebrews left in Israel, mainly farmers and shepherds, continued their old ways of worship to Yahweh, but religious leadership passed to Judah.

Judah at least remained internally stable because its people were loyal to the line of David ruling in Jerusalem. The people of Judah, however, were hard pressed to keep their independence. In 918 B.C. King Shishak of Egypt, in a rare display of energy from that obsolescent kingdom, invaded Palestine, plundered the land and imposed tribute. Judah's vassalage was brief, for Shishak's invasion proved to be a raid and not the preliminary to a lasting occupation. Feeling between Judah and Israel was normally hostile, and border incidents, if not actual war, were frequent. During the reigns of Omri and Ahab in Israel, however, there was a reconciliation. An alliance was concluded and Judah shared to some degree in the prosperity which Omri's policy brought to the northern kingdom. Yet it was not difficult for Judah to become a subject ally of Assyria against Israel in the late eighth century when the Assyrian kings, Tiglath-Pileser III and Sargon II, occupied that land. As a vassal state of Assyria Judah preserved its own kingship until the fall of the Assyrian Empire in 612 B.C. At that time King Josiah, in an attempt to restore the Kingdom of David and Solomon, was caught up in war between Egypt and Babylonia. He perished at Megiddo in 608 B.C., and the state of Judah was destroyed in 586 B.C. by Nebuchadrezzar of Babylon (p. 152). The walls of Jerusalem were dismantled and many members of the governing class were carried into exile to Babylonia.

The significance of Hebrew history throughout the unhappy period of the divided kingdom lies mainly in the development of religious conceptions and practices. By the time of the destruction of Judah in 586 B.C., Hebrew religion was able to hold the people together as a community, so that the Hebrews did not lapse into ultimate anonymity. While discussion of this phenomenon belongs to religious history, it is pertinent to notice briefly some of the main differences between the Hebrew and other religions of this period.

In relation to the polytheistic beliefs of their neighbors, Hebrew religion from the outset was virtually monotheistic and exclusive because of the nature of the Covenant into which the Hebrews had entered with their god Yahweh. He was a national god who had chosen them as his people on certain terms. The articles of the Covenant became the basis both for ethical conceptions and for cult practices, the violation of which involved the loss of Yahweh's goodwill. Accordingly, there were very strong compulsive forces at work in the Hebrew community which were kept alive and developed by the religious leaders, both prophets and priests. The prophets, from the time of Elijah, assumed the role of critics by attacking both the government and society if the people failed to measure up to their ideas of what Yahweh expected. Their teaching deepened conceptions of the divinity of Yahweh, of social justice, and of individual responsibility. The priesthood, in their turn, elaborated the law which governed the ordinary life and religious practice of the Hebrew community. While Hebrew law had much in common with the codes of other Semitic peoples, it differed in being derived continuously from religious revelation. In short, the Hebrews succeeded in divorcing the political fortunes of the state from their religious and personal life as a people. A state was desirable, but the people could keep their identity and survive because of their religious community.

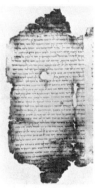

A section of the Dead Sea scrolls, the earliest manuscripts of Biblical materials which have been discovered

The Syro-Hittite Kingdoms

In the Old Testament there are occasional references to Hittites. These people were not the Hittites whose empire was centered in Anatolia during the Late Bronze Age, but those usually referred to by historians as the Syro-

Hittites (p. 97). They were predominantly Luwian in origin and had formed a part of the Hittite Empire, but their period of historical importance lay between 1000 and 700 B.C. By 700 B.C. the Syro-Hittites had been absorbed into the Assyrian Empire, and it is primarily through Assyrian records of conquest and the archaeological investigation of Syro-Hittite cities that something is known of their history and culture.

The Syro-Hittite states were formed in the twelfth and eleventh centuries in eastern Cilicia, northern Syria, and in the mountainous region of southern Anatolia. All the states preserved the traditions of imperial Hittite art and religion, but in northern Syria their culture acquired many Canaanite and Aramaean elements as the consequence of Aramaean infiltration. Each kingdom had as its center a heavily fortified city, the most important of which were Adana in the Cilician plain, Milid (Malatya), Samal (Zingirli), Aleppo, Carchemish, and Hamath. We know little of their history before the ninth and eighth centuries when they were under attack by the Assyrians. At that time the Hittites fought hard to block Assyrian expansion in the west, but failed to unite and were absorbed piecemeal. Once Carchemish, which guarded the crossing of the Euphrates into North Syria, was taken, the road to the west was open; by 700 B.C. the cities had been captured.

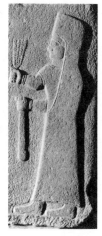

Relief sculpture from Carchemish

The Hittite cities located on the routes from northern Mesopotamia to Syria and Anatolia had become prosperous from their tolls on trade, by the exploitation of their own land and, in some cases, from mineral resources. The kings had the means and labor to build extensively and to procure the luxuries of their period from Phoenician and Aramaean traders or by patronage of their own craftsmen. Thus the cities played an important part in the transmission of cultural influences. Their architecture and sculpture were in the direct traditions of the Hittite Empire which in turn provided models for the Assyrians. The Hittite palaces made a very considerable use of sculptural decoration. The columns of their porticoes rested on bases cut in animal form; the lower courses of the walls were formed by upright slabs of stone, decorated with reliefs of animals, scenes of battle, and religious ceremonies. At Malatya, for example, there are scenes which recall the gods and ceremonies depicted at the imperial Hittite sanctuary at Yazilkaya (p. 96). New elements were also introduced, particularly in North Syria where hunting scenes were popular. Although the style of this Late Hittite work is heavy and blockish and the workmanship often crude, the grim ferocity and power of the best works are compelling. They appealed to the Assyrians, who imitated the motifs and improved on the technique. Assyrian palaces also adapted the plan of the Hittite buildings and their sculptural decoration. The North Syrian area was also an important focal point for the transmission of oriental motifs and techniques to Greece. Mythical creatures of Anatolian and Mesopotamian religious fancy, like sirens and griffins— part animal and part human—were represented on the textiles and metalware exported from Syria to Crete, Rhodes, and Corinth in the Aegean (p. 222). From North Syria trade and stimulation came also to the Anatolian plateau where a more urban type of life was revived in the ninth and eighth centuries.

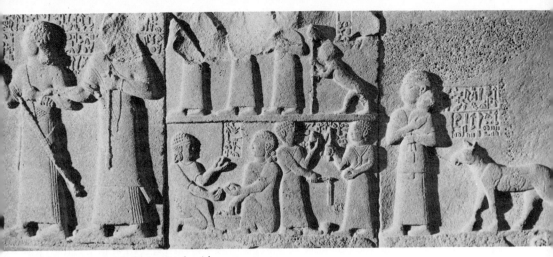

Religious scene on a relief from Carchemish

The Phrygian Kingdom

The history of Asia Minor after the fall of the Hittite Empire is almost entirely obscure until the eighth century B.C. The Aegean coastline was colonized by Greeks in the eleventh and tenth centuries when small settlements were made in the regions later known as Aeolis and Ionia, but their growth was primarily a part of the civilization of Greece (pp. 175–76) and their connections with the Anatolian plateau were tenuous. On the plateau the invaders who had destroyed the Hittite Empire, Thracians and Phrygians from the Balkans, presumably lived a wandering and pastoral life. Naturally it has left few traces, but in the ninth and eighth centuries fortress cities began to rise and to coalesce into the Kingdom of Phrygia, traditionally ruled by the kings of Gordium. Their city was built on the Sangarius River about sixty miles to the west of the modern Turkish capital of Ankara. Some of the Phrygian cities were established on the old Hittite citadels, as at Boghaz-Koy, even using their ruinous buildings, but Phrygian culture seems to have owed little to imperial Hittite traditions. Its origins are obscure and the formative influences disputed. Some scholars argue for strong Greek influences, which would have come to Phrygia from the Greek colonies on the Aegean coast. Others, more plausibly to judge from the material excavated so far, stress the native Anatolian character of Phrygian art and point to connections with the Syro-Hittite cities, with Assyria, and with the equally enigmatic Kingdom of Urartu in southeastern Anatolia.

The Phrygians, however, had a place in Greek tradition. The Homeric poems refer to them as horse-breeders and warriors who lived along the Sangarius in northwestern Asia Minor; legends told of the Phrygian King Midas whose touch turned objects to gold, of his marriage to the daughter of a king of Greek Cyme in Aeolis, and of his suicide by drinking bull's blood. To the Greeks, then, the Phrygians were a remote, barbaric and wealthy people who had a place in their early legends rather than their history. On the other hand

Assyrian inscriptions refer to a King Mita of Muski, plausibly identified with the Greek Midas, who fought with the Assyrians in Cilicia in 716 B.C. and was defeated by Sargon II in 709/08 B.C. Mita was evidently seeking access to the sea through Cilicia and for this purpose had made an alliance with Urartu and some of the Syro-Hittite states of North Syria against the Assyrians. While Midas' touch of gold may be safely assigned to legend, his kingdom was evidently an aggressive and growing state, starting to expand southwards to the older centers of the Fertile Crescent. Its known history, however, was brief because in the early seventh century Phrygia was overrun by a horde of nomads, the Cimmerians, who poured out of the Caucasus and swept across Asia Minor to the Aegean coast. It was in despair at his defeat by the Cimmerians that Midas was reputed to have committed suicide in 696/95 B.C.

Despite the obscurity of Phrygian history, the excavation of its cities, particularly of Gordium by the University of Pennsylvania since 1950, has revealed a culture, distinctive in itself and playing some part in the transmission of new influences in the Early Iron Age. Phrygian life was basically agricultural, but the kings controlled large supplies of labor with which to build massively fortified cities of stone and timber and to heap up great burial mounds. Craftsmen, working for the most part to the order of kings and nobles, became skilled in metal and woodwork, in the weaving of textiles, and in the making of pottery. The latter was decorated, like that of contemporary Greece (p. 220), with geometric motifs and schematized animal designs. By the late eighth century the Phrygians had learned to write their language in alphabetical symbols

The "Midas" Tomb at Gordium, Phrygia. The burial chamber, built of great wooden planks, contained inlaid furniture and bronze vessels.

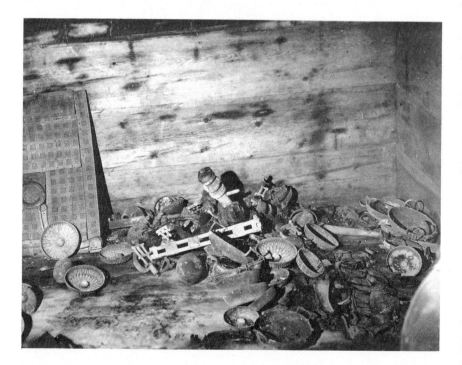

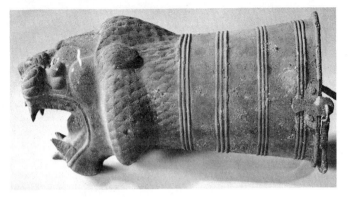

A bronze pail in the shape
of a lion's head.
Gordium, Phrygia

closely resembling those of early Greece. No archives have been found as yet, however, so that we have no information about the organization of Mita's kingdom.

The most impressive remains so far excavated in Gordium are those of the city gates, built of courses of stone tied together vertically and horizontally by heavy wooden beams. The valley of the Sangarius was presumably heavily forested at that time because wood was used also for house construction and for tombs. The tombs of the kings and nobles were built close to the city and their high mounds, *tumuli,* are a feature of the present landscape. The largest, perhaps that of Mita's father, for it is dated between 725 and 700 B.C., was 150 feet in height and nine hundred feet in diameter. The burial chamber was constructed of great squared timbers and then heaped over with stones and clay to fully seal and protect the burial. The tombs, many of which have been excavated, contained quantities of bronze vessels, furniture, textiles, weapons, jewelry, and other precious objects. The quantity of metalware and the discovery of remains of bronze smelters indicate that Gordium was one of the important centers of metalwork in the Early Iron Age. The Phrygian craftsmen received some inspiration from imports brought from Urartu and, in their turn, produced cauldrons and other objects which were exported to the Aegean coast and influenced Greek metalwork. The rise of Phrygia, however, was cut short soon after 700 B.C. by the Cimmerian invasion. Many cities, including Gordium, were plundered and burnt. Others escaped serious damage or revived, but in the sixth century Phrygia was taken over—first, by the new Kingdoms of Lydia and Media, and then by the Persian Empire.

Urartu

The Kingdom of Urartu suffered severely, too, in the Cimmerian invasion and, like Midas, its King Rusas is reported to have committed suicide when his capital city fell. Urartu was apparently an older state than Phrygia and, because of its location, more strongly affected by cultural traditions from Mesopotamia. The kingdom, which probably formed early in the ninth century, was centered around Lake Van in southeastern Anatolia, a country of forested, high mountains, fertile plateaus and valleys, and rich mineral resources. Its later history is known mainly from the records of the wars which the kings of Assyria fought with the rulers of Urartu in the eighth century. Urartu blocked Assyrian control of the routes to the east and north and kept Assyria from access to needed supplies of metals. The Urartian rulers who are sometimes identified as descendants of the Hurrians were powerful and vigorous. They united the tribal groups of the region into a strong state, which pressed Assyria hard, and extended their control into the region of the Upper Tigris and Zab rivers and over the land of the Mannaeans, south of Lake Urmia in northwestern Iran.

The Urartian centers, on which extensive excavation has just begun, were strongly fortified citadels. Although the economy remained agricultural, the kings exploited the mineral resources of their kingdom, and Urartu became an influential center of bronze- and iron-working. Its best-known products are great cauldrons, the rims of which are decorated with the heads of griffins, sirens, and bulls. Some were exported to North Syria and to the Mediterranean coast, thence to Greece, where they, too, formed a part of the orientalizing influences which affected early Greek art. In 714 B.C. Sargon II of Assyria inflicted a heavy defeat on Urartu; then in 707 B.C. the Cimmerians swept over the land. While Urartu soon dropped from history, its cultural traditions were passed on in part to the Medes and Persians.

The Cimmerians

The Cimmerians, whose invasion had such a paralyzing effect in Anatolia, were an Iranian people from southern Russia, driven, according to Greek tradition, by their kindred, the Scythians, into the Caucasus. From the mountains they poured down into eastern Anatolia as a warrior horde, bent on plunder and destruction. Even after ravaging Urartu and Phrygia the roving bands of horsemen continued to terrorize and to raid. In 705 B.C. they were turned from Assyria by Sargon II at the cost of his life, and the Assyrian kings continued to keep them out of the Fertile Crescent. After the destruction of Phrygia the main group turned towards the Black Sea, near which they ultimately settled and were absorbed into the native population. In the seventh century, however, two main descents were made from the plateau to the west. In 668/67 B.C. King Gyges of Lydia (p. 155) defended his kingdom successfully, perhaps with Assyrian aid, but in 652 B.C. he was killed in battle, and his capital city, Sardes, was partially destroyed. Some damage was done also to the Greek cities on the Aegean coast, but the effects of these thrusts were transitory. By the end of the century the Lydians had driven the invaders back to the plateau.

By 700 B.C., as we have noticed in several connections, Assyria had gathered almost all the small states of the Near East under its rule. The petty kingdoms and city-states had played their part in developing trade, in seeking out and distributing metals, and in preserving and developing the traditions of the past. They were too weak and too divided to stand against the military power of Assyria, which formed them into a tributary empire in the course of the ninth and eighth centuries.

VII

The Reorganization of the Near East

(ca. 750–500 B.C.)

IN 745 B.C. TIGLATH-PILESER III became king of Assyria. His kingdom was small and disorganized, despite the successful raids made by Assyrian kings in the preceding century. By the time of his death in 727 B.C., Assyria was the dominant power of the East and the foundations for a wealthy and highly centralized empire had been laid. The warlike and able successors of Tiglath-Pileser III extended it to take in the lands of the Near East from Egypt to western Iran and from southern Anatolia to Arabia and the Persian Gulf. The history of the Assyrian Empire was brief, and the annals of its kings a record of conquest and revolt, but the unity which Assyria had created was not lost when the capital city, Nineveh, fell in 612 B.C. to the combined attack of Babylonians and Medes.

At first the lands of the Empire were divided among new states: a revived Egypt, ruled by kings from Sais in the delta (Saite Egypt), the Kingdom of Media and the New Babylonian Empire. In western Anatolia the Kingdom of Lydia became the chief power and allied itself to Egypt and to Babylonia. Yet, within two generations of the fall of Nineveh, Cyrus the Great of Persia began the campaigns which resulted in the establishment of the Persian Empire. Cyrus' conquest was speedy, for he could build on the organization established by Assyria. While Assyria had been little more than a name to the rising city-states of Greece, the Persian Empire came to symbolize the East, the antithesis to their own European civilization, and its king was the Great King. Persia had drawn together the threads of Near Eastern civilization under its political control. Until Alexander the Great marched east in 334 B.C., the Persian Empire was the framework within which the various peoples of the Near East lived and maintained their separate cultural traditions.

The Assyrian Empire

The Assyrians lived in the region of the Upper Tigris River, a land of hills and upland farms and pastures, which rose from the plain of Babylonia

The reader will find Maps III and VI (pages 74 and 156) useful as he reads this chapter.

to the mountains of Armenia. The people were the product of infiltration and invasion from the plain to the south, predominantly Semitic and akin to the Amorites who had invaded Babylonia in the early part of the second millennium before Christ. Assyria was small, about ten thousand square miles in area, but a key to the communications of Mesopotamia. Although such a key position made the land vulnerable to attack on all sides, it also provided, as the Assyrians demonstrated, a base from which raids could be launched and the movement of trade along the routes converging on Mesopotamia could be controlled.

During the second millennium the Assyrians had absorbed much from Babylonian culture and had played some part in its growth. As we have already noticed (p. 42), Assyrian merchants established trading colonies at Kanesh and at other sites in southern Anatolia in the nineteenth century B.C. to procure copper. They wrote their language, Old Assyrian, in cuneiform symbols. Assyrian law was modeled on the Code of Hammurabi, as we know from the fragmentary remains of a code dating from the Late Bronze Age. The penalties of the Assyrian Code, however, were much more severe than those of Hammurabi and reveal the Assyrians as a harder, even a savage people, in contrast to the Babylonians of the plain. They were mainly herders and farmers, toughened by their life in the hills and by continuous fighting, both against their enemies and among themselves. Yet the kings of the Assyrian Empire regarded themselves as the heirs to Sumerian and Babylonian culture. They collected old inscriptions and founded libraries, in which their scribes copied Babylonian documents—a useful practice to which we owe much of our knowledge of Babylonian civilization.

The first strong Assyrian state was formed in the Late Bronze Age upon the decline of Mitanni, of which the Kingdom Assyria had been a part. In the fourteenth century Ashur-uballit I (1365–30 B.C.) was able to expand to the west, and his successors held a little empire across the arch of the Fertile Crescent for about a century. At the outset of the Iron Age, however, Assyrian power declined rapidly, when repercussions from the ethnic movements in Asia Minor and in the Fertile Crescent were felt. Assyria itself was torn by internal anarchy. Perhaps the disturbances in Asia Minor had cut off supplies of metals at a time when Assyria's strength was needed to ward off new enemies. In the eleventh century Assyria felt the pressure of the Aramaean tribes pushing in from the west and of the Muski (the later Phrygians?) on the north. Tiglath-Pileser I (1105–1070 B.C.) defeated the Muski, but the Aramaeans took over cities on the middle Euphrates, which had belonged to Assyria, and blocked the routes to the west. Continuous fighting, however, trained the Assyrians to war and aided the recoalescence of their kingdom. By 900 B.C. Assyria was a strong, militant state, able to defend itself successfully and to mount long raids (*razzias*) for plunder to the west and south. Yet during this same period Urartu also had become a strong kingdom (pp. 139–40) and the two powers became locked in a lengthy struggle.

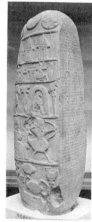

A boundary marker of King Nebuchadrezzar I (1124–03 B.C.). For a time he ruled Assyria, as well as his native Babylonia.

During the ninth century before Christ, Assyria became the chief power of the Near East. The small kingdoms to the west, as far as the Mediterranean coast, were weakened by continuous raids and intimidated by demonstrations of brutal military power. A start was made on the organization of a centralized empire, but Assyria itself was not fully consolidated, and the kings, faced by revolt, had to turn from raiding their neighbors to asserting their own power over would-be usurpers. In the series of raids, however, a purpose is apparent. The Assyrian kings wanted to secure the approaches to their country and to control the main routes of the Fertile Crescent. Apparently they did not wish to engage in trade themselves, but to collect tolls, secure control of the distribution of metals, and to skim off the accumulated wealth of the older trading cities.

Assyrian expansion began in the reign of Adad-nirari II (911–891 B.C.), who advanced to the south below the Lower Zab River and gained control of the routes leading into the mountains to the east of Assyria. He also fought a series of difficult campaigns to the west, where the Assyrian cities on the middle Euphrates were recovered and the frontier was pushed to the Habur River. The new border areas were converted into provinces, tribute was imposed, and military service demanded. Thus a more defensible core of territory was created to serve as a base from which longer campaigns could be mounted.

The most striking military achievements of Assyria in the ninth century were the long campaigns to the west made by Ashur-nasir-pal II (883–59 B.C.) and his son, Shalmaneser III (858–24 B.C.). We know of them in detail through the annals of their reigns found in the excavation of the capital city. In 879 B.C. Ashur-nasir-pal moved from the old Assyrian center at Ashur to Calah (Nimrud) at the junction of the Upper Zab and Tigris rivers. He built a great palace there, which was excavated in the last century by Sir Henry Layard, one of the founders of Assyrian studies. The annals, a yearly chronicle of Ashur-nasir-pal's exploits, were inscribed on the building blocks used for decoration in the palace and other structures and constitute the earliest important body of source material which we have for Assyrian history. They are invaluable both for their historical detail and as a record of the character of Assyrian war and of the aspect which its kings wished to assume.

The annals tell of the Assyrian army advancing relentlessly through wild territory, scaling mountains, crossing rivers and crushing their enemies in battle. Defeated leaders were tortured by mutilation and dismemberment, flayed alive, boiled, or impaled. Their wealth in gold, silver, iron, copper, rare woods, textiles, furniture, and jewelry was carried back to Assyria as plunder. The tribute imposed was listed in itemized detail. Thousands of people were deported to Assyria for settlement on lands which the king wished to develop. The Assyrians were no worse than their contemporaries in waging violent and brutal war, judging from the gory details of Jehu's treatment of the royal family in

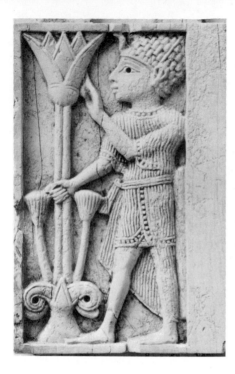

An ivory carving from the Assyrian palace at Nimrud. The carvings were mainly the work of Phoenician craftsmen and were used to inlay furniture.

Israel, but they do seem to have been more systematic in recording the details. Our own twentieth century after Christ is hardly in a position to condemn them, but these annals were first translated in the nineteenth century, when Assyria was revealed in contrast to Victorian England and to Western Europe. Thus Assyrian atrocities in war tended to overshadow the constructive acts of Assyrian kings in developing their country and in breaking the political parochialism of the Near East. The development was an ugly process, but it did build the foundation for a more prosperous unity under the direction of a single great power.

Ashur-nasir-pal opened the routes to Syria and the Mediterranean by the conquest of the Aramaean kingdom of Bit-Adini and by taking the heavily fortified Hittite city of Carchemish on the Euphrates. He marched through Syria to the coast and symbolically commemorated his conquest by dipping his sword in the waters of the Mediterranean. The Phoenician cities were made tributary to Assyria, and soon Damascus and Israel were added by Shalmaneser III. Both Ashur-nasir-pal and Shalmaneser did much to develop Assyria, in addition to raiding and adding to their list of tributary states. New towns were built, the road system was improved, and new land was opened to settlement and cultivation. Both monarchs built on a scale commensurate with their power. At Nimrud the new capital city was laid out on a monumental scale, with parks and gardens irrigated by water brought in channels from the Zab River. Craftsmen were brought from Phoenicia and the Syro-Hittite cities to decorate the palace and to make its furniture. Excavation has revealed the sculpture and discovered the ivory panels, carved in Phoenician style, with which the king's furniture was inlaid.

The conquests made in the ninth century, however, could not be properly consolidated. In the latter part of Shalmaneser's reign, revolt broke out in Assyria, and Urartu began to attack from the north and to expand westwards, threatening control of the routes to Syria and Anatolia. The Assyrians were cut off from supplies of metal, from the tolls on trade, and from the tribute which they had imposed. By the mid-eighth century Assyria had shrunk to its original territory and was beginning to disintegrate as local leaders vied for kingship. The routes to Syria and the west had been blocked by the successful expansion of Urartu, and on the northeast Assyria was similarly barred from the regions south of Lake Urmia. In the Babylonian plain the kings of Babylon were militant and successful in holding Assyria back. Yet Assyria had established a tradition of conquest and possessed a trained and ferocious army. It needed a strong king.

THE GREAT ASSYRIAN KINGS (745–612 B.C.)

Tiglath-Pileser III (745–27 B.C.), who usurped the throne in 745 B.C., was the real founder of the Assyrian Empire, the first of a series of strong kings who continuously extended their frontiers and held the Empire together for over a century. Early in his reign Tiglath-Pileser came to an understanding with the king of Babylon which freed his hands to deal with Urartu. Sardur, the king of Urartu, was defeated and forced to withdraw within the limits of his own kingdom. In the west Tiglath-Pileser thrust through Syria and Palestine as far as the Egyptian frontier. Damascus was retaken and in 734 B.C. Israel made a vassal state. Tiglath-Pileser began the consolidation of his conquests by appointing governors in some territories, using native kings in others, and improving communication throughout the Empire by the establishment of a regular messenger service. In 734 B.C. he himself became king of Babylon upon the death of his former ally and was duly recognized by the great god Marduk as the descendant of the kings of the former Babylonian Empire. Upon Tiglath-Pileser's death his son, Shalmaneser V, was confronted by a coalition in the west between Egypt and Israel and began the reduction of Israel to a province. He died before the capital, Samaria, was taken, but that was accomplished by Sargon II, who came to the throne in 722 B.C. As noticed before (p. 134), many of the leaders of Israel were deported to Assyria at this time, when the state disappeared from history.

Sargon II (722–05 B.C.), like Tiglath-Pileser, came to the throne through usurpation. At the outset of his reign he apparently asserted his claim to a place in Mesopotamian history by taking his name from the great Sargon of Akkad, who had ruled, in legend at least, from the Great Sea, the Mediterranean, to the Persian Gulf. The second Sargon imitated him in a reign filled with war and conquest. At the start Babylon broke away from Assyrian control and could not be recovered for ten years. In the interval Sargon put down revolts in Syria and effectively damaged Assyria's chief rival, Urartu. In 714 B.C. he led his army deep into Urartu, ravaging the land and seizing plunder from its cities. The holy city of Musasir was taken, but Sargon for some reason failed to assault the capital, although the king, Rusas, had fled from it into the mountains. The damage was great, however, and the power of Urartu weakened on the eve of the Cimmerian invasion. Sargon fought successfully, too, against Mita of Muski (Midas of Phrygia) and kept him from penetrating to the coast through Cilicia. It is ironical that Sargon weakened the kingdoms of Anatolia on the eve of the Cimmerian invasion, for in 705 B.C. he had to fight a great battle against their hordes to save his own Empire. Sargon was killed in the fighting, but his army won the battle. The Cimmerians were diverted northward towards Phrygia. Despite the almost continuous warfare of his reign, Sargon found the time to build a new capital north of Nimrud on the Tigris. It was called Dur-Sharrukin (Khorsabad), the city of Sargon.

While Sargon's successful invasion, coupled with the Cimmerian raid, had effectively removed the threat of Urartu from Assyria, the Empire was too new and Assyrian methods of control too harsh to ensure internal peace. Sargon's successor, Sennacherib (704–681 B.C.), did find more time for building and organization than his father but had to cope with serious revolts during his reign. He selected a new capital, Nineveh (Mosul), farther down the Tigris than Dur-Sharrukin and adorned it with a botanical garden and park, for which plants and trees were brought from various parts of the Empire. Sennacherib also cultivated a technical interest in such matters as bronze-casting and irrigation, but like other successful Assyrian kings, he had to assert his power in war. In 703 and in 688 B.C. Babylon revolted. On the latter occasion Sennacherib looted and destroyed the city as an example to his rebellious subjects. Although the revolt was successfully suppressed, Sennacherib had raised a more formidable foe. Since the Elamites had come to the aid of Babylon, Sennacherib felt it necessary to attack their kingdom in the foothills of the Zagros Mountains. The Elamites were well-trained and tough soldiers; consequently the reduction of Elam was to cost Assyria heavily in manpower. In the west Egypt, although not a formidable enemy in itself, intrigued with Judah and the Phoenician cities against Assyria. Sennacherib appeared before Jerusalem and, in the words of his annals, shut up its king, Hezekiah, "like a bird in a cage." Jerusalem itself escaped destruction, but Hezekiah was made a vassal and paid tribute to Assyria. Sennacherib also held the Phoenician cities and even extended the Empire in the west. In 696 B.C., invading Cilicia, he took Tarsus, its chief town. Despite these successes, Sennacherib's reign ended in revolt. His successor, Esarhaddon, came to the throne in a general state of unrest. He proved equal to the challenge and during his reign enlarged the Empire to its greatest extent.

The chief conquest of Esarhaddon's reign (681–69 B.C.) was that of Egypt. The rulers of Egypt had made it their policy to intrigue with the Assyrian vassal kings in the west, and, despite Sennacherib's success, Esarhaddon was threatened again by revolt in that quarter. The king put down the risings and converted Phoenicia into a regular province. Then, to remove the cause of the trouble, in 671 B.C. he invaded Egypt. Although the Egyptian army was defeated in the delta and the city of Memphis captured, Egypt was too large and too far from Assyria to be converted into a province and controlled by a governor with garrison troops. Accordingly, Esarhaddon took the risk of using some of the local Egyptian princes of the delta as vassal kings. Two years after the conquest Esarhaddon died en route to Egypt to suppress a revolt by his vassals. Nevertheless, the Empire was at its height during his reign, and Esarhaddon could afford to plan and build on the grand scale. His most ambitious and useful project was the restoration of Babylon, which was ostentatiously refounded and repopulated.

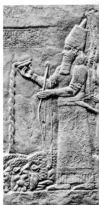

King Ashurbanipal making an offering

Ashurbanipal (669–27 B.C.), who had been proclaimed co-ruler with his father, Esarhaddon, succeeded without difficulty after the latter's death. He was the last of the great kings of Assyria, but even during his reign the dissolution of the Empire began. It was too large to be held by the harsh, terroristic methods of Assyrian control, for Assyrian manpower was small. The Assyrians hired soldiers and used levies from the subject peoples, but in the last analysis the aggressive, violent character of their rule had to be maintained by the Assyrians themselves. In the seventh century, too, new and more dangerous rivals were beginning to appear. In the northeast the Median Kingdom was rising. In Babylonia the Chaldaeans of the south found common cause with the Elamites against Assyria. While Ashurbanipal suppressed the revolt of Egypt at the outset of his reign, its very suppression kindled Egyptian nationalism even more. By 650 B.C. the vassal kings of Sais in the delta had expelled the Assyrian garrisons from Egypt and had begun to consolidate the country under their own control. The Saite kings found a new ally in Gyges, the King of Lydia, who disavowed the alliance with Assyria made in 668/67 B.C. when he needed help against the Cimmerians. Ashurbanipal had granted the alliance disdainfully, as befitted the great king of Assyria, to an upstart of whom he had never heard. While Gyges reaped a proper reward in Assyrian eyes, when he was killed in the Cimmerian attack of 652 B.C., his conduct indicates that Assyria was weakening. In 652 Babylonia and the Elamites revolted. Ashurbanipal had placed his own brother, Shamash-shum-ukin, in charge of Babylon, but the latter conspired with the Elamites, perhaps hoping to gain the Assyrian throne for himself. Ashurbanipal suppressed the revolt by 648 B.C., but the casualties were high and left his Assyrian manpower seriously depleted. In the next decade Media renounced its vassalage to Assyria, and Ashurbanipal's reign ended in political confusion and personal despair. In contrast to the disdain with which he had treated Gyges at the outset of his rule, Ashurbanipal confessed abjectly near the end that all his own endeavors were turning out badly.

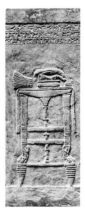

An Assyrian altar

The collapse of the Empire followed quickly upon the death of Ashurbanipal. Babylonia asserted its independence of the Assyrians and made an alliance with the Median Kingdom. In 614 B.C. the two states invaded Assyria.

In 612 they took Nineveh, destroying and plundering the city. Although a remnant of the Assyrians fled to Harran, the Babylonians took that city in 610 and thus ended the last vestige of Assyrian domination.

THE ORGANIZATION OF THE EMPIRE

The Assyrians themselves took little part in the economic life and society of the Empire but remained aloof as a governing group. The ordinary people, most of whom were farmers and shepherds, served in the armies and manned the garrisons which held the Empire by military force. The nobility were a ruling class who acted as administrators and who were moved from post to post at the king's discretion. They took no root in the provinces and vassal states to which they were assigned. The head of state was the king, who ruled absolutely and personally as the chosen representative of Ashur, the warrior god of Assyria, and of Marduk, the great god of Babylon. As the god's representative the king claimed universal dominion and exercised all the functions of political, religious, and military leadership. As high priests of the national god, some Assyrian kings tried to make the worship of Ashur and Marduk supreme in the Empire, but no religious hierarchy was formed under the king's direction; thus the administration of the subject peoples was essentially political and secular.

The absolute role of the king was centralized in the great palaces which were both their residence and administrative center. As we have noticed, almost every king felt it proper to emphasize his dominance by constructing a new palace. Despite the voluminous detail of their annals, we know little of the kings as individuals, for they were described by stereotyped titles: "Esarhaddon, King of the Universe, King of Assyria, Viceroy of Babylon, King of Sumer and Akkad, the exalted prince." In art the kings were represented as strong, fully bearded and dignified figures, wearing elaborate ceremonial costume and bearing the royal insignia of their office. The queen, as principal wife and mother of the heir apparent, had a prominent place at court and at the time of succession might play an important role as regent. The crown prince, who was elaborately trained for his position (judging from Ashurbanipal's training), received instruction not only in war, hunting and religious duties, but in literature and science. An orderly succession, however, was not easy in Assyria since younger sons and members of the lesser branches of the royal family were ambitious and since at all times the kingdom required a strong leader. Perhaps,

Reconstruction of the palace of King Sargon II at Khorsabad

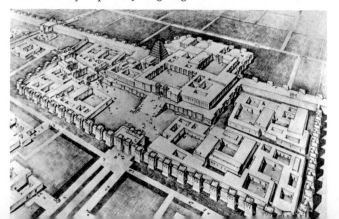

too, an old and primitive custom, which required the removal of the ruler after thirty years of tenure, still had some force at the time of the Assyrian Empire. Such a custom would have been an excuse, at least, to cloak ambition.

The chief officials of state were the prime minister, the general of the armies, and the governors of the provinces. In the palace of the king and in the retinues of the provincial governors there were minor officials and scribes who were able to translate and to write the various languages of the Empire, as well as Assyrian. While there is still much detail to work out about Assyrian administration from the documentary sources, it seems apparent that the kings preferred to set up large units of administration, territorial provinces, in which the formerly independent small states were subordinated as municipalities. The creation of a province was frequently the consequence of revolt by some vassal king who had betrayed his oath of allegiance. The governors were put in general charge of their area of administration and were made responsible for keeping order, collecting the tribute, and carrying out the directives of the king. As we know from the correspondence which has been discovered in the Assyrian palaces, the king's supervision was detailed and strict, and his administration swift to act. He took an overall view of the needs of empire; in many areas roads were improved and messenger services established to link the capital with the governor's residence. Large-scale works of irrigation and agricultural improvement were undertaken, both in Assyria and in the provinces. For example, cotton and indigo were brought to Assyria from Iran, and olive trees and vines were extensively grown in northern Mesopotamia. The parks of the Assyrian kings, like those of their Persian successors, were designed to be botanical and zoological gardens, as well as to give the rulers pleasure.

While Assyrian methods of ensuring order were extremely harsh, it is perhaps worth noting that torture was used primarily for those who had broken their oath of allegiance. It was the penalty for a religious offense. The deportations of peoples did uproot thousands from their homes and obliterated national traditions and ethnic identities, but the movements were carried out with proper regard for the welfare of the people concerned and ultimately resulted in a greater homogeneity of population.

Because war, however, was the most characteristic activity of the Assyrians, they made it as efficient and ruthless as they could. At first the army was mainly a native militia, with the soldiers being imbued with national loyalty. They were hardy, tough and well trained, armed with excellent weapons provided by the large supplies of metal to which the Assyrians had access. In fact, the emphasis on bronze and iron in the booty lists of the kings almost suggests that one of the main purposes of Assyrian war was to acquire those metals.

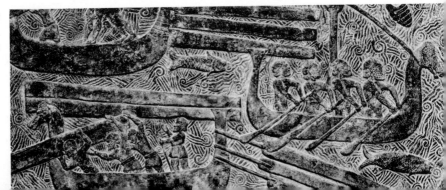

Assyrian soldiers crossing a river. Relief from Khorsabad

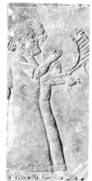

Assyrian soldiers going to battle

The army whose branches were well balanced and coordinated was properly diversified for fighting on various types of terrain. For battle on the plains the Assyrians developed a new type of chariot war. The cars carried three men, a driver, a fighter, and a shield bearer. In the ninth century, when the Assyrians found themselves slow and awkward in mountain warfare, they developed cavalry, making use of both mounted archers and sabre fighters. They probably learned these new techniques from the Aryan invaders of Iran, who were settling in the Zagros Mountains to the northeast of Assyria in this period. From them, the Assyrians also procured their mounts by making long forays to the Iranian plateau. The infantry was heavily armed, highly maneuverable, and it worked closely with the siege troops. The sophisticated art of siege warfare, in fact, was mainly an Assyrian invention. Rams, catapults, techniques of mining under walls, and scaling over them were all employed against the heavily fortified city-states of Syria and the citadels of Urartu.

Musicians

The Assyrian kings, however, were also patrons of art and literature on the grand scale. Their taste in art was eclectic, because the king collected his treasures from the Empire and could use the services of various workmen trained in their native tradition. Yet in relief sculpture, at least, the taste of the kings developed a distinctive Assyrian representation. The practice of decorating their palaces with relief sculptures, cut on a course of upright slabs, was borrowed from the Syro-Hittites, but the Assyrian sculptors developed a new method of presentation and high skill in carving. Scenes were linked in a continuous narrative, which gave unity to the frieze and to the room in which it was displayed. The animal style used by the artists was remarkably powerful and is exemplified, in particular, by the hunting scenes of dying lions tearing at the arrows which have felled them. Evidently a mixture of ferocity and cruelty appealed to Assyrian taste.

The particular contribution of royal patronage to Mesopotamian culture was an almost encyclopaedic summing up of its accumulated knowledge and literature. In the palaces thousands of documents have been found, not only those valuable for the study of Assyrian history and administration, but also copies of older Babylonian records. Those from the library of Ashurbanipal in his palace at Nineveh are an example of this reverence for the past. The king's scribes were set to copying the religious and literary texts of Sumer and Babylonia: the epics, myths, prayers, hymns, astronomical and medical texts, historical chronicles, and royal inscriptions. The scribes also did a considerable amount of scholarly work by compiling vocabularies and dictionaries and making translations into Assyrian. The Assyrian scribes themselves made a significant contribution to historiography by their detailed chronicles of the king's exploits. These annals are voluminous and precise about the events which they record and provide a firm chronology for the Empire. Their bias, of course, wholly Assyrian, the annals condemn the king's enemies as treacherous wretches, deserving of the worst that Assyria can inflict. Yet sometimes, like the annals of Ashur-nasir-pal, their very detail gives a picture of the relentless might of Assyrian conquest. Perhaps the best testimonial to the order and prosperity which the Assyrian Empire had promoted in the Near East was the speed and relative ease with which the new kingdoms, which succeeded it, were able to establish themselves.

Upon the fall of Nineveh in 612 B.C. there was a rush to pick up the spoils by the new states which had developed in reaction to Assyrian pressure. The New Kingdom of Babylonia under its king, Nabopolassar, clashed with Saite Egypt over Syria and Palestine, but emerged as heir to the greater part of the Assyrian Empire, ruling over Babylonia, Assyria, Syria, Palestine and, in its final years, a part of Arabia. Egypt was limited to its own territory, but the Saite kings sponsored a renaissance of Egyptian tradition and brought prosperity to Egypt by encouraging trade with their neighbors and with the rising Greek cities of the Aegean. The Median Kingdom was able to expand into Armenia and Anatolia. There the Medes clashed with Lydia, but the two states agreed upon the Halys River as their frontier. Lydia itself controlled western Asia Minor from the Halys to the Greek cities of the Aegean coast. All these kingdoms were absorbed by Cyrus the Great of Persia, but the interlude between the Assyrian and Persian Empires (612–550 B.C.) was relatively peaceful, during which each kingdom, after initial clashes, accepted the limitations of its power.

The New Babylonian Kingdom (612–539 B.C.)

The chief successor to the Assyrian Empire was the New Babylonian Kingdom, but its rulers had to make good their claim to Syria and Palestine by war with Egypt. In the last days of the Assyrian Empire the Egyptian king, Necho, who had allied himself with Assyria, upon its fall marched in force into Palestine. Nabopolassar of Babylon defeated the Assyrian remnant at Harran in 610 B.C. and wisely maintained good relations with the Medes while he dealt with Necho. The small states of Phoenicia and Palestine, which were a fertile ground for Egyptian intrigue, saw more hope of independence by alliance with Egypt than with Babylonia. The Babylonians made good their claim to the western part of the Empire by defeating the Egyptian army at Carchemish in 605 B.C., but it was not until 568 that a treaty of peace was made between the two powers.

In the interval the little state of Judah, its rulers caught up in the rivalry of their greater neighbors, disappeared. First, King Josiah, in a vain hope of expanding his kingdom, perished in battle with the Egyptians at Megiddo in 608 B.C. Since his successors chose to intrigue with Egypt against Babylonia, the Babylonian king, Nebuchadrezzar, twice took Jerusalem, in 597 and 586 B.C. On the latter occasion the walls of the city were thrown down and many of the governing class were carried off in captivity to Babylonia. There, by the waters of Babylon, as they lamented, the Hebrews of the Exile had to build a new life. In Phoenicia the great fortress city and seaport of Tyre, which played the same game as Judah, resisted siege on several occasions but was taken in 571 B.C. Upon the conclusion of the treaty with Egypt in 568 B.C. Babylon ruled unchecked in the west.

The reign of Nabopolassar's successor, Nebuchadrezzar (605-562 B.C.), was the high point of Babylonian prosperity and power. The king, who proved himself an able administrator and statesman, during his reign built Babylon into the greatest city of the East. Its fortifications were strengthened and a tall ziggurat built, whose stepped construction was misinterpreted in legend as the terraces for the "Hanging Gardens." Nebuchadrezzar, probably by deliberate contrast to Assyria, allowed considerable authority to the priesthoods of the temples in Babylonia, permitting them to make decisions about irrigation and agricultural revenues and, even in some instances about local defense. The Babylonian priesthood regarded their kings as tenants of the gods and demanded that they give a satisfactory account of themselves to Marduk each year. Despite the brilliance of Nebuchadrezzar's reign, he failed to establish the kingship firmly, and three successors reigned between 562 and 556 B.C., when a strong new ruler, Nabonidus, seized the throne.

Nabonidus (556-39) and his son, Belshazzar, who was associated in rule with his father in the latter part of the reign, were the last native rulers of Babylon. Nabonidus was unpopular with the priesthood and people in Babylon, partly because his family was not native to the city but came from Harran, and partly because he attempted to centralize authority in his own hands.

A herd of gazelle. Nineveh, Palace of Ashurbanipal

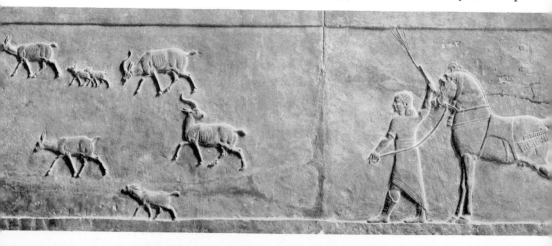

Nabonidus faced a deteriorating economic situation. Nebuchadrezzar had stimulated inflation by spending lavishly on building projects and on the army, while at the same time revenue dropped because the Medes cut the trade routes to the east. Nabonidus, to solve the latter difficulty, made an alliance with Cyrus of Persia about 550 B.C., when the latter was preparing to overthrow the Median Kingdom. This alliance proved of little use, for very soon Cyrus further damaged Babylonian trade by thrusting across Assyria and southern Anatolia to Cilicia. Perhaps to make good these losses Nabonidus devoted ten years of his reign to the conquest of northern Arabia, using the oasis of Temna as a base of operations. To provide a new unifying force for his kingdom, and perhaps to obtain a greater share of temple revenues, Nabonidus tried to make the moon-god, Sin, who had a great temple in Harran and was popular with the Aramaeans, the chief god of the state. The priesthood of Marduk in Babylon turned against Nabonidus and listened to the overtures of Cyrus who was ready by 540 B.C. for the conquest of Babylonia. In 539 B.C. Cyrus attacked and took the city with little resistance. The priesthood recognized him as king of Babylonia, and thus the last native dynasty of Mesopotamia fell. The city of Babylon became one of the important centers of the new Persian Empire.

The Saite Kingdom of Egypt[1] (ca. 650–525 B.C.)

Although Egypt had been in eclipse since the early twelfth century, it had been ruled in part by foreign kings from Nubia and Libya who had adopted Egyptian customs; consequently the traditions of Egypt had endured. The new Egypt, which asserted its independence in the mid-seventh century, was engendered in large part by nationalistic feeling against foreign rule and, in particular, against Assyrian conquest. The Saite kings, who led this renaissance, had begun to rise to prominence in the late eighth century out of the score or more of local princes who ruled in Lower Egypt. At that time their overlords were Nubians who had extended their control from Upper Egypt into the delta. It was against these Nubian kings of Egypt, intriguing among the Assyrian vassals in Palestine and Syria, that Esarhaddon and Ashurbanipal made war. Having defeated them, they selected their vassals from the Egyptian princes of the delta. The princes of the city of Sais, Necho and his son Psammetichus, were among these. Since both proved untrustworthy to Assyria, about 650 B.C., while Ashurbanipal was fighting in Babylonia, Psammetichus expelled the Assyrian garrisons and set about the consolidation of Egypt.

Psammetichus (*ca.* 655–10 B.C.) was able to defeat his rivals and take over Egypt by extensive use of foreign mercenary soldiers whom he obtained through foreign alliances. A pact with Gyges of Lydia provided the chance to hire Carian and Ionian Greek soldiers from western Asia Minor. These were skilled infantry troops, armed and trained in the new heavy-armed infantry

[1] See Map II, page 48.

fashion and tactics which had been introduced into Greece a generation earlier (p. 193). Psammetichus also established trading relations with the Greeks, and by the end of the century a Greek trading post was established at Naukratis on the Canopic mouth of the Nile. The Greeks bought Egyptian wheat, linen and papyrus, as well as minor articles of luxury and paid for them in silver.

While Psammetichus and his successors failed to re-establish an Egyptian Empire in Palestine and Syria, they did restore Egyptian prosperity. Necho II (604–593 B.C.) reviving the trade with Arabia and east Africa, began the construction of a canal from the Nile to the Red Sea. Necho's intrigues with the cities of Phoenicia were accompanied also by a lively trade. Apries (586–69 B.C.) offered refuge in Egypt to the Jews of Palestine after the fall of Jerusalem and hired some as mercenary soldiers. They were quartered at Daphne in the eastern delta and far up the Nile at Elephantine. Apries, however, was too ambitious. He was defeated in an attempt to take over the Greek colony of Cyrene, established in western Libya in the previous century. Revolt in Egypt brought a new king to the throne, Amasis, whose reign marked the height of the Egyptian revival.

Amasis (569–26 B.C.), who cultivated a wide range of foreign alliances, followed a general policy of peace which was inaugurated in 568 B.C. by the treaty with Babylonia and was followed up by the granting of a charter to the Greek colony at Naukratis. The town was made into an international treaty port, in which Greeks of various origins could live and trade. Amasis' connections with western Asia Minor were strengthened by alliances with Croesus of Lydia and with Polycrates, the Greek tyrant of the island of Samos. Within Egypt Amasis restored old temples, began the construction of new ones, and encouraged a revival of the strong, realistic sculptural style of the Old Kingdom. This revival of Egyptian tradition struck a responsive note deep in the hearts of the people. In this period a popular literature, nationalistic in feeling, was developed. Its stories of the heroic days of the rise of the Saite kings were written in the simplified demotic script. The rebirth of Egypt, however, came in a rapidly changing world in which that state could not hold its place. There was no danger from the small Greek city-states, for they were anxious to trade on the terms offered by Amasis, but his reign coincided with the rise of Persia. While Cyrus' conquests stopped at the border of Egypt, his son Cambyses invaded Egypt in 525 B.C. and made it a province of the Persian Empire.

Lydia (ca. 685–547 B.C.)

The Kingdom of Lydia, centered in the valleys of the Hermus and Cayster rivers in western Asia Minor, does not seem to have had any traditions of a civilized past on which to build a nationalistic revival, like that of New Babylonia and Saite Egypt. Hittite relief sculptures, cut high on the cliffs near modern Smyrna, indicate that the land may have been a nominal part of the Hittite Empire, but, as on the Anatolian plateau, the destructive invasions at the outset of the Iron Age cut the continuity of cultural growth. Accordingly, the history of Lydia before the seventh century is very obscure. Probably its coalescence into a kingdom is to be explained by the pressure exerted by the expansion of Phrygia and the attempts of the Greeks on the Aegean coast to penetrate inland up the river valleys. In fact, there are some indications that Lydia was a part of the Phrygian kingdom for a time. Probably it was in this way that influences apparent in early Lydian art came from Assyria and the Syro-Hittite states. Historical Lydia, however, of the seventh and sixth centuries, was strongly affected by its proximity to Greece, when its history became interwoven with that of the Ionian Greek states on the Aegean coast (pp. 187–88).

Whatever the early ties with Phrygia may have been, they were broken by the Cimmerian invasion, at which time our first historical notice of Lydia appears in the annals of Ashurbanipal of Assyria. In 668/67 B.C. the Lydian king, Gyges, appealed to him for help against the Cimmerians. Probably some was given, because Gyges successfully defended himself against the Cimmerians and sent prisoners to Ashurbanipal in acknowledgment. How the kingdom of Gyges was formed and organized is not clear. Greek tradition told of his successful usurpation in the early seventh century from an earlier dynasty of Lydian kings, some of whom may have ruled at Hyde in the Cayster River valley. Gyges, however, made Sardes the center of his kingdom, and that city remained the one great urban center of Lydia. Sardes was located far up the valley of the Hermus River on the banks of a small tributary stream, the Pactolus, which flowed from Mt. Tmolus. Above the city rises a towering, rocky spur of the mountain, which the Lydian kings fortified and made into their citadel. Since Sardes presently is being excavated, it is to be hoped that the earlier history of Lydia will soon be less obscure.

To judge from our present knowledge, the Lydian people lived in peasant and herder villages, cultivating the land and tending the flocks of great landowners. The king himself who was probably the greatest of these at times had difficulty in keeping his nobles in hand. Like the Phrygians of the plateau, the Lydians were renowned as horse breeders in Greek tradition; consequently cavalry formed the most efficient branch of their army. Once organized under a centralized regime, Lydia became a strong and prosperous state. Its wealth was based mainly on agriculture, but there were also deposits of electrum, a natural alloy of gold and silver, in its territory. Discovery of the metal in the Pactolus River, which flowed through Sardes, may have played some part in the rise of that city. In any case, exploitation of the electrum was a royal monopoly which contributed greatly to the power of the kings. To the Greeks of the seventh and sixth centuries Lydia was the chief source of gold (electrum was called "white gold"), and the names of the Lydian kings, like Croesus, were a byword for great wealth.

Gyges and his successors consolidated and expanded their kingdom in hard fighting against the Cimmerian invaders and the Greek cities on the coast. As we have already noticed, the Cimmerians returned about the middle of the cen-

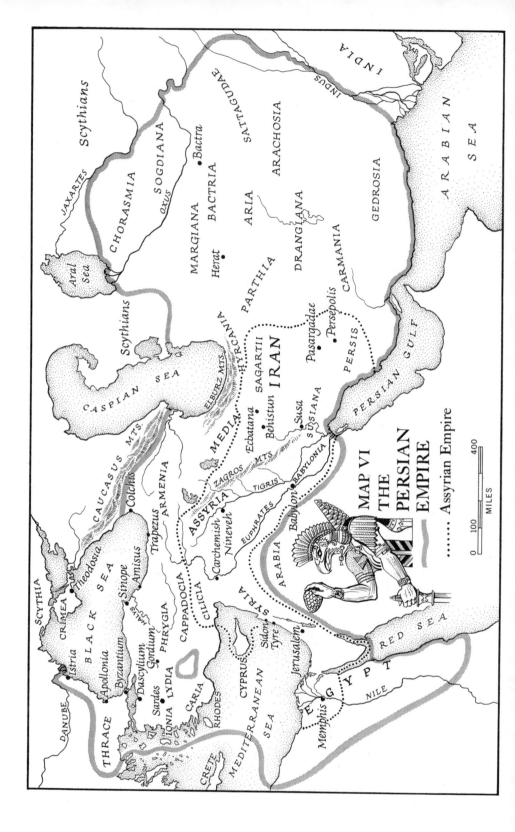

MAP VI
THE
PERSIAN
EMPIRE

.... Assyrian Empire

MILES

0   100   200   400

INDIA

Scythians

JAXARTES

SOGDIANA

CHORASMIA

OXUS

Aral
Sea

MARGIANA

BACTRIA

Bactra

SATTAGUDAE

ARACHOSIA

ARIA

Herat

PARTHIA

DRANGIANA

GEDROSIA

CARMANIA

ARABIAN
SEA

Scythians

CASPIAN
SEA

ELBURZ MTS.

HYRCANIA

SAGARTII

IRAN

Pasargadae

Persepolis

PERSIS

PERSIAN GULF

MEDIA

Ecbatana

Behistun

Susa

SUSIANA

ZAGROS MTS.

CAUCASUS MTS.

ARMENIA

Colchis

Trapezus

ASSYRIA

Carchemish

Nineveh

TIGRIS

EUPHRATES

BABYLONIA

Babylon

ARABIA

SCYTHIA

CRIMEA

Theodosia

BLACK SEA

Sinope

Amisus

HALYS

Byzantium

Apollonia

Istria

DANUBE

THRACE

Dascylium

Gordium

Sardes

PHRYGIA

CAPPADOCIA

CILICIA

SYRIA

Sidon

Tyre

Jerusalem

IONIA

LYDIA

CARIA

RHODES

CYPRUS

MEDITERRANEAN SEA

CRETE

RED SEA

Memphis

EGYPT

NILE

tury to attack Sardes when, although Gyges lost his life and the lower town of Sardes was burnt, they were beaten off. By the end of the century the Cimmerians had been driven back to the plateau, and Alyattes (*ca.* 610–560 B.C.) was able to push inland to take over the former territory of Phrygia up to the Halys River, where the frontier was drawn with the Medes. Since the Lydian hold on the plateau was tenuous, however, the state developed a close relationship with the Greek cities on the coast.

While Lydia never aspired to become a sea power and to take over the Greek cities as ports, the Lydian kings raided the Greeks continuously and in the sixth century Croesus (560–47 B.C.) made them subject allies. Greek soldiers fought in the Lydian army and Greek craftsmen worked for Lydian patronage. Greek merchants exported the agricultural products and electrum of Lydia and brought exotic luxuries from Phoenicia and Egypt to the Lydian market. The two peoples formed a virtual economic union to the great profit of each. Out of their intensive intercourse there developed the first real coinage of the ancient world (p. 187). Croesus took the additional and important step of adopting a bimetallic standard to bring his Lydian coins of electrum into relationship with the silver issues of the Greeks of the Aegean.

During the brief reign of Croesus (560–47 B.C.) the power of Lydia was at its height. His kingdom extended from northwestern Asia Minor to Caria, below the Maeander River, and from the Aegean coast to the Halys. Croesus also established good relations with the Greeks across the Aegean, where he made costly dedications to the oracle of Apollo at Delphi and an alliance with Sparta. Despite his wealth and network of foreign alliances, Croesus was swept up in the Persian conquest. In 547 B.C. Cyrus marched west through Asia Minor and took Sardes by assault. When in 540 B.C. Croesus' Greek allies on the coast had been taken over by one of Cyrus' generals, all of western Asia Minor was in Persian hands.

The Persian Empire

The ancient history of the Near and Middle East culminated in the establishment of the Persian Empire by Cyrus and Darius the Great in the latter part of the sixth century B.C. From their capitals in western Iran the Persian kings ruled over Egypt, Palestine, Syria, Asia Minor, Mesopotamia, Iran itself, and for a time northwestern India and Thrace. The Empire stretched from the Mediterranean to the steppes of central Asia and from the Black and Caspian Seas to the Persian Gulf and Indian Ocean. Its subject peoples included the Greeks of western Asia Minor, the seminomads of the Iranian plateau and the varied ethnic and cultural groups of the Fertile Crescent. All were ruled by the Aryan Medes and Persians who entered Iran about 1000 B.C.

Iran, despite its seeming inaccessibility, is usually described as the land bridge from central to western Asia. It consists of a great central plateau of arid desert rimmed by mountains. On the north the Elburz Mountains form a high

barrier between the plateau and the Caspian Sea, but at each end the mountains
sink into fertile hill country with cultivable valleys. At the west, modern
Azerbaizan, ancient Media, is accessible from the north by the land corridor
west of the Caspian and by routes through the mountains to Anatolia and
northern Mesopotamia. Media was a fertile region with ample rainfall and a
healthy, if severe, climate. On the east the Elburz sink into the hill country of
Parthia, which formed a gateway into Iran for the nomads of central Asia. The
Zagros Mountains closed the west side of the plateau from Mesopotamia, but,
as we have noticed, the Zagros were by no means impassable. The kings of
Sumer, Babylonia and Assyria raided the mountains, and the Kassites and
Mitannians had descended from them. At an early date the Kingdom of Elam
had formed under strong Mesopotamian cultural influence in the region northeast of the Persian Gulf, adjacent to Sumer. The southern part of the plateau,
however, is salt desert and almost untraversable, but passes lead into Baluchistan
and by the Kabul River in the southeast to northwestern India.

The pattern of communication and of habitation followed the mountain
ranges. The chief east-west route through Iran lay along the inner side of the
Elburz from Ecbatana (Hamadan) in Media to Herat in Afghanistan, while the
principal north-south road followed the edge of the plateau along the Zagros.
Agriculture was possible along the edge of the desert with proper irrigation, and
in the Persian Period an elaborate system of underground channels (qanats), to
prevent evaporation, was constructed to bring water from the mountains. There,
rainfall and melting snow provided a good supply. The Zagros Mountains were
cut by long parallel valleys from north to south with fertile soil, timber, and
seasonal pasture. In general, the terrain and the climate of Iran prescribed a seminomadic or locally self-contained type of life in which urbanization and the
formation of centralized authority were slow. While life was primarily pastoral
and agricultural, Iran possessed valuable resources: the timber of the mountains,
iron, copper, tin, lead and semiprecious stones, turquoise and lapis lazuli. Sheep
furnished wool for textiles and, after the coming of the Aryans, there were
horses for cavalry and chariots.

As yet little is known about the early movements and settlement of the
Aryans in Iran. They were warrior horsemen who traveled in bands with their
wives and children in search of good pastureland and favorable locations for
settlement. Probably they came in successive waves of migration on each side of
the Caspian, following the natural routes of communication into the northwestern region of the country, where the Kingdom of Media later coalesced.
Further movement to the west was blocked by the established states of Urartu
and of Mesopotamia, so the Aryans gradually spread and settled in the mountains. At first small bands may have entered the service of local rulers and then
may have taken over control of their citadels and towns. The small Iranian states
so formed were ruled by a chieftain, a local prince, and by a nobility of landowners who made serfs of the native population and established large, virtually
self-sufficient estates. Their society seems to have been much like that of

Homeric Greece (pp. 178–79). The rulers and nobles were warlike and headed kinship groups of retainers, some of whom were dependent on their clan chieftain for livelihood, while others were small-scale farmers. The typical pattern of landholding, however, was the large estate and the way of life mainly pastoral and agricultural. The nobles observed a simple code of behavior, in which the greatest values were skill in war and hunting and the greatest fault, lying and the falsification of an oath.

During the ninth and eighth centuries the Iranians were under heavy pressure from both Urartu and Assyria, whose kings raided, plundered, and exacted tribute when they could. Nevertheless there was a marked growth of urbanization, facilitated by the exploitation of metal resources and by the supplies of labor which the princes could command. The Iranians, too, were influenced by the cultures of Assyria and Urartu from which their workers could learn craft techniques and architecture. Above all, however, defense of their new lands made cooperation in war necessary; thus in the seventh century the Kingdom of Media was formed and freed itself from vassalage to Assyria.

THE KINGDOM OF MEDIA

Although the Medes, or perhaps the territory in which their kingdom later developed, were referred to as early as 836 B.C. in the records of Shalmaneser III of Assyria, the Kingdom of Media did not form until the mid-seventh century. At that time a king, Phraortes, is said to have ruled from Ecbatana (Hamadan) over a territory extending to the east and south. To the north, towards Lake Urmia, the land was held by the Mannaeans and by Scythian nomads who had entered the region in the wake of the Cimmerians. Phraortes made an alliance with these peoples and then boldly struck into Assyria. His Scythian allies, however, proved treacherous. In 653 B.C. they killed Phraortes and claimed lordship over Media. Their hold was evidently loose because Cyaxares, the successor of Phraortes, is said to have built up his army during this period of Scythian rule. Probably he introduced better organization on the model of the Assyrians and taught the Medians to use mounted archers, like the Scythians. In any case, Cyaxares was able to defeat the Scythians. He founded the Median Kingdom by extending his rule over the Mannaeans and over the Persians to the south. The latter had moved down through the Zagros Mountains from Media and formed small states in Elamite territory.

In the latter part of his reign Cyaxares made an alliance with Babylon and, as already described, joined in the attack on Nineveh in 612 B.C. Leaving Mesopotamia and Syria to Babylonia, Cyaxares expanded through Armenia into Asia Minor in the following years. A lengthy conflict with Lydia culminated in 585 B.C. by the conclusion of the alliance which fixed the frontier between the two kingdoms on the Halys River. The Greek historian, Herodotus, told a picturesque story of an eclipse of the sun, forecast by the Greek philosopher, Thales, which was interpreted by both sides as an omen of evil for the final battle of the war; therefore, instead of fighting, the Medes and Lydians made peace. More probably Nebuchadrezzar of Babylon, who was anxious to keep a balance of power, mediated between Cyaxares and Alyattes. To cement the alliance Alyattes' daughter was married to Astyages, the son of Cyaxares. Astyages succeeded to the Median throne in 584 B.C. and, after Nebuchadrezzar's death, began to expand into northern Mesopotamia. War broke out with Nabonidus of Babylon, who found a willing ally for an attack on Media in Astyages' vassal king, Cyrus of Persia. Apparently the Median Kingdom was loosely organized, with its cohesion depending mainly on the personal force of the king and his ability to control the princes of the lesser Iranian states. They felt as well qualified on the score of lineage and quality to rule as the King of the Medes. Accordingly, Cyrus, in 550 B.C., turned on his Median overlord and overthrew the ruling dynasty. This was not so much a conquest as another step in the formation of a strong Aryan state in which the rulers of Persia rather than of Media would be dominant.

THE ACHAEMENIAN KINGDOM OF PERSIA

Those peoples among the Aryan invaders, who were later known as the Persians, seem to have made their way from northwestern Iran along the Zagros Mountains to Elamite territory where about 700 B.C. they formed a state in Parsumash. Its founder was Achaemenes, from whom the Persian kings are called Achaemenids, his descendants. When Assyrian attacks weakened Elam, the successors of Achaemenes were able to extend their rule over the neighboring regions of Anshan and Fars (Persia). They were forced, however, to acknowledge first the sovereignty of Assyria and then of Media. When Cyrus came to the throne of Persia in 559 B.C., he established his capital at Pasargadae, building a royal palace and a temple where subsequent Persian kings were crowned, and began to extend his kingdom over the neighboring Persian princes. His alliance with Nabonidus of Babylon provoked Astyages, Cyrus' nominal overlord and maternal grandfather. In 550 B.C., when Astyages called upon Cyrus to abandon Nabonidus, Cyrus revolted and defeated Astyages. The defeat was almost in the nature of a family quarrel, for Cyrus treated Astyages with consideration and combined the two kingdoms. Both Medes and Persians were used as officials, and Cyrus ruled from Ecbatana, better located than Pasargadae to serve as a base for expansion.

The Persian Empire attained almost its full extent in a single generation with the conquests of Cyrus. The king had the personal force and political genius to hold the loyalty of the Iranian princes and seems to have formed them into a royal council in which he was the "first among equals." He had the military skill to build and lead a devoted army, the élite troops of which were the "Ten Thousand Immortals," a royal bodyguard. Many elements from the subject peoples of the Empire were ultimately drawn into the army, but at the outset the Medes and Persians were hardy, skilled soldiers, familiar with the techniques of war learned from the Assyrians and Scythians and conscious of their own ethnic unity and superiority. Cyrus' attitude towards the Empire which he formed with their aid, however, seems to have been rather more than simply that of a military conqueror. In a Babylonian inscription he caused to be written: "Marduk had visited all lands in search of an upright prince, a king after his own heart, whom he took by the hand. He named his name, 'Cyrus of Anshan' and to the kingdom of the whole world he called him by name." Cyrus proved himself a benevolent and tolerant ruler, sparing the lives of defeated kings and respecting the native beliefs and customs of the people whom he conquered.

As the new king of a united Media and Persia, Cyrus was faced with three problems which had confronted previous Middle Eastern powers: expansion to the Mediterranean Sea was necessary to control the trade routes and communications to the west; as king of Media, Cyrus inherited a traditional quarrel, as well as a common frontier with Lydia; and in the east Iran was open to nomadic raids. Since Croesus of Lydia was the first to offer provocation, Cyrus struck at Lydia. A rapid thrust across Anatolia resulted in the peaceful acquisition of Cilicia and the blocking of aid from Babylonia to Croesus. Then Cyrus marched north to the Halys, capturing Harran from Babylonia en route. An indecisive battle was fought with Croesus on the Halys but, as the latter withdrew towards Sardes in the expectation that Cyrus would break off the war during the winter, Cyrus pursued and inflicted a defeat on the Lydian cavalry with his camel corps. The horses were not used to the smell of camels and panicked. Sardes was taken in 547 B.C. and, according to tradition, Croesus' life was spared. Cyrus called on the Greek cities of the Aegean coast to surrender, but only Miletus came over to him. The conquest was rounded off by the capture of the other cities, left to one of Cyrus' generals, by 540 B.C.

Cyrus himself turned back to the heart of the Empire and spent the following years in securing the eastern approaches to Iran. The land up to the Jaxartes River was annexed and fortified towns constructed to guard against nomad raids. Cyrus seems to have penetrated into northwestern India at this time but set up no organization to govern the land. Next came the turn of Babylonia. As we have noticed, the priesthood of Marduk was hostile to their king, Nabonidus; thus Cyrus was able to secure their goodwill in advance of his attack. In 539 he took the city with little resistance. Cyrus treated Nabonidus well and through the favor of the priesthood was invested with the titles of Babylonian kingship. Marduk had found "a righteous ruler." The fall of Babylon automatically carried with it a claim to the Babylonian possessions in the west. In both Syria and Palestine the native peoples welcomed Cyrus as a liberator; he reciprocated by respecting local traditions and religious practices. The Jews of the Exile were permitted to return to Jerusalem and to rebuild the temple.

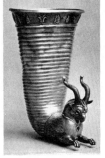

Although the road to Egypt was open, Cyrus left his son Cambyses to prepare an expedition, while returned to the eastern frontier to fight against the nomads. In 530 B.C. he was killed in battle. Cyrus had found little time to organize his conquered territories and made only such arrangements as seemed suitable at the time of victory. In some areas he placed Persians as governors, in

A Persian drinking horn of silver

others maintained native rulers, if they gave promise of loyalty to Persia. Cyrus himself lived at various times in Pasargadae, Ecbatana and Babylon. The Empire still had no real center or organization and had only a military conqueror.

CAMBYSES (530–25 B.C.)

Cyrus had established and maintained his kingship over the Persians by personal force and continued military success, rather than by any recognized sanctions of religion and hereditary descent. When upon his death revolts broke out, his son Cambyses, to whom the army proved loyal, had to postpone the invasion of Egypt. Among other claimants to the throne whom Cambyses put to death was his own brother, Smerdis. By 526 B.C., however, Cambyses was ready to invade Egypt. After the Greek mercenary soldiers of Amasis were defeated at Pelusium in the eastern delta, Cambyses was able to march on Memphis, where he was recognized as a successor to the Pharaohs of Egypt. He then made plans for three great conquests: a march to the famous oracle of Amon in the oasis of that name in the Libyan Desert; the conquest of Carthage; and a march up the valley of the Nile to take over Ethiopia (the land of Kush). All failed. The god Amon, or rather a sandstorm, protected the oasis, but Cambyses did establish control over the Greeks of Cyrene. The Phoenicians refused to contribute naval aid for the attack on Carthage, their own colony, and supply difficulties bogged down the march along the Nile. Towards the end of his stay in Egypt Cambyses seems to have become involved in a dispute with some of the priesthoods in Memphis. In Greek tradition, reported by the historian Herodotus, the king is said to have lapsed into madness and to have insulted the Egyptian gods. Such impiety, so far as we can judge, was uncharacteristic of Cambyses, as well as impolitic. More probably the disgruntled priests slandered him after he had cut down the revenues from some temple estates while favoring others.

While Cambyses was still in Egypt, news came of a revolt far to the east in Iran, where a certain Gaumata, one of the priestly class known as the Magi, had claimed the throne. Gaumata asserted that he was that son of Cyrus, Smerdis, whom Cambyses had secretly put to death. Since Gaumata apparently bore a strong resemblance to Smerdis, which influenced the Persians, and since he remitted taxes liberally, which appealed to the subject peoples, revolt spread rapidly. Cambyses is said to have committed suicide in a fit of despair. The Immortals, however, remained loyal to the name of the Achaemenids and threw their support to a distant relative and one of their officers, Darius, the son of King Hystaspes of Parthia. Darius suppressed the revolts, executed Gaumata, and made good his claim to the throne. In 522 B.C. he began a long reign of thirty-six years, in which time he supplied the systematic organization and care for the whole Empire that Cyrus and Cambyses had been too busy to give.

DARIUS AND THE ORGANIZATION OF THE EMPIRE (522–486 B.C.)

Although the revolts which faced Darius at the outset of his reign were numerous and widespread, they were not concerted, and he was able to deal with them individually. By 522 B.C. Darius had made good his claim to the throne and commemorated his victories in a long inscription, a combination of official autobiography and imperial manifesto. The inscription was cut on a cliff, five hundred feet above the road at Behistun to the south of Ecbatana. It was written in three languages, Old Persian, Elamite, and Babylonian but perhaps was designed to impress the passersby by its setting more than its content. Darius revealed his concern about giving the kingship some sanction of authority, in addition to military success. The latter was important to a warrior people like the Persians, but Darius was at pains to stress his hereditary claim to the throne through the Achaemenid line and his special relationship to Ahura Mazda, the chief god of the Persians. A relief cut at the head of the inscription represented the god, in the form of a winged sun-disk, hovering protectively over Darius' head, and in the inscription Darius spoke of himself as the protégé of Ahura Mazda, charged by the god to bring truth and justice to the Empire. Such association with a national god was, of course, thoroughly in the tradition of Mesopotamian kingship, but in his insistence on the ethical qualities of Ahura Mazda Darius revealed himself as sympathetic to the religious teaching of the reformer Zoroaster. The latter had preached a reform of religion at the time of the rise of the Empire. Darius did not attempt to establish a theocratic state or to make the reformed Persian religion into an imperial worship to promote unity, but his organization of the Empire was characterized by principles of justice and concern for the welfare of the subject peoples.

By the sixth century the Persian religion had become a composite of the beliefs and practices which the Aryan invaders had brought into Iran and those of the people among whom they had settled. Their most important god was Ahura Mazda, a sky-god of the type common to other Indo-European peoples, like the Greek Zeus. There were also Mithras, a sun-god and helper of Ahura Mazda, and Anahita, a fertility goddess who had been adopted from the native

Persepolis. The double-bull capital is from the throne room, or apadana, *of Darius. The column shafts were fluted, showing Greek influence, while the capitals were Assyrian in inspiration. Doorways and windows in the palace of Darius. The lintel is Egyptian in type. The walls of the palace were of sun-dried brick and have not survived.*

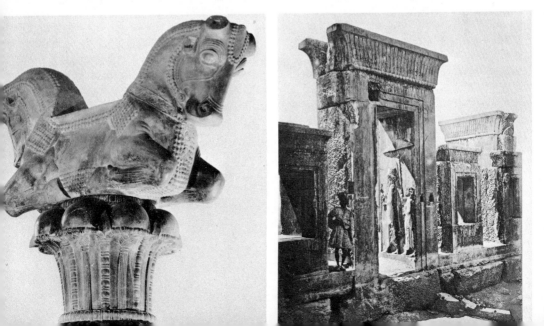

peoples. In addition, the forces of nature—earth, fire and water—were important to the Persians but vaguely conceived. Their gods were worshipped in the open air by blood sacrifices, carried out by a powerful priestly class, known as the Magi. There is some reason to believe that the Magi were priests of the native peoples in origin, but they had become indispensable to the conduct of formal Persian religion. The Magi accompanied the armies to war, performed the sacrifices judged necessary for success, interpreted dreams, and crowned the king. Only they could prepare the sacred and intoxicating drink, *haoma,* used in the rituals of worship. The Magi also tended the fire altars of the Persians, built in the form of a square tower with a room at the top which held the sacred fire. While the great gods, Ahura Mazda and Mithras, were benevolent and helpful to men, the Persians also considered the world to be peopled with evil spirits, *daevas,* the chief of whom was called Ahriman.

During the sixth century, although we are not sure of his dates, the religious reformer and prophet, Zoroaster, appeared in eastern Iran. He was hounded by the established priesthood but found refuge with a king, Vistaspes, probably the father of Darius. Thus it is possible that the revolt of Gaumata may have been sponsored by the Magi to counter the spread of Zoroastrian ideas. We know of Zoroaster's teaching only through later accounts, but he seems to have been like the Hebrew prophets, acting both as a social critic and as a religious reformer. His conception of Ahura Mazda was virtually monotheistic. The god was considered to be all powerful, the creator of the world, and was invested with ethical qualities of truth and justice. He would help man in his struggle against evil, but held human beings responsible for their own acts. The world was thought to be governed by universal principles of justice, sponsored by Ahura Mazda, but was also the scene of conflict with the forces of evil presided over by Ahriman. While victory would ultimately be won by Ahura Mazda, man had to participate individually in the struggle and would be judged by his record. In its later form Zoroastrianism developed these ideas of dualism and of a millennial judgment and multiplied the host of heavenly helpers and evil spirits. Some of these concepts were ultimately incorporated into early Christianity. Darius seems to have shared Zoroaster's monotheistic and ethical conceptions of Ahura Mazda, perhaps through contact with him as a boy at his father's court, but the king made administrative unity for the Empire his chief concern. A reconciliation was effected with the Magi, who incorporated Zoroastrianism into Persian religion and formalized its ideas. These were incorporated ultimately into the sacred book of the Persians, the *Zend-Avesta,* and the worship is still carried on by the Parsees of western India.

An Old Persian inscription, written in cuneiform, from the Palace of Darius at Persepolis

Darius made his office into the Great Kingship known to the Greeks, in which the king seemed to rule absolutely over the Persians and the Empire. There were, however, various limiting factors. The Persian king had to control his unruly relatives and the great nobles by his personal qualities. The inscription said to have been written on Darius' tomb recalls the old Persian virtues: "I was a friend to my friends; as horseman and bowman I proved myself superior to all others; as a hunter I prevailed; I could do everything." While Darius boasted of his personal prowess, he tried also to invest the kingship with appropriate pomp and circumstance and to solidify Persian support. The Persians themselves were made a privileged group, who paid no taxes and from whose nobility the king chose his administrators and generals. But the nobles also remained very powerful, and, despite Darius' emphasis on religion and hereditary sanctions for the kingship, the Persian regime continued to be troubled by attempted usurpations and by the revolts of great provincial governors. The chief nobles and kinsmen of the king also formed a council of state, whose advice the king heeded, even if he was not constrained to follow it.

The subject peoples of the Empire were ruled by a system of provincial government for which the Assyrian Empire had furnished the precedent. The provinces were large territorial units, satrapies, administered by a governor, the satrap, and other officials appointed by the king. While Cyrus and Cambyses had already made a start on the satrapy system, its general application and the detail of organization were the work of Darius. He divided the Empire into about thirty satrapies, each headed by a satrap chosen from the royal family or the important nobles. While the satrap was powerful and in general charge of his province, his authority was not unlimited. Darius also appointed a military commander and a financial official, each individually responsible to the king. The conduct of all these was checked further by the visits, at unannounced and irregular times, of an inspector called the "ear of the king." Despite these measures to centralize authority, the satraps were ambitious and in remote parts of the Empire might rule like lesser kings.

Darius also achieved some degree of administrative unity, at least in the western portion of the Empire, by the establishment of a common code of law administered by royal judges. He collected and revised the existing codes of Babylonia and Assyria and published them in the traditional Mesopotamian form of a casebook. We know of the Persian code only through references in inscriptions, but it is apparent that the conduct of the royal judges was carefully scrutinized and that Darius desired to give some reality to his claim of inaugurating a truthful and just regime.

Darius also introduced a common system of weights and measures for the Empire and began the issuance of a gold coinage, the famous darics. Perhaps his main purpose was to provide a uniform basis for the tax system, but the new standards promoted economic unity within the Empire and the adoption of coinage gradually led to the use of a monetary economy. In each satrapy the tax was fixed in terms of silver, and local metals were discounted according to the king's new standards. When his collectors apparently reckoned their discounts heavily in the king's favor, Darius earned the nickname of "the trader." Much of the actual tax, however, was paid in produce which was used to support the court and the army. The gold and silver so collected came to rest in the king's treasury, with the result that the Persian Empire found itself in the happy position of having a budgetary surplus. The king also spent lavishly on building projects, mainly in Persia, but the provinces were not neglected. For example, irrigation projects to reclaim more land for agriculture were undertaken at the edge of the Syrian Desert, as well as on the Persian plateau, and royal gifts were made as a mark of favor to cities and temples throughout the provinces. The darics were valuable, handsome coins, and in the fifth and fourth centuries they were put to use in diplomacy with Greece, as well as in foreign trade. The Persians themselves, like the Assyrians, took little part in the economic life of the Empire, except in their capacity as owners of great estates. The Phoenicians continued to play their traditional role as middlemen, but trade with the Greeks became lively and the latter made their way throughout the Empire as merchants or to work for the king's patronage. In general, Darius' concern for unity, and the order and peace which Persian rule had brought, resulted in a very considerable development of trade and economic growth both within the Empire and between the lands of the Near East and the developing Greek world.

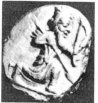

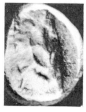

Persian daric

Darius' concern for unity was reflected, too, in his frontier policy and in the improvement of communications between the extremities of the Empire and the centers in Mesopotamia and western Iran. The schemes of conquest in Africa, which Cambyses had contemplated, were given up in favor of finding more defensible frontiers in Asia. The conquest of northwestern India, started by Cyrus, was completed and that land linked to the west by exploration of the sea route. A Greek sea captain from western Asia Minor, Scylax of Caryanda, was placed in charge of a fleet to sail from the mouth of the Indus River to Egypt. After a voyage of thirty months, a new tie of commerce was forged. In Egypt the canal, which Necho had started between the Nile and the Red Sea, was finished.

From the diagonally opposite corner of the Empire, northwestern Asia Minor, Darius led an expedition into southeastern Europe in 513 B.C. Its purpose was interpreted by the Greeks to be the conquest of the Scythians, who lived from the European shore of the Black Sea to the steppes of inner Asia, and Darius did penetrate beyond the Danube into Scythian territory. Justification for such a grandiose plan of conquest may be found in the fact that the Scythian nomads were beginning to coalesce into kingdoms in southern Russia at this time and that their kindred around the Caspian did raid into Iran. Yet Darius was generally more practical, and modern scholars have suggested other purposes. Some consider that Darius hoped to get possession of the gold fields in the Ural Mountains, but this is hardly less ambitious than the conquest of the Scythians. If an economic motive seems reasonable, the conquest of Thrace in southeastern Europe, which Darius did achieve, is plausible. The silver mines in Thrace were the chief source of silver for the Greeks, and, in addition, the possession of Thrace would provide Darius with that beachhead in Europe which has usually seemed desirable to any power holding Asia Minor. Possibly then, Darius' purpose was to find a proper frontier for the Empire in the northwest by making Thrace into a province. His thrust across the Danube was designed to check Scythian raids. Darius' advance into Europe, of course, raised

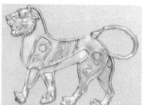

An Achaemenian gold lion, used for appliqué ornament. Iranian craftsmen produced superb work in silver and gold, using animal motifs.

the problem of relations with the Greeks on the west side of the Aegean. That, however, and the wars which they fought with Darius and his successors are best discussed in connection with Greek history (pp. 240–49). It is sufficient to notice here that both Darius and his son Xerxes failed to incorporate Greece into the Empire.

Darius also tied western Asia Minor more closely to his capitals by the development of the famous Royal Road and by the establishment of a messenger service along its course. The road ran from the old Lydian capital of Sardes, which had become the chief center of Persian administration for Asia Minor, up the valley of the Hermus River to the Anatolian plateau. One branch led to Gordium, the former capital of Phrygia, and on to the east, while the other ran southwards over the plateau and the Taurus Mountains to North Syria and Mesopotamia. From Babylon, which was used as a sub-capital by the Persian kings, the roads were improved to Ecbatana and thence to Darius' chief cities, Susa and Persepolis, in western Iran. The distance from Sardes to Persepolis was about sixteen hundred miles, and staging posts were built along the road to provide the king's messengers with fresh mounts. The relay took about a week for the messengers of the king, but for travelers by camel and donkey caravan, about three months. Nevertheless, the road became an important commercial link between the Aegean area of the Empire and its centers. We know little of the measures taken to link the eastern part of the Empire to the capitals, but, judging from the experience of Alexander the Great, communications there remained slow and difficult. The center of gravity in the Empire was Mesopotamia, and its most prosperous, urbanized areas were the older lands of western Asia.

At the outset of his reign Darius chose the Elamite city of Susa as his capital. In 521 B.C. he began to refortify the citadel and to build a large new palace in the Babylonian style. Susa remained an important center of administration, but in 512 B.C. Darius chose a new and more specifically Persian site at Persepolis, the city of the Persians, as the Greeks called it. The palace built

Sculptured balustrade of the monumental stairway to the Palace of Darius at Persepolis

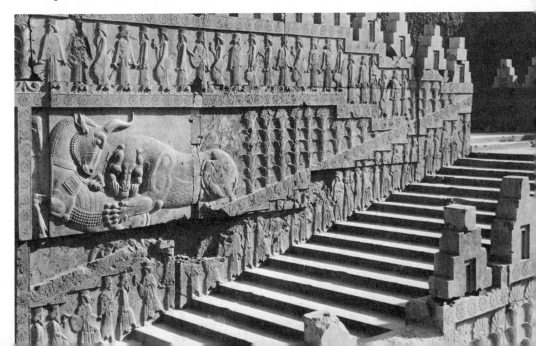

Time	Mesopotamia	Egypt	Syria Palestine	Anatolia	Aegean
Ca. 8000–4500 Neolithic	Agriculture; settled communities	Upper Palaeolithic societies at desert edge	Agriculture; settled communities	Agriculture; settled communities	Agriculture; settled communities
Ca. 4500–3000 Transition	Settlement in delta; Sumerians	Agriculture; settled communities	Chalcolithic	Chalcolithic	Agricultural villages
Ca. 3000 Civilization	Proto-Literate (3200–2800) Urbanization Writing	Archaic (3100–2686) Kingdom Writing	Semitic infiltration (ca. 3500) Urbanization	Urbanization in northwest and southwest (Konya plain)	Urbanization Metallurgy
Ca. 2800–2000 Early Bronze Age	Sumerian Cities Lagash (2500–2340) Akkad (2340–2150) Ur: 3rd Dyn. (2135–2027)	Old Kingdom (2686–2180) Pyramid Age (2600–2500) Anarchy (2180–2080)	Growth of towns Trade with Mesopotamia and Egypt	Local kingdoms Indo-European invasion: Luwians and Hittites (2300–2100)	Early Helladic Early Minoan Growth of towns
Ca. 2000–1600 Middle Bronze Age	Amorite invasion Hammurabi's Empire (1792–ca. 1550)	Middle Kingdom (2080–1640) Hyksos invasion (1720–1570)	Semitic invasion Hyksos invasion (1800–1570)	Assyrian colonies (1900–1800) OLD HITTITE KINGDOM (1650–1500)	Indo-European invasion: Greeks MINOAN CIVILIZATION Trade with Syria, Egypt
Ca. 1600–1200 Late Bronze Age	Kassite rule (1500–1000) Mitanni (1500–1370) Rise of Assyria	EGYPTIAN EMPIRE XVIIIth Dynasty Ikhnaton Clash with Hittites	EGYPTIAN CONTROL Mitanni HITTITE CONTROL Trading cities	HITTITE EMPIRE Clash with: Mittani Hurrians Egypt Achaeans	MYCENAEAN CIVILIZATION (Achaean Greeks) Writing Trade and sea raids
Ca. 1200–1000 Invasions	Aramaean infiltration	Collapse of Empire Peoples of the Sea; Libyans; Nubians.	Raids and settlement: Peoples of the Sea; Aramaeans; Hebrews settle in Palestine	Collapse of Empire Indo-European invasions: Phrygians Thracians	Collapse of Mycenaean civilization Dorian invasion and migrations
Ca. 1000–500 Early Iron Age	ASSYRIAN EMPIRE (900–612) NEW BABYLONIAN EMPIRE (612–539) PERSIAN EMPIRE (539–330)	ASSYRIAN CONQUEST (671–650) SAITE KINGDOM (650–525) PERSIAN CONQUEST (525–332)	Independent Kingdoms and City-states ASSYRIAN, BABYLONIAN CONQUEST PERSIAN CONQUEST (539–332)	Dark Age Urartu: ca. 900? Phrygia: ca. 800? Cimmerian invasion, 700–650 Lydia: 680–547 PERSIAN CONQUEST (547–334)	Dark Age Homeric Greece (9th, 8th cents.) Rise of city-states Colonization PERSIAN WARS (546–479)

Near Eastern Civilizations. Table of relative development

there was not as large as that at Susa, but its architecture was more traditionally Persian. For its construction the king drew lavishly on the resources of the
Empire. A huge terrace was constructed for the palace, approached by a monumental stairway. The sculptured decoration of the staircase was a symbol of
the Empire. A long frieze represented the Immortals of the king's bodyguard,
through whose support he had won the throne, the Persian nobles associated
in its administration, and the varied subject peoples bringing tribute. The columns of the palace were treated in characteristic Assyrian style with sculptured
bull's heads, powerfully and crisply cut by the best workmen of the Empire.
The king needed to draw on the cultural traditions of his subjects throughout
the Empire, for the Persians themselves were still too young to have developed
an individual architectural and sculptural style. Their building was still a reflection of what they found congenial in the older traditions of Babylonia,
Assyria, and Urartu. Perhaps the nomadic traditions apparent in the animal
style of Iranian metalwork might more properly be called Persian, but these
were shared with the nomadic peoples on the fringes of the Empire, where
they are revealed in the burials of Scythian chieftains from South Russia to
the Siberian steppes.

The Persian Empire about 500 B.C. was a new state with a vigorous king
and ruling class. Darius gave it administrative unity rather than homogeneity.
The latter, of course, was scarcely possible because the Persians were few in
number in relation to the subject peoples. Obviously the establishment of a
centralized authority and the improvement of communications and trade with
the eastern Mediterranean stimulated growth over a very wide area. Yet the
main activity of the Empire still was agriculture. The land was held mainly
by large-scale owners, Persians, native nobles, and the great temple establish-

Subjects of the Persian Empire bearing tribute to the king

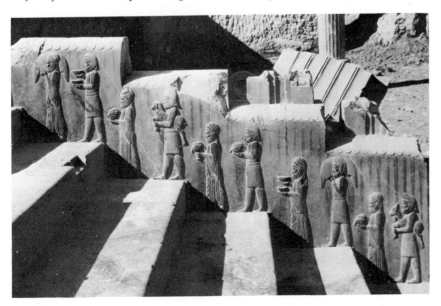

ments. Their fields were worked by serfs and tenants in varying degrees of dependence. Neither did the Persians make any deliberate attempt to urbanize or to alter the systems which they found in existence. Accordingly, there was no development toward a more organic unity through economic and social means and no unification of society through common citizenship and legal privilege, such as characterized the Roman Empire. Instead, Darius made a framework in which the diverse subject peoples could live and maintain their national institutions but received no share in government. Perhaps the general and ready acceptance of Persian rule was partly the result of Assyrian militarism, but the Persian kings exercised a generally benevolent and tolerant rule with some concern for the welfare of their subjects. They scarcely went beyond this, for in the fourth century Alexander the Great found that his enemies were the Persians and the Greek mercenary soldiers in Persian pay, rather than the peoples of the Empire.

The Near East had been reorganized, with its traditions preserved and developed after the invasions of the Early Iron Age. It is now time to turn to Greece, where the rising city-states were to record very different ideas about society and the individual's place in it.

Papyrus of the fifth century B.C. from the Jewish colony on Elephantine Island in the Nile River. The document records the deed of a house from a father to his daughter.

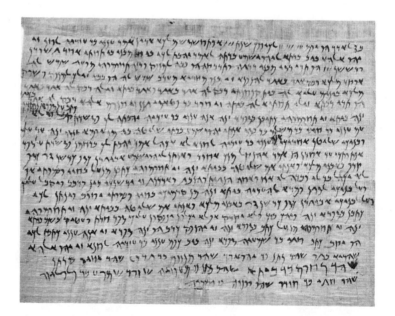

11

Greece

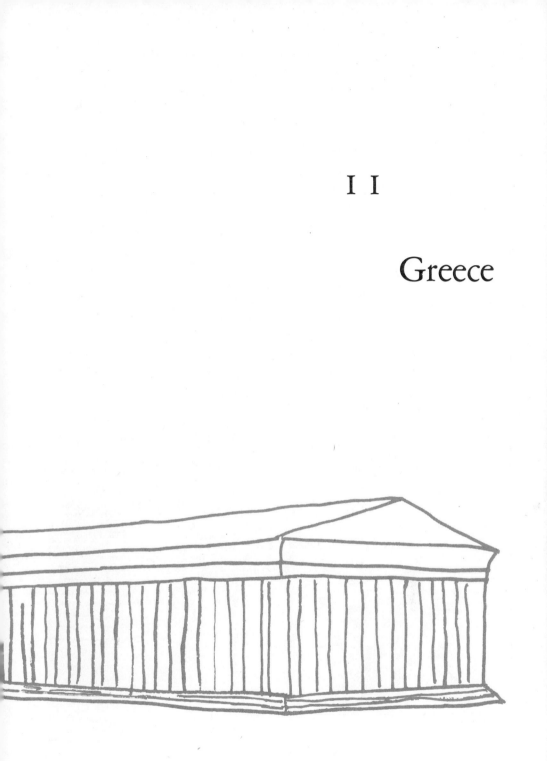

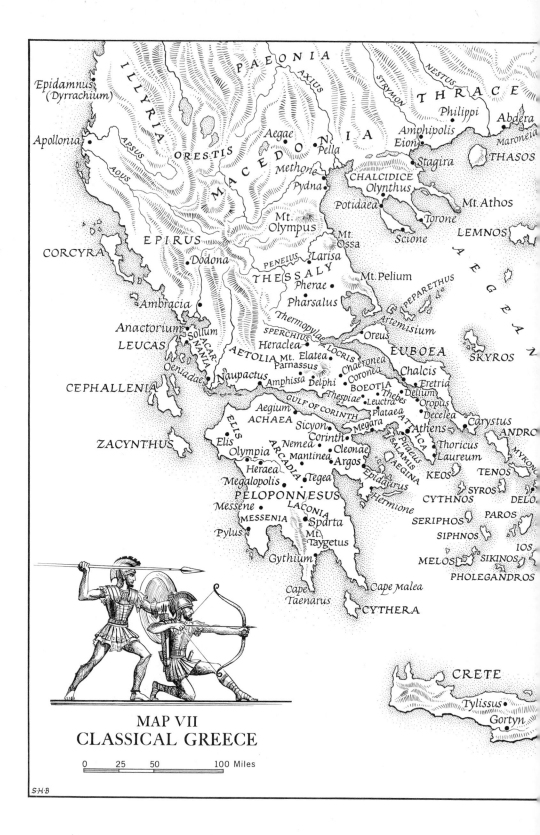

Epidamnus
(Dyrrachium)

ILLYRIA

PAEONIA

THRACE

NESTUS

STRYMON

Philippi

Apollonia

APSUS

AOUS

ORESTIS

Aegae

MACEDONIA

Pella

Abdera

Maroneia

THASOS

Amphipolis

Eion

Methone

Pydna

CHALCIDICE

Olynthus

Stagira

Mt. Athos

Potidaea

CORCYRA

EPIRUS

Dodona

Mt.
Olympus

Mt.
Ossa

Torone

Scione

LEMNOS

PENEIUS

Larisa

THESSALY

Pherae

Pharsalus

Mt. Pelium

AEGEAN

PEPARETHUS

Ambracia

Anactorium

Thermopylae

SPERCHIUS

Artemisium

Oreus

EUBOEA

SKYROS

LEUCAS

ACAR
NANIA

Sollum

Heraclea

Mt. Elatea

Parnassus

LOCRIS

Chaeronea

Oeniadae

Naupactus

Amphissa

Delphi

Coronea

BOEOTIA

Chalcis

Eretria

Delium

Oropus

Decelea

CEPHALLENIA

Aegium

ACHAEA

Sicyon

GULF OF CORINTH

Thespiae

Leuctra

Thebes

Plataea

Carystus

ELIS

Corinth

Megara

ATTICA

Athens

ANDRO

ZACYNTHUS

Elis

Olympia

ARCADIA

Nemea

Mantinea

Cleonae

Argos

SALAMIS

AEGINA

Piraeus

Thoricus

Laureum

KEOS

MYKON

TENOS

Heraea

Megalopolis

Tegea

Epidaurus

Hermione

CYTHNOS

SYROS

DELO

Messene

MESSENIA

PELOPONNESUS

LACONIA

Sparta

SERIPHOS

PAROS

SIPHNOS

Pylus

Mt.
Taygetus

MELOS

SIKINOS

IOS

Gythium

PHOLEGANDROS

Cape
Taenarus

Cape Malea

CYTHERA

CRETE

Tylissus

Gortyn

MAP VII
CLASSICAL GREECE

0   25   50   100 Miles

S·H·B

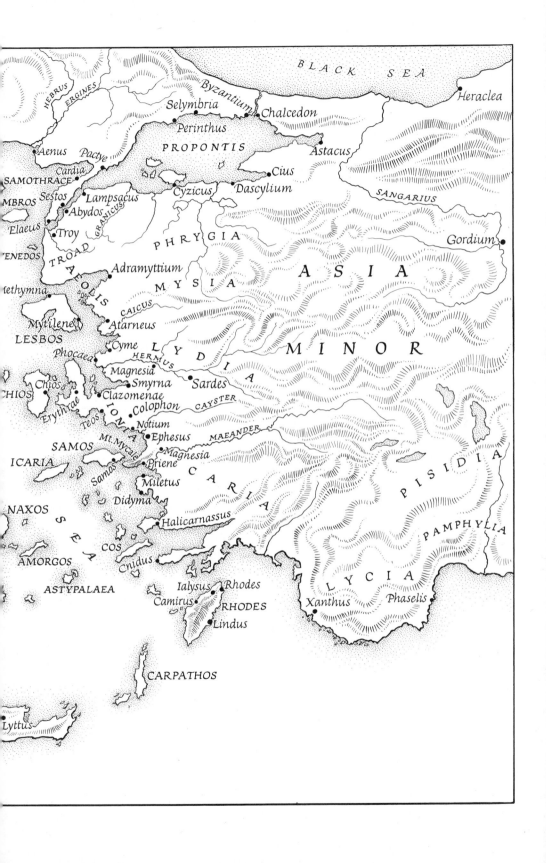

VIII

The Reorganization and Expansion of Greece

(*ca.* 1100–500 B.C.)

THE ADVANCED CIVILIZATION created by the Greeks in the Mycenaean Age was broken by invasions about 1200 B.C. The great citadels were looted and burnt, the rulers killed, and the people enslaved or driven from their lands. When the king's palace, the center of organization, had disappeared, the techniques of administration, of artistic production, and even of writing, perished. A fresh start had to be made in the Aegean area. For several hundred years, until about 750 B.C., Greece reverted to almost complete isolation and to an agrarian and pastoral economy. Connections with the new states of the Near East were slight and their archives have no reference to Greeks. We are confronted with a Dark Age in which archaeology and survivals in dialect and institutions are almost the only guides to historical reconstruction.

Just at the close of the Dark Age the Homeric poems, which are considered usually to have crystallized in their present form in the eighth century, do reflect something of the social organization of the time. Yet we have virtually no other detailed knowledge until about 650 B.C. By that date the city-states familiar in Classical Greece had been established. The Greeks had forged new connections with the Near East and had learned to write and to record. By that time, too, the precarious balance between food supply and population had been reached. Greeks had begun to migrate from the Aegean and to settle along the coasts of the Mediterranean and the Black Sea. This colonizing movement and the growth of trade which accompanied it wrought a profound change in the agrarian towns and laid the foundations of Greek economy for the Classical Period.

The Dark Age (1100–750 B.C.)

The settlement of the Dorian Greeks, which followed upon the invasions of the twelfth century (p. 119), was concentrated mainly in the Peloponnesus

The reader will find Maps VII and VIII (pages 172–173 and 184) useful as he reads this chapter.

and made it the most important Dorian area in Greece. The Dorians settled at Corinth and Sicyon near the Gulf of Corinth, at Argos near the old Mycenaean citadel at Mycenae, and in the southeast at Sparta in Laconia. Achaea, on the south shore of the Gulf of Corinth, Arcadia, in the heart of the Peloponnesus, and Messenia, in the southwest, were left undisturbed for the time being. From the eastern Peloponnesus, however, Dorians crossed the Aegean to Crete, Rhodes, and the adjacent coast of Asia Minor, where they spread as far north as Halicarnassus. The native populations were in some cases reduced to the status of serfs, and the Doric institutions and dialect were imposed. Cyprus remained untouched by the Dorians, so that its Mycenaean colonial settlements long preserved their old style of writing, artistic traditions, and some sporadic trade into the Aegean. But Cyprus was too far from the Aegean to seriously affect its new growth or to share in it. The island's own culture was soon strongly influenced by Phoenician traders and settlers from the nearby coast of Syria.

This Dorian sweep across the old Mycenaean centers and colonial area erected a temporary barrier between the Near East and Greece. It threw those parts of Greece spared in the invasion back on their own resources to build as best they could in a frontier environment. Athens, which had fought off the Dorians, seems to have become a refuge for some Mycenaean groups from Boeotia and the Peloponnesus. According to later tradition the city was regarded as the starting point for a migration in the eleventh century B.C. across the Aegean Islands to the central part of the west coast of Asia Minor. Both archaeological evidence and dialect survival indicate that the tradition was rooted in fact. This migration began the establishment of Ionian Greece, consisting of the Cyclades Islands of the Aegean and the central part of the west coast of Asia Minor. The latter became known as Ionia. The people of the Cyclades and of Ionia used the Ionian dialect of Greek, and on the island of Delos in the middle of the Cyclades a Panionic festival of the god Apollo was celebrated. It is scarcely possible that a large-scale migration was made at one time, for the resources and organization of eleventh and tenth century Greece were incapable of such an effort. Probably a small, compactly organized group, with their Mycenaean traditions still vivid, moved out before 1000 B.C. to Ionia, to be followed by smaller bands of settlers from elsewhere in Greece in the next several centuries.

Across the northern Aegean, another and perhaps even earlier migration from Thessaly and Central Greece established an Aeolic dialect area in the island of Lesbos and the northern part of the west coast of Asia Minor, of Aeolis, as it was called. The traditions of Mycenaean Greece were strong in both Aeolis and Ionia. Ionia, where Homer is reported to have been born, was the scene of the earliest Greek literary and philosophical growth. Throughout the whole of the Aegean, however, communities had to reform or to start afresh.

The chief desires of the people were for land and for security in their new homes. They chose the fertile, easily worked areas, the small plains, mountain valleys, and coastal flats. In the Greek peninsula the districts were rapidly oc-

Greek cup. Geometric style (eighth century B.C.)

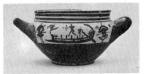

cupied up to the natural frontiers formed by ridges and mountain spurs. The typical form of settlement was a small village, around which lay the farms worked by its inhabitants. The villages were usually situated near some easily defended high point, which could serve as a refuge and house the leaders of the community and the shrines of its gods. The name given the village was *kome* or *asty,* while the high point was called the *polis.* As the two grew together into a larger, unified community, *polis* was applied to the whole to designate the city-state, and the term, *acropolis,* literally "high-town," was used for the old place of refuge. Where the *acropolis* had been well chosen to dominate a fertile plain or valley and to control communication and guard a water supply, it became the nodal point around which population concentrated. On the coast of Asia Minor, the initial settlements took different form. The migrants came in small numbers into a thickly populated area in which they could do little but secure beachheads. A typical settlement has been revealed by the excavation of Old Smyrna. That town was built on a small peninsula, protected from attack by the sea on three sides and by a wall across its connecting isthmus. As their population and strength grew, the Ionian Greeks moved to seize the fertile river estuaries and to push up the valleys as far as they could penetrate. This pressure, however, provoked resistance by the natives and the Greeks were held to the coast.

In Greece the growing towns were cut off from regular intercourse with one another by the mountain barriers. From the outset each community tended to turn inwards upon itself and to cherish a narrow, jealous feeling of loyalty to its own individual traditions and customs. Sometimes, worship of a god, common to several communities, or veneration for a sanctuary prompted the establishment of a religious league, or amphictyony. In Central Greece the important oracle of Apollo at Delphi was administered and protected by its Amphictyonic League of twelve states. In Ionia, where the Greek inhabitants retained some sense of political solidarity from the circumstances of their migration and early settlement, an Ionian League was formed which met to worship the god Poseidon at the Panionium near Priene. In general, however, physical barriers were too strong to be overcome in the early stages of settlement and the new communities of the Aegean grew into hundreds of independent little states. Within each state problems of defense, the need of settling disputes in the common interest, and the advantages of economic diversification all worked to unify the community.

This feeling of loyalty to the local community was fostered at first by the social organization which the Greeks retained from their period of invasion and migration. The society of the city-state was based on the patriarchal family and held together by ties of tribal kinship, characteristic of nomadic groups and necessary for their survival. The single household of father, mother, children, slaves, and possessions, was the basic unit, very firmly under the father's authority and protection. He represented it to the gods in worship and to the other households of the community. As the sons of the family and their male descendants established their own families, a ramifying net of kinship spread to include the group of related households in a clan or *genos* (Roman *gens*). The family of the original ancestor was recognized by the clan as senior, and its head was the clan chieftain. The clan formed a compact group in war and peace for the protection of its members and, conversely, the loyalty of a clan member to his kin transcended other ties.

It is probable that in settled communities membership in the clans was confined to the rulers and leading families and that kinship among the members of groups larger than the clans was fictitious. Yet the Greeks extended this theoretical kinship to the whole society of a state. When a local, territorial group developed from the need of common action in war and peace, it was called a brotherhood, *phratry*. Membership might include several aristocratic clans and a large number of ordinary people such as tenant farmers and craftsmen. Beyond the *phratry* was the tribe, *phyle*, whose members prided themselves on descent from a legendary tribal ancestor and celebrated their affiliation by a religious festival. Several tribes made up a "people," who were similarly regarded as descended from a common forefather. These ideas of family unity were carried over to the newly established territorial states and gave to the political community the cohesiveness of a family group knit together by kinship and religion.

Yet such ties of kinship were essentially inimical to the conception of a territorial state, which served the common good of its individual members. Clan conflict could divide and weaken the state, and the individual, as a clan member, could not be fully responsible to his community as a citizen or to himself as an individual. In time, the development of a common civic loyalty and the emergence of the individual destroyed the reality of these earlier attachments. The forms and the religious associations, however, were preserved for centuries.

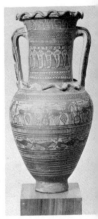

The Homeric State

The earliest Greek society which we can study in some detail is that pictured in the epic poems of Homer, the *Iliad* and the *Odyssey*. The Homeric community had achieved a sense of common identity, but the feeling for clan loyalty was still strong among its citizens. The processes of a settled life and of urbanization had just begun to work.

The stories of the war against Troy (pp. 117–18) and of the aftermath of wandering are placed by Greek tradition at the close of the Mycenaean Age, but we can scarcely use them as historical evidence for that period. Tradition itself placed the life of Homer in the ninth century B.C., and modern scholarship sets the time of composition of the poems in their present form at that time or as late as 700 B.C. For the historian the question is whether the institutions depicted are largely those of Mycenaean Greece or those of the time of composition. On the whole, it seems that the latter is true, although some anachronisms remained in the poems from the manner in which epic themes

Funerary amphora. Geometric style (eighth century B.C. A mourning scene on the neck.

were transmitted and the poetry which embodied them developed. There were several important differences in the Homeric organization from that of the palace-centered economy revealed by the Linear B tablets. Mycenaean Greece had many more and varied craftsmen. The sources of wealth and the resultant prosperity of the Mycenaeans were greater and, as discussed below, Homeric political institutions were of a more informal and primitive character. The names of the heroes, of their cities, and the enterprise against Troy, in which they engaged, were a legacy from the Mycenaean Age, but the actual world of Homer was that of the ninth and eighth centuries. The traditions of Mycenaean times were preserved and elaborated by reciters in a chain of oral transmission, until they were worked into the epics by the poet or poets called Homer in Ionia.

Homeric society was made up of two classes, a nobility, who governed and led in war, and a commons, composed of the nobles' tenant farmers, some freeholding peasants, and a few craftsmen and hired laborers. There were a few slaves, mainly captives of war, but these were attached to the households of the nobles and played no significant part in the economic organization of the community. The process of settlement had produced an economic division, reinforcing that made by seniority in the kinship structure, for the claim of the nobles to position was based on their wealth in land and its products, as well as on their high birth. The start of an urban community is apparent, for we find craftsmen who were woodworkers, employed in ship and house building, potters and blacksmiths. Each household, however, was largely self-sufficient, producing its own food and the textiles which made up a part of its wealth. Each community was virtually isolated from commercial exchange except for the acquisition of metals. The peoples of those towns advantageously situated on the sea, particularly in the islands, had begun to sail, but for piracy rather than for trade. Landowners might exchange their surplus agricultural products for metals and slaves, but the only professional traders were non-Greeks, Phoenicians, or Cypriots, who carried an assortment of trinkets for general trade, a few valuable objects, and perhaps metals for the wealthy.

The government was in the hands of the nobility although a sense of community spirit persisted which is reflected in an assembly of the people. Among the noble families, one was recognized as royal and the kingship normally passed by hereditary descent. The king, however, had to prove himself a successful leader in war and be able to overawe his noble peers in council to hold his position secure. Effective exercise of rule depended very largely on the ruler's personal qualities of forcefulness and achievement. Ideally, the king was responsible for his people in a patriarchal sense, protecting them, sacrificing to the gods and resolving disputes. He might act alone and did have the final decision, but usually he chose to consult a council of nobles. This was a very informal body which met at the king's call and could be elastic in its size, depending on the gravity of the occasion. In meetings, of course, the play of personality was most important, for the council was advisory only and had no clearly defined area of action or rights for itself.

The assembly of the people was similarly limited in power and was used to gain public support for decisions taken by the king and council, rather than to ratify them or to initiate any business of its own. The assembly, however, was composed of the adult males of the community, on whom defense ultimately rested, so that public support for common projects was necessary. Also, there seems to have been a feeling that any member might call a meeting on some question of public concern and was free to speak in the assembly, but in practice such meetings were usually called by the king, and the ordinary man scarcely dared to voice his opposition.

Simple and primitive as these institutions were, they were the prototypes from which the Greek city-state was to develop its organs of government. The overall authority of the king was ultimately divided among magistrates; the council of the nobles became an executive, and at times sovereign body, while the assembly, with its feeling of community, became sovereign in the more democratic governments of Greece.

The people of the Homeric state were just beginning to develop a sense of social responsibility for the ordinary concerns of life. As yet there was no written law to which an injured man might appeal, not even machinery for the making of laws and the regular administration of justice. A wronged man normally turned to his clan for help. Yet people also felt that such unilateral action, if carried too far, might endanger the whole community and they asked for arbitration from nobles other than those of the clans concerned. This arbitration was voluntary, but the verdicts handed out became a part of the body of precedent which formed the customary law of the community. In such a manner models for compromise and recognized compensations for injury were established. While these could only be applied by the king and nobles, public opinion was quick to form and become known in these small communities. This could act as an informal check on too arbitrary action. A seed of growth was present here, and we will find that one of the earliest concerns of the city-state was to obtain social justice and written law codes.

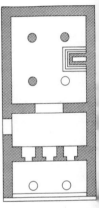

Plan of a megaron

The towns at the end of the Dark Age were still very poor in material wealth when compared to their Mycenaean predecessors, but were growing with increasing acceleration, as exemplified by Old Smyrna. About 900 B.C. the settler there lived in a small, one-room hut, the walls of which were built of sun-dried brick and the roof of thatch. Two centuries later, when the population had increased considerably, the whole town was rebuilt on a modern-looking, checkerboard plan, with rectangular house-blocks of similar size. The houses were of stone, had several rooms, and used the megaron plan, familiar from Bronze Age Greece. Dark Age Greece, however, did not produce any monumental architecture and sculpture because there was not enough wealth and because the men were too unskilled to work properly in stone. Temples of timber and sun-dried brick housed the gods and only small bronze or terracotta figurines were dedicated to them.

Yet two needs were beginning to turn the Greeks to expansion—the scarcity of metals and the nobles' taste for luxuries. The Homeric heroes were sensitive in a somewhat barbaric fashion to the flashing beauty of good arms and armor, to cups of gold, to carved ivory, and to the richness and color of textiles. Greeks acquired such materials mainly by plunder in war and piracy, or as gifts, and they were cherished as heirlooms for generations. Some, however, were purchased from the foreign traders who brought metals, and thus made the possibilities of trade apparent. The Homeric state was ripe for change.

The Age of Hesiod

Homer's nostalgic memories of the Mycenaean Age cast a glow of noble heroism on his characters. The values which the Homeric heroes found important in life became the ideals of aristocratic Greek society. The heroes felt that the worth of a man was in his individual achievement and the qualities which set him apart from his fellows: courage and glory in battle, skill in hunting and sports, and persuasive ability and judgment as a councilor. These activities would change, of course, but the feeling of the prime importance of individual achievement remained, particularly for the aristocratic element in society. The ordinary man, however, had not yet appeared. He found his first spokesman in the poet Hesiod who lived in Boeotia in Central Greece in the seventh century B.C.

Hesiod had grown up on a small farm near the village of Ascra, to which his father had migrated from Aeolis across the Aegean. The farm was left to Hesiod and to his brother, Perses, but Hesiod felt cheated in the disposition of the property. In his poem, the *Works and Days,* he complained that Perses had contrived to get an unfair share through the decision of the nobles who acted as judges for the community. His poem, however, is much more than a personal complaint, for it voices a general feeling of dissatisfaction with society and incorporates age-old maxims of conduct and precepts of farming, which reveal the narrow life of rural Greece.

Government had changed from the patriarchal kingships of the Homeric state to domination by the noble landowners. In the process the feeling of responsibility by the ruler and of trust by the subject had disappeared. A sharper line of economic and social distinction was drawn between the two segments of society; in fact the people may even have lost their right of assembly. Certainly, they had acquired no voice in government, for the political control of the state was in the hands of a small group of ruling families. These aristocrats were designated by such names as Horse Breeders, Land Sharers, and Well-Born. The claim to large estates and to high birth supported their rule, but the common people, even in rural Boeotia, felt the nobles' exercise of power to be unjust and oppressive. Hesiod voiced the ordinary man's protest, but he himself saw no solution, except for individuals to better their own lives or to await the punishment meted out to the unjust by the slow-working justice of Heaven. His indignation marks an austere, new tone in Greek literature, but does not envisage the possibility of reform by political action. The tradition of aristocratic rule was too strong to be easily shaken off.

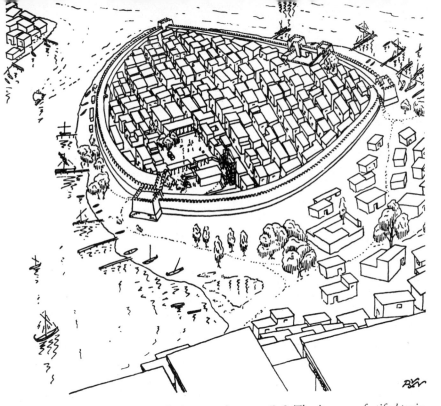

Reconstruction of Old Smyrna in the late seventh century B.C. The city was a fortified penin-sular site, characteristic of Ionian Greece and resembling Homer's description of Phaeacia in the Odyssey.

In Greece, however, a rapid process of expansion was starting. No great power was close at hand to threaten or to interfere with the independence of the city-states until Persia advanced to the Aegean in 547 B.C. Population was increasing to the point of outrunning the local food supply. The system of land tenure made a living by agriculture difficult for all except the noble fam-ilies on large holdings. Apparently property was divisible among the male children, and in a few generations the splitting of holdings had reduced the smaller farms to a mere subsistence level or driven men from them. The number of those who had to live by hiring their labor or by begging, already perceptible in the Homeric community, had increased. These men could not be absorbed by the small craft industries, for craftwork was hereditary in character and the market for its products small. In any case, the thoughts of landless peasants turned primarily to the acquisition of a farm.

As we have noticed, however, the possibility of trade had become apparent and some Greeks had already taken to the sea. Beginning about 775 and for almost three centuries, to about 500 B.C., Greeks migrated to establish trading posts and agricultural colonies around the Mediterranean. As well as draining surplus population from the Greek states, this migration started a social and economic evolution. New elements emerged in society: landholders, who developed the specialized agriculture of vine and olive production for export; merchants who engaged in overseas trade; retailers in the local markets; ship-owners and traders. Alongside the peasants a new urban lower class of crafts-men, artisans, and sailors came into being. The process of urbanization in the agrarian communities was accelerated rapidly, and by 600 B.C. a monetary economy was being introduced through the invention of coinage. The Homeric communities had produced sufficient capital themselves to start the process in action by building ships and providing manpower, but the leaven of coloni-zation was needed to transform society.

The Colonization Movement

Greek expansion is usually explained (and oversimplified) by saying that in the eighth century the precarious balance between population and food sup-ply had been overturned and that men migrated to find new farms. The earliest colonies were trading posts rather than agricultural settlements, and almost everywhere preliminary trading ventures preceded settlement. No doubt many of the migrants, as the movement progressed, were in search of land on which to settle and re-establish the agricultural mode of life familiar to them. Yet the significant result for Greece was to establish an intricate network of trade con-nections, which enabled the Aegean area to import needed food and to develop its industry and special products as payment. Agriculture did remain the basic mode of life for the people of most Greek cities and for the new colonies as well. The leaders of Greek society continued to be drawn from aristocratic land-owners who set the seal of respectability on the practice of agriculture. But, if Greece were to advance beyond the level of a subsistence economy, to in-crease its population, and win the necessary leisure for civilization, grain and metals had to be imported in quantity into the Aegean. It was not enough to simply export the surplus population. The trading activity which accompanied the Greek colonial expansion was vital for the continued growth of the city-states, because through it the Greeks could draw on the resources of the Medi-terranean as well as on their own limited wealth.

The first voyages out of the Aegean were probably made by the islanders of the Cyclades, who found the sea almost literally at their doorsteps and had little cultivable land on their islands. They followed the route of Phoenicians and Cypriots to the southeast and by the ninth century were making trips to the coast of Syria, where luxury products and metals could be obtained. By 750 B.C. a trading post was established at Al Mina near the mouth of the Orontes River. To Al Mina the traders of the Syro-Hittite and Aramaean cities of northern Syria could bring their goods without paying a profit to Phoenician middlemen.

The Greeks bought such articles as metals and metalware, textiles, and carved ivories, carrying them back to the Aegean where their main destinations were Rhodes, Samos, Crete, Corinth, and Athens. Probably, too, small groups of eastern workmen, ivorycarvers and metalworkers, settled in those Greek cities which provided a good market for their skills. For example, on Samos the important sanctuary of the goddess Hera was the recipient of dedications of such products, imported by traders or made on Samos by eastern workmen. The Greeks themselves learned new craft techniques and fresh motifs of design from the newcomers and from the goods of trade. A new wave of oriental influence also began to break on Greek shores. The Greeks adopted the Phoenician alphabet to express their own ideas (pp. 230–31), and the traders speedily disseminated it in the Aegean and to the new colonial areas. The Syrian metrical system and weight standards were taken over.

Just as the Near East had stimulated growth in prehistoric Greece, renewed contacts with its civilization again helped to catalyze Greek ability and energy. Syria, however, was not suitable for large-scale settlement by Greeks, for the land was heavily populated and urbanized, and, after 700 B.C., firmly under Assyrian control. The Assyrians might welcome the Greeks as traders or hire them as mercenary soldiers, but did not want them as independent settlers.

The Aegean islanders, however, found an area for limited settlement closer at hand on the northern shore of the Aegean itself. In the latter part of the eighth century they began to move into the Macedonian Chalcidice, where the three long peninsulas provided harbors and sufficient land to support small towns. About 700 B.C. the big island of Thasos was settled, mainly by men from Paros. Thasos became an important and prosperous little state, partly by its control of the adjacent mainland, partly by serving as a center for the trade carried along the northern Aegean coast. Inland from the coast the broad river valleys were held by barbaric tribal groups, who were willing to trade but resisted Greek settlement and infiltration. In the course of a few generations trade with the interior became profitable, as deposits of silver and gold on Mt. Pangaeus were exploited and exchanged with the Greeks for fine metalwork, textiles, and wine; in addition, the region produced grain and good timber for shipbuilding. All these attractions drew other Greeks to Thrace. Ionians founded colonies and obtained silver with which they could purchase grain in Egypt for their own cities. Corinth founded a colony, Potidaea, by 600 B.C. and Athens, two generations later, began to send colonists to the region.

The new colonies were at first very small in size, with populations numbering only a few score or hundreds of people. The settlement was started under the shield of a mother-city, but the founding cities were themselves so undeveloped politically that the tie of attachment was sentimental and religious in nature, rather than political. An official founder, the *oekist,* was placed in charge of the expedition to divide the land into lots, allocate them to the settlers, and set some aside for the temples and public buildings. The colonists brought the worship of the gods of their own city to the new colony and honored the founder by a special cult. They also imitated the institutions of the mother-city, but the latter assigned no regular governor and did not attempt to collect a tax. The colonies were free to grow and develop independently as new city-

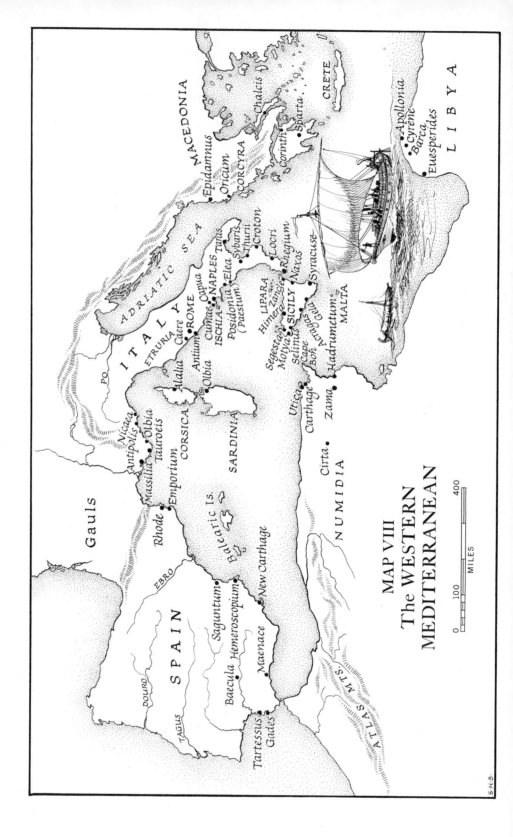

MAP VIII
The WESTERN
MEDITERRANEAN

MILES

0   100   400

S·H·B·

states, and most of them chose to disregard the ties of sentiment and religious affiliation and to work out their own political destinies. Greek colonization was essentially a multiplication of independent city-states and not the beginning of an imperialistic colonial system of the type familiar in modern history.

MAGNA GRAECIA AND THE WESTERN MEDITERRANEAN

The main area of Greek settlement was in South Italy and Sicily, where so many towns were founded that the region came to be known as Magna Graecia, or Great Greece. From about 775 B.C. the Greeks had begun to sail west of the Peloponnesus. They came from Chalcis in Euboea, from the Cyclades and perhaps from Crete. The Chalcidians by-passed the shorelines of South Italy and Sicily and placed a trading colony on the island of Ischia offshore from Naples. Here, apparently, iron and copper could be obtained in exchange for Greek textiles and wine. A generation later the colonists moved across to the fertile coastal plain of modern Naples to establish a colony, Cumae (740 B.C.), which remained the northernmost point of Greek settlement on the west coast of Italy. Cumae served as the main center for trade with the native Italian population and with the Etruscans of central Italy. The Etruscans (p. 422) were themselves migrants from western Asia, and by the time of the Greek settlement had begun to work the iron of their region and to develop the earliest urban civilization of Italy. Their growing wealth provided a market both for Greek goods and for goods from Syria and Phoenicia, which the Greek traders carried. Greek workmen, too, could find employment in Etruria, and the Greek colonists of Magna Graecia enjoyed a profitable role as middlemen in the trade.

In South Italy and Sicily, however, the fertile coastal plains and hill valleys offered good opportunity for agricultural colonies; consequently a heavy influx of settlers set in rapidly. Settlers from Euboea showed the way with a group of colonies founded between 735 and 730 B.C. First, a settlement was placed by Eretrians on the big island of Corcyra to serve as a way station in crossing the Adriatic Sea. Then, Naxos, Zancle, and Rhegium were settled by Chalcidians in the Strait of Messina. The two latter, on opposite sides of the strait, could both control its traffic and serve as transhipment points for cargoes sent on to Cumae. When the way had been thus marked out, further settlement followed quickly. The settlers came mainly from Corinth and Achaea in the overcrowded Peloponnesus, since they had an easy route through the Gulf of Corinth to Corcyra and thence across the Adriatic. Corinthians took over the Eretrian post on Corcyra and went on to found Syracuse (733 B.C.), which ultimately became the most important Greek city of the west. Achaeans settled in a number of small places along the south coast of Italy, the most important of which were Sybaris (about 700 B.C.) and, across the peninsula from it, Posidonia. A land route was developed to connect the two and to supplement the sea route through the Strait of Messina between Sicily and Italy. The most important town of South Italy, Taras (Taranto; 706 B.C.) was founded by Sparta, which sent off a group of political malcontents as colonists. Throughout the seventh century the process of colonization went on and the less desirable sites were occupied, until the Italian coast from Taranto to Naples and the eastern half of Sicily were ringed with Greek settlements. Corinth, in particular, found a good market in the new area for its pottery and manufactured goods and began to import Sicilian grain as the colonists brought their lands under cultivation.

Further Greek expansion in the western Mediterranean was limited. Phoenicians (p. 123) had anticipated the Greeks along the coast of Africa and in the big islands on the way to Gibraltar, where their goal was the tin and copper available in southern Spain. The Phoenician settlement at Carthage grew rapidly, becoming the center of an area of influence which reached out to western Sicily and which closed that part of the island to the Greeks. As Magna Graecia filled up, however, later Greek arrivals, tempted to compete with the Phoenicians for the Spanish metal trade, established a route by southern France and northeastern Spain.

Probably Rhodian traders and Chalcidians had already begun to explore the coast of southern France by the middle of the seventh century, but the lasting settlements were made by Ionians from western Asia Minor. About 635 B.C. a Samian captain, Colaeus, took his ship from Libya in north Africa all the way to the Spanish city, Tartessus, near the Phoenician colony of Gades. He was warmly welcomed by the Tartessians, who probably saw the advantages for themselves of competition between the Phoenicians and Greeks, and so provided Colaeus with a valuable cargo of metal. While other Samians did not follow up Colaeus' venture, Phocaean ships began to make the long voyage to the west and set in motion one of the most interesting processes of Greek trade.

Phocaea itself was a tiny city on the west coast of Asia Minor, supported by a very small agricultural area. Its sailors were apparently attracted to the west, when Colaeus brought his cargo back to Samos. The Phocaeans used a small, light ship, the penteconter, which was rowed by fifty men and built for piracy or swift running with a small cargo. With these vessels they developed a carrying trade to exchange the luxury goods of the eastern Mediterranean for the metals of the west. Tin was brought from the mines of Cornwall in England along the west coast of Europe to Tartessus, where it was picked up by the Phocaean traders. On their way to Tartessus the Phocaeans distributed their cargo of eastern goods in Magna Graecia and Etruria. From Etruria they could supplement the cargo with iron. Thus a trade which extended the length of the Mediterranean was established. Since the route to Spain by Sardinia and the Balearic Islands was made hazardous by the Phoenicians, an alternative course was established along the coast of France. On it colonies were founded at Massilia (Marseilles) and at Emporion (Ampurias) in northeastern Spain about 600 B.C.

The Phocaean traders were active until about 540 B.C. when their city was taken by the Persians after the defeat of Lydia (p. 237), and many Phocaeans left home to try to establish themselves on Corsica. They were defeated at sea and driven from the island by Carthaginians and Etruscans. The tin trade by sea fell again into Phoenician hands, but in this situation the Phocaean colony at Massilia found an opportunity. Greek traders had already begun to travel up the Rhone valley into central France, and now these extended their activities to establish an overland route for the tin. The metal was brought from Cornwall to the French coast, where the valleys of the Loire and Seine rivers provided routes to stations in central France, visited by the Greek merchants. As the population of Massilia grew, the city founded secondary settlements along the Riviera at Nice, Cannes, Monaco and other ports. Thus, in the western Mediterranean there came to be three nests of Greek colonies: in Magna Graecia, the Riviera, and eastern Spain.

THE EASTERN MEDITERRANEAN

In the eastern Mediterranean the Ionian Greeks were particularly active in establishing colonies and developing trade. At first Ionia itself had offered a field for expansion. As control of the coastal plains and river estuaries had been gradually won, the native population was incorporated into the Greek states. Until about 675 B.C. no native power was strong enough to seriously check the Ionians, but by that time Gyges had consolidated the Kingdom of Lydia (pp. 155–56) and had blocked the Greeks from penetrating up the river valleys. The Lydian kings raided Ionian territory and burned the crops, but they showed no desire to incorporate the Greek seaboard into their kingdom. Instead, a very close economic cooperation developed between Ionia and Lydia. Some Ionians served as hired soldiers in the Lydian army, while Lydian kings and nobles commissioned artistic products from Ionian craftsmen. In return, the Ionians exported some of the special products of Lydian agriculture—leather, wine, and textiles. To facilitate this exchange the Lydian kings had developed the mining of electrum. The use of small weights of this metal suggested the invention of coinage; and so between 650 and 625 B.C. the first coins were minted—a fixed weight of electrum guaranteed by the symbol of the issuer. We do not know whether Ionian merchants or the Lydian king began the practice, but its convenience was recognized speedily, and by 600 B.C. those Aegean states which engaged in trade had begun to mint. The Lydian coins were stamped with the royal insignia of Lydia, a lion's head, while the Ionians and the other Greeks used symbols appropriate to the religious cults and legends of their cities, or they even in some instances made puns on the names of their cities. Phocaea, for example, derived from the Greek word for seal, used the device of a seal on its coins, and Rhodes, a rose, to advertise the

From left to right: A Lydian coin of King Croesus (560–547 B.C.). A coin of Rhodes, bearing the state's symbol, a rose. A coin of Cnossus, showing the labyrinth, remembered in tradition from Minoan times

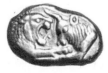
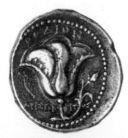
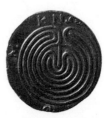

origin of its money. The developing relationship with Lydia absorbed Ionian energies throughout most of the seventh century, but at the same time emigration and overseas trade began, partly as a relief measure for the increase of population and partly under the stimulus of increasing prosperity.

About 700 B.C. the earliest Ionian colony was established at Maroneia on the coast of Thrace by settlers from Chios. The coastal region west of Maroneia was exploited by the existing Greek settlement on Thasos, so Ionian colonization spread eastwards towards the Black Sea. The shores of the Propontis were occupied by agricultural colonies in the course of the seventh century, first by settlers from Miletus, who started the process with a colony at Cyzicus, then by men from Samos and even from Megara across the Aegean. About 625 B.C. a new factor was introduced into the region by the growth of trade into the Black Sea. The colonies in the Propontis perhaps served more as ports of call than as trading centers themselves, but some were very advantageously situated to profit from it. Byzantium, founded on the same site as modern Istanbul, was able to levy tolls and sell provisions to the crews of the ships waiting to make the run through the Bosporus. Sestos, at the head of the Hellespont, the modern Dardanelles, found itself in an equally good position. Thus the trade benefited the stations on the shipping route as well as the Ionians of Asia Minor, who were particularly prominent in the opening of the Black Sea.

The first voyages into the Black Sea were sporadic and exploratory, but from 625 B.C. the process of settlement was rapid and continuous. Although the Greeks found the cold and foggy climate most uncongenial after living in

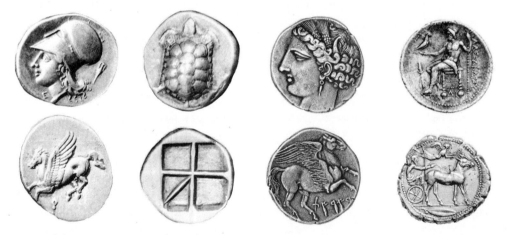

From left to right: A Corinthian didrachm (two-drachma piece) with the helmeted head of Athena and the winged horse Pegasus, the particular symbol of Corinth. An Aeginetan "turtle"; the reverse of these widely circulated coins was stamped only with an incuse square made by the anvil dye. A Carthaginian decadrachm (ten-drachma piece). The winged horse was imitated from Corinthian coins; the inscription is in Phoenician. Top right: reverse of a tetradrachm (four-drachma piece) of Alexander the Great. Zeus enthroned with his eagle Bottom right: reverse of a coin of Sicilian Messana. Victory crowns the mule team of a winner in a chariot race.

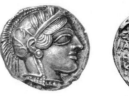

An Athenian tetradrachm, bearing the head of Athena on the front and her sacred bird, the owl, on the back

the Mediterranean and although they met an initially hostile reception from the natives, the economic resources of the region complemented those of the Aegean. The Ionians made their first settlements on small offshore islands or peninsulas, both for safety and to exploit the annual run of tunny fish in the Black Sea. Very soon, however, products other than fish were discovered. Olbia, at the mouth of the Bug River, became a center for the grain trade with the native Scythians, who lived in the fertile area of South Russia. The grain was purchased through the native chieftains, brought down the river, and transshipped at Olbia, where Ionian metalware and textiles were used in payment. On the south shore of the Black Sea, Sinope became an important city, growing from a fishing station into a trading center for the whole adjacent area. To Sinope a mineral earth, *miltos,* used for painting ships, was brought down from Cappadocia in the interior of Anatolia. By the time of the Persian Wars almost every desirable coastal site on the Black Sea had been settled by a Greek colony, and a thriving trade had developed. The Greeks did not penetrate far inland, but established cordial relations with the natives. In many communities fusion between the two groups stimulated further urbanization and, eventually, the coalescence of native kingdoms.

While the Black Sea was being opened and trade developed, Greek contacts were established with Libya and Egypt. The earliest colony was Cyrene in northwestern Libya. Colaeus, the Samian who sailed to Gibraltar, had touched there as it was being founded, about 635 B.C., and had aided the settlers who came from the small island of Thera in the southern Aegean. Cyrene grew rather slowly at first, but in the sixth century fresh colonists came and development of the hinterland began. The land was suitable for sheep grazing and for the cultivation of a plant called *silphium,* which was used as a cooking spice by the Greeks. The colony, because of these products and its strategic position, grew into a large and important city by the time it was taken over by Cambyses in connection with his conquest of Egypt (p. 162).

The Greeks seem to have visited Egypt first as casual traders, perhaps mixing their trade with piracy, then as mercenary soldiers. About 650 B.C. the Saite king of Egypt, Psammetichus I, hired some Ionians and established them in a fort in the delta region. Compatriots came to trade and in the last quarter of the century the Greeks received permission from the Egyptian king to establish a trading colony at Naukratis on the Canopic mouth of the Nile. Various Greeks, mainly Ionians, but also Corinthians, Aeginetans, Rhodians, and Athenians built warehouses, docks, and temples near the existing native town. Naukratis became a depot for the grain which Egypt could supply in quantity, as well as for more specialized products, linen, papyrus, and luxury articles. The Greek settlers bought Greek wine, olive oil, and fine pottery from their compatriots and even established craft industries to imitate Egyptian goods. Since the grain and luxuries, however, had to be paid for with silver, the new device of coinage provided the means. Hoards of Greek coins have been found in the Nile delta where they had been hidden away by Egyptian dealers. The Greeks, seeing the age-old buildings and sculpture of Egypt, began to imitate some of the architectural forms and to carve life-size statues in the manner of the Egyptians (pp. 225–26).

EFFECTS OF COLONIZATION

During the colonization movement which drew to its close about 500 B.C. on the eve of the Persian Wars, the horizons of Greece had been extended to include the whole Mediterranean. The Greek cities in the Aegean still remained basically agricultural in their traditions and activity, but new means of producing wealth had been introduced and new groups had entered their society. As discussed later (pp. 193–97), these groups had a speedy effect in developing new social and political institutions. The difficulties of overpopulation had been temporarily solved by emigration and by the import of grain from Sicily, the Black Sea, and Egypt. Sources of supply for needed metals, iron, tin, and copper had been found and a system of trade worked out to procure them. Greece's own special resources had been developed: olive oil and wine from its farms, and metalwork, textiles, and terracotta products from its craft industries.

Equally significant was the foundation of hundreds of Greek cities in the colonial regions, where new contacts brought a broadening of knowledge. The South Italian and Sicilian colonies, in particular, grew rapidly and became in many cases larger and wealthier than their mother-cities. The fresh start which they enjoyed made them readier to experiment with political and social institutions, so that the colonial areas of Greece contributed much to its cultural growth. In general the colonies remained a part of the Greek world and maintained their ties with the Aegean area through the network of trade. Expansion into the interior of Europe seemed difficult and dangerous. The colonies of the Greek expansion remained, as Plato vividly put it, like frogs sitting around a pond.

Colonization had brought the Greeks of the Aegean into contact with both the uncivilized lands of the West and the Black Sea and with the old, highly developed peoples of the Near East in Syria and Egypt. In the less civilized lands they found mainly a market for selling their own manufactured goods and for procuring needed supplies. Here they spread their own Greek culture. In Syria and Egypt the reverse was true. The Greeks found the stimulus they needed to set their own creativity to work. The minor crafts borrowed new techniques, subject matter, and design motifs, while sculpture found models which would give Greek sculptors a start. Yet the Greeks developed political and social institutions to meet their own particular needs essentially from the forms apparent in the Homeric state. In this respect they owed virtually nothing to the older civilizations.

The Growth of the City-State

(*ca.* 750–500 B.C.)

AT THE SAME TIME as the Greeks were establishing their colonies beyond the Aegean area, they developed their characteristic community, the city-state, or *polis*. Old systems of government by local lords and clan chieftains, like those against whose injustice Hesiod had protested, broke down. The individual citizen became the essential factor of an expanded society and desired to share in and better the political life of his state. His first demand was for the publication of his community's laws, so that he, as well as his aristocratic leaders, might know them. Then, as the new groups created by the economic transformation of Greece leavened society and began to seek political rights, the cities experienced revolution. Since the communities were small and compact, political action was often disconcertingly rapid and direct. Frequently individual leaders seized rule violently and made wholesale changes in the institutions of their city. This age of Greek history, from about 650 to 500 B.C., sometimes called the "Age of the Tyrants," produced a colorful and able group of leaders, whose work helped to bring the city-state into being. By 500 B.C. the Greek states were following two main lines of growth. Sparta remained agrarian and conservative, avoiding revolution and change by imposing a rigid discipline and regimentation upon its citizens. Athens, on the other hand, became volatile and inventive, open to new ideas and experiment. By the eve of the Persian Wars the Athenians had established the fundamental institutions of their democracy, in which the individual could find room for the exercise of his abilities.

Lawgivers

In the seventh century B.C. many of the Greek cities chose men known as Lawgivers to record and publish the customs of the community. The Lawgivers did so by public proclamation or by using the recently disseminated alphabetic

The reader will find Maps VII, IX, and XI (pages 172–173, 202, and 284) useful as he reads this chapter.

writing to inscribe law codes on wooden, bronze, or stone tablets. Many of the newly publicized codes merely recorded existing customs and attempted few innovations to meet changing conditions. Publication itself, however, marked a distinct step towards protecting the position of the individual.

But in the new colonies of South Italy, we hear of the activity of two men, Zaleucus of Locris and Charondas of Catana, who made progressive regulations. Presumably the freer life of the colonies and the clash of customs among migrants from different cities spurred these Lawgivers to new ideas. In their codes old practices are to be found side by side with reform and innovation. For example, it was felt proper to retain fixed penalties of a primitive and retaliatory nature such as blinding, but judicial functions were assigned to regular magistrates. Elaborate precautions were taken to preserve the family by safeguarding the transmission of property through minors and heiresses and prohibiting the alienation of family land by sale or bequest. Yet, the new commercial activity was governed by market regulations, and some humanitarian concern for slaves was shown by penalties for abusing them. In some cases, where the crisis was very grave, the Lawgiver was given authority also to reorganize the social and political institutions of his state. Solon of Athens (pp. 206–10) is the outstanding example of such a reformer.

The early law codes not only had the authority of tradition behind them, but were invested with religious veneration. Lawgivers were frequently regarded as divinely inspired, either by the visitation of a god, or, more frequently, by the approval of the god Apollo given at his oracle in Delphi. The laws were submitted to the oracle, and the god, or rather his priests, had a part in shaping them. Delphi's maxim, "Nothing in excess," was practically applied to encourage sane and moderate regulations. Divine authority, of course, made the laws more readily acceptable, but at the same time made subsequent change more difficult. The Greeks remained curiously reluctant to alter laws, even in the midst of political revolution. They felt that laws were educative and morally formative. Some of the Lawgivers, too, were worshipped as semidivine figures, like Lycurgus of Sparta, and were praised by the Greek philosophers as men whose legislation had fixed the ethical character of their state at a single stroke.

"Tyranny"

While publication of the laws helped to check the arbitrary abuse of authority by the nobles, new leaders, the "tyrants," were most effective in bringing the era of aristocratic government to an end. "Tyranny" was new and the Greeks found this new word for it. "Tyrant" at first had no pejorative meaning in itself, although the modern use of "dictator" perhaps best expresses its significance. Apparently "tyrant" became known to the Greeks as the title of Gyges of Lydia (pp. 155–57), who had usurped the throne by violence and ruled absolutely. His title was appropriate to men who destroyed the aristocratic regimes by violent revolution and held sole power by hiring soldiers and cultivating popular support. The tyrants tried in most cases to make their rule hereditary, but the Greek tyrannies did not last beyond three generations. It was in the democracy of fifth-century Athens, established after the expulsion of a tyrant, that the word gradually acquired its modern connotation. The historian Thucydides used it to distinguish the leader who usurped and held power illegally for his own selfish ends from a king who ruled constitutionally. Plato and Aristotle condemned tyranny as an evil and destructive form of government. Yet in early Greece the tyrants frequently represented the interest of the new middle group in the Greek cities. They worked to unify the whole people in loyalty to the state and to make their cities strong powers. The tyrant usually followed a firm and deliberately planned foreign policy, which laid the foundations for an international political life among the city-states. The older, personal relations of enmity or friendship among nobles of different states were gradually replaced by policies of self-interest for the community as a whole.

The middle class, on which the tyrant's position partly rested, began to appear in the more progressive Greek states when the process of urbanization was stimulated by trade and by the growth of population. The members are to be identified as owners of the small pottery and metalworking manufactures, farmers who turned to olive oil and wine production for export, shipowners, and traders. While the number of those engaged in business was at first small, such economic activity made them independent of the landowning aristocracy. Middle-class interest became centered in the market of the city rather than in the rural villages and the countryside. As early as 700 B.C., some cities began to use men of the middle class for a new type of military formation, the *hoplite* phalanx, which strengthened not only the claim of the middle group to political recognition, but their ability to gain it. This change in the methods of warfare is singled out by Aristotle as a primary cause of revolution.

The Greeks found their model for the new armor and formations in the Assyrian armies, with which Greeks had become familiar in their trading in the east. The *hoplite* was a heavy-armed foot soldier, drawn up for battle in disciplined and maneuverable ranks. He fought at close quarters with thrusting spear and sword. Previously the brunt of battle had been carried by small troops of cavalry and by individual "heroes," who started their fight by throwing spears, then closed to fight a sword duel, like the Homeric champions. The new *hoplite* formations, however, drawn up in line of battle with overlapping shields, were very effective on the defensive and, on level ground or down a slope, could charge with a heavy momentum to break an opposing line. Henceforth, the *hoplite* platoon rather than the individual hero won battles. Some Greeks found a new profession in selling their services as *hoplite* soldiers both in Greece and in the Near Eastern kingdoms when the increasing supply of metal, particularly iron, made the new weapons more readily available. From the citizen *hoplites* or foreign mercenaries came the military power needed by the tyrants to break the aristocratic regimes. A brief survey of the careers of some of the important tyrants will illustrate the factors involved in their rule.

PHEIDON OF ARGOS

The earliest tyranny of which we have some knowledge was that of Pheidon of Argos, who seized power in his native state about 675 B.C. He seems to have been a member of the line of hereditary Dorian kings in Argos, whose power had declined into a formal office under the encroachment of the nobles. Pheidon is said to have expanded this shrunken power into a tyranny, and, since his lifetime coincided with the brief period of Argive military supremacy in the Peloponnesus, is credited with making use of the new *hoplites*. Pheidon defeated Sparta, extended Argive control over his neighbors, Corinth and Sicyon, and even as far as the Olympic sanctuary of Zeus in Elis. To Pheidon are also ascribed the establishment of common standards of weight and measure in the Peloponnesus and the earliest issue of silver coins in Greece.[1] While this last can hardly be true, because the coins formerly ascribed to Pheidon are now dated after 625 B.C., the tyrant may well have been concerned to facilitate commercial exchange in the northeastern Peloponnesus, where Aegean and eastern trade converged.

THE CYPSELIDS OF CORINTH

Pheidon's ability to dominate Corinth indicates that that city's ruling aristocracy, the Bacchiad family, was declining in the early seventh century. The members of the family held the government among themselves, and at the outset of rule, about 750 B.C., had been energetic and efficient. The Corinthian colonies at Corcyra and Syracuse were sponsored by the Bacchiads, and they capitalized on the strategic position of Corinth to develop trade to the west through the Gulf of Corinth and to the east across the Aegean to Rhodes and North Syria. Yet Corcyra had broken away from Corinth and fought the first recorded naval battle in Greek history with its mother-city in 667 B.C. Apparently maritime development promoted the emergence of a middle group in Corinth, which found a champion in Cypselus, the founder of the tyranny, about 650 B.C. His energy and the brilliant rule of his son, Periander, made Corinth the most prosperous city of Greece until its tyrants were deposed about 580 B.C. and the city came under the influence of Sparta.

---

[1]The time of the introduction of coinage in various states of Greece is a subject of current controversy, in which I have chosen to follow the new, low dates for the most part. The problem is important for early Greek history because the time and manner of the transition to a monetary economy is at issue. The chief argument for the low chronology is that the steps leading to coinage are illustrated by the electrum pellets and early coins found in a deposit of precious objects dedicated at the temple of Artemis in Ephesus. The most recent study of the deposit has resulted in the conclusion that the invention of coinage was made in the Ionian-Lydian region between 650 and 600 B.C. The earliest *silver* coins of the cities of the Greek peninsula and the Aegean Islands do not show the preliminary steps to coinage; that is, they are derivative and later and are to be dated at the earliest shortly before 600 B.C. The earliest silver coinage, that of Aegina, is traditionally associated with Pheidon, and some scholars argue that the dates of his career, themselves controversial, allow him to be credited with the Aeginetan coins. In general terms, the dividing line between a natural and a monetary economy in Greece seems to have been about 600 B.C.

The circumstances of Cypselus' seizure of power are obscure, but his policies were plainly designed to break the rule of the Bacchiad clan and their aristocratic supporters. Perhaps personal bitterness towards the Bacchiads was a factor, for Cypselus' mother, a Bacchiad, had married outside the clan, and her kinsmen repudiated and tried to kill Cypselus. Once in control, he executed or exiled the aristocrats and confiscated their property. The land was probably distributed among the poorer peasants to increase popular support for the tyranny, but Cypselus' chief backing was evidently in the new middle group. His regime was mainly peaceful and concerned to expand Corinthian interests in north-western Greece, where timber for shipbuilding was available. Corcyra had become independent, but alternative ports of call for Corinthian ships were established on the island of Leucas and on the Greek coast of the Adriatic Sea. In Corinth itself excavation has revealed that the pottery works were enlarged and something like mass production of a standardized Corinthian style of pottery for export developed. Cypselus was concerned also to develop the city, and the earliest large temple in Corinth, the predecessor of the Temple of Apollo, overlooking the market place, is probably to be dated near the beginning of his rule. Cypselus' death left Corinth in a prosperous and powerful condition which his son, Periander, proceeded to improve.

It is difficult to estimate the methods of internal control used by Periander, for around his name cluster the usual charges made by later Greek historians against tyrants—hiring foreign mercenary troops as a personal bodyguard, and suppression of all freedom in the state and personal brutality. We cannot prove or disprove them, but it is likely that since the rich merchants of the middle group were beginning to demand a share in the government, Periander had to proceed against them as his father had against the aristocrats. Yet he made Corinth the chief city of Greece. Diplomatic relations were extended across the Aegean by his personal friendship with Thrasybulus, the tyrant of Miletus in Ionia. A mark of his own, and of Corinth's prestige, was the request made to him to arbitrate a quarrel between Athens and Mytilene on Lesbos over the town of Sigeum near the Dardanelles. Sigeum had become useful as a port of call when the trade into the Black Sea developed. Periander brought Corinth into that new market and into the new trading center at Naukratis in Egypt. The importance of Corinth was publicized by lavish gifts to the oracle at Delphi and by the development of a sanctuary of the sea-god Poseidon at nearby Isthmia, where a large temple was built and athletic contests established to attract visitors from foreign states.

Periander was able to establish a peaceful succession for his son Psamettichus, but the latter proved unable to retain power. Wealthy commercial families took over the government but were not able to hold the primacy given to Corinth by the tyrants. The pottery trade was lost, particularly to Athens, and in the latter part of the sixth century Corinth entered a league of Peloponnesian states dominated by Sparta.

THE ORTHAGORIDS OF SICYON

In the city of Sicyon, a few miles to the west of Corinth, a different factor, racial inequality, may be recognized as an element in the establishment of tyranny. About 650 B.C. Sicyon's first tyrant, Orthagoras, founded the most enduring of Greek tyrannies. It lasted three full generations and fell to Spartan interference rather than because of internal weakness. This longevity was apparently based on the support of the native people of Sicyon, who had been subjugated by the Dorians at the time of the Dorian invasion. The son of Orthagoras, Cleisthenes, is said to have changed the names of the old Dorian tribes to Pigmen, Assmen, Swinemen, while his own tribe was designated as *Archelaoi*, Leaders of the People. It is doubtful that actual participation in government went beyond Cleisthenes' own family, but the tyranny did stand for an assertion of native power over the Dorian nobles. This situation was reversed after 550 B.C., when Sparta brought Sicyon into its Peloponnesian League and insisted on the restoration of the proper names *Hylleis*, *Pamphyloi* and *Dymanes* to the Dorian tribes. Despite this rather flamboyant childishness, Cleisthenes did give Sicyon a brief span of importance when he helped to protect the oracle at Delphi against Thessalian encroachment in a Sacred War.

THE IONIAN TYRANTS

On the eastern side of the Aegean, whence the word "tyrant" had been borrowed by the Greeks, the appearance of such leaders in the Ionian cities was later than in the Peloponnesus. The hold of the landowning nobility, many of whom were descended from the original colonists, seems to have been very tenacious because many of the cities of Ionia controlled larger and more fertile territories than the cities of the Greek peninsula. Also, the Ionians had grown up in constant war with the Anatolian natives and perhaps felt that political innovation was a dangerous game. But by the end of the seventh century tyrannies appeared at Miletus and Ephesus, and later in the sixth century Polycrates of Samos became the most typical of Greek tyrants.

Polycrates, who came to rule in Samos about 535 B.C., is said to have gained control with the aid of his brothers, but dispossessed them and ruled the island in absolute and picturesque fashion. The position of the island of Samos as the pivot of navigation for cross-Aegean and Asiatic coastal trade was exploited to make Samos the center of a little empire. Polycrates built a fleet of one hundred warships and hired archers and foreign soldiers to protect himself. He seized some of the Aegean Islands and established Samian control over the adjacent coast of Asia Minor. Trade was extended to southern Italy and to Naukratis in Egypt, where Polycrates made a personal friend of King Amasis. In Samos itself the tyrant assembled a group of artists and writers under his patronage and transformed the appearance of his city by monumental building projects. A tunnel was cut through the mountain behind Samos to bring water to the city, harbor works were constructed and the city ringed by a fortification wall. A great new temple was built for the goddess Hera at her sanctuary, the Heraeum, to the west of the city. Polycrates, however, was too close to the new Persian province in western Asia Minor to enjoy his empire for long. The Persian governor at Sardes seems to have contrived his murder in 527 B.C. and brought the island under Persian control.

These examples indicate the role which the tyrants played in the growth of the city-state. The power of the aristocratic governments was broken and the clan system replaced by a class structure, which brought the new middle groups into prominence and aided the peasants and craftsmen. While the careers of the tyrants may have seemed purely selfish to later Greek writers, their age saw the transition of the Greek communities from farming towns to city-states. Physically the city began to assume its characteristic form. The *acropolis* became the religious center, adorned with new temples, prominent among which was that of the patron god of the state. The market place, or *agora,* became the business and political center, housing new civic buildings and political meetings.

The whole *polis* was protected by a fortification wall of stone. Monumental architecture and sculpture were encouraged by this building activity and by the tyrants' gifts to the great sanctuaries of Zeus at Olympia and Apollo at Delphi. The city-state became the focus of loyalty for its citizens and, as its wealth and population increased, began to play a proper part in foreign affairs. The absolute authority of the tyrants, however, prevented the development of free political institutions. The regimes were short-lived once the citizens had developed a sense of civic pride and responsibility.

Toward the close of this brilliant period of the tyrants, the Greek world began to take a new shape. On the east side of the Aegean the cities of Ionia were eclipsed by the imposition of Persian rule. In peninsular Greece Sparta, which had avoided tyranny, if not revolution, became the head of the first important political coalition of Greece, the Peloponnesian League. Athens was molded into a unified state in the sixth century by its tyrants, but rejected them to establish a moderate democracy in 508 B.C. The smaller states began to gravitate to the two poles of Sparta and Athens.

Sparta

It is an interesting paradox that although Sparta seems to have experienced the most effective revolution of all Greek states in the seventh century, two hundred years later the Spartans had become a model of political stability for Greece and resolute foes of all change. The Spartans avoided the absolute rule of a tyrant and won for themselves a considerable degree of popular participation in government. This privilege, however, was confined to a single element in the population, to the Dorian conquerors of Laconia. The pre-Dorian population was denied political rights and a very large part of it compelled to work on the farms of Spartan masters. In fact, Sparta's revolution was partly a means to secure the ruling position of the Spartans over their subjects by an effective regimentation of society. The rewards were great, for Sparta became the foremost military power of Greece, but Spartans had little share in the creation of its literature, art, or philosophy.

EARLY SPARTA

The Dorian invaders occupied the fertile plains of the Eurotas River in Laconia and divided the land into lots, which were distributed among the Dorian families. In later times this was called the "old land" and it could not be alienated from the family. The new owners lived in scattered villages, visiting their estates to supervise the agricultural work carried on for them by the subjugated native population, the *helots,* or serfs of the state. The *helots* were fixed to a lot and shared its produce, one-half at first, with the Spartan master. Intermarriage between the *helots* and Spartans was forbidden, and the Spartans preserved their racial purity by intermarrying only among themselves and by membership in the three Doric tribes. Other pre-Dorian elements, however, retained a relatively favored position. These were the *perioeci,* or dwellers-round, who lived in villages in the mountains bordering the plain of the Eurotas. The *perioeci* were denied political rights and intermarriage into the Spartan community, but retained some local freedom of government and control of their economic activity.

The early government of Sparta was an absolute hereditary kingship, but the office was shared between two families, the Ageadae and the Eurypontides. The two kings acted, sometimes with considerable difficulty, by joint collegiate decision. Probably such a system had originated in a compromise to heal the rivalry between two great Spartan clans. Presumably there was an informal council of clan chieftains to advise the kings as in the Homeric state, but we can only conjecture about other early Spartan institutions.

Since the austere, militaristic character of the Spartans was acquired slowly, early Sparta had a place in the literary and artistic achievement of Greece. In the seventh century, while the Spartans themselves produced few poets, they welcomed foreign artists. The poet Alcman, from Sardes in Lydia, wrote for the religious festivals of Sparta, in which groups of boys and girls sang and performed choral dances. Tyrtaeus, a native Spartan, encouraged his fellow citizens by martial verse in the fighting against Messenia. Excavation of the sanctuary of Artemis in Sparta has revealed a distinctive style of Spartan vase painting, which reached its highest development in the late seventh century. The pottery was exported in some quantity to Ionia and to the colonies of Cyrene and Naukratis. Luxury goods, such as ivory, were imported, but it is striking that this importation virtually ceased about 600 B.C. Evidently the taste for such luxuries was denied when the Spartans militarized their lives and lapsed into economic isolation. The Spartans did not urbanize their state like most of Greece, and a city in the physical sense, with civic buildings and defensive fortifications, never came into being. Instead the "city" of Sparta was formed by a complex of five village settlements, each retaining some identity of its own.

THE MESSENIAN WARS AND THE SPARTAN REVOLUTION

Greek tradition regarded the Spartan system of government and society as the work of the Lawgiver Lycurgus, who is said to have established it at a single stroke in the ninth century B.C. This era lay beyond the horizon of Greek historical knowledge, however, and the system bears the marks of successive innovations, the most significant of which are probably to be dated in the eighth and seventh centuries. At that time the Spartans were trying to conquer and to hold Messenia, their neighbor to the west across Mt. Taygetus, and to defend themselves against Argos. The Spartans had substituted military conquest for overseas migration to solve their need for more land. The large fertile plains of central Messenia, among the richest of Greece, were taken over and divided into lots for distribution among the Spartans, while the Messenians were reduced to the position of *helots*.

Messenian spirit was not broken, and a great revolt, the Second Messenian War, reached its climax in the mid-seventh century. The revolt was crushed, but to hold Messenia the Spartans had to reorganize their own society. Life was regimented and disciplined into a replica of that of a military camp. Apparently the initial conquest of Messenia, about 750 B.C., coincided with the establishment of aristocratic government at the partial expense of the kingship. This aristocratic regime was in turn weakened by the adoption of the *hoplite* formation about 700 B.C. The aristocrats were unable to control the Messenian *helots* and to contain Pheidon of Argos, so that, about 650 B.C., their regime gave way to that of a "*hoplite* government," as it might be called.

This government was characterized by very strong executive officials and an awkward implementation of sovereignty for the ordinary citizens. The dual kingship retained considerable prestige and power in certain areas. Like their predecessors, the kings regularly performed religious service to the gods, exercised judicial functions to preserve the Spartan families intact and led the army in battle. For a time, too, the kings had considerable voice in foreign policy. Their originally complete executive power, however, was greatly limited by the creation of a new office, that of the five *ephors,* or overseers, who were elected annually to represent the five villages of Sparta. If the traditional date of 764 B.C. is correct for the establishment of the ephorate, that office marks a successful encroachment by the nobles on the power of the kings. Ultimately, however, the *ephors* became zealous representatives of the whole citizen body to guard against any absolutist tendencies which the kings might demonstrate. For example, two *ephors* were sent along with the army to supervise the king's generalship, and the whole board took over control of foreign policy. They replaced the kings in presiding over the assembly of the citizens. Beyond their part in Spartan political life, the *ephors* were police officers, with the task of supervising the *helots* to guard against revolt.

The Spartan council of elders, the *gerousia,* was also probably regulated about 750 B.C. to the advantage of the Spartan aristocrats. The council was small, consisting of only thirty members: twenty-eight elders, men over sixty, who were elected for life, and the two kings. At this time the council won certain judicial supervision from the kings, but, like the ephorate, its functions bear marks of further democratization. The council became *probouleutic,* that is, prepared legislation for presentation to the assembly of the citizens. Since this activity presupposes a sovereign assembly, the council presumably only acquired such a task at the time of the *"hoplite* revolution" in the Second Messenian War. The chief product of this revolution, of course, was the establishment of the assembly as the sovereign power in the state.

The assembly was called the *apella* and every Spartan male over twenty years of age was a member. The *apella* elected the *ephors* and councilors, passed on the measures prepared for it by the *gerousia,* declared war, and could impeach the kings. Since the assembly was a meeting of thousands of men, established at a time before the processes of government were refined, its procedures were awkward. Voting was by a shout and, if the noise was ambiguous, a division was made. Legislation could not be initiated by the assembly, and the *ephors* performed committee functions for it. Political privilege stopped short with the Spartans, for citizen rights were held by birth and possession of a family lot. The circle of citizenship was tight, but within it the Spartans themselves had a considerable degree of equality, in token of which they called themselves *homoioi,* or peers. While this degree of participation in government was unusual and progressive for its period, the system tended to freeze in its primary mold. Like the Spartan social organization, it became an anachronism in Classical Greece.

SOCIAL ORGANIZATION

The strict regimentation of their lives, which preserved the identity and helped to secure the domination of the Spartans, was attained by deliberate retention and elaboration of the practices of primitive society. There were similar institutions elsewhere in Greece, particularly in Dorian Crete, but most Greeks modified or abandoned them as city life developed. In Sparta, however, where the Spartans themselves numbered perhaps one in every fifteen of the total population, change was regarded as fatal. The Spartan system was designed to rid the state of weaklings, to train the individual Spartan as a soldier, and to keep him in constant readiness for war. It began at the birth of each child with an examination by a board of inspectors. If the child was found weak or imperfect, it was exposed on the hillside to die from lack of care. Education was carefully designed to prevent the formation of attachments other than to the state and to the child's own age group. At the age of seven, rigorous physical training began, in which the boy was conditioned and taught to shift for himself. He was trained to live off the country, if need be by stealing, and to endure the hardships of route marching and cruel rites of initiation without complaint. Age groups were strictly segregated to build up a strong morale through association and common experience. In the group a harsh discipline was enforced by older boys and special officials, child-trainers. War songs, a few lines from Homer and moralizing maxims were the extent of humanistic training. At twenty the young Spartan became an active soldier in the army and lived in barracks. At thirty, when marriage was permitted, family life was still kept to a minimum. The Spartan joined a military mess of fifteen men, a *syssition,* to which he contributed his share of food from his own farm—a plain diet of bread, cheese, and vegetables, with very little meat and wine. The *syssition* formed a closely knit group of fellow soldiers, who lived and fought together and frequently were bound by ties of an erotic affection which outweighed the Spartan's devotion to wife and children. Only at sixty was the citizen freed from this military life and able to live at home with his family.

This training produced a highly disciplined, tough, and courageous soldier, far more effective in the field than that of any other Greek state, but such a man lacked imagination and proved unable to cope with the political problems of war and occupation. Spartan military skill and courage won the respect and admiration of all Greece, and their single-minded dedication to an end caught the attention of Greek philosophers. Plato, for example, however much he deplored its strictly military aim, respected the stability and controlled working of the Spartan system.

Since the Spartan himself did no work, the economy of the state rested on the labor of the *helots* and *perioeci.* A Spartan lot was worked by several *helot* families who resided on it. Only the state could free or move them, but personal service to their Spartan master was required, as well as farm labor. The *helots* accompanied their masters on campaigns as personal attendants, and some were used as light-armed troops in battle or for labor duties. Unquestioned loyalty and exceptional bravery might bring freedom to an individual *helot,* but even then, complete trust and political privilege were not given. These freed *helots* were used for garrison duty outside Sparta, where they were isolated from their kindred and served under Spartan officers. In Laconia and Messenia the *helots* were continuously watched for signs of revolt. Young Spartans were sent among them in disguise to spy and, if necessary, to arrange secret killings. The *helots,* however, were allowed a free religious life, which kept old traditions alive. Their economic position was not desperate, for the system of paying a fixed proportion of their agricultural production was an inducement to work hard and to use the surplus for themselves.

The commerce and crafts of Sparta were carried on by the *perioeci,* but after 550 B.C. for local use rather than for export. They made the armor and tools, engaged in business, mining, fishing and, in short, performed the nonagricultural labor. They owned their own land and enjoyed a municipal life in their towns, but were liable for military service. In fact, a constantly increasing part of the Spartan army was made up of the *perioeci.* Unlike the *helots,* the *perioeci* seem to have felt that freedom from the Spartan regimen of life was a fair exchange for the lack of political privilege. They remained uniformly loyal, even

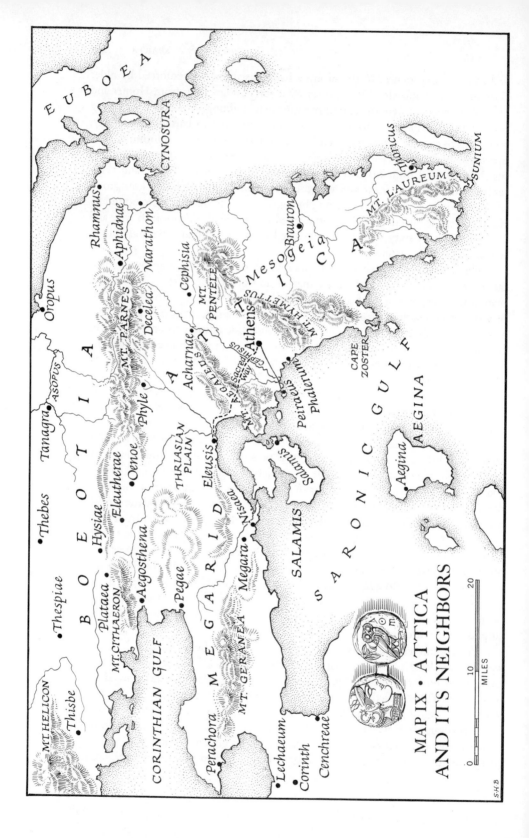

EUBOEA

CYNOSURA

Oropus

Rhamnus

Aphidnae

Marathon

MT. PARNES

Decelea

Cephisia

MT. PENTELE

Brauron

Mesogeia

MT. LAUREUM

Thoricus

SUNIUM

A T T I C A

MT. HYMETTUS

Thebes

Tanagra

Asopus

B O E O T I A

Hysiae

Eleutherae

Oenoe

Phyle

Acharnae

Sacred Way

Athens

CEPHISUS

CAPE ZOSTER

Peiraeus

Phalerum

MT. AEGALEUS

Thespiae

Plataea

MT. CITHAERON

Aegosthena

THRIASIAN PLAIN

Eleusis

Nisaea

SALAMIS

Salamis

S A R O N I C   G U L F

AEGINA

Aegina

MT. HELICON

Thisbe

Pegae

M E G A R I D

Megara

CORINTHIAN GULF

MT. GERANEA

Perachora

Lechaeum

Corinth

Cenchreae

MAP IX · ATTICA
AND ITS NEIGHBORS

0   10   20

MILES

S·H·B

after Sparta lost its military prestige and power by defeat at the battle of Leuctra in 371 B.C.

THE PELOPONNESIAN LEAGUE

Sparta's military predominance in Greece was not based entirely on the quality of its own army. That was a necessary condition, but the fear of *helot* revolt tended to limit the range of its action, and Sparta was reluctant to move outside the Peloponnesus. There, however, Sparta became the leader of the first political coalition of Greek states. About 550 B.C. the Spartans captured the Arcadian city of Tegea near their northern border and established a government favorable to themselves. Tegea was given freedom of local government, but pledged to follow Sparta's lead in foreign affairs and to contribute troops for military service at Sparta's call. On this model Sparta proceeded to form a League among the main states of the Peloponnesus. All states were brought in except Argos, and the League, when fully mobilized, could put an army of fifty thousand men in the field.

The Peloponnesian League remained an instrument of Spartan policy until the opposition of Corinth forced a liberalization of its structure. In 506 B.C. the Spartan king, Cleomenes, called for full-scale war against Athens. Corinth refused to cooperate and, through fear of the absolutism of Cleomenes, was backed both by the Spartan *ephors* and the other Peloponnesian states. The League was converted from a group of subject allies to a military coalition of free states. They determined their foreign policy collectively by assemblies to which each state sent delegates. Nevertheless, Sparta remained dominant in League affairs and continued to hold the military command of its forces in war. The League could move with Sparta, but hardly without it. By 500 B.C. the Peloponnesian League was the most powerful military force in Greece and, when the Persian attack came, the Greeks looked to Sparta for leadership.

Athens

Athens, ultimately the most famous of Greek city-states, grew to prominence rather slowly. It had little share in the colonization movement and, only after a thorough reorganization of society in 594 B.C. by the statesman Solon, began to develop rapidly. Since Athens became the intellectual and, for a time in the fifth century, the political center of Greece, its history was always of more interest than that of any other Greek state. We can trace the evolution of its institutions from a hereditary monarchy in the Dark Age through aristocracy and tyranny to democracy.

ATHENS IN THE DARK AGE

The slow start of Athens was caused in part by its relatively unfavorable position for trade in early Greece and by the lengthy process of uniting the land of Attica into a city-state. Attica lay beside, rather than on, the main land route from Central Greece to the Peloponnesus. Megara, not Athens, was the chief control point for land traffic. In the Saronic Gulf the island of Aegina was better situated for trade, while to the east of Attica the Cyclades and Euboea controlled the approaches from the Aegean. Attica, too, was large for a Greek state, with a territory of about a thousand square miles. That the people remained farmers for a long period tended to consolidate the position of the landowning nobility and to slow the process of change.

While the city of Athens was plainly the most important center in Attica in the Mycenaean Period, we do not know whether its kings ruled all the land and, if so, how much unity was preserved throughout the Dark Age. Athenian tradition assigned the unification of Attica to the hero, Theseus, but apparently the cohesion of the Mycenaean kingdom was shattered by the invasions at the outset of the Dark Age. The local regions of Attica developed independent political and religious traditions, and so reunification had to start from the city of Athens. The city itself grew up again around its old citadel, the Acropolis, which was able to dominate the plain of Athens. There were harbor towns, Phalerum and Peiraeus, but maritime growth waited on the incorporation of the districts beyond the mountain ridges rimming the Athenian plain.

Probably the first district to be added was the plain of Mesogeia, the center-land across Mt. Hymettus to the east. The Mesogeia, in its turn, gave access to the rocky tip of the Attic promontory, Sunium. In Laureum in this area were silver mines, which the Athenians began to work only about 600 B.C., when a monetary economy was being established in Greece. The second district added, probably in the eighth century, was the coastal plain of Marathon beyond Mt. Pentele, from which came the marble for Athenian architecture and sculpture. Finally, about 700 B.C., the important sanctuary and town of Eleusis to the west of Athens across Mt. Aegaleus was incorporated into the state. Eleusis' earlier independence is attested in a hymn to the harvest-goddess, Demeter, which tells the story of her daughter Persephone, whose abduction to the underworld by Pluto symbolized the death of vegetation. The old agricultural cult at the shrine was developed into the famous Eleusinian Mysteries for all the citizens of the unified city-state. While the unification of Attica destroyed the independence of the separate regions and concentrated government in Athens, it did not involve the subjection of the people or large-scale removal to the city. Athens had no *helots* or *perioeci*. While the nobles went to the city to share in the government, they also retained their land elsewhere in Attica. The towns and villages of the countryside remained local centers and became the basic unit, *demes,* in the later democratic organization. Since a large part of the Athenian population remained rural, it was difficult at times to reconcile rural and urban interests in the unified city-state.

ARISTOCRATIC GOVERNMENT

Before the unification of Attica was completed, the government of the growing state had been taken over from its hereditary kings by the Athenian nobility, the *Eupatrids,* or Well-Born. Their noble birth was indicated by affiliation to clans, *gene,* each member of which traced his lineage from a divine ancestor. The stability of these great family groups was maintained by ownership of large tracts of land which remained inalienable. Presumably the collective power of the clan chieftains was increased when they moved to Athens and they were able to strip the kingship of its authority. About 750 B.C. separate administrative offices were established, for which the clan chiefs vied in annual elections. The most important office was that of the *archon,* the leader who held broad and undefined administrative and judicial functions. The title of the king, *basileus,* was retained for an office, but its holder was limited mainly to religious duties. A third office, that of the *polemarch,* war leader, was created in this early period, but the *archon* remained Athens' most important magistrate until the time of the Persian Wars. All these offices were probably annual and elective from the outset, although the *archon* list, which recorded the annual holders of that office, was kept only from 683/82 B.C.

Like other aristocratic states of Greece, early Athens must have had a council of nobles, probably elective for life from the *Eupatrids.* It is plausibly identified as the Council of the Areopagus, known only from a later date, but marked as old and once powerful by its prestige and retention of religious and judicial authority. The council probably elected the magistrates and heard appeals from their verdicts.

Because the political assembly of the citizens was weak, the ordinary citizen would have felt his attachment to the state primarily through ties of religion and kinship. These ordinary Athenians, numbering at least three-quarters of the population, were small-scale farmers, a few craftsmen who worked for local markets, and a group of landless men, the *thetes.* Probably only the landowners were recognized as assembly members, but all would have been dependent on the clan chieftains, the local magnates, for protection and help in an emergency. Their link to the state was through local associations, the *phratries,* brotherhoods, which included both members of the clans and ordinary Athenians (p. 177). Each *phratry* held an annual festival, the *Apaturia,* to worship its protecting gods and to enroll new members of its families into the community by a sort of parish registration. Citizenship was thus exclusive and hereditary, jealously guarded by feelings of kinship and religious tradition. In this sense the state was a large family group. Its nature was represented by a new architectural symbol, the *prytaneum,* or town hall, which replaced the king's palace. The *prytaneum* was both the office of the *archon* and a house of the goddess Hestia where her fire was kept continuously burning on the hearth of the state. As in a well-regulated family, the senior members held authority.

In the course of the seventh century the aristocratic state began to disintegrate. Offices were few in number, so that rivalry for them among the noble families was intense. This pressure might have been met by the creation of new magistracies, but statesmen were needed too, not merely officials. Athens was subjected to new stresses—demands for codification of the law, protests against the injustice and greed of the nobles, and most important, an agrarian crisis. One mark of the growing complexity of administration was the establishment, about 650 B.C., of new judicial officers, the *thesmothetai*, law setters, which increased the important magistracies to nine. This may have temporarily satisfied the demands of the nobles for office and helped to still the demands for better administration of justice, but twenty years later, in 632 B.C., the clans were thrown into conflict by the attempt of a young nobleman, Cylon, to establish a tyranny.

Cylon had obtained some popular acclaim by a victory in the chariot race at the Olympic Games. He won further acclaim by marrying the daughter of Theagenes, the powerful tyrant of Megara. Cylon's ambition to become a tyrant seems to have exceeded his judgment, for he interpreted popular applause as political support and counted on Megarian military intervention to help him gain the tyranny. He did succeed in seizing the Acropolis with a small group of his clansmen, but the people favored the *archon*, Megacles, head of the powerful Alcmeonid clan. Before Theagenes could intervene in force, if he really wanted to, Cylon was besieged in a sanctuary on the Acropolis by Megacles. A safe-conduct permitted Cylon to leave, but some of his followers were killed near the altars of the shrine. Public opinion could not condone this sacrilege, and the solidarity of the noble clans was split when Cylon's relatives demanded expulsion of the Alcmeonids from Attica to purge the state of bloodguilt. The Alcmeonids were exiled but the damage to Athens was great. Megara was estranged and began to raid Athenian territory; the clans were quarreling among themselves; and public opinion demanded that the state take greater responsibility in family feuds. The affair of Cylon then, trivial in itself, was the prelude to a generation of crisis.

In 621 B.C. the homicide laws of Athens were reformed and perhaps a part of its law codified by a Lawgiver, Draco. In later tradition Draco was credited with a complete law code and even reorganization of the state, but in reality he seems to have concerned himself only with homicide. Certainly, that was the most pressing issue of the day. He drew a distinction between justifiable and non-justifiable killing and recognized the common interest by making it necessary to submit such cases to public trial. Prosecution, however, was still left to the victim's family or to his *phratry*. While this marked a distinct step in the extension of the responsibility of the state, it did not, of course, meet Athens' other problems.

SOLON

An obvious shortcoming of the *Eupatrid* government was its inability to defend Attica against Megarian raids and to take the island of Salamis, which lay offshore from Peiraeus and Eleusis. Probably the nobles clung to outmoded methods of warfare and failed to make use of the new *hoplite* tactics. Perhaps the supply of *hoplites* in Attica was limited by a small middle group, for the city was not fully urbanized. In any case, *Eupatrid* direction proved faulty, and the more progressive elements among them began to think in terms of a thoroughgoing reorganization of Athens. Their concern was deepened by a dangerous agrarian crisis which threatened revolution.

Many of the small-scale farmers of Attica were being reduced to a serflike condition or to actual slavery. The cause of this desperate condition was essentially the general change in Greek economy, which was beginning to affect Athens. The *Eupatrid* nobles could export their surplus olive oil, wine, and grain to obtain the luxuries which the growing carrying trade of other states made available, but the small-scale farmer had to use all his land to raise the grain needed for his family. Population pressure was great, because Athens had sought no relief in colonization and had long since brought all its available land under cultivation. In this situation the nobles seem to have greedily exploited their opportunities for obtaining more land. The small-scale farmers, faced with a crop loss in a poor year or through a Megarian raid, could apply only to the nobles for grain to last until the next harvest. Apparently the nobles demanded one-sixth of the farmer's produce as payment on the loan. While this in itself was not an excessive percentage, payment seems to have been perpetual, and failure to meet it resulted in the use of the land by the lender and in slavery for its former owner. The precise conditions of such loans are obscure, but, even if perpetual payment were not included in them, the small holdings of the Athenian farmer could hardly produce enough grain to feed his family and to pay the sixth. Thus some Athenians were becoming sixth-parters, *hektemors,* and others were being sold into slavery. To them cancellation of debts and a fresh start seemed the only solution. To the clamor of the distressed was added the voice of the *thetes* asking for redistribution of land.

This crisis was resolved by the genius of the statesman, Solon. He was a member of the Athenian aristocracy but is said to have engaged in trade and to have won public confidence by advocating vigorous prosecution of the war against Megara. In the late 590's, probably in 594 B.C., Solon was elected *archon* and given a mandate to reorganize the state. We may assume that he had the support of all but a small group of the most conservative nobles, for the alternative was violent revolution. No doubt the farmers and *thetes* hoped for more than the nobles were prepared to give, but Solon, a moderate man, held the state together and was able to start Athens on its remarkable development of the next two centuries.

Solon described his reforms in his own poetry as the establishment of good law and impartial justice for all. In later ages he was regarded as the wise founder of the Athenian democracy. Propaganda and adulatory tradition have probably credited him, as they do all great figures, with too much and have made it difficult to assess his work accurately. It is clear, however, that he gave a fundamental stability of law and order to the Athenians at a critical period, probably by complete codification, and firmly oriented the trend of Athenian growth towards democracy.

First, a proclamation was issued to correct the agrarian distress. This *seisachtheia,* disburdenment, cancelled existing agrarian debts and forbade the pledging of a debtor's person and those of his family as security on a loan. The *hektemors* were relieved of their burden of debt to the loss of the nobles, those who had been enslaved were freed, and the recurrence of such conditions was prevented. There was, however, no confiscation and general redistribution of land. The *thetes'* hopes of becoming landowners were dashed, and the chief benefactors of the disburdenment were the small-scale farmers. Solon went on to give them a place in the government by a reorganization of Athenian society.

The basis of political privilege was shifted from birth to wealth, and so the circle of those who shared in government was widened considerably. The shift was accomplished by making a fourfold classification of the citizens according to the produce from their land and by allowing graduated participation in government according to class. Possibly some such classification had been used previously for military service, but Solon refined and extended it. The four classes established were:

(1) *Pentakosiomedimni*   500 bushel-men: those whose land produced an annual minimum of 500 *medimni* (about 750 bushels) of grain or 500 measures of wine.

(2) *Hippeis*   Knights: those whose land produced an annual minimum of 300 *medimni* of grain or 300 measures of wine.

(3) *Zeugitae*   Owners of a yoke of oxen: those whose minimum annual production was 200 *medimni* of grain or measures of wine.

(4) *Thetes*   Those whose production was below 200 *medimni* of grain or measures of wine.

Wealth was thus substituted for noble birth as a qualification for political privilege. In fact, the nobility easily qualified for the first two classes and continued to have a larger share in government than the small-scale farmers, who made up the third class, and the landless men in the fourth group. It is noteworthy that the standards are expressed in terms of produce without monetary equivalents and that possession of about seventy acres of productive land, the acreage necessary, it is calculated, to yield five hundred *medimni* of grain, qualified a man for the highest rank of society in Athens. As yet the middle class was negligible.

The political institutions already developed by the aristocratic state were not abolished, but their nature changed as the new qualifications began to work. The nine *archons* were elected from only the upper two classes, although minor officials might be drawn from the upper three. This restriction still limited the leadership of Athens to wealthy landowners, but began to give the ordinary small-scale farmer some training in administration. It is disputed whether Solon established a Council of Four Hundred, with one hundred men elected from each of the four old tribes. On the whole this seems unlikely, for there does not seem to be any evidence of activity by this council throughout the sixth century. The Council of the Areopagus was retained, apparently confined to the two upper classes and with its functions more clearly defined. It heard cases of deliberate homicide, of impiety, and of other religious offenses and cases of treason to the state. The popular assembly may have included the *thetes* as well as the three upper classes, but that is not entirely certain. The assembly's functions, however, were defined and regularized, so that the body acquired greater power. The assembly elected the officials and had final voice in decisions of war and peace. While it could not initiate legislation, it passed on the laws submitted to it by the *archon*.

The most effective check on any arbitrary tendencies displayed by the magistrates was provided by the establishment of a popular court of appeal, the *heliaea*. This was really the popular assembly in judicial function to hear appeals by citizens from the decisions of the magistrates. While its procedure must have been awkward, and the mass of the people at a loss about the fine points of the law, the *heliaea* could redress flagrant abuse and safeguard the individual citizen.

This type of government, called a timocracy from its use of wealth as a qualification for office, was a compromise. The leadership of the state was kept in the hands of the wealthy landowners, but they were made partly responsible to the people. Election to office had to be sought by cultivating the goodwill of the ordinary citizens, and the officials' verdicts might be reversed by an appeal. For the first time the largest part of the Athenian population, the small-scale farmers, began to play an active part in government as they voted in elections and decided on the merits of legislation and appeals presented to them. Yet neither the disburdenment nor the timocracy corrected the economic conditions which had plunged the farmers into the plight from which they had been extricated. Athens was still too exclusively agrarian to be at ease in the changing economy of Greece. Solon seems to have sensed this, because he issued a series of regulations which gave a new direction to Athenian economic growth.

Athenian trade was oriented with that of Corinth and Euboea, and directed away from Aegina, by the issuance of a coinage and adjustment of the metrical standards to those of Corinth. Export of all agricultural products, except olive oil, was forbidden. Perhaps this had the immediate aim of making Athenian grain available to the Athenians, but, as the production of olive oil for export proved profitable, land was withdrawn from grain production and Athens soon became dependent on imported grain for its food supply. Before 550 B.C. the Athenians began to seek a share in the grain exporting markets of Magna Graecia, the Black Sea, and Egypt. Under this spur industry enlarged. Also, Solon is said to have encouraged foreign workmen to come to Athens. Some Corinthians evidently did so, for in the following decade Athenian pottery improved its techniques of manufacture under Corinthian influence. The Athenians learned too well for Corinth's good, because by 550 B.C. their wares had virtually driven Corinthian pottery from the Mediterranean markets.

Solon, as we have noticed, regarded his legal reforms as most significant.

In a sense he was correct, for his code was probably the first complete publication of Athenian law and custom. The code remained in use for generations, to judge by later references to it and by the archaic language employed in the fragments of law attributed to Solon. Like most Greek codes, Solon's was conservative, with careful regard for the preservation of the family and property rights.

When his term of office was over, Solon is said to have left Athens to travel, extracting a promise from the people that his reforms would be left unchanged for ten years. He was wise, for the political privileges given to the people stimulated the formation of rival factions. By 560 B.C. Athens was experiencing its first tyranny.

THE TYRANNY OF THE PEISISTRATIDS

The new political system of Solon had made it necessary for the *Eupatrids* to seek voting support among the people in candidacy for office. In the generation after Solon's archonship three factions emerged whose views seem to have been formed largely by economic interest and their attitude to the Solonian program. Those *Eupatrids* who were unreconciled to Solon's reforms and hurt by the cancellation of debts formed a group called the *Pedieis,* Plainsmen, because their estates and followers were concentrated in the plains of Athens and Eleusis. Opposed to them was a moderate group, who had supported Solon, but whose leaders had probably opposed the redistribution of land. They were called the *Paraloi,* Shoremen, and were led by Megacles of the Alcmeonid family, a descendant of the *archon* who had suppressed Cylon. This faction contained a radical element made up of the *thetes* who had hoped for land in 594 B.C. and were prepared to support revolution to get it. About 560 B.C. they found a leader in Peisistratus, a *Eupatrid,* who split them off into a separate faction called the *Hyperakrioi,* or Men of the Mountain Slopes.

Peisistratus decided that the way to power lay through tyranny rather than the archonship. In 560 B.C. he seized the Acropolis with a small bodyguard allowed him by the assembly on the plea of protection from his rivals. Because the force was too small, however, and Peisistratus' popular following limited to his own faction, they proved unable to stand against a combination of the other two groups. Peisistratus was forced to give up his plan. Once out of power he made a coalition with the *Paraloi* and Megacles by which he was reinstated. Tyranny, however, did not allow two masters; consequently in 556 B.C. Megacles withdrew his support, thus forcing Peisistratus into exile. For ten years he lived abroad, making personal alliances with the state of Argos and with Lygdamis, the tyrant of the island of Naxos. Peisistratus prepared carefully for a return by raising money from silver mines in Thrace, hiring mercenary soldiers, and cultivating his followers in Attica. In 546 B.C. he landed near Marathon, defeated his enemies in battle and established a tyranny which lasted under his own rule until 527 B.C. and under that of his sons until 510 B.C.

In Athenian tradition, despite the unpopular label of tyranny, the Peisistratid period was regarded as the Golden Age of archaic Athens. The verdict was deserved, for Peisistratus and his sons improved the well-being of the ordinary Athenians, continued to break down the power of the *Eupatrids,* which Solon had weakened, and gave Athens a recognized position of importance among Greek states. In the battle by which Attica was gained, some of the nobles had been killed. Others were forced into exile, among them the Alcmeonids, and Peisistratus was able to confiscate their land. The *thetes* profited by a distribution of the land and were established as small-scale farmers by a program of loans. The hold of the clan leaders in the rural areas was further shaken by the creation of district judges who heard minor, local cases as representatives of the central government. Even a new tax of one-twentieth of the produce from the farms did not seem to have cost Peisistratus any loss of support from the farmers. The Solonian system of government was not altered, but Peisistratus arranged that men of his own choice were elected to the important offices. Probably no actual compulsion was used, for Peisistratus' popular following was large, and even the lukewarm had to admit that Athens was growing rapidly in wealth and power.

Peisistratus carefully maintained the foreign relations which he had established and extended Athenian influence where opportunity allowed. In Boeotia the large city of Thebes became an Athenian ally and helped to guard the northern frontier of Attica. The trading interest of Athenians in the northern Aegean and in the Black Sea was developed by the foundation of two colonies. Sigeum, over which Athens and Mytilene on Lesbos had quarreled two generations earlier, was strengthened, and across the Hellespont the Thracian Chersonesus opened up in the Athenian interest. Peisistratus sent Miltiades, the head of an important Athenian clan friendly to himself, to govern it.

In Athens stimulus was given to cultural growth by the hospitality extended to Ionians who fled their homes when Ionia was taken over by Persia in 545–40 B.C. Among them were writers and artists. Other new residents were attracted as Athens emerged from its provinciality. By some device which we do not know, Peisistratus was able to make these aliens Athenian citizens. This liberality indicates that the bars to citizenship, set by religion and ties of kinship, were weakening as the power of the aristocratic clans declined. Peisistratus stimulated feelings of patriotism to the city by various devices. A new coinage was issued, bearing the civic symbols of the goddess Athena: on the front, Athena's head and an olive twig, on the back, her bird, the little owl which makes its nest in the cliffs of the Athenian Acropolis. The Acropolis itself was remodeled to fit the new dignity of the city. A gateway was built at the west end, and on the highest point a great temple of Athena started. In the lower city a large temple to Olympian Zeus, designed to be one of the largest structures in Greece, was begun. It proved rather too large for the resources of Athens, for the building was not finished until the reign of the Roman Emperor Hadrian, who provided funds for its completion almost seven hundred years later.

The two sons of Peisistratus, Hippias and Hipparchus, succeeded to their father's position in 527 B.C., the elder of whom, Hippias, exercised political authority. Hippias, although a vigorous and able ruler with a policy similar to that of his father, failed to maintain good connections abroad and to keep his internal support at home. He was confronted with rather more difficult problems. The Athenian people were themselves growing to political maturity and readier to assert their authority if the opportunity came. A new Spartan king, Cleomenes, who came to the throne in 519 B.C., was aggressive and planned to extend Sparta's influence beyond the Peloponnesus. Athens' Peloponnesian ally, Argos, became relatively weaker under threat of attack by Cleomenes. In Boeotia Thebes had begun to bring the smaller Boeotian cities under its control.

Perhaps fearful of Theban expansion Hippias made a serious mistake in 517 B.C. In that year Plataea, a small city controlling the Boeotian end of the main pass over Mt. Parnes, was threatened by Thebes. The Plataeans asked Cleomenes for help, but the latter adroitly referred them to Hippias as better situated to give aid. Hippias pledged Athenian support, which saved Plataea, but at the cost of enmity with the bigger state of Thebes. That city welcomed the Athenian political exiles and provided a base for intrigue against Hippias. The oracle at Delphi, where Spartan and Theban influence was strong, began a propaganda campaign for the downfall of the Athenian tyranny. A handsome gift to Delphi by the Alcmeonids no doubt played its part in prompting Apollo to advocate Spartan interference in Athens.

The first attack upon the tyranny of Hippias, however, came in 514 B.C. from inside Athens itself. Two men, Harmodius and Aristogeiton, later celebrated by the Athenian democracy as tyrannicides, conspired to kill the tyrants. The democracy's adulation was misplaced, for the tyrannicides' motives were personal, not political, and they assassinated only Hipparchus. No popular support appeared for the liberators, but Hippias tightened his precautions against the Athenian upper classes and even disarmed part of the army. Next came an attempt of the Alcmeonids to invade Attica. They, too, found no support from the people and were repulsed. The conservative nobles, however, remnants of the old faction of the *Pedieis,* had better success. Their leader, Isagoras, intrigued with Cleomenes, and in 510 B.C. the Spartans invaded Attica, expelled Hippias and his chief supporters, and allowed the Athenian exiles to return. Since the people had remained apathetic during this interference, Isagoras apparently felt the occasion was proper for a return to aristocratic government. The citizen lists were revised to exclude the new citizens whom Peisistratus had enrolled. Isagoras had in mind to establish a Council of Three Hundred to rule the state, but there was little support for such conservatism among the Athenians. Its only hope of success lay in Spartan aid. That, however, would have reduced Athens to the role of a subject ally of Sparta. In this situation Cleisthenes, the leader of the Alcmeonids, found his opportunity.

CLEISTHENES AND DEMOCRACY

The Alcmeonids, by family tradition, had always been ready to oppose other *Eupatrids,* but it is not likely that Cleisthenes had thought of becoming a popular champion. In the situation after the expulsion of Hippias, however, his only chance of political power lay in turning to the people and opposing the schemes of Isagoras. Whatever his motives, subsequently Cleisthenes showed a quality of statesmanship which could continue the work of Solon and Peisistratus. Isagoras' policy would have made Athens subservient to Sparta, whereas Cleisthenes not only established democracy, but kept his city independent and ready to play its own part in the struggle against Persia.

The sequence of events which brought Cleisthenes to power is not entirely clear. Presumably Cleisthenes' cultivation of the people compelled Isagoras to ask Cleomenes of Sparta for support. Cleomenes came with a small force and obliged Cleisthenes and seven hundred other Athenian families to leave Athens. Isagoras then proposed to establish his new Council of Three Hundred. The existing Council, either the Areopagus or Solon's Council of Four Hundred, refused to be dissolved. Instead, it rallied the people, beseiged Cleomenes on the Acropolis, and called on Cleisthenes and the exiles to return. They did so and granted Cleomenes a safe-conduct out of Attica to avoid an all-out war with Sparta. Cleisthenes was able to proceed with his reorganization of the state.

The vital issue of the moment was to provide a new basis for citizenship, which would bring the disenfranchised back into the state and break the power of the *Eupatrids* once and for all. Cleisthenes achieved this by adopting the principle of residence as the qualification for citizenship and by carrying out a thoroughgoing reorganization of government. The means were at hand in the *demes,* the old towns and villages of Attica which retained a strong local tradition of their own. A few new *demes* were created in the city of Athens, which were artificial, but the Cleisthenean system had the initial advantage of being able to build on a familiar institution. In each *deme* a registration was made of all the males of eighteen years and older. These *deme* rolls were the citizen rolls. The process cut squarely across the kinship lines of family and clan since members of the same clan resided by this time in different *demes* as a consequence of the natural spread of population in Attica. Henceforth a man voted and participated in the government as a member of his *deme.* Its interests rather than those of his clan or *phratry* predominated. *Deme* membership was made hereditary and the *demotic,* or *deme,* designation, gradually became a part of the citizen's name. The clans and *phratries* survived as family and religious associations only.

The *demes* enjoyed local self-government, electing a *demarch,* or mayor, assembling for discussion of *deme* affairs, worshipping patron gods and erecting buildings for their various activities. A vigorous political life existed locally along with that of the city-state of Athens. To link the *demes* into the government of the state Cleisthenes used a unit called the *trittys,* or third. The *trittys* had been a geographical section of the *phratries* but Cleisthenes altered its character by making a *trittys* out of a small and varying number of *demes* from each of the broad economic regions of Attica—the city of Athens, the coastal region, and the interior. Three such thirds were grouped into a new tribe. There were ten tribes, thirty *trittyes,* and at this time perhaps about one hundred and seventy *demes*. The number of *demes* was increased as Athens grew, but the number of *trittyes* and tribes remained unchanged, except that the population of each increased. The ten tribes were entirely new, roughly equal in population at the outset. Just as registration in the *demes* had destroyed the cohesion of the clans in political life, the tribal system was designed to prevent regional loyalties from having too much influence. Each tribe contained a cross section or fair sample of the Athenian population. To cloak the artificial character of the tribes, an ancestor was found for each among the legendary figures of Athens' past and the selection sealed with the approval of the Delphic oracle. Since the tribes were used as the basis for military service, by levying tribal regiments, cohesion and loyalty developed quickly in each tribe. A new organ of government, the *boule,* a Council of Five Hundred, was established and linked closely to the tribal organization.

The Council of Five Hundred was to play a very large role in the working of the Athenian democracy. Each of the ten tribes elected fifty members, in proportion to the population of its *demes,* to represent it in the council. Service was widely spread among the citizens, for nobody was allowed to serve more than twice as a councilor and the terms were to be noncontinuous. The council met as a whole at regular times, but its business was prepared and carried on in the interval by a further application of the principle of rotation through the *prytany* system. Each tribal group of fifty councilors (the *prytaneis*) met daily for one-tenth of the year. To preside as chairman of the *prytaneis,* a different member was chosen each day by lot. It is calculated that by this ingenious system about two-thirds of the Athenian citizens of every generation would get very direct experience in governing their state.

The main function of the council was *probouleutic.* It prepared and drafted the legislation for the *ecclesia,* the popular assembly. In addition, the council checked the abuse of magisterial power by reviewing the officials' record in office at the conclusion of the term. It also took over a large part of the financial administration of Athens and the conduct of foreign affairs. As time progressed, more and more executive and administrative functions were performed by the committees of the council. In short, the routine running of the state depended very largely upon it, for the sovereign assembly was too large to handle detail efficiently.

The functions of the *ecclesia* were more clearly defined, although no significant additions needed to be made to them. Solon had given it the right of electing magistrates, legislating and, through the *heliaea,* judicial power. It was the final authority in the state, the people meeting to discuss and vote directly on all vital issues. The meeting was potentially very large, for the number of citizens in the Athenian population was probably about thirty thousand at this time.[1] In practice, however, attendance tended to be largely urban, since the meetings were held in the city of Athens. This vitiated to some degree the elaborate precautions made by Cleisthenes to guard against regional interest, but meetings were held regularly and a routine order of business eventually established for them. If the rural citizens complained, they might be properly blamed for disinterest. Probably, too, Cleisthenes counted on the support of urban voters, for his own following was in the city rather than the countryside.

Other institutions seem to have been little changed. Perhaps, if Peisistratus had not already done so, possession of land as a qualification for membership in the assembly was removed. It is probable, too, that the Solonian property qualifications for the four classes were stated in terms of money in the Cleisthenean period, if that was not done by Cleisthenes himself. The Areopagus continued in existence, exercising its time-honored functions in religious and homicide cases. The *heliaea* continued to hear appeals from the decisions of the magistrates.

This system of Cleisthenes is usually described as moderate democracy, but its emphasis was on equalizing the power of the Athenian leadership with that of the people. It removed the group influence of clan and *phratry* from the political working of the state and substituted that of the individual citizen. The magistrates were made more responsible to the people through the review of their conduct by the new council. The archonship itself was broadened by setting the standard of qualification in monetary terms as well as landed property. Perhaps the best means for curtailing the powers of the magistrates was the broad functions given to the Council of Five Hundred, chosen by the people from their own *demes*. There was, however, continuing apprehension among the Athenians that leadership in itself was suspect, for in the following generation several steps were taken to further weaken the important offices.

The ingenious device of *ostracism,* ascribed to Cleisthenes by Aristotle, was first used in 487 B.C. It was designed to remove for a period of ten years leaders who were thought to be dangerous to the state. In the sixth *prytany* of the year the assembly was asked if it wished to hold an *ostracism.* If so, provision was made for voting in the market place, and at the proper time the citizens presented themselves for an unpopularity contest. Each wrote the name of the man whom he wished to ostracize, that is, to banish from the state for ten years without loss of property, on an *ostrakon,* a piece of broken pottery. To

---

[1] This particular figure for the Athenian citizen body, the adult males, is given by Herodotus, but we do not know how he obtained it or how accurate it is. The number seems reasonable when compared to other information about the population of Athens. The figures given by ancient historians for the size of armies, battle casualties, slaves and the population of cities are frequently suspect, for they had no statistical base. Also, numerals are particularly liable to faulty copying from manuscript to manuscript. For many places and times we have no information at all, but for others, such as Athens in the Classical Period, estimates may be made from army figures and other data, which seem reasonably sure. These, at least, give a scale against which other cities may be compared, because Athens was one of the largest of Greek city-states.

make the process valid at least six thousand votes had to be cast, but a simple plurality ostracized the "winner." Perhaps *ostracism* was a useful device against revolution and tyranny when it was first introduced, but it was easy to abuse. The quorum of six thousand was low, and so organized blocks of comparatively few votes might have great effect. Such abuse appeared, for example, in an *ostracism* in 478 B.C. From that occasion groups of ballots have been found written by the same hand with the name of Themistocles. They were evidently prepared for distribution at the polls. At times, too, Athens would have profited by the continued presence of a leader of the loyal opposition.

In 501 B.C. an important new elective office, the *strategia,* generalship, was established. The citizens of each tribe elected a general, thus making up a board of ten, which served as a council of war and took charge of campaigns. The *polemarch* seems to have retained an overall control for ten years, but after the battle of Marathon in 490 B.C. his duties became ceremonial, and the way was open for one general of the group to rise to special prominence by his ability. Since re-election over an indefinite term was allowed, the generalship speedily became the most important Athenian office because the history of the state was one of almost constant war and crisis. The *strategia* thus pushed the archonship into the background, and in 488/87 B.C. this subordination was recognized by a change in the system of election. The tribes selected a panel of five hundred men from which the nine *archons* were chosen by lot. Although the candidates had to meet certain qualifications, only chance governed the final selection. This state of affairs has been represented as an application of the principle that any Athenian was qualified by nature to hold office, but it really indicates that the office was not sufficiently important for the process of direct election.

Such were the historical experience and institutions which Athens brought to the critical period of the Persian Wars. The state was by no means as powerful or tried in war as Sparta, but its new government was supported by the majority of its people, who proved that they could work their democratic system successfully in war as well as in peace.

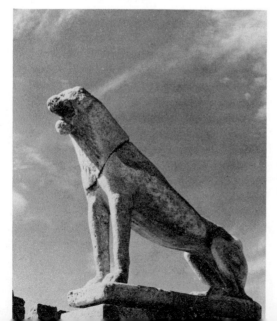

Lion from Delos (sixth century B.C.). This was one of a row of lions facing the sacred lake in the Sanctuary of Apollo.

The Greek Cultural Renaissance

(750–500 B.C.)

IN THE SPRING of 479 B.C. the Persians offered peace on very favorable terms to the Athenians in an attempt to detach them from the Greek coalition fighting against Persia. The historian Herodotus reported the Athenian reasons for continued loyalty to the cause of Greece as follows: "the kinship of all Greeks in blood and speech, and the shrines of gods and the sacrifices that we have in common, and the likeness of our ways of life, to all which it would ill become Athenians to be false." This unity of race, language, religion, and custom was consciously expressed by the Greeks for the first time during the Persian Wars.

Although Greek civilization was partly a heritage from the Mycenaean Period and the Dark Age, its character was largely formed in the centuries which elapsed from the time of Homer to the Persian Wars. During that period the Greeks worked out new forms in literature and art and developed a new manner of thinking about nature and man's place in it. The renewed influence of the Near East brought by the contacts of trade and travel acted as a catalyst, but the Greek achievement was unique and should be understood in relation to the emergence of the Greek city-state and of the individual. The Greeks revealed a new attitude of mind, lyrical in expression, curiously searching and rational. This burgeoning is called frequently the Greek Renaissance, for, while its roots lay in the past, it was the prelude to the flowering of Classical Greece.

Heritage

The most obvious legacies from prehistoric Greece were the Greek people themselves and their language. At the outset of the Dark Age, Greece received its last substantial influx of population by the Dorian settlement. The Dorians

The reader will find Map VII (pages 172–173) useful as he reads this chapter.

were Indo-Europeans who strengthened that element in the racial blend which we call Greek. Included in it were the Mediterranean people, who had developed Minoan culture, the Achaean Greeks, who had entered the peninsula about 1900 B.C., and finally the Dorians. The Indo-European invaders had imposed their own Greek language, which, as noticed above, came eventually to be regarded as a mark of homogeneity. They had taken over many words from the speech of the original inhabitants, particularly the names of places and of indigenous plants. Words for exotic products had been borrowed from the Near East in the Mycenaean Period. Such additions to vocabulary were made, of course, throughout the history of the language, but the political domination of the Indo-Europeans killed the earlier speech as a living tongue. The regional isolation of the Dark Age led to the growth of marked dialectal differences, but these were mainly matters of pronunciation and minor usage. There was no real barrier to mutual understanding, so that the linguistic basis for a common culture was established. Men could discuss and transmit their experience when intercourse between the parts of Greece developed, and gradually the differences in dialect also disappeared.

The epic poetry, known to us mainly by the *Iliad* and *Odyssey* of Homer, was the first great expression in literature of Greek culture. The language of the epics was not the language of daily use but was an amalgam of different periods, even of different dialects, developed in Aeolis and Ionia by successive generations of reciters. It was designed to express the legendary material of their heroic traditions and could be understood wherever the poems were recited. In the eighth century knowledge of the epics was rapidly diffused throughout Greece. Embodied in them were religious traditions of the great gods recognized by all the Greek people. Homer's poems thus linked the Greece of his own age to the Mycenaean past and helped to make the Olympian deities, as they were called, a common possession.

The name, Olympian, was applied to the gods from their presumed residence on the summit of Mt. Olympus in Thessaly. The divine group was believed to live together there in a great household, like that of a king on earth, but each god was sharply characterized and presided over his own particular province. Probably in Mycenaean times a pantheon had been formed from the gods of the Indo-European invaders and those of Minoan Crete. For example, the Linear B inscriptions record offerings to Zeus, Hera, Poseidon, Hermes, and Athena. Zeus, the sky-god and king of the gods, seems to have been the chief god of the invaders, but the conception of his wife, Hera, may be affected by the ideas associated with the Minoan Mother-Goddess. Athena, who became the protectress of Athens, and Demeter, the harvest-goddess, seem to have had their origin in the chthonic beliefs of Minoan religion. To Homer, however, the gods were fully humanized and set above mankind only by the possession of immortality and superhuman power. Sometimes they displayed all the meanness of ordinary mortals. They quarreled jealously, played favorites, resorted to trickery and deceit, or hid to escape the anger of Zeus, patriarchal lord of the heavenly establishment. Men had to worship all the gods by prayer and sacrifice, for each deity controlled some province of human action and could help or harm men directly and speedily. Zeus and Apollo, however, moved in greater dignity and revealed certain qualities which were to make them the greatest of the gods to later Greeks.

Zeus not only composed quarrels among his family as a father, but presided over all of heaven and earth as a king to mete out justice. Hesiod, for example, appealed to him for retribution on the greedy nobles. Apollo was a fierce god who struck down his enemies ruthlessly with arrows from his bow, but he was also a god of purity and healing. Later, at his shrine in Delphi, Apollo became a moral force for order and moderation in Greece.

In addition to the Olympians, the Greeks worshipped a bewildering variety of other deities, ranging from the vaguely conceived powers living in woodlands, rivers, and the countryside to the powerful local gods of tribe and clan. As the worship of the Olympians spread, identifications were often made between them and a local god when a kindred conception was recognized. This hardly simplified the religious complexity, for each locality had its heroes and demigods, its clan, and tribal ancestors. About them all Greek mythopoetic fancy played, linking the gods and heroes together in stories which mirror the religious tone of successive ages. Old myths, such as that in which Zeus was said to have killed his father, reveal the savagery of primitive times. There was no standard teaching or dogma in Greek religion and no regular clergy to impose it. Greek thought was free to range beyond religion or to reject it, as well as to work within its framework. As the city-state came into being, the role of the gods became social and political, to protect their communities and promote the welfare of their people. Religion was inseparable from political life, but priests did not control or direct the community, for the priesthood was only one among the other civic offices.

While legend, myth, and religious practice had been transmitted by folk memory and oral tradition through the Dark Age, the practice of art was interrupted, for it had been closely associated with the patronage of the Mycenaean kings. In the Dark Age the techniques of monumental architecture, of fresco-painting, and of the skilled crafts of ivory-carving and metalwork were lost. Although a continuous tradition may be traced in the craft of pottery making, the Greeks very speedily developed a new vase decoration in geometric forms, which was far removed in spirit from the products of the late Mycenaean Period.

The pottery of the Dark Age is best known from the excavation of the graves in the cemetery at Athens, the Cerameicus. By 1000 B.C. a new style, Protogeometric, had been developed from the stereotyped and lifeless representations of late Mycenaean vase decoration. The pots themselves had new shapes, which are clear and taut in line. The geometric designs used on them are simple, but clearly drawn and arranged in an austere, balanced composition. Already the characteristic Greek sense of form and balance had appeared. In the ninth century this Protogeometric style changed to the richer and more elaborate Geometric composition. The fully developed Geometric vases give the impression of a richly variegated tapestry, interwoven with geometric motifs. About 750 B.C. some artists began to represent schematic human and animal figures. The scenes picture funerals and battles, seafaring, or rows of animals and birds. They are bold and pleasing in effect, but Greek art, once concerned with human action as its subject matter, needed the technical knowledge which was to come from the renewal of contacts with the Near East.

New Influences

A rapid growth of Greek culture commenced in the eighth century as new influences began to work. Probably the catalyst was the renewal of closer contacts with the more highly developed civilizations of the Near East, but this influence can easily be exaggerated. It is more obvious in the art products than in the area of literature and thought. Yet, while Greek craftsmen learned much from eastern models and techniques, they quickly applied their knowledge to their own needs and produced articles which are individual and Greek rather than imitative.

Less apparent, but more potent than eastern influences, were the society of the city-state and the growth of individualism. The city-state called forth new ideas of social responsibility, which demanded expression in literature and changed men's ways of thinking about themselves and their gods. Early Greek poets, such as Tyrtaeus of Sparta and Solon of Athens, were concerned with justice and order in their communities. It is significant, too, that the revival of monumental architecture found its first expression in the temple of the god who protected the city. Individualism demanded a new literary form, lyric poetry, in which the writer could express his personal emotions. The cultural growth of archaic Greece was rapid and complex, and its various phases may be seen in the interaction of the different forces at work in the period. The rapidity of progress is most apparent in Greek art, above all in vase painting.

A Protogeometric pitcher

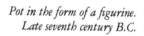
A Late Geometric pitcher, showing a mixture of geometric and orientalizing decoration

Pot in the form of a figurine. Late seventh century B.C.

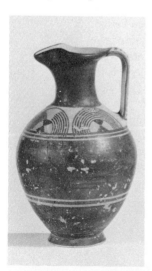

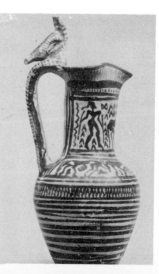

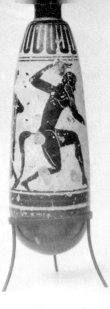

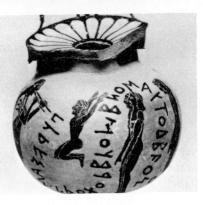

A Corinthian aryballos. *Boys' group
in a dancing contest.* Ca. 580 B.C.

A Corinthian alabastron. *Satyr. Sixth century B.C.*

Early Greek Civilization

PAINTING

In the Archaic Period successive generations of painters, whose work we
know from the great quantity of Greek vases which have been preserved, converted the stiff, schematized figures of Late Geometric drawing into fluid and
lively representations of the human figure. They worked on pottery by tradition
and their painting is not a great art, but its various styles reflect vividly the
growth of the new Greek spirit and the rapid mastery of technique.

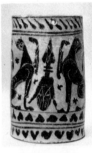

*An orientalizing
plaque. Early
sixth century B.C.*

The most important early centers of pottery production were Corinth and
Athens on the Greek peninsula, and Rhodes and the Cyclades in the Aegean.
Since the potters of Athens worked primarily for their local market, many of
their colorful vases have been found in the graves of the Athenian nobility of
the period. The wares of the Cyclades, Corinth and Rhodes, however, were exported widely to the new colonies. At first the painters of the vases used new
motifs from the East almost exclusively, but soon after 700 B.C. they turned
their growing technical skill to representations from Greek myth and heroic
legends. For example, the labors of Herakles and scenes from the *Odyssey,* such
as the blinding of Polyphemus by Odysseus and his men, were popular. Greek
representational art began with a zest and ambitious gusto that for a time exceeded the skill with which it solved its problems.

The organization of the pottery industry was also a significant factor in the
development of the Greek economy, for the volume of export from the Aegean
was impressively great. The craft grew rapidly, attracting good potters and
painters whose fine products were purchased not only in Greece and the colonies,
but in foreign areas such as Etruria. In addition, terracotta vessels carried wine,
olive oil, and luxury products like perfume and salves. For example, Corinth
developed special types of vases, the *aryballos* and *alabastron,* to contain these
products. Study of the vase forms and of their places of origin, identified by the

221

distinctive local styles of painting and clays, allows the lines of trade and the growth of commerce to be worked out.

From about 750 until 575 B.C. Corinth was plainly the leading commercial city of Greece, with Rhodes a good second. When the Corinthian pottery began to degenerate into a product of mass manufacture, the finer Athenian and Ionian vases replaced it in the markets. In Corinth excavation of the potters' quarter of the city offers an example of the role of that industry in the process of urbanization. The beds of fine pottery clay on the western edge of the city offered a location conveniently near the growing town. Small workshops were built near the clay beds, each individually owned and employing several to a dozen workmen. The little "factories" were made of sun-dried brick and consisted only of the necessary washing basins, drying floors and kilns. From them and others like them in the other manufacturing centers came the thousands of vases exported to help pay for the grain and metals needed in the Aegean.

The quickening influence of new ideas is apparent in the Late Geometric painting of the latter part of the eighth century. At that time trade goods from the North Syrian area stimulated a wave of eastern influence, which was so strong that the term "Orientalizing" is used to characterize Greek art in the seventh century B.C. These goods were the metalware, jewelry, textiles, and ivory carvings brought by traders from such ports as Al Mina or obtained from the Phoenicians. They were decorated with elaborate floral and curvilinear ornament, with friezes and heraldic designs of lions and panthers, or the half-human, half-animal creations of eastern myth, such as sphinxes and sirens. At first the Greeks were overwhelmed and abandoned the principles of their tidy geometric designing. Potters shaped their vessels after elaborate metal vessels, and the painters decorated the pots with sprawling motifs from the eastern repertoire. In place of Late Geometric design throughout the Aegean, each center developed its own particular version of the orientalizing style.

By 625 B.C. the orientalizing influences began to lose their initial appeal and a transition was made to the black-figure technique of painting, in which the native Greek sense of order reasserted itself. The lush floral ornament was converted into a neat frame for panels which presented the main scene directly and clearly to the viewer. The new technique used black silhouettes for the figures against a ground reserved in the color of the clay, greenish yellow in Corinthian vases, orange red in the Athenian. The figures were enlivened with details incised in the fabric by a sharp, pointed tool and by added vivid colors,

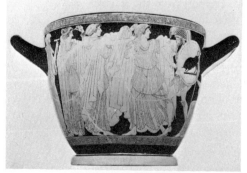

Left: Athenian red-figured cup (490–475 B.C.)

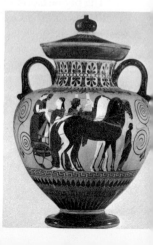

Right: Athenian black-figured amphora (540–525 B.C.)

purple, white, blue and yellow. The repertoire of subject matter was greatly enlarged to include scenes of almost every human activity, ranging from everyday life to great religious festivals and elaborate narratives from myth. In the hands of the Athenian artist Exekias, about 550 B.C., the craft rose almost to the height of great art, as his simple poignant scene of the suicide of Ajax indicates. The despair of the hero, which led him to fall on his sword, is implied with a restraint and dignity which causes us to forget the still-primitive technique of the drawing. Work in black-figure had, however, very definite limitations. The line made by the engraving tool was stiff and better suited for the elaboration of ornament than for the expression of movement or emotion. Within a century the possibilities had been exploited, and about 525 B.C. artists in Athens began to experiment with a new method of drawing, red-figure, which reached its climax about the middle of the fifth century.

Red-figure decoration was the reverse of black-figure. The panels for the scenes were left in the color of the clay background, and the remainder of the vase was covered with a lustrous black glaze. The outlines and details of the figures and ornament were drawn with a fine, single-hair brush, which made a firm, supple line. The artists were thus able to concentrate on the problems of drawing. By 450 B.C. the problems of foreshortening and perspective and the representation of movement and emotion were largely solved. Red-figure technique had reached its climax. At this point the decoration of pottery began to drop to the level of a minor art, since the better artists turned to monumental painting. Architecture and sculpture, too, which had made a later start than vase painting, had by that time mastered their own techniques.

ARCHITECTURE

The revival of monumental architecture in Greece was intimately linked with the growth of the city-state because such architecture needed capital and the training of skilled workmen to plan the structures and to cut and fit the stone. The tyrants, in particular, sought to develop the physical form of the city, just as they unified its society. They not only built temples to house the patron gods and serve as a tangible symbol of unity, but they were concerned, too, with such facilities as water supply and fortifications. The art of building, however, concentrated mainly on the temple, and by the time of the Persian Wars the typical ground plan of that structure was standardized, and the Doric and Ionic orders, or styles of building, had achieved their essential forms.

The Greeks regarded the temple as the house of the god to whom it was dedicated, rather than as the meeting place of his worshippers. The building housed the god's statue and property, the gifts from worshippers and sometimes the treasury of the city. The ritual of worship was carried on outside, where a long altar across the front of the temple was built for sacrifice. Perhaps because of this conception of the temple as a house, the plan chosen for it was adapted from the megaron, the most prominent and typical element of the Mycenaean palaces. Perhaps some continuity existed between the house of the king and the

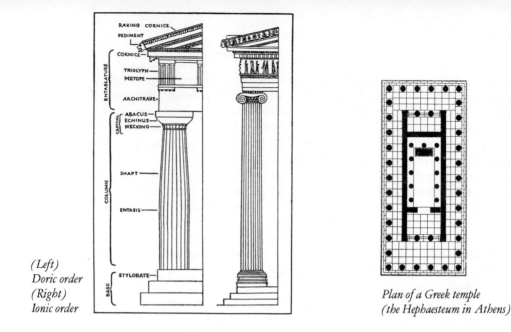

Plan of a Greek temple
(the Hephaesteum in Athens)

house of the god. The architectural links, however, cannot be traced through the Dark Age, and the developed Greek temple seems to owe little to Minoan or Mycenaean forms. The earliest remains of large temples, dated about 650 B.C., were built of sun-dried brick and timber on a stone foundation. They were long, narrow rectangular structures, low and heavy in appearance, probably with a pitched roof and a gable, at least at one end. By 600 B.C. progressive builders had converted the original brick and timber elements into stone.

In peninsular Greece and the western colonies of Magna Graecia the Doric style of building became standard. The ground plan consisted of three elements: a foreporch, *pronaos;* a large room, the *naos* or *cella,* in which the statue of the god was set; and, at the rear, a smaller, normally separate chamber, the *opistho-domos.* Around the structure a narrow colonnade was built to afford shelter. Characteristic of the Doric order are the column capitals and the triglyph frieze, which seem to be obvious transformations into stone of originally functional elements of wooden construction.

The Ionic order, as the name indicates, was developed in the Ionian area of Greece and betrays some marks of eastern influence. The early Ionian temples have more variation in plan than the Doric and were from the outset richer and lighter in appearance. The typical column capital, with volutes, only became standard after various floral capitals adapted from Asiatic models had been tried in different parts of the East Greek area. The Ionian frieze consisted of three plain horizontal bands, but column bases and moldings were carved with rich and intricate floral and leaf designs.

The quality of Greek building lay in the balance and proportion of its elements, attained by constant modification and experiment, and in the beauty of the stonework, rather than in techniques of construction. The blocks were carefully cut and jointed, without mortar, but bonded by metal clamps and dowels. Weight was carried by a post and lintel construction, so that buildings were normally simple: one story in height and rectangular in shape, with narrow rooms, unless additional rows of columns were set to carry the spanning beams. The structures were saved from too great severity, however, by the use of architectural sculpture and bright color. The triangular gables, pediments, at each end of a temple and the metopes of the Doric frieze offered fields for the display of high relief sculpture. Vivid red, blue, and green served to articulate the various elements of the building. Otherwise, the delicate contrasts of form would have been lost in the bright sunlight of Greece.

During the Archaic Period the *acropolis* was increasingly reserved for sacred purposes, although it might be used in time of need as a place of refuge. The important temples were usually set on its top, oriented to the east. The *agora* remained an open area for political assembly, markets, and informal meetings. Some shrines and small buildings might be concentrated near it, but development of specialized buildings for the various civic activities was accomplished mainly in the Classical and Hellenistic Periods. Private houses were also simple and utilitarian. Most cities fortified only their *acropolis,* but a few were sufficiently wealthy to wall much of their built-up area. The development of sophisticated fortification techniques also lay in the future.

SCULPTURE

Early Greek sculptors, who began to carve statues in stone in the latter part of the seventh century B.C., had little native tradition to call on. Craftsmen in the eighth century had made skillful use of geometric forms to cast small bronze figurines of men and horses. Perhaps, too, they had carved larger figures from wood, but such statues, *xoana,* were apparently little more than roughly trimmed tree trunks or slabs draped with clothing. The art for which Greece is best known owed much at first to the Near East, particularly Egypt, for its inspiration. The Egyptian male and female standing figures are the obvious prototypes of the two chief Greek types of the Archaic Period, the *kouros* (male) and *kore* (female). By concentration on the problems involved in these and other simple forms, Greek sculptors succeeded in the course of a few generations in creating an individual Greek art.

The early *kouroi* (male figures), like their Egyptian models, stand stiffly erect, staring straight ahead. The arms, with fists clenched, are extended along the body, and the only hint of movement is given by the slight advance of the left leg. The *korai* are slablike figures with little hint of the female body under the tight casing of drapery. The sculptors were reluctant to cut into their stone and drew on the surface of the block rather than carving it plastically. The surface was treated as a field for decoration, and schematic formulas were used for the hair, features, and muscles. Yet, by striving towards a more naturalistic representation, the artists gave their figures an inner movement and life.

As in architecture and vase painting, there were in the beginning local schools of sculptors. Peloponnesian work, as in the group of Kleobis and Biton from Delphi, was distinguished by its massive strength, but the style used in the islands and Ionia was more graceful and decorative. The quality of Ionian

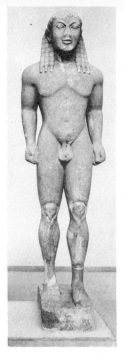

Archaic kouros. *One of the group of Kleobis and Biton from Delphi* (ca. 600 B.C.)

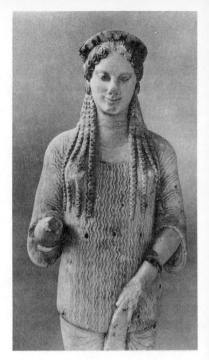

Archaic kore. *Found on the Athenian Acropolis* (No. 670; ca. 520 B.C.)

workmanship is well exemplified by the group of *korai* which were dedicated on the Athenian Acropolis in the latter part of the sixth century. Some were probably carved by Ionian artists who came to Athens after the Persian occupation of their homeland in 540 B.C. Sculptors, in fact, tended to move from place to place to work on commissions, and gradually a more homogeneous style was developed. Athenian sculptors, in particular, profited from the influx of the Ionian artists to produce, by the time of the Persian Wars, a blend of Peloponnesian and Ionian characteristics in their work. The figures which they carved were strong, but with grace and beauty of line and modeling, with the heads thoughtful and dignified expressing an inner strength and life. Greek art had almost achieved its characteristic ideal representation of humanity at the outset of the Classical Period.

Sculpture was used primarily for religious purposes throughout the Archaic Period, although its patrons were private individuals, as well as the city-states and the sanctuaries of the gods. The *kouroi* and *korai* probably represented worshippers who were dedicating themselves to the god in effigy. Perhaps this conception, too, had some effect in directing the artists to carve an idealized figure rather than an individual portrait. Although the pediments and the metopes of the temples were soon used to display sculpture, from about 600 B.C., attempts were made to work out narrative compositions which might use an appropriate subject from myth or local legend. Religious feeling also prompted the carving of grave monuments, but early sculpture was little used for other commemorative purposes or to decorate private homes. The great arts of architecture and sculpture in early Greece were thus associated intimately with the religious life of the community, rather than designed for the individual's aesthetic pleasure.

RELIGION

The practice of religion was primarily an activity for the whole community in the seventh and sixth centuries. The people of the city felt themselves to be under the particular care of one deity whose worship was developed as a focal point of loyalty to the state. The attention given in Athens to the cult of Athena is a case in point. The tyrant Peisistratus made the goddess the special protectress of Athens and even associated her closely with himself. According to Herodotus, Peisistratus, on his first return from exile in 560 B.C., staged an impressive pageant in which he dressed a tall and dignified Athenian girl in armor to represent the goddess and had her ride with him in a chariot into the city. When he established himself firmly in power, the worship of Athena was made the chief cult. The goddess' portrait was stamped on the Athenian coins, a large new temple was started for her on the Acropolis, and her local festival, the Panathenaea, developed into a great pageant and celebration held every four years. Contestants were invited from all parts of Greece to compete in poetry and music, as well as athletic sports, and the culmination of the festival was a procession of the people of Athens to Athena's temple on the Acropolis. There the daughters of the *Eupatrid* families presented a new dress to their goddess.

The state cults were administered by elected priests, who were concerned with the ritual of worship and care for the sanctuaries, rather than with theology or ministering to the worshippers. The cults were supported by state funds or the revenues from property set aside for such a purpose. Every citizen was expected to participate in worship as part of his civic duty. Thus atheism was the failure to perform such religious duties and not essentially a matter of belief. In addition to the official gods of the city, each Greek also worshipped the spirits who protected his household, presided over the activity by which he made a living, and were associated with the locality in which he lived. A web of religious feeling and association thus bound the citizen to his community.

At the same time, however, certain shrines of the great gods became centers for all the Greek people. These centers not only fostered feelings of national unity, but their festivals also provided opportunities for international meeting. Most important were Olympia in Elis, sacred to Zeus, and Delphi in Phocis, the chief shrine of Apollo. Both became the scene of great international festivals, the Olympic Games of Zeus and the Pythian Games of Apollo. In addition, Delphi, the principal oracle of Greece, even spread its reputation to Lydia, whose kings made generous gifts of gold and silver. Zeus, too, had an oracular shrine at Dodona in western Greece, but it was too remote and difficult to reach to become as popular as Delphi.

The Olympic Games were first celebrated, according to Greek tradition, in the year 776 B.C. Until the seventh century they had only a local importance and drew their contestants only from the Peloponnesian states, but by the time of the Persian Wars visitors were coming from all parts of the Greek world, from Magna Graecia to Ionia. An Olympic victory conferred great prestige on both the contestant and his city. The victor's prize was only an olive wreath, but on his return home he was fêted by his city, poems were written in his honor, and public maintenance in the city *prytaneum* was granted. The program of the games expanded as the festival grew, from simple footraces, boxing, and wrestling matches to four-horse chariot races, in which only tyrants or members of the great aristocratic families could afford to enter. In addition to the athletic sports, there were recitations, musical contests, and declamations. The festival was a fair to which traders also brought goods to sell as souvenirs or for dedication to the god. The Olympic Games were held every four years and for their duration a sacred truce was proclaimed to enable contestants and visitors to attend in safety. The sanctuary was administered by local Elian officials, but its international character was emphasized by the publication of official victor lists, which in time became recognized by Greek historians as offering a convenient chronological frame for Greek history.

The reputation of Delphi rested mainly on the oracular character of the shrine, which seems to have been taken over by Apollo from an original chthonic cult, extending back to Mycenaean times. The prophecies of Apollo were made known through the inspiration of a local priestess, the Pythia, whose unintelligible babblings were translated by the priests into verse. The priesthood was intelligent and perspicacious, making use of information received from visitors, and they were evidently motivated by a sincere conviction that Apollo stood for a principle of moderation and order. The Delphic motto, "Nothing in excess," was applied in Apollo's sanction of the law codes submitted to him. For example, the Lycurgan institutions of Sparta received the god's blessing, and the excesses of the worship of Dionysus were tamed when the cults of that god were brought into the religious organization of the city-states. Delphi's political advice seems to have been unduly favorable to such Doric states as Sparta, but, on the whole, the shrine was a salutary and restraining influence in Greece both for individuals and communities.

While the Delphic priesthood was local, drawn from the town of Delphi, the shrine came under the protection of a league of twelve states, the Delphic Amphictyony. Each member-state sent delegates to a meeting of the league

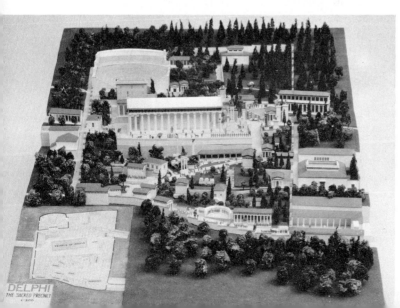

Model of the Sanctuary of Apollo at Delphi. A Sacred Way, bordered with monuments and the "treasuries" (to hold dedications) of various Greek cities, zigzags up to the Temple of Apollo. Behind Apollo's Temple is the theater.

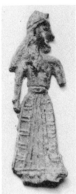

council and pledged to protect the sanctuary from attack. The members even went beyond this to pledge to establish rules of warfare among themselves, by agreeing not to cut off the water supply of a city under attack and to respect the rights of prisoners of war.

In the early sixth century other festivals were developed on the Olympian model—at Nemea for the worship of Herakles, and at Isthmia, also near Corinth, for Poseidon. The Ionian Greeks of Athens, the Cyclades and the coast of Asia Minor met at Delos, the traditional birthplace of Apollo and Artemis, in an annual festival. At all these sanctuaries a great temple was built to the god under whose patronage the festival was held. Around the temple various special buildings were constructed at the expense of city-states and individuals. These "treasuries" housed the dedications of city-states and of their citizens. Stadiums, shrines to the less important deities, and buildings to house the visitors were constructed.

Both civic cult and international festival, however, had a public character which prevented them from satisfying the private religious feelings of individuals, who were better cared for by the growth of the mystery religions, such as the Eleusinian Mysteries of the goddess Demeter and the worship of Dionysus and by Orphism.

The Eleusinian Mysteries were essentially local in character, for they were celebrated at the shrine of the harvest-goddess, Demeter, in Eleusis and open only to Athenian citizens. A procession of initiates walked along a Sacred Way from Athens to Eleusis, where the revelation of the Mysteries was made. While the secrecy was so well kept that we are not certain in what the revelation consisted, it is probable that some representation of the myth of Demeter was performed, in which the initiates might identify themselves and experience the emotions which the drama evoked. The myth itself was a story to explain the age-old phenomenon of the death and birth of vegetation. As the worshipper became more sophisticated, he might identify the course of human life, of birth, death, and the hope of immortality with the old agricultural rites. The mystery thus had the appeal of an esoteric ceremony and communicated a sense of hope and warmth. As the Hymn to Demeter expressed it: "Happy is he among men upon earth who has seen these mysteries; but he who is uninitiate and has no part in them, never has lot (portion) of like good things once he is dead, down in the darkness and gloom."

The worship of Dionysus, the god who presided over natural fertility, provoked a wilder and more hysterical feeling of identification with nature. Dionysus was thought of as accompanied by his troop of silens and satyrs, part-human and part-animal, and by maenads, female devotees, who, crazed with religious frenzy, might rend and tear any creature they encountered. Because the rites of worship were associated with the vintage festival, drunkenness freed the celebrants from ordinary restraints and led them to a wild carnival. When these rural rites were brought into the religious organization of the city-state, they were modified and associated with other worships. In particular, they were

Lead figurines dedicated in the shrine of Artemis Orthia in Sparta (seventh century B.C.). (See also page 231.)

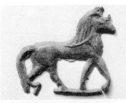

linked to local hero cults in which mimetic ceremonies celebrated episodes of the hero's life. Out of this union the drama seems to have been born. In Athens a dramatic representation was added to the festival of Dionysus in 534 B.C., and a generation later the first of the great Athenian tragedians, Aeschylus, was writing plays for the festival.

Orphism converted the savage legend of the death of Dionysus into a religious worship. The legend told how Dionysus was eaten alive by the Titans, giants born of Earth, who challenged the primacy of Zeus. Zeus blasted them with his thunderbolt, and from their ashes sprang mankind who inherited a two-fold nature, the divinity of Dionysus and the animality of the Titans. Orpheus was a legendary bard of Thrace who sang of this myth, but the teaching associated with his name was the work of wandering devotees, the Orphists, who explained the legend as a mystery: man had a divine soul and an impure body; by living a life of purity he could fight against the pollution of his body, while death would release the soul of the good man to live in happiness and of the evil man to punishment.

LITERATURE AND PHILOSOPHY

During the eighth century, judging by the earliest preserved inscriptions, the Greeks began to write in a new alphabetic script, which had evidently been learned from the Phoenicians or at some of the Greek trading posts in northern Syria, such as Al Mina, for the letter forms were derived from those of north-western Semitic. Alphabetic writing, as we have noticed (p. 100), already had had a long history, coming into use in Palestine and Syria in the Late Bronze Age. The Phoenician characters were modified for the sounds of the Greek language by the invention of signs for vowels. At first there was variation in the separate Greek dialect areas, for the symbols were disseminated along the Aegean trading routes, but ultimately an alphabet of twenty-four signs became standard. One early variant, the Chalcidian alphabet, was carried to the Chalcidian colonies in Italy. Perhaps the Romans learned it in Cumae, and in time the letter forms were further modified for the Latin language, thus becoming the prototypes for subsequent writing in the languages of Western Europe.

The use of alphabetic writing by the Greeks not only enabled them to record and to establish the archives and communication without which a complex society could not perpetuate itself, but also to approach general literacy. The old Linear B system, like cuneiform and hieroglyphics, had been the possession only of trained scribes because of the number and complexity of the symbols. The relatively few alphabetic signs could be learned and used by anyone, and so they spread rapidly to all levels of society in the more progressive city-states. In the late seventh and early sixth century, vase painters began to identify the figures on their pottery by names and to sign their better vases. The introduction of *ostracism* into Athens presupposed at least an elementary knowledge of writing, although the spelling of the candidates' names was highly individual. Literature no longer depended entirely on oral transmission; thus it was not only easier for the Greeks to transmit their reflections on a rapidly changing society to posterity but also to their own generation. Material for writing was available at first in parchment, made from sheepskin, but, as soon as the trade with Phoenicia and Egypt was well established, in Egyptian papyrus. For more permanent record and display, tablets of stone or bronze were used. Our knowledge of the works of Greek literature comes through a long chain of manuscript copyists, but we possess thousands of public documents recovered in excavations, which were cut on stone to be a permanent record of publication in the Greek cities.

While the techniques for recording literature came from the Near East to Greece, Greek literature and thought owed little to eastern models, but were evoked by Greek experience itself. The lead in developing literature in the seventh century, and philosophy in the sixth, was taken by Ionian Greeks in the eastern Aegean. The Ionians not only enjoyed possessing traditional epic poetry, but also had sufficient wealth to provide the necessary leisure for literary creation. Although Homeric epics had revealed a high degree of sophistication, Homer himself was anonymous. The later Ionian writers and thinkers were very individual, more concerned with their personal feelings and ideas than with their community. Across the Aegean, however, writers were more interested in the new society and problems of the city-state.

The new literature of Ionia was personal lyric poetry. Its origins are probably to be sought in local folk song, to which a stimulus was given by musical scales learned in Anatolia. The poet was both musician and literary composer, for his work was sung or recited to the accompaniment of the lyre. The rhythm was highly complex and refined, and its metrical patterns set the models for Greek lyrical composition. The earliest writer known to us with some intimacy was Archilochus, who moved from his native island of Paros to the colony on Thasos about 670 B.C. The wars of the colonists with the Thracian natives engaged his attention to some extent, but his own career seemed much more significant. Unlike the Homeric heroes, Archilochus was not only unashamed to fling his shield away and run for his life, but to tell about it. His scathing satire on an unfaithful girl and her father is said to have driven them to suicide. His literary fragments also reveal the wide geographical knowledge of the Cycladic sailors of this period. They ranged from Sicily to the Black Sea, and Archilochus himself probably wandered restlessly, making his living as a mercenary soldier. As he pointed out, new shields could be bought, but his life was unique.

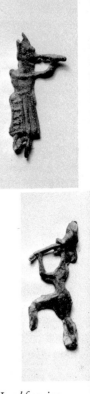

Lead figurines from the shrine of Artemis Orthia in Sparta. (See also page 229.)

An important center of this new personal poetry was the island of Lesbos, where the poetess, Sappho, and her contemporary, Alcaeus, lived and wrote about 600 B.C. Sappho was born into an aristocratic family and enjoyed a refined and luxurious life, gathering about her a circle of young women and girls in whose company she found the main inspiration for her poetry. The feeling in her verse is intensely feminine, so delicately sensitive in feeling that translation is almost impossible. Despite the rather formidable Aeolian dialect in

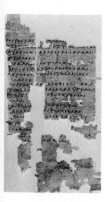

which it was written, Sappho's poetry continued to be read until the seventh century after Christ, as fragments on papyri found in Egypt indicate.

Alcaeus, in contrast to Sappho, was actively engaged in the political struggles of his native city and forced into exile for a time. His poetry heaped scorn on his political opponent, the "tyrant" Pittacus, and also gave a vivid picture of the banquets, drinking, and seafaring of aristocratic East Greeks. The themes of drinking, banqueting, and the pleasures and pains of love were developed by Anacreon of Teos and Simonides of Keos in the latter part of the sixth century. We possess only fragments of all this personal lyric poetry, but they are sufficient to reveal the intense enjoyment and beauty, or despair, which the Ionian aristocracy found in life.

Other Ionians in the sixth century began to reflect on their own traditions and on the world around them. The old explanations of nature by myth and of history by legend were summarily rejected, when the first essays in scientific observation and rational deduction were attempted. The results of this early scientific thought were crude and speedily given up by the Greeks themselves, but the method was all important since it formed the basis for subsequent western thought. The Ionian natural scientists observed the world around them and attempted to deduce an explanation for its multiform phenomena. Thales of Miletus (early sixth century B.C.) propounded the thesis that water was the basic element in the universe. His successors, Anaximander and Anaximenes, suggested earth and air. This search for a primary element and, perhaps, the growth of order and law in the city-states, ultimately led Heracleitus in the late sixth century to the proposition that behind the cosmos was a rational principle, *logos,* which ordered the world, even if phenomena were in constant change.

The conceptions of the gods and their myths could hardly escape unscathed in this critical environment. Xenophanes, born in Colophon about 570 B.C., who settled at Elea in South Italy, attacked the Greek anthropomorphic conceptions of deity, observing that the gods of the Ethiopians were black and those of the Thracians had blue eyes and red hair. If cows had hands, they would paint their gods as cows. Myths seemed savage and brutish when compared to the new-found workings of law and justice in the cities; consequently some myths were explained as allegory and others were half-forgotten or changed in conformity with the spirit of the age.

This intellectual growth extended to pragmatic science. Perhaps the practical knowledge of Babylonia and Egypt had some influence in this respect. Thales is said to have been able to predict an eclipse of the sun in 585 B.C., but that story may be apocryphal, like that of his tumble into a well as he was striding across a field looking at the stars. Anaximander, however, drew a map of the known world about 540 B.C., and Ionian engineers were used by Darius of Persia when he bridged rivers in his thrust into Scythia in 513 B.C. The Greeks probably learned from the Phoenicians how to write nautical guides for navigation. Descriptive handbooks of the Mediterranean coastline, describing landfalls and prominent physical features were produced. Along with the geographical descriptions were observations and legends of peoples, which gave birth to the science of ethnography.

The first synthesis of this new knowledge was composed by Hecataeus of Miletus about 500 B.C. His work described the whole Mediterranean and was prefaced with a dictum reflecting the new spirit of critical enquiry: "I have found the myths of the Greeks many and ridiculous." In the book were included local history and genealogy. A body of knowledge, subject to criticism and expansion, was coming into existence.

To mathematics the philosopher Pythagoras, perhaps the most influential of the early thinkers, gave a philosophical direction. Pythagoras was born in Samos about 580 B.C. and later moved to South Italy, to the city of Croton. He explained the order of the universe as a mystical system of numbers, which to his mind were realities whose harmonious interrelation regulated the cosmos. The inspiration for this hypothesis lay in the discovery of the mathematical laws embodying the relation of the strings of the lyre to the pitch of the tone which it made. Pythagoras organized his following into a school, whose members taught not only his esoteric philosophy, but also engaged in political criticism of the governments of their period. The Pythagoreans seem to have advocated the earliest principles of "mixed" government, which Aristotelian political theory was later to develop. They also directed attention to psychology and ethics, for man's soul was regarded as dwelling in harmony within him and attaining self-fulfillment by the practice of virtue, in itself a harmony. This particular line of thought was to have a profound influence on Plato.

These new ideas were carried from Ionia to mainland Greece and the western colonies to become an element in the common Greek civilization which was coming into being. They were the possession of the relatively few who constituted its intelligentsia and did not affect the mind of ordinary Greeks for generations. The ordinary Greek believed devoutly in the great Olympian gods and in the deities who protected his city or directed his daily activity. His consciousness of cultural unity was expressed by the unity of language and by conventional religion rather than in the new intellectual life.

In the cities of peninsular Greece, the new lyric expression was concerned to a greater degree with the society of the city-states than with the feelings of its individual members. In Sparta, for example, before 600 B.C. the poet Alcman wrote choral songs for the religious dances and songs of Spartan girls. His poetry caught their spirit and grace, and his compositions were elaborately complex to express the song and movement of the chorus as it danced. Tyrtaeus encouraged the Spartan army with his marching songs and praised the new Lycurgan institutions as embodying a principle of order and justice for the state. In Athens Solon recorded his political reforms in general terms of praise for the good order (*eunomia*) which his work had brought (p. 207).

Most revealing of the aristocratic character of Archaic Greece was the poetry of Theognis of Megara and Pindar of Thebes. Both were the spokesmen of aristocratic society, but Theognis bitterly felt its passing, while Pindar expressed its ideals. Theognis lived in Megara in the mid-sixth century, when the aristocratic leaders were overturned by a tyrant in the interests of the new middle group and of the common people. He savagely attacked the newly rich and money, "the root of all evil," as Alcaeus had already called it. They were turning his world upside down; aristocrats were marrying the daughters of the newly rich for their money, while noblewomen were taking rich farmers as husbands. Because the old order was on its way out, Theognis was savage and bitter.

Pindar, however, was conscious only of the golden tradition of aristocratic Greece. In long, complex choral odes, written in honor of the victors at the national festivals, he sang of the lineage of his heroes, the glorious achievements of their forefathers and the myths and legends of their cities. All his themes are woven together in odes, whose structure and language could only have been appreciated by a select and aristocratic audience. Pindar wrote from 498 to 446 B.C., but his spirit is that of the Greece which vanished with the Persian Wars and the rise of the common man in fifth-century Athens.

Panhellenism and Separatism

By the eve of the Persian Wars the Greeks had developed the basic elements of a common language, religion, and traditions into a uniform civilization. It might be said that Greece even had a national conscience as well as a consciousness of cultural unity. When the Ionian states were attacked by Persia in 546 B.C. and again when they revolted in 499 B.C., Ionian leaders appealed to Sparta and to other Greek states to observe the ties of Panhellenism and to send military help. Sparta did rebuke Cyrus of Persia in 546 B.C., and Athens and Eretria sent small military forces in 498 B.C. Again, as noticed before, Athens refused to play the traitor to Greece by making a separate peace with Persia in 479 B.C. These manifestations of political Panhellenism, however, were prompted by the threat of Persian aggression. The conditions of political growth in Greece had made each city-state autonomous and separate. In general, the Greek world was a microcosm of small powers whose citizens were linked far more closely to their own state than to the conceptions of Panhellenism. The latter, in fact, by 500 B.C. had hardly acquired the force of an idea, let alone any political form. The Greeks, however, had made some advances toward cooperation among their city-states which helped to break down the barriers of separatism.

Just as arbitration had seemed a proper method of settling disputes between individuals, cities occasionally made use of arbitration by a powerful third party. In the late seventh century Athens and Mytilene referred their quarrel over Sigeum to Periander of Corinth. Treaties of peace and terms of alliance between states had replaced the older personal relationships between prominent clan chieftains and tyrants. The latter had, in fact, given their states the continuous direction needed for a foreign policy. The efforts of the tyrants did not lead to unity, but specific ideas about the welfare and interests of the whole community were a necessary preliminary to any firm relations among the states.

Some permanent coalitions had been made among the cities of Greece and were having an effect in international relations. The Ionian League had a quasi-political character, as well as the function of a religious league for worship of Poseidon. The delegates sent by the Ionian states to the council of the League were able to organize resistance under joint leadership at the time of the Persian attack and more effectively in the Ionian Revolt. Thales even offered a sophisticated plan of federal unity, under which the Ionian states would give up their independence and form a federation, but his idea could not prevail against the desire of each state for autonomy. In peninsular Greece the Peloponnesian League, headed by Sparta, had worked out machinery for cooperation among its members, by which they decided on joint action and were led in the field by the Spartans. Unfortunately the policy of King Cleomenes had tried to make the League an instrument of Sparta. He embittered relations between Athens and Thebes and made understanding between Sparta and Argos impossible. The members of the League, too, felt that their primary interest was the welfare of the Peloponnesus. Yet, when the threat of attack by Persia became real enough to alarm the Greeks, the nucleus for a war coalition existed. The Peloponnesian League was the core around which a successful defense was formed.

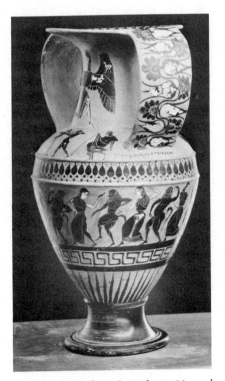

Athenian black-figured amphora. Maenads and satyrs dancing (550–525 B.C.)

XI

The Wars with Persia

(*ca.* 550–479 B.C.)

WHEN CYRUS OF PERSIA defeated Croesus of Lydia and took over the Ionian cities on the Aegean coast of Asia Minor (546–40 B.C.), the hitherto separate courses of Greek and Near Eastern political history were drawn together. Up to this time the city-states of Greece had been able to grow without even a threat of interference by the great powers of the Near East. Assyria's expansion had been directed to the lands of the Fertile Crescent, and its western horizon reached only to Cyprus. While Croesus had systematically reduced the Ionian cities to the position of subject allies, he envisaged Lydia as a land power and made no attempt to take over the Aegean Islands or to cross to Greece. Cyrus, too, was concerned only to round out his new Lydian province by incorporating the Greeks of Asia Minor.

Darius and Xerxes, however, realized that entry into Europe was necessary to hold Asia Minor securely and that a free Greece across the Aegean was disturbing to a subject Ionia. Although both kings failed in their attacks on Greece, their action brought Persia permanently into Greek considerations, and a new epoch in Greek history opened with the Persian Wars. The Greek victories over Xerxes in 480–79 B.C. enabled Greece to fulfill the promise of its early growth, for no Persian king again attempted open attack across the Aegean. Throughout the fifth and fourth centuries, however, the Greeks had to reckon with the policy of this powerful foreign state, which sometimes became a decisive factor in their own political action.

Persia and Ionia

The Persian conquest of Ionia was a corollary to Cyrus' occupation of Lydia (p. 161), for the Ionian cities, with the exception of Miletus, had aided Croesus and continued to resist Cyrus. Cyrus made a treaty of alliance with

The reader will find Maps VII and X (pages 172–173 and 241) useful as he reads this chapter.

Miletus but entrusted the reduction of the other cities to his general, Harpagus. The efforts of the Ionian League to offer a joint resistance were ineffectual. The defection of Miletus crippled their war effort, and a plea for help to Sparta, in the name of their common Hellenic race, brought little response. Sparta is said to have protested to Cyrus, but even the latter's contemptuous reply, "Who are the Spartans?" provoked no military action. The philosopher Thales proposed that the Ionians form a unified state, but the plea was futile, for each Ionian city wished to maintain its autonomy. More desperately, another Ionian sage, Bias of Priene, advocated the establishment of a new Ionia on the island of Sardinia in the far west. The suggestion perhaps had some result in Phocaea and Teos. Many Phocaeans sailed west to attempt, unsuccessfully, the colonization of Corsica (pp. 186–87), and some Teans migrated to Abdera in Thrace. Appeals to unity, however, were fruitless, and by 540 B.C. Harpagus had reduced the Asiatic Greek cities and established Persian control along the eastern shoreline of the Aegean Sea. Western Asia Minor was divided into three satrapies: Phrygia, comprising the area south of the Hellespont, with its capital at Dascylium, Ionia and Lydia, jointly administered by a single satrap from Sardes, the former Lydian capital.

The framework of Persian organization was loose, and the satraps followed the usual Persian policy of allowing a very considerable degree of freedom to their subjects. The cities were controlled by Greek "tyrants," who were allowed a free hand in local administration, in return for their loyalty to Persia. A moderate tribute was imposed, for Asia Minor was now the King's Land, and military service was demanded for the king's wars. These conditions of subjection were neither very oppressive nor vindictive, but they were imposed at a particularly critical time. The Ionian cities, like Athens, had been moving towards more democratic forms of government. When free experiment was cut short by the "tyrants," the eclipse of Ionia began. Many intellectual leaders, such as Xenophanes and Pythagoras, migrated to Magna Graecia. Artists and craftsmen followed them or moved to Athens; thus within a generation Ionia had lost its cultural primacy in Greece.

Persian control, however, did not at first seriously affect the economic well-being of Ionia. The patronage given by Lydian kings to Greek craftsmen was replaced by that of the Persian satraps. Although the Persian capitals, Susa and Persepolis, were remote, Ionian traders had good access to the Anatolian plateau by the Royal Road, which the Persians developed as a link to their western satrapies (p. 167). Political stability in western Asia was assured, and Persian economic policy continued to follow that of Croesus. Lydian gold was coined into the famous Persian darics, named for King Darius, issued on a bimetallic standard, which facilitated exchange with the silver of the Aegean area. Persia placed no barriers to Ionian trade by sea, although perhaps the Ionians suffered more from Phoenician competition in the southeastern Mediterranean than previously. On the other hand, Ionian trade with South Italy was intensified, while the merchants of Miletus and Chios, in particular, were very active in Thrace and the Black Sea. The Aegean and the East began to grow more closely together through economic ties, but the Ionians chafed at the loss of independence and the minor role for which they were cast in Darius' plans for his northwestern frontier.

DARIUS' SCYTHIAN EXPEDITION

In 513 B.C. Darius launched an expedition across the Hellespont into Thrace and Scythia. To the Greek historian Herodotus the aim of the attack seemed to be the addition of Scythia to the Persian Empire. It appeared an arrogant and miscalculated flight in the face of heaven, for Scythia stretched vaguely north and east of the Danube, across South Russia to the Caucasus and beyond. Darius, however, probably aimed at little more than he actually achieved (pp. 166–67): a new satrapy of Thrace, bounded by the Danube on the north and the Strymon on the west, with a friendly territory lying beyond each frontier. Such an acquisition would have guarded the approaches from Europe to Asia Minor and brought the gold and silver mining areas of Thrace into the Empire. On the west the Strymon was secured by a pledge of allegiance from the king of Macedonia. The thrust across the Danube, however, failed in its purpose of cowing the Scythians and preventing their raids. As Darius advanced, the Scythians fell back, burning their fields of grain until lack of supplies forced the Persians to retreat. In the campaigns the Ionians cooperated fully and loyally with Darius. An Ionian fleet sailed along the west coast of the Black Sea to support the land forces. Ionian engineers bridged the Danube with pontoons, and the "tyrants" protected the causeway, while Darius operated north of the river.

In the settlement of Thrace, however, difficulties arose between the Persian governor and the Ionians. Darius offered Histiaeus, the tyrant of Miletus, a town in west Thrace as a reward for his services. Histiaeus' authority, or ambition, proved incompatible with the administration of the Persian governor, so that Darius invited Histiaeus to reside in Susa. This episode seems symptomatic of Ionian and Persian relations in the new province. The Ionian merchants had long regarded Thrace as their particular trading area, using its silver to pay for grain from Egypt. The Persians, of course, would regard their own treasury as the proper destination for Thracian gold and silver. To the political resentment felt by Ionians at the loss of their independence were added restrictions in acquiring silver and the political disgrace of one of their leaders, Histiaeus. The latter's son-in-law, Aristagoras, who succeeded him in Miletus, triggered revolt in 499 B.C.

THE IONIAN REVOLT

At first Aristagoras seems to have aimed at becoming the tyrant of a new Persian province in the Aegean, but his scheming resulted in a fiasco, from which he could only extricate himself by defying Persia. He proposed to the Persian satrap at Sardes, Artaphernes, that advantage be taken of civil strife in the big island of Naxos. It might be annexed and Persian control extended over the Aegean. A fleet of two hundred ships was authorized for the purpose, and a Persian general, Megabates, appointed to direct the campaign. Aristagoras and Megabates not only failed to agree on tactics, but found a remarkably stiff resistance on Naxos. The attack failed and Aristagoras was faced with political disgrace. To save himself, he played on Ionian resentment and engineered a general revolt against Persian authority. The rapidity with which defection spread from the Hellespont to Cyprus indicates a general and deep resentment of Persian control. Evidently the Greeks of western Asia felt that their freedom and livelihood were at stake. As the revolt progressed, the people of the Ionian cities took its direction out of the hands of Aristagoras and his fellow tyrants. Democratic governments were formed, and the Ionian League displayed the unity of planning and action which it had failed to show at the time of Cyrus' conquest. The situation was initially favorable to the Greeks, for Persia had few troops in the area and needed time to mobilize and to concentrate a fleet from Egypt and Phoenicia.

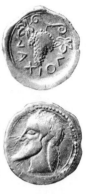

A coin of Naxos

Aristagoras tried to turn the revolt into a general Greek war on Persia by appealing to states across the Aegean for help. In Greece, however, the major states had not yet developed any compelling fear of Persia. They had made no move to save Ionia from Cyrus and had watched with apparent indifference the establishment of a Persian province in Thrace. Aristagoras' appeal got little response. King Cleomenes of Sparta, while tempted, refused on the grounds that Persia was too vast and powerful. Athens did offer a force of twenty ships. This, it is to be suspected, was prompted more by the consideration that their former tyrant, Hippias, had taken refuge in Asia Minor, where he was intriguing for Persian help, than by a feeling of kinship with the Ionians. Eretria, in acknowledgment of an old favor done by Miletus, sent five ships. Evidently the brunt of war was going to be carried by the Ionians themselves.

The military action opened in 498 B.C. with a daring raid on Sardes. Accompanied by the Athenians and Eretrians the Ionians marched up the valley of the Cayster River, crossed the mountains and burst on the town unexpectedly. They failed to take the citadel held by the Persian garrison, but burnt the lower town. On the way back to the coast the force was ambushed, but the success at Sardes spread the revolt. At this point, however, the Athenians and Eretrians withdrew. The Athenian defection is usually explained by internal politics in Athens. The *archon* of that year, who seems to have been a supporter of the exiled Hippias, wished to avoid irritating Persia. Yet the people elected him, and it may be assumed that Athens felt its duty had been done and it had little to fear from Persia. In Ionia, however, the revolt was prosecuted vigorously. The cities of the Hellespont, the people of Caria and Lycia and the Greeks along the coast as far as Cyprus joined.

Persia, however, far superior in potential strength, by 495 B.C. had mobilized an overwhelming army and concentrated its fleet from Phoenicia and Egypt. The Persians took the initiative and closed in on Miletus. The city was besieged, and the Ionian fleet brought to battle at the island of Lade off the harbor. Since the last hope of the Ionians lay in their fleet, a total mobilization of 353 ships was made for the battle. No aid came from across the Aegean, and as the Persian army besieged Miletus, discouragement began to grow. Discipline, at first strictly enforced by the commander, Dionysius, suffered, and in the battle the substantial Samian and Lesbian contingents deserted. The Chiots and Milesians fought particularly well, but the odds were too great. The battle was lost. The Persian commanders discouraged further resistance by burning Miletus and deporting its population to Persia. The revolt had failed, but Darius was faced with the need of a wholesale reorganization of the northwestern satrapies.

The settlement of Ionia was sensible and tolerant. Darius, stopping further reprisals by the Persian commanders, recognized the new democratic governments in the Ionian cities. Probably he felt that the former tyrants had been too personally ambitious and that broader governments would help to remove the causes of dissatisfaction. The tribute was reassessed, but still moderately, and more stability provided in Ionia by arrangements for settling disputes among the cities by arbitration.

It remained to reorganize Thrace. Mardonius, the king's son-in-law, was sent with a small army and fleet to make his way through Thrace to Macedonia. Persian authority was re-established in the satrapy, and the last Greek holdings liquidated. Miltiades, the leader of the Athenian settlement in Thrace founded in the Peisistratid regime, sought refuge in Athens. Although Mardonius' fleet was wrecked off the rocky coast of Mt. Athos, his purpose was achieved. In 491 he returned to Asia.

Darius' Attack on Athens (490 B.C.)

The restoration of Persian authority in Asia Minor and Thrace provoked slight reaction in Greece. Even when it became apparent in 491 B.C. that Darius was going to strike directly across the Aegean, the major city-states were indifferent or could not agree upon any joint defense. Cleomenes of Sparta was anti-Persian, but his direction of policy was made difficult by the jealousy of the Spartan *ephors* and of his fellow king. The members of the Peloponnesian League for their part felt no apprehension, since the attack seemed to be aimed at Athens and Eretria. In Athens the new democracy established by Cleisthenes had not yet firmly jelled. Athenian foreign policy reflected internal friction, which arose from the circumstances of the expulsion of the Peisistratids, and the former tyrant Hippias still had friends in Athens who worked for his restoration. While the conservative *Eupatrids* and the democrats were united in their opposition to the tyrant, they were divided on the issue of policy towards Sparta. The *Eupatrids* favored Panhellenism and following a Spartan lead, but the democrats remembered that Sparta had tried to prevent the establishment of the democracy in 508 B.C. At that time Cleisthenes had even gone

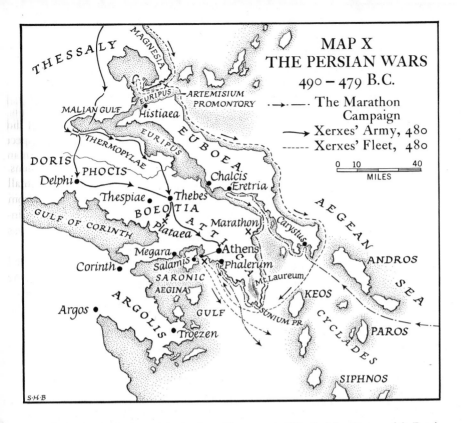

so far as to seek Persian help against Cleomenes. Hippias' intrigues with Persia changed this attitude, but, even so, Athens had not supported the Ionian Revolt wholeheartedly. By the time the revolt ended, new leaders had appeared in Athens who realized the danger of Persian aggression and perhaps saw in it the necessary pressure to unite the Athenians.

Foremost among these new men was Themistocles, whose foresight and ingenuity were to establish Athens as a great power in Greece. He estimated that Athens' future lay in the development of sea power and, even before the Persian threat of attack, had begun to improve Peiraeus as a more secure and commodious harbor for the city than the roadstead at Phalerum. Themistocles found a useful, if not entirely congenial, ally in Miltiades, when the latter returned from Thrace and began to advocate a policy of strong resistance against Persia. Coming into prominence, too, was Aristides the *Eupatrid,* a loyal Athenian, if not an ardent democrat like his rival, Themistocles. On the eve of the Persian attack a change in Athenian temper was apparent. The people demanded that the dramatist Phrynichus be tried for presenting the play, *The Taking of Miletus,* which was an uncomfortable reminder of the failure of the Ionian Revolt.

Darius prepared for his attack by an attempt to divide and weaken the Greeks, although they had given little indication of a will to unity. Envoys were sent to the main islands of the Aegean and to the cities of Greece to demand earth and water as tokens of surrender. The most important island state, Aegina, submitted, "medized," as the Greeks put it, which indicated that naval resistance to the attack would be negligible, if not impossible. Sparta brusquely refused, as did Athens and Eretria, but these cities still did not work out plans for joint resistance. Darius was encouraged by the prospect of a short war and a weak defense. Among his advisers the former Athenian tyrant Hippias held out the prospect of a betrayal by supporters in Athens. The king decided to strike directly at Athens and Eretria with a relatively small but efficient force. Victory would give him a hold in Central Greece, from which Persian control could be extended relatively easily over the whole peninsula. The expedition, estimated at about 200 warships and 25,000 men, was placed under the command of Datis and Artaphernes.

The fleet sailed from its concentration point on Samos and encountered no serious resistance from the Aegean islanders on the crossing to Euboea. At Naxos the Persians made an object lesson by burning the town, but in Delos the shrine of Apollo was respected and a gesture of goodwill made to the islanders by a generous dedication. Since no opposition was offered by the Greeks at sea, the Persians proceeded to their first objective, Eretria, taking the Euboean town of Carystus en route. Whether Athens was unable to help effectively or had neglected to plan aid for the Eretrians is not clear, but Eretria fought alone. The city held out for six days and was then betrayed. The Persians burnt the temples and sent the surviving inhabitants off to Susa—a fate hardly justified by the Eretrians' small contribution to the Ionian Revolt, but probably designed to impress Athens with the penalty of resistance.

The Athenians, faced with the prospect of such a fate, hurriedly sent for aid to Sparta and to the little city of Plataea, which they had helped against Thebes in 517 B.C. Plataea responded by sending its army of a thousand men, but Sparta had to defer its help. The Spartans were celebrating a religious festival, which they could not break off without offending the gods. Aid was promised, however, as soon as they could properly march to war. Meanwhile, the Persians debarked on the coastal plain of Marathon, where Peisistratus had landed in 546 B.C., when he established his tyranny in Athens. Perhaps the strategy was suggested by Hippias, who hoped that memories would be stirred, but the plain at Marathon offered the Persians a chance to deploy their army and exercise the cavalry. The city of Athens was only a day's march across the spurs of Mt. Pentele, and an approach across the Athenian plain would allow the Persians to use their cavalry, an arm in which the Athenians were most deficient. The Athenians, confronted with the choice of marching to Marathon or waiting to risk a battle before Athens, were persuaded by Miltiades to send the army to Marathon.

The scene of the first great victory of the Greeks against a foreign invader was a small, semicircular plain, closed by the foothills of Mt. Pentele at the rear and by a marsh on the north side. The Athenian soldiers, ten thousand *hoplites,* were drawn up on the hills overlooking the Persian camp on the shore. For several days the Athenian generals debated the advisability of attack, then, with the decision taken, watched for the proper moment. In the meantime the small Plataean force, numbering a thousand men, arrived. At a time when the Persian cavalry was unprepared, Miltiades ordered the advance. The Greek wings, deliberately strengthened, broke the Persian lines, turned in to the center and killed 6400 of the enemy with a loss of only 192 men. The Persians were chased back across the plain and lost some of their ships, but the greater part of the force got safely on board. While the Athenians had won at Marathon, there was still danger to the city if the Persians could round Cape Sunium and land troops before the Athenian army returned to its defense. As the Persians sailed off to the south towards Sunium, Miltiades hurried his army back to Athens. The Athenians won the race, and when the Persians came to Phalerum to anchor, the Athenian soldiers were ready to repel a landing. The Persian commanders decided that the risk was too great and turned to sail across the Aegean. Persia's main purpose of securing a beachhead in Greece had failed and its prestige was damaged, but only a battle, not the war, was lost. The Persians still held the eastern islands of the Aegean and their satrapy in Thrace, from which another attack might be launched.

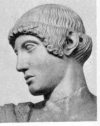

To the Athenians, the victory at Marathon, their own first important victory, gave tremendous stimulus and confidence. They had demonstrated to Greece that Persians could be defeated. The rest of Greece was impressed, and, when the Spartans arrived too late for the battle, they made a special trip to Marathon to view the Persian dead. Marathon, marking the start of Athens' rise to power, in later Greek tradition became the symbol of the Greek will to freedom. For the time being the Athenians rendered their proper thanks to heaven by dedicating a new *stoa* to Apollo at Delphi and by beginning work on a temple to Athena on their own Acropolis. The democrats under Themistocles' aggressive leadership had their way. In 488/87 B.C. the series of constitutional changes which weakened the archonship were made, and the new device of *ostracism* was used against suspect or too conservative leaders (p. 216).

Apollo. From the Temple of Zeus at Olympia

Miltiades, whose tactics won the victory at Marathon, fared badly at the hands of his countrymen. In 489 B.C. the Athenians decided to punish Aegina, Paros, and other islands which had medized. Perhaps Miltiades was thinking of establishing an island line of defense against renewed Persian attack, but the scheme failed. He was unable to take Paros and was suspected of having been bribed by the Parians, despite a wound incurred in the action. Even when he was brought to trial on a stretcher, a large fine was imposed, but Miltiades died before the sentence was executed, a victim of factional politics in Athens. The action against Aegina was abortive, too, for Cleomenes of Sparta, who had cooperated with Athens in the venture, died in 489 B.C. Athens and Aegina began a futile war of mutual raiding parties and diplomatic squabbling. While Athens achieved little success in the war, Themistocles did use it as an excuse to make Athens a naval power and indirectly to further the defense of Greece.

In 483 B.C., when a rich vein of silver was found in the state mines at

Laureum, Themistocles urged that the proceeds be used to build an up-to-date fleet of triremes. The war against Aegina scarcely needed such an armament, but the fleet would make Athens the strongest naval power of Greece. Themistocles was aware that the Persians were starting to prepare another attack against Greece, even if many Athenians were slow to credit the rumors. Some Athenians wished to divide the new-found wealth among the citizen body. Themistocles was also opposed by Aristides, the conservative *Eupatrid* leader. The pretext of war against Aegina, however, persuaded the Athenians and in a final contest for control Aristides was ostracized. The building of a hundred new vessels started in 482. The Athenians still had much to learn about naval war, but they had introduced a new element of power into Greece. Two generations later Thucydides, the historian of the Peloponnesian Wars, gave Themistocles his due: "For Themistocles was a man whose natural force was unmistakable, . . . from his own native acuteness, . . . he was the ablest judge of the course to be pursued in a sudden emergency, and could best divine what was likely to happen in the remotest future."

Xerxes' Attack on Greece (481–79 B.C.)

Until 483 B.C. circumstances delayed any plans which the Persians may have had for a renewal of the attack on Greece. Revolt had broken out in Egypt which drew the king's attention to that quarter of the Empire. When Darius died in 486 B.C., his successor, Xerxes, had to familiarize himself with rule and assert his position among the Persian nobles. Perhaps his decision to resume the attack on Greece was contrived to confirm his position, as much as to solve the still unsatisfactory condition of the northwestern frontier. In 483 Xerxes began to prepare for a large-scale campaign by land and sea, designed to reduce the whole of peninsular Greece to subjection. The plan was to strike from the north, from the satrapy of Thrace. The army could be supported and supplied by a great fleet moving along the coast from the Hellespont to Athens and the Peloponnesus.

The route was prepared painstakingly. A pontoon bridge was thrown across the Hellespont, and a canal cut through the peninsula of Mt. Athos to avoid the disaster which had overtaken Mardonius' fleet in 492. In Thrace roads were built and the towns stocked with grain. Naval forces were levied from Egypt, Phoenicia and the Greek coastal cities of western Asia Minor. The land army, with a well-trained core of Persian archers and cavalry, was drawn from the varied peoples of the Empire. The size of the expedition so surpassed the experience of the Greeks that they could form no rational estimate of it. Herodotus reported their impressions: 1207 warships and 3000 auxiliary vessels, a total fighting force of 2,317,000, with as many servants and camp followers. Modern historians suggest, as a reasonable estimate, about 600 warships and three Persian army corps of 60,000 men each. Potential Greek naval power was outweighed about two to one and the land force, about three to one.

When Xerxes came to Sardes to organize his army, the gravity of the Persian threat came home to the Greeks. The king sent envoys to all the important Greek states, except Sparta and Athens, to ask for surrender with a promise of immunity. Sparta and Athens, thus marked as the chief objectives of the war, took steps to prepare the defense. In the autumn of 481 B.C. a Panhellenic Congress was convoked at Corinth to form a war coalition. Although thirty-one states responded, there were vital absentees. Thessaly and most of the small states of Northern and Central Greece were absent. Both the Greeks and Xerxes calculated, rightly, that the zeal of the northern states to defend Greece would diminish in relation to the proximity of the Persian army. At the same time the northern Greeks were correct in judging that the main desire of the Peloponnesian League would be to protect the Peloponnesus at the Isthmus of Corinth.

The Congress proceeded vigorously to form a Panhellenic coalition and to work out plans for defense. Old quarrels, most notably that between Athens and Aegina, were patched up. (Aegina was to play a useful part in the naval war.) Wavering cities were warned by a threat that the property of all those states which submitted to Persia without a struggle would be confiscated, while Delphi's moral encouragement was invited by the vow to dedicate one-tenth of such property to Apollo. Old hostilities and fear of Persia outweighed this manifesto, however, for several states and even Delphi itself hedged or remained neutral. Argos could not bring itself to work with Sparta and left a dangerously weak spot in the general unity of the Peloponnesus. Crete, too, felt far enough removed to declare its neutrality. Both secured oracles favorable to their stand from Delphi. That shrine itself was pessimistically cautious about the chances for a Greek victory. Throughout the war it failed to give the moral support which might have been expected from the foremost oracle of Greece. Corcyra, which could have furnished a sizeable fleet, pledged help, but later discovered convenient delaying winds off the southern Peloponnesus, at a time when the fleet might have played a part at Salamis. Gelon, the tyrant of Syracuse, sent no aid, but at least he had a valid excuse. Sicily was threatened by Carthaginian attack, perhaps stimulated at this particular time by Xerxes through his Phoenician subjects. Gelon had to defend western Greek freedom at the same time that Athens and Sparta fought for Aegean Greece. Despite the discouragement of these diplomatic failures and the ambiguous attitude of Northern Greece, the Congress proceeded with its plans for defense.

The overall command was given to Sparta, with King Leonidas in charge of the land forces and Eurybiades of the Greek fleet. Athens yielded its claim to naval command, although its new ships numbered 200 of the combined Greek fleet of 334 warships. Themistocles, however, came to have a very influential and at times decisive role in the planning. Probably the general strategy of defense was discussed in the Congress, but the decisions were left to a council of the various allied commanders meeting, as occasion demanded, under the presidency of the Spartan generals. The Congress itself was a landmark of Panhellenism. It achieved a coalition for defense and created a working organization for fighting the war. As in any such coalition of free states the selfish interests of each member for its own security had to be adjusted to the common good and changes of plan made as the fighting developed. Such adjustments could hardly be understood by those who suffered from the decisions. Yet the overall direction was firm and held the coalition together until the Persians were driven from Greece and the Aegean in 479 B.C.

Xerxes' plan of campaign seems to have been simple but too inflexible in its execution. Army and fleet were to advance side by side from the north, winning submission by the threat of occupation or crushing any force which stood against them. Xerxes seems to have given little thought to naval war or amphibious action, for the fleet served only for supply and communication.

The Greeks could do little but adjust their defense as the Persians advanced. They planned to meet the land army in terrain where a narrow corridor would permit a holding action, while the fleet fought in narrow waters and perhaps inflicted telling damage on the Persian ships. Political considerations, of course, played their part in the selection of the appropriate battleground. If Northern Greece were to be held, it was necessary to stand in the mountains between Thessaly and Macedonia. Yet this would involve committing large forces far to the north of both Athens and the Peloponnesus, and an initial defeat might well be fatal. Between Thessaly and the Isthmus of Corinth the most favorable places were in the pass of Thermopylae and the channel off Cape Artemisium, the northern tip of Euboea. This selection, however, would entail the loss of Thessaly and a threat to much of Central Greece. The final line would have to be the Isthmus of Corinth itself, but to hold that meant the surrender of Athens. Also, unless the Persian fleet were defeated, the Isthmus could be bypassed by landings on the coast of Argos, which remained suspiciously neutral. We do not know how the generals estimated all these factors and contingencies, but at least some effort was made to hold each position and to defend as much of Greece as successive circumstances permitted.

While Xerxes was advancing, a force of ten thousand men was sent to the pass of Tempe in northern Thessaly, where the mountains were close to the sea. The men had to be pulled out before contact was made with the enemy, for, without complete Thessalian loyalty, the position at Tempe was weak. The adjacent coastal waters were not suitable for the type of naval action desired by the Greeks, and Tempe could be turned by passes farther west. As Xerxes drew nearer, it became apparent that the Thessalians would go over to the enemy, to medize and betray the passes. Accordingly, the Greeks decided to hold the narrow coastal passage at Thermopylae and stationed their fleet at Artemisium.

Thermopylae became, like Marathon, one of the famous battles of Greek history, but, in this case, the Spartans under their king, Leonidas, won the laurels. According to Greek tradition the defense of the pass terminated in a last-ditch stand by a small band of three hundred Spartans, four hundred

Ballots (ostraka) *cast to ostracize* Aristides, Themistocles, Pericles, *and* Cimon (p. 247 *at bottom right*)

Thebans, and seven hundred men from Boeotian Thespiae. It seems questionable, however, whether the final sacrifice was necessary. The operation was apparently designed to hold ground only until the fleets engaged off Artemisium. The position at Thermopylae was prematurely endangered by the treachery of a Phocian, Ephialtes, who showed the Persians a way around the Greek rear which made Thermopylae untenable. Leonidas dismissed most of the Greek force before the final action was joined, but chose to sacrifice himself and the small force of men whom he retained. The French comment on the charge of the Light Brigade at Balaclava seems to apply here too: it was magnificent, but it was not war.

The Greek fleet did inflict damage on the Persians at Artemisium, although here, too, the Greeks were forced to retreat. Heaven first aided them by a storm which scattered the enemy, and in the fighting some Persian ships were sunk or captured. The odds at sea were narrowed, for the Greeks sailed back to Salamis with little damage to their own ships. They had hoped to encourage the Ionians serving in the Persian fleet to desert but were disappointed. Evidently the Ionians still thought Persian victory certain, for the land route to Athens and the Isthmus of Corinth lay open.

The states of Central Greece, except for Phocis, went over to the Persian side. The Phocian towns and religious shrines were plundered and burnt, except for the oracle at Delphi. Apollo is said to have protected his own sanctuary, but we may suspect that Xerxes was aware of the god's equivocal attitude and of the propaganda effect to be obtained by sparing the shrine.

The Greeks had now to make their most important decision of the war, and there seems to have been very considerable difference of opinion on the action to be taken. The Peloponnesian League forces wished to prepare a line of defense at the Isthmus of Corinth. In fact, the whole army fell back to the Peloponnesus and started to build a wall across the Isthmus. Athens was ex-

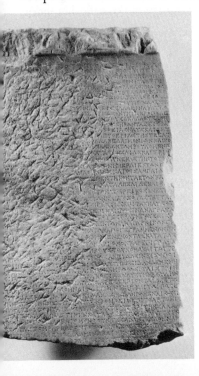

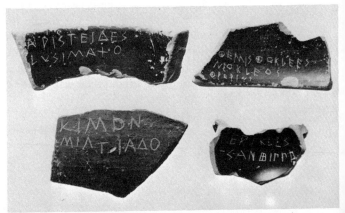

The "Themistocles Decree." This inscription, found in Troezen and dated to the latter part of the fourth century B. C. by its letter forms and orthography, records a decree apparently moved by Themistocles in 480 B.C. It provided for the evacuation of the Athenians to Troezen and Salamis and for deploying the Athenian fleet before the battle of Artemisium. Many scholars regard the decree as a later fabrication, and so its subject matter has not been used in the text.

posed, but the evacuation of its citizens to the island of Salamis and across the Saronic Gulf to Troezen was covered by the Greek fleet. As the evacuation was carried on, leaving the city to be occupied by Xerxes, there was fierce debate whether the fleet should remain in the waters off Salamis to protect the Athenians and offer battle to the Persian fleet or sail to the Peloponnesus and protect its coasts. Themistocles, by argument and threat—he even asserted that the Athenians would go on board their ships and sail off to Magna Graecia—won agreement to stay at Salamis. It remained to make the Persians fight and to avoid a blockade, which would have demoralized the non-Athenian elements among the Greeks. Themistocles contrived to play on Xerxes' desire for a quick victory before the campaigning season came to an end by sending him a message which represented Greek morale as on the verge of collapse. The king was tempted and ordered the Persian fleet to close in on the Greek ships stationed in the narrow strait between Salamis and the Athenian coast. The ground was of the Greeks' own choosing, and in the mêlée which followed they inflicted a crushing defeat. The Persian ships could not maneuver properly and bring their greater numbers to bear. The victory at Salamis was the turning point of the war, for it gave the Greeks control of the Aegean, threatened Xerxes' lines of communication and raised the possibility of revolt in Ionia.

Salamis was fought in September, too late in the year for Xerxes to try the issue again, but the king acted decisively and rapidly to protect his position. The remnants of the Persian fleet, still substantial, were dispatched to the Hellespont to protect the crossing point from Europe. One army corps was withdrawn to Ionia to prevent revolt and another stationed along the roads in Thrace to guard communication. Mardonius was left in Greece with the remainder of the force, still able to meet the Greeks on slightly superior terms in a land battle. He was directed to split the Greek war coalition by diplomatic means during the winter and to prepare for a campaign in the following spring. The Greeks were limited to punishing those states which had gone over to the Persians, but the whole complexion of the war and its prospects had changed.

In the course of the winter Mardonius attempted to exploit the resentment felt by the Athenian people at the evacuation of their city before Salamis. Through Alexander, the king of Macedonia, Mardonius offered very favorable terms which would have made Athens the Persian agent for the control of Greece: equal alliance with Persia, funds to rebuild the temples on the Acropolis, torn down when the Persians occupied the city, and enlargement of Athenian territory. Sparta, alarmed at the prospect of fighting on without Athenian aid, countered by an offer to provide help for the Athenian refugees. Both the Persians and the Spartans were turned down by the Athenians. The Persian overture, however, provided leverage by which the Peloponnesians might be brought out from behind their wall on the Isthmus to fight a land battle against Mardonius' army.

The issue was finally decided at Plataea in the late summer of 479 B.C., but not before Mardonius had again invaded Attica and renewed the offer of alliance. Sparta, perhaps apprehensive at the continued neutrality of Argos, took a long time in its preparations, but, finally, in early summer the commander, Pausanias, had marshalled a force of about 100,000 men. Mardonius fell back into Boeotia so as to have room for maneuver and use of his cavalry. The battle was fought on the slopes before Plataea and skillfully decided in the Greek favor. Mardonius was killed in the fighting, and the Persians fled north to make good their retreat to Asia, before the Greeks could occupy the cities along the Hellespont.

At the same time the Greek fleet had acted decisively in the Aegean. Its commander received assurances of Ionian aid, if he would bring the fleet to Samos, where the Persian navy had taken up position. Xerxes had reorganized his naval forces and was supporting them with an army stationed near the peninsula of Mycale. When the Greek fleet advanced from Delos, the Persian commanders refused naval action and sailed back to the rocky coast of Mycale, where their sailors were landed and fortified themselves. The Greeks moved in and, by a well-planned and rapid landing, defeated the troops and destroyed the Persian fleet. On shore the Milesians betrayed their Persian officers, and at sea the Samians rendered substantial help. But little could be done to liberate the Ionian coastal cities so long as the Persian army remained in the area. At this point the Spartans decided that the immediate Persian threat was dispelled and the Peloponnesian units returned home. The Athenians and islanders, however, more alive to Aegean interests, sailed north to besiege Sestos on the Hellespont and block the main crossing point from Europe.

While the Greeks in the Aegean were engaged in the defeat of Xerxes, their kindred in Sicily were attacked by the Carthaginians. The latter had held the western part of the island since the early period of Phoenician colonization and, as their trading empire grew, desired to expand into the eastern part held by the Greek colonies. There, Syracuse had grown into a great and prosperous city, led by its tyrant, Gelon. His aggressive policy had incurred the hostility of some of the smaller Greek towns, and Himera, one of them, incited the Carthaginians to try to free the island from Syracuse. Perhaps, too, Carthage was encouraged by Xerxes to act at this particular time. While the battle of Plataea was being fought in Boeotia, Gelon met and defeated the Carthaginians at Himera. Magna Graecia, like Aegean Greece, was free to develop independently.

The Problem of Greek Political Unity

During the war the political balance within Greece had shifted. At the Congress of Corinth in 481 B.C. Sparta had been recognized by all as the proper leader of the war coalition. Themistocles' insight and vigor, however, and the naval victories at Salamis and Mycale brought recognition to Athens and at the same time proved the value of sea power as a new factor in the science of war. In the course of the war relations between Athens and Sparta had been strained and some ill-feeling bred. Probably the Athenian leadership realized the need of withdrawing the army to the Isthmus after Thermopylae, but the ordinary Athenian, judging by the account of Herodotus, felt deserted or even betrayed. The sight of the ruined temples on the Athenian Acropolis and the cost of two evacuations made the Athenians feel, with some justification, that they had suffered most in the war, while at the same time their fleet had contributed most to the ultimate victory.

Beneath the flush of enthusiasm and joy which followed the battle of Plataea, there were strong tensions. On the surface Panhellenism prevailed, and the Greeks took steps to convert their war coalition into a permanent Hellenic League. The allies pledged to send representatives to an annual meeting and festival of commemoration at Plataea. They decided to carry the war to Asia Minor and again chose a Spartan, Pausanias, as their leader. There was little thought that such a prosecution of the war would necessarily be naval and carried out far from the Peloponnesus in a theater where action would depend on Athens and its fleet. As early as the following year, in 478 B.C., Athens and Sparta began to go their separate ways. There was no open break, but the new Hellenic League was strained. By 461 B.C. the war-born unity of Greece had collapsed into a destructive rivalry between its two great powers.

Herodotus

The wars with Persia were the first great historical experience in which almost all Greeks shared. Their decisive victories against great odds shaped Greek history in the fifth and fourth centuries. There was a natural stir of speculation after the events of 481–79 B.C. about the origin of the conflict and how victory had been achieved. Within a generation, as perspective was gained, some appreciation of the significance of the victory and of the course of events to which it had led was felt. Fortunately this period of the mid-fifth century produced a historian worthy of his subject. Herodotus realized the significance of his theme, the Persian Wars, and mirrored the reflection and knowledge of his times. His *History of the Persian Wars* represents this vital transition between the older culture of Archaic Greece with its aristocratic values and the new era just beginning.

Herodotus was born about 484 B.C. in Halicarnassus on the Carian coast of Asia Minor. He died about 425 B.C., a few years after the Peloponnesian War between Athens and Sparta had begun. We know little of his life, except what can be deduced from the book itself. His culture was Ionian, sophisticated, rational and inquiring, but he shared the common disdain of Classical Greeks for Ionia which resulted from Ionia's failure against Persia. Halicarnassus, too, was a Persian possession, but he left it for Samos with his family soon after 467 B.C., when a revolt led by his cousin, Panyassis, was unsuccessful. Presumably the family property was confiscated, for Herodotus seems to have made his living as a merchant. He traveled very widely, partly on business, partly to observe, to talk and gather the material ultimately used in the history. He knew Samos and Aegean Greece extremely well, and made his home for a time in Periclean Athens, where he was on intimate terms with the tragedian Sophocles and with Pericles himself. Presumably Herodotus' enjoyment and admiration of Athens prompted the very favorable account in his history of the Athenian part in the war and the political gossip about such figures as Themistocles. Journeys to the Black Sea, Egypt and Cyrene furnished the material for the detailed accounts of those lands, which comprise the second and fourth books of the history. He did not, however, visit Persia or write an account of Babylonia, promised in connection with his visit to Babylon. The history seems to have been composed after 450 B.C. and was probably written in part in Magna Graecia, for in 443 B.C. he moved there as a member of the new Athenian colony of Thurii in South Italy. The book was first published piecemeal by public readings. Its apparent discursiveness is the result of an epic conception of his theme rather than of any looseness of composition and failure of revision.

Herodotus had an example of historical writing in the work of Hecataeus (p. 233), who had insisted that history be truthful and critical. Hecataeus, however, had lacked a meaningful theme, one in which the experience of a whole generation of men was involved or on which the creative imagination of its interpreter could work. Herodotus conceived his history on a broad scale, designed to show the contrasting character and civilization of the peoples who fought, as well as to give an account of the events of the wars.

Herodotus' conception of historiography is an interesting example of the transitional period of thought in which he lived: "What Herodotus the Halicarnassian has learned by inquiry [*historie*] is here set forth: in order that the memory of the past may not be blotted out from among men by time, and that great and marvelous deeds done by Greeks and foreigners and especially the reason why they warred against each other may not lack renown." The "inquiry" is thoroughly in the spirit of Ionian natural science. Herodotus carried it out by personal observation of the lands and peoples in whom he was interested, by talking with them, by asking questions and drawing inferences. The material was sifted with a keen and honest mind and a very considerable amount of common sense. If he could not reconcile various stories, the several versions were set down, often with a quietly ironic comment to indicate his own opinion. Part of the "inquiry," however, was to preserve the great deeds of the men who fought the wars. The spirit is that of Homer and of aristocratic Greece, which held that the proper end of human activity was excellence and glory. Herodotus made no necessary distinction in quality between Greek and foreigner and did not exhibit the racial contempt for non-Greeks which frequently is found in later Greek writers. He gives a fresh and sympathetic account of the lands and peoples of the Persian Empire and finds as much to criticize in Greece as he does among the "barbarians." Yet the Greeks did win the war, and Herodotus found in them certain qualities beyond the common courage and humanity found in all men.

Near the beginning of the history a contrast is drawn between Greek and barbarian by the story of a meeting between Croesus of Lydia and Solon of Athens. The meeting was unhistorical, which did not bother Herodotus, because he used it as an illustrative parable. Croesus, the "barbarian," showed Solon, the wise man of Greece, his treasury stocked with gold, a symbol of wealth and power, and asked Solon to name the happiest man of his experience. Contrary to Croesus' expectation of being so designated, Solon listed several relatively obscure Greeks. All had lived a sane, moderate life in comfortable circumstances and had died before disaster fell upon them, admired for some exploit by their fellows. To the Greeks of Herodotus' time the gods were jealous of human prosperity, so that a man had to walk carefully and not pronounce himself happy until death had come.

Herodotus' explanation of the Persian disaster lay in this conventional Greek outlook. The gods had given Asia to the Persians as their land. Darius' thrust into Scythia and Xerxes' invasion of Greece were arrogant transgressions. Xerxes had further flouted nature by bridging the Hellespont and cutting a canal through the peninsula of Mt. Athos. Herodotus represented the king as blinded by presumption, arrogant and seized by fits of unreasoning anger, in which he behaved like a typical despot. The gods had blinded Xerxes and would strike him down.

The book is delightful to read, but its moralizing framework of thought seems unsatisfactory to the historian looking for a rational explanation of the events of the war. Herodotus explains too much by personal feelings of hate, revenge, and ambition. He was also limited in his account by the sources of information available. The "inquiry," written a generation after the war, was largely based on information supplied by combatants and their descendants. While this was very congenial to Herodotus' own taste for anecdote and colorful personality, it resulted in confused accounts of most battles and provided no real information about the overall plans of the Greek and Persian high councils of war. Perhaps the gossip of the ordinary soldiers and a picture of the average Athenian's feeling about Sparta's apparent callousness to Athenian interest are fair balance. Herodotus is properly called the "Father of History" from the universal meaning which he gave to his subject matter, the breadth and shrewdness of his treatment, and his essential honesty of thought and search for the truth.

A decadrachm of Syracuse. These commemorative issues of Syracuse are among the finest of Greek coins.

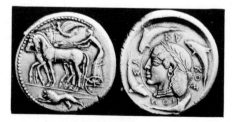

XII

The Athenian Empire

(478–431 B.C.)

DURING THE FIFTH CENTURY B.C. the most significant new factor in Greek history was the establishment of an Athenian Empire. After the Greek victories over Persia, Athens rapidly became the political, commercial and cultural center of the Greek world. With their new navy the Athenians were able to control the islands and the coastal cities of the Aegean Sea. The profits from trade and Empire allowed the lower and middle classes to participate fully in government. The development of a more complete democracy in Athens and of an Empire in the Aegean was accompanied by a surge of creativity in art and literature. The Parthenon and the Propylaea, which still crown the Athenian Acropolis, were erected, and Athenian drama, begun by Aeschylus, was developed to its classic form by Sophocles. In 431 B.C., at the outset of the Peloponnesian War, Pericles, the greatest statesman of Athenian history, could appropriately describe his city as "The school of Hellas."

Pericles, more than any other Athenian, was the architect of the Empire and the real founder of Athenian democracy. A token of his work is the name, Periclean Period, given to this most important phase of Athenian history. Pericles was a member of the Alcmeonid family, which had given Athens a statesman in almost every generation since his ancestor Megacles had blocked Cylon's attempt at tyranny in 632 B.C. Following the tradition of his ancestors, Pericles identified himself as a young man with the democratic groups in Athens. Like his kinsman Cleisthenes, he may have seen political opportunity in opposition, but he well understood the shifting in gravity to the middle group in Athenian society which had been in process since the time of Solon, and, like Themistocles, realized the intimate connection between Athenian sea power and the prosperity of the state. It was Pericles' radical innovation of pay for state service which permitted the middle and lower classes to participate so fully in government, and his pride and confidence in the quality of his fellow

The reader will find Maps VII and IX (pages 172–173 and 202) useful as he reads this chapter.

Athenians that justified in his mind the Empire which they founded. As a person Pericles was aloof and dignified, finding his private pleasure in an intimate intellectual circle, of which Herodotus and Sophocles were members, but able to win support from the people by his remarkable power of oratory. He won their loyalty by his sincere concern for their interests and by his ambitious plans for Athens.

Yet Pericles was largely responsible for the defeat of Panhellenism in Greece and, in a sense, of Athens itself by bringing on the disastrous Peloponnesian War between Athens and Sparta. As the wealth and power of Athens grew, Sparta and its allies began to fear that they would be forced into the Athenian Empire. The member-states of the Empire, transformed from free partners of Athens into subjects, became embittered by the loss of their autonomy, however much they might benefit materially from close association with Athens. By 461 B.C. Greece was divided into two coalitions, headed by Athens and Sparta. A generation later the Greeks tried to resolve the issue in the Peloponnesian War (431–04 B.C.). Athens lost its Empire, and the city itself narrowly escaped destruction, but Sparta and the other states of Greece were too weakened and embittered by the strain of war to establish a firm peace. The war had its great historian, Thucydides, whose penetrating study of power and its abuse interpreted the political failure of Classical Greece. The Greeks, despite their achievements in art, literature and thought, were unable to solve the problem of living together in peace.

The Delian League (478–61 B.C.)

Greek unity, cemented by the formation of the Hellenic League after the victory at Plataea in 479 B.C., began to crack almost immediately. Within two years Athens had been recognized as the leader of a new Greek coalition, the Delian League, in which Sparta had no part. The explanation for the split lies mainly in the very different stakes which the various Greek allies had in continuing the war across the Aegean Sea. To Sparta and its Peloponnesian allies their own interests did not seem to be really involved, although Sparta liked the prestige of command. The Aegean islanders and Ionians, some of whom were not yet liberated, rightly felt that Persia was a continuing threat to their independence. The Athenians, conscious of themselves as a naval power with Aegean interests and smarting from the Persian destruction of their city, were anxious to carry the war to victory in Asia Minor. They were ready to assert their independence of Spartan leadership.

The Athenians felt that it was necessary for Athens' security and dignity to rebuild the city's walls, thrown down during the Persian occupation. To a Greek city-state its walls were a symbol of independence as well as a means of defense. Despite the argument of Sparta that new defenses would give Persia a fortified base, if the invasion were renewed, the Athenians persisted. While Themistocles spun out an explanation in Sparta, the people of Athens worked

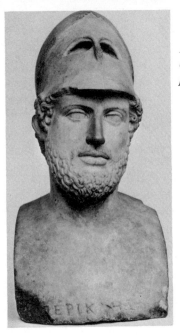

Pericles. Roman copy
of the original
portrait by
Cresilas

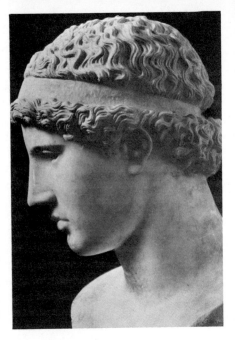

The Lemnian Athena.
Roman copy of the
original by Pheidias,
once standing
on the Athenian
Acropolis

night and day to complete the new fortifications, dragging blocks from the debris of Persian destruction. In a few weeks the walls were ready and Athens faced Sparta as an equal. The Spartans could only acquiesce, for they were committed to the war against Persia and the Spartan general Pausanias was in command of the allied troops in the Hellespont.

THE FORMATION OF THE LEAGUE

Pausanias' conduct of the command there proved unacceptable, not only to the allies, but to Sparta itself. The victory at Plataea had so inflated him with vanity and stimulated his ambition that he was arrogant and unapproachable by his officers and men. He even intrigued to upset his own superiors in Sparta. Even worse, he was suspected of plotting with the Persian commanders in northern Asia Minor, probably contemplating an appointment by Xerxes to take charge of operations against the Greeks. The Spartan government was forced to recall Pausanias to Sparta for trial and to allow the command in the Hellespont to devolve on Athens. The Aegean allies gravitated to Athens as a kindred and sympathetic power, whose new fleet could offer protection against Persia. When Sparta sent out another commander, Dorcis, the situation had grown not only beyond his control, but the new Delian League was coming into being. This was conceived as the military arm of the larger Hellenic League. While the members did not want Spartan leadership for their war against Persia, they did not wish to break away completely. Sparta could once more acquiesce in the situation without too much loss of prestige.

The Delian League was formed in 477 B.C. to liberate the Greek cities still under Persian control and to get compensation by ravaging the king's lands. The objectives were limited, but naturally enough in the flush of successful war

255

no thought was given to the eventual dissolution of the League. The members swore an oath to abide by their agreements in a picturesque ceremony, in which iron weights were sunk into the sea. The organization would endure until the iron rose again. The League was a free association between Athens and the group of independent allies. Each member-state cast one vote in a general assembly held annually on the island of Delos, the traditional religious center of the Ionian Greeks. League policy was determined by the vote of the assembly and by Athens in agreement, for Athens was the *hegemon,* or military leader, of the League. It was Athens' responsibility to command military operations and provide a large part of the fleet, to set the members' contributions in ships and manpower or money, and to appoint the financial officers, the *Hellenotamiae,* Treasurers of the Greeks. In 477 B.C. the basic contributions were set by Aristides at 460 talents.[1] The sum was large, but it presumably included both payments in money and the monetary equivalent of contributions in military service. The League had made a promising start, for this difficult task of assessment had been settled to the satisfaction of all by Aristides, who received the nickname, "the Just," for his good work.

There were, however, latent difficulties and ambiguities in the arrangements, which continuous military activity gradually brought into the open. The *hegemony* of Athens gave that city great influence, which hardened into a natural assumption of control. Both Athens and a small member-state might come to feel that the small state's contribution was better made by money than service, thus eroding away independence. The trend of development was for Athens to make the decisions and to carry the brunt of the military burden.

CIMONIAN IMPERIALISM

At the outset Athenian policy had a reassuringly Panhellenic character. The dangerous opportunism of Themistocles was replaced by conservatism at home and Panhellenism abroad under a new leader, Cimon, the son of Miltiades, the victor at Marathon. Cimon had won Athenian confidence by his bravery and ability in the Persian Wars and retained it by genial and upright political conduct in Athens. His stable conservatism and simple policy of friendship to Sparta and hostility to Persia appealed to Athenians after their hardships and the disturbance of the war. Themistocles had skirted dangerously near to an open break with Sparta; furthermore his secret dealings with Xerxes during the war acquired the color of treason in the innuendo of postwar Athenian politics. He had been a close associate of Pausanias, whose intrigues with Persia seem to

---

[1] It is very difficult to give the modern values of Greek monetary units because of our extremely limited knowledge of ancient prices and of their fluctuations. The modern value in *gold* of the Athenian drachma is about twenty cents and of the talent $1,200, but its purchasing power in antiquity would have been many times that and would, of course, have varied in different places and at different times. The standard daily wage in the late fifth century B.C. was one drachma and the cost of living probably about half as much. The Athenian currency scale was as follows: 6 obols = 1 drachma; 100 drachmas = 1 mina; 60 minas = 1 talent. Fractional currency, below 1 drachma, usually had only a local circulation, and the coins used in foreign trade and for large transactions were 4 drachma pieces, *tetradrachms.* A few states issued 10 drachma pieces, but the mina and the talent were expressions of value.

have implicated Themistocles. In the 470's both the great war leaders were disgraced. Pausanias was starved to the point of death in a sanctuary in Sparta where he had taken refuge to avoid trial. Themistocles was ostracized from Athens, then driven from Greece to find a hospitable refuge in Persian Asia Minor. The field was then left free for Cimon to direct Athenian and League policy. Ironically, Cimon's success against Persia prepared the ground for the conversion of the Delian League into the Athenian Empire.

In the action against Persia, while the interests of the League and of Greece were generally served, Athens found opportunity for its own advantage. At first attacks were made against the Persian garrisons remaining in Thrace which might be used in a renewal of the Persian invasion. One such town, Eion on the Strymon River, was made available for Athenian settlement. Then a pirate's lair on the island of Skyros was cleared out. This was to the profit of Aegean commerce, but Skyros, too, was settled by Athenians. The small city of Carystus on Euboea was forced into the League without apparent cause, but no large-scale attack was mounted against Persian Asia Minor. Accordingly, in 468 B.C. the island of Naxos decided to withdraw from the League. Naxos was attacked by Athens and compelled to re-enter under penalty of losing its vote in the assembly. As Thucydides noted, this was the first allied city to be "enslaved." Perhaps partly to reassure the other members of the League, Cimon, about 467 B.C., prepared a large expedition of 300 ships, two-thirds of which were Athenian, to attack the Persians in the southeastern Mediterranean where they were concentrating a fleet.

The Persians had mustered their ships at the mouth of the Eurymedon River in Pamphylia, apparently to strike into the Aegean. Cimon defeated them decisively and followed up his victory by advancing to Cyprus, where a squadron of Phoenician ships was shattered. These victories effectively dispelled the Persian threat and opened the area to the extension of the League. Many towns along the coast and in Caria were brought into the organization as nonvoting, contributory members. Athenian trade into the southeastern Mediterranean was developed, as indicated by the merchants' hoards of Athenian silver coins, found by excavation on the Syrian coast and in the Nile delta.

Cimon followed up his victory in southern Asia Minor by sailing northwards to clear the last Persian troops out of the region of the Hellespont and of Thrace. In that area, too, as the Persians were cleared out, Athenian interests were substituted. Athenian settlers and traders began to encroach upon the traditional influence of the island of Thasos. In 465 B.C. when Thasos determined to challenge Athens by withdrawing from the League, Athenian reprisal was swift. Thasos was attacked, and a large group of Athenian colonists put into the Strymon River valley to found a new town, Amphipolis. Evidently Athens intended to control the mining and timber lands of the northern Aegean. When the Athenian colonists were attacked by Thracian natives and forced to abandon their enterprise, Athens pressed the siege of Thasos. In 462 B.C. the city surrendered. Thasos was compelled to tear down its walls, surrender the fleet and give up all possessions on the adjacent Thracian shore. Contribution to the League was fixed in terms of money, and the once-powerful little state became a subject ally of Athens. The harshness of the terms gave warning that no League member was free to withdraw. Here then was demonstrated a change of temper in the Athenians.

THE DISGRACE OF CIMON

In the 460's an increasing number of Athenians had begun to realize the usefulness of the League for Athens. The lower class, the *thetes*, who served in the Athenian fleet as rowers, found a new livelihood as sailors on merchant ships. The middle groups profited from the growth of trade and local industry since employment was high and material well-being increasing. As these benefits of sea power were realized, the conservative influence of Cimon and of the Athenian upper class declined. The political interests of the middle and lower classes in Athens became identified with greater democratic privilege at home and with a more deliberate and aggressive Athenian imperialism abroad. The vacuum in popular leadership, left by Themistocles, was filled by the rise of new men, Ephialtes and Pericles. Opportunity was found to repudiate Cimon and Panhellenism in a crisis of foreign policy when a request came from Sparta for aid against the *helots*.

In 464 B.C. when a disastrous earthquake had shaken the southern Peloponnesus, the city of Sparta was leveled, many Spartans killed, and the government so disorganized that control was relaxed over the *helots* in Laconia and Messenia. Revolt broke out on a broad scale and, while Sparta recovered Laconia, the Messenians who seized the natural stronghold of Mt. Ithome in central Messenia defied attempts to reduce them by siege. Cimon persuaded the Athenians to send help to Sparta, putting his policy of Panhellenism at stake. But at Mt. Ithome ill-feeling broke out between Spartans and Athenians, and Sparta complained of Athenian sympathy for the *helots*. Finally the Athenians were brusquely invited to go home. The fiasco left Cimon vulnerable to attack by his political opponents who, in 461 B.C., secured his *ostracism*. Ephialtes was assassinated, for reasons unknown, by a Boeotian visitor in Athens, and Pericles began to make himself the leading political figure in Athens and Athens the dominant state in Greece.

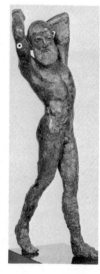

*Bronze
figurine of
Hephaestus(?).
Ca. 460 B.C.*

Athens and the Empire (461-31 B.C.)

PERICLEAN POLITICS

Before the disgrace of Cimon, Ephialtes and Pericles had removed a constitutional block to more complete popular sovereignty by discrediting the Council of the Areopagus and stripping away much of its remaining political power. Charges of corruption had been brought against individual Areopagites to create an impression of the unworthiness of the council. While Cimon was out of Athens, a decree was pushed through the assembly which deprived the

Areopagus of its "guardianship of the law," as Aristotle phrased it. Apparently the council lost its right to supervise the conduct of the magistrates and to safeguard the law against illegal decrees, that is, to prosecute the movers of such decrees. The new arrangement transferred supervision of the magistrates to the Council of Five Hundred and protection of the law to the *heliaea,* the popular courts.

This was the opening stroke of a legislative program by which Pericles extended the democracy and consolidated his popular support. In 457 B.C. the lower middle class gained access to the archonship when the property qualification for that office was lowered to Solon's third class, the *zeugitae.* The privileged area of archonship and, through it, the Areopagus, was now open to many more Athenians, for by the mid-fifth century the formal qualification for the third class, an income of 200 drachmas, had been greatly cheapened through inflation. It remained to make participation in government easier for the lower class. In the late 450's Pericles introduced the most significant of his measures, pay for the Athenian jurymen, who were drawn by lot from a panel of six thousand citizens to staff the law courts. Pay for service to the state was a new principle in Greece. When it was extended in the following years to officials, to members of the council, to soldiers and sailors, it attracted trenchant criticism from antidemocratic politicians. The pay was not large, only one-half drachma per day for jurors, and a drachma for councilors, but it did enable the poor Athenian citizen to serve his government without sacrificing his livelihood. Since Athenian citizenship had become more valuable, it had to be safeguarded. Consequently in 451 B.C. Pericles passed legislation limiting citizenship to those of Athenian birth on both sides of the family, not merely through the father, as previously. By these measures Pericles won solid support for his ambitious plans to extend Athenian power abroad.

PERICLEAN IMPERIALISM

In 461 B.C. the prospects for Athenian aggrandizement were promising. In Greece Sparta had been weakened by the *helot* revolt and its army was tied down at Mt. Ithome. Persia was threatened by revolt in Egypt, following upon the temporary dislocation of naval power by Cimon's victory at the Eurymedon River. Accordingly, Pericles tried to exploit every opening, straining Athenian resources to the limit and calling on the League forces for continuous service. His first move was to isolate Central Greece, where he hoped to replace Theban control by Athenian influence and occupation. Adroit alliances were made with Argos and Megara to hamper Spartan action beyond the Peloponnesus, while support was obtained in Northern Greece by alliance with Thessaly. At the same time Pericles began a large building plan to increase Athens' own security. The harbor system of the Peiraeus was improved and construction started on the Long Walls, which were to stretch from Peiraeus to the fortifications of Athens. The Long Walls would form a corridor, through which grain and other supplies could be brought when Athens was under siege. Athens also secured a useful port of call at the entrance of the Corinthian Gulf by sponsoring a new settlement at Naupactus. The settlers there were the same Messenian *helots* who had defended Mt. Ithome. Sparta, making the best of a bad situation, finally had allowed them to leave under safe-conduct. Despite the provocative character of all these moves, Pericles ordered an Athenian fleet of 200 ships to advance from Cyprus to Egypt to help the Egyptian rebels against Persia.

Greek reaction was fast, but at first ineffective, as Pericles had anticipated. Corinth and Aegina, who felt their sea trade threatened, declared war on Athens. In the naval fighting Athens captured Aegina and added it to the League as a tributary state. In 457 B.C. Sparta joined Thebes in declaring war on Athens. The Athenians were defeated at Tanagra in Boeotia, but Sparta was not able to follow up the victory. When the Spartan army withdrew, Athens advanced again into Boeotia taking over many of the smaller cities and installing governments favorable to itself.

In Egypt the Athenians were initially successful, but found themselves committed to a desperate struggle in the marshes of the Nile delta and the waters off Egypt against continuously increasing Persian forces. By 453 B.C. the Athenian expedition had collapsed in a disaster from which Athens extricated only a few hundred men. Already in the previous year the worsening situation in Egypt had been used as an excuse by Pericles to move the treasury of the Delian League from Delos to Athens. The Persians made no attempt to enter the Aegean, but Pericles was forced to reorient his policy of expansion.

The intensive military activity in Central Greece and Egypt had been carried on partly with the levies from the Delian League, but largely by Athens itself. The cost had been very high in casualties and money, with the result that Pericles' leadership was shaken. Since he evidently felt the need for consolidation, in 456 B.C. he had sponsored a motion to recall Cimon from exile. Both leaders, whatever their differences in outlook, were concerned for Athens' well-being and worked to strengthen Athenian control of the Delian League, which was done by shifting the treasury, the large sum of five thousand talents, from Delos to Athens. The Athenian assembly then began to decide how the funds should be spent. The five thousand talents became an Athenian reserve from which the state might borrow. The Council of Five Hundred henceforth set the assessments on the states of the League at four-year periods. An annual quota of one-sixtieth of each state's contribution was allocated to the treasury of Athens' patron goddess, Athena. The annual tribute after 454 B.C., amounting to almost four hundred talents in cash, was used not only to pay the expenses of the Empire but also for specifically Athenian expenses. These financial measures marked an important step in the formation of an Athenian subject empire, but the organization was still regarded by Athens as the instrument for the joint Greek war against Persia.

In Athens the people's dejection at the disaster in Egypt and their fear of Spartan re-entry into Central Greece favored a more Panhellenic policy. In 451

B.C. Cimon was able to make a truce for five years with Sparta, at the cost of the alliance with Argos, but retaining the Athenian gains in Central Greece. To counter a possible Persian attack, he prepared another great League expedition into the southeastern Mediterranean. For this purpose many of the small states of the Delian League changed their contributions in ships to money, leaving only the big islands of Samos, Chios, and Lesbos as military contributors. The League fleet struck at the Persian concentration in Cyprus and won a victory, but Cimon was killed in the action. When the victory was not followed up, Pericles apparently took the momentous step of using his temporary advantage to conclude a peace with Persia in 448 B.C.

While there is some dispute about the authenticity of the peace, called the Peace of Callias from the Athenian envoy who is supposed to have negotiated it, major hostilities between Athens and Persia did cease after 448 B.C. There seems to have been a mutual recognition of each other's territorial limits and a decision of noninterference. With the cessation of war against Persia the aim of the Delian League had been achieved, so that its members felt a natural disinclination to pay their contributions. The Athenians had to use coercion. Pericles seized on the opportunity offered by the end of war with Persia to forestall the impending lapse of the truce with Sparta and to promote Athenian leadership in Greek affairs. He planned a Panhellenic Congress in Athens to discuss the restoration of Greek temples destroyed by the Persians and to work out a scheme for the policing of the seas. But Athenian aggression in Greece had killed the feeling for Panhellenism. Pericles' invitation to the Congress evoked no response. Instead of rebuilding temples throughout Greece, he proposed to the Athenians that the city rebuild her own ruined structures by using League funds.

Soon Pericles was forced to yield most of Central Greece. In Boeotia, Thebes successfully instigated revolt in the cities which Athens had taken over, and an Athenian force sent to recover them was ambushed and captured. This disaster encouraged the Euboeans to revolt against Athens and Megara to declare its independence. Before Euboea could be recovered, the truce with Sparta lapsed and a Spartan army invaded Attica. While Pericles extricated what he could from the situation, his project for an Athenian land empire in Greece had failed. Only Plataea and the Messenian *helot* settlement at Naupactus remained Athenian allies. The islands of Euboea and Aegina, however, were held, for Athens could not be effectively challenged at sea.

In 445 B.C. Sparta and Athens recognized the stalemate by arranging a peace for thirty years. Greece was formally divided into two power zones, when Sparta recognized the Athenian maritime empire and pledged not to interfere with its members, and Athens agreed not to interfere with the Peloponnesian League and the allies of Sparta. Provision was made for the settlement of disputes by arbitration, but no clear procedure was laid down for the process. While Pericles had failed in his grandiose schemes to put Athens in control of Central Greece and the whole of the eastern Mediterranean, he had established an Athenian Empire which was recognized by Persia and Sparta. The peace was an uneasy stalemate, but it provided the opportunity for reorganization of the Empire and the further development of Athens itself.

THE ORGANIZATION OF THE EMPIRE

After the peace with Sparta, Pericles extended the influence and power of Athens by diplomacy and the founding of Athenian colonies. Control of Thrace was secured by new settlements at Brea in 444 B.C. and at Amphipolis in 437 B.C. When the latter venture was successful that time, Athens gained access to the timber, grain and metals of the northern Aegean and could supervise shipping along the coast from the Hellespont. Also in 437 B.C. a detachment of the Athenian fleet paraded along the shore of the Black Sea in a goodwill tour. Alliances were made with the larger Greek city-states there, and a small Athenian colony was placed at Amisus on the south coast. Since Persian interest in the Black Sea was evidently slight at this time, the result of these ventures was that Athens had control of the grain shipped from Thrace and the Black Sea.

In South Italy and Sicily, where Athenian trade had been growing since the early sixth century, the power of Syracuse prevented any real extension of Athenian political influence, but Pericles established a new and interesting settlement at Thurii in South Italy. In 443 B.C. a colonizing expedition was sent out as a Panhellenic venture under Athenian auspices. Prominent Greek intellectuals, among them Herodotus, the historian, and Hippodamus, the architect and town planner, were invited to participate in a model foundation. The colonists, however, rejected Athenian leadership in a few years, and Athens' interest in the west had to remain commercial for the time being. The Empire itself was disturbed in 441 B.C. by the revolt of Samos, which was joined by Byzantium on the Bosporus. The reduction of Samos required a major effort by Athens, but in 439 B.C. the island was forced to surrender and became a subject ally. Only Lesbos and Chios then remained as free partners of Athens. Pericles also took steps to tighten the organization of the Empire and link it more closely to Athens.

After 445 B.C. the Empire included about three hundred members, fanning out in a great semicircle from Athens along the coastline of the Aegean, from Macedonia to the southern coast of Asia Minor. Athenian sea power held the small scattered subject states easily and without excessive administrative expense. We know a considerable amount about the Empire from a series of documents called the tribute lists. From 454 to 415 B.C. the Athenians recorded the annual quota of money paid to Athena's treasury by each state on marble slabs, which were set up on the Athenian Acropolis. Many have survived, and their study throws a useful light on the administrative history of the Empire. In 443 B.C. a reorganization was made which grouped the members into five districts: Ionia, the Islands of the Aegean, Thrace, the Hellespont and Caria. Within each district large cities were assessed individually, but the smaller grouped into a single tribute unit. In 438 B.C. Caria and Ionia were merged into a single district, with some inland cities given up to Persian control. Athens exercised care to make adjustments in the assessments, according to changing circumstance. The money was collected by the member-states themselves and paid over to Athens, except when the exaction of arrears made Athenian intervention necessary. An annual sum of 350 to 400 talents was collected, which left a useful excess above the costs of administration for the use of Athens.

Not only the states of the Empire but all of Greece received very tangible benefits, when the Aegean area was knitted together under the protection of Athenian sea power. The Aegean was kept clear of Persian ships and pirates. The city of Athens became an important metropolitan market, to which traders and craftsmen flocked to make a good living. Athens had agreed to the freedom of the seas for all Greeks in the peace with Sparta in 445 B.C., but, despite this, the Athenians drew the Empire together into a close economic unit. Commercial treaties were made with their subject states, which guaranteed protection of commerce on favorable terms and turned their trade to Athens. In 425 B.C., in the course of the Peloponnesian War, the Athenians issued a decree to standardize the weights and measures of the Empire to Athenian standards and closed local mints. This, of course, was partly a war measure and, when Athens' position deteriorated in the course of the fighting, did not prove effective. Yet Athenian silver coinage did become the medium for general Greek exchange and for trade into the Persian Empire. Despite the very real benefits of economic integration, both the subject states of the Empire and the free trading states of Greece realized the threat latent in Athenian naval power and resented Athenian leadership. They knew that Athens could close the sea lanes and control the flow of grain, timber, and metals into the Aegean. So long as Athens observed the peace, however, the chief difficulties were with the members of the Empire, who desired complete autonomy.

The degree of Athenian interference in the local affairs of the subject states varied, but, when Athens felt her own security was involved, her control was very far-reaching. For example, in Erythrae and Miletus in Ionia, Athenian garrisons were stationed and a governor appointed, whose task it was to install a system of government patterned on that of Athens. Important law suits, where cases involved tribute, treason and murder, had to be referred to Athenian courts. After a revolt Athens imposed severe penalties, as she did in Euboea in 445. The opponents of Athens were exiled and their lands confiscated to be made available for Athenian *cleruch* colonists. Athenians were invited to enroll for such a colony and to the members of the group so formed lots of land, *kleroi*, were assigned. The *cleruch* thus became a member of a privileged Athenian community in the territory of a subject state, retaining Athenian citizenship and helping to protect Athenian interests.

These harsh methods by which Athens assured its control of the Empire bulked large among the complaints of the subject states and seem to have outweighed the material benefits which they enjoyed, although in each state a pro-Athenian faction formed. The supporters of Athens were the middle- and lower-class citizens, who favored a democratic system of government and were alive to the benefits of increased trade. Opposed to them and to Athenian control were the conservative upper-class landowners. Athenian aggressiveness was producing a revolution in Greece, but it could not break out into fighting until the Peloponnesian War gave the anti-Athenian groups some expectation of aid from Sparta. Athens is sometimes criticized in modern accounts of the Empire for the failure to extend its own citizenship. Yet it is only fair to observe that such a device had no tradition in Greek experience and that the subject states did not expect it or want it. They wished to be autonomous.

As the pattern of Empire became established, political thinking sought justification or condemnation for it along traditional Greek lines. To an Athenian patriot like Pericles, Athens' services to Greece against Persia and the example of Athenian courage, energy, and use of its opportunities seemed sufficient justification for the Empire. To the enemies of Athens and to the embittered subject states Athens was a tyrant who had destroyed Greek freedom, but Sparta could appear in a somewhat anomalous role as a defender of liberty. In Athens itself the aristocratic upper class protested the diversion of Empire funds to Athenian uses. In the critical years between 449 and 445 B.C., when the conversion to Empire was completed, a rival to Pericles appeared in the person of Thucydides, the son of Melesias. He publicly challenged Pericles' proposal to use the revenues from the Empire for the construction of the Parthenon. Athens was "as it were, some vain woman, hung round with precious stones and figures and temples, which cost a world of money," but the material benefits of Empire were too great to be abandoned, and Pericles obtained the *ostracism* of Thucydides in 443 B.C.

THE SOCIETY AND ECONOMY OF ATHENS

At the outbreak of the Peloponnesian War in 431 B.C. Athens had changed profoundly from what it was at the time of the Persian Wars. It was probably the largest city-state in Greece, with a population estimated at well over 300,000 people. The most marked change was the increase in the number of *metics*, resident aliens, and of slaves. The *metics* numbered about 35,000 and the slaves perhaps as many as 115,000. There would have been about 168,000 Athenians of whom 40,000, the adult men, formed the active citizen body. Some notion of the rise in social status may be formed by comparing the number of 10,000 *hoplites* which Athens mustered for Marathon and the 23,000 which the state could mobilize in 431 B.C. Evidently the middle class, from which the *hoplites* would have been drawn, had grown markedly and formed the bulk of the population. About 50 percent of the total population seems to have resided in the city of Athens and the harbor town of Peiraeus, with the result that in numbers the urban group predominated in the affairs of the state as a whole.

The growth of population and prosperity had not changed the traditional methods of making a living as much as might be expected. The ordinary Athenian found new activity in government and administration of the Empire rather than in a change of occupation. It is calculated that about 20,000

Athenians, fifty percent of the adult citizen body, received state pay for part or the whole of the year. Service as jurymen, councilors, officials, as soldiers and sailors, was not only available, but obligatory. For the Athenian, however, agriculture still remained the traditional and dignified manner of life. The upper-class families still possessed large estates, but the characteristic Athenian farmer was the small freeholder, who worked his farm with the members of his family and two or three slaves. The crops had become more specialized as the advantages of exporting olive oil and wine were realized, but the techniques of agriculture remained static. So long as imported grain was available, there was probably little incentive to change from the old method of cultivation which left one-third of the land lie fallow each year, and Athens probably raised only twenty-five percent of the cereals necessary to feed its population. The increased opportunities of employment in the city benefited the landless *thetes* most, for work was available on the Periclean building projects, in the flourishing craft industries, in small-scale retailing, and odd jobs. But the development of Athenian commerce and industry seems to have been largely in the hands of the resident aliens.

The position of the *metic,* resident alien, in Athens was particularly favorable, and they were loyal and useful members of the community. While the *metic* could not become an Athenian citizen by any regular process, such as naturalization, he did share some of the privileges and obligations of citizenship. He could engage in his trade or craft freely and was protected in his enterprises and person by Athenian law. As in modern America, the alien was liable to military service and the payment of taxes. The *metics* fought well for Athens, and some were rewarded by special grants of citizenship for their services.

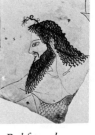

Red-figured cup fragment. Triton (early fifth century B.C.)

The position of the slave in Athenian society is somewhat debatable. The slaves were numerous and extensively used, but Athens is hardly to be regarded as a slave state, essentially dependent for its well-being on their labor. The state itself employed slaves for clerical work and used them as a police force in the city. Slave labor was also used indirectly by the state in the silver mines at Laureum and on other state projects by leasing contracts for such work to the owners of gangs of slaves. Most slaves, however, seem to have been in family and domestic service where, as on the farms, they worked alongside their master. Except for the slaves in the mines where conditions of work were harsh and where slaves were regarded as expendable, they seem to have been well treated and received legal protection against personal abuse. While there was a growth of humanitarian feeling among Athenians which condemned slavery as incompatible with the dignity of man, it did not result in practical programs for emancipation. Although the individual slaveowner showed a paternal attitude to his slaves and Athenian writers occasionally protested against slavery as an institution, this liberality was extended no farther than the consideration of believing it improper to enslave Greeks. Accordingly, most slaves originated from the lands on the fringes of the Greek world, and great repugnance was felt at selling Greek prisoners of war into slavery.

In general the increase in material well-being included free Athenian, *metic* and slave alike. There seems to have been no great difference in the conditions of labor for the ordinary member of any one of these groups. An inscription of 409/8 B.C., which recorded construction work on the Temple of Erechtheus (p. 272), is particularly enlightening, although it may reflect some abnormality in the labor force since Athens was at war. (Athens, however, was usually at war.) The labor force on the Temple of Erechtheus consisted of 24 Athenians, 40 *metics* and 17 slaves engaged in work as stonecutters, carpenters and ordinary laborers. The men were hired individually or in small groups of two or three for their specific jobs. Apparently hiring was quite informal and agreements made only for the performance of a particular piece of work. The state took no interest in regulating conditions of work or wages. Rather surprisingly a standard rate of one drachma per day was paid, without any differential for the different types of work involved. In fact, the architect and a stonecutter received the same wage.

The real meaning of the wage is difficult to determine. Probably a man could find employment for about 250 to 280 days per year, thus earning an annual income of 280 drachmas. His living expenses would amount to about 125 drachmas. An industrious bachelor would fare very well, a married man with two or three children would have no margin over subsistence. The ordinary Athenian, however, lived simply in a small, unpretentious house. His recreation was found in the festivals and public facilities like gymnasiums which were provided by the city. Luxuries of diet, clothing and furniture were for the very rich, although they, too, lived relatively simply. In democratic Athens extravagance and ostentation were quick to attract attention and draw censure.

The financing employed by the Athenian state was simple. The tribute from the Empire and from other imperial profits, war booty, reparations and rent from leased land in the subject states formed the greater part of Athenian revenues, perhaps about six hundred talents a year. In addition Athens leased its silver mines and public land, taxed aliens and collected tolls from the shipping in Athenian harbors. These revenues and those from the Empire amounted in all to about one thousand talents. While no direct tax was levied on Athenian citizens before the Peloponnesian War, the wealthy were subject to regular *liturgies,* a form of capital levy. The most important were the maintenance of a warship for a year and the subsidization of events like the production costs of a drama in the public festivals. Expenditures had to be made for the building of ships, of fortifications, payment of state service and the rearing of war orphans. The Empire revenues made the difference between living hand to mouth and living luxuriously, with a margin for public building on a large-scale and the accumulation of a reserve. In 431 B.C. Athens had a reserve of 6000 talents. This excess was unique for a Greek city-state because most states lived within their annual incomes and had to forego any extraordinary expense. For example, Sparta was able to build a large fleet and to hire sailors in the Peloponnesian War only by direct subsidies in cash from Persia. Athens was the envy of fifth-century Greece for its solvency, expenditures on public buildings and festivals, and for its cash reserve.

Periclean Athens

THE DEMOCRACY

Pericles' system of pay for state service provided the means by which the ordinary Athenian could participate directly in his government. Athenians wished to participate and it was expected of them. "We (Athenians) alone regard a man who takes no interest in public affairs, not as a harmless, but as a useless character," observed Pericles in his famous Funeral Speech in honor of the Athenians killed in war in 431 B.C. Virtually every Athenian citizen acquired familiarity at first-hand both with the routine of governing Athens and with the problems of administering the Empire.

The *ecclesia,* or assembly, was the sovereign political body in the state which included all the citizens. Meeting regularly for discussion and the passage of legislation, it was well organized to deal with business speedily. A speaker presided, a herald made announcements and a secretary kept record of the proceedings. The meeting usually began with the reading of a report from the Council of the Five Hundred. This was debated with full right of amendment and the introduction of motions. Any citizen could speak, but usually the leaders of various small groups or some generally recognized statesman, such as Pericles, carried the discussion. Athens had no regular party system which divided the citizens into several large, well-defined groups with specific policies. A vital question, such as the diversion of the Empire funds or, at a later date, the question of war or peace with Sparta, might force definite alignments. Usually decisions were made by the jockeying and adjustment of small, temporary groupings. The vote was taken after debate by a show of hands, except for *ostracism* and cases of treason, where the ballot was used. Potentially, of course, assembly meetings could be very large, but, in practice, a quorum of six thousand was set for important business. That number was considered to be a "full" assembly. There were factors which tended to affect the decisions. Meetings were held in the city of Athens, which entailed some difficulty for the attendance of farmers from outlying districts. A regular order of business throughout the year corrected this urban weighting to some degree, but a common criticism by the opponents of democracy was that the urban poor dominated the meeting. This criticism was exaggerated, but through the assembly the mass of Athenians, middle and lower class, made the important decisions for Athens.

The *heliaea,* law courts, gave the ordinary Athenians control of the administration of justice. From the panel of six thousand names, changed yearly, juries of varying size were drawn by lot. A magistrate presided at the trial, but the jury decided the question of guilt and set the penalty. An Athenian trial was essentially a legal contest between two citizens before their fellows, since the state took no initiatory action, and any citizen was free to start a suit in his own or the public interest. He presented his own case, although the speech might be written for him by a professional speechwriter. Although legal procedure was speedy once the trial was set, the speeches limited, and the verdict taken as soon as the jury had heard the speeches, the pressure of legal business was great. The delay involved in receiving a prompt hearing was a common complaint. The addition of legal business from the Empire was partly the cause; another was that Athenians enjoyed litigation. Some relief was possible for the Athenian citizens by a system of traveling judges, who heard cases in the *demes,* and by recourse to arbitration. More serious were the complaints about the quality of Athenian justice which referred to the susceptibility of the jurymen to emotional pleas and hasty decisions and the tendency of Athenian politicians to use the courts for political purposes.

Service in the *boule* (the Council of Five Hundred) and in the higher magistracies was limited, but the democratic principles of rotation of office and a low property qualification enabled many Athenians to obtain first-hand administrative and executive experience. The council kept the government functioning by virtually continuous session under the *prytany* system (p. 214). It prepared business for the assembly and supervised the execution of the latter's decrees. In addition, much of the detailed work of supervision and administration, which would be carried on by departments in a modern government, was handled by the council and its committees. The conduct of magistrates was scrutinized, finance and building programs administered, the tribute assessed and matters of military and diplomatic urgency weighed. Election to the council was a mark of confidence and recognition from an Athenian's fellow citizens.

The higher magistracies, which had been very powerful in Athens before the time of Cleisthenes, were weak under the democratic system. The only exception was the chief generalship. Partly as a legacy from aristocratic government and tyranny, partly from the newness of the system, the ordinary Athenian had a profound distrust of superiority. The accounts and conduct of the civil magistrates were closely and regularly scrutinized by the council. Even generals in the field were hampered by fear of political prosecution for failure or for a too-heavy casualty list, and during the Peloponnesian War their strategy was often daring in conception but timid in execution. While use of the lot governed the final selection of the *archons,* those offices which required technical knowledge, such as finance and the generalships, were filled by election. In the whole Athenian system, however, there was room only in the election of generals for a continuity of strong leadership. In the fifth century the Athenians elected a panel of ten generals, of whom one was chief commander, *strategos autokrator.* This latter office might be held any number of times. It was through this chief generalship, which Pericles held fifteen times, that he was able to develop his policy for Athens.

While Athenian democracy allowed a very full participation in government to each Athenian, it is usually charged with several serious defects. In the assembly and in the *heliaea* decisions were taken quickly under the immediate impact of emotion, which could be stirred easily by an able speaker. The Athenians were a quick and volatile people, susceptible to the spoken, rather than the written, word as a result of their education and way of life. They were un-usually well informed and experienced in public affairs, but the success of government depended, too, on the quality of leadership in the assembly. An able and sincere statesman, like Pericles, concerned for the whole state, could give the necessary continuity of direction. An unscrupulous demagogue, devoted to his own or to sectional interest, could do immense damage, as the events of the Peloponnesian War were to demonstrate.

In 431 B.C. Pericles made a funeral speech to honor those Athenians who had died in the fighting during the first year of the Peloponnesian War. It was reported by Thucydides and remains the best statement for democracy from antiquity. There was much that Pericles did not need to enlarge upon, for certain principles, recognized by all, had been established in the course of Athenian political experience from the time of Solon: personal liberty, equality before the law, freedom of speech and action. Pericles himself, although he did not mention his service specifically, had added equality of opportunity for political office. He was chiefly concerned to demonstrate the quality of democracy as a system of government. To Pericles democracy represented the collective interest of the whole state, not that of the lower class, as the enemies of democracy charged, for in the democracy class interest was reconciled, and each citizen had an opportunity to make his contribution to the welfare of the whole. Above all, democracy was educative and liberative, by providing the proper environment for the human spirit to fulfill its potential ability. Life in democratic Athens was marked by freedom and mutual tolerance in private affairs, by openness and free discussion in public matters, and by respect for law and tradition. Democracy was rooted implicitly in trust in the essential goodness of human nature and in the individual's capacity for judgement. The Periclean state, then, could leave much to the individual—his moral conduct, religious beliefs, intellectual life and cultural values—while the government concerned itself with concrete measures for the welfare of the people, whose collective voice was final.

The Athenian Acropolis. Visible on the Acropolis (left to right) are the Propylaea, the Erechtheum, and the Parthenon. At the foot is the Odeum (theater) of Herodes Atticus, built in the second century after Christ.

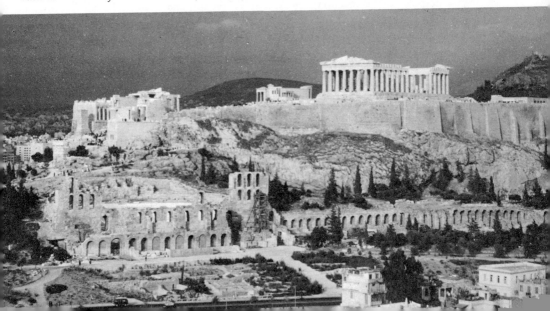

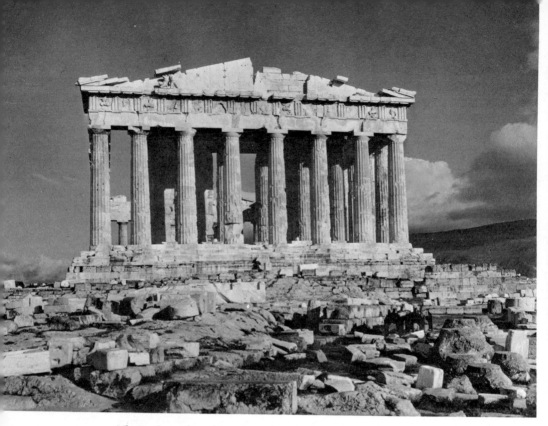

The Parthenon from the west

THE ACROPOLIS

Pericles left a tangible monument of Athens' greatness and of Athenian artistic skill and taste in the group of buildings which still crowns the Athenian Acropolis. Persian destruction of its temples provided the opportunity, and tribute from the Empire helped supply the money, for construction. The walls which surround the Acropolis had been rebuilt by Cimon, so Pericles was able to proceed with the buildings which they enclose. Most important was a new temple, the Parthenon, for Athena Parthenos, the Maiden Goddess who was the patron deity of the state. The Parthenon was begun in 447 B.C. and dedicated in 438 B.C., although its sculpture was not completed until five years later. The architects were Ictinus and Callicrates, and the master-sculptor, Pheidias. The building was of Pentelic marble and Doric in style. It was set on the high point of the Acropolis to dominate not only the other structures but the whole city of Athens and to be an emblem of Athenian history and greatness.

The Parthenon was a large temple, measuring 100 feet by 230 feet and contained two main rooms. The western room, the Parthenon, was used as a treasury, while the eastern, the Hekatompedon or 100-foot room, held the statue of Athena made by Pheidias. The image, of gold and ivory, represented

Athena in the full panoply of war as the patroness of Athenian power and victory. The sculpture on the exterior of the building was similarly appropriate. Presumably Pheidias drew the designs although many sculptors did the work. Around the exterior of the temple, to be viewed from the colonnade, was a frieze, 523 feet in length, representing the Panathenaic Procession, in which the citizens of Athens went up to the Acropolis each year to dedicate a new robe to the goddess. From the west end of the building the procession of knights, maidens and elders was represented as making its way to the gods of Olympus seated in dignity at the east end. The panels of the metopes represented a traditional Greek myth intended to symbolize the victory of civilization over barbarism, the struggle between the human Lapiths and the brute Centaurs who had carried off the Lapith women at a wedding feast. The gables held scenes from Athenian legend. At the east end the birth of Athena from the head of Zeus was depicted and given universal significance by the horses of the Sun rising in one corner and those of the Moon setting in the other. The west gable represented the contest of Athena and the sea-god, Poseidon, for the land of Attica. Just as the institutions of the democracy gave scope to the human spirit, the style of the sculpture represented the ideal dignity of men and the gods.

Upon the dedication of the Parthenon, construction was started on the monumental gateway to the Acropolis, the Propylaea. Under the direction of the architect Mnesicles work was begun in 437 B.C. and terminated in 432 B.C. The gateway was designed to bring traffic through a central corridor, flanked by projecting wings. Apparently the vested interest of older sanctuaries prevented the design from being completely followed out, for the southwest and east wings are abbreviated. The Propylaea was also Doric on the exterior, but the corridor was heightened by the use of more slender Ionic columns. Pericles

Goddesses from the west pediment of the Parthenon (identified as Persephone, Demeter, and Iris)

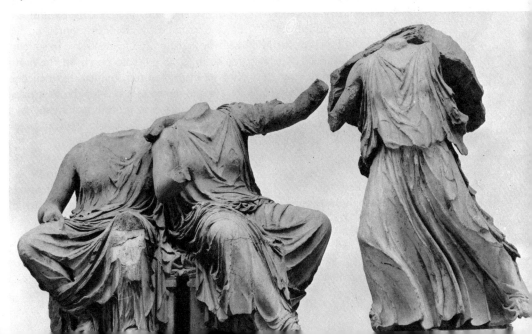

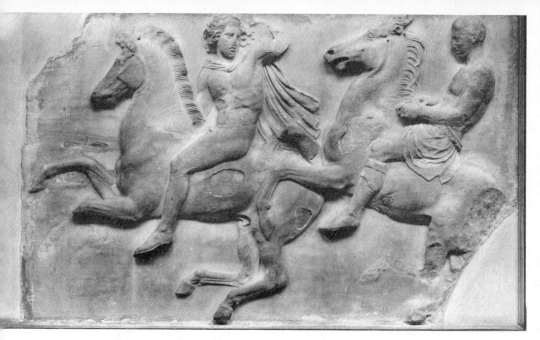

Horsemen in the Panathenaic Procession from the Parthenon frieze

died in 429 B.C., before his design for the Acropolis could be completed. His successors, despite the costs of war, followed the plans and erected the Temple of Athena Nike and the Erechtheum before the defeat of Athens in 404 B.C.

Between 427-24 B.C. the little Ionic Temple of Athena Nike, Victory, was built on the bastion south of the Propylaea to commemorate Athens' victories in war and to be a hopeful augury for the future. Its small size and Ionic delicacy provided a foil for the Doric Propylaea. Construction was begun also on the Erechtheum, north of the Parthenon, but completion was delayed by the vicissitudes of the Peloponnesian War until 406 B.C. The plan of the Erechtheum was unusually complicated, for it had to house three deities and bow to the needs for space of existing sanctuaries. The temple contained the shrines of Athena Polias, the age-old city goddess of the Acropolis, of Erechtheus, a legendary Mycenaean king of Athens, and of Poseidon. Skillful use was made of the difficulties of siting the building by giving it a porch on the south side, the Porch of the Maidens, whose sculptured figures serve to support the porch roof and, as a balance for them, a very ornate porch on the north side. The Erechtheum relieved the heavier majesty of the dominating Parthenon to the south, somewhat as the Nike Temple served as a foil for the Propylaea. The achievement of Athens in the fifth century was fittingly commemorated in this complex of buildings, which became the models of Classical Greek sculpture and architecture for succeeding generations.

DRAMA

In the Periclean Age Athens became an intellectual center, drawing writers and philosophers from all the cities of Greece to enjoy the hospitality of

Pericles, but the city's most vital intellectual force was its own tragic drama. The origin of the drama is obscure, like that of other genres growing from folk practice, although the presentations presumably developed from a religious performance of song and dance by a large chorus. Perhaps in the sixth century this choral recitation of heroic legends, with some mimetic action, was made a part of the Dionysiac cult festivals, which were very popular at that time. In Athens Peisistratus made the Dionysiac festival a regular part of the civic religion, and the playwright, Thespis, is said to have combined the chorus with an actor delivering set speeches. While this innovation would allow comment and description, the dramatic tension of two or more confronting figures was still absent. The real founder of tragedy was Aeschylus, who is credited with the introduction of a second actor and with the use of serious subject matter, drawn from the whole range of Greek myth and legend.

In the fifth century, the Athenians enlarged the dramatic festivals by adding the presentation of comedy in 487 B.C. The earliest comedies extant, however, are those of Aristophanes, dating from the period of the Peloponnesian War (p. 298). For the tragic festival, the competitors entered a set of three plays, a trilogy, to which was added a satyr play, a piece of buffoonery, to serve as comic relief. From the entries three works were selected for the final round, which was judged by a committee selected from the Athenian citizens. Costs of production were borne by a wealthy citizen as a regular liturgy for the state, similar to the outfitting of a trireme for war. Since the prestige of victory was great for both writer and patron, regular records were kept of the winners of the contests, which give us some idea of what the Athenians thought of the plays we now possess. Most of them won prizes, but we have only a very small selection of the large number of plays performed. The drama was regarded, of course, as a means of serious religious instruction, dealing with moral and theological problems, and Athenian citizens attended the presentations as part of their religious life. In the hands of the great tragedians, Aeschylus, Sophocles and Euripides, drama also became a great literary form. In these few pages only a brief idea of its formal nature can be given and the writers set in their historical background.

A caryatid from the Erechtheum

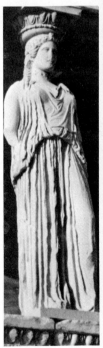

Greek tragedy had the combined effect of modern opera and drama, since the choral parts were sung and danced, while the dialogue was spoken. Although the part of the chorus declined steadily, until it was little more than musical interlude, the chorus at its best was an intelligent spectator, commenting appropriately on the progress of the action and reflecting the emotional development of the play. There was relatively little direct representation of action, and the spoken parts consisted of monologue, set speeches and dialogue, with reports of the action as needed. Consequently, diction and language were supremely important in the presentation, while stage effects and elaborate scenery could be kept to a minimum. The form of the Greek theater, familiar to us from the well-preserved examples in Athens and at Epidaurus (p. 330), belongs to the period subsequent to the great period of the drama.

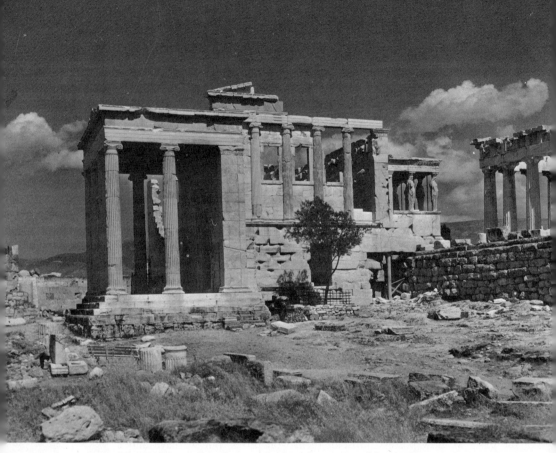

The Erechtheum from the west. On the right a corner of the Parthenon

Aeschylus (525–456 B.C.) lived in the generation of the Persian Wars and of Cimonian Panhellenism, during which Athens rose to greatness. He fought as a soldier at Marathon and in the battles against Xerxes. Most of Aeschylus' life was spent in Athens, but in 467 B.C. he was a guest at the court of Hiero I, the tyrant of Syracuse, for whom he wrote a play, and in 456 he died in Gela, while on another visit to Sicily. Aeschylus was an extremely prolific playwright and is credited with writing ninety plays, seven of which have survived. Some of these refer to contemporary events. Aeschylus' earliest surviving play, the *Persians,* produced in 472 B.C., is the only Greek drama extant which has a theme directly from contemporary history. It contains a spirited description of the sea battle at Salamis in 480 B.C., recounted by a messenger to the Persian court, and the whole play extols the glory of Athens. The *Oresteia,* our only surviving trilogy, performed in 458 B.C., deals with the expiation of blood guilt in the family of Agamemnon and praises the new role which had just been assigned to the Areopagus. Since the play was written shortly after the time when Ephialtes and Pericles reformed that body, we might conclude that Aeschylus felt sympathy with the new, Periclean, type of democracy.

The value of Aeschylus' plays, of course, lies not in their response to contemporary history, but in the quality of Aeschylus as a dramatist and religious thinker. He is considered the most powerful of Greek tragedians, with a unique ability to build up a slowly growing suspense to the breaking point and a mastery of imaginative diction to express the deep conceptions of his thought. As noticed before, Aeschylus set the tone of Greek drama as a profoundly serious teaching of the problems of theology and morality. He was concerned to present the gods in all their terrifying power and mystery, with Zeus as the arbiter of destiny and justice for mankind.

Sophocles' life (*ca.* 497–06 B.C.) covers virtually the whole of the fifth century, but he is regarded as the particular dramatist of Periclean Athens, for nearly all his surviving plays were written before the Peloponnesian War. Like Aeschylus, Sophocles played a full and distinguished part as an Athenian citizen, being elected to the board of *Hellenotamiae* in 443 B.C. and to a generalship at the time of the Samian revolt in 440 B.C. He was a friend of Pericles and of Herodotus and, certainly, a sympathetic admirer of Euripides, whose death he publicly mourned, although their conceptions of drama were very different. Sophocles was also a voluminous writer, credited with about 120 plays, of which we possess only seven. He is said to have made numerous minor technical innovations in the drama and the important one of adding a third actor, by which he was able to increase the complexity of his plots. Rather than long trilogies Sophocles wrote plays complete in themselves, in which he concentrated on character and plot. Sophocles is praised for the fine balance between choral and dramatic elements in his plays and for the use of the choral odes to weave action and emotional development together. His plays are on a more human plane of interest than those of Aeschylus, being more concerned with human conduct than with divine principles. He is regarded as the most "classic" of the three great dramatists of Athens, writing with a mastery of the dramatic form and with subtle harmony of language and structure. Aristotle pronounced the *Oedipus Tyrannus* the most perfect of plays.

The proof, as for all the Greek drama, is in the reading or performance, rather than in a brief description. The dramatic conceptions of Euripides and of Aristophanes were very different from those of their two predecessors and are better understood in the context of intellectual change which the Athenians experienced in the course of the Peloponnesian War (pp. 295-301).

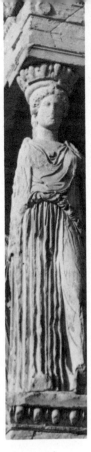

A caryatid from the Erechtheum

XIII

The Peloponnesian War

(431–404 B.C.)

THE GENERAL PEACE established with Persia (448 B.C.) and Sparta (445 B.C.) proved brief for the Athenians, since in 431 B.C. war broke out again with Sparta and its allies. The Peloponnesian War, as it is called, ultimately drew in most of the Greek city-states and Persia. The two great coalitions fought for ten years to a virtual stalemate. In 421 B.C. they made a nominal peace, but six years later the Athenians invaded Sicily in a reckless attempt to add Magna Graecia to the Empire. When the invasion failed at great cost to Athens, the subject states of the Empire were encouraged to revolt. Persia, too, was encouraged to subsidize the construction of a fleet for Sparta, and the combination was too great for Athens to bear. In 404 B.C. the Athenians surrendered and gave up the remnants of their Empire.

The Peloponnesian War was a turning point in the history of Greece, for the struggle between Athens and Sparta encouraged revolution and civil war in many states where democrats and oligarchs fought for control. The internal unity and stability of the city-state were shattered. Men's minds, too, were transformed when a new generation, accustomed to the excitement and the rapid change of war, questioned traditional beliefs and customs. A revolution in thought and education, the Sophistic Movement, laid the groundwork for the philosophies of Plato and Aristotle in the next century. These more profound aspects of the war, as well as its military events, were well understood by the historian Thucydides who wrote its history.

Thucydides and His History

Thucydides (*ca.* 460–400 B.C.) was an Athenian, born about 460 B.C., when Pericles was winning the political leadership of Athens. As a young man

The reader will find Maps VII, IX, XI, XII (pages 172–173, 202, 284, and 293) useful as he reads this chapter.

Thucydides saw the fruits of the Periclean policy in the well-being and confidence of Athens which came during the years of peace after 445 B.C. He expressed his admiration in the Funeral Speech of Pericles (p. 269) and in passages praising the quality of Pericles' political wisdom. Little is known about Thucydides' life, but he fought for Athens until 424 B.C. with considerable skill and courage. We know that he was elected general for that year and assigned to a command in Thrace. Through no fault of his own he failed to prevent the loss of Amphipolis to the enemy and was penalized by banishment. Thucydides then turned his exile to advantage by visits to Sparta and elsewhere in Greece to collect material for his history of the war. Although he probably lived to 400 B.C., the history was not finished but breaks off in the events of 411 B.C. Neither Thucydides' loyalty to Periclean Athens nor banishment by the Athenians affected his remarkable impartiality. His primary concern was to give as true an account of the war as he could and to relate its particular occurrences to the general pattern of human behavior.

Thucydides recognized the war as the greatest conflict ever fought in Greece, since Athens and Sparta were at the height of their power. Athens, in particular, had made itself great by exploiting the very factors which had stimulated the development of Greece—sea power and the accumulation of capital wealth. To demonstrate this point, Thucydides wrote a sketch of early Greek history as an introduction to his book. He laid aside the framework of myth, in which the Greeks had set their past, and, by a remarkable exercise of rationalizing historical judgment, reconstructed the early history of Greece in real terms. This was also the approach he used in his history of the war—first, collecting and appraising information carefully; then, studying this material in the light of the behavior of human beings and of states.

Thucydides described the events of the war year by year, but the narrative moves on two levels of meaning. The detailed military action is written in a vivid fashion, through which the reader can relive the event and feel the sudden impact of unexpected turns of fortune. The deeper meaning and political movement of the war is presented dramatically by the use of paired speeches. In them Thucydides mingles what was actually said by the speakers with what he felt appropriate to show the elements involved in a critical situation. The speeches are not strictly historical but serve as a means of analysis or presenting differing points of view. In this manner the national psychology of Athenians and Spartans is contrasted, and the fear of Athens felt by other Greek states is revealed. The changing temper of the Athenians themselves is demonstrated by appropriate speeches at critical moments throughout the war's course.

Unlike Herodotus, Thucydides conceived of history as occurring in a world of purely human action, without divine direction or interference. In his view men are responsible for their history, can shape it by their intelligence, and avoid being its victims. Thus, the Athenians, who had established the Empire by energy and opportunism, and the Spartans, who naturally resented and envied Athens' rise to prominence, were themselves responsible for the conflict. The war was inevitable from the course of action which each, Athens in particular, had chosen to follow. Their choice was made because they acted as men will in such circumstances, but the intelligent man could assess such situations and, perhaps, avoid them. He could estimate the force of human instincts to dominate the weak, to defend possessions and cherish prestige. Thucydides tried to single out the psychological factors which are operative in men and show how they work. In his thinking history could be instructive, for, while it does not repeat itself, the causes of political behavior are constant, even if the context changes. Thucydides examined the war with an awesome clarity and the realization that Greece was experiencing a tragedy of its own making.

The Steps to War

In the period after the peace treaty with Sparta in 445 B.C. the success of Pericles' diplomacy and his skill in organizing the Empire had heightened the atmosphere of distrust with which the rest of Greece regarded Athens. In 433 B.C. Pericles began to act more provocatively and hastened the coming of war. First, Athens accepted an offer of alliance with Corcyra, despite the warning of Corinth that such an act was hostile and would break the peace.

Corcyra, founded by Corinth three hundred years previously, had grown into a moderately powerful maritime state by exploiting its strategic position on the crossing from Greece to Magna Graecia. While the Corcyreans had long since rebuffed Corinthian attempts at control, they had joined Corinth in founding colonies along the coast of northwestern Greece. Corcyra provided some of the settlers, while Corinth had furnished the founder. In one of these colonies, Epidamnus, factional strife broke out between democrats and oligarchs in 435 B.C. The factions turned for help to Corinth and Corcyra respectively, and a full-scale war developed in which Corinth enlisted the help of some of the smaller Peloponnesian states. Sparta remained aloof and vainly urged arbitration to settle the dispute. The Corcyreans, who had hitherto prided themselves on their political isolation, now turned to Athens for help. They pointed out how useful it would be to Athens to acquire such a strategically situated ally as themselves, and to add the Corcyrean fleet—the third largest in Greece—to the Athenian navy. These considerations outweighed the warning given by Corinth, and Athens made a defensive alliance with Corcyra in 433 B.C. Legally, the Athenian action was defensible, for Corcyra was not a member of the Peloponnesian League, protected by treaty from Athenian interference, but the new alliance certainly threatened the position of Corinth in the Adriatic Sea. Almost immediately Athens demonstrated that it would support Corcyra, for an Athenian naval squadron forced the Corinthian fleet to break off a successful engagement with the Corcyreans. Corinth began to urge Sparta and the other members of the Peloponnesian League to war.

In the following year the Corinthians were aggravated still further, when Athens issued an ultimatum to Potidaea in the Macedonian Chalcidice which was once a Corinthian colony but had been taken over by Athens into the Delian League after the Persian Wars. Although the city was tributary to Athens, the Athenians had concurred up to this time in a traditional practice by which Corinth sent an official annually to its former colony. In 432 B.C. the Athenian ultimatum ordered the people of Potidaea to expel the official, give hostages to Athens, and tear down their city walls. In desperation Potidaea turned to Corinth and, through the good offices of that city, got a secret promise from the Spartan government to invade Attica, if Athens attacked Potidaea. The Corinthians aided by sending a force of two thousand Peloponnesian "volunteers" to Potidaea and by helping to stir revolt among other Athenian tributaries of the district in collusion with Perdiccas, the king of Macedonia. Perdiccas' aim was simply to increase his own territory, but his sudden action forced Athens to put a large force into the area. Potidaea was besieged and unofficially Athens and Corinth were at war.

Pericles' next move against the Peloponnesian League created a situation from which there could be no withdrawal without the disintegration of the League itself. Athens issued the Megarian Decrees, by which Megara was excluded from the use of any port in the Athenian Empire. The purpose of the Decrees was not so much to hurt Megara as to warn Athens' enemies of what to expect. Megara refused to be intimidated and added its voice to that of Corinth in urging Sparta to declare war on Athens. Their pleas were heeded. The Spartan assembly itself decided for war and then convoked a meeting of the Peloponnesian League, in which the whole Spartan alliance was brought into line. The Athenian actions were branded as deliberately provocative, and the decision for war was taken in the conviction that Greek freedom was at stake.

Pericles' confidence in taking the risk of war seemed justified by his careful estimate of Athenian resources and of the strategy to be based on them. The financial position of the state was excellent, with a reserve of six thousand talents in the treasury. Since the Athenian fleet was in full control of the Aegean Sea, the Empire could be held, and the importation of grain from the Black Sea and from Egypt assured without difficulty. Although the Spartan and Boeotian armies could invade Attica almost at will, the Athenians would be safe behind the walls of the city and would be able to get their supplies in from Peiraeus through the Long Walls. The Athenians could not hope to defeat their enemies in a full-scale land battle, for they could muster only about 23,000 *hoplites* against the 50,000 or more which Sparta could call upon. Accordingly, Pericles planned to bring the citizens into the city from their farms and to avoid battle. Pericles' strategy, however, was not entirely defensive. The alliance with Corcyra opened up the possibility of successful action in northwestern Greece, where Corinthian sea power, effective in the Gulf of Corinth and the Adriatic Sea, might be defeated, thus hampering the import of grain from Sicily to the Peloponnesus. Raids were planned also along the coast of the Peloponnesus. Yet, even if it had been possible to blockade the whole Peloponnesus, the Spartan coalition could hardly be starved into defeat, for some of its members produced a surplus of grain, and all of them could communicate freely by land. Hope of victory for Athens lay in making the war seem endless to the enemy and wearying the Spartan alliance into disintegration.

The Spartan king, Archidamus, reasoned along much the same lines. He hoped that the volatile Athenians would lose their patience and send the army out of the city to fight for the Athenian countryside. On land the position and resources of the Spartan alliance were very strong. All the major states of the Peloponnesus, except Argos, belonged to the Peloponnesian League, and the neutrality of Argos was assured by a treaty for ten years. Boeotia, headed by Thebes, was solidly on the Spartan side except for Plataea, and the Boeotians placed it under siege at the outset of the war. So long as the Peloponnesian League held Megara, communication from the Peloponnesus to Boeotia was easy, and they could join in laying Attica waste.

There was little hope of fighting Athens at sea. The Corinthian navy was too small to offer battle in the Aegean, and the Peloponnesian states lacked money to build a fleet. Early in the war Sparta made an attempt to get financial help from the Persians, but the latter judged that at that time Athens was too strong to be attacked. At the outset, then, the war seemed likely to be a contest in staying power, with neither Athens nor Sparta in a position to do vital damage. In general the conflict maintained this character for the first ten years, during the so-called Archidamian phase, because Archidamus, the king of Sparta, had estimated its nature correctly.

The Archidamian War (431–21 B.C.)

In the first two years the war developed as each side had anticipated. The Peloponnesian army invaded Attica to destroy the standing crop and to burn farmhouses and orchards, while the Athenians crowded into the city to find an uncomfortable security. The open areas of Athens mushroomed with shacks and water was scarce, but grain came in from Peiraeus, and the Athenians could derive some comfort from their successful raids on the Peloponnesian coast and by guaranteeing control of Aegina through the installation of a *cleruch* settlement.

Both sides revealed a bitter temper in their fighting and largely ignored the conventions of war in pressing the sieges of Potidaea and Plataea to extremes. The Athenians grimly tightened the siege of Potidaea and forced the garrison to cannibalism before it surrendered in the winter of 429 B.C. The Potidaeans were turned loose to find what refuge they could among the native people of the district. The Plataeans, cut off from effective Athenian help, held out until 428 B.C. Then the people surrendered on condition of a fair trial, but the Spartan judges asked only one question—whether the Plataeans had helped the Spartan alliance in the war. Because there could be no answer, Sparta allowed the Thebans to execute the men and sell the women and children into slavery.

THE PLAGUE

On the whole the Athenians could be satisfied with the progress of the war until 430/29 B.C., when a paralyzing blow struck Athens. A mysterious plague, brought by ship from Egypt, began to rage violently in the city, crowded with refugees and suffering from lack of sanitation and water. Thucydides himself was attacked but recovered and included in his history a clinical description of the symptoms and course of the disease, along with a telling account of its effect on Athenian morale: "The crowding of the people out of the country into the city aggravated the misery; and the newly arrived suffered most. For having no houses of their own, but inhabiting in the heat of summer stifling huts, the mortality among them was dreadful, and they perished in wild disorder. . . . the violence of the calamity was such that men, not knowing where to turn, grew reckless of all law, human and divine. . . . they reflected that life and riches were alike transitory, and they resolved to enjoy themselves while they could, and to think only of pleasure." In the depth of their suffering the Athenians even asked for peace from Sparta but were refused. The winter of 429 B.C. marked the climax of the plague, but it lasted for three years in all and had left Athens shaken and demoralized, without the steadying leadership of Pericles. He had died of the plague in the autumn of 429 B.C.

The results of the plague were lasting. Although the Spartans were afraid to approach Athens while the disease was at its height and failed to press their temporary advantage, Athens was hard hit. It is estimated that about one-third of the population died, and this not only depleted the existing military force, but thinned out the recruits for a generation. The psychological effects of the disease were even more telling. Because medicine could not account rationally for the appearance and disappearance of the plague, the feeling persisted that Athens had offended heaven and could do little but hope for a reversal of fortune. The temper of the Athenians, naturally volatile, began to swing from despair and vindictive hatred to exaggerated optimism, as the events of the war turned out badly or well. That collective judgment of the assembly, on which Pericles had taught Athens to pride itself, was badly impaired. The Athenian fleet, however, was not damaged, and in 429 B.C. an Athenian admiral, Phormio, won a brilliant victory in the Corinthian Gulf against superior forces. Athens took a firmer grip on the war in the following year, and a new leader, Cleon, replaced Pericles.

THE LEADERSHIP OF CLEON

The weakness of Athens encouraged thoughts of revolt among the members of the Empire. In 428 the oligarchical leaders of Mytilene, the largest city on Lesbos and one of the remaining two free allies of Athens, plotted to withdraw. The oligarchs received a promise of help from Sparta, but when the plan was leaked to Athens the Athenians promptly blockaded the city. The Spartans had been faster with their promises than with help, and Mytilene surrendered a week before a small Peloponnesian fleet arrived off the coast of Asia Minor.

The Spartan commander, instead of trying to help Mytilene or to spread the revolt, by scurrying back to the Peloponnesus lost the chance to shake Athens' hold on the islands. The Athenians, smarting with anger, proceeded to discuss the punishment of Mytilene.

In Athens the hurt of war and of the plague was beginning to split that unity of feeling which Pericles had fostered. The war bore heavily on the conservative upper class through *liturgies* and the damage done to their estates, and on the small-scale farmers, whose sole source of livelihood was from their farms. These men thought naturally of the pleasant days before the war and of the prospects of a fair peace. They were not disloyal to Athens, but the war was stretching out, and fate had disclosed its ugly side. On the other hand, war had brought profit to the shopkeepers, pedlars and keepers of lodging houses in the city when the farmers poured in. Craftsmen and traders could still sell their goods in Athens and throughout the Empire, while the sailors of the fleet had steady pay and little fighting. This urban group was numerically superior and found new leaders to fill the place of Pericles. Chief among these was a wealthy tanner, Cleon, an unscrupulous and able demagogue, who knew how to play on the moods of the assembly.

Cleon exploited the desire of the Athenians to exact vengeance from Mytilene for its treachery and argued that Athens should exercise only expediency in dealing with members of the Empire. In the circumstances he called for a terrifying example, putting the men of Mytilene to death and enslaving the women and children. After Cleon's proposal carried in the assembly, a ship was sent off to notify the Athenian commander at Mytilene to proceed with the work. On the following morning, however, a change of heart was perceptible among the citizens, and Diodotus, a leader of the conservative group, urged that the penalty be revoked. He, too, had to talk in terms of expediency to get a hearing, but he argued that control of the Empire could be assured better by calculated leniency. He suggested that they let Mytilene's walls be dismantled, its ships surrendered, and the land be confiscated for Athenian *cleruchs*. The Mytilenians could work the land and pay one hundred talents as an annual rent. This cynical compassion appealed to the assembly, and a second ship was sent off to rescind the original order. The vessel arrived in time to prevent the massacre. The episode is illustrative of the changing temper of the Athenian assembly and of the political methods of its demagogues. While it is scarcely possible to distinguish between a war and a peace party at this time, the Athenians were beginning to divide on vital matters of policy concerning the war and the Empire. Cleon and the "war group" were prepared to extend the fighting recklessly to force a successful conclusion and, as the passage of the coinage decree in 425 indicates, to tighten Athenian economic control of the Empire.

Under Cleon's militant leadership, which discarded the prudence of Pericles, the Athenians almost won the war as they turned to the offensive in the next three years. In 427 B.C. an opportunity was offered for interference in

Sicily. Leontini and Rhegium invited Athenian help against Syracuse, and Athens responded with a small force of twenty ships. That was sufficient to keep Sicily in disorder and to cut down the supply of grain to the Peloponnesus. In 424 B.C., however, when Athens made no further substantial commitment, Syracuse induced its enemies to form a united front and invite the Athenians to go home. Perhaps Athens had lost a good chance, but the city was too weak to support a major war in two theaters, and after 427 B.C. it had to keep a watchful eye on Corcyra.

In Corcyra revolution erupted. Thucydides singles this out as typical of the internal division growing among all the allies and subjects of Athens as the war stretched on. The oligarchical group, who identified freedom with the Spartan cause, gathered strength, waiting a chance to take over the city. Civil war began when the oligarchs killed off sixty of their opponents in the council house and seized the government. The Athenians had to intervene to help the democrats, who, in their turn, initiated a pitiless massacre of the oligarchs. Corcyra was retained as an ally, but its people were embittered and could give little help to Athens.

Although Corcyra's revolution had impaired Athenian action across the Adriatic, a new Athenian general, Demosthenes, gave Athens its first victory over the Peloponnesians on land. In 426 B.C. Demosthenes was assigned to command in northwestern Greece. His first campaign—an ambitious plan to march through Aetolia and attack Boeotia from the west—was a failure because he had too few men and underestimated the ability of the Aetolians to conduct a guerilla war in the mountains. In the next year, however, when a Peloponnesian force crossed the Gulf of Corinth to take advantage of Demosthenes' losses and occupy Naupactus, he defeated them heavily and won Athens' first triumph over front-line Peloponnesian troops in the war. Athenian morale soared again, and the assembly sent a fleet to Corcyra and Sicily, with Demosthenes on board, mysteriously entrusted to take whatever action he wished around the Peloponnesus. He chose to fortify the rocky, uninhabited promontory of Pylus in western Messenia.

The Athenian occupation of Pylus and the resultant victory over the Spartans has an almost comic opera atmosphere of success by blundering good luck. Pylus closed the north end of the Bay of Navarino, the best harbor in the western Peloponnesus. At that time the area was unprotected and sparsely inhabited, for the *helot* farms of Messenia lay to the east of the hills which enclosed the bay. Across the harbor entrance was the island of Sphacteria. As the Athenian fleet was sailing north along the Peloponnesian coast, a storm arose and the fleet put into Pylus for shelter. Demosthenes wanted to fortify the promontory, but the generals in charge refused. The soldiers and sailors, bored by waiting around, began to throw up a rough wall of clay and rocks. When the fleet sailed, Demosthenes was left with five ships to defend his little fortress. Presumably he expected to use it as a base for raiding and as a refuge for *helot* deserters. He was speedily attacked by a Spartan force, which stationed

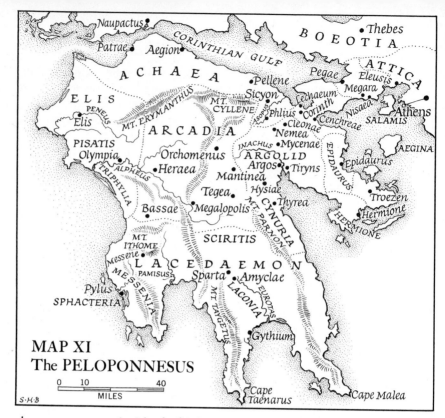

MAP XI
The PELOPONNESUS

0   10   40
MILES

S·H·B

about 420 men on the island of Sphacteria to hold the harbor entrance. Demosthenes recalled the Athenian fleet, which arrived in time to relieve him, and he was able to blockade the men on Sphacteria.

The effect of this small operation on the Spartans was astonishing. They judged that rescue of the men on Sphacteria was hopeless and arranged a truce, during which negotiations for peace could be carried on without consultation of their allies. Although about half of the force on the island were Spartan citizens whose capture would bring great disgrace to Sparta, Spartans had fought to the death before this at Thermopylae. Probably the real aim of Sparta was to recover the Athenian fort on Pylus, from which a *helot* revolt might be stirred up. In any case, they were prepared to go to a considerable length to get peace, but not as far as Athens demanded.

On Cleon's advice the Athenians made a series of demands which Sparta could not accept without the consent of its allies, so that the negotiations broke down. Athens sent reinforcements to Pylus, bringing the number of troops there up to fourteen thousand. This should have been enough to overwhelm the island's garrison of about four hundred, but the Athenians were strangely reluctant to attack. Athenian lives were also precious, or, as Cleon suspected, the Athenian generals were dragging their feet and were more anxious to gain a negotiated peace than to win a hard-fought victory.

Cleon demanded action, boasting that he could take Sphacteria and get back to Athens within twenty days. By way of answer the assembly assigned

284

him to command the operation and allowed him to name Demosthenes as his colleague. On Cleon's arrival in Pylus a fire was started by chance on the island, which burned off the cover and exposed the Spartan positions. The situation of the garrison was hopeless, cut off from food and water and exposed to Athenian arrows and spears. The Spartan government authorized the men to surrender, despite their offer to fight to the end, and Cleon returned to Athens within the promised twenty days.

Athens' refusal to negotiate seriously with Sparta at this time is regarded by Thucydides as the turning point of the war. Neither side had suffered beyond the possibility of recovery, and in each there were substantial groups favoring peace. Athens, in fact, would have profited greatly by accepting the Spartan offer of peace and alliance. In addition to gaining prestige, Athens would have been the dominant partner of a pact made in such circumstances, and Sparta would have lost its coalition. Instead, Cleon tried for complete military victory and failed.

After the success at Pylus, Cleon planned a far-reaching series of operations. The Peloponnesus was almost besieged by attacks on all sides. Messenians from Naupactus were stationed at Pylus, and an Athenian force was sent to occupy the island of Cythera, off the southeast tip of the Peloponnesus, from which shipping could be controlled. A successful raid was made on the Corinthian coast and a garrison left to harass the Peloponnesians. Then the tide of war turned. The Athenians planned both a full-scale assault on Megara, to cut the road from the Peloponnesus, and also an invasion of Boeotia simultaneously from the west and the east. The attack on Megara failed, thanks to the speedy action of a new and brilliant Spartan general, Brasidas. Success against Boeotia depended on secrecy and proper timing, both of which were bungled. The attack from the west was driven off before the force from Attica arrived at its proper destination, forewarning the Boeotians and allowing them to inflict a very heavy defeat on the Athenian army at Delium. Cleon had failed to capitalize on his opportunity, and the initiative passed again to Sparta.

The Spartans, at the urging of Brasidas, decided to create a diversion in Thrace, where Perdiccas of Macedonia was pleased to cooperate in upsetting Athenian influence. Brasidas, with a small force, slipped skillfully through Thessaly, which was allied to Athens, and arrived safely in Thrace. There he soon posed a serious threat to the Athenians, for, in addition to his military skill, Brasidas showed an unusual political finesse and personal integrity. He kept his pledge of freedom to those towns which revolted from Athens, although Perdiccas had expected to add them to his kingdom. Brasidas' chief prize was Amphipolis which he detached from the Athenians in 424 B.C., before Thucydides could arrive on the scene. Back in Athens news of Brasidas' success, coupled with the heavy loss at Delium, had weakened Cleon's position, and the Athenians began to negotiate with Sparta for a truce. The Spartans, too, now that they had Brasidas' achievements to bargain with, were agreeable, and in 423 B.C. a truce was made for one year, during which the advocates of peace on each side hoped to negotiate a treaty. The negotiations failed, since dispute arose over the time at which Brasidas had captured certain towns, and, in disgust at Sparta's lack of support for him, he kept on fighting. When the truce expired, Athens had to make a full-scale effort to recover the losses in Thrace and named Cleon as general. He rashly attacked Amphipolis and his force was driven off, but both he and Brasidas were killed in the fighting. With the war leaders on each side dead, the proponents of peace were able to negotiate once more, and in 421 B.C. a settlement was worked out, largely by the Athenian conservative leader, Nicias. He was a representative of the landed groups in Athens, and his election as general revealed the swing of opinion for a negotiated settlement.

The Peace of Nicias (421–15 B.C.)

The Peace of Nicias resolved none of the basic issues for which the war had started, but was the result of war-weariness and of the realization that neither side could achieve a complete victory. Sparta wished to recover the men on Sphacteria and be free to act when the alliance with Argos terminated, for the Argives did not seem disposed to renew it. Athens had suffered severe losses at the battle of Delium and exhausted its finances in the extensive operations of the past few years. Neither side was in a position to demand much from the other, but, on the whole, Athens emerged in the stronger position.

The settlement made peace for fifty years, but with the proviso that the oaths guaranteeing the treaty had to be renewed annually. Disputes were to be settled by arbitration, and each side pledged to restore its prisoners of war and to hand over the places which had been captured. The latter clause caused great dispute and, indeed, was never fully carried out. For example, those towns freed by Brasidas showed no disposition to re-enter the Athenian Empire, and Athens felt that it was Sparta's duty to recapture them. Pending that unlikely eventuality, the Athenians would not give up Pylus. Also, the claims of Sparta's allies were ignored. Thebes and Corinth were particularly dissatisfied, for Thebes would have to forego the pleasures of raiding Attica, and the Corinthians did not recover their colonies in northwestern Greece which had been taken by Athens. When the treaty was presented to the Spartan allies for ratification, Thebes, Megara, Corinth, and Elis rejected it and, in effect, broke up the Spartan alliance. To protect herself, Sparta made a defensive pact with Athens, by which each pledged to aid the other in the event of attack. The fighting had stopped, and each state was concerned to restore and strengthen its position.

In the diplomatic struggles of the years immediately following the Peace, Sparta contrived to reform its alliance, while Athens again committed itself to imperialistic aggrandizement and war. Argos, upon the lapse of its treaty with Sparta, began to form a new coalition with the disgruntled Spartan allies. While Sparta had formally provided against Athenian entry into this coalition, the opportunity to join Argos and to renew the war was tempting to the Athenians and became a matter of party politics. Nicias and the "peace" groups firmly supported the Spartan alliance, but the democratic "war" party found a new leader in Alcibiades the Alcmeonid and regarded Athens' chances optimistically once more.

Alcibiades was destined to have one of the most picturesque careers in antiquity. In 420 B.C. he was young, wealthy, strikingly handsome, with abilities on the order of genius, but completely undisciplined. Like his Alcmeonid ancestors, Alcibiades became a popular leader, but his democratic colleagues suspected that his real aim was a personal tyranny in Athens rather than preservation of the democratic system. He made friends and enemies easily and through sheer charm or insolence as the occasion required got away with escapades which would have ruined an ordinary man's career. When Argos approached Athens directly with an invitation to join its coalition, the infectious enthusiasm of Alcibiades persuaded the Athenians to accept and to embarrass Sparta with a demand for the restoration of the Thracian towns.

The alliance with Argos was Athens' first step on the road back to war, but the peace groups were still sufficiently strong to keep the city from sending military aid to Argos when hostilities began in the Peloponnesus. "Volunteers" appeared on the Argive side, but Sparta ignored their presence and acted only against the Peloponnesian allies of Argos. At the battle of Mantinea in 418 B.C. Sparta decisively defeated the Argive coalition and brought the Peloponnesians back into line. Athenian energy was diverted from meddling in the Peloponnesus to strengthening the Empire and putting its finances in order. The Athenian farms were soon back in production, although the olive groves were crippled for a generation. As trade recovered and the tribute came in regularly, the well-being of the prewar period seemed to be returning.

The Athenian people were ready for action and decided to bring the small island of Melos in the southwestern Aegean into the Empire. Melos had been settled by Dorians at a very early date and was of no particular strategic importance, but it had flouted Athens. In 425 B.C., under the drive of Cleon's imperialism, Athens seems to have assessed Melos for tribute and included it in the Empire. The Melians had apparently disregarded this one-sided assertion of control and had pursued a course of neutrality in the war with impunity. In 416 B.C. the Athenians felt that Melian neutrality could be tolerated no longer and issued an ultimatum to the Melians to join the Empire voluntarily or be brought in by force.

Thucydides developed the episode at some length in his Melian Dialogue, to illustrate the nature of Athenian imperialism on the eve of the Sicilian expedition. The Melian officials pleaded their case with adroitness and dignity, but the arguments fell on deaf ears. The Athenian generals stated that Athens had no cause to fear reprisal from Sparta and Melos none to hope for it. Athens would seek only its own advantage, the incorporation of Melos into the Empire, and would pay no heed to the feelings of conventional morality, decency, or religion. Upon the Melian refusal to surrender the island was attacked and taken, the men were killed, the women and children were enslaved, and the land was given to Athenian *cleruchs*. In this mood of deliberate aggrandizement, the Athenians listened to a request for aid from their Sicilian allies.

The Sicilian Expedition (415–12 B.C.)

In 416 B.C. the Sicilian city of Segesta, at war with its neighbor, Selinus, invited Athenian help, offering to pay the costs. The Athenians, at first properly cautious, sent envoys to investigate, but the men were deceived and brought back a favorable report on Segesta's ability to pay. The opportunity to fight a war which would cost nothing and to add new tribute-paying members to the Empire caught the fancy of the Athenian assembly. To Alcibiades Segesta's invitation seemed to be the key which would unlock Magna Graecia and the western Mediterranean to Athenian conquest. The assembly quickly passed a resolution: "to assist the Segestans, . . . to restore the Leontines (a former ally), and generally to further in such manner as they deemed best the Athenian interests in Sicily." Athenian knowledge of affairs in Sicily and consideration of their own position in Greece was as vague as the last clause of their resolution. At the least, an attack on Selinus would involve war with Syracuse, to which Selinus was allied. The Athenians forgot that Syracuse had been able to form a united front against them in 424 B.C. Also, in Greece Athenian behavior toward Sparta since the Peace of Nicias gave that state cause for war at any time, and Athens was already fighting with Corinth as the result of a raid on the latter's territory in the previous year. All these considerations, as well as the great cost of supplying a force by sea hundreds of miles distant, were ignored.

Nicias alone, who represented the more cautious feeling in Athens, tried to dissuade the assembly by representing the situation realistically. He attacked the irresponsibility of Alcibiades and finally urged, if the Athenians must go to Sicily, that they send a much larger force. Only the latter argument made any impression, and that was not what Nicias had expected, for the assembly authorized a force which amounted to 94 warships, 4500 *hoplite* soldiers, several thousands of light-armed troops, and several hundred small ships. This was a substantial part of the Athenian military establishment and was paid for out of their own treasury, since Segesta was going to pay on arrival. The selection of generals to lead the expedition was as ill-considered as the project itself. Three men were appointed, Alcibiades, Nicias and Lamachus. Between Nicias and Alcibiades there could be no agreement because they were divided on the feasibility of the expedition, on its purpose, and by political principles and temperament. Lamachus was an experienced and competent soldier, but had no political influence to weigh against the two most important political leaders of Athens.

Before the fleet sailed an ugly incident occurred which boded ill for the future. During the night busts of the god Hermes, set up before the doors of buildings throughout the city, were mutilated. Public opinion considered the sacrilege an insult to the city by some minor political group, and Alcibiades' enemies turned suspicion upon him. Drunken frolics in his past gave some grounds for suspicion, perhaps, but it is hardly likely that he would have risked disgrace on the eve of his own great project. Unfortunately Alcibiades was given no chance to clear himself in a public trial, as he asked, and the expedition sailed with the threat of prosecution hanging over its most ardent advocate.

As the fleet coasted along southern Italy, the people of the Greek cities made their lack of enthusiasm for Athenian interference obvious, and the Athenian generals had to work out some plan of unilateral action. Nicias proposed that they sail to Segesta, settle its affairs quickly and then, after a show of force along the coast of Sicily, return to Athens. Alcibiades, apparently unable to believe that Athens was not welcome, wished to invite the cities of Magna Graecia into alliance and then attack Syracuse. Lamachus, probably soundly, suggested attacking Syracuse immediately, since it was known to be unprepared. When his proposal met with no support, Lamachus sided with Alcibiades. While Alcibiades' plan was being put into action, a summons came for him to return home to stand trial for his alleged sacrilege. Fearing condemnation, he slipped off to Sparta on the way back, and the fortunes of the expedition were left to Nicias, the senior general, and to Lamachus. Since it was too late in the year for extensive action, both the Athenians and Syracuse settled down to prepare their campaigns for 414 B.C.

Nicias and Lamachus sent to Athens for money and reinforcements and began to seek help from the native Sicels, since the Greeks of Magna Graecia were proving uncooperative. Syracuse put its defenses in order and requested aid from Corinth and Sparta. In Sparta Alcibiades added his voice to the Syracusan plea and represented the Athenian purpose as nothing less than the complete conquest of the west, where great armies of mercenaries would be raised and unleashed on the Spartan alliance. More realistically, he urged Sparta to invade Attica and establish a fortified base at Decelea in the hills north of Athens, whence raids could be launched at will. For the moment the Spartans sent a small force to Syracuse under the command of an experienced Spartan officer, Gylippus.

While neither Athens nor Syracuse was able to prepare a decisive action for 414 B.C., the odds began to favor Syracuse. The Athenians, with their reinforcements, were able to land near Syracuse and almost succeeded in blockading the city, but Lamachus was killed in the fighting and Gylippus got through the Athenian lines into Syracuse with a force of three thousand men. In the lull of the following winter, Nicias advised Athens either to withdraw his force or to send substantial reinforcements. Time was short, for in Greece the pressure was heavy on Sparta to renew the war, and Athens had to decide whether to risk war in two great theaters. The assembly voted to take the chance and authorized another large fleet with five thousand *hoplites* to sail under the command of Demosthenes, who had brought them victory at Pylus. The Athenians miscalculated, for in 413 B.C. Sparta reopened the war by fortifying Decelea and sending more help to Syracuse.

In the summer of 413 B.C. the battle for Syracuse reached its climax, and the Athenian expedition collapsed in complete defeat. Thucydides' narrative is at its best when describing the Athenian attempts to extend their siege lines and break into the city, the Syracusan counter-attacks, and the eventual blockade of the Athenian forces. Much of the Athenian fleet might have been extricated by sea at the time it became apparent that Syracuse could not be taken. The Athenian lines around their encampment still held, and the Syracusans had not been able to blockade the harbor entrance. Demosthenes advised embarking the troops and setting sail for Athens while they could, when an eclipse of the moon occurred. Nicias, his senior officer, became superstitious and heeded the warning of soothsayers that thrice nine days must elapse before the fleet should sail. Within that time the Syracusans put a line of ships across the harbor mouth and hemmed in the Athenian ships. Despite a valiant effort to break through, the fleet was destroyed and the survivors were forced to try an escape by land across enemy territory in the intense heat of early autumn.

The Athenian columns were harassed and driven along on their march until they finally ground to a halt at a mud-filled stream bed. Many soldiers considered scooping up water to slake their thirst more important than fighting. As a result the remnants of two Athenian armies surrendered and were put to death or sold into slavery. Athens had lost 200 warships, about 4500 of its own *hoplites* and more than 40,000 men levied from the subject states or hired for the war at Athens' expense. In two years the Athenian vision of a Mediterranean Empire had changed to the bleak prospect of a war for their very survival.

Revolution and Defeat in Athens (411–400 B.C.)

However much Athens is to be criticized for the Sicilian Expedition, the behavior of the Athenians in defeat was remarkably steady. The nature of the war had changed almost overnight. The establishment of a garrison at Decelea both relieved the Spartans of their annual invasion of Attica and provided a refuge for Athenian slaves, who deserted in continuously increasing numbers. The Athenian fleet had lost two-thirds of its warships in Sicily, and the treasury had only a thousand talents for new construction. The long-awaited opportunity for the subject states of the Empire to revolt seemed at hand. Persia could see a chance to recover the Ionian Greek cities and, when Sparta asked for assistance, agreed to furnish money.

The Athenians faced the situation manfully. A special committee was appointed to deal with the financial problems of the state, and construction started on a new fleet immediately. To hold the Aegean, Athens stationed the remainder of the fleet at Samos, from which cross-Aegean communication and traffic along the coast of Asia Minor could be controlled. Nevertheless, many of the smaller coastal towns of Ionia revolted successfully, and, most seriously, Chios, Athens' last remaining free ally, broke away. The Athenians managed to hold the grain route from the Black Sea and to establish at least a balance of naval power, since a disagreement over the terms of Persian subsidization to Sparta prevented the latter from building up rapidly at sea. Athens had weathered the immediate storm, but worse was to come.

While the war was in this delicate balance, revolution broke out in Athens and an oligarchical group seized control of the government. This oligarchical movement had grown out of the opposition of the conservative upper class and of the farmers to the aggressive war policies of the democrats. So long as the war went successfully or not too badly, which was the case until 421 B.C., the peace groups had been able to influence action on occasion, but not to control it. In these circumstances extremists, who favored not only peace with Sparta but a change to oligarchy in Athens, had gone underground to form small, secret clubs which plotted revolution and attacked democratic leaders by prosecution in the courts. After the disaster in Sicily, the extremists came out into the open to denounce the war policy of the democrats, which had brought Athens to defeat. Since there was justice in the criticism, the extremists attracted a following among the middle class, who had served Athens as *hoplites* and who had suffered severely at Delium and in Sicily. As the Empire fell apart, the financial burden of war fell more heavily on them. These moderates wanted to place a limitation on citizenship by establishing a property qualification which would disfranchise the lower class, where the democratic leaders found their chief support. The extremists, however, wished a very narrow control of government by a selected few. Such was the state of affairs in Athens in 411 B.C. when Alcibiades again took a hand in Athenian affairs. As usual where he was concerned, action followed quickly.

Alcibiades fled from Sparta, where he allegedly had seduced the king's wife, to the Persians in Asia Minor, as a means of reintroducing himself into the good graces of Athens. He seems to have persuaded the Persian satraps to cut their subsidies to the Spartans and then to have gone to Samos, where he represented himself as able to secure a Persian alliance for Athens, if Athens would change its form of government to an oligarchy. The higher officers of the fleet were persuaded to enter into negotiations with the oligarchical extremists in Athens. A *coup* was planned for both the city and the fleet in Samos.

At first events developed as planned. In Athens the oligarchs got control of affairs by contriving to hold an assembly meeting outside the walls of the city, where only the *hoplites* and upper class felt safe in attending because of the Spartan raiders in the neighborhood. At the meeting the constitutional safeguards to the democratic system were suspended, and a committee of four hundred, with its personnel prearranged, was selected to draw up a new form of government. Moderate support was obtained by holding out the promise of a limit on citizenship, which would create a citizen body of about five thousand, by setting a qualification essentially the same as that for *hoplite* service. Thus it is usually referred to as the *"hoplite census."* The committee of four hundred were to take charge of the government, while this list of citizens and a new constitution were prepared. The "400" had no intention of going through with the plan, but their announced intention to do so held the moderates in line for the time being. But in Samos the *coup* failed miserably. The sailors, who would have been among the disfranchised, found out what was in the wind and declared themselves to be the true democratic government of Athens and elected generals to carry on the war. Alcibiades, despite his failure to produce a Persian alliance and his plots with the oligarchs, adroitly emerged as a democratic general, entrusted with important naval operations.

The oligarchical government in Athens made overtures of peace to Sparta and began to arrest and execute the leaders of the democratic groups. The Spartans, rightly suspicious of the ability of the "400" to surrender Athens, were slow to respond and, as the war continued, the grip of the "400" became more insecure. When the news came from Samos that the fleet had remained democratic, quarrels broke out and the moderates withdrew their support. They deposed the extremists and established a moderate oligarchy, "the government of the 5000," to rule in Athens. This government continued the war against Sparta and managed to defend Athens successfully, although the island of Euboea was lost. When it became apparent that Athens would not be surrendered, the Spartans moved across the Aegean to try to cut the grain route from the Black Sea, and the onus of war thus passed to the democratic fleet in Samos under the leadership of Alcibiades. The fleet was in difficulties for a time, but in 410 B.C. won a decisive victory at Cyzicus and gained the Athenians a breathing spell.

During the naval struggle the "5000" had loyally cooperated with the fleet and in the summer of 410 B.C. each government lapsed of its own volition in order to restore the regular democratic system in Athens. The restored democracy was prepared to use the moderate leaders but turned violently on those extremists left in Athens. Each citizen took an oath, "I will kill with my own hand anyone who overthrows the democracy at Athens, holds office under an undemocratic regime, seeks to establish a tyranny, or collaborates with a tyrant." The extremists were hounded from Athens, exiled, and fined. Such reprisal was understandable, but it deepened the disunity of the state when Athens needed the full loyalty of all its citizens to prosecute the war. Alcibiades, understandably, did not return to the city at this time, although he continued to serve Athens in the Aegean.

The action of the war slowed indecisively for the next two years, while Athens tried to recover the subject states, for the Persian satraps had begun to refuse subsidies to Sparta in the hope that each side would wear down the other. Perhaps the most striking event of the period was the eventual return of the conquering hero, Alcibiades, to his native city. He carefully waited offshore until assured that he would be greeted by a triumphal procession and not a warrant for arrest. Athens, however, received him back with a fête and re-elected him general.

In 407 B.C. the last act of the war began. Sparta sent out an exceptionally able and energetic commander, Lysander, to the Aegean, and the king of Persia, disturbed by the recovery of Athens, sent his younger son, Cyrus, to revive the

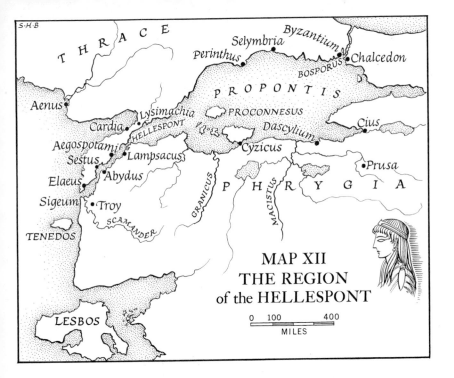

THRACE

Byzantium
Selymbria
Perinthus
Chalcedon
BOSPORUS

PROPONTIS

Aenus

PROCONNESUS

Lysimachia
Cardia
Dascylium
Cius

HELLESPONT
Cyzicus

Aegospotami
Lampsacus
Sestus
Prusa

Elaeus
Abydus
PHRYGIA

GRANICUS

Sigeum
Troy

MACISTUS

SCAMANDER

TENEDOS

MAP XII
THE REGION
of the HELLESPONT

0   100   400
MILES

LESBOS

policy of subsidization. Lysander and Cyrus not only had a common purpose, but worked together on easy personal terms. They agreed that, in exchange for generous subsidies, Persia should acquire the Ionian Greek cities. It is difficult to say how seriously Sparta meant this seeming reversal of its avowed purpose in fighting the war, because, for the Greeks to exchange subjection to Athens for subjection to Persia was hardly a gain. But for the moment Sparta had to have a fleet to win the war, and with Cyrus' cooperation the Spartan naval buildup proceeded rapidly.

The Athenians found that it became increasingly harder to win their naval victories. Although Alcibiades was absent at the battle of Notium in 407 B.C., his deputy lost so many ships that Alcibiades judged it better to retire to his private castle on the shores of the Hellespont than to continue as an Athenian general. In the following year the Athenians again won at the Arginusae Islands, but many ships were damaged and many crew members lost in a storm. The victory had a tragic sequel in Athens, where the outraged assembly demanded that the generals be put on trial as a group and executed for the loss of the sailors. No attempt was made to determine the degree of individual responsibility. One unfortunate general, in fact, had been struggling in the water when the order to return to harbor was given. But Athenian nerves were on the ragged edge, and the people could not face a reverse steadily. The final battle of the war came in 405 B.C. at Aegospotami in the Hellespont, where, despite a warning from Alcibiades, who tried to do Athens a last good service, the Athenians relaxed their guard and were taken unprepared by the Spartan fleet. The Spartans destroyed Athens' ships and cut the vital grain route from the

Black Sea. It remained only to take Athens itself. Lysander sailed for the Peiraeus and laid siege to the city. Although the Athenians held out doggedly through the autumn and winter of 404 B.C., they finally were starved into surrender. Corinth and Thebes wished to destroy the city and to treat the people as the Athenians had treated other Greeks, to kill the men and sell the women and children as slaves, but Sparta was more lenient. The terms imposed were crippling, yet the state survived. The Athenians were required to renounce their claims to the Empire (most of the states had already revolted), to limit the navy to twelve ships, to demolish the Long Walls and to become a subject ally of Sparta. A Spartan garrison was installed, and the victorious allies stayed to watch the demolition of the Long Walls to the music of flutes. After twenty-seven years of war the Spartan coalition had achieved its avowed war aim and could announce that freedom had been restored to Greece.

Athens, however, was not to obtain internal peace for several years, for the disastrous end of the war, like the defeat in Sicily, bred another oligarchic revolution. The oligarchic extremists who had gone into exile when the democracy was restored in 410 B.C. were allowed to return and began to scheme once more. Foremost among them was the aristocrat, Critias, who engineered a *coup* on lines like that in 411 B.C. The situation in the city was favorable to change, for the democratic leaders had been killed in the war or discredited by the defeat. The moderates, led by Theramenes, who had been prominent in the government of the "5000," hoped again for a moderate oligarchy, but in 404/3 B.C. Lysander and the Spartan garrison were on the spot to give support to whichever group seemed best for Spartan interests. The history of 411 B.C. began to repeat itself. Critias and the extremists pretended to collaborate with the moderates while insinuating themselves into power. A committee of thirty, among them Critias and Theramenes, was appointed to draft a new constitution on conservative lines and to establish a citizen body of three thousand. With the approval of Lysander and general public support, the committee began a purge of obvious wrongdoers in Athens. When the purge went beyond this and began to serve the political aims of the extremists, the moderates tried to call a halt and get on with the framing of a constitution. In the power struggle which followed, Critias, by armed force and the tacit consent of the Spartan garrison, secured the condemnation of Theramenes and turned the purge into a reign of terror. About fifteen hundred Athenians were put to death, while many fled to the hills. The situation rapidly descended into chaos and Sparta had to step in. The Spartans might prefer that Athens have an oligarchical government but above all they wished for a quiet, cooperative ally. When a new democratic leader, Thrasyboulos, began guerilla war from the hills, and the "thirty" in the city lost all public support, the Spartan king appeared before Athens with an army. He arranged a compromise between Thrasyboulos and the moderates, by which an amnesty was declared for all except the extreme oligarchs. The Athenians restored their traditional democracy and overhauled the legal system to correct the political abuses from which it had suffered. Athens was once more a whole state and could turn to the necessary tasks of recovery from the damage of war.

The Intellectual Transformation of Athens

During the Peloponnesian War Athenian society underwent a far-reaching change, for the stability which it had enjoyed in the Periclean Period was undermined. Although the city retained its democratic form of government after the war, the principles and institutions of Periclean democracy had been repudiated or trenchantly questioned by the upper and middle classes. The oligarchs, by discussion of their ideas and the attempt to apply them practically, developed a theory of oligarchy, which appealed to the better educated and more articulate part of the Athenian population and eventually had a very potent influence on the political philosophy of Plato and Aristotle. In fact, the theory of oligarchy, rather than of Periclean democracy, became the normal frame of reference for Greek political thought. The democracy had been too closely linked with the Athenian Empire to be generally accepted, and after the war, partly as a result of oligarchical pressure, partly because of the concentration of wealth in relatively few hands, democracy tended to be sectional, a government by the lower class, not by the people as a whole. Plato discussed democracy in this sense, and it is useful to examine the ground from which his ideas grew.

An interesting product of about 420 B.C., when the oligarchical clubs were coming into being in Athens, is a political pamphlet, which apparently represented the type of discussion carried on in them. The author is unknown and usually referred to as the "Old Oligarch." He criticized the democracy from the point of view of an upper-class Athenian, who found its workings most distasteful, but the author realized its source of strength very clearly. The basic premise was that only the "best" men were fit to rule, while in democratic Athens the "best" were exploited in the interests of the "people," the lower class. The roots of the idea went back, of course, to the aristocratic city-state, which tended to be compact, isolated, and self-sufficient, with its wealth drawn from agriculture and its society held together in a moral union based on aristocratic values. To the oligarchs, the Athenian democracy seemed to have destroyed this traditional society and to have substituted anarchic misgovernment by the urban mob.

The "Old Oligarch" castigated the "people" as ignorant and disorderly and their magistrates as selfish, unscrupulous demagogues, since any man had the right to hold office and could obtain it by pandering to the people for their votes. The assembly, in his thought, had no sense of responsibility and paid for its luxuries by exploiting the rich and living on the profits of empire. The oligarchs were anti-imperialistic, partly because they desired peace and close collaboration with Sparta and partly on more theoretical grounds. The metropolitan character of Athens was regarded as corruptive to the simon-pure ethos, the individual character of the Athenians, because of the influences of resident aliens and the pampered insolence of slaves. Such was the ordinary material of oligarchic criticism, but its political implications are more apparent from the revolution of 411 B.C.

In the revolution two trends of political opinion appeared. The extremists sought to establish a dictatorial government of the few, whose claim to rule lay in their definition of themselves as the "best." By "best" the oligarch wistfully identified himself with a moral, social, and intellectual ideal, but in fact he tended to be representative of old, upper-class families whose wealth still lay in land. These ideas were repudiated in practice both in 411 and in 403 B.C. On the other hand, the moderate oligarchs produced a government in 411 B.C. which won the praise of Aristotle and Thucydides. In his account of the Athenian Constitution, Aristotle observed: "It would appear that in this period Athens had a good form of government, when, in a time of war, the government was in the hands of those able to serve with full equipment." Thucydides said "This government during its early days was the best which the Athenians ever enjoyed within my memory."

The moderate oligarchs desired a system in which the politically active citizens were defined by a proper property qualification, in this case, the *"hoplite census."* The political principle involved was that the right to hold office and to make decisions should be given to those who had a substantial amount of property. Other members of the state should have legal and personal rights only. In Athens the *hoplite* line of qualification would have enfranchised less than half of the citizens. Within this selected group an intricate system of rotation allocated the executive tasks of government to the officials and members of the council, the few, and the important decisions to the rest of the politically eligible, the many, who in due time would themselves hold office. The moderates also accepted the democratic principles of election to office, use of the lot, and the familiar governmental organs of the magistracy, council, and assembly. They did, however, abolish pay for state service and raised the eligible age limits for the exercise of political rights to thirty. Such a system could not last in wartime Athens, where the disfranchised citizens carried the brunt of war, but its principles provided a fruitful source for the theory of mixed government developed by Aristotle and applied to Rome by later theorists.

These new political ideas were only a part of the change in education and thought during the latter part of the fifth century, which is known as the Sophistic Movement. The Sophists, professional providers of wisdom, lectured and taught in the cities of Greece but in particular gravitated to Athens. That branch of their teaching which attracted most public attention, and which probably resulted in the highest fees for instruction, was the art of communication, both spoken and written. The Sophists developed oratory as an art and laid the basis of Greek prose writing. Such studies were particularly useful in the democratic states of Greece, where political success depended primarily on the ability to influence the assembly and to hold one's own in argument. The "inventor" of rhetoric is said to have been Corax, a Sicilian, who lived in the middle of the fifth century. Evidently oratory received particular attention in Sicily, for, when Gorgias of Leontini came as an envoy to Athens in 427 B.C., he gave a dazzling display which amazed and impressed the Athenian assembly. In Athens such an aid to political leadership was not to be disdained; consequently many Sophists came to the city during the war. The history of Thucydides provides an early example of the newly developed prose style which employed rhetorical devices to persuade and excite emotion.

Thucydides' humanistic view of history, too, was a reflection of the intellectual attitudes of the Sophistic Movement. They were the originators of Humanism in western thought. In the latter part of the fifth century, men were more conscious of their role as responsible members of their communities, and so more concerned about their rights in society and about society itself. The Sophists in their role as teachers attempted to prepare their students for political life by teaching a knowledge of society, politics, and history. As thinkers they developed the view that the city-state and its institutions were the product of man's intelligence and created by man-made law. Justice, for example, was not the personal decision of Zeus, but the result of an agreement among men. "Justice only exists where there is equal power to enforce it," as the Athenian envoys to Melos had stated.

A typical Sophist, and a very influential one, was Protagoras of Ceus (ca. 485-10 B.C.), who taught ethics, politics, and mathematics, drafted a set of laws for Pericles' colony at Thurii, and developed a characteristic Sophistic philosophy. His dictum, "Man is the measure of all things," indicated the focus of Sophistic teaching—man as an individual and man in society and nature. Because they regarded truth as relative to the individual, the Sophists measured the traditions and conventional beliefs of their society and those of foreign states, compared them, and found much in each to be wanting. Most Sophists were agnostics or, at least, they denied the existence of the gods and substituted conventions among men for divine sanctions. They had no set dogma but unleashed a variety of opinion and criticism which shook the traditional life of Greece.

In Athens the Sophists found a particularly receptive audience among the wealthy young men of the city because no system of public education existed and because the war dissolved family life to a considerable degree. Instead of acquiring traditional instruction from their fathers or the elder members of the family, the young men flocked to the Sophists where they learned to argue, quibble, and display their new knowledge. Since the Sophists taught for a fee, sometimes a very sizable one, the benefits of higher education were confined to the wealthy. The ordinary Athenian, however, did acquire some familiarity, usually distorted, with the new education. He listened to public declamations, to the speeches of political leaders, and in the theater to the plays of Aristophanes and Euripides. The ordinary man of Athens was bewildered and displeased, and he came to identify the new rationalism as one of the forces which was destroying his traditional life and weakening Athens.

This popular rejection of rationalism resulted partly from the Sophistic challenge to religious beliefs and superstition and partly from political change. The Athenian democrat saw that the wealthy young men were members of the oligarchic clubs whose leaders were among the intelligentsia of Athens. Antiphon, for example, the most sinister of the extremists in 411 B.C., was also one of the leaders in the development of Greek prose writing and a consummate orator in the new style. Alcibiades, suspected of aiming at a tyranny, was an intimate of Socrates, who was identified as a Sophist in the popular mind. Critias, the extremist of 404 B.C., was also a member of the Socratic circle. Because the new learning seemed to go hand in hand with oligarchy or tyranny in the later stages of the war, its devotees were sometimes driven from Athens. In 415 B.C. the suspicion of sacrilege motivated the prosecution of Alcibiades. Protagoras fled Athens about 412 B.C., and in 409 Euripides moved to Macedonia. The tolerance and freedom of speech which had characterized Periclean Athens was disappearing. Our best mirror of Athenian thought, next to the history of Thucydides, is the contemporary theater of Aristophanes and Euripides. The former was a conservative and opposed to the Sophists, the latter sympathetic at least to some of their ideas.

Aristophanes (*ca.* 450–388 B.C.) lived almost half of his life under the duress of the Peloponnesian War, and many of his eleven extant plays have specific themes of war and politics, while others satirize aspects of Athenian life. He was a conservative, peace-loving Athenian, who remembered the good days of peace before the war, and, during its early stages, attacked Cleon and praised the benefits of peace. As early as 426 B.C. his *Babylonians* satirized the Athenian Empire by representing the subject states of Athens as slaves of the tyrant *Demos,* the Athenian people. Although Cleon impeached him for this representation, Aristophanes evidently got off lightly, for he returned to the attack in the *Hippeis* (*Knights*) in 424 B.C. and castigated Cleon as an unscrupulous demagogue. In the same period the delights of peace were praised in the *Acharnians* (425 B.C.) and in the *Peace* (421 B.C.). While the tradition of Old Comedy encouraged trenchant criticism of public figures and of state policy, the performance of such plays is indicative both of the wide freedom of speech still allowed in Athens and the fact that Aristophanes' themes were congenial to many of the audience that saw his plays. It is noteworthy that, in the latter part of the war, he turned more to fancy (*Birds,* 414 B.C.) and farcical political satire (*Women in Parliament, Lysistrata*). As a staunch conservative of the old school, Aristophanes was opposed to the new education and to the Sophists. In the *Clouds* (423 B.C.) he lampooned Socrates as a Sophist who ran a Think-Factory in which the young men of Athens and the old traditions of Athenian society were perverted. Aristophanes' humor was usually good-natured and meant in fun, except against Cleon and Euripides, where he was deadly serious.

Euripides (*ca.* 485–07 B.C.) was appropriately singled out for attack by a conservative like Aristophanes, for his plays broke with the traditions of Athenian tragedy and found much to criticize in the accepted theology of the Olympian gods. Perhaps our conception of Euripides is inadequate, for almost all of his nineteen extant plays were written during the war and they reveal a variety of themes and attitudes which reflect a restless and growing mind.

Euripides' life was not typical of Periclean Athens, for he seems to have been austere and withdrawn and took little part in public affairs. Evidently he found the city uncongenial after the restoration of the democracy and retired to Macedonia, where he died in 407 B.C. while a guest at the court of its king, Archelaus. Euripides considered the traditional myths about the Olympians as little more than a collection of stories, which were not only out of date but pernicious, if given authority, and was interested in human beings, whose conduct he found superior to that of the gods. Two of his most famous plays, the *Medea* and the *Hippolytus,* show the conflict of will and passion, while the character of Admetus in the *Alcestis* is a study in selfishness. Although Euripides denied the gods, the elemental forces which some of them represented were depicted as terrifyingly real—erotic passion in the *Phaedra* and the religious hysteria of Dionysiac worship in his most powerful play, the *Bacchae.* The plays show the obvious influence of the intellectual debates of his period, but Euripides scarcely fell into any school of thought. He would deny that justice came from heaven but was by no means certain that it was the product of rational convention. Human nature, as Phaedra observed in the *Hippolytus,* was irrational: "That which is good we learn and recognize, yet practice not the lesson, some from sloth, and some professing pleasure in the stead of duty."

During the early part of the war Euripides showed himself as a loyal Athenian. The *Heracleidae* (430 B.C.) hymned the glorification of Athens, and in other early plays there were long passages celebrating the city. By 415 B.C., however, he had acquired a thorough distaste for war as the cause of much human distress. The *Trojan Women,* perhaps with a reminiscence of the brutality of Athens to Melos, represented the pathos and suffering in a captured city and condemned imperialism:

> Fool, that in the sack of towns lays temples waste,
> And tombs, the sanctuaries of the dead.
> He, sowing desolation, reaps destruction.

In the plays of this period Euripides criticized the Athenian fault of making hasty decisions under the impact of emotion and apparently preferred control of the state by the middle class. As in the case of Aristophanes, his later plays, such as the *Iphigenia in Aulis* and the *Ion,* departed from tradition to introduce new, romantic themes. Euripides' focus of life remained the city-state, but he evidently found it increasingly less satisfactory.

In 399 B.C. Athens' earliest native philosopher, Socrates (*ca.* 470–399 B.C.), was tried on charges of corrupting the young men of Athens and of neglecting the city's gods and introducing other new gods. He was found guilty and condemned to death. In the report of his trial by Plato, the *Apology,* Socrates scorned to make a proper defense, but instead gave a typical display of Sophistic techniques of argument and then a sincere justification of his purpose in life—to know himself and to persuade others to know themselves. Before devoting his later years to this mission, Socrates had served Athens well in the war, fighting

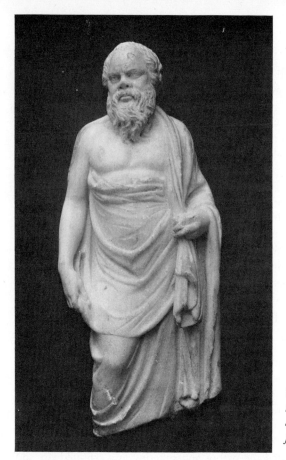

*Socrates. A statuette of
the Hellenistic Period,
after an original of the
fourth century B.C.*

as a *hoplite* in the revolt of Samos, at Potidaea, Delium, and Amphipolis. He was elected once to the Council of Five Hundred, for 406/5 B.C., and took an unpopular stand at the trial of the generals after the battle of Arginusae. Socrates insisted that they be tried individually, as the law required, not as a group to satisfy the anger of the Athenian assembly. Usually, however, Socrates had stood aloof from public life to avoid, as he stated in the *Apology,* compromising his own principles of individual conduct.

About twenty-five years before he was condemned to death, Socrates had been pilloried as a Sophist by Aristophanes in the *Clouds,* and probably he was identified as such by many Athenians. Certainly the cross-examination of his accuser in the *Apology* indicates a mastery of Sophistic verbal techniques. Aristophanes' attack probably came soon after Socrates had undertaken his mission and when he was becoming a notorious figure in the city. Earlier in his career he had been interested in the physical theories of Ionian philosophers about the universe, but had turned to this search for truth as a result of the famous answer of the Delphic oracle that no man was wiser than Socrates. Conscious of his own ignorance Socrates began to test the oracle. The Athenians who crossed his path were cross-examined to ascertain whether they acted and thought from opinion and convention or from knowledge. By adroit and, it must be said, leading questions, Socrates reduced his hapless subjects to helplessness or anger. He also must have offended many Athenians who merely observed. His argument rejected the conventional goods of society, wealth and material well-being as proper ends of life, and rejected the idea of being a good man according to the conventions of society. Unlike the Sophists he also rejected the idea that goodness could be learned, like a technical accomplishment.

Yet destructive argument was only a preliminary part of the Socratic method. With those who cared to continue the discussion he would make a fresh start and build up truthful concepts in their minds. Socrates sought to establish an absolute morality by the exercise of reason and, ultimately, by the individual's intuition of the good. Happiness was virtue and virtue, knowledge. Men could attain to knowledge by the rejection of opinion but would understand the truth only in their own souls. He himself could take no other course in his life than his search for the truth, because he had acted in the knowledge that he was right.

Socrates' wholehearted attention to this nonmaterial purpose and the impressive personality of the man made his influence directly personal. He wrote nothing, but through the members of his intimate circle of friends made a deeper mark than any other man of his period on the subsequent development of Greek thought. This influence is most obvious, of course, in the dialogues of Plato, but Socrates was also father to the hedonistic philosophy of Aristippus of Cyrene and to the ascetic teaching of Antisthenes the Cynic. If in the last analysis Socrates considered that man himself is the right judge of his own conduct and must establish an absolute standard within himself, he stands with the Sophists as one of the founders of Humanism.

The ordinary Athenians could not understand Socrates' almost mystical quality of leadership and the purpose of his cross-examination. They saw him as the brilliant verbalist, who turned conventional opinion inside out and was suspect politically because his intimates were the chief enemies of Athenian democracy, Alcibiades, Critias, and many of the oligarchs. In 399 B.C. it was not only Socrates who was on trial, but also the new education and the intelligentsia of Athens, for they had moved beyond the popular norms of thought and conduct.

XIV

The Fourth Century

(404–336 B.C.)

DURING THE FOURTH CENTURY before Christ the focus of history began to shift from the older Greek city-states of the Aegean to strong new powers coming into being in the regions on the edge of Greek civilization. In the western Mediterranean Syracuse exploited the prestige of its victory over Athens in 412 B.C. to dominate much of Magna Graecia, and in a long series of wars successfully defended the Western Greeks from Carthage. Carthage itself became the great sea power of the West, ruling a wide empire of trading colonies. In Italy the native Italic peoples pressed down into the fertile coastal plains from the hills, encroaching upon the land of the Greek colonies and of Etruria. They were met, however, by the growing power of Rome, which by the end of the century had forged a Roman Confederacy out of the diverse elements of Italy (pp. 454–56). As yet Rome's path was separate from those of Carthage and of the Greeks, so that the growth of Rome attracted little attention.

In Greece itself the peoples of the hinterland in the west and north began to form federal leagues and kingdoms and to enter into the international politics of the older Greek states. Most significant was the rise of Macedonia into a strongly centralized national state under King Philip II. Philip extended Macedonian territory to the natural mountain barriers on the west and north and eastwards through Thrace to the Hellespont, where he confronted Persian Asia Minor. The Persians regained control of Ionia, but their Empire was disturbed by intrigue and revolt, and the Great King did not attempt to resume invasion of European Greece. The rise of the new states was spurred in large part by the urbanization and political coalescence which had been encouraged by trade and contact with the Aegean centers over several centuries. The energy of the great city-states, particularly of Athens, had been sapped by the long, hard fighting of the Peloponnesian War, and they were less able to interfere effectively.

The reader will find Maps VII and VIII (pages 172–173 and 184) useful as he reads this chapter.

Political and Economic Change

The relatively great size and undeveloped character of many of the new states gave rise to different types of political organization than those in the autonomous city-states of old Greece. In the fourth century there was a considerable growth of federal associations, in which cantons and towns were linked together by common citizenship and government. For example, the Aetolian League was formed in the mountainous, unurbanized country of Aetolia, where the people had a sense of ethnic unity, and in the Macedonian Chalcidice the small cities, formerly subject states of Athens, grouped together in a league. They were able to resist foreign domination, until Philip incorporated the region into Macedonia in 348 B.C. Monarchy again became a characteristic form of government, the best example of which was the national state of Macedonia, whose people centered their loyalty on the king. This turn, in an unstable age, to the strength provided by absolutism was paralleled in many of the older Greek cities by the reappearance of tyranny. The rise of Syracuse, for example, was engineered by its great tyrant, Dionysius I, whose regime was studied by Plato on a visit to the tyrant's court.

For the most part, however, the older Greek city-states clung to their traditional organization and modes of political behavior, even when these failed to cope with the new and complex problems confronting Greece. Sparta, Athens, and Thebes sought, as in the fifth century, to extend their power by imperialistic aggression and to form alliances and coalitions for their own advantage. But in the fourth century no one state possessed the resources in fighting power and wealth to establish a marked superiority, and so the political scene was characterized by a shifting kaleidoscope of attempts at empire, the formation of counteralliances, and by almost continuous war. Each state was ready, like Sparta in the Peloponnesian War, to accept Persian help, while Persian interest could be satisfied by keeping Greece divided and its major powers weak. As stability proved harder to obtain, the more desirable a general and permanent peace seemed. The Greeks groped for peace, but failed to find a formula which could reconcile the traditional desire of each state for autonomy with the existence of a power strong enough to guarantee the peace. In the end the formula was provided by Philip II of Macedonia, who formed a united states of Greece under his personal leadership.

The political difficulties of Greece were aggravated by economic stress, partly from war damage, and partly from the change in their relation to the rest of the Mediterranean. Athens, in particular, was hard hit for some years by the results of defeat. Farmhouses had to be rebuilt and vineyards and olive groves put back into operation, but such damage was reparable and recovery fairly quick. More serious was the loss of revenue from the Empire, which had provided a margin of ease in the Periclean Period. Athens was dependent on its own resources in the fourth century and to attain some prosperity had to re-establish the trade which had been disrupted in the later stages of the war. While this was achieved to a considerable degree, the city was no longer the one great, metropolitan center of Greece. Instead, trade and wealth became more generally diffused throughout the whole of the Aegean. At the same time the markets for Aegean products began to diminish, so that Greece found it more difficult to pay for needed imports of grain.

Local industries had grown up in the colonial regions of southern France, Magna Graecia, and the Black Sea to supply the pottery, metalware, and other goods needed in everyday life. The colonists, by setting out vines and olive trees where local conditions were favorable, could grow their own staples of wine and oil. Traders from the colonies worked up connections with the native peoples in their hinterland and, as the natives began to urbanize, were able to supply needed goods. For example, merchants from Massilia traveled far up the Rhone valley into central France to trade with the Celts, and in southern Italy a locally manufactured red-figured pottery, known as Campanian ware, was produced. There was still a good market for the high-grade olive oil, fine wine, luxury textiles, costly metalware, and jewelry of the older Aegean farms and workshops, but mass production for export declined. The Aegean Greeks still could make a considerable amount of money from trade and industry, but since wealth came to the more aggressive and businesslike few, opportunity for employment declined. Nevertheless, there were more mouths to feed in Greece than there had been in the fifth century because a rising birth rate had speedily replaced and exceeded the casualties of the war. Furthermore many more slaves were imported, for they were readily available, cheaper, and easier to control than free labor.

Greek society had been unsettled by the long war, and men found it difficult to return to their previous activity or to find new work. Since there was no room for agricultural expansion in the older states of Greece, a drift began from countryside to city, but in the cities the free man faced the competition of slave labor and the decline in production. Men began to move from city to city and to seek employment as mercenary soldiers. The market for their services was good in the constant warfare of the fourth century, and thousands were hired by Persia and the Greek cities to fight their wars. War, in fact, was made easier, although more expensive, by the facility with which groups of mercenaries could shift from one paymaster to another. In these economic conditions men developed new social attitudes. The feeling grew that a free man should not perform manual labor. That was *banausic* and to be done by slaves. Agriculture was still respectable but seemed boorish to the sophisticated city dweller. The unity and stability of society in the city-state began to disintegrate, for the drifting soldier and laborer formed no attachment beyond the term of his pay, and the individual citizen became more detached and egocentric, as society became more cosmopolitan.

While the Greeks were unable to vie with these great trends of change, they were aware of them and made numerous piecemeal advances of a technical nature. Methods of agriculture were studied and improved, but the amount of cultivable land could not be increased, except by emigration or conquest, for which Greece did not have the opportunity or strength. In commerce and business Greece moved into a semicapitalistic economy. Men with money were prepared to make loans and investments in trading ventures, as well as to purchase land, and to organize banks which accepted deposits for reinvestment. In response to these activities, techniques and practices of financing were developed, and the economic organization of the Aegean, temporarily dislocated by the defeat of Athens, was formed this time by private enterprise rather than by political interest. City finance, too, was carefully scrutinized, but, since the resources of the small city-states could not be expanded, money was found by more ingenious systems of taxation or by capital levy. The fourth century was not a period of overall decline, but a time of shifting and change, in which the older city-states found themselves in difficulty as Greece moved into a new and larger world.

The Political Scene in Greece (404–362 B.C.)

THE SPARTAN EMPIRE

At the conclusion of the Peloponnesian War, Greece needed imaginative leadership to recover political stability. The balance of power between Athens and Sparta, which, at least, had provided fifteen years of peace before the war, was lost, but Sparta had gained the prestige and power to make a thorough reorganization. The problems were difficult. The former subject states of the Athenian Empire expected freedom, but Sparta had promised those states in Ionia to Persia as a *quid pro quo* for financial help. The Spartan allies were anxious to get complete compensation for their losses and a generous share of the booty. In almost all Greek cities a sharp cleavage had grown between oligarch and democrat, which increasingly reflected the distinction between rich and poor. While Sparta favored oligarchies, which looked to Sparta for support, some of the newly freed states retained democratic systems of government. Sparta was singularly ill-equipped to deal with these problems. Its own institutions were obsolete, and the Spartan had shown little flair for political tasks in the past. As a result of his education and training he tended to seek an easy solution in the military terms of order and discipline and as a person was usually brusque and harsh, greedy for money and the good things of life which were not available in Sparta. The prospects for a successful reorganization of Greece were not promising.

Spartan policy in the immediate aftermath of the war was made largely by Lysander, an exceptionally able soldier, but proud, personally ambitious, and reluctant to take advice. He dealt with the former subject states of Athens in purely military terms and quickly substituted a system of Spartan control for that of Athens. The cities seemed to have fallen out of the frying pan into the fire. In some states Lysander supported oligarchies as he had in Athens.

In others Spartan governors, *harmosts,* were appointed and backed up by garrisons. Tribute was imposed, amounting eventually to a thousand talents, to pay the costs of operating by land and sea on a wide scale outside the Peloponnesus. Some of these measures were undoubtedly necessary to keep order, but Sparta soon found itself committed to the direction of a large empire. The Spartan allies, particularly Thebes and Corinth, those who had hoped to share in the spoils, felt cheated and disappointed just as after the Peace of Nicias in 421 B.C. Accordingly, the coalition, which had contributed much to victory, began to disintegrate, and Sparta was increasingly thrown back on its own resources.

Sparta's chief problem was to find the manpower for its commitments. By the early fourth century the number of Spartan citizens in good standing had declined to a few thousand men of military age, who showed no disposition to enlarge their number by relaxing the rigid social organization. Accordingly, more *perioeci* were put in the Spartan army, *helots* were used on garrison duty where their safety would depend on loyalty to Sparta, and thousands of mercenaries were hired to serve in the army and with the fleet. The Spartan king, Agesilaus, as able a soldier as Lysander and more politically astute, realized the insecurity of Sparta's position and tried to enlist Greek support by reversing Sparta's attitude to Persia and moving to liberate the Ionian Greeks.

At first, events in Persia played into Agesilaus' hands. In 405 B.C. King Darius died and left his kingdom to his elder son, Artaxerxes. The new king appointed Cyrus, his younger brother, as viceroy for Asia Minor, which was proper and reasonable in view of Cyrus' experience and close cooperation with Lysander. Cyrus, however, was ambitious to take over the whole Persian Empire and grasped at the chance to form a large army from the demobilized Greek soldiers who were seeking employment. He enlisted an army of fourteen thousand Greeks under the command of a Spartan, Clearchus, and added the men to his own native troops. Naval support in the Aegean was provided by the cooperation of the Spartan fleet. Perhaps Cyrus' payment for Spartan help was a tacit agreement to forget the Persian claim to the Ionian cities or, perhaps, the Spartans hoped that Cyrus would be tied down by a long war in the heart of western Asia. In any case Cyrus started east from Sardes in 401 B.C. to gain the throne of Persia. In his army was a young Athenian, Xenophon (p. 333), who had been a member of the Socratic circle and had found Athens most uncongenial after the war. While neither he nor his fellow soldiers, who elected him as one of their generals, found the fortunes for which they had hoped, Xenophon wrote an account of their remarkable march in his *Anabasis.*

Cyrus led his army inland through Lydia and Phrygia to strike across the Taurus Mountains and reach the Euphrates River in North Syria near Thapsacus. From this point they marched along the Euphrates to Cunaxa, north of Babylon, where the Tigris and Euphrates come close together. At Cunaxa Artaxerxes' army blocked the roads which led south into Babylonia and eastwards towards Iran. In the ensuing battle the native troops in Cyrus' army were defeated and Cyrus killed, but the Greek mercenaries won an easy victory, preserving their formations intact and, eventually, cutting their way through to the Tigris River. The Greeks decided to strike north for the Black Sea through lands unknown to them, rather than to fight their way back to Sardes and the Aegean. Accordingly, they started off to the north along the Tigris, marching through Kurdistan and Armenia to the great plateau of Erzerum in eastern Anatolia, cut off by mountains from the Black Sea. The Greeks fought, cajoled and bribed their way through the nomadic and mountain tribesmen finally to burst out above the Greek colony of Trapezus with a cry of "*thalassa, thalassa,* the sea, the sea.*" In the spring of 400 B.C. they made their way back to the Aegean, partly by ship, partly by land along the coast. They found that the Persians had reoccupied the Ionian coastal cities, and that Sparta was engaged in a war of liberation, and, therefore, that ready and congenial employment was at hand. Their exploit had been remarkable, both as a demonstration of military skill and as a revelation that Greek armies might operate far inland from the sea. Some Greeks began to think of Asia Minor as a field for new Greek settlement, but first Ionia had to be won.

Sparta was well prepared to undertake an invasion of western Asia Minor at this time, for the army was large and well trained and could be supported by a sizable fleet. Also, Persia was hampered by revolt in Egypt and had to build a fleet for service in the Aegean. Unfortunately general Greek sentiment for the liberation of Ionia was lukewarm, to say the least, and to some states the Spartan engagement in Asia Minor seemed an opportunity to attack Sparta in Greece. Also Agesilaus conducted the campaign more as a series of raids by the army for booty than as a well-coordinated enterprise by land and sea to seize strategic areas and prevent Persian concentration. He was unable to win decisively before hostilities started against Sparta in Greece. There, Thebes, Corinth, Athens, Argos, and some of the minor states formed a coalition and struck into the Peloponnesus in 395 B.C., opening the Corinthian War, as it was called. While the Greeks moved too slowly to defeat Sparta before Agesilaus' return from Asia Minor, Persia had been relieved, and the Great King now began to subsidize the anti-Spartan coalition to keep the war going. The Persians hired an Athenian admiral, Conon, who won a victory over the Spartan fleet at Cnidus in 394 B.C. With Persian money Athens was able to reconstruct the Long Walls and to build a new navy, and the anti-Spartan coalition was able to hire mercenaries. Even so, the war dragged along in Greece without decisive result. In 392 B.C. Sparta tried to redress the situation by sending an envoy, Antalcidas, to King Artaxerxes to persuade him to arrange a peace settlement for Greece, by which Ionia would be left to Persian control and Sparta to recover her leadership. The Great King allowed the situation to deteriorate until 387 B.C., when, perhaps disturbed by the speed of Athens' recovery, he summoned the Greeks to send delegates to him and read to them the terms of a general peace.

The King's Peace was drafted purely in the interests of Persia and made a skillful appeal to the traditional Greek feeling that each city-state should be autonomous. By this time all were prepared to abandon Ionia for their own interests and readily subscribed to a pledge to recognize the Persian claim to the Ionian cities. All other Greek cities were to be free and all leagues to be dissolved. Athens was allowed to retain several islands, Lemnos, Imbros, and Skyros, in which there was a predominantly Athenian *cleruch* population. Throughout Aegean Greece a general peace was established. Since the Great King had dictated the terms, he was in effect the guarantor of the agreement, but his only interest in peace was to increase the available supply of mercenaries for the Persian army. Accordingly, Sparta, whose envoys had arranged the peace, assumed that its role was to act as Persian agent in enforcing the terms. Naturally the Spartans felt that the prohibition against leagues did not apply to themselves and under the shield of the King's Peace embarked on a policy of imperialistic aggression.

In the Peloponnesus the Spartans tightened their control of the Peloponnesian League by establishing oligarchical governments favorable to themselves in most of the member states and discontinuing the assembly meetings. These arrangements converted the free states into virtual subjects and destroyed loyalty to Sparta, except in a very small segment of the people. As occasion offered, the Spartans treated the rest of Greece in the same way. In 382 B.C. Theban oligarchs betrayed their city to a Spartan force camped nearby and, as a reward, were supported by a Spartan garrison. During the same year Sparta, in collusion with the king of Macedonia, broke up the Chalcidian League, and made the former members subject allies. These operations marked the wide extent of Spartan control, but its real power had become increasingly hollow. As cities lost their independence and many citizens fled into exile, a tide of ill will rose against the Spartans. In 378 B.C. the reaction began.

THE LEADERSHIP OF THEBES AND ATHENS

Some Theban exiles slipped back into Thebes in disguise and through the collusion of a minor official came to a banquet of the Theban oligarchical officials as flute girls and dancers. When the party was well advanced, the "women" killed their hosts, rallied their townsmen against the Spartan garrison and succeeded in freeing the city. Unofficial help came from Athens, and Sparta was threatened by the breakdown of its authority in Boeotia. Although Athens had not aided Thebes officially, the Spartan garrison commander at Thespiae, a small Boeotian town, took it upon himself to capture Peiraeus. When he miscalculated the distance of his night march through the mountains, dawn found him well inside Athenian territory but far from his objective. Faced with apparent attack by Sparta, Athens made an alliance with Thebes and proceeded to organize a new Athenian League directed specifically against Sparta.

In Boeotia the Theban leaders, Pelopidas and Epaminondas, reorganized the Theban army and began to free the Boeotian towns, one by one, from their Spartan garrisons and to incorporate them into the Boeotian League. The élite of the new army was a company of three hundred men under the command of Pelopidas, known as the Sacred Band, whose members were sworn to die or conquer in their battles. While their devotion to Thebes and to each other set a tone of uncompromising loyalty in the army, Epaminondas introduced innovations into the *hoplite* phalanx which were to be of longstanding importance. He brigaded the heavy-armed men into massive wedges, fifty deep, supported by light-armed troops and cavalry. Even before these technical changes were complete, the skill and spirit of the Boeotians unpleasantly surprised the Spartans and discouraged a full-scale attempt to retake Thebes.

The antagonism to Sparta was a unifying force in the reorganization of the Boeotian League, and Epaminondas demonstrated an unusual quality of statesmanship in constituting it along more democratic lines than previously. He was a rare combination of expert soldier, man of action and idealist, determined to break Sparta and establish Thebes as a great power in Greece. The new League, which included seven districts of Boeotia, brought all the citizens together in regular assembly meetings to elect their officials and decide on matters of policy. The chief officials, known as *Boeotarchs*, leaders of Boeotia, were representatives of each district who led the Boeotian army on their League enterprises. Under the imaginative leadership of Epaminondas, Thebes had cleared all the Spartan garrisons from Boeotia by 374 B.C. and began to extend its influence to nearby areas.

Athens, spurred by the Boeotian example, rapidly extended its new alliance, the Second Athenian League, among the islands and coastal states of the Aegean. Athens was again able to offer protection by her navy but was careful to avoid the mistakes of the past. In the new organization emphasis was placed on the full autonomy of the prospective members. As previously Athens held the military leadership of the League's forces, but policy was made by agreement between a general assembly of the allies, in which each state had one vote, and the Athenians. Athens had no share in the League assembly and the members, in fact, selected their own presiding officers. Because the meetings were held in Athens, the wishes of the Athenians were made known easily to the delegates. Athens soon became the dominant partner in the League but at the outset made a genuine attempt to avoid infringing on the autonomy of the member states. For example, the Athenians pledged that they would not make *cleruch* settlements or hold land in them. Athenians who did so might be tried by the League assembly. Other cases arising from betrayal of the League arrangements were to be tried by a system of two courts, one Athenian and the other the League assembly itself. Payments and military service by the allies to the common cause were called euphemistically contributions. The organization made a promising start when Chios and some of the smaller islands of the Aegean joined the small nucleus of allies which Athens had acquired prior to the King's Peace. Thebes, too, was a nominal member of the League, but occupied primarily with its problems of reorganization in Central Greece.

While the alliance of Athens and Thebes confronted Sparta with a formidable combination on land and sea, which did check that state's aggression, relations between the new allies became uneasy. When Thebes began to interfere in the politics of its neighbor, Phocis, and destroyed Plataea, the old ally of Athens, Athens began to draw closer to Sparta. By 371 B.C. both states felt that a reaffirmation of the King's Peace was necessary to halt the expansion of Thebes. Persia, too, was anxious that Greece be at peace, for mercenaries were needed to deal with a new revolt in Egypt. Accordingly, Sparta convoked a peace conference at which delegates were present from the Great King, Athens, Thebes, and the minor Peloponnesian states. Once again a general peace was proclaimed, and its guarantee stiffened by a proviso that any signatory of the peace might attack a state which did not observe the terms. Athens signed for her own League and Sparta signed for the Peloponnesian League, but objections were raised to Thebes' signing for her allies. To permit her to do so would have been tantamount to Sparta's recognition of the Boeotian League. Accordingly, Thebes walked out of the conference, laying herself open to attack by the others.

The Spartans precipitately rushed an army to Boeotia, where Epaminondas had prepared to fight at Leuctra. When the two armies met in 371 B.C. Epaminondas inflicted a crushing defeat on the Spartan forces with his new tactics. The Theban victory, which ended the long history of Spartan military prestige and domination in Greece, opened the way for a Theban Empire.

Although there was some opposition among the Boeotians themselves, because they were beginning to learn the high cost of extensive military action, Pelopidas and Epaminondas generally had their way in establishing Theban power abroad. In the years immediately following Leuctra, Epaminondas marched his army twice into the Peloponnesus and invaded the fertile river plain of the Eurotas. Sparta itself was not attacked, when he saw that the Spartans were prepared to defend their city to the death, but Epaminondas created a new order in the Peloponnesus to hold Sparta in check. He encouraged the cities of Arcadia to build a new center, Megalopolis, the Big City, for their Arcadian League and freed the *helots* of Messenia. Their kindred were invited from Naupactus and even from Sicily, where some had gone after the Peloponnesian War, to found a new city-state, Messene on the slopes of Mt. Ithome. Ithome had been the chief center of Messenia before the Spartan conquest in the eighth century, and time and again its rugged slopes had offered protection to the leaders of revolt against Sparta. The mountain was almost impregnable in itself, but to accommodate the new city, a large and well-engineered circuit wall was built. The wall is still one of the most impressive fortifications in Greece. To protect the new states and to confine Sparta, Epaminondas arranged alliances between Arcadia, Messene, and Argos, thus blocking the roads leading from Sparta to the west and north. Sparta was deprived of more than half of her farming land by the loss of Messenia and was reduced to the rank of a second-rate power. Even so, the Spartans made no effort to integrate their *perioeci* and remaining *helots* into the state, and consequently revolution in Sparta was delayed for almost another hundred and fifty years.

Circumstances were favorable to Theban expansion in Central and Northern Greece, and Thebes rapidly extended control over Thessaly to the frontier of Macedonia. During the Theban fight to reorganize the Boeotian League against Sparta, a tyrant of Pherae in Thessaly, Jason, had taken advantage of Spartan preoccupation to organize Thessaly under his domination by hiring a strong force of mercenaries and developing the Thessalian cavalry. Jason had ambitions to challenge Theban leadership, but he was assassinated in 370 B.C. and succeeded by a brutal and treacherous ruler, Alexander. The Thessalian cities turned to Thebes for help. Pelopidas led an army against Alexander, defeated the tyrant and confined him to his own city of Pherae. While Pelopidas was killed in the operations, Epaminondas took over the organization of Thessaly and molded its towns into a League under Theban influence. He extended alliances also to the small states of western Greece and in 363 B.C. began to make Thebes a naval power. To secure the south shore of the Corinthian Gulf the cities of Achaea were forced to make alliances with Thebes and to change their oligarchic governments, which had favored Sparta, into democracies. A fleet of a hundred warships was planned to challenge Athenian control in the Aegean.

But, just as the domination of Sparta had encouraged reaction, so, too, the other Greek states began at this time to unite against Thebes. Already in 371 B.C. Athens had tried to turn the abortive peace of that year into a tool of the Athenian League but failed to enlist support. Now, in 367, Sparta and Athens tried the device of getting Persian support for a new declaration of Greek independence and a common peace. Theban delegates, however, convinced the Great King that his best interest lay in using Thebes as a Persian agent in Greece, and the conference broke up in heated disagreement. Athens and Sparta were thrown back on their own resources, but found support for an anti-Theban policy among the members of the Arcadian League. The new Theban order in the Peloponnesus was disturbed, and by 363 B.C. a coalition was formed against Thebes, consisting of Sparta, Athens, Elis, Mantinea, and Achaea. Epaminondas marched into the Peloponnesus once again to save the situation and met his enemies at the battle of Mantinea in Arcadia in 362 B.C. His army won the battle handily, but in its closing moments Epaminondas was killed. As his last advice to Thebes, he urged that peace be made, using the advantage of his victory.

All the Greeks, except Sparta, which had hoped to recover Messenia, were weary of war and willing to accept the current state of affairs. Accordingly, a general peace was made, with Sparta abstaining but impotent, and a manifesto issued to reject Persian interference in Greece. The peace left the Theban and Athenian systems of alliance intact for the moment, but each began to disintegrate quickly. Neither Thebes nor Athens had the power for further aggrandizement, and among the minor states compulsion to seek protection had vanished with the military collapse of Sparta and the death of Epaminondas. Theban power shrank to its own Boeotian League, and in 357 B.C. many of Athens' Aegean allies revolted successfully against her. Greece had finally obtained a general peace, but had failed to establish any real unanimity or leadership among the separate city-states.

Carthage and the Western Greeks

CARTHAGE

In the western Mediterranean Carthage, rising to the height of its power in the fourth and third centuries, pressed hard against the Greeks in Sicily and tried to take over the whole island. Of all the Phoenician foundations made in the western Mediterranean (p. 123), Carthage enjoyed the most strategic situation for trade and sea power. The city was located on the African coast across from Sicily, where shipping through the channel between the eastern and western basins of the Mediterranean could be controlled readily. It had a strong defensible position, good harborage on the peninsula on which it was built, and ready access to the fertile coastal plain of Tunisia. When ties with Tyre were weakened by the incorporation of Phoenicia into the Assyrian and, later, the Persian Empire, Carthage had become independent and extended its own control along the coast of North 'Africa and throughout the western Mediterranean.

The wealth of Carthage was derived partly from exploitation of its fertile hinterland and partly from industry and trade. The African natives were subjugated, and a very profitable system of agriculture based on their labor was developed. The semiarid land next to the Sahara was used for sheep raising, which provided wool for a textile industry, and the well-watered coastal strip was intensively developed for cereal, fruit, and garden produce. The wealthy merchant families owned large tracts of land, and from their experience Carthaginians produced handbooks on estate management and agricultural techniques, which were of use to Rome at a later date. Although the natives were never given any share in government and were ready for revolt whenever an enemy of Carthage could gain access to them, the shield of Carthaginian sea power was strong and very widely spread.

Carthage gradually took over the other Phoenician colonies along the African coast, such as nearby Utica, the Balearic Islands, Malta, Sardinia, Corsica, and southern Spain. At first these were free allies, but in the course of time were reduced to subject status, liable for military service and tribute. In addition, the Carthaginians founded trading posts at strategic points to control the shipping of the western Mediterranean outside of Magna Graecia in an effort to establish a complete monopoly of trade. The trade was varied and extensive, linking Western Europe and North Africa to the eastern Mediterranean. To the metals of Spain which had been the primary goal of the Phoenician traders, the Carthaginians added European furs and amber, African exotics from caravan trade in the desert and even from the Atlantic, where merchants sailed as far as the Guinea Coast. This wealth from trade and agriculture supported a mercantile society in which political control was held by wealthy merchant families, as in Venice at the time of the Renaissance.

The Carthaginian system of government was praised by Aristotle for its stability, but rivalry for office seems to have been intense among the wealthy families. At the head of state were two magistrates, elected annually, the *suffetes*, who worked closely with a council of three hundred members elected for life. This council had a directive subcommittee of thirty members, but decisions seem to have been made by the magistrates in consultation with the whole group. In case of disagreement the disputes were resolved by a popular assembly of all the Carthaginian citizens, but this occasional function and the election of magistrates and councilors from those properly qualified by wealth marked the limits of popular sovereignty. During the fifth century the power of the magistrates was further curbed by the council when a judicial body of 104 judges, made up of councilors, was established to examine the conduct and accounts of the magistrates.

The chief weakness of Carthage lay in its military system. The army was manned by mercenaries and by levies drawn from the subject peoples, while the ships were rowed by hired men or slaves. The Carthaginians themselves acted as officers and were extremely skillful sailors, but the state used its citizens as regular soldiers only in case of extreme emergency. While the great wealth drawn from tribute and tolls on trade permitted the hiring of thousands of men and the use of good equipment, the city was vulnerable, for as soon as Carthaginian naval power was defeated, the natives of the Carthaginian hinterland were ready to turn against their masters.

Carthage remained typically Phoenician and thoroughly materialistic in culture. The Phoenician gods of the early colonists, Astarte, Melkart, and the Baals, remained the great gods of the state, worshipped by the practice of temple prostitution and, in moments of extreme peril, by human sacrifice. Carthaginian art was a blend of Phoenician and Greek influences, lacking taste and originality, but goods were produced in quantity for export in the western Mediterranean. While Carthage was one of the great cities of antiquity, with a population of about three-quarters of a million in its heyday, we know little of its physical character, for Rome destroyed it completely in 148 B.C. In the fourth century, however, Carthage was just reaching the zenith of its prosperity, grasping at the Greek part of Sicily and at control of the waters around southern Italy.

DIONYSIUS I AND SYRACUSE

Among the Greek cities of the West, Syracuse had risen to first place in size and wealth. Its prosperity was built on trade and sea power, and its prestige had been won by the victories over Carthage at Himera in 480 B.C. and over the Athenians in 413/12. Like Athens, Syracuse had become a democracy in the fifth century, but its stability was even more troubled by extremists of both oligarchic and democratic views whose hatreds ran deep. In the fourth century, when Carthage was trying to take over all Sicily, Syracuse was weakened by jealousy among its leaders. Out of the crises of invasion and internal strife emerged one of the most famous of Greek tyrants, Dionysius I, who brought Syracuse to the height of its power from 405 to 367 B.C.

After the repulse of Athens from Sicily, Carthage attempted to improve its holdings on the island by playing much the same game as Alcibiades had advocated for the Athenians. An occasion was found to invade the Greek part of Sicily by aiding Segesta against its enemy, Selinus. Among the Syracusan generals selected to deal with the invasion was Dionysius, an exceedingly able and thoroughly unscrupulous man. By accusing his fellow generals of treason and incompetence, he was advanced by the people to the position of commander-in-chief, whence, with the support of his bodyguard, it was but a step to tyranny. Dionysius obtained a reasonable peace from Carthage, more by good fortune than generalship, because a plague attacked the Carthaginian army after it had won decisive victories over Selinus and Himera. Dionysius used the time gained to consolidate his tyranny.

Dionysius retained a democratic form of government in Syracuse but saw to it that members of his family and close friends were elected to the important offices. He cultivated popular goodwill by the distribution of land confiscated from the Syracusan oligarchs, and by freeing the slaves to increase the number of citizens. But the main basis of Dionysius' authority was a large mercenary army of over ten thousand men. With it Dionysius garrisoned the citadel at Syracuse and extended his control over native and Greek towns in eastern Sicily. Syracuse itself was enlarged, fortified, and its harbor facilities improved. Like Epaminondas, Dionysius was one of the great military innovators of his age who developed weapons for siege warfare, a type of armament in which Greece had been deficient hitherto.

In 398 B.C. Dionysius, with considerable Greek support, issued an ultimatum to the Carthaginians to withdraw from the island. When the latter were unimpressed, Dionysius advanced to western Sicily to besiege the Carthaginian base at Motya, a fortified island, where he put his new siege machinery to use. After a causeway was built from the shore, battering rams, catapults and towers were dragged out to breach the wall. Despite a long, hard-fought defense, Motya was taken, but the siege had given the Carthaginians time to mobilize. In the resulting war Dionysius was outmatched by sea and lost the support of the native Sicels. In 393 the Carthaginians were able to besiege Syracuse but once again were decimated by the plague and forced to make an inconclusive peace. In preparation for the next round they built a fortified base at Lilybaeum in western Sicily and undermined the position of Dionysius among the Greeks by intrigue.

Dionysius used this interlude of peace to expand across the Strait of Messina into southern Italy and to add the Greek cities of that region to his little empire. He hired native Italians, Gauls or Greeks, as the occasion demanded, and achieved his purpose by playing city against city and faction against faction. Control of the Strait of Messina allowed him to move freely about the coast of Italy. Dionysius sent ships into the Adriatic where he founded trading posts as far north as the estuary of the Po. The western coast of Italy was raided and Carthaginian shipping harassed in the Tyrrhenian Sea. While Dionysius was never able to drive the Carthaginians from Sicily, he had made Syracuse the most important city of Magna Graecia and the center of commercial exchange between Aegean Greece and the West. Tyranny, violence, and intrigue, however, destroyed internal freedom in the Greek cities under his control and pent up a tide of anarchy. His son and successor, Dionysius II, reaped the harvest of revolt and war which spread over Sicily and South Italy in the latter part of the fourth century.

When Dionysius II succeeded in 367 B.C. at the age of thirty, his reign was made difficult by the ambitions of his uncle, Dion, who had played a prominent part in the previous reign. Perhaps to make the young Dionysius more tractable, Dion invited his friend Plato to become Dionysius' teacher, for the young man was interested in philosophical speculation and wished to become the patron of intellectual life in western Greece. Plato had high hopes of making his pupil a philosopher-king, but soon after his arrival in Syracuse in 366 B.C., he became enmeshed in the court intrigue between the supporters of Dion and Dionysius. Despite Plato's attempts on this and a later occasion in 361 to reconcile uncle and nephew, civil war broke out. Dionysius had to deal with the realities of Sicilian politics in the harsh, practical way of his father, rather than by philosophical theories. He gave up the project of expelling the Carthaginians and made a settlement with them by which the Halycus River was recognized as the frontier between Greek and Carthaginian Sicily. In the Greek area Dion and Dionysius tore the Syracusan Empire apart in war and massacre, as bands of unemployed mercenaries roved from city to city, killing and looting. Finally, in 344 B.C. the people of Syracuse appealed for help to their old mother-city and ally in Greece, Corinth. The Corinthians sent out Timoleon, an able soldier and known man of integrity, who could be trusted not to establish a tyranny of his own.

Timoleon skillfully insinuated himself into the web of political plot and counterplot in Sicily, first using Dionysius to expel the Carthaginians from Syracusan territory, then securing the exile of Dionysius. When Syracuse had been freed, Timoleon proceeded against Carthaginians, local tyrants and mercenary captains. By 339 B.C. Carthage was content to make peace on the same terms as previously, and two years later Timoleon captured and put to death the last of the petty tyrants. Settlers were invited from Greece to repopulate the Sicilian cities, and for a generation the island recovered its stability and prosperity. Timoleon himself, unselfish and idealistic to the last, retired to private life and died in Syracuse, where the people properly honored him by a public tomb and the establishment of a festival.

Unfortunately the people of the Sicilian cities proved unable to work their free governments, so that disorder and anarchy burst out once more. In 317 B.C. a new strong man, Agathocles, seized power in Syracuse and, like Dionysius I, got control of Greek Sicily and the cities in the toe of Italy. He waged war successfully against Carthage, on one occasion landing in North Africa and coming close to capturing the city. Agathocles' regime restored stability until his death

Syracusan coin, using Corinthian symbols

in 279 B.C., when he declared Syracuse free in his will. By that time Rome had fallen heir to the problems of Magna Graecia. The Romans found Carthage in firm control of western Sicily and ready to move into the Greek cities when opportunity offered. In the interval Syracuse had held the Greek position and maintained Hellenism as a vital cultural force. Underneath the political turmoil, urbanization was proceeding, and the Greek language and customs were making steady headway among the native people of Sicily and South Italy.

The Rise of Macedonia (359–36 B.C.)

Until the reign of Philip II (359–36 B.C.) Macedonia had been of only intermittent interest to the Greeks. The Macedonians, although of the same Indo-European stock as the invaders of Greece, had not shared a similar historical experience. City-states had not developed, the Macedonians spoke an obscure dialect of Greek, and only the nobles regarded themselves as Greeks. Thus, to the Greeks of the mid-fourth century, Macedonia seemed a barbarian land, from which they procured some timber for shipbuilding and in whose political affairs they meddled when their own interests were concerned. At that time Macedonia was about half as large as the present Macedonian district of Greece. The richest land lay in the valleys of the Haliacmon and Axius (Vardar) rivers, but the plateaus and mountains to the west and north had good pasture and supported a numerous population. Passes led westward through the mountains to Illyria and the Adriatic Sea and north to the Danube River, but Macedonia was oriented east to Thrace and south to the Aegean. A line of hills along the Strymon River formed the frontier with western Thrace, with its big trading center of Amphipolis and the gold and silver mines of Mt. Pangaeus. To the south the Greek colonies of the Macedonian Chalcidice, formed into the Chalcidian League in the fourth century, possessed some good agricultural land and exploited the trade by sea which Macedonia might have had. Before the time of Philip, the Macedonian kings had built some roads and established a capital at Pella, but had scarcely been able to consolidate their country into a strong kingdom because of its almost Homeric conditions of life.

The people of Macedonia were conscious of themselves as a distinctive people, "the Macedonians," and met in a military assembly of the free and arms-bearing men to acclaim their king and to hear important judicial cases, such as treason. At the head of the people was the king, usually attaining his position by hereditary descent, but with the need of popular acclamation because the king's primary responsibility was to lead in war. A weak or child ruler might be rejected in time of crisis. Like the Homeric kings, the Macedonian ruler was helped, or checked, by his nobles. They were the tribal and clan chieftains, mainly from upland Macedonia, who controlled their people by ties of kinship and personal loyalty. The organization, from king to peasant and shepherd, was still personal and patriarchal in character. Under a strong and successful king, Macedonia might be a very formidable state, but under a weak leader the people could fall apart in chaotic disunity. Philip II provided the leadership which welded the country into a national state, the first which had developed in the Aegean area.

THE CONSOLIDATION OF MACEDONIA (359–46 B.C.)

In 359 B.C. Philip became regent of Macedonia for his young nephew, Amyntas, but in a short time was acclaimed king in his own right and established the succession in his family. Like all the royal family, Philip had received a Greek education and spoke Greek fluently because the royal house had Hellenized and claimed a family connection with the early Doric kings of Argos. Although only twenty-two years of age, Philip was thoroughly familiar with the Greek political scene since he had spent three years, 367–64 B.C., as a hostage in Thebes. Despite an educated familiarity and admiration for Greek culture, Philip remained Macedonian and considered the interests of Macedonia and of his own dynasty paramount. He followed the policy of his predecessors, such as Perdiccas and Archelaus in the Peloponnesian War, in trying to consolidate and expand Macedonia, but he succeeded beyond their highest ambitions. The explanation lies partly in the fact that his reign coincided with a period of weakness in Greece and partly in his own qualities. His qualities are difficult to estimate, for we see Philip mainly through Greek eyes. In the mouths of his enemies, like Demosthenes of Athens (pp. 334–35), terms such as barbarian, drunkard, and scoundrel were normal. Even his friends, like the Panhellenist Isocrates (pp. 342–43), recognized a barbarian element of irrational passion in Philip. Their standard of judgment, however, was that of philosophical ethics, not that of the practical politics of Greece in the fourth century. Judging from his career, Philip was able to assess the basic factors of a situation clearly and coldly, make up his mind quickly, and carry out his plans by whatever means seemed appropriate. He preferred diplomacy to force and was a more skillful master of diplomatic half-truths and implications than the Greeks. When bribery was useful, he would use it. If force were necessary, Philip turned to that, but as a last resort and, then, decisively, for he built up the superb army which Alexander later turned against Persia. Above all, Philip was a statesman, who desired to direct the chief trends of his period to the end of a strong Macedonia and Greece.

In 359 B.C. Philip began to win over the clan chieftains of the Macedonian highlands by a mixture of persuasion and force. The advantages of close cooperation were demonstrated by campaigns against the Illyrians and Paeonians to the west and north. Against Illyria Philip found an ally in the Kingdom of Epirus, with which he cemented an alliance in 358 B.C. by marriage to the Epirote princess, Olympias, who became the mother of Alexander two years later. When temporary peace had been obtained on the frontiers, Philip turned in 357 B.C. to the Strymon valley. The moment was well chosen, for Athens, which might have opposed this move into its trading region, was involved in war with some of the members of the Athenian League. Philip gave the Athenians to understand that he would hand over Amphipolis to them in exchange for Pydna, a coastal town in Athenian possession. Amphipolis was captured, but, instead of giving it to Athens, Philip made another adroit move to lessen the chance of effective Athenian reprisal. He captured the town of Potidaea in the Macedonian Chalcidice and gave it to Olynthus, the largest city of the Chalcidian League, thus aligning the League firmly with himself. Athens' only recourse was to intrigue with the tribal chieftains on the Macedonian frontiers, while Philip and the Chalcidian League tampered with the loyalty of the remaining possessions of Athens. Philip had won time to begin the internal consolidation of his kingdom.

The metal from the mines of the Pangaeus region provided Philip with a good silver coinage and the means to build roads and to found new towns. The coins were used in diplomacy and trade, which brought Macedonia gradually into the network of Aegean commerce. Colonies of Macedonians and of landless men from Greece were founded in the good farming land of the Strymon River valley and one of its villages, Crenides, built into a proper city, Philippi. It was the prototype of the numerous "Philippis," "Alexandrias," and the like, which Macedonian kings were to found in the Hellenistic Period. Philippi was a municipality of the Macedonian Kingdom, not an independent city-state. Roads were also built to connect the centers of Macedonia, and the little army which Philip had inherited was expanded and reorganized.

The Macedonian farmers and shepherds, tough, hardy men, made excellent military material for Philip's army. In it he adapted the professional techniques of war developed by the Greek mercenary captains and the Theban phalanx, familiar to him from his stay in Thebes as a hostage. The infantry was arranged into heavy formations of sixteen ranks, armed with long pikes, and spaced more widely than Greek *hoplites*. Thus, the Macedonians were more maneuverable and almost as powerful on attack as the more cumbrous Theban phalanx. In addition, a heavy, armored cavalry force was organized as a striking unit, which gave Philip a great edge over Greek opponents. From Greek mercenary tactics came the use of companies of light-armed troops to support the heavy infantry and cavalry. Philip was familiar also with the new type of siege machinery used by Dionysius I in Sicily but had little occasion to employ it. The particular quality of his army lay in its national character. Recruiting was done on a territorial basis, with men from the same district, often from the same tribe, being brigaded together into regiments which were given special titles and battle honors to establish a continuous tradition. They possessed a spirit and stubborn loyalty paralleled only by that of the Theban and Spartan armies in their prime. Leadership was provided by the clan chieftains and nobles of Macedonia, whom Philip developed as special troops, the "Companions," fighting and living with the king and centering their loyalty and that of their clansmen on his person. Since Macedonian manpower was limited to about forty thousand men at the most, Philip hired mercenaries and levied troops from his allies. These, too, were integrated with the Macedonians, and the whole formed into a fighting force of a caliber hitherto unknown in Greek warfare, a trained and disciplined army of professional skill and national spirit.

In 352 B.C. Philip was able to establish control over Thessaly by taking advantage of the dislocation caused in Central Greece by a Sacred War, proclaimed three years earlier by Thebes and Thessaly against Phocis. The Phocians, who had been outraged by a Theban attempt to use the Amphictyonic Council for purely selfish political ends against them, in defiance had seized the shrine of Delphi and used its temple treasures to hire an army. Although the treasures were valuable, Phocian scruples against their sale were slight. Consequently the war turned out to be unexpectedly difficult and protracted for Thebes and its allies. In the course of operations Thessaly was defeated, and some of its cities called on Philip to come to their aid. At first the Phocian mercenaries defeated him, but Philip returned to the attack, drove the Phocians from Thessaly and reorganized the Thessalian League in his own interest. That land was made an adjunct to Macedonia by the election of Philip as general of the Thessalian League, with the right to levy soldiers from its members. Philip was thus thoroughly entrenched in Northern Greece and retained a cause for war against Phocis, should the need arise to invoke it.

In the next year Macedonian authority was extended to the Hebrus River in eastern Thrace, and in 349 B.C. Philip felt ready to deal with the Chalcidian League. This operation involved danger of war with Athens, already irritated by Philip's action against its ally, Phocis, and by his expansion into eastern Thrace. The latter threatened Athens' grain route through the Hellespont. Philip guarded against Athenian intervention by fomenting a revolt in Euboea against Athenian authority. Then in 349 B.C. he issued an ultimatum to Olynthus, the acceptance of which would have broken up the Chalcidian League and made Olynthus subject to Macedonia. The people of Olynthus chose to fight and appealed to Athens for help. Despite the powerful argument of Demosthenes that Athens should attack Philip in Macedonia, the Athenians could not do so effectively. There was division in Athens itself about Philip's intentions, for some regarded his attack on Olynthus as a local matter, of no concern to Athens' future safety. The revolt in Euboea required attention, and Athens did not have the strength to undertake a major war at such a distance. Philip captured Olynthus, destroyed the city, and took over the Chalcidice with its good harbors and connections for trade into the Aegean. After some ineffectual raiding and futile diplomatic maneuvers to embarrass Philip, Athens began to negotiate for a settlement in 346 B.C.

The Peace of Philocrates, as it was called from the principal Athenian negotiator, was a victory for Philip. He succeeded in convincing the Athenian envoys that Macedonia had no quarrel with Athens and that it was unnecessary to include Athens' ally, Phocis, in the peace. The Athenians signed and, almost on the morrow, Philip invaded Phocis to finish the Sacred War. The towns of Phocis were burnt and plundered, and its political organization, the Phocian League, dissolved. Philip was voted the seat on the Amphictyonic Council vacated by Phocis, thus taking a place among the older states of Greece in its most venerable religious association. Athens, Thebes, and the minor city-states had to reckon with the new power which had appeared in their midst and to try to gauge Philip's aims.

THE CONQUEST OF GREECE (346–38 B.C.)

There was still considerable room for debate about the intentions of Philip, for he had made peace with Athens and re-established order in Central Greece. Like a proper Greek, he had made gifts to Delphi to restore its depleted treasury. Thebes preferred to take Philip's actions at their face value and demonstrated friendship by voting with Philip on the Amphictyonic Council. Isocrates of Athens wrote to Philip, suggesting that he unite the states of Greece and lead them against Persia, throwing open Asia Minor to Greek settlement. In Athens, however, chagrin at being outwitted in the Peace of Philocrates began to swing that state to hostility. Demosthenes made headway in his attempt to prepare Athens for eventual war.

Nevertheless, Demosthenes' struggle to put Athens on a proper war footing and to rouse the rest of Greece against Philip was a long, uphill fight. Some of his opponents in Athens, who sincerely believed that Philip wanted peace and alliance with Athens, regarded Demosthenes' attacks on Philip as prejudicing a real understanding. They reflected, too, that Demosthenes had to make his own political career by opposition to Athenian leaders who had already done much to restore Athens' position after the near collapse of the League in 355 B.C. These men, Eubulus and Aeschines, had followed a cautious foreign policy which avoided all-out war, but still opposed and harassed Philip in the northern Aegean. They had restored Athenian finances to a healthy condition, built up the fleet, and diverted some money for military purposes from the Theoric Fund, from which state payments and welfare came. They believed, with some justification, that Demosthenes' militancy would lead to an unnecessary war in which Athens would be defeated. To Demosthenes, Philip's purpose seemed to be the enslavement of Greece to Macedonia, a process in which the annexation of Thessaly and the destruction of Phocis and Olynthus were but the first steps. Accordingly, Demosthenes attacked his opponents in the courts on charges of treason and corruption and advocated that Athens accelerate its military buildup and raise a Greek coalition against Philip. Slowly Athens began to prepare for the final struggle.

To rouse Greece against Philip was even more difficult than to stir Athens. The reputation of Athens as a protector of Greek freedom had been tarnished twice, and to most Greek states there seemed little to chose between Philip and Athens. Philip spent money freely and established virtual "fifth columns" in the Greek cities, men who supported him either from self-interest or from a sincere conviction that Philip could do more for their city than could Athens. The paramount consideration to many was not the preservation of Greek freedom, as Demosthenes argued, but under whose patronage, that of Athens or Philip, they could find security and support for their own political interests. The action of the anti-Spartan coalition in the Peloponnesus was typical. Messene and Arcadia made alliances with both Philip and Athens, hoping to sit on the fence until the issue was decided.

Yet in the diplomatic contest Athens had reasonable success, for the Peloponnesus was at least neutralized, the Athenian allies in the Hellespont held in line to protect the vital grain route, and Megara and Euboea won over. By 340 B.C. a coalition had been formed to defend Greece against Philip, but Thebes still remained aloof. Overtures were made also to Persia, for Philip's advance in Thrace was alarming to the Great King. Probably the Persian officials gave some financial aid to the Athenian allies in the Hellespont, but the Great King judged it preferable to follow the usual Persian policy of allowing the Greek powers to wear themselves out.

In 340 B.C. the diplomatic sparring came to an end when Philip forced the war. He attacked the Athenian allies, Byzantium and Perinthus, whose loss would cut off the grain supply from Athens. The Athenians had to declare war and send aid against Philip, but neither Athens nor Philip had sufficiently large fleets to fight a naval war or to make landings on each other's coasts. Philip, to win decisively, had to set up a land battle in Greece. He used his position in the Amphictyonic Council to stir up trouble and obtain a pretext for marching into Central Greece. Since Thebes, more than ever, was the key to the situation, both Philip and Athens sent envoys to bargain for support. Demosthenes, acting for Athens, offered to pay two-thirds of the Theban war expenses and to give up some towns on the Boeotian-Attic border, which Thebes had long claimed. Whether moved by Demosthenes' eloquence and the profit he held out or by apprehension of Philip is not clear, but Thebes elected to join Athens and threw the army of the Boeotian League into the battle. Philip skillfully contrived to outmaneuver the combined Greek forces and to force battle on ground where his heavy cavalry could be used to advantage, near the town of Chaeronea in Boeotia. In the autumn of 338 B.C. the Macedonian army won a complete victory, and Philip became the political arbiter of Greece, to do with it as he wished.

THE LEAGUE OF CORINTH

After the victory at Chaeronea, Philip worked very rapidly to put his plans into execution. Evidently he had given much thought to them and wished to prevent bitterness and despair from growing out of delay. First Philip made a series of separate peace settlements with his enemies and adjustments with his allies, which were designed to remove old causes of war between the Greek states and to ensure support for his own ideas. In some cities, upon report of the news from Chaeronea, the pro-Macedonian parties seized control of their local governments, killing and exiling opponents. Philip allowed this up to a point, but, except in the case of Thebes, he himself did not encourage such change. In Athens, for example, young Alexander negotiated a fair settlement with the anti-Macedonian leaders and permitted Demosthenes to continue in political life. The general effect of the separate settlements was to destroy the previous systems of control—of Thebes in Central Greece, of Athens in the Aegean, and of Sparta in the Peloponnesus. In Central Greece the Phocian League was re-organized, and the influence of the Amphictyonic Council was increased to counter Thebes. In the Peloponnesus Philip revived the policy of Epaminondas by strengthening Messenia, Arcadia and Argos with allocations of territory from the Spartan frontiers. It is likely that the detailed and extensive knowledge of Greek politics required for this wholesale remodeling was supplied by Aristotle. He had been the tutor of Alexander and is known to have written a sort of diplomatic handbook, the *Dikaiomata* (*Justifications*). Philip, however, did safeguard his military control of Greece by putting Macedonian garrisons into Thebes, Chalcis and Corinth. This provoked resentment, but was a reasonable precaution for the early stages of a new order.

When the settlements were well started, Philip, in the winter of 337 B.C., put the crowning touch on his program by the formation of a new League, the League of Corinth, named from its place of meeting. All the states of Greece were invited to send delegates to discuss the arrangements, and at the same time rumors of a great war against Persia were circulated. Philip planned that the League would conduct the affairs of Greece in a peaceful fashion under his personal presidency and that it would become the tool for a joint Macedonian-Greek war on Persia. The delegates came from every state (except Sparta, which sulked in isolation) and worked out their covenants. Philip and his successors were to be personal *hegemons* of the League, to command its military forces and to be a link to Macedonia. All the Greek states, former Macedonian allies and enemies alike, were placed on the same footing and grouped into new units for representation, which were based on military strength. Perhaps Philip intended these divisions to be a start on a new map of Greece, but that was as far as he could safely go at the moment. The principles of individual autonomy, freedom from tribute and freedom from Macedonian garrisons were asserted for each Greek state. Warfare was forbidden among the members of the League, and arrangements made to arbitrate disputes, whose settlement would be guaranteed by the League collectively. In an effort to eradicate civil war and revolution, each member pledged to maintain the system of government in operation at the time of signing the League agreements. This political freeze was unrealistic, but perhaps was designed to serve as a warning rather than a firm principle. The delegates to the League were to make its foreign policy without referral to their own states or to Philip. This somewhat surprising surrender of control by Philip was presumably designed to serve his advantage indirectly. His wishes could be made known through agents, from Thessaly, for example, and thus Philip could not be blocked by delegates who used communicating with the home government as an excuse for delay and obstruction.

At the outset this ambitious blueprint for a new Greece was little more than a paper model. Behind Philip's wishes, of course, was the coercive force of the Macedonian army, but he preferred to keep that argument in the background. The League had to be infused with a spirit of cooperation and given a cause with some appeal to Greek tradition. War against Persia seemed to be the best possibility, since the Greeks themselves in the common peace at Mantinea in 362 B.C. had sworn to reject Persian interference in their affairs and had talked of such a war for almost half a century (p. 342). When the motion for war was presented, the delegates approved enthusiastically and elected Philip as commander-in-chief, promising a large force of 35,000 men from their states.

This thoroughgoing attempt to reorient Greek political life and to make a strong Greek-Macedonian union was to fail, but Philip may be credited with a more complete vision than any statesman of his century. He was constructive in that he attempted to end the futile and endless warfare which was destroying the Greek city-states. Fundamentally the Greeks themselves wished to stop their wars, as the various attempts at a common peace indicate. The economic malaise of Greece might have been corrected by peace, expansion of trade, and a renewal of emigration on a large scale. So far as we can tell, Philip contemplated war against Persia in Asia Minor only and did not originate the adventurous dreams of Alexander to conquer the whole Empire. Philip, too, was aware of the half-formulated wish among the Greeks to establish federal organizations and unions larger than the single city-state. He respected and encouraged those which existed and offered a model in the League of Corinth. To make the organization durable, however, the Greeks would have had to lay aside their centuries-old tradition of the fully independent city-state and to transform the urge to imperialistic aggrandizement, which was a part of it, to mutual cooperation. Such cooperation might have been accomplished by a long period of firm and understanding direction by Philip, but history did not provide the opportunity.

In 337 B.C. Philip returned to Macedonia to prepare the projected invasion of Persia. In the following year he was assassinated at a festival by a young Macedonian officer with a personal grudge. Alexander succeeded to the throne, but had to reassert his authority in Greece, and left, never to return, in 334 B.C. Alexander's conquest of the whole Persian Empire, and the rise of Rome in the western Mediterranean, created a new world in which the independent city-state was an anachronism, in which only a united Greece could have played a decisive political role.

XV

The Civilization of Greece
in the Fourth Century

WHILE THE VICTORY OF PHILIP II over the Greeks at Chaeronea in 338 B.C. virtually ended the political independence of the city-states of Greece, their mold was stamped on the rest of antiquity in significant fashion. To Plato and Aristotle life in a city-state seemed the only proper way of existence for civilized man. Both philosophers were acutely aware that the cities which they knew fell short of providing a suitable environment, and each, in his own way, was deeply concerned with reform. Nevertheless, they could conceive of no other framework than that of the city-state for the ideal communities which they described. Thus, at the time when the city was losing its political importance, Greek philosophy examined its society thoroughly and established the city as the ideal form of community.

By the fourth century, too, the Greek city had developed the characteristic elements of its physical form, temples, civic, and recreational buildings. These architectural forms, along with Greek institutions and customs, had begun already to spread into native, non-Greek areas. This remarkable germinative quality of Greek culture was to flower luxuriantly in the Near East in the period after Alexander. He and most of his successors considered that the Greek city was the best type of community for their new lands. Even if the new cities were not independent states, they preserved the urban mode of life developed in Aegean Greece, and it was ready for wholesale transplantation by the fourth century. We will look first at the physical form of a Greek city.

The City-State

As city life became more complex and varied, the *agora*, the open square used as a place of gathering, increasingly replaced the *acropolis* as the heart of the city. In the *agora* the citizens gathered for political and commercial business or

The reader will find Map VII (pages 172–173) useful as he reads this chapter.

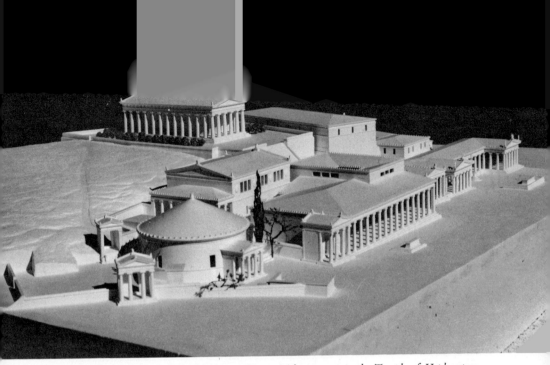

The Athenian agora. *Model of the buildings on the west side: top center, the Temple of Hephaestus; left to right, the round* tholos, Bouleuterion, *shrine of the Mother of the Gods, and the* Stoa *of Zeus*

for social meeting and talk, matters of almost equal importance to the gregarious Greeks. In the cities of Classical Greece the *agoras* were of various forms, for each developed to fit the particular needs of its own city, but all shared certain general characteristics, well exemplified by the *agora* of Athens. Despite its very imperfect preservation, we know a considerable amount about the Athenian *agora,* thanks to the thorough excavations carried on by the American School of Classical Studies at Athens since the nineteen thirties.

An *agora,* of course, had to occupy a central position in the city, where it could easily be reached by the important roadways leading from the main gates. In Athens the *agora* was located just to the northwest of the Acropolis, from which the ancient city fanned out. From the early sixth century this region had acquired an increasingly public and monumental character, reflecting the growth of the city. As on the Acropolis, damage to the buildings by the Persians in 480–79 B.C. provided an opportunity for rebuilding and reorganization, and by the fourth century special types of buildings had been developed for the various functions of the *agora.*

The main civic buildings of Athens were constructed along the west side of the *agora* from the southwest corner, where a round building, the *tholos,* was built in the period of Cimon's leadership (*ca.* 465 B.C.). There the *prytaneis,* the committee of the Council of Five Hundred, met and dined. To the north were the council buildings, an Old *Bouleuterion,* which was used as an archives office, and its successor, the New *Bouleuterion,* erected in the late fifth century. This

325

structure was typical of later Greek council houses, a small, compact auditorium with the seats built like a horseshoe around a speaker's place. It is an interesting comment on the attendance of the Athenian councilors that there was not enough space to seat all five hundred. Since political activity might be aided by the gods, this part of the *agora* was also the site of small temples and shrines. In front of the Old *Bouleuterion* was a long pedestal, on which were erected statues of those ten heroes of Athens who had been pressed into service as divine ancestors for the Athenian tribes. The pedestal itself served as a notice board to which public announcements were fixed. North of the council houses were small shrines of the Mother of the Gods, of Apollo Patroos, the progenitor of the Ionian Greeks, and of Zeus and Athena in their capacities as protectors of the *phratries*.

The row of civic structures on the west side of the *agora* was completed by the *Stoa* of Zeus (Royal *Stoa*), which honored Zeus as the protector of Athens' freedom and contained the offices of the king *archon* and exhibited the law code of Solon. The Royal *Stoa* was of the same high quality of construction as the buildings on the Athenian Acropolis and was the earliest example of the type

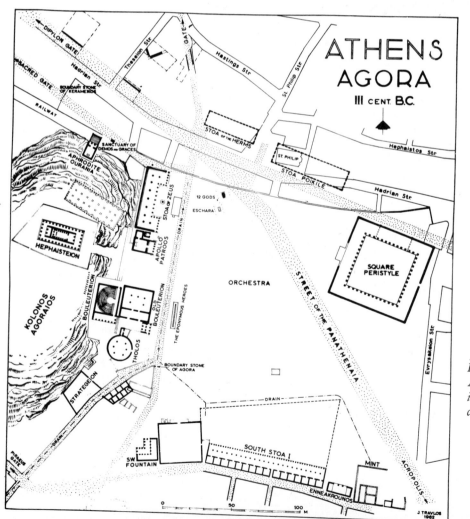

Plan of the Athenian ag in the third century B.C.

of *stoa* with shallow, projecting wings at each end to break the straight façade. Dominating the buildings on the west side of the *agora* was the Temple of Hephaestus on the slope to the west—the best preserved of Athenian temples, because it was used as a church in the medieval period.

The *agora* proper, the open area lying to the east of the major civic buildings, was used for the political purpose of balloting for *ostracism,* but regular assembly meetings were moved from the *agora* in the fifth century for lack of adequate space. The activity of the law courts was provided for by the *heliaea* on the south side and a square structure in the northeastern corner of the *agora.* To take care of the commercial and social activity of the *agora* the Athenians used *stoas,* colonnades, happily described as the general-purpose buildings of Greek architecture. The *stoa* was simply a wall tied to a row of columns by a roof, admirably designed for easy access and for shelter from the hot Greek sun in summer and the rain in winter. The space might be doubled easily by the introduction of an inner row of columns or by the addition of a second story. In the fifth and fourth centuries the north and south ends of the *agora* were provided with *stoas,* of which that on the south has been excavated. In the Hellenistic Period it became the practice to frame the sides of an *agora* with colonnades and to regularize its shape into a rectangle. This was done for the Athenian *agora* in the second century B.C., when King Attalus of Pergamum provided funds for the construction of the *stoa* along the east side of the *agora.* The colonnades also contained small shops, the tables of money changers, and the offices of bankers. They were thronged by shoppers, slaves, and traders, or men who simply came to look and talk.

The meetings of the Athenian assembly were held on a hill, the Pnyx, to the southwest of the *agora.* The slope of the hill was built up artificially to form an auditorium sloping to the rock-cut *bema,* the speaker's platform. Apparently, as in the case of the council, the space was not adequate for a "full (6000) assembly," since the capacity of the Pnyx in the fifth century is estimated at about five thousand people. Since no permanent seats were installed and since these meetings involved some discomfort, perhaps we should not be too critical of their decisions. About 330 B.C. a drastic remodeling of the auditorium provided space for about twice as many citizens. But in the fourth century the Athenians were paid a fee to attend assemblies.

Except for recreational facilities, like gymnasiums in the suburbs, a Greek city was compactly built around its *acropolis* and *agora.* Residence in the suburbs was hardly safe under conditions of almost continuous warfare, so that the urban population crowded inside the city walls. The course of the walls was dictated primarily by the needs of defense and sometimes did not permit good areas for residence to be utilized. Greek skill was high in military architecture, and much money and care went into the construction of the long circuit walls around the cities. Around some cities, like those of Messene, founded in 369 B.C., walls were constructed of large, beautifully dressed stone blocks with a full use of towers, parapets, archer slots, and loopholes to permit crossfire on

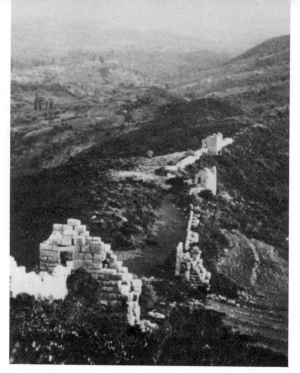

A stretch of the fortification wall of Messene, built in the fourth century B.C.

the attacking force. Most walls, however, were of cheaper construction, with a roughly cut stone facing over a core of sun-dried brick or packed earth and rubble.

The most complete remains of the residential quarters of a Classical Greek city are in Olynthus, which Philip II destroyed in 348 B.C. A large part of Olynthus was a "new" town, deliberately laid out on a checkerboard plan, in contrast to older Greek cities which had grown haphazardly. This type of planning probably originated in Ionia, where regularly planned blocks were used in Old Smyrna as early as the seventh century and in Miletus, rebuilt in 479 B.C., after its destruction at the end of the Ionian Revolt. The spread of town planning from Ionia is associated with Hippodamus, who is said to have planned the Periclean building in the Peiraeus about 450 B.C. and Pericles' colony at Thurii in 443 B.C. Systematic town planning was well known by the outset of the Peloponnesian War, when construction began on the north hill at Olynthus. The area to be developed there was laid out with long avenues running along the ridge to give level thoroughfares and narrower cross streets running up the slope. These formed blocks, which were built up with two rows of five houses of uniform size, 60 feet by 60 feet, divided by a narrow alley. They were the dwellings of middle-class citizens and give a good idea of the appearance of a Greek city and the living conditions of that class.

Since the cities put most of their wealth and available artistic skill into sacred and public construction, the private residential quarters presented a monotonous, even drab, appearance. Because space was at a premium, the houses were built compactly, fronting on narrow streets and without garden areas. Doorways were simple and the windows set high in blank, stuccoed walls.

The houses at Olynthus, however, were reasonably commodious, with five to seven rooms, and show considerable variety in their interior arrangements. They were built two stories in height around a central courtyard, which usually had a partial colonnade and stairway to the second floor. The amenities of living were simple, compared to middle-class houses in Roman cities of a later age, but by no means inadequate. Water was provided by a cistern in the courtyard and public fountain houses in the city. The latter offered to the women of the household all the opportunity for gossip provided by an American laundromat. Heating was provided by portable charcoal braziers. Most houses had a bathroom with a terracotta tub and a dining room, recognizable by its bench for the diners and, usually, by a special floor of pebble mosaic. The bedrooms were upstairs, where a pleasing feature was provided by a gallery overlooking the courtyard.

The homes of the wealthy were, of course, larger and better furnished, as we know from an inventory of Alcibiades' household effects, sold at auction after his exile. For the poor, living conditions were desperately crowded and uncomfortable, but all Greeks spent a large part of their life in the public quarters of the city, in the *agora* and temple precincts and, from the fourth century, in the recreational buildings which the cities began to construct on a considerable scale.

The Theater of Dionysus at Athens and that at Epidaurus in the Argolid provide examples of the familiar form of Greek theater which had evolved.

*Olynthus. Model of the Villa of
Good Fortune (fourth century B.C.)*

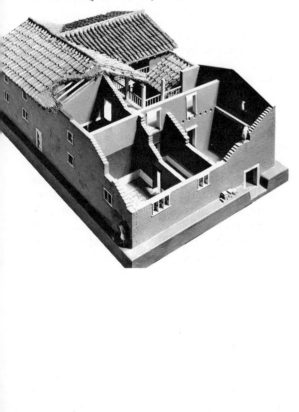

*Olynthus. Plan of city blocks,
showing typical checkerboard
layout*

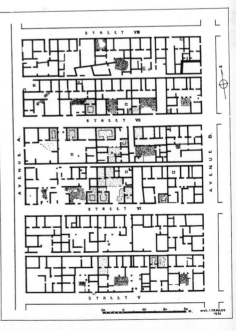

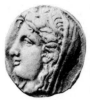

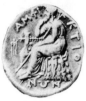

The earliest element was the *orchestra,* or circular dancing floor, the shape of which was probably originally determined by the spectators crowding around to see the spectacle. In the center there was an altar for Dionysus, around which the action of the plays was staged. It is likely that the earliest "theater" was performed in the *agora,* but soon transferred to a convenient hillside, where a large crowd could be accommodated. This natural auditorium was called the *theatron,* or viewing place. To convert it into monumental form, the hillslope was cut out in a great semicircle and provided with rows of stone benches. The scene building (so-called because at first a tent, *skene,* was used) furnished an architectural background for the action, as well as dressing rooms for the actors. At a later date, in Hellenistic times, the action was transferred to a raised stage, but the *orchestra* was retained for the chorus and musicians. The Greek theater was never roofed, and use of the natural hillsides saved the cost of the enormous vaulted construction developed by Roman architecture. Although the capacity of the large Greek theaters was about seventeen thousand, the acoustics were excellent; thus the theater could be used for large public meetings as well as for the drama.

In the fourth century the gymnasiums were developed from suburban parks into more formal athletic and school grounds, used for general social and educational purposes. This dual character as exercise ground and school is well exemplified by the famous old gymnasiums of Athens. The Academy, located about three-quarters of a mile to the northwest of the city, had been used since the sixth century for athletic practice, sports and lounging. In 387 B.C., however, when Plato took over a house near its shrines for his lectures, the name, Academy, became synonymous with his school of philosophy. Some lines in Aristophanes' *Clouds* picture the pre-Platonic Academy:

> "But you will below to the Academe go, and under the olives contend
> With your chaplet of reed, in a contest of speed with some excellent rival and friend;
> All fragrant with woodbine and peaceful content, and the leaf which the lime-blossoms fling,
> When the plane whispers love to the elm in the grove in the beautiful season of Spring."

The gymnasiums were usually located in the leafy quiet of the suburbs and offered a welcome contrast to the bustle and noise of the *agora.* To the east of Athens another famous gymnasium, the Lyceum, became the site of Aristotle's philosophical school in 335 B.C. In addition, Athens had several other gymnasiums, as did any Greek city, for they were a regular part of the city's educational activity and were supervised by an elected official, the *gymnasiarch.*

By the latter part of the fourth century a regular type of building had been devised for the gymnasium, which is exemplified by that in the sanctuary of Asclepius at Epidaurus. It consisted of a large colonnaded court, where boxing, wrestling, and jumping could be carried on, surrounded by rows of rooms for

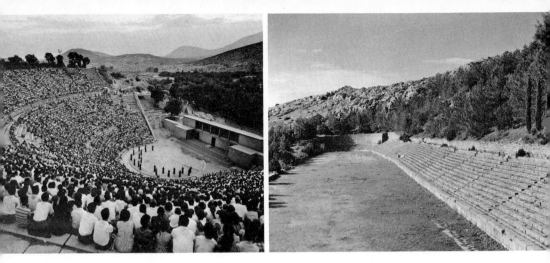

Epidaurus. Modern performance of
a classical drama in the theater

The stadium at Delphi

washing, massage, class and lecture use. Usually set close to the gymnasium was the stadium for footraces. The Greek word *stadion* had several meanings: it was a measure of about two hundred yards; it was the footrace over that distance; and it was also the ground where the race was held. The footrace was probably the oldest of Greek contests, and at first the stadium was only a level piece of ground with the distance for the race marked off. In the stadium at Epidaurus arrangements were more permanent. A row of stone blocks was set flush to the ground, with grooves cut into their surface to give footing for a standing start, and stone benches were placed along the course for the spectators.

Intellectual Life

RELIGION

As Greek society became more individual and cosmopolitan, there was, of course, a corresponding change in men's ideas. Some clung to their old traditional beliefs and the seeming safety offered by conservatism, while others discussed reform or sought the completely new. Superficially there seemed to be no marked decline in the civic religions because the cults and rituals of sacrifice were properly maintained, the priests were duly elected, and the festivals were as well attended as they had been previously. No city undertook a building program of the magnitude which Pericles had conceived for the Athenian Acropolis, but in the fourth century many new temples were constructed in the more prosperous regions of Greece. The new Peloponnesian cities, like Messene, needed shrines and temples to house their civic gods. In Asia Minor the Greek cities enjoyed more prosperity under Persian than under Athenian control, as the result of more intensive trade with the hinterland. At Ephesus and at Didyma, near Miletus, grandiose temples, which took their place among the most famous of antiquity, were built for Artemis and Apollo respectively. In the mid-fourth century international contributions paid for a new temple of Apollo at Delphi. Nevertheless, the cities seem to have spent more on secular buildings and their fortifications than on religious architecture.

Although men supported their civic religion as a matter of form and tradition, they turned increasingly to superstition and exotic forms of worship for their personal needs. To the mercenary soldiers and those who drifted from city to city, the religious beliefs intimately linked with their family life and to the city of their birth seemed outworn. "Luck" was personified as a goddess who seemed to many to rule their own and their city's fortunes. As the mystery religions increased in popularity, Orphism (p. 230), in particular, acquired many adherents. Oracles were sought from Delphi as before, but in the cities sellers of oracles and interpreters of dreams made a living by selling their occult knowledge.

Perhaps the most striking example of mass adherence to a cult with the appeal of the miraculous is that given to Asclepius, the god of healing, previously an obscure, local deity. During the fourth century his sanctuary at Epidaurus became the chief healing shrine of Greece, where miraculous cures might be made overnight. The sick, victims of almost every disease or accident, prepared themselves with prayer and purification to sleep in the temple of the god where he or his associate deities might appear in a dream to heal or advise them. The grateful patients left written records of their cures for exhibition in the sanctuary and made very generous donations to the god. Around the temple a whole complex of buildings was constructed to entertain visitors and adorn the shrine. In addition to the theater, stadium, and gymnasium mentioned above, guest houses were erected at Epidaurus for those patients who made a prolonged stay. Athletic facilities might seem incompatible with a hospital, but they were used for contests in the festival of Asclepius and for genuine, if simple, medical treatment which accompanied the faith healing. Since Asclepius was the god of Greek medicine, doctors were attached to his shrine, who performed simple operations and prescribed special diets and limited exercise for the patients. This combination of psychological and physical treatment worked so well that Epidaurus became the center from which cults of Asclepius were disseminated to other Greek cities and even, in 218 B.C., to Rome. An interesting branch-cult was that at Corinth, where the grateful patients dedicated models in terracotta of their eyes, ears, legs, arms, and other parts of their bodies which Asclepius had cured.

LITERATURE AND ORATORY

The fourth century was the great age of Greek prose writing in which the new schools of rhetoric, oratory, and philosophy developed various styles and genres which began to replace the free-lance teaching of the Sophists. The problems with which Greek tragedy had dealt in the fifth century were discussed by philosophy in the fourth, and reproductions of old plays seem to have been more popular than the new. Comedy, as exemplified by Aristophanes' last play, *Ploutos* (*Wealth*), tended to become a wry mirror of everyday life and manners, while political leaders themselves dealt in invective and scurrilous attacks on their fellows.

Historiography was more notable for its new interests than for the penetration of its writers. The historians recognized the new individualism of society and paid attention to biography and to the characterization of prominent figures, like Philip of Macedonia. They were increasingly aware, too, of the world beyond Greece. Ephorus of Cyme in Aeolis wrote a voluminous universal history, in which his account of Greece from the time of the Dorian invasion was the central theme, but long sections were devoted to Egypt and to Persia. One historian, Ctesias of Cnidus in Caria, wrote a history of India and of Persia, but this was premature in the light of Greek knowledge of central Asia, and Ctesias had to rely on fantasy. Time, too, had placed the greatness of Athens in perspective, and its past was treated in a series of local histories, the earliest of which was by Hellanicus of Lesbos. These works survive only in fragments which were excerpted by later writers, and for most of our knowledge of the early fourth century we are dependent on the Athenian Xenophon (430–354 B.C.)

Xenophon's long list of books reveals the wide range of activity which appealed to his individual interests. He had been a member of the Socratic circle and acknowledged the influence of Socrates on his education by a lengthy account of Socrates' life, the *Memorabilia*. The study reveals the mediocrity of Xenophon's mind more than it revealed the unique character of Socrates, since Xenophon did Socrates the disservice of trying to establish him as a plaster saint. Xenophon was more at home with his own interests as a country gentleman and ex-soldier. The *Anabasis* (pp. 306–07) described the far hinterland of Anatolia for the Greeks, and the *Hellenica* gave an account of Greek history from 411 B.C., where Thucydides had broken off, to the battle of Mantinea in 362 B.C. Xenophon wrote well and vividly of colorful personalities, like Theramenes and Agesilaus, and of single episodes, such as the regime of the "thirty" in Athens, but he lacked the power of penetrating analysis and of coordinating his material, which Thucydides had possessed. His essays on hunting, cavalry, estate management, education (in which Cyrus the Great of Persia was the protagonist), and on the revenues of Athens are of interest for the views and pursuits of a conservative, upper-class Greek, who admired the discipline and order of Spartan society in contrast to that of his own Athens.

The conditions of life in Athens under the restored democracy were particularly favorable for the development of political oratory. Men who "went into politics" almost as an avocation, needed a mastery of public speaking for success. Some of the new leaders were wealthy men who wanted prestige and recognition, while others were poor, equally ambitious, but hoped to improve their financial position through public office. Perhaps competition for the assembly's favor was no keener than it had been in the fifth century, but political methods seem to have been more unscrupulous. The usual tools of the politician were fierce invective in public speech and charges of corruption and treason in the law courts. He not only had to be thoroughly familiar with public finance, law and court techniques, but also a would-be statesman. Under these conditions, since the ordinary citizen also had to plead efficiently in the courts, he provided himself with ready-made speeches written by professional speech writers. The most interesting among these was a *metic,* Lysias, who tailored his speeches to the character of his clients. Even though the Sophists continued to supply most of the training for these activities, a new development of the period was the rise of more permanent schools of oratory, of which the most successful was that of Isocrates, who began his career as a professional speech writer (pp. 342–43) and became one of the most influential political figures of his age.

In the political crisis produced by the rise of Macedonia, a galaxy of very able political orators came into prominence in Athens, the chief of whom was Demosthenes (384–22 B.C.), the protagonist of Greek freedom against Philip II. He had acquired training in speaking by long practice, even overcoming a speech defect, and by suing his guardians for the waste of his inheritance. His first political speech, in 355 B.C., *On the Symmories,* was on public finance, a sensible recommendation about raising money for naval expenses. In 350 B.C., when it was apparent that Philip would attack the Chalcidian League, Demosthenes delivered his *First Philippic,* a fine, carefully considered speech in which he showed an appreciative understanding of Philip's adroit diplomacy and maneuver and advocated Athenian aid to Olynthus. In the *Olynthiacs* of the following year Demosthenes turned to vilification of Philip and began his long effort to divert money from the Theoric Fund to military expenditures. From this point until his death in 322 B.C. Demosthenes was identified with a policy of hostility to Philip and Alexander, in the course of which he delivered some of the most impassioned and finest political speeches of antiquity, making himself and Athens the champions of Greek freedom against the Macedonian tyrants, as he branded Philip and Alexander.

Demosthenes could not see freedom, as Philip did, existing within the framework of the League of Corinth, but only in the traditional pattern of independent Greek states, among which Athens held primacy. He fought for his conception of freedom, perhaps the only one which could stimulate the creative activity of Greece, with all the weapons at his disposal. Demosthenes was unscrupulous in political attack and a vindictive hater. When news of Philip's assassination came to Athens, he put on festive garlands and joined the assembly in a message of congratulation to the assassin. Yet Philip's death did not bring

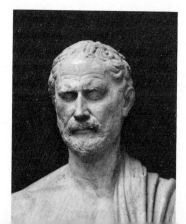

Demosthenes. Roman copy of an original of the Hellenistic Period

the freedom for which Demosthenes and his party hoped. Demosthenes transferred his attacks to Alexander, perhaps not realizing how insignificant they seemed to the conqueror of the Persian Empire, far off in the heart of Asia. In 332 B.C. Demosthenes' fellow citizens enthusiastically endorsed his career, when his rival, Aeschines, sued him in the courts. Demosthenes delivered a long, reasoned defense of his lifework in the *Crown*. Aeschines, as a prosecutor, obtained less than the necessary one-fifth of the jury's votes and had to depart from Athens. After Alexander's death in 323 B.C. Demosthenes helped to bring Athens into the Lamian War, in which the Greeks attempted to throw off Macedonian control. The revolt failed, and a pro-Macedonian government was installed in Athens. When Demosthenes was condemned to death, he fled for refuge to a small shrine at Calauria across the Saronic Gulf. After Macedonian soldiers surrounded the temple, Demosthenes took poison and died, crawling from the altar, lest he pollute the sacred ground with death. Demosthenes' colleague Lycurgus had already pronounced a fitting epitaph on Demosthenes' career when he spoke in 330 B.C. of the dead at Chaeronea: "They alone in all Greece had the freedom of Greece in their bones; for they died as Greece fell into slavery. With their bodies the freedom of Greece was buried."

PHILOSOPHY

The fourth century was particularly rich in the growth of Greek philosophical speculation, for the intellectuals of Greece turned to philosophy and scholarship when their belief in the civic religion and the anthropomorphic gods of Olympus declined. Plato and Aristotle founded the great philosophical systems of antiquity which were to direct the thought of Greece and Rome for centuries. It is impossible, of course, to sketch their thought and that of their contemporaries in a few pages, but perhaps useful to notice some of the criticism and suggestion which were developed for the political and social conditions of their period. Although Plato and Aristotle put their faith in the city-state, other philosophers, notably Diogenes the Cynic, turned from society to emphasize the value of a private, ascetic life for man.

Diogenes came to Athens and Corinth from Sinope, his birthplace on the Black Sea, to spread his ascetic and asocial philosophy of life by example, as well as precept. He and a contemporary, Antisthenes, were regarded as the founders of the Cynic school of philosophy, perhaps so-called from the shameless, aggressive character of its adherents' way of life, which was considered to resemble that of a homeless dog (*kunos* is the Greek word for dog). Diogenes' philosophy has been well described as that of the "displaced man" of the fourth century. He considered that the individual should be self-sufficient, devoting himself to a life of virtue, which denied the ties of family, society, and the state. The material comforts of life and its familiar conventions seemed to Diogenes to give a false sense of well-being and satisfaction. Diogenes, however, needed an audience, and his way of life was anything but a withdrawal from the contamination of urban society. He wore a beggar's costume, begged for his living and found shelter where he could, in public buildings and, according to one story, in a wooden tub in Corinth, where he became something of a tourist attraction. His wit was astringent, designed to attract publicity. On one occasion, when observed walking about Athens in the bright daylight, carrying a lighted lantern, Diogenes answered the obvious question by replying that he was searching for an honest man.

Plato (429–347 B.C.), on the other hand, was deeply and responsibly concerned that society, without which man could not live, be reformed. Plato belonged to an old upper-class Athenian family and, as a young man, looked forward to the normal political life, in which a man of his connections would engage. He wrote in one of his letters, however, that the spectacle of oligarchic and democratic conflict in Athens convinced him that practical politics was impossible for a man of principle. The condemnation of Socrates made a profound impression on Plato and perhaps was most effective in turning him to teaching and philosophy. He is said to have traveled widely after Socrates' death. He visited Sicily, where he became a friend of Dion, the uncle of Dionysius II. About 387 B.C. Plato established his school at the Academy in Athens and, aside from his unfortunate visits to Sicily (p. 315) when he failed to make Dionysius II into a philosopher-king, lived in Athens until his death in 347 B.C. The Academy became known particularly for its work in mathematics and jurisprudence, as well as for the philosophical development of Platonism. From Plato's death until A.D. 529, when the Byzantine emperor, Justinian I, closed the pagan schools of philosophy, the Academy was one of the great intellectual centers of Greek and Roman civilization.

Plato, like his teacher Socrates, regarded the contact of living minds as essential for the process of teaching, but, fortunately for posterity, also developed his ideas in written form. The various dialogues were appropriately set in lively debate, with historical characters, chief among them Socrates, as the protagonists. The dialogues, in addition to being philosophic in content, are literary masterpieces of Greek prose, in which the dramatic form is essential to the thought. They cover the whole range of ethical, metaphysical, and political philosophy, discuss education, theology and, to some degree, technical mathematics and science. In the wide range of material covering all of Plato's working life of fifty years, the *Republic* and the *Laws* embody the most important political ideas.

Plato considered that the individual could achieve a good and truly happy life, the aim of all men, only through membership in a good and just society. Thus in the *Republic* he began with the question, "What is justice," and answered in a long, intricate discussion during which the form of an ideal city-state was gradually created. The social structure of the ideal state was so organized that the individual would find true happiness only through his work as a member of the community. While an individual's social function should be the expression of his own abilities and psychological aptitudes, the state was to provide the opportunity for such expression by its system of education and by its power of government. Thus the psychological nature of man and his desire for social justice was linked with the organization of the state.

Plato believed that three basic elements in the nature of man were revealed by the ordinary behavior of human beings. As this idea is usually expressed, man had a tripartite soul. On the lowest level there was his appetite, desire, for food, shelter, and the good things of life in a material sense. The satisfaction of this appetite occupied the attention and time of most men; in some degree such satisfaction was necessary for all men. But preoccupation with appetite conflicted with the other two elements of the soul, spirit and wisdom. Spirit might be exemplified by the courage and loyalty of a good soldier fighting for his state or revealed by rebellion against some infringement of a man's rights. Spirit would appear, too, in the conflict among the three elements of the soul. Wisdom, the highest element and regulative power, was the clear and sure knowledge which comes from considered, rational judgment of what is good. Every man would have some share of these three elements, but not in equal measure; they were bestowed by heredity and might be cultivated and directed by education.

The ideal state was the expression in political form of the human soul, since in it each individual would find his happiness by the proper and regulated exercise of his chief aptitude for the common good. The society of the state, then, was stratified into three classes, which correspond to the three divisions of the tripartite soul. Most men, in whose souls the element of appetite was strongest, were engaged in the economic activities necessary for the existence of the community. But Plato distrusted such activity as too stimulative to man's appetite for wealth and material comfort; accordingly, in the *Republic* only the necessary minimum of trade, business and agriculture was allowed, in order to prevent men from selfish exploitation of their appetite. While Plato considered peace desirable, he thought that it was hardly attainable, so that his state needed a class of soldiers. For this purpose he proposed to use the men in whose souls the element of spirit predominated. The community would be protected by their courage and loyalty, and they would be educated by special training. That small élite in whose souls wisdom was the chief element would form a highly educated and trained governing class of "philosopher-kings." Their function would be to supervise the working of the whole community, to select and allocate its citizens in accordance with individual aptitudes, and to make sure that each man received a training proper for his function.

It is obvious that in the ideal state much that had been familiar and cherished in Greek life was to be rejected. In addition to eliminating excessive economic activity for the lowest class, Plato also proposed to discard the family as an institution for the governing group. To him the family seemed pernicious, since the affection and energy of its members were directed largely to their own small circle. Also, woman's role as a mother and housewife prevented her from being a useful member of society in her own right. Accordingly, Plato was going to emancipate women from the household, if not from work. The ruling class was to live a communal life in barrack-like quarters, without private possessions or concern about their families and livelihood. The rulers would be supported by the labor of the workers and were thus entirely free to carry on their duties of government and education. From the educational system, most of the great poetry of Greece, Homeric epic and the drama, were to be excluded, rather wistfully, for Plato considered poetry to be untrue and harmful to the young. It presented the gods and men in immoral and humiliating behavior. There was little need for formal organs of government in the *Republic,* since each individual was allocated to his function by its authoritarian rulers, who supervised the system at every stage.

But in the ideal state justice was attained. Each type of man had his proper function—labor, war, or rule, and each individual found his happiness in the fulfillment of his function. He knew his abilities and was happy in the knowledge that he was doing for the whole community that for which he was best fitted and trained. There was no room for the feelings of injustice and exploitation which gave rise to personal unhappiness and bred revolution and anarchy in the actual states of Greece.

Plato measured the political systems of his own day against the standards of the *Republic* and found them wanting. The model of Sparta, with its regulated system of education and sharply defined class structure of *helots, perioeci,* and Spartan citizens, must have suggested some of the features of the *Republic* to Plato, but his aim for his community was social justice, not war. He admitted that aristocratic governments were good, in that aristocracy had love of honor and excellence as its purpose, but these were lesser goods than wisdom. Oligarchy was set farther down the scale than aristocracy, since the aim of oligarchical rulers was to obtain wealth. Wealth introduced the harmful effects of appetite into the state: personal rivalry and class strife. Plato condemned democracy, as he knew it in fourth-century Athens, because there was no connection between political power and individual quality in the democratic state. Each citizen's appetite ruled him in a society without controls. The result was political chaos. Even more destructive than democracy, however, was tyranny, for a tyrant was entirely selfish, seeking power and wealth for his private gratification and ruling without law or restraint. The tyrannical state had returned to the jungle law, "Might is right," and was the complete abnegation of the principle of justice which underlay human life and society.

It is easy, of course, to criticize Plato's ideal state for its assumptions about the psychological nature of man, the excessively high demands made on human nature and for the authoritarian character of its government. But Plato was almost passionately concerned to give a meaning to human life in terms of absolute standards and verities. He, of course, was wryly aware that his state was an ideal, hardly possible of fulfillment, but discussed his ideas confidently and cheerfully in the *Republic.* They were something to which men might aspire.

In his last and more systematic political study, the *Laws,* Plato turned to more practical, but still authoritarian ideas of reform. The book was designed, perhaps, more as a practical handbook for his students than a statement of principle. All citizens could own private property, but their incomes were taxed at the rate of almost 100 percent, over a fixed, modest limit. The family was reinstated, but women were to share in the educational system. A considerable amount of physical education was prescribed for the primary stages of education, and, interestingly enough, full educational use made of the child's instinct to play. In secondary education Plato advocated a coordinated curriculum of the various branches of learning to provide a broad basis for those who would advance to higher education. For the *Laws* Plato modified his criticism of democracy and prescribed a system of mixed government which used the principles of popular and personal control, but selected as a governing group only a small council. The laws of the state were considered to be as important as the council in forming the kind of citizen who was deemed desirable. An important innovation of the *Laws,* destined to have a very long history in thought and practice, was the rigid prescription of a state theology, deviation from which was regarded as criminal.

Aristotle (384-22 B.C.) was more detached and clinical in his political studies than Plato, but he, too, conceived of the environment of a city-state as the only proper setting for the "good" life. This more dispassionate attitude is perhaps to be explained in part by the circumstances of his life, most of which was spent as an alien in Athens. Aristotle was born at Stagira in the Macedonian Chalcidice in 384 B.C. and came to Athens at the age of seventeen to be a student at Plato's Academy. He remained until Plato's death, probably serving as a sort of research assistant on the compilation of the large amount of material needed for the *Laws*. In 347 B.C. he joined some fellow Platonists at the city of Assus in the Troad, which was under the control of a nearby tyrant, Hermias, whose daughter Aristotle married. In Assus Aristotle acquired some first-hand knowledge of government and, in 344 B.C., moved to the nearby island of Lesbos, where he indulged an interest in marine biology. His general interest in science and, in particular, biology may be explained by the professional interests of his father, who was court physician to the king of Macedonia. Probably this old association also accounted for Philip's selection of Aristotle as a tutor to Alexander about 342 B.C. We know little of the detail of Aristotle's teaching, but it probably gave Alexander ideas about the use to which the techniques of Greek civilization might be put and a taste for scientific investigation, which prompted him to take along a group of scientists on his campaign into the Persian Empire. When Alexander became king in 336 B.C., Aristotle returned to Athens to found his own school, the Lyceum, where he remained until 323 B.C. During this period Aristotle was a close friend of the Macedonian general Antipater who had been left by Alexander to supervise Greece. But the Athenians thought that Aristotle was too good a friend of Macedonia; consequently when Athens joined in the Lamian War after Alexander's death, Aristotle had to flee for safety to Chalcis in Euboea, where he died in 322 B.C.

The Aristotelian school had a different function than Plato's Academy since it was concerned with the classification of Greek knowledge as well as the education of individuals. In addition to his philosophical works, Aristotle himself made a zoological classification, wrote the *Poetics* on literary criticism and prepared the material for his work on political science. Under his direction memoranda were made of 158 Greek and non-Greek constitutions, of which the *Constitution of Athens* alone survives. These provided part of the material for his major book, the *Politics,* in which his views on the state are expressed. The *Politics* is a collection of essays and notes on political topics, perhaps lecture notes collected and published after Aristotle's death. The students at the Lyceum continued this type of scholarly work, and Theophrastus, who became head of the school, made a classification for botany, and Aristoxenus wrote a book on musicology. They were typical of this age, which showed an astounding intellectual vitality and curiosity, further stimulated by the opening up of the East to the Greeks in the generation following Aristotle.

The inductive method used by Aristotle for the study of political philosophy was very different from Plato's approach. Aristotle assiduously collected the data of historical and current institutions and studied his material to elucidate a general law applicable to human experience. In his political thinking, as elsewhere, he adhered to the doctrine of the "mean," favoring moderation and a balance between extremes. Accordingly, his ideas of reform and his critical observations were much more practical and closer to reality than those of Plato. Perhaps Aristotle might be described as a moderate reformer with a hope for the impossible.

Aristotle's conception of an ideal city was a small, largely self-sufficient, agricultural state, which could be taken in by a single view. Thus, all the citizens could participate directly in its government and share the intimate unity which mutual knowledge of one another encouraged. The purpose of this state was to enable its members to achieve the "good" life, only possible in a developed community. This end of moral perfection for the individual was to be attained by a proper system of education, law, and political institutions. Aristotle, however, with his more developed sense of history, admitted as necessary and valuable many of the institutions discarded by Plato in the *Republic.*

For example, Aristotle considered that the city-state had developed from the household, through the clan village, to the complex urban organization which was familiar in Classical Greece. The household, then, was a natural form of association, traditional, and valuable to the developed community. The bonds of affection felt by its members for one another could be developed into a warm loyalty towards the state, of which the household was a part. Further, the structure of authority in the household, where the father was a ruling patriarch, conditioned men for the political structure of the state. Wife and children accepted the father's authority as reasonable and good, while the slave accepted him as absolute master. Slavery was a natural social institution in Aristotle's thinking, although he felt that only barbarians, unfit for a free life, should be enslaved. Aristotle also recognized the value of private property, provided its source was a natural one, such as agriculture. Wealth from the use of money was vigorously condemned and, in all cases, should be moderate and properly used. So derived and used, property provided the leisure necessary for the "good" life and contributed to the well-being of its owner as an extension of his personality.

Aristotle, like Plato, believed that government should be in the hands only of those properly qualified to rule. The best arrangement would be rule by a supremely qualified individual, a "great" man, but that was scarcely possible in the existing conditions of life. Accordingly, Aristotle advocated that the citizen entrusted with authority should possess virtue, that is, be excellent at his function, have moderate wealth, and live in a condition of liberty which would enable him to enjoy ease and personal freedom for the "good" life. Automatically, this definition excluded those who earned their living by manual labor. These would be members of the state, but would not possess the rights of active citizenship. The best practicable state, then, was not very dissimilar from the moderate oligarchy of the Athenian revolution of 411 B.C., which Aristotle had praised. There should be a large middle class, which would balance the extremes of the very rich and the very poor, thus avoiding class strife and making the state stable. The government should be mixed by a careful selection of democratic and oligarchic institutions. Aristotle recognized much good in democracy, particularly its high quality of collective judgment and the practice of popular election in which this was exercised. Like the oligarchs, however, he condemned the equal opportunity for office offered by democracy and the principle of pay for state service. Aristotle subscribed thoroughly to the view of law as formative and educative, able to condition the type of citizen desirable for the community.

Both Plato and Aristotle were very conscious of the common civilization of Greece and convinced that the small autonomous city-state was necessary for its continuance. Neither seems to have been particularly interested in the political panaceas of the period: union among the Greek states, common peace, and a joint war against Persia. In a sense both were extremely conservative, looking back to the tradition of aristocracy, to the ideas of oligarchy and the model of stability which Sparta seemed to provide. Since stability seemed of the greatest importance to them, they were inclined to put their faith in authoritarian government by an intellectual élite or by a "great" man. Perhaps from the nature of the city-state itself, which they so carefully examined, an authoritarian government seemed necessary. Periclean democracy was the result of a happy conjunction between democracy in Athens and empire abroad and was described by the historian, Thucydides, as nominally a democracy, but really coming under the rule of her greatest citizen. The Athenian democracy, too, had failed to protect Athens in war. While Plato and Aristotle were studying the city-state so intensively, their contemporary, Isocrates, was attempting to revive the political character of Panhellenism and was searching for a leader of the united states of Greece.

Panhellenism and New Directions

The Greeks had been conscious of the unity of their culture since the time of the Persian Wars, when the invasions of Darius and Xerxes first brought home the desirability of close military alliance. The war coalition against Persia grew briefly into a Hellenic League, but the possibility of closer political union was destroyed by the rise of the Athenian Empire and the rivalry between Athens and Sparta. The Athenian Empire itself had united much of Greece, but in an unacceptable relationship which impaired the autonomy of its members. These political developments, however, had not destroyed the feeling that all Greeks shared their civilization in common, although Athenians showed an undue tendency to take the credit for Greek civilization.

In the fifth century this general consciousness of being Greek was reinforced by the contrasts drawn between Greek and barbarian. Regrettably, but perhaps understandably, as a result of the victories over Persia against great numerical odds and wealth, contempt for the non-Greek world grew rapidly. While the gods had been on the side of Greece in the wars and Xerxes' arrogance had offended heaven, the fighting proved the Greeks to be better men. Ionian science could account for this by the theory that environment, both geographical and institutional, determined the quality of men. "Soft lands bred soft people." In Asia the climate was warm and the lands fruitful, but the people were effeminate; in Europe, where the climate was harsh and cold and the country uncleared, men were rough and uncivilized. Aegean Greece, however, was the middle land, where the physical conditions spurred the development of a free and courageous people, who had developed a superior way of life. It became a commonplace to observe that all Greeks were free and all barbarians slaves, except one, the Great King. Aristotle is said to have advised Alexander to distinguish between Greek and non-Greek, and to deal with the former as a leader of free men, the latter as a master of slaves. Alexander was to develop different ideas of his own, but many Greeks shared the view of Aristotle.

In the political and economic stress of the fourth century, when Persia actively interfered in Greek affairs once more, the advantages of political union again became apparent. Now the idea was strengthened by the consciousness of Greek superiority because it seemed improper that Greece, which deserved so well of fortune, should be weaker and poorer than Persia. Some of the leading orators of Greece, in public declamations at the international festivals, advocated war on Persia to preserve and enrich Greek civilization. Their arguments, however splendidly rhetorical, were generalized and occasional. The cause of Panhellenism in the fourth century was associated in particular with one man, Isocrates of Athens.

Isocrates (436–338 B.C.), impoverished by the Peloponnesian War, began his professional life as a speech writer for the law courts, and in 392 B.C. was able to establish a school in Athens. It rivalled Plato's in popularity, and, through Isocrates' own writing and that of his students, probably had more contemporary influence. Unlike Plato, Isocrates was concerned to teach practical politics and oratory, not philosophical speculation, and consequently was branded as a Sophist by his rival. Although Isocrates did collect fees and teach practical subjects, he was genuinely concerned with the conditions of international politics in Greece and with the interests of Greek culture as a whole. In the school, instruction was divided into a basic training in grammar, debate, literature, and more advanced work in rhetoric. Isocrates favored the traditional ethics of Greek society as a whole, while locally, in Athens, he advocated a return to more conservative government by strengthening the power of the Areopagus and reviving a moderate, pre-Periclean type of democracy. His Panhellenic interests affected historians, in particular, and Ephorus' history (p. 333) helped to spread his ideas. Isocrates, too, influenced the development of Greek prose writing, by introducing a rich diction and involved type of expression, which became a model in the later schools of rhetoric.

Isocrates' argument for Panhellenism was simple. The political disorder and weakness of Greece could be cured by the establishment of a common peace and political union among the separate states. When united, Greece was strong enough to defeat Persia and find a new field for emigration in Asia Minor. The propriety of the war was justified by the superiority of Greek civilization, for Isocrates did not envisage Greek culture as extensible to barbarians. Perhaps wisely, he did not attempt to explain how the perennial dilemma of Greek union, reconciliation of separate autonomy with firm leadership, was to be solved. Instead, in a succession of essays, he appealed to various states and political leaders to undertake the task, addressing Athens first in 380 B.C. in his *Panegyricus* and finally Philip of Macedonia in a letter in 346 B.C. Despite his hopes in the leadership of Philip, Isocrates remained a patriotic Athenian to the end, since he envisaged a special place for Athens, justified by its cultural achievement, in the new Greece.

Isocrates' plea to Philip called upon him to reconcile the Greek states and to lead them against Persia. Philip did so, but he had his own ideas about Macedonia's relation to Greece and about his own quarrel with Persia. Isocrates can scarcely be credited with first suggesting these ideas to him. It was more significant for the future that Isocrates turned to the idea of a personal leader for Greece. In his thought, as in that of Plato and Aristotle, the "great" man, who could take hold and inaugurate a new era, was prominent. Isocrates assured Philip that, if he could unite Greece, he could become a god. Alexander and his successors did so, combining the Macedonian monarchy with the old Greek concept of hero worship.

ART

The new interests of the fourth century are reflected particularly well in its sculpture, which changed from the grandeur and dignity of fifth-century art to a simpler, more human level. Elaborate works were still commissioned for sacred

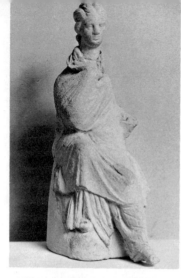

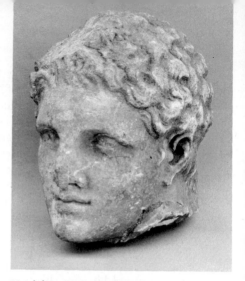

A Tanagra figurine; fashionable
lady of the fourth century B.C.

Head from Tegea, in the style
of Scopas (370–50 B.C.)

buildings and for dedication in the sanctuaries, but the individual interests of
private patrons in all classes of society are apparent. For the poor, dainty terracotta figurines were turned out in quantity. The best known are those from
Tanagra in Boeotia, which represented fashionably dressed and elegant women
from daily life, rather than gods and goddesses. The middle- and upper-class
Athenian families chose quiet scenes of family life for their carved grave monuments in the Cerameicus, which expressed the pathos of grief. A new interest in
individual portraiture is apparent, particularly of the great men of the period:
athletes, orators, statesmen, and rulers. Stylistic emphasis was on the rendering
of sensuous grace, emotion, charm, and even humor.

The best-known work of the period is an original group by the sculptor
Praxiteles, found at Olympia, where it was dedicated in the sanctuary of Hera.
Praxiteles represented the god Hermes, holding the baby Dionysus and catch-
ing his attention by some object, probably a bunch of grapes, held in the missing hand. Like much fourth-century work, the group is symbolic in meaning, to
commemorate an alliance made in 343 B.C. between Arcadia and Elis, the states
which the two gods were connected with in myth. The formal political symbol-
ism is well masked by the beauty and quiet humor of the scene. Its appeal lies
primarily in the contrast between man and child, nude body and swag of
drapery, and in the strong, but gracefully sinuous body of Hermes. This graceful
stance is characteristic of all the figures carved by Praxiteles and appears in
copies of his other well-known works, the *Sauroctonus,* the boy killing the lizard,
and the Aphrodite of Cnidus.

In strong contrast to the style of Praxiteles was that of his contemporary,
Scopas, which is known from the work in a temple at Tegea in Arcadia and
from two of the great buildings of the fourth century, the Temple of Artemis at
Ephesus and the Mausoleum at Halicarnassus. Scopas' heads are distinctive for
their almost melodramatic emotion, rendered by wide, staring eyes and open

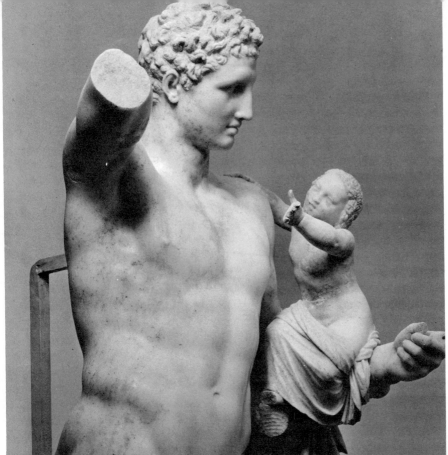

Hermes with the baby Dionysus,
probably by Praxiteles (350–30 B.C.)

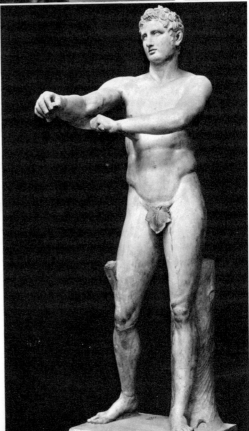

The Apoxyomenos by Lysippus. An athlete
scraping oil from his arm. Roman copy
of the late fourth century original

mouths. They indicate a new tendency of Greek sculpture, to break out of its self-contained envelope into another dimension.

The Mausoleum, on which Scopas and others worked on the frieze, was one of the remarkable buildings of antiquity. It was constructed by Artemisia as a tomb for her husband Mausolus, the Persian satrap of Caria. The form of the building was unique, a pyramid resting on a colonnade, itself supported on a great square base. The purpose of the monument, a commemoration of the greatness of an individual ruler, was also new in Greek art, and reflects a fusion of Greek and Eastern tastes which foreshadowed the Hellenistic Age.

Lysippus, the last great sculptor of the century, reveals its final, transitional phase. His usual subject matter was conventional, the nude male figure, but he devised a new set of proportions, with smaller heads on slender firm bodies, which reach out into the third dimension. Lysippus was almost a court sculptor for Alexander. He made portraits of the conqueror and created hunting and battle scenes of Alexander's friends. With artists working on commission for rulers such as Alexander and Artemisia, we are moving into an age of courts and kings, toward the East and away from the city-states of the Aegean.

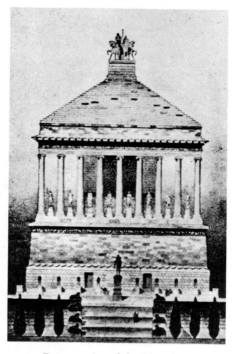

Reconstruction of the Mausoleum at Halicarnassus in Caria, built ca. 350 B.C.

III

The Hellenistic East

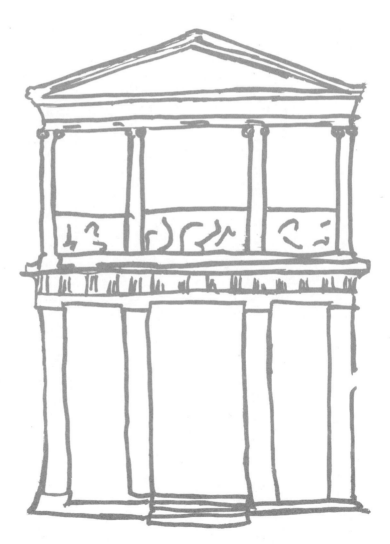

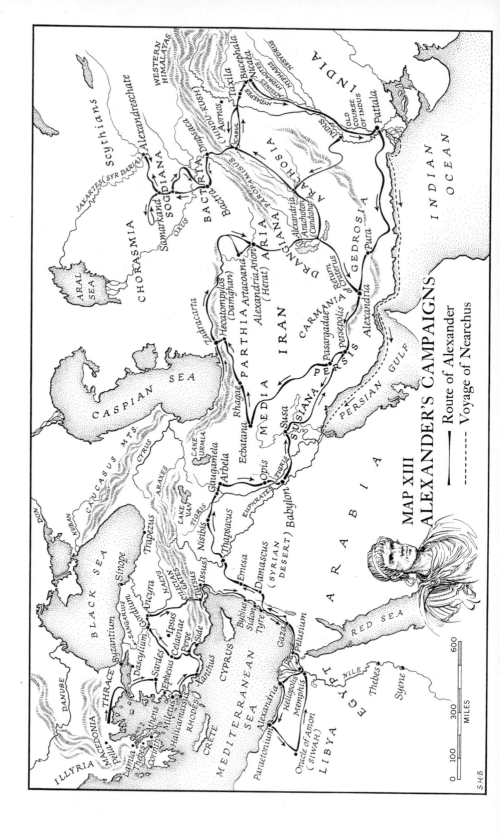

MAP XIII
ALEXANDER'S CAMPAIGNS

Route of Alexander ———
Voyage of Nearchus -------

XVI

Alexander the Great and His Successors

(336–275 B.C.)

ALEXANDER WAS ONE of the pivotal figures of ancient history, whose career marked the beginning of a new epoch, the Hellenistic Age. In 336 B.C. he inherited the Kingdom of Macedonia and the leadership of the Greek League of Corinth from his father, Philip II. Thirteen years later, in 323 B.C., Alexander died in Babylon, the ruler of an Empire which stretched from Greece and Egypt across the land mass of western Asia to Turkestan and northwestern India. Not only was his military conquest spectacular enough in itself to place Alexander among the world's great generals, but the effects of these conquests also shaped subsequent history. Alexander broke the separate molds, already crumbling, which Greeks and Persians had made, to bring the West and East of his day into union. The Empire which he established was soon torn apart by the wars of his successors, the Macedonian generals, who fought to set up kingdoms of their own. Yet, the political barrier between Greece and the Persian Empire was down, and the long process of cultural interpenetration on a large scale had started.

At first the Macedonians and Greeks went into the East as a governing class and imposed a pattern of Hellenization, which slowly changed the face of western Asia. In the long run the religious ideas of the East made their way West and helped to transform the Roman Empire and medieval Europe. After Alexander men could think in terms of the whole world as the home of civilized men living together in concord. By some scholars Alexander is credited with the conception of this idea. It could have grown out of his experience, but perhaps, he, himself, thought no farther than of the needs of administration and peace for his Empire. Yet he did establish the condition which inspired men to think in terms of common brotherhood and universal law, no matter whether they thought as philosophers and religious teachers, or whether they were rulers, who might implement this condition.

Alexander—The War Against Persia

Alexander's career was to show a remarkable combination of very practical military and administrative ability and an almost romantic idealism and taste for heroic adventure. While, of course, his ideas grew with experience and achievement, he was oriented in these directions by his early training and education. When he took over the throne of Macedonia at the age of twenty, Alexander had already helped his father for several years to weld Macedonia into a strong state and had profited from six years of association with Aristotle. Philip gave Alexander military experience against the Thracians and a responsible command at Chaeronea. Also, Alexander had founded a new settlement at Alexandropolis in Thrace and negotiated successfully with Athens after the battle of Chaeronea. He was known and trusted by Philip's generals and the Macedonian people, who speedily saw their support confirmed by his decisive handling of the situation after Philip's assassination.

Alexander's obvious enthusiasm for Greek culture and his appreciation of the use to which its techniques might be put are usually attributed to Aristotle's teaching, but the philosopher must have found his student unusually firm-minded and selective. Alexander discovered in himself a particular affinity for the Heroic Age of Greece. He read the *Iliad* avidly and venerated Achilles as a kindred spirit. When he landed in Asia, his first act was to offer a sacrifice at Troy, as if he were renewing Agamemnon's war against the barbarians. In fact, until he had taken the Persian capital, Persepolis, and burned the palace of Xerxes, the war was publicized as an act of revenge for the Persian attacks on Greece. From the outset the campaign also had the character of an exploratory and colonizing expedition, for which Alexander took along botanists, zoologists, geographers, and Aristotle's nephew, Callisthenes, a self-appointed historian. Alexander, however, showed from the start a disposition to disregard Aristotle's disdain for barbarians (pp. 340–41). He might publicize the conflict as a war of revenge, but he organized his conquests in his own interest as the new ruler of the Persian Empire, whose people were to have their place along with Macedonians and Greeks under his rule.

Although Philip had planned the war as a joint enterprise with the Greek states and had been promised considerable help by them, Alexander received very little aid and was hampered by revolt. After Philip's death the League of Corinth at first accepted Alexander as its new commander-in-chief, so that he felt free to complete preparations in Macedonia. Philip had secured a bridgehead on the Asiatic side of the Hellespont, but the tribal peoples on the north and west of Macedonia were again proving troublesome. In swift campaigns Alexander advanced to the Danube, where he established Macedonian control along the south bank, and into Illyria, where the mountain tribes were brought into line. These successes won the loyalty and admiration of the Macedonians, but in the course of the campaign against Illyria, a rumor arose in Greece that Alexander had been killed.

Thebes and Athens rose in revolt to dissolve the League of Corinth, but Alexander swiftly appeared in Central Greece with a Macedonian army. In one week Thebes was captured and his authority was re-established. Alexander chose to make an example of Thebes and insisted that the League authorize the complete destruction of the city (except for the house of Pindar), that the men be put to death, and that the women and children be sold into slavery. While some Greeks favored this, such savagery was hateful to most and, from Alexander's best interests, injudicious. The destruction of one of the leading cities of Greece probably prevented the growth of any real cooperation between Alexander and the Greeks. On his departure for Asia Alexander felt that it was necessary to leave a large force in Macedonia under the experienced general Antipater. Fear of a Greek revolt aided by the existence of a Persian fleet was a primary consideration in the campaign until the fleet could be broken up. Alexander asked for only seven thousand men from the Greek states and a fleet of 160 warships. But he never fully trusted this force; consequently the army had to be made up almost entirely from Macedonians and allies in whom Alexander had confidence.

The army with which Alexander started was small, about 35,000 in all, but was exceptionally well trained and coordinated. Its strength lay primarily in the heavily armed Macedonian cavalry, two thousand in number, and in the phalanxes of Macedonian foot soldiers, about twelve thousand men. From the tribal peoples on the Macedonian frontiers came five thousand light-armed troops and from Thessaly three thousand excellently trained cavalry. The Greek contingent of seven thousand plus five thousand mercenaries made up the remainder. Alexander could not afford to hire more mercenaries, for his treasury was almost empty. Since he expected that the fruits of the war would support him, he set up no supply bases in advance; he did not even develop a scheme of overall strategy and worked out further plans only as a new vista opened up after each victory. Alexander, however, was always careful to organize newly acquired territory as he went along and to keep a line of communication to Macedonia intact. His generals, experienced and loyal, were the men trained by Philip and, despite the fact that they were by age contemporaries of his father, they were ready to obey their young king. The most important generals were Parmenion, who acted as chief-of-staff, and Antigonus Monophthalmus, the One-eyed, who was to hold Anatolia as Alexander advanced into the Persian Empire. Young men were also advanced by Alexander and by the end of the campaigns the names of the generals form the roster of the early Hellenistic kings. Not the least tribute to the force of Alexander's personality was his ability to command the respect of these very able, aggressive officers.

Alexander could not envisage his problems of supply and communication in advance, for the extent and physical character of the Persian Empire was only partly known to the Greeks of his age. They were familiar with western Asia Minor and knew something of its hinterland from Herodotus and Xenophon's *Anabasis*. Some had traveled along the Royal Road, which ran from Sardes to the Fertile Crescent and on to the great cities of Mesopotamia and western Iran.

Syria and Egypt, of course, had long been familiar, and Greeks had visited Babylon. But for lands beyond Mesopotamia—western Iran and Media, the Iranian plateau, and the mountains to the east rising to the Himalayas—information was proportionately vague. Somewhere to the east, out on the edge of the Empire, were the limits of the world and the great stream of Ocean, which encircled the three "islands," Europe, Asia, and Libya (Africa). The Greeks thought that the edge of the habitable world was desert and dry steppe land where, at best, nomads wandered about, and, at worst, a desert of sand and rock like the Sahara, formed the shore of Ocean. The nomadic peoples, who lived beyond the Scythians in central Asia, seemed the last of mankind to the northeast, while northwestern India was the limit in the east. Nothing was known of the subcontinent of India, China, or southeastern Asia.

The hold of Persia on the Empire had weakened in the fourth century, but the state was still immensely wealthy and powerful in contrast to Greece and Macedonia. The royal family had experienced more than its usual intrigue, and in 334 B.C., when Alexander's campaign began, the young king, Darius III, had reigned for only two years. He obtained the throne after a series of murders which left bitter dissension among the high nobles of the court. The powerful satraps, who ruled their great provinces almost as private kingdoms, had shaken the central authority in the course of the century by successive revolts. They felt as well qualified as the king to hold the throne and, even while they prepared to fight against a foreign invader, they insisted that their advice be heeded and concessions be made by Darius. In an effort to consolidate the Empire, Darius' predecessors had abandoned the traditional policy of religious tolerance for the subject peoples, so that the latter had revolted frequently and felt no loyalty to the Persian government. To the Jews of Palestine, to the Egyptians and Babylonians, Alexander was to appear as a liberator who would restore their traditional way of life.

Darius had a formidable army, particularly strong in Persian cavalry, archers, and Greek mercenaries, who formed the companies of heavy infantry. He also had the money and manpower to organize successive armies as Alexander shattered them in battle. We have no way of estimating the size of any one of them, but it is likely that Alexander's forces were always outnumbered in the great battles of the war. The potential Persian naval strength, also far greater than Alexander's small Macedonian and Greek fleets, occupied the foreground of his thought for the first two years of fighting. Persian weakness lay in the divided counsels of their command and in the need of Darius, for the sake of his own authority, to win a single, smashing victory. At the outset he thought about the war in terms of the historic policy the Persians had developed for Greek affairs. The Macedonian invasion seemed to be another attack on Asia Minor, like that of Agesilaus. Persia had dealt with the latter by subsidizing opposition in Greece. Accordingly, in 335 B.C. Darius sent some money to Thebes and Athens but failed to capitalize on Alexander's preoccupation by military aid or by attacking Thrace and Macedonia from the east. Darius failed, too, to use the fleet to stir revolt in Greece after Alexander had started his campaign. The Persians still thought primarily in terms of land warfare, even after their experience in the invasions of Greece and at the hands of Cimon in the fifth century.

THE WAR—GRANICUS TO PERSEPOLIS

When Alexander crossed the Hellespont in 334 B.C., he found a Persian army commanded by the satraps of Anatolia ready to block his advance. Memnon, the commander of the Greek mercenaries in Persian service, knew the quality of the Macedonian troops and the latent danger to Alexander of revolt in Greece. He advised the Persians to fall back, devastate the country, and harass Alexander by guerilla war. The satraps preferred to rely on their greater numbers and their good cavalry to stop the invasion at the outset. They drew up on the far bank of the Granicus River, which looped inland behind the Hellespont, but lost the advantage of their numbers in a faulty deployment. Alexander was able to get his men across the river and concentrate his attack on smashing the Persian forces with heavy casualties. He, himself, set a pattern of behavior which was to secure the loyalty of his men and to keep their morale high. He fought in the thick of battle where he narrowly escaped death, and made it a point to praise the soldiers individually and to visit the wounded after the battle. Three hundred complete suits of Persian armor were sent as a dedication to Athena in Athens to stress the victory as part of the war of revenge and to stir Greek enthusiasm.

After the victory at the Granicus opened the way to western Asia Minor, Alexander marched down the west coast where he freed the Greek cities and occupied Sardes, the chief Persian city of Anatolia, where the Royal Road began. From there Parmenion was sent inland to Gordium in Phrygia to hold the flank in western Anatolia, while Alexander proceeded along the coast. The threat offered by the Persian fleet had become very real, since Memnon had brought it into the Aegean and was attacking the islands. Alexander, although he might have struck into the heart of the Empire by the Royal Road, decided to defeat the fleet on land by occupying all its bases and making sure of his communications. Accordingly, after taking Miletus and Halicarnassus which could have offered good harborage to the Persians, he spent the winter in administrative work and in clearing Lycia and Pamphylia in the southwest, while Darius concentrated another army at Babylon.

Alexander restored the independence of the Greek cities in western Asia Minor by removing their pro-Persian governments, usually headed by landowning oligarchs, and canceling the tribute which they paid to Persia. Contributions to his own war chest were accepted and given gratefully. Possibly the island cities, like Chios, became members of the League of Corinth, but those on the mainland were allied directly to Alexander and hailed him as their liberator and patron. He did not, however, enlarge their territories at the expense of the native Anatolians. The Persian satrapy system was retained for the native areas although Alexander appointed Macedonians as governors and, of course, collected the tribute for himself as the successor to the Great King. To establish peace and to indicate his respect for the non-Greek peoples, Alexander allowed them to practice their own customs and religious rites freely and had himself adopted by the Carian queen, Ada.

In the spring of 333 B.C. Alexander moved back to Gordium to assure his hold on Phrygia and, as legend has it, to cut the Gordian knot, which had hitherto defied untying. The man who untied the knot, a complicated attachment of the yoke to the tongue of an old Phrygian king's chariot, would become master of Asia. From Gordium Alexander turned south to Tarsus in Cilicia, where he paused to prepare for entering Syria. Darius marched his army northwestward from Babylon and, after a halt near the modern city of Aleppo, crossed behind Alexander, who was now in Syria, to take up his position at Issus, at the head of the Gulf of Iskanderun. Darius thus got between Alexander and the road to the north and placed his army on ground of his own choosing. The terrain was narrow, however, for the proper use of cavalry, and once again Alexander's impetuous charge broke the Persian formations and sent Darius into headlong flight from the battlefield. The rest of the Persian army, particularly the Greek mercenaries, fought well but could not defeat the Macedonian phalanxes. The Macedonians captured all Darius' luxurious baggage, as well as his wife, mother, and two daughters, who had accompanied the king. They were well treated by Alexander, who assured them that his war was with Darius, not women. He had won possession of all the land west of the Euphrates River, but some of Darius' generals had extricated themselves with a sizable force and retreated into central Anatolia, whence they could harass the communications. Accordingly, Alexander assigned Antigonus with a substantial force to operate in Phrygia.

Alexander himself continued methodically down the coast of Phoenicia to capture the harbors which might be used by the Persian fleet. Most of the

Alexander the Great, fighting in the battle of Issus. A mosaic from Pompeii, after a Hellenistic painting of ca. 300 B.C.

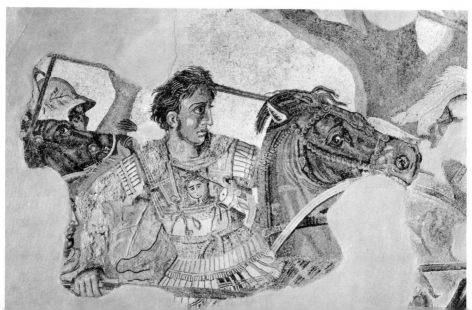

Phoenician cities surrendered, but Tyre, the great port city of the southeastern Mediterranean, proved a formidable obstacle and delayed Alexander for over seven months. Its offshore island, on which were the main docks and harbor installations, had been converted into a fortress which was considered impregnable. Alexander, scraping together what ships he could, tried to take it by sea, but the walls were too massive and well defended. Accordingly, he had to build a causeway, half a mile in length, to the island, pull heavy siege machinery to the walls and batter them down. When the wall was breached, a great assault was made on the whole fortress across the causeway and by naval attack from the sea. The Macedonians poured in and massacred the inhabitants. The fall of Tyre justified the long delay, for it ended Alexander's fear of the Persian fleet. Many ships had surrendered to him in the course of the siege; by the end of the siege he was free to advance to Egypt and round off his conquest of the southeastern Mediterranean.

During the siege of Tyre, Darius, who had retired beyond the Euphrates, proposed peace to Alexander. The king offered to yield all the Empire west of the Euphrates and to give his daughter in marriage to Alexander in exchange for peace and alliance. Alexander considered, however, that his victory at Issus had already established him as king of Persia and that the whole Empire was rightfully his. His rejection of the offer was significant for the history of the Near East because the territory which Darius offered was what Rome eventually found could be held safely. Asia Minor and a line along the Euphrates were defensible, and the area could be administered properly by a Mediterranean power and brought into fruitful economic and political union with the Aegean and the West. Beyond the Euphrates lay the vast reaches of Asia, where Rome found that even Mesopotamia was too difficult to govern. "When Parmenion told him that, for his part, if he were Alexander, he should readily embrace the terms, 'So would I,' said Alexander, 'if I were Parmenion.'" He had resolved to take the whole Empire as his own, but for the moment kept on with his plan to secure the coast.

The fortress of Gaza, the gateway to Egypt, required a siege of two months to force the Persian garrison into surrender, but the Persian governor of Egypt made no attempt to hold the Nile valley, where he would have had to control a hostile population. After he surrendered, and Alexander entered Egypt as a liberator, the Egyptians made Alexander their Pharaoh, the protector and god of Egypt. The Macedonian king thus took his place in the line of tradition that reached back for almost three thousand years. As a dutiful Pharaoh and curious visitor, Alexander paid a visit to the famous oracle of Amon in the Oasis of Siwah, where the priests greeted him as "Son of Re." Rumors began to circulate among the Greeks that Alexander had been recognized as the son of Zeus, with whom they identified Amon. As Pharaoh, Alexander was the son of Re, but the new idea appealed to those Greeks who wished to flatter him. Whatever Alexander thought of it he concealed and went about the more urgent business of organizing Egypt. Several officials were appointed in order to split the military, civil, and financial administration of the country. The military command was entrusted to three Macedonians; Cleomenes, a Greek, was to administer the finances, and two others, Egyptians, were to exercise civil jurisdiction. Alexander was disposed evidently to use talent where he found it. A new city, Alexandria, was founded, which was designed to become the commercial and shipping center of the southeastern Mediterranean to supplement Tyre. Alexander was curious, too, about the cause of the Nile floods and is said to have sent an exploratory party up the Nile, while he himself turned back to lead his army along the Fertile Crescent into Mesopotamia.

Alexander paused again in Tyre to make arrangements for the western section of the Empire and then pushed on to meet Darius. The latter, with a great imperial army, was blocking the way to Babylon and Persia at Gaugamela near ancient Nineveh. Darius' army was weak in heavy infantry because after the battle of Issus the Greek mercenaries in Persian employ had decided that the Persian cause was desperate and had deserted in large numbers. Nevertheless, his cavalry was as formidable as ever, and he hoped for much from two hundred chariots armed with scythe blades on their wheel hubs. Alexander had increased his own force to about forty thousand men, taking care to enlarge the cavalry, but, even so, he was outnumbered as usual. The battle was narrowly won by Alexander, but in the ensuing rout the Persians not only lost many men but also lost their last opportunity for organized resistance. Darius escaped into Media, but Alexander struck south to secure the great cities in the heart of the Empire.

First Alexander came to Babylon where he was welcomed by the people as their liberator and was invested with all the titles of the Mesopotamian kingship. Then the new Pharaoh of Egypt, Great King of Persia, King of Sumer and Akkad, Lord of the Universe, entered Persia to take over Susa, Persepolis and Pasargadae, the Persian capitals. At Persepolis he formally symbolized the attainment of Greek revenge by demolishing and burning the palace of Xerxes. For himself he took possession of the gold and silver bullion and precious objects accumulated in the palaces and treasuries, estimated at the fantastic amount of 180,000 talents, that is, several billion dollars in purchasing power. Three years previously Alexander had left Macedonia with about seventy talents remaining in his treasury.

The destruction of the royal palace at Persepolis had symbolized the Greek revenge on Persia. Thereafter Alexander made the expedition entirely his own and began to act more and more as the Great King, before whom all subjects were equal. Certainly the Greeks had remained unresponsive to his gestures of goodwill and to his concern to preserve the League of Corinth. The member states regarded the League as a Macedonian device that was to control them. In Athens, which was particularly favored by Alexander, Lycurgus, a new leader, while correct in his relations with Alexander, was very cool. Sparta, which had remained outside the League, was openly hostile, and in 331 B.C. the Spartan king, Agis, started a war against Macedonia. Athens toyed with the idea of joining, but discretion won out, and Agis was helped by only a few Peloponnesian states. Nevertheless, Antipater had to intervene in force with his Macedonian army, with the result that the whole affair, coming as it did after Alexander's great victories, was an affront to his achievement. Upon Alexander's recommendation the League penalized Sparta's ringleaders with heavy fines and compelled her to enter the League. While the settlement was reasonably mild, Greek opinion that the League was Alexander's instrument, not theirs, was confirmed. Alexander decided to dispense with his Greek allies as such and dismissed the League contingents from service. The men were amply rewarded, and, while some chose to serve Alexander as individual mercenary soldiers, in 330 B.C. formal Greek participation in the war was terminated.

THE WAR—ECBATANA TO INDIA

At Ecbatana, the old capital of Media, Alexander made administrative arrangements for the western part of the Empire before starting east in pursuit of Darius. Control of the eastern Mediterranean allowed Alexander to supplement the road from Macedonia through Asia Minor by sea transport to Ephesus and Tyre. From these cities the Royal Road and the routes of the Fertile Crescent carried communication to Babylon and thence to Ecbatana. Along the routes Alexander stationed a few garrisons at strategic control points and placed a general in charge of each main sector. Far to the north in Phrygia Antigonus the One-eyed kept watch, and at Ecbatana Alexander stationed Parmenion to guard the lines running through Media to the east. Harpalus, a Greek, was entrusted with the treasury and financial administration, which later proved to be a poor choice. Alexander felt it expedient, perhaps from the lack of trained personnel, to appoint several Persian nobles to govern satrapies. The most important of these nobles was Mazaeus, who was reappointed as satrap of Babylon.

As the conversion of Persian bullion into coinage had already started, the new coins were flowing back along the lines of communication to pay for soldiers, supplies, and the multifarious needs of the new regime. Alexander continued to coin on the Athenian standard in silver, demonetizing the Persian gold, evidently intending to link more closely the Aegean with Near Eastern commerce. Greece began to recover rapidly and many individual Greeks moved into the East in the trail of Alexander's army as opportunities for trade and settlement appeared. Alexander, himself, was freed from all financial concern for the rest of his career, except for the integrity of his officials.

Alexander's pursuit of Darius led him into a new and very different type of war for the next three years, 330–27 B.C. He had broken the organized resistance of Persia, but there still remained the need to get the allegiance of the Persian nobles who might aspire to the throne and re-establish the monarchy. Since they lived in fortified castles in the mountainous area of eastern Iran, war against them involved a whole series of separate forays, and since there were no great cities and properly developed road systems, Alexander had to march and fight in difficult desert and mountain country—in a maze of valleys, streams and mountain passes. The land they gained was difficult to hold securely and required more men than Alexander could afford, but as king of Persia, he considered the eastern provinces within his realm. In addition, his curiosity was aroused by the land beyond them—by the prospect of the edge of the world and the Ocean stream.

Alexander's first aim was to capture Darius. In the course of the latter's flight, however, he was killed by Bessus, a Bactrian prince who was one of the nobles in his entourage. Alexander came upon the body of the dead king in the desert near Damghan and sent it back to Persepolis for a royal burial; then he hurried on after Bessus, who had fled into his native Bactria across the mountains. But Alexander was forced to turn south and impose his authority on Aria and Drangiana before entering Bactria in order to prevent uprisings in his rear.

By this time some of the Macedonians had marched too far and were disturbed at the prospect of chasing another will-o'-the-wisp king, as well as being disgruntled at Alexander's apparent favoritism to Persians and Persian customs. Their Macedonian king seemed to be turning into a Persian despot. Philotas, the son of Parmenion, conspired with a small group against Alexander, but the plot was discovered and Philotas was tried and executed. According to Macedonian practice, since a man's family was guilty for his treason, Alexander sent orders back to Ecbatana for the execution of Parmenion. While Parmenion had been outspoken in opposition to Alexander on occasion, there is no reason to believe that he was involved in his son's plot, and Alexander could surely have found a way to save his own and his father's old general from a disgraceful death. Perhaps as the problems of reigning came home to Alexander, he decided that the time had come to begin putting the Macedonians in their place among his new peoples. For the moment there was no additional trouble, since the conspiracy was small and Alexander's hold on the loyalty of his men was too great to be disturbed by a palace intrigue.

In Drangiana Alexander received the formal submission of the satraps of Carmania and Gedrosia and was able to turn north again through Arachosia to the Hindu Kush Mountains, across which lay Bactria. The army crossed by the Khawak Pass, 11,600 feet in elevation, in order to come out to the north of Bessus' position and cut him off from potential support in northern Bactria and Sogdiana. The men had to eat their mules raw in the high mountains for lack of other food and firewood, but came through without severe loss and prepared to deal with Bessus.

Bessus had fled across the Oxus River but was soon captured and sent to Bactra (Balkh), the chief town of Bactria, which Alexander made the next center in his communication line. A Sogdianian noble, Spitamenes, took up the conflict with Alexander and led the chase into Sogdiana (Turkestan)across the Oxus. Spitamenes was an able and dogged opponent, who defied Alexander for well over a year, drawing support from Sogdiana and from the nomads who lived across the Jaxartes River. Finally, in the winter of 328 B.C., after Spitamenes was defeated, his nomad allies put him to death and sent his head as a peace offering to Alexander. In the course of the campaigns, Alexander pushed on through the town of Samarkand and came to the limit of the Persian Empire in Ferghana on the Jaxartes River. Beyond it lay the steppe land of central Asia. Alexander identified the Jaxartes (Syr Daria) as the Don River, which he knew flowed into the Sea of Azov in South Russia, and thought that he had come to the edge of Europe, the land of the nomads who lived beyond the Scythians. He wondered how the Caspian Sea, which he had passed in the pursuit of Darius, fitted into this picture (which was quite distorted), but put aside the temptation to find out for the time being. Instead, he founded another Alexandria on the Jaxartes, Alexandreschate, the "Farthest," and turned to the winning of Bactria and Sogdiana. To facilitate the conquest, he married Roxane, the daughter of a Bactrian prince, and began to take more Persians into the army and his administration. In all, thirty thousand young Bactrians were enlisted for training and sent back to the heart of the Empire for future use in the army.

Another crisis developed in his circle of intimates when Alexander tried to get the Macedonians and Greeks of his "court" to observe the Persian practice of *proskynesis,* full prostration in his presence. In their minds the ceremony was appropriate only for a god and, whatever Alexander's intentions were, the practice was not to their liking. After Aristotle's nephew Callisthenes blocked the attempt, Alexander gave up the idea, but Callisthenes was soon executed for alleged complicity in another plot, this time by the Macedonian page boys, one of whom was piqued at Alexander. These episodes indicated a growing dissatisfaction among some of the Macedonian intimates of Alexander as he became less of a Macedonian and more of a Persian king, but his hold remained firm on the ordinary soldiers.

In 327 B.C. Alexander led his army into the land that is now Pakistan, to which Persia had a shadowy claim and which the Greeks considered to be the last inhabited part of the world. Conquest of India, the land of the Indus River, would round off Alexander's occupation of the whole of Persian Asia. The army advanced to the Cabul River, where Alexander sent off his baggage train to enter India by the Khyber Pass, while he subjugated the hill tribes en route to the Indus River. The first contacts with India were reassuring, for Taxiles, the king of Taxila, made an alliance with Alexander and entertained the army, giving the men time to survey the wonders of India. Alexander felt, however, that he must push on before the melting snow from the Himalayas flooded the rivers in his path. Taxiles was made a vassal prince and a garrison was left in Taxila.

Through his alliance with Taxiles, Alexander had automatically acquired a new enemy, Porus, the king of the Punjab, with whom Taxiles was at war. Alexander led his army, augmented by five thousand Indian troops, to the area of Haranpur on the Hydaspes River (Jhelum), where he found the army of Porus drawn up on the far bank. There was also a new enemy, a force of war elephants, against which his cavalry horses would be useless. After considerable maneuvering to extend Porus' troops, Alexander crossed the Hydaspes in a thunderstorm and successfully dealt with the elephants. He rolled back part of Porus's army upon them and sent in his infantry in extended order to hurl javelins at the animals and their riders until the maddened beasts ran amok through their own troops. Although this took care of the elephants, the battle was more difficult to win than Gaugamela. Porus's army was routed, however, and the advance could continue. Porus was made a vassal king by Alexander, who took title to the Punjab and founded two new cities to commemorate his victory, Alexandria Nicaea and Alexandria Bucephala, the latter named for his war horse, Bucephalus.

From the Hydaspes Alexander marched on to the east to find the elusive stream of Ocean, but, as the miles stretched on, the weary army heard only of more peoples and farther lands. Finally, on the bank of the Hyphasis River (Beas), the men refused to proceed. For three days Alexander sulked in his tent, like his venerated Achilles, but then started the long march back. His thrust into the Punjab left little trace in the region, for the territory was too large and too far from the centers in Persia to be organized. A few Greeks and Macedonians were left behind, but Alexander set up only nominal control through the client kings, Taxiles and Porus.

The retreat, if such it is to be called, had a triumphal air. Alexander built a fleet on the Hydaspes River, by which part of the army was floated down to the Indus and thence to the sea, while the others marched along the banks. Towns were captured, in one of which Alexander nearly lost his life in battle, and more people were added for the moment to the Empire. At Pattala, in the apex of the delta of the Indus River, a city was built to serve as the Indian terminus for a sea route to the Gulf of Persia. Alexander had reached an ocean at last and realized that he could use it to link the parts of his Empire together. He directed Nearchus, in charge of the fleet, to coast along from Pattala to the Persian Gulf, to explore the sea route and to keep in touch with the main body of the army which he would lead along the coast. A third, and smaller force, under Craterus (whom Alexander had made his second in command since the death of Parmenion), had already been detached to explore an inland route by Candahar to the Gulf.

Nearchus' fleet and Alexander's army set off as planned, but soon lost touch with each other when the army had to detour inland to avoid the coastal mountains, the existence of which had not been suspected. Nearchus' fleet was challenged by a school of whales. The men valiantly drove them off by blowing trumpets but had a relatively easy time in contrast to the army's march through the Gedrosian Desert. Guides lost the way, the men had to march by night because of the heat, water was scarce, and Alexander only kept up morale in the thinning ranks by dismounting and trudging alongside the soldiers. In the spring of 324 B.C. Nearchus, Alexander and Craterus made their rendezvous near the entrance to the Persian Gulf. An appropriately Bacchanalian celebration was held and then Alexander proceeded to Susa, which he had left six years previously en route to Ecbatana and the east.

Alexander—The Empire

Since Alexander's communications with the West had been very tenuous during the campaign in India, he had to repair the damage of maladministration by some of his officials and consider the larger problems of empire and plans for the future. Some of the Persian satraps, whom he had appointed, had misgoverned so crassly that they were put to death. Harpalus, who had embezzled money from the treasury in the expectation that Alexander would not return, departed hurriedly for the Aegean. In Egypt, Cleomenes, the Greek financial official, had cornered the wheat market for his own profit and was marked for removal. Above all there was need to reorganize the army, since the Macedonian veterans, who had served so well, were past their prime or weakened by wounds and the strain of long marches and fighting. Although much of the personnel had been replaced since the army left the Hellespont, the force probably remained largely European until the Bactrian and Indian campaigns. It had been necessary then to take in many native troops, and the whole force needed combing out and reintegration.

For the future Alexander planned a joint Macedonian-Persian army, for which he had on hand the thirty thousand Persian youths whom he had sent from Bactria. To bring Macedonian and Persian together in concord, Alexander set an example by taking a Persian second wife, Barsine, and by arranging marriages for eighty of his officers with daughters of the Persian nobility. In addition, more than ten thousand Greek and Macedonian soldiers were required to legalize their casual unions with native women. Alexander then discharged ten thousand Macedonian veterans, paying them liberal bonuses and arranging to send them back to Macedonia. The men, however, refused to go and were supported by a meeting of the whole Macedonian army. Alexander discharged them all and retired to his tent, but, when the men pressed around, weeping and begging to be reinstated, he relented and held a great feast of reconciliation at Opis on the Tigris River.

When nine thousand Greeks, Macedonians, and Persians sat down to dinner together at Opis, Greek priests and Persian Magi offered prayer and made the invocations. Each guest poured a libation from a single great mixing bowl, and Alexander prayed for concord and partnership in his kingdom between Macedonians and Persians. After the reconciliation was effected, Alexander made a start on a new, mixed army, while the Macedonian veterans prepared for their long march homeward.

Alexander also tried to adjust his relations with the Greek states. In 324 B.C. he made two requests of the members of the League of Corinth: that each state restore its political exiles, and that he be deified by the Greeks. The first provoked much resentment, partly because restoration of political rights and property would have been very difficult to arrange, but mainly because Alexander seemed to be arbitrarily interfering again with the internal autonomy of the states. Force would have been necessary to restore the exiles, but Alexander died before the situation came to that point. His request for deification was received much more indifferently. Sparta's response was typical, if more laconic, than that of most states. The assembly passed a motion that if Alexander wished to become a god, he might do so. It is usually considered that Alexander's purpose in asking for deification was political and designed to establish a new relationship by which his authority was strengthened. Possibly it would have been more difficult for the Greeks to challenge Alexander the god than Alexander the king, but Alexander may have been asking for no more than traditional Greek recognition of his achievement and services. Many individual Greeks were genuinely impressed by the conquest and realized that Alexander had opened new opportunities to them. He was appealing to a common Greek religious attitude, that the highest honor, as for a god, should be paid to a man whom heaven obviously favored and who had performed a great service. For example, the founders of colonies were so honored by the colonists, and Lysander and Agesilaus had been deified by various communities earlier in the fourth century. Alexander, of course, had always shown himself ready to take advantage of any religious attitude which would facilitate his authority.

For the immediate future Alexander seems to have planned a very large number of building projects in the Empire, ranging from roads, harbors and irrigation canals to whole new cities. He himself was keenly anxious to send out more exploratory expeditions, partly from curiosity, and partly to lay the groundwork for better communication and trade. Most important to him were the long-deferred exploration of the Caspian Sea and a circumnavigation of Arabia from the Persian Gulf to the Red Sea. He wished to colonize the coasts and islands of the Gulf and make it the central link in routes to India and to Egypt. Money was still available for all these projects, but it is calculated that in 323 B.C. he was nearing the end of the Persian bullion. Alexander was not the type of man to make or live by a budget, and he never needed to. In June, 323 B.C., he contracted a fever in Babylon and died, at not quite thirty-three years of age.

Alexander died at a time when he was only beginning to deal with the immense problems of organizing his Empire as a whole, so that it is difficult to estimate his qualities and ideas as a ruler. He had begun to use Greeks, Macedonians and Persians in the army and in administration. Probably his own marriages and those he sponsored for his officers indicate that he contemplated the establishment of a single ruling class formed from Hellenic and native elements. This idea of mixing his peoples, of fusion, is evident also in the type of city which he founded, although we have little knowledge of their organization. Alexander is credited with the foundation of seventy cities, of which only two, Alexandria in Egypt and Alexandretta in the Gulf of Iskanderun, were west of the Tigris River. The number is certainly exaggerated, but enough certain foundations are known to indicate that urbanization had a place in his plans. These cities were only garrison towns at first, but they were new foundations. A few replaced native villages. The population was a mixture of Greek and

Macedonian soldiers, Greek traders and settlers and natives from the vicinity. To judge from Alexandria, the cities were designed to be Greek in physical character and, to some degree, in institutions. Alexander, however, had no intention of creating a new world of independent city-states—those in Greece were troublesome enough—or of imposing Hellenization to the detriment of native institutions. He did not break up the great temple estates of the East nor interfere with the property rights of the Persian nobles. Instead, he tried to win their cooperation. The cities apparently were to become urban centers for their districts and to establish the Greek practices of urban life. Many generations of peace and continuous pressure from the central government would have been necessary to develop them and, as it was, the cities had little effect on the life of the eastern part of the Empire.

Alexander also showed concern to unify his Empire by economic and political ties. The minting of the Persian silver on the Athenian weight standard tied Mediterranean and Near Eastern commerce together, and the projects for long sea routes would have supplemented the slow and tedious movement on land by caravan. In general, Alexander simply took over the Persian satrapy system for his administrative purposes, but he made several significant changes which show an awareness of its defects. For example, in Egypt, where revolt had been endemic, Alexander became the Pharaoh, the people's own king and god. In the Asian satrapies, where the satrap had been almost a local king and too powerful for central control, Alexander divided authority. His satraps were in charge of civil administration only, while separate military and financial officials were directly responsible to Alexander himself. As we have already noticed, Alexander did not establish a budget and proper accounting system. The money taken in tribute, taxes, and booty was paid into his purse, and he spent it as he wished.

Beyond these ideas of limited fusion and of economic and administrative unity, it is difficult to conjecture. Alexander was the personal, absolute ruler of his Empire, but he appeared in a different aspect to each of its major peoples. They had no common denominator but Alexander. Perhaps, as some scholars have argued, Alexander conceived of his function as ruler in a different way than his predecessors: thus he thought it the business of the ruler to promote union among his people without distinction of race. It is argued that this idea was based on a vision of the brotherhood of mankind. Be that as it may, Alexander's career opened a new epoch in history.

The almost immediate result of Alexander's death, however, was war and political chaos. The new monarchy was only as strong as its ruler, and Alexander made no provision for the succession. In his family there were Philip Arrhidaeus, a half-brother, but mentally defective, and Roxane who was pregnant. The Macedonians felt that the monarchy should be kept in Alexander's family and that the unity of Empire should be preserved. Given these circumstances, a regency seemed the only solution, and by agreement one of the older generals, Perdiccas, was selected to be regent. Arrhidaeus was to be king in name and, if

Roxane's child were a boy, he would become a joint ruler. The organized power of the Empire, however, lay in the Macedonian elements of the army and the able, vigorous generals of Alexander's staff. They were ambitious, and the spoils were too great to wait long.

The Establishment of the Hellenistic Kingdoms

The generals who suddenly emerged from the shadow cast by the stature of Alexander were a striking group. They had been trained to command in war, to organize long communication lines and to administer large territories. As the generals of an army which had never lost a battle, they were extraordinarily competent. But they did not share the plans and ideas of Alexander, for one of their first acts was to give up the projects for which he was preparing. They might pay lip service to the idea of a united empire, but their aim was personal power, and they fought for the factors which contributed to it—strategic cities and routes and, above all, the trained soldiers and technicians needed for their armies and new territories. The generals were not concerned about political principles, except when these could be turned into useful slogans, but they struggled to get a kingdom by whatever means they could, since none felt safe from another's ambition.

In 323 B.C., when the regency was established, the generals, known as the Successors, agreed on a division of the satrapies for administrative purposes, and each retired to make what he could of his own territory. Perdiccas, the regent, whose duties were increased by the birth of a boy to Roxane, was left to administer Asia with the help of Craterus. The latter, for the present, was assigned to lead home the veterans discharged by Alexander. Antipater continued in his position as administrator of Macedonia and Greece, as did Antigonus in central Asia Minor. Ptolemy, with an eye to the potential wealth and easy defensibility of Egypt, contrived to get that assignment. Minor figures received the less important districts, of which the most important was Thrace, assigned to Lysimachus.

Almost immediately revolt broke out on the fringes of the Empire, in Greece and Bactria, which stirred a general flare-up. The Greek states of the League of Corinth, led by Athens, seized the occasion of Alexander's death to abolish the League and form a new coalition for war against Macedonia. The means to fight were provided in part by Harpalus, who conveniently arrived in Athens with some of the money embezzled from Alexander's treasury. Antipater was besieged in the Thessalian city of Lamia, from which the Lamian War took its name, and had to appeal to the other generals for help. Craterus arrived with the Macedonian veterans and Cleitus came with the fleet. The Greeks were speedily suppressed, and Antipater worked out a new formula to control Greece. Instead of dealing with the states collectively through the League of Corinth, he made individual settlements with them and installed pro-Macedonian governments and garrisons. The Peiraeus was garrisoned, and the democratic government in Athens was replaced by an oligarchy, which condemned Demosthenes to death (p. 335). In Bactria the garrisons which Alexander had left felt themselves cut off and were profoundly dissatisfied with their life on the frontier of the Empire. Accordingly, they packed up and started west to civilization. Perdiccas dealt with the situation by directing Peithon, the satrap of Media, to round up the men, many of whom were put to death.

Meanwhile, relations among the generals began to deteriorate rapidly. Perdiccas was envied for his possession of Asia and his position as regent since the latter gave him some claim to the loyalty of the Macedonian soldiers, who were still responsive to the memory of Alexander. Antipater felt that the wards should be kept in Macedonia, where Olympias, Alexander's mother lived. She wanted some influence in the direction of affairs for herself. The other generals began to intrigue and to form alignments to strengthen their positions. Ptolemy saw an opportunity to improve his standing among the soldiers by a clever piece of body snatching in which he got hold of the corpse of Alexander. Perdiccas had sent the body to be buried in the royal cemetery at Aegae in Macedonia. When the funeral cortege was crossing from Babylon to Damascus, Ptolemy induced the officer in charge to turn off to Egypt, alleging that Alexander had expressed a wish to be buried in the Oasis of Siwah. Ptolemy, however, held the body at Memphis until a great tomb could be constructed in Alexandria. This trick was designed to put him in the light of a successor to Alexander, looking after the conqueror's burial, like a dutiful son.

Ptolemy's successful attempt to improve his position began the struggle for power. For fifty years the Wars of the Successors swept over Greece and the lands of the Near and Middle East. In their course the royal line of Philip and Alexander perished, for Philip Arrhidaeus and Roxane's son were put to death when their usefulness as pawns had vanished. The unity of Alexander's Empire was preserved in name only through successive reshufflings of power among the generals until they felt strong enough to declare themselves independent kings. Many of Alexander's generals perished in the fighting, but by 275 B.C. the new Hellenistic East had taken shape and Macedonian kings were established in the lands of the former Persian Empire.

Macedonia itself came to be ruled by the descendants of Antigonus, who had been placed in charge of central Asia Minor. First, Antigonus and his son Demetrius Poliorcetes (the Besieger) tried to get control of the whole Empire by launching offensives in Asia and building up their influence in the Aegean. There Antipater had died in 319 B.C., and a dispute over the succession to his position provided a favorable opportunity. In the course of the wars Antigonus and Demetrius built up a powerful navy, and in 305 B.C. Demetrius made a tremendous attack on the city of Rhodes. At that time the island was entering a phase of prosperity as a distributor of goods from the southeastern Mediterranean to the Aegean. The fame of Demetrius' siege of Rhodes rivaled that of Alexander's attack on Tyre, but the Rhodians beat Demetrius off. Their victory was commemorated by the erection of the Colossus of Rhodes, a great statue of bronze, over 100 feet in height, which stood beside the harbor entrance until 227 B.C. when it was toppled by an earthquake. The offensive of Antigonus and Demetrius was brought to an end in 302 B.C. at the battle of Ipsus in Phrygia which was lost by Demetrius' impetuosity. He rode off in pursuit of the enemy's cavalry, weakening his father's position. Antigonus was killed and Demetrius became a glorified pirate, operating from the Aegean Islands and hanging on to a few cities in Greece. Nevertheless, in 297 B.C. he was able to move in on Macedonia. While Demetrius himself was defeated by Lysimachus, who had succeeded in holding Thrace throughout the wars, his son Antigonus Gonatas firmly established the Antigonid Dynasty as rulers of Macedonia in 279 B.C.

Gonatas found his opportunity in the confusion which followed upon the irruption of a horde of barbarians from the Danube valley into Thrace and Macedonia. These were the Gauls, a Celtic people from Central Europe. One large group crossed into Asia Minor, where they settled in the district known as Galatia in the center of Anatolia. Another group thrust into Greece and advanced towards Delphi with the intention of plundering the shrine. They were checked by the Aetolian League and turned back to the north, where Gonatas defeated their bands in Macedonia, winning popular support for his kingship.

Perdiccas, who had held a very strong position at the outset of the wars as regent for Alexander's heirs, was removed from the scene very early. In 321 B.C. he was defeated by Ptolemy, whom he tried to punish for the snatching of Alexander's body, and was murdered by some of his own officers. One of them, Seleucus, obtained the satrapy of Babylonia as a reward in the redistribution of territory made at Triparadeisos in Syria after Perdiccas' death. While Seleucus held Babylonia only with considerable difficulty until the defeat of Antigonus and Demetrius at Ipsus, he was then able to proclaim himself king. A rapid extension of control brought him into conflict with Lysimachus of Thrace, but the defeat of the latter at the battle of Corupedion in 281 B.C. made Seleucus master of western Asia Minor. Seleucus and his son, Antiochus, also advanced eastwards into Iran to the borders of India. Thus the Seleucid Dynasty became the heir to the greater part of the territory which had comprised the Persian Empire.

Of all the generals of Alexander, Ptolemy emerged in the strongest position. He held Egypt successfully from the first division of the satrapies in 323 B.C. and extended his control into southern Syria and even into the Aegean by adroit diplomacy and war. In 306 B.C. he proclaimed himself king of Egypt. His descendants, the Ptolemies, were to rule the land until the suicide of Cleopatra in 31 B.C. after the defeat inflicted upon her and Mark Antony by Augustus Caesar.

By 275 B.C. political equilibrium had been restored. The new kingdoms of Egypt, Macedonia, and Seleucid Asia were stabilized and had begun to proceed with their tasks of consolidation. The old order of the Persian Empire had been swept away in the East, and in place of the Great King the descendants of the Macedonian generals of Alexander reigned. The subsequent era of comparative peace permitted a rapid development of their kingdoms, and the cultural unity of the Hellenistic epoch was established before Rome entered the East.

The impact of the Wars of the Successors was not as damaging as might be supposed from their duration. The wars which had been waged by professionals, generals and soldiers alike, did not involve the loyalties of the peoples through whose countries they fought. The professional soldier wanted good pay, plunder and, on discharge, a liberal bonus of land or money. The best mercenaries came from the Greek cities and Macedonia, so the impact of war fell mostly on the Aegean area, where the generals wanted to control the source of supply. Also, they could levy contributions of money and material on the established cities of the Aegean, which had found a new prosperity after Alexander's conquests. Some soldiers returned to their homelands upon discharge, but most settled in veterans' colonies in the new kingdoms, where they formed a relatively privileged part of the population and a reservoir of manpower for the king's army. In the course of the wars, too, many individual Greeks moved into Asia and Egypt as settlers, where they could profit from the business and trading opportunities offered by the movement of the armies and the new settlements. Greek technicians, engineers, accountants, architects, and craftsmen were in particular demand. Greeks and Macedonians spilled over into the East to form a governing class and to impose a pattern of Hellenization which stretched over the political frontiers of the new states. This had not been Alexander's plan but was imposed by the Successors' aggressive drives for power.

XVII

The Hellenistic Kingdoms

(*ca.* 275–200 B.C.)

ABOUT 275 B.C. RELATIVE STABILITY was attained in the Aegean and the Near East with the establishment of the three great Hellenistic Kingdoms, Antigonid Macedonia, Seleucid Asia, and Ptolemaic Egypt. No one of them was strong enough to dominate the others and to restore Alexander's Empire. Accordingly, they maintained a balance of power by limited war and diplomacy until about 220 B.C., when young, ambitious rulers came to the thrones of Macedonia and Seleucid Asia and when Rome began to take a part in the political affairs of the eastern Mediterranean. In the interval the Hellenistic rulers worked with great energy and skill to consolidate their new kingdoms internally and to establish zones of influence and commercial markets abroad. Friction was particularly intense between the Seleucids and Ptolemies over Phoenicia and Palestine, through which ran the road from Seleucid Syria to Egypt, and between all the kingdoms for access to the Greek cities of the Aegean. These cities offered a market for their products and supplied the skilled Greek soldiers, settlers, and technicians needed to build and maintain the new kingdoms. The history of the third century is complicated, and there are great gaps in our information, so that it is easier to consider each of the great states separately and then turn, in the following chapter, to the cultural unity of Hellenism, which bound them all together.

Ptolemaic Egypt

The new Macedonian rulers skillfully seized on the peculiar geographical character and traditional organization of Egypt to make their state the strongest and most prosperous of the Hellenistic Kingdoms. They found that in general the Egyptians had continued in the way of life that had been established over thousands of years. The Assyrian and Persian occupations and the presence of

The reader will find Map II (page 48) and the Front Endpaper useful as he reads this chapter.

the few foreigners, mainly Greeks and Jews, who resided there, had had slight influence. The mass of peasants and artisans, almost seven million in number, lived in the towns and villages of the Nile valley and worked in the age-old manner, paying much of their produce to the government and temples and taking no part in the rule of their country. To the Greeks, Egypt had always seemed a very wealthy country from which they bought wheat, linen, papyrus, and some of the products of Egyptian craftsmen, trained by centuries of hereditary skill. Most of Egypt's wealth, of course, was drawn from the intensive agriculture based on the annual alluviation of the Nile and the elaborate artificial system of irrigation.

The Ptolemies, like Alexander, were careful to win the cooperation of the priests and the lower classes among the scribes, which made their task of government much easier, but it was the hard work and ability of the rulers which restored Egypt to a place of power. The first Ptolemy, Alexander's general, regarded his satrapy as a potential kingdom from 323 B.C., when he took it over, and he began the work of organization. But Ptolemy's time was largely preoccupied with the defense of his kingdom, so that the internal organization of Hellenistic Egypt was chiefly the work of his successors, Ptolemy II Philadelphus (285–46 B.C.), and Ptolemy III Euergetes (246–21 B.C.). All were concerned to protect Egypt and to amplify its resources by the establishment of a foreign empire.

FOREIGN POLICY

The first Ptolemy sized up the strategic advantages of his satrapy with a trained military eye and took steps to protect the weak points. Since the valley of the Nile was bordered by desert on the east, south, and west, the only organized power in Africa within striking distance of Egypt was the old Greek colony of Cyrene. While Cyrene offered no real threat to Egypt, possession of the Cyrenaica would secure the western desert and amplify Egypt's revenues. Accordingly, in 322 B.C. Ptolemy took over the Cyrenaica and made it an appendage to Egypt, generally ruled by a member of the Ptolemaic family. Both rulers and people were successful on occasion in breaking away from Egypt but, in the main, Cyrene remained a part of the kingdom until 116 B.C.

Coin of Philip V

Egypt, however, was vulnerable from the north, whence attack could come by sea or by invasion through Palestine and the Isthmus of Suez. Accordingly, the Ptolemies initiated an aggressive naval program by which they gained almost complete control of the Aegean Sea and the southeastern Mediterranean. The Egyptian fleet was based on the new city of Alexandria, and a screen of

Hellenistic rulers (left to right): Antiochus III; Alexander the Great; Ptolemy II and Arsinoë, his wife.

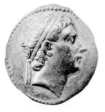 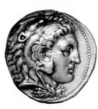 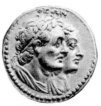

advanced positions was established in the Aegean and western Asia Minor by alliances and occupation. In the Aegean the larger islands, which had formed an Island League during the Wars of the Successors, became allies of Egypt, pledged to contribute naval help. Along the coast of Greece some small ports were garrisoned and used as bases, from which the Ptolemies could interfere in Greek politics against Macedonia. In western Asia Minor the Ptolemies contested with the Seleucids for control of the big port cities of Smyrna, Ephesus, and Miletus. This naval power in the Aegean and an active diplomacy, liberally supplied with money, secured access to soldiers and settlers whom the Ptolemies wished to recruit and to the markets of the Greek cities. The approaches to the Aegean were held by the establishment of vassal kingdoms in Lycia and Cyprus and by close cooperation with the big island of Rhodes, which rapidly grew to prosperity as a distributor for eastern trade into the Aegean. This aggressive policy resulted, of course, in constant war with Macedonia and the Seleucids, but the Ptolemies held their own with Macedonia until 258 B.C., when they were defeated in the naval battle of Cos (p. 388), and with the Seleucids until the end of the third century. The main bone of contention with the Seleucids was the land approach to Egypt from Syria.

Ptolemy I had seized Phoenicia and southern Syria in 319 B.C. and thus raised an issue with the Seleucids which was disputed throughout the third century in a series of five Syrian Wars. The Ptolemies regarded possession of Palestine and the Isthmus of Suez as vital to Egyptian security. They also wanted to control the Phoenician ports which were the termini of caravan routes from Arabia and Mesopotamia. Ptolemaic control of Phoenicia and lower Syria, however, posed a threat to the Seleucid corridor to the sea through the valley of the Orontes River and to their harbors in North Syria at Seleucia and Laodicea. The difficulty of finding an acceptable frontier, analogous to the quarrel between New Kingdom Egypt and the Hittite Empire, was not resolved until the Seleucids took over Phoenicia and Palestine in 198/97 B.C. in the Fifth Syrian War. Throughout the third century, however, the Ptolemies generally remained in possession and scored notable successes over the Seleucids, once in 243 B.C. by a strike into the heart of the Seleucid Empire, in which they took Antioch, and once at the battle of Raphia in 217 B.C.

The Ptolemaic occupation of Phoenicia and Palestine had a lasting effect, for Phoenician Sidon became a thoroughly Hellenized city, and even Palestine was urbanized to a considerable degree. The Ptolemies placed numerous garrisons, manned by Greek soldiers, throughout Palestine and introduced a strong Greek element of soldier-settlers, traders, and businessmen. Palestine was organized on the model of Egypt. The king was represented by a military governor, an economic manager, and subordinate officials in charge of the local divisions of the land. The Jewish upper classes began to Hellenize, although the farmers and shepherds remained stubbornly conservative and lived by the Law.

The Ptolemaic Empire well served its primary function of guarding Egypt and also contributed to commercial and fiscal purposes. Considerable revenue was drawn from the possessions in the form of taxes or tribute, and requisitions of food and billets were made for the garrisons. These charges defrayed much of the cost of defense and administration, while some products, like the copper of Cyprus, supplied an important need in Egypt itself. There the Ptolemies worked out an elaborately planned economy administered by the ruling group of Greco-Macedonians.

GOVERNMENT

Since the first Ptolemy was a Hellenized Macedonian general who established his kingdom in the stress of war, it was natural for him to reign as an absolute monarch and to create a governing class of Greeks and Macedonians, congenial and useful to himself. The monarchy, however, had a double aspect because the Ptolemies wished to find a basis of loyalty for both the Greek and Egyptian elements of their people. Like Alexander, they became Pharaohs, bearing the traditional titles and reigning over their Egyptian subjects as native kings.

For the Greeks the practice of worship of the king as a god was gradually established. In 311 B.C. Ptolemy founded a cult in Alexandria to worship the deified Alexander, for whose body he had built a magnificent tomb. A priesthood, in which only the new Hellenic aristocracy of Alexandria could serve, was set up, a temple was built, and state funds were provided for regular worship. Ptolemy thus associated himself with Alexander and shared in the magic of his name, which was still potent at that time in winning the loyalty of Macedonian soldiers. In the following years Ptolemy himself was hailed as a god and worshipped under the title Soter (Savior) by several Greek communities outside of Egypt, notably by the Rhodians in 304 B.C. after he had given them help during the siege of Demetrius Poliorcetes. When Ptolemy died in 283 B.C., his son established worship for the dead king in Alexandria and, two years later upon her death, he associated Ptolemy's wife, Berenice, in the cult. The final step, to include the living members of the royal family with the dead, was taken in 271 B.C., when Ptolemy II established worship for himself and his sister, whom he had married, taking the title, Philadelphus (lover of his sister). Thus, the divine character and continuity of the whole Macedonian line, from Alexander to himself, were emphasized. The practice was continued by subsequent kings who chose titles to emphasize the character in which they wished to appear to their Greek subjects and to the Greek world in general. For example, the third Ptolemy was deified under the title, Euergetes (Benefactor) since the king wished to appear as a responsible ruler who served and protected his state as a true king should.

The rule of the Ptolemies, however, whether as Pharaoh of Egypt or Savior and Benefactor of Greeks, was absolute and personal. For several generations the monarchy retained the traces of its origin. The kings worked extremely hard, lived in relative simplicity, and kept Macedonian habits. They preserved their Macedonian blood line by dynastic intermarriage with the other Hellenistic royal families and their own collateral branches. Occasionally the Egyptian practice of brother and sister marriage was used, as by Philadelphus, but the motive was political and not simply "Egyptianizing." Yet Egypt was a very wealthy country, and in the second and first centuries B.C. the kings slipped easily into a luxurious and more Egyptian type of court life. But even the last of the Ptolemies, Cleopatra, a name synonymous with Egypt, retained the political ambition and flair of her ancestors in whose courts the queens were a potent political influence.

ECONOMY

Like the former Pharaohs, the Ptolemies were the owners of Egypt and managed the land as a great private estate in which they had personal control of production and labor. Their purpose was to make the land as productive and self-sufficient as possible. The traditional economic organization of Egypt, which had been devised for this purpose, was retained and improved by the introduction of Greek techniques of accounting, tax collection and an elaborate system of paper work. In fact, the remains of such materials, the papyri discovered by excavation, provide our knowledge of the system. The center of administration was in Alexandria, where the first Ptolemy moved his residence from Memphis. After the king, the most important official was the *dioecetes,* the financial and economic director. The old division of Egypt into nomes, departments, was retained, with a district capital and local steward of the king in each. The important officials were Greeks or Macedonians, but the backbone of the bureaucracy at the lower level was the Egyptian lower class of scribes. The latter adjusted to the new regime, learned Greek, and carried on the multifarious tasks of registration and the writing of reports to their superior officers. The basis of wealth was the land, and the method of its exploitation was carefully planned to drain off the greater part of production into the king's hands. The Ptolemies had little place for the free economy and system of private enterprise which had characterized the Greek city-states.

All Egypt belonged to the king, and most of the productive land was worked directly for him by tenants on a contract system. Large tracts, the traditional sacred land, were released to the temples and, in addition, the kings gave estates as gifts to the high officials of the administration and allocated small lots to the soldiers for settlement, the *cleruch* land. The "royal land," along with the personnel who worked it, was carefully registered each year by the village officials, who forwarded the reports to Alexandria where the schedules of production were made up. Cultivation was assigned to the tenants by contracts, in which the rent was set, usually in accord with the growing conditions of the year, and the crop specified. The king furnished the seed and collected his rent in produce. Very careful supervision was exercised at seed time and again at harvest, when that portion designated as "rent" was taken from the yield, collected in the district capitals, and then shipped to the granaries in Alexandria. The main crops were wheat and barley, but all agricultural production from which a profit might be made was similarly regulated. In addition to rent, the tenants paid various taxes in produce and were liable for labor on the irrigation canals and other public projects. Since in all probably over 50 percent of their production was paid over to the king, the tenants were left with little margin beyond a subsistence level. The tenants, however, were regarded as free men who could, and sometimes did, move from their villages, although there was little incentive to change residence, for everywhere in Egypt the work and production of the natives were similarly organized.

The sacred land, the god's estate, was worked on a similar system by the "slaves of the god," as the temple tenants were called, under the supervision of the priests, but the king appointed a representative to each temple and collected rent from the produce. Much of the rent might be paid back in the form of gifts, but the Ptolemies wanted to underline the fact of their ownership of the land and to make sure that the temples paid for themselves. It was to the mutual advantage of kings and priests to cooperate, but there were many points of friction in the system of supervision; thus one may suspect that priestly influence sometimes contributed to revolt and strikes among the peasants. On the whole, however, during the third century, the Egyptians, peasants and priests alike, seem to have been reasonably satisfied. The system was traditional, even if the Ptolemies ran it more efficiently than it was operated in the past, the attitude of the kings was benevolent, and a new atmosphere of energetic growth pervaded Egypt.

The use of *cleruch* land was a new phenomenon in Egypt, and its Greek holders were privileged in contrast to the natives. Because the Ptolemies were dependent on a foreign army, mostly Greek and Macedonian, they wished to tie the soldiers to Egypt, both to foster their loyalty and to have a supply of trained men available for war. Instead of maintaining a standing army in barracks, the king granted a lot, a *kleros,* to each soldier, which was sufficient to maintain a family. Most of the lots so allocated were on newly reclaimed land, but the general practice was to scatter the holdings and thus prevent the formation of locally autonomous communities. The Ptolemies wished the interest of the soldier-settler to be in his holding, not in a city-state of the Greek type. Quarters were provided for the settlers, often by the construction of new houses, but sometimes by billets in a native village. The latter practice naturally caused considerable friction since the villages were crowded and the natives resented the greater privileges of the Greek *cleruchs*. Although the latter paid taxes and had only the use, not the right of sale of their holdings, the soldiers could plant what they wished and worked the lots conscientiously with their families. While the system was designed to maintain a privileged military group, separate from the natives, many of the soldier-settlers tended to Egyptianize because they married Egyptian wives and lived much of their lives in a native environment.

The Ptolemies also bestowed huge estates on valued and favored officials.

We know a great deal about the estate of Apollonius, the *dioecetes* of Ptolemy Philadelphus, for some of the records kept by his manager, Zenon, have survived. Apollonius' operations were elaborately planned, for not only was the estate an experimental farm, in which new crops and methods of agriculture were tried out, but was also a very luxurious private residence. These big estates were theoretically revocable by the king, but they tended to become hereditary, as did the lots of the *cleruchs*.

The Ptolemies also increased the production and self-sufficiency of Egypt by programs to reclaim land and to introduce new crops, particularly to satisfy the tastes of their Greek population. Since the Greeks used wine and olive oil, rather than the beer and sesame oil of the Egyptians, vines were introduced from the Aegean, and olive groves started. The new vineyards produced a satisfactory wine, but the olive culture was a failure because the trees could not adjust to the soil and climate. The Greeks in Egypt continued to pay a high price for their oil, since there was a fifty percent tariff on the imported product. Since the Greeks also ate pork and preferred to use wool for their clothing, the Ptolemies imported pigs from Sicily and a species of sheep from Arabia that adapted well to the climate of Egypt. Many of these new crops were tried out on the land given to the Greeks in the Fayoum, where large-scale reclamation was carried on. The work of drainage and irrigation, of which we have very technical records, was done by Greek engineers. New land was also made along the edge of the desert by extensions of the irrigation system. No doubt familiar foods kept the Greek population happier, but the aim of the Ptolemies was to protect their favorable balance of trade by making Egypt as self-sufficient as possible.

As a consequence of this system of planned production, great stocks of raw materials accumulated in the king's warehouses. The large supply of skilled labor in Egypt made it possible to regulate processing and, in addition, distribution was controlled by a system of state monopolies. For example, the vegetable oils, used extensively by the native population, were processed in oil mills under state supervision and sold only by licensed merchants at a fixed price. The production and sale of textiles, salt, and even the national beverage, beer, were similarly regulated as government monopolies.

The economic planning, of course, included a careful regulation of foreign trade to obtain a favorable balance for Egypt. The Ptolemies had to buy metals, timber and exotic products such as ivory, incense, spices, precious stones, and rare woods. They procured the exotics by a vigorous program of exploration and development of the routes through the Red Sea (p. 393), both for use in Egypt and for resale to the Aegean. In addition to natural products the special products of Egyptian craftwork—fine glass, jewelry, and *objets d'art*— were exported, but grain was the chief commodity. Ptolemaic Egypt became the most important supplier to the Greek cities of the Aegean, where virtual control of the grain supply brought political returns, as well as commercial profits. The trade from Egypt was funneled mainly through Alexandria. We do not know the details of its organization, but we do know that foreign traders gathered to the city in great numbers to buy goods and ship them on their own vessels.

This commerce was supported by an excellent coinage of gold, silver, and copper, more for use abroad and in Alexandria than in rural Egypt, where payment in produce and exchange by barter remained the practice. The Ptolemies obtained their gold from mines in the Nubian Desert, which were worked under conditions of terrible hardship by gangs of criminals and prisoners of war. The silver came from the Aegean, as payment for the grain, and the copper from the vassal state of Cyprus. From the outset Ptolemy I departed from the minting practice of Alexander to issue lighter coins, close to those of Rhodes in weight, and his successors lightened the standard still more to bring it in line with that of the Phoenician cities, where it was used for the caravan trade. The result was to establish an exclusive area of Ptolemaic trade in Egypt and its dependencies, for Seleucid coinage, minted on the Attic standard which Alexander had adopted, was excluded.

In addition to the revenues derived from the planned economy, taxation yielded a very considerable amount to the kings because taxes were heavy, extensive and ingenious. Taxes were levied on property, sales, legal acts and, neatly, on exemptions from another tax. Historically the most significant part of the tax system was the method of collection, which probably became the model for Roman practice. Taxes were collected by awarding contracts to individuals who guaranteed the calculated amount of yield to the government and who were allowed a certain percentage for the expenses of collection and for profit. Thus the government was not only sure of its tax monies, but the system also provided a very considerable business for tax contractors, who were mostly Greek businessmen. This system seems to have been introduced in the third century from Egypt into Sicily, where the Romans learned of it when they made Sicily a province.

HELLENIZATION

The Ptolemies, the wealthiest of the Hellenistic rulers, spent large sums on diplomacy among the Greek city-states and in making Alexandria one of the great cities of the Mediterranean. Since modern Alexandria lies directly over the ancient city, there is little of Ptolemaic or Roman Alexandria to be seen, but numerous references in literature reflect the impression which the city made on contemporaries. The most famous structure was the Pharos, a lighthouse, built by the first two Ptolemies, which towered more than four hundred feet in height. The light, reflected in a metal mirror, could be seen about twenty miles at sea. Alexandria contained the famous buildings of Hellenistic Egypt: the royal palaces, Alexander's Mausoleum, the Library and Museum, where writers and scholars were supported by the kings' patronage (pp. 402, 406). The buildings rivaled those of the ancient Pharaohs but were built in Greek style. The broad avenues, lit by torches at night, were lined with long colonnades. The city was famous for its parks, gardens, a zoo, and the various recreational buildings familiar from the cities of the Aegean. The population was a polyglot mixture of Greeks, Egyptians, Hebrews, and other nationalities, drawn to Alexandria by its wealth and opportunities. Society, of course, was headed by the court and the high officials of the administration, who deliberately cultivated Greek traditions. Alexandria, however, was not a true Greek city-state. The Greeks were reckoned as the active citizens, who elected civic officials and preserved the institutions of Greek life, but each sizable foreign group, like the Jews, had a separate corporative existence, and the whole city was under the direction of a governor appointed by the king. The Greek life of Egypt was largely concentrated in Alexandria, for the only other Greek cities were the old colony at Naukratis and a military foundation, Ptolemais, far up the Nile in the Thebaid.

The Greeks in Egypt held a privileged position as a governing class, somewhat like that of Europeans in the early period of foreign colonization. The high administrative officials lived luxuriously in Alexandria and took their ease on estates and villas in the suburbs. Greek traders, businessmen, accountants, architects, and engineers found ample employment and a good living. The Greek farmer-soldiers were privileged, too, in their freedom and the possibility of some profit in their economic life. Among the natives the priesthood held its traditional position of eminence, but the mass of the native population enjoyed none of the Greeks' privileges and had little time and energy to work for themselves. They remained Egyptian and, as we have noticed, began to Egyptianize the Greek settlers who lived in proximity to them. Many *cleruchs* married native wives, and although the children were counted as Greeks, the mother's culture had a stronger influence than that of the father. The rural Greek population turned to the religious customs and superstitions of the Egyptian peasants and grew into a mixed, bilingual group, more Egyptian than Greek.

The elaborate organization began to break down after the death of Ptolemy III (Euergetes) in 221 B.C. His successor, Ptolemy IV (Philopater) did win a decisive victory over the Seleucids in 217 B.C. at Raphia, but only by strengthening the army with native Egyptian troops because he was lacking in Greek soldiers. Since the victory had the effect of fostering Egyptian nationalism, a serious revolt soon broke out, in which the newly trained native troops joined. This outburst was the forerunner of a series of revolts and peasant strikes which weakened Egypt throughout the following century. The kings began to indulge a luxurious indolence, leaving the government to their officials, who were often competent men but self-seeking and jealous of one another. As central authority slackened, corruption and laxity grew in the bureaucracy, whose intricate machinery needed close, continuous supervision. The kings also neglected their foreign possessions; thus from the end of the third century the Empire began to crumble. Aegean Greece came under the protection of Rome, and in 198–97 B.C. Palestine and Phoenicia were lost to the Seleucids. The Ptolemies found

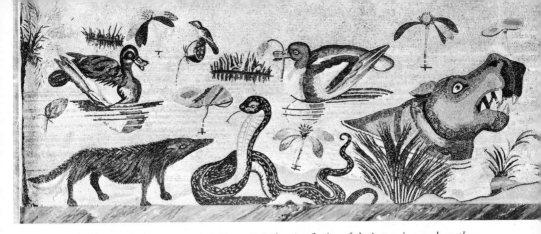

Birds and beasts of the Nile. From a mosaic at Pompeii, Italy. A reflection of the impression made on the Romans by the exotic scenery of Egypt

in Rome a prop against further Seleucid encroachment, but were increasingly harassed by their internal problems. The temple estates and privileges of the priests were increased to gain the latter's support, but since no possibility existed of drawing the two parts of Egypt, Greek and native, into a close union the ruling class of Greeks dwindled away.

The Seleucid Kingdom

Seleucus I, the founder of the Seleucid Kingdom, was the real successor of Alexander in the sense that he acquired the bulk of the old Persian Empire in western Asia and followed Alexander's general policy of working with the native elements and founding cities. Seleucus' heritage was not a defensible and compact state, like Egypt, but the diverse parts were acquired piecemeal in the Wars of the Successors. Seleucus became governor of Babylonia after the murder of Perdiccas in 321 B.C. but did not consolidate his hold on the satrapy until 308 B.C. In the following years he added the eastern satrapies of the Empire, including India, but yielded that in 303 B.C. to the Maurya king, Chandragupta, in exchange for five hundred war elephants. Victory over Antigonus and Demetrius at the battle of Ipsus enabled Seleucus to expand into their territory. Northern Syria was taken and, in 296 B.C., Cilicia. Seleucus next advanced into Asia Minor, where he conquered Lysimachus at Corupedion in 281 B.C. He took over all of western Asia Minor and laid claim to Thrace and Macedonia. While Seleucus' successor, Antiochus I, had to forego entry into Europe, he fought hard and successfully to hold on to the Asiatic part of the Empire. This, in fact, became the main purpose of the Seleucids, simply to hold on to the vast area of their kingdom, with its varied peoples and long lines of communication.

THE EMPIRE

In western Asia Minor the Seleucids had to control or, at least, establish favorable relations with the Greek cities to recruit the manpower needed for their armies and program of settlement. They claimed suzerainty over the Greek cities by virtue of Seleucus' conquest, but the Greeks, asserting that independence had been restored to them by Alexander, contrived to play off Ptolemy against Seleucid whenever possible. Since the cities were strong and well fortified, they found a renewed prosperity in the development of trade with the hinterland of Anatolia. Accordingly, Seleucid influence was maintained with difficulty by a mixture of threats, force, diplomacy, and outright gifts or exemptions from taxation. In northwestern Asia Minor the rise of Pergamum (p. 385) into a separate, small kingdom in the third century further undermined the Seleucid position, since the new state found an ally in the Ptolemies and made a considerable show of posing as the champion of Hellenism. In northern and central Anatolia, which Alexander had bypassed, the Seleucids were forced to permit the rise of Hellenized native states in Bithynia, Pontus, Cappadocia, and Galatia. Dynastic marriages were made into the royal families of Pontus and Cappadocia, which claimed descent from the old Iranian kings, but the Seleucid kings fought the Gauls in the interest of their Greek allies.

The heart of the Empire was Seleucid Syria, which stretched along the Orontes River and the Amuk plain across the arch of the Fertile Crescent to Mesopotamia. The region was very fertile, well populated, and strategically located to control the routes into Asia Minor and to keep a watchful eye on the activities of the Ptolemies in Phoenicia and Palestine. In Mesopotamia particularly cordial relations were established with the Babylonian priesthood and people as a counterweight to Iranian influence, so that Babylonia was held long after the eastern, Iranian section of the Empire was lost.

Iran, in fact, broke away in the middle of the third century when the Seleucid hold was relaxed by family quarrels over the succession. A new Iranian state, Parthia, began to form under King Arsaces, and in Bactria the Seleucid governors renounced Seleucid authority to form a new kingdom of their own (pp. 382–84). While the East was nominally recovered by Antiochus III in the latter part of the third century by a series of campaigns which rivaled Alexander's, Antiochus' authority was short-lived. Thus, the political history of the Seleucid regime is largely a record of its valiant, but ultimately unsuccessful, attempt to hold the outlying provinces. The kings worked hard, ruling personally and conducting a difficult and extensive diplomacy, but because the combination of dynastic quarrels, the nationalism of their subject peoples, and Roman pressure was too great to support, the kingdom melted away. Nevertheless, in the region west of the Euphrates, the Seleucids left a foundation of Hellenized city life on which Rome could build its eastern provinces.

GOVERNMENT

The Seleucid administration was necessarily much less centralized than that of the Ptolemies because of the unwieldy variety of the Empire. Seleucus established a monarchy of the Macedonian type, in which he ruled personally with the assistance of his kinsmen, friends, and high administrative officials, such as the director of finance, who was a virtual prime minister. It was the personal ambition of these kinsmen and friends which led to the internal quarrels that so weakened the kingdom. To secure the allegiance of their Greek subjects the Seleucid kings encouraged the establishment of ruler cults in the Greek cities and established state worship of the king in their provinces. Many Greek cities voluntarily recognized the king as a divine benefactor and worshipped him in return for signal services and acts, such as the remission of taxes or a victory over their enemies. These voluntary city cults should be distinguished from the state cult which was deliberately fostered by the kings and extended on occasion to the native peoples. Antiochus I initiated the cult by building a temple and sanctuary near the tomb of his father, Seleucus. When the later kings extended the practice, there was a state cult in the chief city of each of the provinces by the end of the third century. The dignitaries of the province were chosen for the priesthood and carried on official worship of the dead and living Seleucids.

In their administration of the Empire the Seleucids followed the general practice of Alexander. The former Persian satrapies were retained, with a Greek or Macedonian as governor, but the big satrapies were subdivided for more efficient government, and financial administration was kept directly under the king's control. For the more remote areas and those where national feeling was very strong, native rulers were given full local autonomy in exchange for some military assistance and an occasional payment of tribute. In this manner Antiochus III restored his nominal title to the eastern part of the Empire. In the satrapies, however, native unrest was avoided to a considerable extent by a policy of religious tolerance and in many cases substantial encouragement of native religious practices. The Seleucids made gifts to the local temples in the native cities of Mesopotamia, and in Babylon restored the great temple of the god, Esagila. The notorious interference of Antiochus IV in Palestine in 167 B.C., when he confiscated the treasures of the temple in Jerusalem and attempted to force the Jews to worship Zeus, was a part of his general program of Hellenization to strengthen the state. He was supported by that segment of upper-class Jewish society which had Hellenized (pp. 476–77).

URBANIZATION AND HELLENIZATION

The Seleucid purposes in settling thousands of Greek and Macedonian immigrants were essentially political and military: to provide a homogeneous group of subjects on whose loyalty the kings could rely, and whose settlements would provide a defensive shield for the vital parts of the Empire. The settlers were grouped in organized communities, ranging from rural colonies and garrison towns to new cities uniformly of Greek type. In Seleucid Syria, which formed the nodal point for communication and control of the western part of the Empire, four main urban centers were founded by Seleucus I.

The most important of these was the city of Antioch, at the southwest corner of the plain of Amuk on the Orontes River. Antioch was designed to be the political capital, housing the palace and the court of the kings. The population was formed from Greeks, Macedonians, Jews, and Syrians. At the outset the town had two quarters, one for the Europeans, the other for the Syrians and Jews. The whole city was laid out on the familiar gridiron plan of new Greek cities and, like Alexandria, was Greek in appearance. The population, starting from a modest twenty thousand in 300 B.C., grew rapidly, and Antioch became one of the great cities of the Roman and Byzantine Empires, as well as the Seleucid capital. In early Roman times the population seems to have been about 600,000. About five miles to the south a villa resort was developed at Daphnae, which became famous in antiquity for its gardens, springs, and groves. It still preserves some magnificent mosaics of the Late Roman Period. Little, however, is preserved of Seleucid Antioch because of continuous growth and habitation. To the south of Antioch, along the Orontes River, was Apamea, the chief military base of the Seleucids. On the coast new ports, Seleucia in the delta of the Orontes River, and Laodicea, farther to the south, carried most of the Seleucid trade with the eastern Mediterranean. In addition to these main cities Syria was protected by a ring of new settlements on a more modest scale, most of which bore Macedonian names and give a map of the land the appearance of a new Macedonia.

In western Asia Minor, where urbanization was well advanced, the Seleucids sometimes enlarged the older Greek cities by additional land, but their main effort went into the establishment of rural colonies, *katoikiai*. Immigrant soldiers formed the population and guarded the routes and the rich agricultural areas of native Phrygia, Lydia, and Caria.

In Mesopotamia, which had been urbanized since the third millennium, an extensive program of city foundation was hardly necessary, but the Seleucids built a new, Greek subcapital, Seleucia on the Tigris, on the site of Opis, where Alexander had held his famous feast of reconciliation. Also, a string of settlements was founded along the roads of the Tigris and Euphrates River valleys to the north and west. Seleucia became a large and prosperous city, as big as Antioch, for it was the terminus of the caravan roads from India and eastern Iran. One of the Seleucid cities on the Euphrates, Dura-Europus, has been excavated and reveals the general type of city foundation. The city was Greek, with the familiar buildings and political institutions of a city-state of the Aegean. The citizens possessed a locally autonomous political life, but there was a garrison commander and various royal officials to represent the king. Like a proper *polis,* Dura-Europus administered an adjacent rural territory, in which lots of land were assigned to the settlers, active soldiers, veterans, immigrants from the Aegean and natives of the locality.

We know little of Seleucid activity in the eastern satrapies, but apparently a screen of settlements was placed in the mountains of Media and Persis to protect Mesopotamia on the east, with garrisons strung along the roads across Iran. The Seleucids did not have the manpower to thoroughly settle the eastern portion of the Empire and were confronted there by a homogeneous Iranian population, which cherished its nationalism and was difficult to reconcile.

The land on which the new settlements were established was chiefly "King's Land," to which the Seleucids had taken title by right of conquest. Large tracts, mainly in Asia Minor and Syria, were confiscated from the great temple estates and wealthy native landlords for the same purpose. The kings also gave land of this origin to existing cities to enlarge their rural territories, and they made gifts of estates to favored administrators and friends. Work on the land had been performed by hereditary "serfs" for the most part, so that the general effect of urbanization was to transfer the obligations of the peasants from the king, temples and native landlords to the cities, and to withdraw vast areas from their former owners' exploitation. The "serfs" did not become full citizens of the new communities but, being exposed to Hellenization, might expect a rise of status in the course of time. The very considerable amount of land retained by the kings was still worked through a system of hereditary tenantry by which the "royal peasants" paid their rent in produce. The system, however, was not as systematic and oppressive as that of the Ptolemies because rents and taxes were lighter and the general effects of urbanization gradually spread. Nevertheless, the gulf remained wide between the privileged class of Greek and Macedonian rulers and settlers in the cities and the mass of natives in the countryside. To bridge it would have taken generations of peace and stability which the Seleucids could not win.

The Seleucids also worked towards a more complete economic unification of their Empire and competed with the Ptolemies in foreign trade. While the Empire was too diverse to be welded into a single economic unit, a good, plentiful coinage was issued which circulated widely and freely and which replaced barter over much of western Asia. Since the Seleucids coined on the Attic weight standard adopted by Alexander, for a time their coins were stamped with his portrait to emphasize the continuity of rule. The monetary and trading monopoly of the Ptolemies was countered by excluding Ptolemaic coinage from Seleucid possessions, and by developing the routes which Alexander had contemplated to India and southern Arabia for exotics and luxury products (p. 394). Because Ptolemaic control of the sea, however, made marketing difficult, the Seleucids also used Rhodes as a distributing agent and, when possible, the Greek cities on the west coast of Asia Minor. The products of Syrian industry and some grain were exported, but the volume of trade was probably less than that of Egypt. Although we do not know the details of their organization of trade as fully as Egypt's, we do know that much of the handling was in Greek hands, for Greek became established as a language of trade in the Empire, along with Aramaic.

The Seleucid social policy of urbanization and the attraction exerted by the Greek ruling class resulted in a very considerable degree of Hellenization. Greek was the official language of the Empire, and those natives of the upper class, particularly in the cities, who wished to be on cordial terms with their governors, learned Greek and adopted some measure of Greek habits. The Syrians who wished to trade into the Aegean and with Rhodes became "Greek Syrians." The slaves in the Greek households Hellenized rapidly, too, but throughout the countryside, on the great temple estates and in the villages, the natives clung to their traditional customs. Since the Greek settlers lived a familiar urban type of life, there was not so great a tendency, as in Egypt, to forget their Greek traditions, but intermarriage with native women and the attraction of native religious beliefs and practices affected them. In general, the effect of the new regime was to stimulate a rapid economic advance, particularly in Asia Minor and Syria, in which the Greeks profited more than the natives, but which also benefited the latter.

While dynastic quarrels and the Iranian resurgence cost the Seleucids the eastern part of the Empire in the mid-third century, an energetic attempt was made to restore the kingdom in its entirety by Antiochus III, who came to the throne in 223 B.C. He had first to recover part of Seleucid Asia Minor, which was held by a rebellious cousin, Achaeus, and to put down a revolt by Molon, the governor of Media, who had detached Babylonia and western Persia from Antiochus. Antiochus defeated Molon and came to terms with Achaeus, then turned south to win Phoenicia and Palestine. Antiochus' army was defeated by the Egyptians at Raphia in 217 B.C., but a follow-up of the victory was prevented by native revolts in Egypt. Accordingly, Antiochus marched east to bring the Iranians to terms and the Bactrian kings into the Seleucid fold. He reduced the Iranians to tributary status for the time being and made an agreement with Euthydemus, the king of Bactria, by which each pledged to do what he could for Hellenization in the East, where it was seriously endangered. When Antiochus returned to the West in 204 B.C., something of Alexander's aura of greatness hung about him. Men began to talk of a new Alexander.

Antiochus proceeded to restore Seleucid authority in the West by making an agreement with Philip V of Macedon to divide up the foreign possessions of the Ptolemies. In 198/97 B.C. he gained Phoenicia and Palestine from Egypt and turned his attention to the Greek cities of Asia Minor. At that point he was confronted by a Roman ultimatum to respect the freedom of the Greeks (p. 473). Bewildered by this unexpected Roman interest in Asia Minor and angered at the Roman tone, Antiochus challenged the Romans, but was defeated in Greece in 190 and in Asia Minor in 189 B.C. By the terms of the settlement the Seleucids were excluded from Greek Asia Minor and the Aegean. Perforce, Antiochus and his successors turned their attention eastward and tried, without access to fresh Greek manpower, to curb native revolt and to resist Roman interference.

The Greeks in Bactria and India

One of the most remarkable demonstrations of the energy and ability of the Greco-Macedonian conquerors of the Persian Empire was the establishment of Greek kingdoms in Bactria (Afghanistan) and northern India. The life of these kingdoms was short, for they flourished only during the first half of the second century B.C. Their subsequent historical influence was slight, but the

Greek rulers revealed an unexpected ability to enlist native cooperation which was a necessary condition for even their temporary success. There was moreover no possibility of recruiting soldiers and settlers from the West since Seleucid assistance was precluded by the rise of Parthia between Seleucid Babylonia and Bactria. The Seleucids also demanded acknowledgment of their authority, which the Bactrian Greeks repudiated soon after the middle of the third century.

The governor of Bactria, Diodotus, took advantage of the family quarrels of the Seleucids about 250 B.C. to regard himself as the king's ally, rather than his governor, but the real founders of the Kingdom of Bactria were Euthydemus, a Greek soldier from Magnesia in western Asia Minor, and his son, Demetrius. In the latter part of the third century Euthydemus consolidated Bactria and Sogdiana under his authority, ruling from the fortified city of Bactra. He resisted nomadic raids from the steppe land across the Jaxartes River, held the Parthians in check from the west and fought stoutly against Antiochus, when the latter besieged Bactra in 208 B.C. Their treaty of mutual support left Euthydemus and Demetrius a free hand to proceed with the consolidation of the kingdom.

The rulers came to terms with the Iranian nobility, who lived in fortified castles, and sponsored a policy of urbanization throughout Bactria. The villages were expanded into the walled towns characteristic of central Asia, which gave protection from the nomads, and new communities were formed. The good grazing land of Bactria and the rich agricultural plains of Sogdiana supported the economy of the kingdom. Bactria also became known in tradition as the "land of a thousand cities." Such a description was probably a hyperbole, reflecting the impression made by the foundation of towns where there had been none before. In addition to the revenues from agriculture, the rulers of Bactria profited from their location at the crossroads of Asiatic caravan routes. The roads from India ran through their territory to Bactra and thence across Iran to the Seleucid markets in Seleucia and Babylon. Probably, too, trade was carried on with the nomadic peoples of western Siberia and, perhaps, with western China. To service the caravan routes and their own economy, the Bactrian kings issued a fine series of coins bearing the portraits of their kings. The quality of the workmanship used on them is a testimony to the skill of the Greek craftsmen who worked in the Bactrian cities. The coins themselves are an invaluable aid in the reconstruction of Bactrian history.

By 189 B.C. when the new kingdom was strong enough to expand southwards, the Seleucid satrapies which lay between Bactria and India were taken over. This conquest further consolidated the Bactrian hold on the trade routes and led the kings on into India. In 183 B.C. Demetrius crossed the mountains and marched down the valley of the Cabul River into Taxila, as Alexander had done 150 years previously. In the interval, however, the Maurya Kingdom, extending across northern India, had grown into a strong power under the kings Chandragupta and his grandson, Asoka. By the second century the

Buddhist religion had developed rapidly and was a strong rival to Brahmanism. Since Demetrius and his Greeks seem to have ranged themselves on the side of the Buddhists, they were thus able to gain Indian allies for the invasion. Demetrius took Taxila and advanced to the Indus River, where he turned downstream to the delta, incorporating the area into his kingdom and refounding Pattala as a new city, Demetrias.

Demetrius' general, Menander, was dispatched east through the Punjab, where he occupied Sagala and the Maurya capital, Patra, on the upper Ganges River. The Greeks cooperated closely with their Indian allies and took the princes into council to form a joint government. Greek craftsmen were brought into the kingdom, and a new series of coins, with Indian legends, was issued. The sea route from the Indus to South Arabia was developed to supplement the land routes, now made difficult by the growth of Parthia.

The united Kingdom of Bactria and India proved difficult to hold under a single authority, and after 169 B.C. the stability of Bactria itself was weakened by Seleucid interference. Antiochus IV, excluded from action in the West by Roman fiat and concerned about the expansion of Parthia in Iran, tried to regain Bactria. He sent his cousin, Eucratides, with a small force to bring Bactria back to Seleucid rule. Eucratides incited some of the Bactrian Greeks to rebellion against Demetrius and undermined the authority of the royal family. Apparently, the rebels preferred Antiochus' policy of Hellenic supremacy to their own king's collaboration with natives. Eucratides was killed by the son of Demetrius, but the damage to the Greek position was fatal, and the Bactrian Kingdom began to crumble.

The Parthians consolidated all of Iran from Mesopotamia eastwards by 141 B.C. As nomadic pressure increased from the steppes, the Kingdom of Bactria vanished by 128 B.C. In that year a Chinese general, Chang K'ien, wrote a report describing his tour of inspection across central Asia to the Han emperor, Wu-ti. Chang K'ien visited Bactria and found it occupied by the Yueh-Chi, who had pushed west across the steppes from northwestern China. In India Menander continued to rule the Indian Kingdom until his death in 150 B.C. Much of the region was overrun by the Saca invaders a generation later, and the small pockets of Greek authority remaining in northern India vanished in the following century. From Iran the Parthians, expanding their kingdom into northern Mesopotamia, by 100 B.C. had pushed the Seleucids to the west of the Euphrates River. The Euphrates became the eastern frontier of the Roman Empire, and the Kingdom of Parthia supplanted the Seleucids as the great power of the Middle East.

Pergamum and the Native Kingdoms of Asia Minor

In northern and central Asia Minor, where the Seleucids were unable to assert their authority, a group of native kingdoms arose in the third century. Their rulers were particularly ardent promoters of Hellenism. The most important of these was Pergamum in northwestern Asia Minor, which ruled the native districts of that region and the old Greek cities of Aeolis. The city of Pergamum was strategically situated to control the main routes of the region. During the Wars of the Successors Lysimachus of Thrace used the town as a base for military operations. The garrison commander, Philetaerus, betrayed Pergamum to Seleucus I when the latter was attacking Lysimachus, and he contrived to retain Lysimachus' war fund of about nine thousand talents. Philetaerus ruled as a nominal vassal of the Seleucids from 283 to 263 B.C. Upon his death his successors, Eumenes (263–41 B.C.) and Attalus (241–197 B.C.), asserted independence and expanded the little kingdom into a strong and wealthy state. The Pergamene kings assumed the role of protectors of Hellenism against the raids of the Galatians from the east and scored notable successes, which they commemorated in sculpture (p. 411) and which won the loyalty of the Greek cities of Aeolis. The Attalids of Pergamum were able to protect themselves against the Seleucids by their own good army and by alliance with the Ptolemies. They developed a considerable trade in the products of their region through the Aeolic Greek ports.

The Pergamene kings exploited the rich agricultural land of the adjacent Caicus River valley and from the revenues made lavish gifts to the older cities of Greece, such as Athens, and built their own Pergamum into a spectacularly beautiful city. The towering fortress of its *acropolis* was crowned with the royal palace and adorned by a theater and a great altar of Zeus (p. 411). The Attalids were also patrons of literature who established a library and entertained writers at their court. The city, built on the level ground at the foot of the *acropolis,* was organized as a Greek city-state, with the familiar institutions of council and magistrates, but political life was directed in all essentials by the kings. In the rural hinterland the kings retained the traditional life of the native villages which was centered around their temples, so that the city of Pergamum, like Alexandria, was essentially the Greek façade of a native state. When the Romans entered Greece, the Attalids adroitly allied themselves to Rome against Macedonia and the Seleucids, thus prolonging independence until 133 B.C., when the last king bequeathed his kingdom to Rome.

Along the south coast of the Black Sea the Persian satrapies of Bithynia and Pontus coalesced into kingdoms under the rule of native dynasts after Alexander's death. The kings claimed descent from the former rulers of Iran, but pursued a policy of Hellenization. The court and the upper class learned Greek. The kings promoted urbanization, transforming their rural, backward regions into thriving states, which played a role in the trade and diplomacy of the Hellenistic world. The king of Bithynia had done an initial disservice to Hellenism by allowing the Gauls to enter Asia Minor in 279 B.C. and by directing their settlement to the region of central Phrygia, which became known as Galatia. The Gallic community, however, acted as Bithynia's buffer against the Seleucids.

Galatia remained purely Celtic throughout the Hellenistic Period and had a tribal and cantonal organization like that of the Celtic states of Gaul in Western

Europe. Beyond Galatia, in central Anatolia, another native kingdom, Cappadocia, was formed in the early third century. The Cappadocian rulers claimed descent from the Persian kings, but maintained a Hellenic court and intermarried with the Seleucids. These native Anatolian kingdoms grew in power and wealth and in the first century B.C. were combined under King Mithridates of Pontus, who made the last stand of the Hellenistic East against the armies of Sulla, Lucullus, and Pompey (pp. 523–27, 533–34, 537).

Macedonia and Greece

THE POSITION OF THE GREEK CITY-STATES

The need of the Hellenistic rulers for Greek manpower placed the city-states of the Aegean under continuous political tension. Because Macedonia was closed to the recruiting of Seleucids and Ptolemies after Antigonus Gonatas established a stable kingdom in 279 B.C., the older cities of Greece and western Asia Minor were the particular objects of their attention. As we have noticed above, the Seleucids vied with Egypt and Pergamum over the Greeks of Asia Minor. In the Aegean and Greece the Ptolemies made an effort to upset the protectorate which Macedonia claimed as its traditional right. The Greek cities themselves were in a most uneasy situation because their desire for independence persisted without the capacity to attain it or to defend themselves successfully. The Ptolemies supported the Greek cities against Macedonia by money, gifts, and the provision of grain, but not with full-scale military aid. Under these pressures Greek cities were drawn closer together for protection and in the Hellenistic Period they combined into leagues and federal associations even more readily than in the fourth century. Two large Leagues developed, the Aetolian League in western Greece and the Achaean League in the Peloponnesus. These two were mutually hostile, however, and to the tension produced by conflict between the Ptolemies and Antigonids that of the Leagues was added. Thus, Greek political life in the third century was characterized by its usual instability and war. Nevertheless, the political exclusiveness which had characterized the city-states began to dissolve. Instead of fighting each other over a trivial dispute, there was more recourse to arbitration by a third party. The autonomy of the states was breached by grants of mutual citizenship and by the frequent invitations to judges from other cities to hear cases. The city-state was declining into a municipality but was not yet ready to acknowledge the fact.

Alexander's conquest and the establishment of the Hellenistic Kingdoms had brought economic growth and prosperity to Greece for a time. Although the great kings threatened and interfered, they also cultivated good will by direct gifts of money, grain, and buildings. The supply of money in the Aegean was greatly increased by Alexander's coinage of the Persian bullion and by the expenditures of the kings. New markets were not only provided for Greek wine, olive oil and manufactured goods in the growing kingdoms of the East, but there were also opportunities for Greek emigrants. This renewed prosperity in the Aegean made its cities a market for eastern goods, and a flourishing trade developed. Corinth and Athens enjoyed a considerable share, but there was a general tendency for the tide of prosperity to shift across the Aegean. As the big port cities of Asia Minor grew rapidly, Rhodes, too, became a commercial and maritime power of primary importance in the Aegean (pp. 394–95).

This revival in the Aegean, however, began to slacken about the middle of the third century when the economies of the new kingdoms had become established and the market for Greek goods declined. Migration from Greece fell off, and Greek social distress became apparent once again as wealth became concentrated in the hands of the middle-class landowners and businessmen while farmers and craftsmen became poorer. After 250 B.C. an increasingly sharp contrast divided rich and poor. To the clamor for the cancellation of debts and redistribution of land there was added political tension between the states, internal revolution, and civil war.

POLITICAL DIVISION AND SOCIAL STRIFE

When Antigonus Gonatas took over Macedonia after the Gallic invasion, he already controlled a considerable part of Greece, including the key military fortresses of Corinth, the Athenian Peiraeus, Chalcis in Euboea, and Demetrias in Thessaly, a new city founded by his father. These "fetters of Greece" were held by Macedonian garrisons, while other cities were controlled by pro-Macedonian governments supported and subsidized by Gonatas. Even if he had wished to abandon this direct control in favor of a "free" League, like that of Philip II, Gonatas had no opportunity to do so, for Ptolemy II Philadelphus instigated uprisings and war.

In 278 B.C. Ptolemy persuaded the Spartan king, Areus, to start a war in the Peloponnesus against Gonatas. Gonatas held on to the key fortress of Corinth, but most of the other Macedonian holdings won their independence. The war of Areus, however, had been confined to the Peloponnesus, and Ptolemy soon devised a more ambitious policy to upset Macedonia, using King Pyrrhus of Epirus. Pyrrhus, who had been unsuccessful in attacking Macedonia in the 280's and who had been driven from Italy by the Romans in 275 B.C., was still in search of a kingdom more worthy than Epirus for his not inconsiderable talents. Pyrrhus attacked Macedonia from the west, but was driven off and transferred his attention to the Peloponnesus. He invaded with a small force, offering protection to the Peloponnesian cities, most of whom were no longer in need of it, and was ingloriously killed in street fighting in Argos. According to tradition an old woman hit him on the head with a roof tile thrown from her house. In 267 B.C. Ptolemy provoked a more serious threat to the Macedonian position by instigating Athens and Sparta to rise in the Chremonidean War. The conflict which lasted until 261 B.C. is noteworthy as Athens' last attempt to regain some measure of political power and prestige. The war was lost, and Athens eschewed politics in favor of trade and intellectual fame as the seat of the philosophical schools.

Since these efforts of Ptolemy to shake the hold of Macedonia were designed more to check Gonatas' suspected ambition as the son of Demetrius than to acquire territory, Ptolemy sent no troops to help his allies. The Ptolemaic hold on the Aegean, however, was a serious threat to the Macedonian protectorate, for by it Ptolemy controlled the import of grain to the Greek cities. After his success in the Chremonidean War, Gonatas attacked in the Aegean and defeated the Ptolemaic fleet off the island of Cos in 258 B.C. While the net result of the conflict was in favor of Gonatas, his hold on the Peloponnesus and Central Greece had been disturbed, and he had been diverted from necessary reorganization in Macedonia itself. Accordingly, until his death in 243 B.C. Gonatas turned his attention to Macedonia and to strengthening his frontiers against the barbarian peoples to the north. The need to contain the barbarians also engaged the attention of his successor, Demetrius, who reigned until 225 B.C. In this interval conditions were favorable to the growth of the Leagues and to a stronger assertion of independence by the Greek cities, which may have understood the function which Macedonia performed in shielding them on the north, but saw only their own opportunity for rejecting Macedonian control in the situation.

The Aetolian League had come into existence in the early fourth century as a national union of the tribal cantons of Aetolia but played little part in Greek affairs until after the death of Alexander. Then the Aetolians who had identified themselves as anti-Macedonian by joining in the Lamian War against Antipater had acquired considerable prestige in Central Greece by their successful stand against the Gauls in 279 B.C. They became the patrons of the Delphic oracle and worked against Macedonia to extend their own political influence. After Gonatas and Demetrius devoted their attention to Macedonia itself, the Aetolians, ready to profit by any occasion, began to collaborate occasionally with Macedonia against the Achaean League which was growing to power in the Peloponnesus.

The Aetolian League remained essentially national in character, and its citizens, linked by federal citizenship, met in a general assembly to elect officials and determine policy. Each canton, however, retained local autonomy, and the League did not take in foreign states as such. Instead, Aetolian influence was extended by alliances and by the interesting device of *isopolity,* which was an exchange of citizenship between Aetolia and individuals of a foreign state. The latter could exercise the rights of citizenship when in Aetolia and worked for Aetolian interests in their own cities. The League had a bad reputation for piracy and banditry in the more civilized parts of Greece. We hear of this through the historian Polybius (p. 408), a citizen of the Achaean League, which was the target of much Aetolian raiding.

The Achaean League began as a union of the small city-states of Achaea in the northern Peloponnesus, which were freed in the wake of Areus' war against Gonatas, and grew into a true federal organization by extending citizenship to foreign states. The citizens of its member-states who had both federal and local citizenship assembled to elect officials and to determine important matters of

League policy. Each member-state also sent delegates to a federal council, which conducted the affairs of the League in the intervals between the assembly meetings. The Achaean League was one of the more fruitful experiments of Greek political practice, for its truly federal nature resolved the difficulty experienced by other Greek leagues in which one state was supreme and suppressed the rights of the other members.

The main architect of the Achaean League was Aratus of Sicyon, who displayed considerable political skill by maintaining himself in office as League president (*strategos*) or as a member of the council for about thirty years from 245 to 215 B.C. Aratus' greatest exploit was the capture of the great Macedonian fortress of Acrocorinth, the citadel of Corinth, by a surprise attack at night. The capture of Corinth released the Peloponnesus from Macedonian control and made the Achaean League its chief power. Aratus, however, proved to be a better statesman than general, for in attacks on Athens and Argos he failed to bring them into the League by force. The Achaean League, in fact, united only a part of the Peloponnesus, since ideas of separatism died hard in the smaller states, and Aratus' ambitions received a rude check by the revival of a militant and nationalistic Sparta.

The Spartans, until the latter part of the third century B.C., had maintained their obsolete social system in Laconia, despite the continuous shrinkage in the number of properly qualified citizens. In 240 B.C. a young king, Agis, came to the throne with ideas for a revival of monarchical power against the Spartan *ephors* and of expansion in the Peloponnesus. He may have been affected, too, by familiarity with ideas of Cynic asceticism, for the revolution, which he and his successor engineered, was colored with a specious stress on the old Lycurgan Sparta and the value of its discipline. The basis of a new Sparta, however, was to be an expansion of citizenship; its propaganda slogan was cancellation of debts and redistribution of property. Since these proposals had a very real appeal to the lower classes of Greece, the Spartan revival was soon regarded as a social revolution which threatened the propertied classes of other cities.

Agis tried to implement his ideas from above by use of his royal power but was assassinated by the *ephors*. His successor, Cleomenes, deemed a safe young man by the magistrates, proved more adroit. Cleomenes hired soldiers, deposed the *ephors*, and put social reform into effect. When a surge of national feeling made the small Spartan army a formidable fighting force, through its ability and his revolutionary slogan, Cleomenes began to break up the Achaean League. At this juncture Aratus reversed his policy to Macedonia and called upon its regent, Antigonus Doson, for help. Doson, acting for the young king, Philip V, invaded the Peloponnesus in 222 B.C. and defeated the Spartan forces at the battle of Sellasia. The Achaean League was saved, but the price of Macedonian aid was the re-establishment of the protectorate.

Doson and Philip made the last statesmanlike effort to unite Macedonia with the Greek city-states. They revived and liberalized the old League of Corinth and allowed a very considerable measure of freedom to the Greeks. In the new organization it was necessary for the decisions of the general assembly to be ratified by the member-states separately, so that individual members might abstain from joint undertakings of the League. While this weakened the potential strength of the organization, the concession was the limit of cooperation which Doson could demand from his Greek allies. The League did not include all Greece, for Aetolia remained outside, and many small cities preferred to stand aloof. Yet the combination of Greek and Macedonian strength could have been formidable. By 220 B.C. thoughtful Greeks were already conscious that a new great power, Rome, was rising, as one Greek put it, like a cloud in the west. When the test of unity came, in Rome's wars against Macedonia, the League broke apart and Roman conquest was facilitated by division in Greece.

The political division of Greece and Macedonia in the third century was a picture in miniature of that which existed throughout the Hellenistic world. The great powers were divided in political policy and commercial rivalry. In the new kingdoms of the East there was a gulf between the privileged ruling classes of Greeks and Macedonians and the native peoples, which kept them from becoming organically unified states, just as Greece and Macedonia were prevented by other causes. The fragmentation caused by Alexander's successors was to be mended by Rome rather than by a Hellenistic power. In the Hellenistic world, however, there was a new and fruitful unity of culture among the Greeks from the Aegean to Alexandria and Babylon. A new vigor and energy emerged when Aegean Greece and the Near East were drawn together by ties of trade and mutual intercourse.

XVIII

The Hellenistic World

THE NEW WORLD WHICH ALEXANDER and his successors had established was linked together by continuous movement and intercourse among its various parts. The Greeks traveled, not only as soldiers and settlers to new homes, but as traders, officials on their government's business, and for their own private interest and pleasure. A very considerable stock of historical and geographical knowledge was accumulated which became the ordinary fund of information possessed by educated people. Men's intellectual interests transcended the political frontiers delimiting their countries and were not impeded, among the Greeks at least, by differences in language and culture. A new form of Greek, the *koine* or common tongue, came into general use in the Hellenistic countries. It could be learned relatively easily by those natives who became Hellenized, for the *koine* was simpler and less subtle than the Greek of the Classical Period.

This intellectual unity was not only confined to practical knowledge but was also reflected in the whole cultural life of the period. The new philosophical systems were concerned with universal standards of conduct for the cosmopolitan individuals who were intellectual citizens of the inhabited world, the *oikumene*. Although literature and art represented the great variety of individual tastes in the new society, they also clung tenaciously to the heritage of classical tradition from the past, while science burgeoned rapidly with the extension of men's horizons. During most of the third century the general atmosphere was one of hope and of rapid growth. First we will discuss the growth of communication and trade, which was so important for the extension of Hellenistic culture, then the culture itself.

Communications and Trade

The general ease of travel, as well as the transport of goods, was considerably facilitated on both land and sea in the Hellenistic Period. The Seleucid

The reader will find Map II (page 48) and the Front Endpaper useful as he reads this chapter.

kings added to the existing road system inherited from the Persian Empire to link the new cities of their kingdom. The new settlements in the more developed regions offered accommodations; desert roads were provided with stopping places and supplies of water; main routes were patrolled and made safe for the traveler, although brigandage seems to have been common in the mountains and more unsettled areas. Travel was fast for the government messenger who used horses or camels and who could get fresh mounts at the regular posting stops. The ordinary traveler and merchant, however, proceeding at donkey and camel caravan pace at the rate of about thirty miles a day, would not be able to do much better than this in the Near East until the twentieth century. But in Egypt and Mesopotamia he could use the river boats on the Nile and the Euphrates, by which most of the traffic was carried in those countries.

Travel by sea in the eastern Mediterranean increased greatly in volume. While there were no marked technical improvements in navigation, cargo ships were built larger (a standard vessel had about 250 tons capacity) and they multiplied in number with the development of trade between Egypt, Syria, and the Aegean. The most notable improvement was made in harbor construction, which included building breakwaters to protect and deepen the anchorages. Large docks and warehouses were also constructed to accommodate the shipping.

With one notable exception the geographical horizons of the Hellenistic world remained much the same as they were for Alexander. In the latter part of the fourth century Pytheas, a Greek from Massilia in southern France, set out in search of the source of tin, jealously guarded by the Carthaginians. Pytheas slipped through the Strait of Gibraltar, past the Carthaginian colony of Gades, and then coasted along Spain and France as far as Brittany. In Brittany he evidently heard of the tin mines of Cornwall, for he crossed the English Channel, examined the Cornwall workings, and wrote an account of them in the record of his voyage. Continuing on from Cornwall Pytheas seems to have circumnavigated most of Britain and then crossed the North Sea to the coast of Europe, where he sailed northwards beyond Jutland. In these northern waters Pytheas encountered thick fog and sea ice from the Arctic which impeded his ship. It was a voyage which perhaps gives him the distinction of being the first Arctic explorer. Pytheas returned to Massilia to tell tales, which were not believed. Neither could they be checked because the Carthaginians continued to keep their tin route into the Atlantic well guarded.

The Hellenistic rulers of the East, however, were primarily interested in the exploration and development of their own territories. Both Ptolemies and Seleucids established new commercial contacts to procure the costly, exotic products of east Africa, Arabia, and India.

PTOLEMAIC TRADE

The Ptolemies, like the native Pharaohs of Egypt before them, were attracted southwards by the commerce with eastern Africa and Arabia. They wanted ivory, spices, incense, pearls, coral, and rare woods, both for their own use and for re-export to the Aegean markets. Accordingly, the early Ptolemies occupied the valley of the Nile beyond the First Cataract where the famous Temple of Philae was built and the land of Nubia was taken over. Trade was thereby promoted with the Ethiopian Kingdom of Meroë, which lay beyond Khartum in the Sudan, but the increase in trade only resulted in the excessive strengthening of Meroe. When the Ethiopians began to interfere with Egyptian outposts, Ptolemy VI advanced to the Second Cataract. Some goods were brought down the Nile valley by this route, but the main effort of the Ptolemies was made in the Red Sea. About 280 B.C. Ptolemy II Philadelphus sent Admiral Ariston to explore the west coast of the Red Sea as far as the Strait of Bab-el-Mandeb. The king also reopened the old Pharaonic Canal which ran from the apex of the Nile delta to the north end of the Gulf of Suez. Since the canal soon silted in, the trade goods had to be obtained by a combination of sea and desert transport. Forts were built along the Red Sea coast from Arsinoe (Suez) to the "Cinnamon Land" (Somaliland) and a sea patrol was established. The goods were brought to the fort Berenice on the Aelantic Gulf and then taken by desert road to Koptos on the Nile.

While these projects placed the African trade in the hands of the Ptolemies, the Arabian goods, and some which came by sea to South Arabia from India, had been carried for centuries by a caravan route along the west coast of Arabia. The road, controlled by the Nabataean Arabs, terminated in Petra, whence goods were sent on to the ports of Phoenicia. Although the early Ptolemies held Phoenicia, they tried to develop alternate routes to get a firmer grip on the whole traffic. Philadelphus first attacked the Nabataeans, then coming to an agreement with them, he concentrated his attention on securing the northern end of the route. Forts were placed in Transjordania and in the desert area of southern Palestine in order to guard the traffic en route to Phoenicia. Although the costs of this trade were high and the volume slight, the demand in the Mediterranean was great and the profits very considerable.

About 120 B.C. the Ptolemies established a direct connection to India from the Red Sea, but probably no regular traffic resulted until the time of the Roman Empire. According to legend the connection was the result of chance. A Hindu sailor, found shipwrecked on the coast of the Red Sea, was taken to Alexandria, where he was questioned and induced to guide a Greek captain, Eudoxus, by open sea to India. Eudoxus made two successful voyages, but after he quarreled with the Ptolemies about his share of the profits, he gave up his voyaging. It is not clear whether the discovery of the monsoons, which were regularly used in Roman times, is to be connected with the voyages of Eudoxus. Their "discoverer" is said to have been a certain Hippalus, and although the date of his voyage is unknown, it may perhaps be placed in the time of Augustus, rather than in the time of Eudoxus.

SELEUCID TRADE

The Seleucids, in their turn, succeeded in funneling considerable eastern trade through Antioch, and from there they could re-export through their own

Syrian ports or send goods north through Asia Minor to the Greek cities on the Aegean coast. The Seleucids contrived to get a share of the trade with South Arabia in much the same manner as the Ptolemies. A caravan route, controlled by the Gerrhaean Arabs, ran along the west shore of the Persian Gulf. The Seleucids garrisoned some of the islands in the Gulf, established a few forts along both shores and protected these positions with a flotilla. They were thus able to control the Gerrhaeans to some extent and divert goods by sea to the head of the Persian Gulf and then by river to Seleucia.

Their main connections with India were by the long caravan roads which started from Babylonia and Seleucia. One road led through Media, Iran, and Bactria; another led through the territory which Alexander had traversed on his return from India, by Susiana, Persis, Carmania, and across Gedrosia (Baluchistan). These roads seem to have been used more than the sea route, which Nearchus had explored, until the second century B.C., when land connections with the east became difficult because of the rise of Parthia. The Seleucids were thus able to offer the exotic products of India and Arabia in competition with the Ptolemies. There may have been some contact with western China, but the "Silk Routes" were not well established until the time of the Parthian and Roman Empires, when Parthia took the place of the Seleucid Kingdom as an intermediary between the Far East and the Mediterranean.

Ptolemies and Seleucids exported these exotics, along with their own products, into the markets of the Aegean and bought heavily from the Greek cities in return. We cannot estimate the volume of trade very precisely, but it was far greater than that of the Athenian Empire or of Carthage. Many factors contributed to its growth: the plentiful circulation of coinage, the general replacement of barter in western Asia by a monetary economy, the tremendous spurt in urbanization, better transport and communication, and the establishment of uniform business methods patterned on those of earlier Greek merchants. The Greek *koine* was the language used for international commerce, and Greek law and business forms regulated exchange. Trade was generally free, subject to the law of supply and demand in circumstances favorable to growth and expansion. The best example of the effect of the trade is offered by Rhodes, which became the wealthiest and most influential of Greek city-states in the third and early second centuries.

RHODES

The location of Rhodes at the focal point of traffic between the Aegean and the southeastern Mediterranean made the island a natural clearing center for trade. The Rhodians who had been experienced merchants and sailors for generations were well able to capitalize on their new opportunity. They themselves carried on a trade in wine, the wide extent of which is indicated by the wine jar handles stamped with the insignia of Rhodian magistrates, which are found throughout the Black Sea and the Mediterranean. Rhodes' particular function in the Hellenistic Period, however, was to act as a clearing house and distributing agent for general trade. For this purpose the Rhodians acted as bankers or agents, buying up goods and reshipping, offering credit and facilities for handling cargoes. Many foreign merchants and bankers, particularly from Syria, Phoenicia and Alexandria, came to live in Rhodes and carry on their business. The volume of trade, according to the Rhodians when they complained to Rome of its shrinkage, was fifty million drachmas a year, almost five times that of Athens at about 400 B.C. Rhodes collected a 2 percent tax on the goods handled in the port and from that income alone was a very wealthy city. In addition, the Rhodians drew revenues from the territory which they controlled in southwestern Asia Minor and could count on their wealthy citizens and foreign residents for liturgies and gifts.

From all these sources Rhodes was able to maintain a strong, well-trained navy, which enforced the Rhodian doctrine of freedom of the seas by clearing the trade routes of pirates. Perhaps the greatest marks of Rhodes' maritime repute were the general adoption of its sea law by other seafarers of the Mediterranean and the help given voluntarily to the city in 227 B.C., when Rhodes was severely damaged by earthquake. Gifts came from Sicily, Egypt, the Seleucids, Pontus, Pergamum, and various Greek cities of the Aegean and Black seas.

The great period of Rhodes' maritime supremacy was in the latter part of the third and in the early second century B.C. After 167 the city's trade shrank drastically. At that time Rhodes was penalized by Rome for suspected cooperation with Macedonia. Rhodian possessions in southwestern Asia Minor were taken away and trade was diminished by the establishment of a free port at Delos. The Eastern traders and Italian merchants, who were just beginning to take a direct part in Eastern commerce, moved to Delos and made that island a center for trade in grain and the transhipment of slaves, then a valuable com-

Hellenistic trade goods: (left) wine amphora; (middle) a Megarian bowl; (right) a silver pitcher

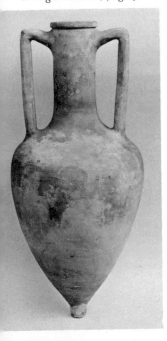
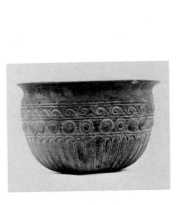
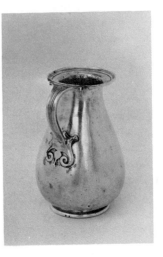

modity on the Italian market. While Rhodes profited most from the trade of
the early Hellenistic Period, all the large port cities of western Asia had their
share, from Alexandria, through Phoenicia and Syria, to the old Ionian cities in
western Asia Minor and on the approaches to the Black Sea. From the time of
Alexander's campaigns until early in the first century, when Roman wars dislocated the East, the trade brought prosperity and new vigor to the Hellenistic
cities.

Hellenistic Society and Culture

While the whole of Hellenistic society shared common tastes and cultural
values, there were differences between the older cities of the Aegean and the
new cities of the Hellenistic Kingdoms. In the older cities the characteristic citizen, whose ideas and behavior set the tone of society, was the reasonably well-
to-do man of the middle class. He might own land or workshops or be engaged
in commerce and banking. Professional men, such as doctors and architects,
however, did not belong to this group but were usually migratory and made
their living by fees. These middle-class citizens were the magistrates and
councilors of their cities who contributed money loyally to public buildings, religious festivals, and to education. They were conservative and materialistic in
outlook, engrossed in their own community and their own business and family
affairs, but they were not distinguished for their intellectual interests. Towards
the lower class of free men, who earned a living by daily wages and piecework
on the farms and in the cities, the middle class was essentially antagonistic. In
order to protect its economic position, it opposed the demands for cancellation
of debts and redistribution of land. Yet the cities did try to provide an ample
supply of grain, which was distributed free or at a low cost to the poor, and to
extend recreational and educational facilities for the benefit of all citizens. Many
cities also provided a public doctor and some measure of medical care.

The middle-class citizens lived better than their counterparts in Classical
Greece. They enjoyed more varied food, had better clothing, more personal possessions, and better houses. We have some idea of the type of home which became popular in the late third and second centuries B.C. by virtue of the well-
preserved houses of wealthy merchants on Delos. The houses were spacious, had
a large number of rooms, and were characterized by a pleasing colonnaded court
or peristyle, off of which the main living room opened. The living rooms were
decorated with wall paintings of an architectural type and had elaborate mosaic
floors. The households evidently used more slaves then than they had in the
past and lived more comfortably, with attention to family life. The attitude to
slaves was humane. We find, for example, that in some cities the slaves were
included in the distribution of food and that they were allowed to form their
own social associations. Slaves were frequently freed and, to judge from the
comedies of the period (p. 407), they might enjoy very familiar places in the
household. Women and children, too, were more prominent in society and were

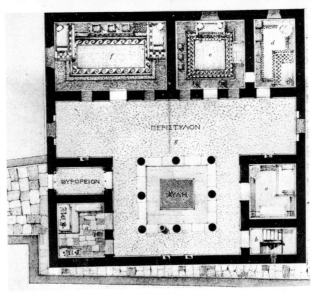

A Delian house of the peristyle type: the living rooms, with mosaic floors, open off the colonnaded court.

treated sentimentally in literature and art. Thus the tone of Hellenistic life has a more familiar, modern character than that of Classical Greece.

In the eastern kingdoms the situation was somewhat different. The historian Michael Rostovtzeff in his *Social and Economic History of the Hellenistic World* (II, 1107) has characterized the society of the kingdoms in these words: "Externally the Hellenistic world was a unit, internally it was split into two unequal parts, one Greek, the other native, one centered in the cities and city-like settlements, the other spread over the country, in its villages, hamlets, and temples."

The Greeks, with whom we should include the Macedonians, formed a privileged class which was able to maintain its Hellenic way of life in the cities and, to a considerable degree also, in the less developed military and rural colonies of the Seleucid Kingdom. The life of the Greeks was modeled on that of the older cities from which they had come and with which they kept up connections. The educational system was public and centered on the gymnasium, in which classes were held for children and which served as a social club for adults. The gymnasiums were supported at public expense and by regular gifts from the wealthier citizens and kings. The familiar political institutions of the city-state were also retained: magistrates, councils, and assemblies, through which the citizens administered their local affairs. Greek law was used and a general uniformity of practice established that was based on the Athenian code and on the royal decrees issued from time to time. The public religious worship and the physical appearance of the cities were Greek although they were usually divided into separate residential quarters for Europeans and for natives. Royal money built and helped to maintain these cities, and their citizens were subjects of the king as fully as the rural natives, but the cities were a transplantation of Greek life to the Near East.

Within Greek society there was a hierarchy, most apparent in the capitals, in which an upper class was formed by the high officials of the administration,

Antiochus IV
Epiphanes

The city of
Antioch on
the Orontes River
personified as
Tyche *(Fortune)*

the generals of the army, and the specialists needed for the tasks of government and finance. Below this there was the middle class of merchants and professional men, for architects and doctors ranked higher in the new cities than they did in the Aegean. The middle class, however, was just as civic-minded and loyal to the communities as its Aegean counterpart. The lower class of Greeks was made up of ordinary soldiers and settlers who might rise to the middle group by taking advantage of economic opportunity because in the new countries the chances of economic betterment were greater. All these Greeks were marked off by privilege and way of life from the mass of the natives who lived in the countryside.

Upper-class natives were attracted generally to urban Greek life by the material and social advantages which it offered, but Hellenization was a condition for their association with Greek society. Native merchants, Syrians and Phoenicians in particular, tended to Hellenize rapidly, because of their desire to do business in the Greek cities and to join in the trade to the Aegean. Despite all this, there was a counterpull, by the sheer mass of native population, towards orientalization, and lower-class Greeks were affected by the ideas and practices of their native wives and associates. Nevertheless, the founding of cities and the reluctance of the kings to alter the old economic systems kept the Greek privileges largely intact. The Romans at first shattered the political order of the Hellenistic states, but ended by supporting urban life and Hellenization. The pattern of Greek city life thus became characteristic of western Asia Minor under the Seleucid regime and in the Roman Empire.

RELIGION AND PHILOSOPHY

In the cities of the Aegean area the traditional worship and festivals of the great Olympian gods and of the civic cults were carried on with as much intensity as they had before, but there was also a rapid growth of private associations of individuals for religious and social purposes. Fewer temples were built, because most deities were already well provided for, but the great international sanctuaries at Olympia and Delphi were enlarged with new buildings. A minor mystery cult in the island of Samothrace was favored by the patronage of the kings of Macedonia and the nearby city-states in northwestern Asia Minor. In fact those worships, like the mysteries and the healing cult of Asclepius, which catered specifically to the individual, were very popular. This feeling of individual need presumably accounts for the formation of private associations. Their members were usually men of the same trade, who selected a patron deity, met frequently, and in most cases looked after the welfare of their individual members in adversity. The associations provided the warm intimacy of a small group, in contrast to the formal worships of the great gods and of the city deities. The ordinary man did not deny the latter but merely added the worship of his private god to them. The social aspects of religion were much the same as in the fourth century: the unsophisticated people in both country and city were sincere in their worship, the intelligentsia turned to philosophy, and the more unreflective sophisticates devoted themselves to chance, superstition, or some of the new Eastern cults which began to spread to the Greek cities.

The Greeks who came as soldiers and settlers into the Hellenistic Kingdoms brought their Greek gods with them, built temples, established worships, and elected boards of priests as they had done in their former city-states. In this sense there was a very considerable extension of Greek religion in the Hellenistic Period. Yet, because the new worships were delocalized from their original settings, they were weaker, and those aspects of divinity which represented natural and universal forces tended to predominate. As a consequence it was easy for the Greeks to see resemblances in their own gods to native deities, to make identifications, and to conceive new hybrid deities in whose worship Greeks and Hellenized natives both could join. This was true of the gods associated with the astrological pseudo-science of Babylonia and with the magic of Egypt. These gods began to enjoy a great vogue in the eastern Mediterranean, but the oriental cults which appealed most to the Greeks at this time were the Egyptian worships of Serapis and Isis.

The Egyptian god Serapis was worshipped in Memphis especially but in his native form would seem to have little appeal for the Greeks. Serapis was the bull calf Apis who upon his death had merged with the god of the afterlife, Osiris. Ptolemy I transplanted and remodeled the cult in Alexandria with the intention of attracting the worship of both Greeks and natives. A temple was built and a cult statue representing Serapis in the form of the Greek Pluto, the most obvious counterpart of Osiris, was set up, but the Egyptians soon returned to their native conception of Serapis. On the other hand the Greeks became enthusiastic, but conceived of Serapis under the aspects of a healing god and a patron of sailors. From Alexandria his worship was carried by seamen and traders to the ports of the Aegean where it became well established. Private missionary work of the same nature also disseminated the worship of Isis, the old Egyptian fertility goddess and wife of Osiris. Her worship had an appeal similar to that of the Greek mystery cults, for it involved a ritual of initiation and purification, by which the initiate entered a better life on earth and attained a promise of future happiness. When Italian traders entered the commerce of the eastern Mediterranean, the cult became popular with them and was taken back to Italy.

In the long run the most important result of the Greek contact with oriental religions was the ordinary man's familiarity with the idea of a god who might be worshipped by all and who was generally benevolent to mankind. While a similar idea was developed on a different level by the new Greek philosophy of Stoicism, which had its own concepts of universal law and justice, Greek philosophy showed little interest in the thought of oriental religions. The more thoughtful Greeks, from pride of race and of their own intellectual tradition, followed one or another of the new Greek philosophical schools rather than any of the religions of the East. The Hebrew testament was translated into Hellenistic Greek, in the version of the Septuagint, so-called from the seventy scholars who were supposed to have worked on it, but the translation was for the use of Hellenized Jews since the Greeks did not read it.

Athens remained the center of philosophical study throughout the Hellenistic Period, with the older schools established by Aristotle and Plato still influential and popular. The work in each school tended toward a narrower specialization than their founders had envisaged. The Peripatetics of the Lyceum, after a brief foray into natural science, concentrated on historiography, while the Academy became concerned, in a destructive, critical manner with logic and the theory of knowledge. Its important leaders, Arcesilaus and Carneades, were adept in pointing out the flaws in the new philosophical systems which were developed. The new philosophies were primarily concerned in providing standards of conduct and a rationale of life for the cosmopolitan society of the period. The old, simple rules of behavior, based on traditional Greek education and the social customs of the city-state, were even more unsatisfactory in the Hellenistic Age than in the fourth century. Individual men wanted answers from philosophy, and philosophers were very ready to supply them in the form of tracts, lectures, street-corner harangues, treatises, and whole new systems of thought, such as Epicureanism and Stoicism.

There were, of course, the negative answers, already given, of Scepticism and Cynicism. The Sceptics thought that nothing was known or could be known and armed the individual with indifference—nothing really mattered. In ordinary life, however, there had to be some rule of conduct, so the Sceptics contradicted themselves by advocating a morality based on empiricism, that is, the ordinary conventions of society. The Cynics continued to advocate that all convention be discarded and that man return to nature. They practiced what they preached and found considerable ammunition for diatribes against the comforts of luxury and the pursuit of wealth in the materialistic life of the cities. These attacks, and the doctrine of a return to the simple life, were preached on the street corners by wandering Cynics, who lived as they could, often in rags and eating little more than bread. While this teaching did suggest a course of conduct for the individual, it offered no real help in grappling with the problems of social life in the highly urbanized communities of the Hellenistic states. Cynicism remained a useful irritant, but not a popular solution, for the universal practice of Cynicism would have dissolved society.

Epicureanism was formulated by Epicurus (*ca.* 341–270 B.C.) as a thorough-going system of philosophy with its main emphasis on conduct and its basis in natural science. The latter was experiencing a rapid development in his day but Epicurus turned back to the old theories of Leucippus and Democritus of the fifth century B.C. to explain the world as a fortuitous concourse of atoms and to develop a mechanistic explanation of the universe. The existence of the gods was not denied, but divine action and concern in human affairs were rejected. Man stood alone and had the freedom of will to pursue whatever aim in life he considered most important. To Epicurus that was pleasure, but pleasures should be selected according to their relative quality by the exercise of reason, with the sensual pleasures of the body and of appetite subjected to those of the mind. Thus the Epicurean was not a slave to the material pleasures of a luxurious life but a man of refined tastes, who took his enjoyment thoughtfully in art or literature or some other private pursuit. Ideally he was a man of means who could live without engaging in business or public life. While Epicureanism did not deny the obligations of an individual to society, like Cynicism, its teaching tended to encourage withdrawal.

Stoicism did face, rather grimly, the problems of duty and responsibility in public life and appealed to the pride and dignity of man in adversity. The founder of Stoicism was Zeno (*ca.* 330–260 B.C.), from the city of Citium in Cyprus, part Greek and part Phoenician, who went to Athens in 311 B.C. and talked mainly in the *Stoa Poikile* (the Painted *Stoa*) from which the name *Stoa* was applied to his philosophy. He and his successor, Cleanthes (*ca.* 305–230 B.C.), taught orally, and the principles of Stoicism were written down and publicized more widely by Chrysippus (*ca.* 280–07 B.C.). The early Stoics were concerned mainly with morality and laid down rules of conduct, by which man should live according to nature and triumph over the trials of life. They believed in the brotherhood of man and advocated an ascetic life. To the Stoics "nature" was governed by a universal principle of justice or, in theological terms, by a god immanent in matter and guiding the universe. Of all the Greek philosophical systems, Stoicism was to have special appeal for the Romans, who found its rigorous insistence on duty in public life congenial to their own traditions.

The new, monarchical forms of government were justified by philosophical arguments, which were developed mainly by the Stoics. While the older Greek city-states remained staunchly republican and opposed to the rule of any Hellenistic king, the Greek population of the new cities had to come to terms with kingship. As we have seen, the kings used the device of ruler cult, which was associated with the Greek attitude of hero worship, to win the loyalty of their Greek subjects. The philosophers argued that the best form of government was kingship and delineated the ideal king as the "best" man, who ruled in the interest of his subjects. In theory the king was the state, and the law of the realm expressed his will. The kings naturally subscribed to these conceptions of their position and stressed their care for the people of their kingdoms by titles such as Savior and Benefactor. In the monarchical states a new definition of freedom of the subject had to be found because the term could no longer be applied to political action, except in a local and limited autonomy. Accordingly, freedom tended to be thought of as a possession of the individual, expressed in his personal conduct rather than in public action. Philosophy thus accommodated itself to the altered social conditions of the period.

SCIENCE

At the outset of the Hellenistic Period Greek science had been given a new method: it was the systematic observation applied both by Aristotle to the classification of animals, and by his successor, Theophrastus, to the classification of plants. Alexander's enthusiasm for science, which prompted him to take along a group of scientists on his campaigns, was shared by the Ptolemies, who established the Museum in Alexandria and made that city the chief center for scientific work in the third century B.C. The Museum was an institute for research. Dedicated to the Muses, it housed about one hundred scholars, who lived and worked together in its buildings and took their ease in its gardens, all at the expense of the Ptolemies. Science was also stimulated by the opening up of new lands to the Greeks. They learned something of practical methods from the Egyptians and a very great amount from the astronomical data collected by the Babylonian priests. As a consequence Hellenistic scientists made tremendous advances in some fields, particularly geography, mathematics, astronomy and medicine. Their work brought them almost to the point where modern science began. In fact the work of Hellenistic scientists formed the body of knowledge which supplied information to society throughout the remainder of antiquity.

Mathematics, of course, was basic to work in geography and astronomy, and in geometry, in particular, great advances were made. Euclid worked in Alexandria in the early third century and wrote his famous book, the *Elements,* on plane and solid geometry, which remained a standard text until a few generations ago. The book was a model of clear, compact organization in the demonstration of his theorems. Archimedes (*ca.* 287–212 B.C.) of Syracuse, also a genius of practical mechanics, advanced solid geometry and plane curves by measuring the sphere, the cone and the cylinder, and arrived very close to the measurement of *pi.* The most useful of Archimedes' mechanical devices was his screw for raising water, which was put to use in irrigation projects and in pumping water from mines. During the siege of Syracuse by the Romans, in which he was killed, Archimedes delayed the capture of the city by devising several ingenious war machines.

The Hellenistic work in geometry marked the limit of pure mathematics for the Greeks, for they did not devise an algebraic notation. Geometry and careful observation, however, were applied to astronomy with striking results. Aristarchus of Samos (*ca.* 310–230 B.C.) concluded that the sun was the center of the planetary system, a discovery which shocked his contemporaries, who were geocentric in their views, and drew a charge of impiety from Cleanthes, the Stoic philosopher. A lively debate was carried on, but since Aristarchus' conclusion could not be proved by Hellenistic methods, the geocentric theory became firmly re-established. Its chief proponent in the second century B.C. was Hipparchus of Nicaea, who did, however, measure the length of the solar year and of the lunar month very accurately. Hipparchus based his work to some degree on the records of Babylonian astronomy. In the second century after Christ Hellenistic work in astronomy was synthesized by Claudius Ptolemaeus (Ptolemy) of Alexandria, whose book, known as the *Almagest,* was used by Arab scholars. It was translated into Latin in A.D. 1496 and became the starting point for modern astronomy, even though Copernicus completely rejected some of its conclusions.

The great name in mathematical geography is that of Eratosthenes (*ca.* 275–195 B.C.), who measured the circumference of the earth as 24,662 miles, a figure which is in error only by about two hundred miles, according to modern calculation. His method was to place sundials at Syene and Alexandria to determine the positions of the sun and then compute the distance by the angle which he thus obtained. Eratosthenes also drew a map of the inhabited world with a grid of latitudes, calculated by comparing the known points of latitude and of longitudes by surface mensuration. He concluded from the ebb and flow of tides in the Atlantic and Indian oceans (the tides of the Indian Ocean had been reported by Nearchus, Alexander's admiral) that the seas were one and that the inhabited world of Asia, Africa, and Europe was a huge island. Eratosthenes' book of descriptive geography, based on his own mathematics and the reports of travelers, was the first scientific geography of the world. Further work in descriptive geography was done by Posidonius in the later Hellenistic Period, who was able to visit the Atlantic coast of Spain, made accessible by Roman conquest, and by Strabo, whose book describing the Roman Empire in the time of Augustus is our chief source of geographical information for that period. Ptolemy made a synthesis of both geography and astronomy, which became a standard work for centuries.

The science of medicine continued to be associated with the great sanctuary of Asclepius on the island of Cos, where Hippocrates had established a sound tradition of training and had written on medicine in the fifth century B.C. Alexandria, however, became an important center for anatomy since vivisection was carried on there; thus the resulting knowledge advanced surgery to a relatively sure procedure in the more simple types of operation. The most potent anaesthetic was opium. Several important discoveries were made by Herophilus of Chalcedon, who traced the nervous system from the brain and discovered the value of pulsation in diagnosis. The social aspects of medicine, already well established in Classical Greece, were extended in the Hellenistic Period. Most cities maintained a public physician, as well as several private practitioners, and some kind of state medical care seems to have existed in Ptolemaic Egypt, although we know little of its working. Specialization, of course, developed in such favorable circumstances because we know of specialists being brought from Cos to other cities in cases of epidemic. The royal courts, too, had their own special physicians who quite naturally were doctors of the highest reputation and who were maintained in the palaces. In building cities such matters as siting to take advantage of the sun and wind, drainage, and shelter were considered. Along with valid medical practice there existed a considerable amount of quackery and magic, which used both housewives' remedies and a varied and frequently useless (if not harmful) pharmacopeia.

Little progress was made, however, in some fields where we might have expected it. The scientific work of Aristotle and Theophrastus in zoology and botany was not advanced although considerable attention was given to the introduction of new animals and plants in the eastern kingdoms. Unfortunately Ptolemaic interest in zoology seems to have been limited to the acquisition of rare specimens for the Alexandrian zoo and for display in festivals. There was little geology, except for rudimentary prospecting, and chemistry was mainly used in the extensive pharmacopeia of medicine and magic alike.

The great scientific advances which were made in the course of the third

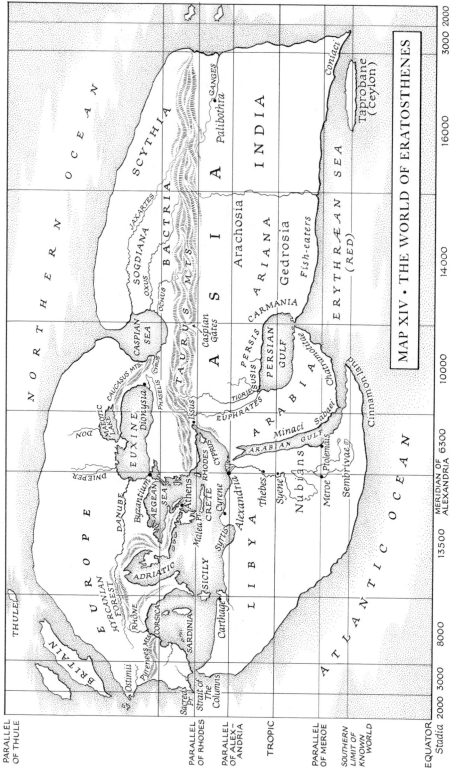

MAP XIV · THE WORLD OF ERATOSTHENES

century, when the energy of the Hellenistic Period was at its height, were not developed in theory, nor were their principles extensively applied in practice. Several explanations are advanced to account for this halt at a critical point: there was little incentive to make significant applications of scientific discoveries in an age when labor, both free and slave, was cheap; the new method of systematic observation could not go very far without the development of scientific apparatus, which was not made; the Roman conquest brought a temporary shock and dislocation to the Hellenistic world and resulted in apathy or an eager attention to the new patron, Rome.

LITERATURE

Hellenistic writing was tremendous in quantity, for it reflected all the varied interests of a society which was engaged in building new cities and kingdoms and at the same time was striving to preserve its older Greek tradition. There was much technical writing on science, warfare, government, and geography. Biography and history were also popular in an era of colorful personalities and rapid change. But it is striking that the Greeks themselves showed little interest in the history and in the thought of the unknown peoples with whom they came in contact; it is also striking that those peoples took little interest in Greek literature and philosophy. The chief exception was the Jewish community in Alexandria. Jewish scholars began to read and to compare Greek philosophy with their own thought, and a school of Greco-Jewish learning came into existence, the chief representative of which was Philo in the first century after Christ. Apart from this, however, there was little real blending or even mutual interest. Greek science learned much from Babylonia, but Greek philosophers ignored Hebraic and Indian thought. India was very remote, but the Seleucid envoy to the court of Chandragupta, a man called Megasthenes, wrote an account of the court and of Hinduism. His book seems to have been superficial but was reasonably accurate and might have served as a start. Histories of Egypt and Babylonia were written in Greek, but by an Egyptian named Manetho and by a Babylonian named Berossus, both books probably at the request of their respective kings, Ptolemy I and Antiochus I. This strange lack of interest on the part of the Greeks was apparently a facet of their pride of race and of the very deliberate attempt to preserve their own traditions. Hellenized natives, for their part, evidently felt that it was sufficient to learn the Greek *koine* as a practical tool and to imitate the manners of contemporary Greek society, but that it was unnecessary to study its traditions.

The overwhelming interest of the Greeks in their own traditions did result in much constructive scholarship. The foundations of literary history and of criticism were established, yet imaginative writing, particularly poetry, was academic and imitative. Scholarly and literary activity was concentrated largely in the new capital cities where the writers could enjoy the patronage of the kings and find a community of other scholars. Alexandria was the chief center, but the Seleucids invited some writers to Antioch, and the Attalids tried to establish a lesser Alexandria in Pergamum. The Library in Alexandria, off to an early start with funds liberally supplied by Ptolemy II Philadelphus ultimately became the largest institution of its type in the ancient world, with a collection of well over a half million manuscript rolls. Among them were the treasures of Greek literature: texts of Homer, the lyric poets, the tragedians, historians, and orators. The manuscripts were copied, edited, commented on for their language, grammar, subject matter, and metrics, and biographies were written of their authors. One product of this work, which is familiar to modern readers of these authors, is the division of works into "books," as in Homer and Herodotus. The kings of Pergamum also built up a substantial library, and private individuals everywhere formed collections. The distribution of books, both new and "classic," was much wider than it had been previously, and special establishments for publishing, that is, copying by hand, were set up in the big cities.

Hellenistic poetry was very closely associated with Alexandria, from which the term, Alexandrianism, is borrowed. The poetry was highly polished and erudite, smacking of the study rather than the garret. The most famous Hellenistic poet, however, Theocritus (*ca.* 315-250 B.C.), avoided extensive artificiality. Theocritus was born in Sicily, went to Alexandria to live for a time and then moved to the island of Cos. His idylls established the literary form of pastoral poetry, in which rustic shepherds sing of their loves and enjoy their wine on the warm hillsides but neglect their flocks. This rustic, but artful, simplicity had a great appeal, of course, to the oversophisticated, urban society of the Hellenistic Age. Theocritus found a vivacious theme in city life also in his fifteenth idyll which depicts two chattering women of Alexandria on their way to a festival of Adonis.

Theocritus' contemporary poets in Alexandria were more "Alexandrian." The erudition of Callimachus is understandable, for he was a librarian and scholar, as well as a poet. He wrote hymns for the Ptolemaic festivals, *epyllions,* or little epics, which concentrated on a single episode in a legend, and epigrams. In defense of his penchant for short poems, Callimachus coined the useful epigram, "A great book is a great evil," and carried on a fierce verbal polemic with Apollonius of Rhodes, who preferred the long epic poem. Apollonius' best-known work is the *Argonautica,* the story of Jason's quest for the Golden Fleece. It is perhaps a better argument for Callimachus' point of view than for his own, because the poem is best in treatment of single episodes and in describing the romantic love of Jason and Medea, but weak in composition. Callimachus' preference for the short poem prevailed since the most appealing Hellenistic poetry, after the third century, consists of epigrams collected in the *Greek Anthology*. Hellenistic poetry had a very considerable influence on Latin writers of the Late Republic and Augustan periods, on Catullus, Ovid, Propertius, and Vergil.

Drama was extremely popular as entertainment in the cities of the Hellenistic Period, but in tragedy much of the repertoire was the classic theater of the fifth century, Euripides above all, or plays written in imitating him. Comedy, however, was given a new form by the Athenian Menander (*ca.* 342–291 B.C.), the principal writer of the New Comedy. His was a social comedy of manners, which depicted the typical middle-class life of the Greek cities. The characters were stock types, a gruff father who did not understand his children, a young playboy hero, an unfortunate heroine, and sly, insolent slaves. The plots were stereotyped, usually dealing with the trials of a foundling of good birth, who was ultimately recognized, restored to a rightful position, and properly married off. Menander's characterization and large stock of devices for complicating the plot gave the plays considerable variety. Until 1957 his work was known only by fragments and by the adaptation of his plays for the Roman stage by Plautus and Terence, but in that year a virtually complete play, *The Dysculus* (*Difficult Man*), written on papyrus, was found. The mime, an indecent farce with scenes of lower-class urban life, became a popular form of entertainment, but our best examples of the type, by Herondas of Cos, are Alexandrian in nature. Their scene and characters are drawn from contemporary life; however, Herondas wrote in the archaic and difficult Ionic dialect used by Hipponax of Ephesus for similar material in the sixth century B.C.

The historiography of the Hellenistic Period was voluminous and dealt thoroughly with contemporary events, but unfortunately much of it has been lost entirely or survives piecemeal by being incorporated in the books of later writers. For example, Ptolemy I wrote an account of Alexander's campaigns, but we know it through adaptation of the material by Arrian, a writer of the second century after Christ, who wrote the *Anabasis of Alexander*. Arrian was a competent Roman administrator in the Near East who made good use of Ptolemy's book. His *Anabasis* is our chief source for Alexander's career. Many biographies and accounts of Alexander were written, some laudatory and some using hostile gossip, for Alexander was not liked by the Peripatetic school of historiography, which he had offended by putting Aristotle's nephew, Callisthenes, to death. A considerable amount of this type of material appears in Plutarch's biography of Alexander. Many biographies of other famous men were produced during the period, which were used by Plutarch for his Greek *Lives of Famous Men,* but Plutarch's shaping of the material reflects his own interest and the interest of his time, the second century after Christ (pp. 659–60). Chronology, too, was studied with useful results. Eratosthenes, the geographer, made a calendar of famous events from the Trojan War, while Apollodorus of Athens wrote a chronology of history in verse.

Continuous historical accounts of the events from Alexander's death were written by a series of able, contemporary historians of whose works we have only a fragmentary selection. Thus much of the work of Hieronymus of Cardia who described the Wars of the Successors was excerpted almost verbatim by Diodorus in the late first century B.C. in the latter's universal history. Phylarchus wrote of the period which modern historians call the Balance of Power, 275–220 B.C., but he is known chiefly from the account of the revolution in

Sparta, which Plutarch used for his *Lives of Agis and Cleomenes*. The great wars of the Roman conquest, from 221 to 146 B.C., were described by Polybius (201–120 B.C.), whose history stands comparison with the works of Herodotus and Thucydides. Polybius' *History* consisted originally of forty books of which we have the first five entire and fragments from the remainder. The Roman historian Livy, however, made extensive use of Polybius, of whose work excerpts may be read in Livy's *History of Rome* (p. 586).

Polybius was a citizen of the Achaean League, in whose affairs both he and his father were prominent. In 167 B.C. he was taken as a hostage to Rome, where he became a house guest of the great Scipio family, was entertained as befitted a man of his education and standing, and was introduced to the political figures and life of Rome. He thoroughly realized the historical implications of Rome's conquest of the Mediterranean, by which its western and eastern parts were brought together under Roman rule, and he was concerned to explain the causes of Roman success and the character and purpose of the Roman people to the Greeks of his age. For his account of the wars and diplomacy of the conquest Polybius drew upon his considerable knowledge of the countries over which the wars were fought, and of the peoples and personages engaged in them. He conceived of historiography in the didactic tradition of Thucydides as a course of instruction for statesmen. While his history showed a perceptible bias in favor of the Achaean League, and some misunderstanding of the working and character of Roman political institutions, it is of first-rate importance for understanding the history of the period in which Rome and the Hellenistic East began to mesh.

ART

The establishment of the Hellenistic Kingdoms opened a new world of opportunity to Greek architects, builders, and artists. The social policies of the kings required the construction of scores of new cities and the improvement of old ones. The kings and the wealthy men of the period were patrons of art who collected old masterpieces, when they could get them, and commissioned new works for their cities or for their private pleasure. Generally speaking, the Greek art of the Hellenistic world, like its literature, remained firmly in the Greek tradition and borrowed relatively little, at least in the earlier stages, from Egypt and Persia. There was more floridity, even a baroque grandeur, in the more important buildings and the great cities which may have been due to Eastern influence or, perhaps, merely expressed the desire of the kings and patrons to impress. But for the most part the new cities tended to be uniform in design and their buildings stereotyped. Hippodamian planning (p. 328) offered a very satisfactory layout and allowed rapid building and provision for future needs, so that, with due regard to local topography, the checkerboard plans were used ubiquitously. The sculptors responded to the varied tastes of the new age by equally varied work. Some imitated and adapted the types of the Classical Period, while others developed the trends noticed in the art of the

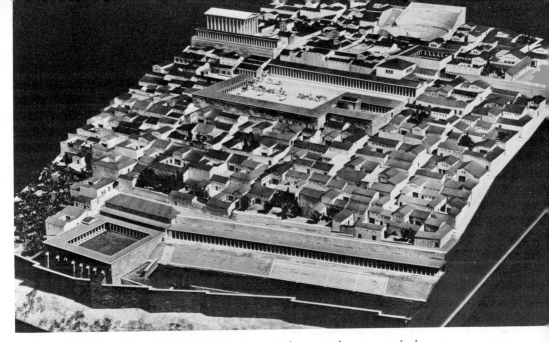

Priene: in the foreground, the gymnasium and stadium; in the center, the agora, *and, above, the Temple of Athena.*

fourth century: emotion, sentimentality, sensuous beauty, and realism. In an age of individualism when portraiture was important, kings ran the whole gamut of representation from being depicted as heroic conquerors to looking like battered old men. Hellenistic sculpture was technically adept. Much of its appeal lies in the variety of expression, which is in contrast to the limited repertoire of Classical Greek art.

The best example of a small Hellenistic city is given by the well-preserved remains of Priene in western Asia Minor, near the delta of the Maeander River. About 350 B.C. the people of Priene moved from their original city, since its harbor had silted up, to a new location farther inland where their economy was based entirely on agriculture. Alexander contributed some money for construction, and further building was done in the third and second centuries B.C., all of which the original gridiron plan accommodated efficiently. Although Priene was a small city of only a few thousand population, the citizens felt that their town should possess all the physical facilities proper to a great city and built them solidly and well. The site chosen was high up on the ridge along the north side of the Maeander River plain, to catch the sun with a southern exposure and with the wind blowing in from the sea to the west. The fortification wall was skillfully engineered and strongly built to resist the siege machinery of the Hellenistic Period, and a good supply of water was piped down from a source in the ridge to a reservoir, from which it was distributed in public fountains.

The streets of the town formed the usual checkerboard, in which the main avenues ran across the slope. Blocks of appropriate size were planned for the

409

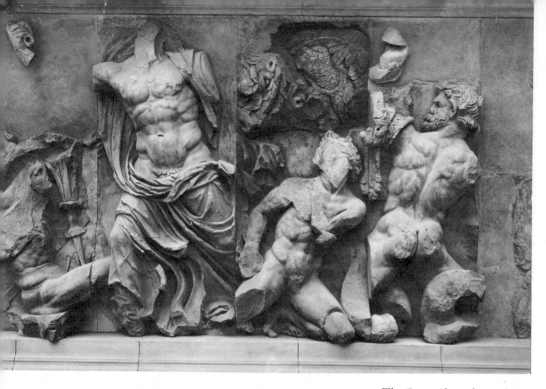

The Great Altar of Zeus from Pergamum. Scene from the battle of gods and giants

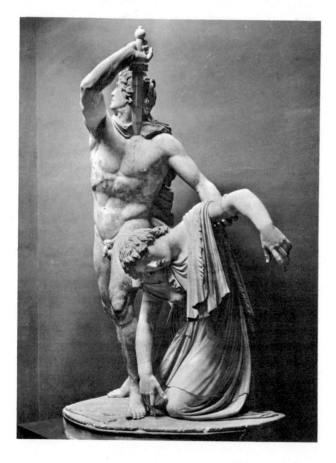

A Galatian killing himself and his wife. Roman copy from the group commemorating the victory of Attalus I over the Galatians, ca. 240 B.C.

houses, set four to a block, and multiple block units accommodated the public buildings. The north side of the *agora* bordered the main avenue. Along it were constructed the main civic buildings, while the other three sides were enclosed with colonnades for business and lounging. In this manner the whole business and political life of the city was concentrated in a regularly planned area, which was easily accessible by means of the principal street. The temple of the city goddess, Athena, and the theater were set higher up the slope, where they dominated the city and were remote from the bustle of the *agora*. The Temple of Athena, despite the small size of Priene, was built by one of the leading architects of Greek Asia Minor and was regarded as a classic model in ancient handbooks of architecture. On the lower side of the town the gymnasium and stadium formed a single complex, well situated apart from the business area.

The sculptors of the Hellenistic Period tended to be mobile, moving from city to city to seek commissions or to work on some special project. While this practice made for considerable homogeneity of style, there were distinctive schools of art at Rhodes and Pergamum, where there was continuous opportunity for work. The kings of Pergamum, who were anxious to publicize their city as a champion of Hellenism, found a fruitful subject in their victories over the Gauls. About 240 B.C., to celebrate the first great triumph, a series of works was commissioned which we know through Roman copies. They were distinctive in style and subject and achieved considerable popularity. The best known are the Dying Gaul, in which a Gallic warrior is represented, slowly sinking in death, and the group of a Gaul and his wife. He has killed her and is about to commit suicide rather than surrender to the Pergamenes. The artist has suggested the Pergamene victory only by implication, for his purpose was to universalize the suffering and pathos in defeat of the Gallic warriors. Victory over the Gauls was also the occasion for the *tour de force* of Hellenistic sculpture, the frieze of the Great Altar of Zeus built on the Pergamene *acropolis* by Eumenes II in the early second century B.C. The theme was traditional—the victory of the gods over the giants—but the style and feeling were thoroughly Hellenistic. The writhing bodies of gods and giants locked in violent combat evoked the chaos out of which the gods won victory for civilization.

Another circle of sculptors worked in Rhodes, where they could find patronage in the city or from the various foreigners who visited the port. Among their best-known works is a representation of the *Tyche* (*Fortune*) of Antioch, in which the city is personified as a goddess wearing a turreted crown to symbolize the battlements of the city, and with a youthful river-god below her throne to personify the Orontes River which flowed past Antioch. The famous Winged Victory of Samothrace in the Louvre was also the work of Rhodian sculptors. The goddess is represented settling down on the prow of a warship to commemorate a Rhodian victory over Antiochus III in 190 B.C. An example of later Rhodian work (*ca.* 25 B.C.) is the famous group of Laocoön and his sons struggling in the coils of snakes which rise out of the ground

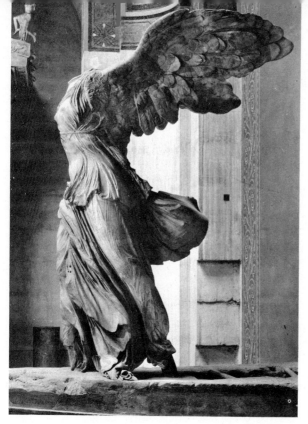

The Nike (Victory) of Samothrace.
The sculpture commemorated a Rhodian
victory over Antiochus III, ca. *190 B.C.*

at the moment of sacrifice. Its violence, pathos and strong contrasts, which stir emotion, recall the work of Pergamene artists and indicate how the currents of Hellenistic art were blended together.

The genre work of the Hellenistic Period strikes a fresh and surprising note after the idealization familiar from Classical Greek art. The subjects were bizarre figures drawn from the daily life of the cities, represented in grimly realistic or sentimental fashion: an old, drunken woman, a fisherman and a professional boxer, or there are charming groups, like the boy and the goose and the engaging boy jockey. Sculptors, like poets, found a theme in the nymphs and fauns who frequented the groves and springs of the countryside.

The patronage of the kings demanded a considerable amount of portraiture, both for statues and for the splendid series of coins, issued by the rulers. Usually the royal portrait was idealized by representing the king as a strong, youthful heroic figure, for which Alexander had set the fashion, but some portraits are strongly realistic, like the portrait heads of the Bactrian kings. In general, Hellenistic sculpture, to a much greater degree than the work of the Classical Period, represented the extremes of taste and variety of the age. The Greek artists had descended from the level of the gods to that of men and lost little in the process. Hellenistic painting is almost unknown by original works, but, to judge from the copies made for Roman patrons, it exhibited the same virtuosity and treatment of subject matter as did the sculpture.

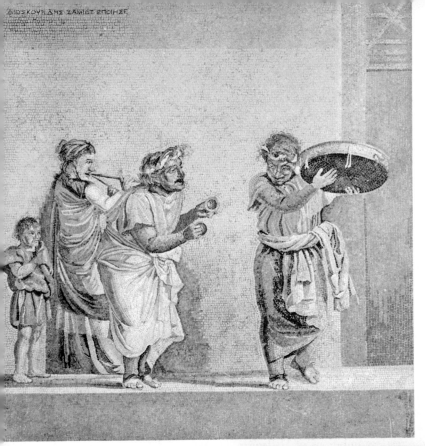

Street musicians. A mosaic from
Pompeii, after a Hellenistic painting
by Dioskourides of Samos

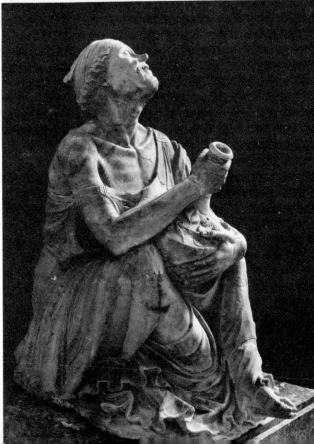

A drunken old woman. Roman copy
of a Hellenistic bronze of the second
century B.C. Such genre scenes
were popular in that period.

Rome and the Hellenistic States

In the third century B.C. the courses of Greek and Roman history came together when Rome and the Hellenistic Kingdoms entered into direct political contact. Rome had already been affected by cultural and commercial contacts, mainly indirect, with the Greek colonies of Magna Graecia (pp. 185–87), but in the 270's the Romans were drawn into war with King Pyrrhus of Epirus and in the last quarter of the century were fighting in western Greece. Neither Rome nor the Hellenistic kings knew very much about each other. Rome had rapidly established her domination over most of Italy in the latter part of the fourth century and combined its peoples into a confederation. The strength of the ties which held that organization together and the stubborn Roman tenacity of purpose were alike unknown to the Hellenistic kings. Rome, for its part, had been wholly engrossed in Italy and left foreign commerce to the Etruscans, Italian Greeks, and Carthaginians. Rome's first direct contact with Hellenistic Greece came through the interference of Pyrrhus in southern Italy at the invitation of Tarentum to help that city against Rome. Pyrrhus, ambitious to extend his rule to Italy, responded by appearing with an army of twenty thousand men. Despite his famous "Pyrrhic" (excessively costly) victories at the outset, the Romans drove Pyrrhus from Italy in 275 B.C. He sailed back to Epirus to try his fortunes again in Greece, but did leave Rome with a healthy respect for the fighting qualities of Hellenistic armies and a profound distrust of the restless ambitions of Hellenistic kings.

This check to the ambition of a second-rate Greek power caused no particular reaction in the great Hellenistic rulers, except perhaps in the astute mind of Ptolemy II Philadelphus. In 273 B.C. Ptolemy sent an embassy to Rome to establish friendly relations between the two powers. Ptolemy's motives are unknown, but it is reasonably suggested that, since he had commercial relations with Syracuse and Carthage, he presumably hoped to extend his western trade. Through these contacts he would have been aware of Rome's growing power in Italy. Friendly relations with Rome would have seemed desirable, even if no immediate trade resulted, and in the long run Egypt did indeed benefit considerably from Ptolemy's overture.

In 230 B.C. Rome itself intervened directly in the affairs of Greece in response to an appeal from the Greeks of South Italy to protect their shipping from Illyrian pirates. Fifteen years later, when Rome was fighting for survival against Hannibal of Carthage, Philip V of Macedonia joined Hannibal. The political history of the eastern and western Mediterranean had merged for the rest of antiquity, and it is time to turn back to trace the growth of Rome to this point, when it entered the Hellenistic world as a new, major power.

I V

Rome

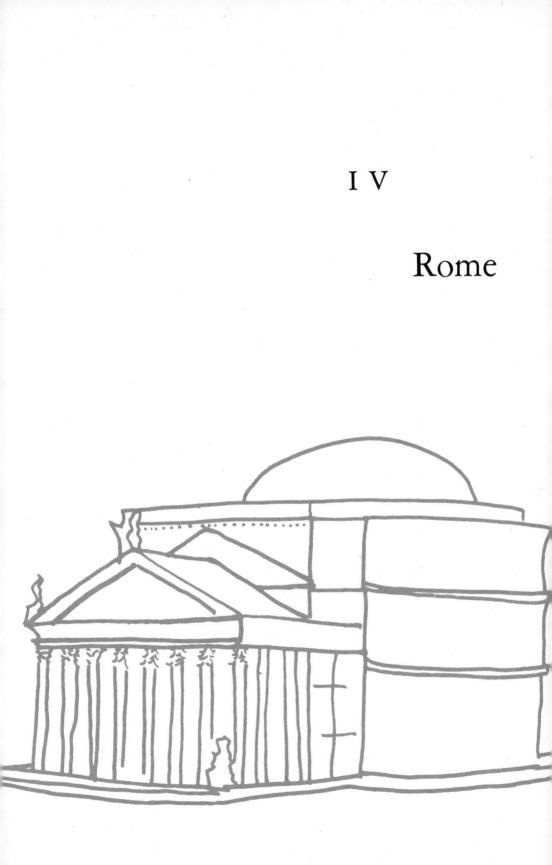

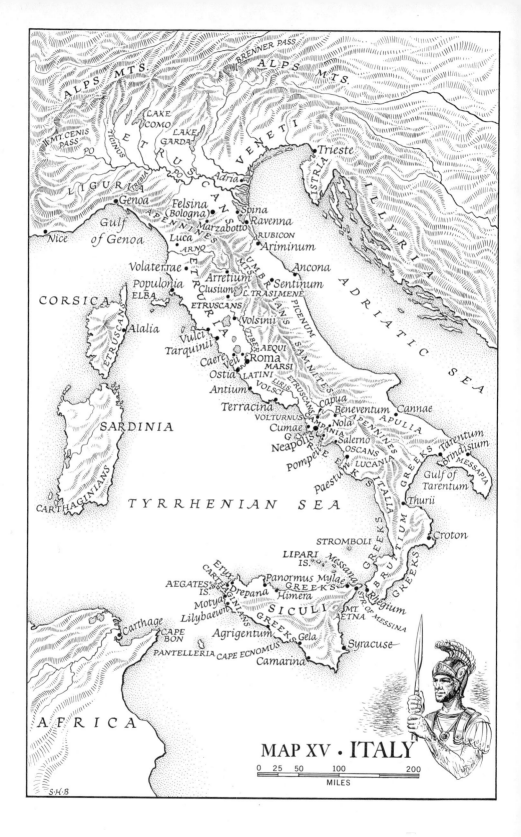

MAP XV · ITALY

0   25   50   100   200

MILES

S·H·B

X I X

The Etruscans and Early Rome

(*ca.* 800–500 B.C.)

IN THE PERSPECTIVE OF HISTORY, Rome's particular achievement was to organize a stable and acceptable form of government for the ancient world. The Roman Empire included not only the Mediterranean and the Near East but much of continental Europe as well, from the Atlantic Ocean and the North Sea, along the Rhine and the Danube rivers, to the Black Sea. Over this vast area Rome established general conditions of peace and prosperity for several centuries, during which a highly organized society, of very different origins and customs, accepted with some enthusiasm Rome's imperial government. The cultural traditions of Greece and the Near East were gathered up and blended with those of Rome itself into a form in which they could be passed on to Western Europe and to the Byzantine Empire. The political ideas and legal institutions, the philosophy, literature, and art, which form the basis of the western tradition, were developed and preserved. Christianity also spread in the community of the Roman Empire. For a time the Roman government attempted to stamp out the Christian Church, but in the fourth century after Christ the emperors became Christians and placed the weight of their authority behind the Church. New ideas and institutions were then engrafted into the pagan tradition and the Medieval Period began.

The Romans, who established the Empire and worked out its government, had a very insignificant beginning in a group of shepherd villages on the hills of Rome beside the Tiber River. We hardly hear of them in history until after the time of Alexander the Great. During the early period of Rome's growth it was the Etruscans who dominated Italy, while the Greek colonies of Magna Graecia were the chief link with the more civilized world of the East. By the beginning of the third century B.C., however, Rome had become the chief power of Italy and by 133 B.C. was the dominant power of the Mediterranean

The reader will find Maps XV, XVI (pages 416 and 430) and the illustration on page 502 useful as he reads this chapter.

and committed to the governing of this area. While the central position of Rome in Italy and of Italy in the Mediterranean might seem to have marked out the Roman people for such a role, their achievement rested on their own unique military and political abilities to mold Italy into a nation and the Empire into an organic community.

Italy and the Italian Peoples

The history of Italy, as distinguished from its prehistory, began in the seventh century B.C., when the names of its peoples and some events were recorded by the Greeks. Throughout the prehistoric period Italian culture was slow to develop in contrast to the early civilizations of the Near East and to the Minoan-Mycenaean civilization of Greece, but the Italian peoples established a stable, agricultural economy and began to exploit the metal resources of Central Italy. The native population was formed from the Mediterranean migrants, who came to Italy in the New Stone Age, and Indo-Europeans, who came during the Italian Bronze Age, from about 1500 to 1000 B.C. The latter imposed their language on Italy, just as their kindred had on Greece, so that the dialects of Italy were predominantly Indo-European. In the ninth and eighth centuries B.C. Italian growth was quickened with the arrival of new immigrants from the eastern Mediterranean, the Etruscans and the Greek colonists. In the Etruscan regions of Italy urbanization proceeded rapidly as writing and other techniques of civilization were introduced. Apparently the Greek colonists fixed the name Italy on the land, first applying it to the southern part of the toe of the Italian peninsula where they had settled. The natives of that area referred to their land as Vitelia, "land of cattle." The application was gradually extended until in the late second century, from the time of Polybius, it designated the whole of the peninsula from the Alps southwards.

THE PHYSICAL CHARACTER OF ITALY

The relative slowness of growth in prehistoric Italy is largely explained by the location and physical characteristics of the peninsula, which tended to cut its people off from the eastern Mediterranean and to link them to continental Europe. In fact, the long peninsula of Italy, from the Alps to the Strait of Messina and Sicily, is considerably less Mediterranean than its two thousand miles of coastline might suggest. Northern and Central Italy, as far south as Rome, which is more continental than Mediterranean in climate and vegetation, has always tended to be affected by developments in Europe. Southern Italy and Sicily, which are more thoroughly Mediterranean, were close to Greece in their contacts. The Alps, which form an arc from Nice to Trieste, despite their height and the difficulty of the high passes, were not a complete shield from Europe. The Riviera offered access to France, and the routes at the head of the Adriatic, to Central Europe and the Balkans. Also, the rich lands of the Po River valley, from which the Alps rise abruptly on the north, are cut off to some degree from the rest of the peninsula by the Apennine Mountains. The Apennines form a somewhat misplaced vertebral system for the Italian peninsula, since the mountains are close to the east coast, leaving little room for cultivation and making the climate on that side cold and uncomfortable. These factors, combined with the lack of harborage and good beaches from Trieste to Brindisi, directed settlement and trade to the west coast. Thus the fertile coastal plains of Etruria, Latium, and Campania, and the tablelands and valleys of the central Apennines became the chief areas of settlement. While the west coast had only one good harbor, Naples, the shelving beaches and partially navigable rivers, like the Tiber, provided landing ground for ancient ships. In the interior, communication by land was not particularly difficult, so that settlement could spread throughout the peninsula.

The agricultural resources of Italy were much richer than those of Greece, and its peoples freer from scarcity of food, which had spurred the Greeks to take to the sea and to trade for a living. The soil along much of the west coast is volcanic in origin, enriched with humus and is well watered, so that a variety of crops could be grown with proper cultivation—grain, garden produce, fruit, vines, and olives. The forest growth was abundant on the mountain slopes, ranging from the deciduous trees of the continental region to the evergreens of the south. In addition to timber for building and firewood, the forests yielded nut crops of acorns, beechnuts and chestnuts, which provided food for pigs. In north central Italy there were deposits of iron, tin, and copper. In most areas there was good stone for building and abundant beds of clay for bricks and pottery. While the metals were extensively used in local production and for trade, Italy was characteristically an agricultural and pastoral country. Thus the early inhabitants were farmers and herders who predominated in early times because land for agriculture had to be cleared and drained, a process which required centuries. The big islands near Italy also added to its wealth. In historical times Sicily became a large-scale producer of grain, Elba had deposits of iron, and Corsica had a heavy forest growth. Because of the open character of the hills and mountains, a network of roads could be established to link the regions and cities more closely together than they had been in Greece. Nevertheless, the diversity of area and difficulty of communication were such that the ultimate coalescence of the whole peninsula depended on a political process that was to be engineered only by one power, Rome.

SETTLEMENT

While there are numerous traces of Old Stone Age man in Italy, the substratum of the population was probably formed in the New Stone Age by immigration of a Mediterranean people, who had established their culture over the peninsula by 2500 B.C. Some came by land from Spain and France into northern Italy, where they settled in the caves of Liguria, while others crossed from North Africa into Sicily and South Italy, and from there they spread northwards. While some agriculture was carried on the neolithic peoples lived mainly by herding and hunting, for the land was still heavily forested and the work of clearing slow. Caves were extensively used for dwellings, particularly in Liguria. The people of a single cave formed a small community, living with their animals and burying their dead in the cave itself. Small villages of huts have also been found, where the people fortified their settlements with a ditch and practiced more agriculture than the cave dwellers. The typical hut dwelling in the colder regions of Italy was ingeniously designed to withstand the climate, somewhat in the manner of a sod hut on our own prairies. A pit, several feet in depth, was excavated, above which the framework of the hut was erected and entwined with branches or reeds plastered with clay.

The burial grounds of the neolithic peoples are rather better known than their settlements and reveal a standard type of burial. The bodies were placed in a contracted position, with knees drawn up and arms folded across the chest, while in the grave were placed ornaments, pottery jars originally filled with food and drink, and small trinkets. Since there was some navigation and trade along the coast, the large islands of Sardinia and Corsica were populated in the New Stone Age. Towards 2000 B.C. the use of copper was introduced, probably by migration of small groups from the Danube valley into northern Italy and by contacts from sea trade in the southern part of the peninsula.

In the period of transition between the Stone and the Bronze Ages, a culture akin to that of the Swiss Lake Dwellers was developed in the Italian lake district and lasted until about 1000 B.C. The settlements were like those of their Swiss counterparts and were probably established by migrants from across the Alps. The houses were built on wooden platforms along the shore and were supported by stakes driven into the soft lake bottom. In addition to fishing and hunting, the people practiced an extensive agriculture, sowing wheat and barley and growing some vegetables and fruit. Northern Italy also attracted small groups of migrants from Western and Central Europe, who brought their knowledge of metallurgy and helped to establish the Bronze Age towards 1500 B.C.

Perhaps the most interesting of the cultures of the Bronze Age was that known as *Terremare* (Black Earth) along the south bank of the Po River. The name was applied because of the dark soil which had resulted from the decay of debris in the course of living for generations in the same settlements. The villages were built of huts, sometimes surrounded by a ditch and palisades for protection, and with an open area, probably a market place, in the central part. During the latter part of the Bronze Age, when there seems to have been frequent flooding along the river, stakes were used to support the huts, somewhat in the manner of the settlements of the Lake Dwellers, but there was no cultural connection between the two. *Terremare* was a fully developed Bronze Age culture, whose people used horses and carts and displayed considerable skill in making their tools and weapons. The latter indicate that the *Terremare* people were linked with western Hungary and Central Europe, probably as the result of migration rather than trade.

Southern Italy and Sicily also flourished in the Bronze Age, but drew their inspiration mainly from trade with Mycenaean Greece, as imported objects indicate—Aegean swords, daggers, and pottery. Probably Mycenaean trading posts were established on the coasts of Sicily and South Italy, but after the collapse of the main centers in Greece, these connections became very tenuous. There may have been some trade during the Dark Age, but the early Hellenic influences in historical Italy were the result of the intensive Greek colonization of the eighth and seventh centuries (pp. 185-87).

The prehistoric cultures of Sardinia and Malta reached their height in the Bronze Age and have left some impressive remains in the megalithic architecture of the tombs and towers. The tombs are similar to the dolmens of Western Europe. They were built above ground of great stone slabs which form the sides and roof, and among them were *menhirs* (markers). A *menhir* was a slab of stone set upright in the ground. The groups of dolmens were collective burial places used over a long period of time by a single community. The *nuraghes* (towers) are massively built structures which were evidently used in defending the community and suggest that the islands had been subjected to raids by pirates.

Towards the end of the Bronze Age there was a large-scale migration into Italy of Indo-European peoples. The migrants came from the north and east, through the Alpine passes or around the head of the Adriatic and across the sea from Illyria. Their movement is probably to be connected with those into Asia Minor and Greece, where the invaders destroyed the Hittite and Mycenaean civilizations. In Italy, however, since none of the cultural groups had established a strong political power during the Bronze Age, the invasion took the form of infiltration and mingling with the older peoples. Yet the Indo-European tribes were warlike and domineering and imposed their speech and typical patriarchal social organization over most of the peninsula.

Soon after the arrival of the Indo-Europeans a marked change started in north central Italy, which was characterized by the development of the local metal resources and by the gradual establishment of an advanced metallurgy. Iron came into use for weapons and tools, but there was also a distinct advance in the techniques of bronzeworking for armor and utensils. The introduction of the Iron Age apparently resulted from contacts established with the peoples of the Danube valley and of the Balkans in the wake of the migrations. Distinctive regional cultures arose, the most representative of which is Villanovan, named from a village near Bologna. The Villanovans, like their predecessors, lived in irregular hut villages, but were turbulent and warlike, judging from the stocks of weapons and armor in their tombs. The typical form of burial was cremation, in which the ashes were placed in a large biconical jar, decorated with geometric patterns. The earlier jars were of polished black pottery, but the later ones were of bronze. This local exploitation of Italian metals evidently attracted the notice of traders, for in the ninth and eighth centuries the Etruscans and Greeks appeared in the waters off western Italy to trade and to found settlements.

The Etruscan Civilization

SETTLEMENT AND EXPANSION

The most formative influence in early Italy was that of the Etruscan civilization, which came into being in Etruria, the region west of the Apennine Mountains between the Tiber and Arno rivers. The civilization is known reasonably well from the remains of the cities and tombs, but the origin of the Etruscan people themselves is enigmatic. Since there were very strong Italic elements in early Etruscan culture, some scholars regard it as a native Italian growth which, like early Greek civilization, was strongly affected at first by Orientalizing influences from trade contacts and then by Greek civilization itself. Yet there were elements which could hardly result from trade and which point to western Asia Minor as the place from which the Etruscans came. Their language, which was distinctive in Italy, is not Indo-European and has affinities with a pre-Indo-European language in northwestern Asia Minor. Although Etruscan was written in Greek alphabetic characters, possibly learned from the Greek colonists of Cumae in the seventh century B.C., it is very imperfectly understood. Certain features of Etruscan architecture, the plan of their temples and the types of tomb, seem Asiatic, not Italian in inspiration. Also, some religious practices, such as divination of the future from the livers of sacrificed animals, were Asiatic. Since none of these social traits was likely to have developed from casual contacts, it seems likely that the Etruscans were a people who left Asia Minor after the collapse of the Mycenaean and Hittite civilizations to find new homes in Italy. Perhaps their traders knew of the metal available in Etruria and led their people to the source of supply in the course of the ninth century B.C.

The number of Etruscan migrants must have been small, but they were superior in arms and fighting ability to the native Italians and seized strong points along the coast, making their early settlements at Tarquinii, Caere, and Vulci. From the coast they pushed inland to occupy strategic hill settlements, from which the adjacent territory and the native people could be controlled. In all, about eighteen such fortified cities were founded in Etruria, each ruled by an Etruscan king and a small group of nobles. The cities were independent of one another, but the twelve most important formed a confederation for common worship in an annual festival and, occasionally, for collaboration in war. While the Etruscans intermarried with the Italians and in the course of time a class of merchants arose in the Etruscan cities, the character of their regime remained that of a dominant, military and landowning aristocracy. As in Greece the original monarchies soon gave way to aristocratic rule, in which the noble landowners, *lucumones,* formed a governing council and elected annual magistrates. The Italian natives cultivated the fertile lands of Etruria and worked its metals for their masters. Trade was soon established with the Carthaginians and Greeks and in the seventh century the Etruscans themselves expanded throughout Italy by land and sea.

By 600 B.C., when all of Etruria was occupied and its cities had become prosperous and populous, the Etruscans advanced southwards from Tarquinii and Caere to take over the towns of Latium, including Rome, and to conquer Campania as far south as Salerno. The Greek colony at Cumae was occupied but soon revolted successfully, and the southern limit of Etruscan occupation remained the cities of Capua and Nola, which they founded at the eastern edge of the Campanian plain. Etruscan ships controlled the Tyrrhenian Sea, preying on Greek commerce and defeating the Phocaeans from Ionia about 535 B.C. in the battle of Alalia, where Carthage joined them to oust the Greeks. After Corsica and Elba were brought under Etruscan control, iron was procured from Elba and copper from Sardinia to supply the metalworking center at Populonia on the Italian coast. In the last quarter of the sixth century the Etruscans pushed across the Apennines into the valley of the Po River, where they established a number of outposts and garrison towns, among which the most important were Felsina, near Bologna, and Spina on the Adriatic Sea. This penetration to the north was the high-water mark of Etruscan expansion, for about 500 B.C. their power began to crumble. The conquests had been made by individual Etruscan nobles leading small bands of warriors and some native Italian troops. The leaders set themselves up as kings in the conquered communities and ruled by military domination and exactions of tribute. Because the warrior-kings acknowledged no central authority and made no firm alliance among themselves, their control was narrowly based and vulnerable.

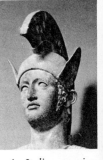

An Italian warrior or the god Mars

According to tradition Rome was the first Italian city to renounce Etruscan control, when the Roman nobles rebelled against their Etruscan king in 509 B.C. and established a republican form of government. This Roman revolt, however, which was only a part of the general rejection of Etruscan authority by the Latins, some scholars would place after the other Latins had obtained their freedom. In 505 B.C. the other towns of Latium defeated the Etruscans at Aricia with the help of the Greeks from Cumae and thus blocked Etruscan access to Campania. In 474 B.C. Etruscan sea power was broken by Hieron, the tyrant of Syracuse, and a generation later in 438 B.C. Capua was taken by the Samnite hill people. This completed the destruction of Etruscan control in the regions south of Etruria. Although their sea trade was largely taken over by Carthaginians and Greeks, Etruscan traders continued to cross the Alps into the Rhineland and Central Europe. Their towns in the Po valley lasted until after 400 B.C. About that time hordes of Gauls poured into Italy from the north and raided down into the peninsula as far as Rome, which they occupied briefly. Although the Gauls retreated from Central Italy, they remained in the Po valley and gave a Celtic character to the region, which was called by the Romans Cisalpine Gaul, the Gaul on the nearer side of the Alps. Thus, soon after 400 B.C. the Etruscans were reduced again to Etruria, which became a part of the Roman Confederacy in the early third century B.C. From then on the Etruscans gradually lost their identity in the general Romanization of Italy. The Etruscan language was forgotten, and their individual culture survived only as a part of that of Rome, a condition indicated by the antiquarian interest of the Emperor Claudius (A.D. 41–54), who devoted a lengthy study to Etruscan history. He was among the last who knew the language.

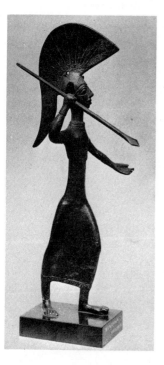

An Etruscan inscription from Perugia

CIVILIZATION

Despite the aggressive and domineering character of their conquest, the Etruscans exerted a strong civilizing influence in Italy. Their nobles based a luxurious life on intensive development of Italian agriculture, metalwork and trade. New tracts of farming land were cleared and drained by the construction of channels and dams, and Italian crops were amplified by the introduction of vines and olive trees. The breeding of horses was skillfully practiced, since, as befitted a military aristocracy, the Etruscans were fond of horse and chariot racing. The metal industry was enlarged by thorough mining of the deposits in Etruria and the importation of metals from Sardinia and Elba. Etruscan metalwork was technically very competent and of high artistic quality, so that Etruria became an exporter of metal products to Western and Central Europe, to the Aegean and western Mediterranean. While the Etruscans did not want Greek settlement on their coasts, they did trade extensively with the Greek colonies in southern France, Spain and, through the cities of Magna Graecia, with Greece itself. Greek vases, fine wines and olive oil were imported, and Greek workmen came to Etruria to execute artistic commissions. The result, of course, was a very strong Greek influence on Etruscan art. This extensive Etruscan trade was carried on by barter until about 500 B.C., at which time the

Minerva, a warrior goddess.

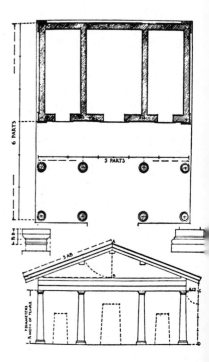

Ground plan and façade of a typical Etruscan temple

Etruscans began to use the coins of the Ionian cities as a medium of exchange, but within a generation they issued a coinage of their own. Although much of this seaborne commerce was lost after Hieron's victory in 474 B.C., local agriculture and metalwork maintained the well-being of the Etruscans until the first century B.C.

Italy's earliest monumental architecture was developed in the fortified hill towns of the Etruscans, but apparently regular checkerboard planning, which some of them exhibit, was borrowed from the Greeks after the fifth century. A typical example of a late Etruscan town is furnished by Marzabotto, south of Bologna. It was laid out on a checkerboard plan, with emphasis on the two main streets crossing at right angles; it had regular blocks of houses and an excellently engineered drainage system. The Etruscans, in fact, excelled in the construction of drainage channels, bridges, and gateways. In the third century they adopted the use of the true arch, which made a type of construction very durable as well as pleasing in appearance.

The most important structure in an Etruscan town was the temple, broad and heavy in appearance, with a very deep porch in front, occupying almost half of the structure. The *cella* was divided into three long narrow chambers to provide for a triad of deities. The temples were raised on a stone basis, which necessitated a flight of steps up to floor level, and the superstructure was built of brick with wooden beams and roof timbers. To protect the latter from the weather and to serve as ornament, a heavy revetment of terra cotta was attached to the eaves. As the low horizontal lines of the temple drew the eye to the center, the brightly painted ornament concentrated attention on the façade. Whereas the Greek temple attracted people to visit the house of their god and to loiter in the colonnades, the Etruscan temple emphasized the awful majesty of the deities by the impressive façade and by screening them from the worshippers by the deep porch and dark closed rooms of the *cella*.

Etruscans made elaborate provision for a life after death by constructing great tombs, filling them with furniture and precious possessions and by painting vivid, realistic pictures on the walls. The most impressive type of tombs were large *tumuli*, in which a mound of earth was heaped over the burial chamber, like the burial mounds of Lydia and Phrygia in Asia Minor. Others were in the form of an elaborate underground house, where a series of rooms and corridors were tunneled through the rock. These were used for family burials over a period of several generations and were filled with costly articles, imported Greek vases, and objects of gold, silver and ivory. More fine Greek vases, in fact, have been found in Etruscan tombs than in Greece itself.

The wall paintings of the tombs cover a wide range of time, from the latter part of the sixth century to the second century B.C., and collectively form the most important group of paintings which we possess from Greece or Italy before those in the houses of Roman Pompeii. The paintings of the sixth and fifth centuries were strongly under the influence, first of Ionian, then of Athenian art, but drew most of their subject matter from Etruscan life. A few scenes from

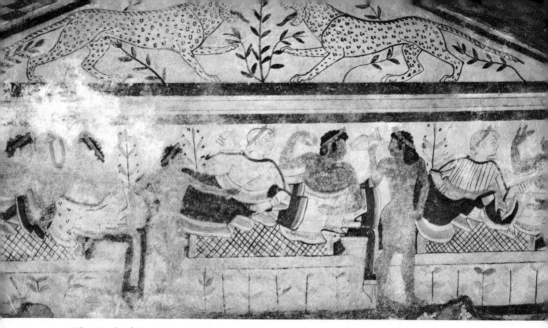

The Tomb of the Leopards at Tarquinii (early fifth century B.C.). Such banquet scenes were standard decoration on Etruscan tombs of that period.

Greek myth probably reproduced motifs of a type used in Etruscan houses, but most paintings represented the funeral games and banquet which accompanied the burial of the dead. Perhaps it was hoped that the paintings would prolong the magical effects of the funeral for the dead man living in his grave below ground who was represented as reclining on a funeral couch, surrounded by the ceremonies of the funeral. There was spirited dancing and flute playing, wrestling and combats between armed men. These Etruscan funeral combats, fought to the death by prisoners of war and slaves, were regarded as a sort of human sacrifice and were the prototypes of the Roman gladiatorial exhibitions. Scenes of the everyday life of the Etruscans, hunting, fishing in the sea, horse and chariot racing gave a more cheerful tone. In fact the effect given to all the earlier paintings by the bright colors and the strong, vital figures was one of exuberant, prosperous life.

But by the third century B.C., when Etruscan civilization was dying, this earlier exuberance was replaced by mournful and gloomy introspection. Perhaps

Funeral dance in a tomb at Ruvo, Apulia (fifth century B.C.). Greco-Italian painting

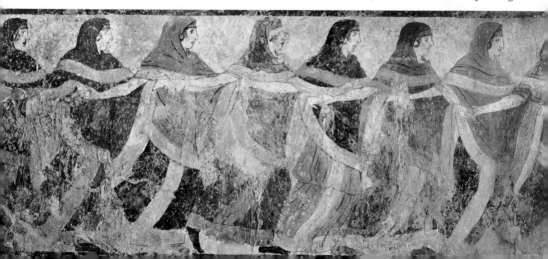

the emotionalism, characteristic of Greek art in that period, had some influence in bringing this change of tone, but more probably the Etruscans themselves had experienced a change of mood. The banquet scenes painted in the tombs became quiet, the faces of the banqueters withdrawn and still, while scenes from the underworld, with fierce and ugly demons, replaced the former scenes of cheerful, everyday life.

Etruscan sculptors, unlike the sculptors of early Greece, used terra cotta and bronze rather than stone and were extremely proficient technically in these media. The pediments of the temples were filled with terra-cotta groups, usually representing a scene from Greek myth but showing some striking differences in the conception of the deities. For example, a fine pedimental group of the late sixth century B.C. from the Temple of Veii represents Apollo, Hermes, Diana, and other gods striking down a deer. The figure of Apollo is richly treated in the manner of the Ionian work of this period, but the god himself is a vital, almost sinister, figure. This same strength and latent ferocity appears in the best known of the bronze sculptures, the Capitoline Wolf and the Chimaera, which date from the early fifth century. The wolf was originally placed on the Capitoline Hill in Rome, where it was a dedication to Jupiter. The figure shows a striking combination of richly patterned and meticulously executed work on the hairy ruff and of lean, tense ferocity in the body and head. The Chimaera, an eastern fancy which was part lion, goat, and snake, shows the same characteristics. Etruscan portrait sculpture, which also was rendered in both bronze and terra cotta, was strongly realistic. Probably this feeling for realism in portraiture is to be linked with the belief in individual survival after death, which is apparent in the tomb paintings.

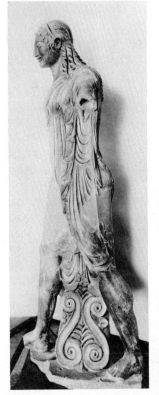

The Apollo of Veii (ca. 500 B.C.). Painted terra-cotta statue from the pediment of the temple.

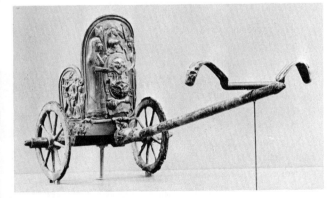

An Etruscan bronze chariot
(sixth century B.C.)

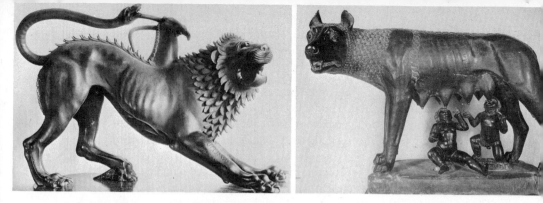

Left: The Chimaera (early fifth century B.C.). Right: The Capitoline Wolf (early fifth century B.C.). The children, Romulus and Remus, were added in the Renaissance.

The Etruscans conceived of nature and of human activity as governed by numerous gods and spirits, among which the more malevolent had a prominent place. The triad of deities, for which the temples provided, were Juno, Minerva and Tinia, who was identified by the Romans with their Jupiter. Among the demons Charun, the conductor of souls to the underworld, held a dubious primacy, being conceived as a repulsive, blue-skinned creature in human form, with snakes twisting about his shoulders. Since living in a world peopled so extensively with spirits ready to harm mankind was hazardous, the Etruscans developed an elaborate set of procedures for telling the future and for warding off evil. Most characteristic was liver divination, the inspection of the livers of sacrificed animals, to detect and interpret any abnormality. This practice, which linked the Etruscans with the people of western Asia, was adopted by the Romans, along with other methods, which may have been more specifically Italian. Thunder and lightning, the flight of birds from a particular quarter of the sky, freaks of nature, all had some particular relevance to human activities as signs from the gods and required interpretation by experts. Since the Etruscan priesthood seems to have been authoritarian, the public lives of the Etruscans were hedged about by strict rules of ritual and procedure. Ordinary social life, however, was shared on equal terms by men and women, as the wall paintings reveal. They show women attending games and funeral banquets and taking part in scenes of daily life.

Italian civilization owed much to the Etruscans: urbanization and monumental architecture, advanced methods of agriculture, a wide range of trade and foreign contacts, and a highly expressive and technically competent art. Early Greek influence in Central Italy came largely through an Etruscan medium. The Romans, for example, began to use writing in the sixth century, while they were ruled by Etruscan kings. The Etruscan language is still a barrier to understanding their life more fully. There are about ten thousand inscriptions, but all are very short and seem to record little more than burials, official titles, and dedications to the gods. One of the longest documents is part of a religious calendar. Latin borrowed some Etruscan words, which are explained by ancient scholars, but since we know little more than the parts of speech, numerals, the titles of officials, and proper names, the language is not yet fully understood.

428

Rome of the Kings

LATIUM

The region of Latium, the land of the Latin peoples, of whom the Romans were one, was a small coastal plain, lying between the sea and the Apennine Mountains and bounded by the Tiber River on the north and the Volscian Hills on the south. The northern part of Latium, near Rome, was dominated by the Alban Hills, an extinct volcanic mass, the highest point of which rose to about three thousand feet. As a result of earlier volcanic activity and the decay of vegetation the soil of Latium was very fertile and, together with the hill slopes, could support a relatively large population by agriculture and grazing. The Latins were Italic, descendants of the neolithic population and of the Indo-Europeans, who had entered the country from the northeast in the Late Bronze Age. They were divided into peoples, *populi,* each of which inhabited a district, *pagus,* of its own, in which the inhabitants lived in scattered villages. The more powerful peoples raided and expanded into their neighbor's territory, but did not establish an overall political union or central authority. A large number of the Latin villages around the Alban Hills had formed a loosely organized league at an early date to celebrate the annual festival of Jupiter, but the organization seems to have had no political significance. In the sixth century, when Rome under its Etruscan kings may have become a threat to other Latin towns, eight of the Latin communities formed their own association, the Arician League, which warred against the Romans and met to worship Diana in the town of Aricia. In 505 B.C., as we have noticed, the coalition, aided by the Greeks from Cumae, was able to defeat the Etruscans and assert Latin independence.

EARLY ROME

The beginnings of Rome were insignificant and obscure. The early Romans were not distinguishable among their Latin neighbors, and neither did they provoke the curiosity of literate Greeks, who might have told us something of early Rome, until after Rome's victories over Pyrrhus and the Carthaginians in the third century B.C. In the interval the Romans had learned to write but kept only a few official records: their religious calendars, lists of magistrates, and some laws and treaties. These provided the bare bones of history, but no Roman historian appeared until the late third century B.C., when Quintus Fabius Pictor wrote Rome's first history in Greek. He and his successors were able to amplify their accounts with legends and stories which had been passed down orally from generation to generation. Some of these were popular folk tales, while others were the traditions of great Roman families, who proudly kept the exploits of their ancestors alive. Yet such a record hardly befitted the dignity of the world power which Rome was then becoming, so that, to supply the deficiency, a national myth was gradually formed, which could explain Rome's origin and account for its greatness.

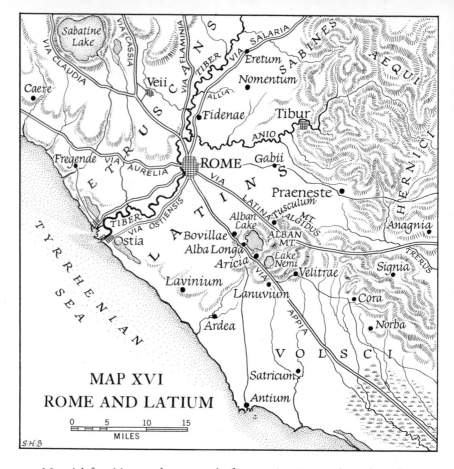

MAP XVI
ROME AND LATIUM

0   5   10   15
MILES

S·H·B

Material for this was drawn partly from native Roman legends and partly invented or inflated by Greek writers. In the native Roman material we may distinguish the story of Romulus, who seems to have been named from the city, Rome, but was made into its founder in Greek fashion, like the founders of Greek colonies. Among the early kings there was Numa, who gave religious customs to Rome and who was ranked with Lycurgus of Sparta. The vivid story of the rape of the Sabine women was designed to explain the fact that there was a Sabine element, that is, people from the Sabine Hills to the east, among the early Romans.

The origins of Rome were connected neatly to the Heroic Age of Greece by the story of Aeneas and his descendants, the theme of Vergil's epic poem, the *Aeneid* (p. 584). According to the story Aeneas himself did not found Rome but came to nearby Lavinium; Aeneas' son, Ascanius, moved a step nearer by founding Alba Longa, the site of the Alban festival of Jupiter, and at an appropriate interval among Aeneas' descendants was Romulus. Thus the awkward gap between the Trojan War and the founding of Rome was bridged, and Greek fiction and native Roman tradition were woven together.

The myths are of value in understanding the Roman pride of race, and the shaping of the myths demonstrates the influence of Greek thinking about history, but the content is not factual. No more factual is the traditional date of the "founding" of Rome, 753 B.C., from which the Romans later reckoned the chronology of their history. To reconstruct the early history of Rome it is necessary to utilize archaeological data, to study carefully the survivals of customs and institutions, and to sift the legends for the core of truth which some of them may contain. The results are uncertain and conjectural until we come to the firmer ground of the third century B.C.

Rome was advantageously located to dominate Latium and the Italian peninsula, but this factor played its part only after the Roman villages had grown into a city. The initial settlements were made on a group of hills by the Tiber River, about fifteen miles from its mouth. The hills marked the limit of navigation from the sea, but even that was difficult against the current and through the sand bars, so at a later date Rome developed a port, Ostia, at the river mouth. In the Tiber at Rome, however, there was an island, near which the river could be forded. As a result the location was important for communications by land, both in Latium itself and into Central Italy along the valley of the Tiber. The early settlement at Rome seems to have had some importance for the distribution of salt, since an ancient road, the *Via Salaria* (Salt Road) ran along the Tiber.

The people of early Rome were farmers and herders, like their Latin kindred, and settled on the hills as a defensible and reasonably healthy site. Some traces of inhabitation during the Bronze Age have been found, but our earliest, and very fragmentary, picture of Rome is from the Early Iron Age, between about 900 and 600 B.C. At that time there were separate villages on the Palatine, Quirinal and Viminal hills. The people lived in small huts and buried their dead in several cemeteries which have been excavated. Two types of burial were in use: cremation, in which the ashes were placed in urns, and inhumation, where the dead were laid in hollowed-out tree trunks. Presumably this divergence of practice represented two different groups among the population (Latins and Sabines ?), but, since the types of burial were mixed in the same cemetery, some intermingling had started. While the villages were still individual political units, their inhabitants joined together in religious rites, which were perpetuated in the Festival of the *Septimontium* (Seven Mounts) apparently dating from the early seventh century.

While Rome experienced a considerable development under its Etruscan rulers in the sixth century, the agricultural villages seem to have coalesced into a city before that time. For example, early huts on the low ground which later became the Roman Forum were replaced by a public shrine before 575 B.C., and before 600 B.C. a sanctuary had been built on the Capitoline Hill. Other archaeological evidence indicates that by 600 Rome contained workers and traders, as well as farmers, and was a flourishing town. Under Etruscan rule it developed still further. The shrine on the Capitoline Hill was replaced by a large temple on the Etruscan model for Jupiter Capitolinus, and various Etruscan religious rites and customs were introduced. Rome was given a formal, sacred boundary line, the *pomoerium,* as well as a defensive wall of stone and earth. This wall was built for defense, not as a sacred boundary, since the course of the two was not identical. The Capitoline Hill was separately fortified to serve as a citadel or *arx,* and the communities of the four hills and the intervening low ground were included in the city, which came to be known as the City of the Four Regions: the Palatina, Esquilina, Collina, and Suburana. A cattle market, the Forum Boarium, and the Roman Forum, in the low ground below the Palatine Hill, began to develop. It is likely that the name Roma, which is apparently Etruscan, was applied to the community at this time.

According to Roman tradition seven kings ruled in Rome between the foundation of the city and the revolution which overthrew the monarchy in 509 B.C. While Romulus does not seem to have been an historical figure, it is probable that the names of the remaining six were correctly preserved: Numa Pompilius, Tullus Hostilius, Ancus Marcius, Lucius Tarquinius Priscus, Servius Tullius, and Lucius Tarquinius Superbus. The name Tarquin, of course, suggests that at least its bearers were Etruscans, and the odium attached in tradition to Tarquin the Proud is what might be expected for the last king of a dynasty overthrown by revolution. It is scarcely possible to credit the detailed accounts of any one of the kings, however, for Roman historians have evidently used the names as tags, to which they could attach a wholesale range of activity. It is a very difficult and technical task to sort out the probable from the false and the later from the earlier, but the general nature of Roman institutions in the period of the kings seems clear.

EARLY ROMAN GOVERNMENT

The system of government was much the same as that which we have seen in Homeric Greece or in Macedonia before the time of Alexander the Great. The king ruled with the advice of a council of the nobles, called the Senate, and the consent of an assembly of the arms-bearing citizens. The office was elective, although it tended to remain in a single royal family. When a new king was created, the Senate made the selection according to the proper religious procedures and presented the candidate to the assembly for approval. The authority of the king, his *imperium,* was absolute and all-embracing, since he was the leader of the people in war, their chief priest, and supreme judge. As military leader the king could act for his people in foreign affairs, as well as lead them in battle. His judicial power was exercised mainly in enforcing the ancestral custom of the Roman community, the *mos maiorum,* for which he could impose punishments, levy fines, and in extreme cases use the death penalty. As religious head of the state the king offered sacrifices to the great gods and supervised the regular performance of religious ceremonies. His actions, however, as in the Homeric state, were tempered by the pressure of the Senate and the need for public support in any major undertaking like war on another people. Above all traditional custom was a compelling influence in Rome, which the king had to observe and guard.

The Senate, probably a council of elders originally, consisted of leaders from the important families of Rome, selected by the king to serve for life. While the Senate did not have legislative or executive powers, the members possessed the more intangible authority of their dignity and position in the community, which was reinforced by the continuity of their group and by individual life tenure. Since each senator was the head of a large group of kinsmen and retainers, the combined will of the Senate was potent.

The people of Rome had been divided into thirty groups, called *curiae*, from a very early period. These met in a general assembly, the Curiate, or *Comitia Curiata*. The *curiae* were apparently pseudokinship divisions, like the Greek *phratries*, in which membership was hereditary and which included all the arms-bearing men of the state, nobles and ordinary citizens, rich and poor alike. In the assembly the citizens voted in their curial groups and a majority of the curial units determined the decisions. Thus in Rome individuals counted as members of their groups, rather than in their own right. Each *curia* also had its own religious worships and contributed a specific quota to the army, ten cavalrymen and one hundred foot soldiers. The *curiae* were more basic to the organization of Rome than the three early tribes which were formed from them: the Ramnes, Tities, and Luceres. The assembly was called by the king to hear business concerning the whole community, such as adoptions and the reading of wills, and to approve declarations of war and the selection of a new king.

The strong conception of authority and seniority which appeared in the *imperium* of the king and in the influence of the Senate was characteristic of Roman society. In the single family the authority of the father, the *paterfamilias*, was absolute. He was the head of the household, which included the immediate members related by blood and marriage, the slaves, and property. The father represented this group to the community and to the spirits and the ancestors of the household who guarded its welfare. In Roman society, however, as in Homeric Greece, women had a respected and influential place. Those families which claimed descent from a common ancestor through the male line formed the larger unit of the *gens* or clan. Clan members were marked as such by their use of the clan name, the *nomen*, in addition to a personal name, the *praenomen*. At a later date, as the families comprising a *gens* multiplied, family names were devised to mark the particular branch of the *gens* to which a man belonged. For example, Julius Caesar's full name was Gaius Julius Caesar, which designated him as the individual, Gaius, of the Caesar family in the Julian clan. In the sixth century B.C. there were perhaps sixty clans in Rome, which formed great vertical divisions in society. The heads of the clans were wealthy landowners, leaders in war, by virtue of their superior arms, and in political life, by their position in the Senate and by the influence which they wielded among the families of their own clan and over their dependents. The dependents, *clients*, worked the land of their patrons as tenant farmers, followed them in war and gave them political support in the assembly. In return the patron provided a livelihood for his *client* and protected his interest in public and private life. Since the relationship was hereditary and guaranteed by religious feeling, the great clan, together with its component families and *clients,* formed a solid block in Roman society, whose members usually acted in concert.

Just as in the aristocratic Greek states, economic development in Rome brought a horizontal class structure into existence, which began to cut across the older lines of kinship. The upper class of Rome, the patricians, were members of the families and descendants of the men who formed the Senate, known as *patres,* fathers. The patricians alone possessed the political privileges of Rome, the right to hold office and to carry out the religious and political business of the state. The patricians maintained themselves for a long time as a strictly closed caste, for marriage outside their own ranks was forbidden. Social rank, wealth in land, and political privilege distinguished the patricians from the lower class, the plebeians. The plebeian group was made up of various elements. There were the new lower class in the city of Rome, traders, artisans and laborers, free farmers, who owned small plots of land, and probably the *clients* of the great families. The latter normally followed the political lead of the clan head, but economically and socially they were plebeians. Among the plebeians there were also some wealthy families, who were excluded from the patrician group because they were of recent foreign extraction or because they lacked the badge of ennoblement, membership in the Senate. The gulf between patrician and plebeian was very deep and broad, and until it was closed Rome remained thoroughly under the direction of the patrician families.

EARLY ROMAN RELIGION

By the end of the Monarchical Period Roman religion had already absorbed some Etruscan and Greek conceptions and practices, which were blended with the older beliefs which Romans shared with other Italic peoples. This native substratum of belief was animistic, that is, the Romans believed that nature was filled with impersonal spiritual forces whose power (or *numen*) was revealed in actions affecting man. As the Romans became more sophisticated, they thought of these powers as belonging to deities who had personal traits and names, but they did not arrange the gods into a pattern or make up myths to explain their relations to one another and to mankind. The major deities and spirits were, of course, closely linked with the activities and institutions important in early Roman life—the household, agriculture, herding, war, and the general welfare of the community. The household religion was most warm and individual because the spirits of the household were very much a part of the family group and their worship was carried on by its members. Among the household deities there were Janus, who guarded the doorway; Vesta, the goddess of the hearth; the Penates, who presided over the storehouse; the Lar, who was the spirit of the family fields; and the household Genius, a sort of shadowy double of the father. These and the spirits of the family ancestors looked after the welfare of the whole group.

The gods of the community were, of course, concerned with the welfare of the whole state and were the object of its civic worship. The Roman attitude to the gods is expressed by their word *religio*, which meant primarily the feeling of respect and awe towards what was sacred and, more technically, the strict observance of the ritual of worship. The term did not at first have any moral or theological connotation but indicated the contractual basis of Roman religion. The worshippers, in return for the due observance of the rites of worship and sacrifice, expected the gods to do their part in looking after the community. Also, the will of the gods towards any activity might be ascertained beforehand by interpretation of the auspices. Thus, it was extremely important for the welfare of Rome that the proper men, who knew the ritual and the technical formalities of religious observance, should represent the state toward the gods. For this purpose boards of priests were chosen, drawn only from the patrician element of society.

The most important priestly college, that of the *pontifices*, headed by the *pontifex maximus*, protected and supervised the sacred law of the state. The *pontifices* drew up the religious calendar of festivals and designated which days were proper for the conduct of public business. They knew the right formulas for legal action, without which cases could not be heard. The *pontifex maximus* was elected by the whole people, but his colleagues and members of the other priestly colleges were, for the most part, appointed by him. The boards of priests were in charge of the various religious activities of the state: the *flamines* carried out the ritual acts of worship; and the *fetiales* were entrusted with the formal conduct of foreign relations, to ensure that Rome always entered upon a negotiation or war with the approval of the gods. This convenient technique of foreign policy ensured that all Rome's wars were "just." The *augures*, who consulted the auspices before assembly meetings and other important legal acts, were most important for political action. In battle the kings and later on the generals consulted the auspices before engaging in action. The various priests might also be state officials in a political capacity and their religious duties were essentially administrative. Accordingly, Roman public religion was political in character and its practice was a very important part of the political action of the state.

The great gods of the Roman state, established as a triad in the sixth century under Etruscan influence, were Jupiter, Juno, and Minerva. Jupiter was an Indo-European sky-god in origin, who controlled the power of thunder and lightning, and was regarded as the especial guardian of Rome. Juno, conceived later under Greek influence as his wife, was the patroness of women, while Minerva was the goddess of craftsmen. Mars, who had originally been an agricultural god, developed into the god of war who protected the farms of Rome and gave his name to the parade ground of the Roman army, the Field of Mars. Ceres, the goddess of the harvest, and Liber, the god of vines, were equivalent to the Greek Demeter and Dionysus who were propitiated to ensure the agricultural success of the Romans. The great festivals of Rome were also intimately linked to agricultural life and gave color and warmth to the civic religion. The Saturnalia, in particular, which came in December, was a gay and cheerful carnival for the old agricultural god Saturnus. Banquets were held, gifts exchanged, and slaves were waited upon by their masters.

The influence of Etruscan religious practices on Rome has already been noticed, that is, the introduction of temples, of deities, divination, and the funeral games. From the Greeks, mainly through an Etruscan medium, the Romans borrowed conceptions of the personal appearance of their gods and identified them with their Greek counterparts. Apollo, Mercury (Hermes), and Diana (Artemis) were represented in Greek fashion and given temples in Rome. From the Greeks of Cumae a collection of oracles, the Sibylline Books, was brought to Rome for consultation by the priests in time of crisis. The Romans were prepared to adopt what was useful to them from the religious life of their neighbors and to blend their borrowings with their own beliefs.

While Roman religion was legalistic and concerned with the groups of household and state rather than with the individual, its practice did have a profound effect on Roman social values. The highest Roman virtue was *pietas,* the proper observance of obligations to the gods, to the state and to the family, and the most important quality of Roman character was *gravitas,* a serious, dignified attitude to life. Material and practical as they were, the Romans learned from their religion and the regimen of their household a sense of personal duty, responsibility, and a profound respect for ancestral custom. The Romans did not embark on action lightly, but once a decision was made, they held to it with stubborn tenacity.

The Tomb of the Lionesses at Tarquinii (ca. 520 B.C.). Ritual dance

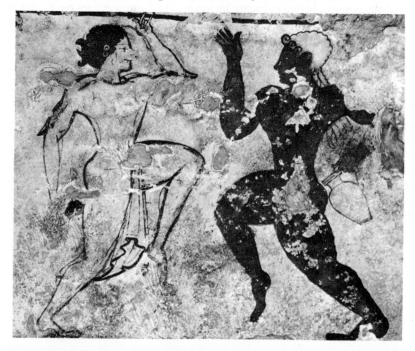

X X

The Early Roman Republic

(*ca.* 500–264 B.C.)

BETWEEN 509 B.C., when, according to tradition, the Romans expelled their last king, Tarquin, and 264 B.C., when the First Punic War with Carthage began, Rome grew from a city-state of local importance in Latium to become the chief power in Italy. At first the Romans and their Latin kindred had difficulty in holding back the Etruscans and the Italic hill people from Latium. In 391 B.C. Rome itself was occupied briefly by Celtic invaders, who swept across the Alps into Italy. In the following century, however, the Romans were able to knit the diverse peoples of Italy together into a confederation under Roman leadership. Unlike the Greek city-states, Rome worked out a formula for bringing foreign peoples into loyal union with itself and laid the foundation for an Italian nation.

During this period of expansion in Italy the Romans also developed their Republic into a strong, unified state. The Roman constitution did not come into being at a single stroke in 509 B.C. as a statement of principles and practice written by the founders of the Republic, but was the product of a lengthy, complicated growth. The political institutions grew partly from the continuous pressure exerted by military needs for defense and expansion, and partly from the struggle of the plebeians for political privilege and economic relief. At times the plebeian leaders made skillful use of a military crisis to obtain what they wanted; at other times the dominant patricians abused their privileges and evaded their responsibilities, but each group remained loyal to Rome and both groups were steadily brought closer to each other by successive adjustments. When finally, in 287 B.C., the principle of popular sovereignty was asserted, the first phase of Rome's long political history came to an end. The course of growth is often obscure for the same reasons as it is for monarchical Rome, and, when we can see the Romans in political action by the third century B.C., their institutions seem to be very awkward and full of duplication and overlapping. Yet

The reader will find Map XV (page 416) useful as he reads this chapter.

the institutions worked with surprising flexibility through almost two centuries of large-scale and continuous war, when Rome came into conflict with Carthage and the Hellenistic Kingdoms.

The Constitution of the Early Republic

According to Roman tradition, the revolution which overthrew the monarchy was engineered by the patrician families of Rome. We cannot be sure whether they were rudely provoked by the tyranny of Tarquin or whether their "revolution" was the final act of a long process of change in which the monarchy had weakened gradually. Perhaps Tarquin's rule was broken by his rivalry with another famous Etruscan king, Lars Porsenna of Clusium. The latter seems to have occupied Rome for a brief time and perhaps was overthrown by the general Latin uprising against the Etruscan overlords. If so, an opportunity was provided for the Roman patricians. Whatever the process, the patricians emerged in the early fifth century in firm control of Rome. They held the new magisterial offices which replaced the kingship, and they continued to serve as priests and members of the Senate. They also continued to control the Curiate Assembly by the predominance of their clan members and *clients* in the *curiae*. There was good reason for this patrician domination, in addition to their part in establishing the Republic. The new state was threatened by Etruscan attack and harassed by the raids of the hill peoples, so that the fighting qualities and leadership of the great patrician chieftains were needed. The revolution also consolidated the economic position of the patrician landowners, because trade, encouraged by the Etruscans, dwindled and agricultural interests prevailed once more.

PATRICIAN GOVERNMENT

The new heads of state, who took the place of the king, were two patrician magistrates, ultimately called consuls, who were elected annually by the assembly. They retained the symbols of kingship, sitting in state on an official (*curule*) chair, inlaid with ivory, and were accompanied in public by *lictors,* who carried the *fasces,* a bundle of rods fastened together containing an axe with its blade projecting from the bundle. The consuls possessed a broad, undefined power to carry out their duties as the executive heads of the state, but careful provision was made to prevent any permanent consolidation of power in their hands. The consul's authority in military affairs outside of Rome was absolute because he retained the *imperium* of the king, which gave him command of the army, authority in foreign affairs, and the power to impose the death sentence on Roman soldiers. The consuls also took the auspices before political action, but the *pontifex maximus* and an official who retained the king's title, *rex sacrificorum,* took over much of the routine practice of religious supervision. The consular *imperium* was limited in Rome itself, where citizens might appeal his verdict in capital cases to the assembly.

The most important curbs on consular power were the limitation of tenure to one year and the right of veto exercised by each consul on the public acts of his colleague. That is, each consul could say, "No," to his fellow and the action stopped. This principle of the veto between consuls was also extended to other Roman magistracies as they were created. At times this could and did result in paralysis, which was both embarrassing and dangerous. Various devices were tried to avoid such situations, but the principle remained a firm tenet of Roman practice. In Rome consuls came to exercise authority in alternate months, if both were in the city at the same time, and, if the two consuls were present on the field of battle, each exercised command on alternate days. At least such an arrangement imposed the need for joint consultation, and no great damage seems to have been done. In extremely critical conditions of war and sedition, however, a solution was found by the appointment of a dictator. The consuls, with the advice of the Senate, designated some tried and loyal man, who was invested with the sole and absolute authority in the state for a period of six months. He held *imperium* and was permitted to appoint an assistant, the *magister equitum* (master of the cavalry).

The Senate, recruited from prominent patricians, grew in prestige and authority because it possessed a continuity of existence through the life tenure of its members, while magistrates held office only for a year. In time, too, it became the regular practice for the consuls and other senior magistrates to enter the ranks of the Senate after their term of office. Obviously few would think seriously of challenging the advice of a body into which they were to enter as junior members. Thus, while the Senate could not legislate for the state, its expressions of opinion (*consulta*) acquired great force. The Senate, too, assumed the power of ratifying the acts of the assembly. The Curiate Assembly continued in existence, formally acting on proposals submitted to it, but its real functions were soon taken over by other assemblies which were developed to meet new situations as Rome grew.

While the power of the patricians had increased by the removal of the kingship, the plebeians lost ground, for they had almost no voice in government and no king to favor their cause. Soon after the founding of the Republic they began a struggle for political equality with the patricians, known as the Struggle of the Orders. While political privilege was the main goal, the different groups among the plebeians suffered from various disadvantages. The wealthy plebeian families, from whom leadership came, were primarily concerned to get political and social equality, the right to hold office and to enter the Senate. The urban plebeians, traders, craftsmen and laborers, had been hurt economically by the hostile attitude of their patrician government toward trade, but in this early period thought more of legal protection against the arbitrary conduct of patrician magistrates than of a general change in the tone of life in Rome. The rural plebeians, mainly the free farmers, but to an increasing degree the *clients* also, were concerned with their difficulties in making a living at farming, because of Rome's agrarian situation and harsh laws of debt.

The position of the farmer in Rome at this time was similar in many respects to that of the Athenian peasants in the pre-Solonian period (p. 207). Since land was scarce, the farmer's holding was small, consisting of two *iugera*, about one and one-third acres. He could probably graze his animals on public commons and was able theoretically to rent public land, the *ager publicus*. Usually, however, the farmer did not have the means to rent and to develop public land and, in fact, there was little available until Rome acquired new tracts by conquest. In the meantime his own holding might suffer from the continuous raiding by Rome's neighbors. Since there was much written about famine in fifth-century Rome, the farmer must have had to borrow grain frequently for seed and food from the wealthier landowners. As security he could pledge only his labor because the land itself was inalienable according to ancestral custom. Failure to pay the debt could result in being sold into slavery. To the rural plebeian, then, distribution of land, protection of his person, and amelioration of the laws of debt would seem most important.

All these factors played their part in stirring the plebeians to agitation. The traditional accounts of the Struggle of the Orders emphasize the use made by the plebeians of a walkout (*secessio*) in which they would withdraw from the city *en masse* and refuse to return until their demands were met. These walkouts did win specific gains, but the condition which allowed them to be effective was the result of a reorganization of the state to meet the needs of war. Plebeian help was needed to win Rome's battles.

THE SERVIAN REFORM

This reorganization of the state is known as the Servian Reform, since Roman tradition assigned it to Servius Tullius, the king who ruled before Tarquin the Proud. Possibly Servius did make the Roman army more up-to-date, but the resultant political developments seem to have taken place in the late sixth and fifth centuries. The new system replaced the old kinship grouping of Roman society by a territorial division into tribes and classified the citizens into five groups by a schedule of their wealth. Thus in Rome the Servian Reform had somewhat the same role as the Solonian property groupings in Athens. The new division separated the Romans into four urban tribes in the city of Rome and sixteen rural tribes in Roman land outside the city. As Roman territory increased, the number of rural tribes was multiplied until, in the third century, there were thirty-five in all. A complete registration of the citizens, patricians and plebeians alike, was made, both to assign individuals to the tribes and to classify them according to wealth. Five property classes were set up, presumably at first on the basis of land, although, later, monetary qualifications were substituted. Outside the classification were men of great wealth, who could serve in war as cavalry and maintain their own mounts, and men of no wealth, who were of little use in the warfare of the sixth and fifth centuries. For military service the tribes contributed an equal number of men, drawn mainly from the upper, wealthy class.

The system reflected the general change in the conditions of war in Italy during the late sixth and fifth centuries. As in early Greece there was a change over from cavalry and individual fighting to the disciplined phalanx of infantry, equipped with heavy body-armor. Accordingly, the Servian Reform replaced the old curial levy by the new *classis,* as it was called. For the purposes of the conscription the members of each class were divided into companies of about one hundred each, *centuries,* with each class having an equal number of senior *centuries,* men beyond military age (47–60) and junior *centuries* (17–46) of fighting men. Since the impact of war had to be borne by the wealthy, who could provide their own equipment, the cavalry, mainly made up of patricians, and the first class contained a greater number of *centuries,* who might be called for service in the field.

The following table indicates the allocation of *centuries* according to the schedule of wealth. The actual number of men in the cavalry and first class would be far less than of those in the poorer classes.

Cavalry	18 centuries
First Class	80 centuries
Second Class	20 centuries
Third Class	20 centuries
Fourth Class	20 centuries
Fifth Class	30 centuries
Supernumerary (proletarians)	5 centuries
	193 centuries

This system of levying the army developed into a political assembly, the Centuriate Assembly (*Comitia Centuriata,* "the nation in arms"), analogous to the army assembly of Macedonia. The assembly met at the sound of a trumpet blast in the Field of Mars and in its voting followed the order of classification. The votes were counted by *centuries;* each *century* determined its own vote, and a majority of the *centuries* carried the decision. Voting began with the cavalry *centuries* and proceeded down the schedule, *century* by *century,* until a majority was reached. A glance at the table indicates that a majority could be attained by the end of the first class. The Centuriate Assembly, then, was dominated by the wealthy citizens of Rome, who would usually vote in agreement, particularly on any matter touching their class interest. The system was by no means unfair for its period because the wealthy carried the actual burden of war, and the voting did give political voice to the wealthy plebeians whose means put them in the first class.

The new assembly took over the important functions of the older Curiate Assembly: to elect the consuls, to declare war, and to vote on the proposals which the consuls submitted to it. This legislative right was curtailed, however, by the need for senatorial ratification. Since the Romans were reluctant to discard any institution, the Curiate Assembly remained in existence, formally ratifying elected consuls and religious decisions. In a sense the assembly even became representative, for thirty members, one from each *curia,* were deemed a full assembly in the first century B.C.

Another important product of the Servian Reform was a new magistrate, the censor, who first appeared in 443 B.C. when he relieved the consuls of the task of classification. The censors, two in number, were elected normally every five years to conduct a registration, although their actual term of office was eighteen months. This was not merely a clerical duty because reassignment of individuals to lower classes might be involved, a result by no means pleasing to the vanity of those being demoted. The censorship soon added other duties—scrutiny of the senators' records and conduct, which might be made grounds for expulsion from the Senate, the letting of contracts for public works, and the enrollment of new members in the Senate and tribes. The censors were elected by the Centuriate Assembly but did not hold the *imperium*. Nevertheless the office was powerful and dignified and came to be regarded as the crown of a man's public career.

While this gradual reorganization of the whole state brought political voice to wealthy plebeians, it neither gave them access to the high offices of state nor secured legal and economic benefits for the poor. Early in the fifth century the plebeians began to organize to secure rights for themselves. They established a sort of state within the state, forming an assembly and electing officers of their own. These plebeian institutions were effective in gaining privileges and were finally brought into the structure of the state to become a regular part of the constitution when sovereignty of the whole people was recognized in 287 B.C.

The new Servian tribal arrangement seemed a convenient frame for organization to the urban plebeians which they soon used to establish a purely plebeian meeting of the four urban tribes, the *Concilium Plebis Tributum* (the Council of the Plebs by Tribes). In it the plebeians could discuss their grievances, form plans and select their own officers—the tribunes of the people—to protect their interests. Recognition of these officers was won from the patricians in 471 B.C., when the plebeians swore to put anyone to death who interfered with a tribune in the course of his duty. For the time being this duty was to protect plebeians from summary arrest by the patrician magistrates. The persons of the tribunes thus became sacrosanct and their *ius auxilii* (right of help) was established. Later in the fifth century this urban council was extended to include the rural tribes as well, and the number of tribunes was increased from four to ten. Their right of help developed into a veto on political action by which they could stop the working of the state.

The enlargement of the plebeian council to include all the tribes, probably twenty at this time, had the effect of converting it into an assembly of the people, although it is likely that patricians did not take part in the meetings at first. Even if they did, the plebeians outnumbered them and the meeting was recognized essentially as a plebeian assembly. While its primary function was to elect the tribunes, the assembly acquired a quasi-legislative right by registering expressions of popular opinion, which were called plebiscites. These did not have the force of law without senatorial approval but did carry great weight. The voting in the assembly, which became known as the *Comitia Tributa* (Tribal Assembly) was carried out by the usual group system, with each tribe reaching its own vote and a majority of the tribes determining the will of the assembly.

In the fourth century, when the relative ease of voting in the Tribal Assembly became apparent, it was consulted more and more frequently on important matters affecting the whole people and began to take a place alongside the Centuriate Assembly as one of the regular meetings of the Roman people.

The protection which the plebeians had won through their tribunes was the prelude to an agitation for codification of Roman custom, which in 451-50 B.C. culminated in the publication of the Twelve Tables. These twelve paragraphs, setting out the customs and legal practices of early Rome, became the basis of Roman law and a continuing source for its interpretation. In Cicero's day, four centuries later, young lawyers still learned the Tables by heart and appealed to them for precedents. There is a story that, preliminary to the drafting of the Tables, a commission was sent to Greece to study Greek law codes, but the content of the Twelve Tables seems to be purely local and Roman. Apparently the story is another of the type noticed before; it was intended to bring the beginnings of Rome into connection with Greece, in this case to give the Tables a prestige similar to that of the codes of the Greek Lawgivers.

The Tables were a mixture of primitive practice and of regulations to meet the needs which had forced their publication. Their significance lies partly in making the law known to all for the first time and partly in establishing all free men as equal before it. There was much detailed regulation of family and testamentary rights and of contracts and debt, with elaborate definition, if not amelioration, of the penalties for the latter. The Tables also defined the rights of association in Rome. This was helpful to the plebeians, because trade guilds (*collegia*) were recognized as legal organizations, although clubs which met in secrecy were prohibited as politically suspect. Since the formulas used in court procedure were not published, this important area of law remained the preserve of the priests; that is, they were veiled in religious secrecy and kept plebeians from free use of the courts.

PLEBEIAN EQUALITY

After these successes the plebeians turned their attention to other needs: access to the magistracies, social equality, and betterment of economic conditions for the poor. Perhaps their ambitions played some part in the temporary shelving of the consulship, which was used only sporadically between 445 and 366 B.C. Instead, some military tribunes, commanders of the tribal contingents in the army, were elected to hold consular power. Although this might be considered a patrician move to protect the consulship from plebeian encroachment, it may simply reflect the fact that Rome was engaged in several military operations at the same time in the late fifth and early fourth centuries. The dictatorship, too, was frequently used during this period.

But new minor offices, established about 420 B.C., were made available to plebeians. The consuls had been assisted by two officials, the quaestors, appointed by the consuls themselves. The number of quaestors was now increased to four and the office made elective. Two were assigned to help the consuls in war, where they served as quartermasters, while two remained in Rome as officials of the treasury. In this same period a new office, the aedileship, was established as a purely plebeian magistracy. Two aediles were elected to supervise the markets and public works and to act as police commissioners in the city. The establishment of their office was a mark of the growth of Rome, which by the late fifth century was beginning to regain its previous importance as a center of Latium and western Italy. Following upon the creation of these offices, there was a lull in plebeian agitation, while the Romans were engaged in continuous war, first on Etruscan Veii (p. 449) and then against the Gauls (pp. 449–50). The shock of the Gallic invasion evidently lessened confidence in patrician leadership. Not only were more plebeians elected as military tribunes, but a fierce struggle began which culminated in a series of measures passed in 367 B.C., the Licinian-Sextian laws, which breached the patrician hold on the high offices.

The Licinian-Sextian legislation restored the consulship, which became regular from 366 B.C., and allowed the plebeians to hold one position annually. At the same time, however, a new office with *imperium* was created, that of praetor, to be in charge of the civil administration in Rome and specifically of the law courts. There was ample need for an additional magistracy in Rome, but the creation of the praetorship has the mark of patrician counterthrust, because the office was reserved for patricians until 337 B.C. Also, the patricians secured for themselves the two new aedileships established at this time. Nevertheless, the plebeian wedge had been driven in, and in the remaining years of the fourth century all the high offices became available to plebeians: the dictatorship in 356 B.C., the censorship in 351 B.C., and, finally, the last to yield, the priestly colleges in 300 B.C. In effect, access to the important offices with *imperium* opened the way into the Senate, and the composition of that body changed.

The wealthy plebeians, once members of the Senate, rapidly acquired the outlook of their patrician colleagues and subscribed to the tradition of senatorial dignity and authority. The two orders had, in fact, been permitted to intermarry since 445 B.C. by the passage of the *Lex Canuleia*. Patricians and wealthy plebeians grew together into an oligarchy of wealth and position in which the holding of political office conferred ennoblement. In this new nobility the descendants of the great patrician houses were recognized as leaders, but the plebeian nobles supported the senatorial traditions, and thus the social conflict shifted to a struggle between all those privileged by wealth and position and those who remained poor.

In the fourth century the grievances of both the urban and the rural poor were aggravated. Although Roman territory had been increased by conquest and the state had made some public land available, the people complained that large tracts were rented to the wealthy while the people still suffered from debt. The number of urban plebeians had increased by immigration to Rome as the city grew in importance, but the newcomers were enrolled in the four urban

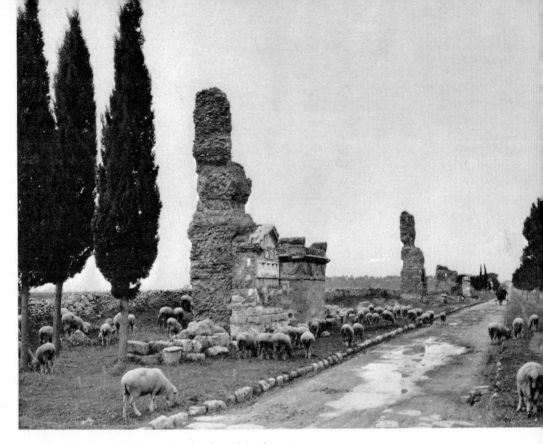

A stretch of the Appian Way, bordered with tombs and cypresses

tribes and were outvoted in the assembly by the rural tribes under the domination of the wealthy landowners. To add to the unrest, demands for military service increased because Rome had become involved in the Samnite Wars with the peoples of Central Italy (pp. 451-53).

The struggle entered its final stages in the closing years of the fourth century. First a series of new regulations softened the harshness of the laws of debt. These set interest charges, permitted property to be accepted as security on loans and forbade the imprisonment of debtors. In 312 B.C. a censor of liberal views, Appius Claudius, initiated other measures to relieve the urban poor. He began great public-works projects, mainly from military considerations, but the work provided considerable employment. An aqueduct, Rome's first, was built to bring water to the city, and a road, the Appian Way, was constructed to link Rome with Capua in Campania. Appius alarmed his colleagues in the government by enrolling some of the urban poor in the rural tribes, where their votes would count more. Fuel was added to the plebeian anger when the Senate unwisely reversed these classifications in 304 B.C. Although some concessions were hastily made—a handbook of legal formulas was published and the right of appeal to the assembly defined—plebeian demands focused on full political equality for all.

In 287 B.C. the plebeians withdrew from Rome and refused their cooperation until their demands were met. They had chosen the moment well, for Rome was just winding up the Samnite Wars, in which plebeian soldiers had played a large part. When they marched back into the city, the political fight had been won. The Senate approved a dictator, Hortensius, to deal with the situation, who sponsored the famous Hortensian Law. The Law recognized the plebiscites of the Tribal Assembly as valid and binding on the whole state, without senatorial ratification, so that the will of the people as a whole became sovereign. The tribunes, who could preside over the Tribal Assembly, soon were brought into the working of the state. They could sit with the Senate and their right to veto official actions was enlarged, thus putting them in a better position to paralyze the functioning of governmental machinery. Rome was far from being a democracy in practice, but the means had been won to implement popular sovereignty, if the people continued to care enough about it to use and extend their power.

The Romans, however, in the early third century B.C. did not think of their political struggle in these theoretical terms. The plebeians had suffered from certain practical disadvantages which they had corrected, but they had not discussed the relative values and principles of different forms of government. The upper class, too, was still unacquainted with the political debates carried on by Greek philosophers and with the practical experience of the Greek states. Thus, after 287 B.C. no deliberate effort was made to attain a more complete democratic system by removing the obstacles which stood in the way. These were not seen as obstacles, but simply as part of the Roman system, and the people's interest continued to focus on more immediate, practical problems.

There were many elements in the system of government which tended to consolidate the power of the upper class, and in Rome tradition was not lightly challenged. The magistracies were few in number and required continuous hard work. They were considered as honors which brought prestige, if no pay, to their holders. Only the wealthy could afford to serve, and so in practice the high magistracies became confined to a relatively few great families, whose generations of experience and social connections were at the disposal of their own members. A regular course of office (*cursus honorum*) established the steps by which a young man would rise in a political career from the minor posts of quaestor and aedile to the important offices with *imperium,* the praetorship and the consulship. Although Rome's tasks of government increased with the expansion of the state, there was great reluctance to increase the number of magistrates. Tenure of office was limited to one year, and it was felt improper to repeat a term until a long period of time, ten years, had elapsed, but in 327 B.C. an innovation of great significance for the future was made. A consulship was extended beyond its term to allow the holder to continue in military command by the device of proconsulship—he continued to act with consular powers in the field but without being re-elected. In this area where new offices might have been created none was made. The practice could provide governors for Rome's overseas provinces and continuity of generalship in war, but it also prevented extension of the number of offices and tended to consolidate the power of the governing class.

The authoritative position of the Senate as the real governing body in Rome was also inimical to the growth of democracy. The senators had had extensive experience in administration, knew the technicalities of Roman political practice, and had an intense corporate loyalty. An embassy sent by Pyrrhus to Rome reported that the Roman Senate was like an assembly of kings. While the Senate could not pass laws, senatorial resolutions, taken after debate, directed the conduct of the magistrates and formed the policy of the state. All continuing, important business was the province of the Senate: the strategy of wars, the allocation of monies, foreign policy, and the day-by-day task of keeping Rome in equilibrium. The assemblies, by contrast, were limited, since they could act only on the business submitted to them by their presiding officers, the consuls and the tribunes. The new formal sovereignty of the assembly was impaired in practice by lack of a secret ballot and by the control exercised over their *clients* by the senatorial families. When Rome entered upon great wars of conquest beyond the borders of Italy after 264 B.C., the momentum towards popular sovereignty was prolonged for a time, but by the end of the third century the pendulum moved back towards senatorial oligarchy. The conduct of overseas wars involved quick decisions and continuity of direction which only the Senate could give.

Roman Expansion in Italy

The revolt of Rome and the Latin people against their Etruscan rulers at the end of the sixth century B.C. heralded a general change in the organization of Italy in favor of the Italic peoples. The latter did possess some cultural basis for unity among themselves in their common Indo-European dialects and social organization. While this in itself did not result in political cohesion, it facilitated the coalescence of their tribes and peoples into larger units in response to Etruscan political pressure and to the civilizing influences from Etruria and the Greek colonies. Throughout the fifth century, as the Italic peoples gained strength, the Etruscans and Greeks were placed more and more on the defensive.

Those Italians, Umbrians and Samnites, who lived in the northern and central Apennines, pressed southwards, pushing some tribes into the coastal plains and encroaching on the territories of the Greek colonies in the southern part of Italy. The fields of Latium were raided by the Aequi and the Volsci from the nearby hills, when these peoples felt the pressure of the Samnites. The Samnites themselves moved down into the mountains east of Campania and after 450 B.C. forced their way into the rich Campanian plain. Capua was taken from its Etruscan rulers in 445 B.C. and Cumae from the Greeks in 426.

The new Samnite rulers of the coastal plain speedily learned city life and settled down to enjoy the wealth and luxurious living which Campania provided. Capua became the center of a league of Campanian towns and one of the richest cities of Italy. The Samnites of the hills, however, continued to live in scattered villages but gradually formed larger units and joined together in raids into the plain. Another group of Italic peoples, the Lucanians, moved into the south of the peninsula and pressed hard against the Greek colonies.

To unite the peoples of Italy, Rome had first to join with its own Latin neighbors in common defense against the Etruscans, the Aequi, and the Volsci; then, by military conquest, colonization and astute political settlements, it had to extend its authority over the Etruscans, the Italic peoples of Central Italy and the Greek cities of the south.

THE LATIN LEAGUE

According to Roman tradition union between Rome and the Latins was forged by an agreement, the *Foedus Cassianum*, after a Roman victory over the Latins at Lake Regillus in 493 B.C. There is reason to doubt the victory, for the terms of the treaty represent the Latins and Romans as equal parties, and it was perhaps against Etruscan Rome that the Latins fought (p. 438). The agreement, in fact, probably represents the culmination of a period of cooperation by Rome and the Latins against their mutual enemies rather than a start. It is to be dated later than 493 B.C. In any case, the ultimate union was very close and provided not only for common action in war but also for social unification. The two parties were to observe perpetual peace, to give mutual aid in war, and to divide their spoils in equal shares. Of more significance in the long run than the military agreement was the sharing of private rights of citizenship. A Latin could do business and hold property in Rome with full legal protection (*commercium*) and, if he married a Roman, his children could inherit his property and citizenship (*conubium*). Conversely a Roman had the same privilege in Latin towns. This exchange fostered the social and economic unification of Latium and ultimately became one of the regular devices by which the people of Italy were linked together.

Following the agreement between Rome and the Latins, a similar pact is said to have been concluded by them with the Hernici, who lived in the mountains behind the Aequi and Volsci. This early example of the principle "divide and conquer," which was to characterize Roman foreign policy, facilitated the wars in which Rome immediately became engaged. Perhaps war is too strong a term, because military action against the Aequi and Volsci was little more than a series of raids in the campaigning season to destroy crops and seize booty. Both Rome and the Latins, however, acquired additional territory and founded small colonies. Overpopulation in Latium was relieved to some extent and Roman soldiers gained experience and confidence. Roman tradition preserved and improved many stories about the wars. Perhaps the most familiar is that of Coriolanus, told by Plutarch and Shakespeare, who, from injured pride, turned traitor to Rome and led the Volsci against his city. There is also the story of Cincinnatus, taken from his ploughing to become dictator and lead Rome to victory against the Aequi, only to return with ostentatious modesty to his interrupted work.

Although the Etruscan Confederacy made no concerted effort to recover Rome, the Etruscan city of Veii, a few miles up the Tiber from Rome, remained a bitter foe. Veii was built on a seemingly impregnable precipice overhanging the river, from which vantage it controlled the road into southern Etruria and held a large and fertile territory, extending to Fidenae on the Latin side of the river. The Veians tried to force their way down the Tiber to the sea and for a time occupied the Janiculum Hill, where Vatican City now stands. Rome fought three wars against the Veians in the course of the fifth century, the first of which ended in Roman defeat. But in 425 B.C. the Romans took Fidenae, and after a lengthy, difficult siege Veii itself fell in 396 B.C. Despite Veii's importance, no help came from other Etruscan cities. Perhaps the Etruscans were already preoccupied with the threat of Gallic invasion, but more likely this lack of cooperation was a sign of decline.

The final war on Veii was an important landmark in Roman development. Since the siege of the city was protracted, the Romans introduced regular pay for their soldiers and began to change the army from a temporary levy of citizens into a force for more regular service. The victory also brought Rome its first large addition of territory. The city of Veii was destroyed and the people killed or enslaved, so that Veian territory was left free for Roman use. The land was declared public property and a large part distributed among the plebeians to quiet their agitation for agrarian relief. The Romans followed up the conquest by taking over the southern approaches to Etruria, where Satricum and Nepete were granted to the Latins for colonization, although Rome had kept all the Veian land for itself. The war had, in fact, been a Roman enterprise and was indicative of the more aggressive, dominating position which Rome had begun to take toward its Latin allies. Before this altered relationship could develop into open hostility, however, the Romans received a rude shock by the invasion of the Gauls who began to sweep down through Italy *ca.* 400 B.C.

THE GALLIC INVASION

This movement of the Celts or Gauls, as the Romans called them, was one of the thrusts of Celtic migration which took them by successive stages into Western Europe and the British Isles. They were peoples of Indo-European speech living in Central Europe from the Rhineland to the middle Danube who in the Early Iron Age had apparently developed the Hallstatt culture, so-called from the typical site at Hallstatt near Salzburg in Austria. The Celts lived in tribal groups, the chieftains in heavily walled towns, which served as refuge places for the population, and the ordinary people in farming villages. The culture is known, in particular, from the elaborate burials of the rulers, whose house-like tombs were covered by mounds containing weapons, chariots, tools, and precious objects. The metalware and art were distinctive, the latter showing considerable affinity to the animal-style work of the Scythians in southern Russia. Apparently population pressure and the movement of Germanic peoples into their homeland from the north and east set the Celts in motion. Some moved eastwards down the Danube and broke into Greece and Asia Minor in 279 B.C. (p. 366), but most settled in France and Britain. This particular group which came into Italy probably crossed the Alps to seek plunder in Italy, a place they may have heard of from Etruscan traders who had traveled into Celtic country since the seventh century.

The Gauls rapidly spread through the valley of the Po River between the Alps and the Apennines. While some remained to attack the Etruscan settlements in the region, a large force of about forty thousand crossed the mountains and pushed south towards Rome. They moved in tribal bands, men, women, children and animals, pressing on to plunder and burn rather than to seize the land and settle down. In battle the Gauls were a terrifying spectacle. The men fought naked with long, iron swords in a wild, shouting melée, spurred on by the cries of their women, and killing without mercy. A Roman army of about thirteen thousand men marched out of Rome to stop them at the Allia River before they could reach the city but were defeated and scattered with heavy loss. Rome was plundered and burnt, except for the Capitoline Hill, which held out under siege, and, when the Gauls began to tire of their relative inactivity, the Romans bribed them to move off to the north again. Some returned to the Po valley, but others stayed in the lower peninsula to sell their services as mercenary soldiers or to settle in small groups. In the north the Etruscan garrison towns, like that at Marzabotto, were overrun about 350 B.C. by the Gauls, who then began to settle down on Etruscan lands and who combined farming with raids south of the mountains. The Romans not only lost their city and property in the raid but their control of Latium as well and had to make a fresh start.

Rome was made defensible again by the construction of a new fortification wall of stone, the so-called Servian Wall, parts of which are still standing. The state was strengthened internally by the concessions to the plebeians in the Licinian-Sextian laws (p. 444), and control over Latium was recovered and extended. Rome resumed its domineering attitude, denying a share in some Volscian territory to the Latins and alarming them by extending its political interest to the Samnites and the towns of Campania to the south. In 354 B.C. Rome made a treaty with the Samnites, ostensibly against the Gauls, but to the Latins it seemed as if Rome were encircling them. Six years later, in 348 B.C., the Latins were again affronted by a Roman treaty with Carthage, in which Rome acted for the Latin coastal towns without consulting its allies.

THE LATIN REVOLT

By 340 B.C. the Latins had determined to make a stand against Rome. The time seemed propitious because Rome was disturbed by plebeian agitation and because help was promised by the Campanians. Accordingly, the Latin League demanded independence from Rome or full equality. The Romans refused to negotiate and in several swift campaigns defeated the Latin and Campanian forces by 338 B.C. The Latin League was dissolved, but the ensuing settlement was thoroughly fair and marked an important step in the establishment of the Roman Confederacy in Italy. Several of the Latin towns nearest to Rome were granted full Roman citizenship, while retaining their local self-government. In 322 B.C. one of their citizens, a man of Tusculum, was elected consul. Other towns, farther from Rome, were granted half-citizenship (*civitas sine suffragio*) by which they enjoyed the private rights of *commercium* and *conubium,* and their citizens could attain Roman citizenship by moving their residence to Rome. These towns, too, retained local independence but followed the Roman lead in foreign affairs and provided troops for Rome's wars. Still other Latin towns, those farthest from Rome, were made equal allies but tied closely to Rome by the retention of private rights with that city although these were terminated among themselves. The town of Antium on the coast did receive a small garrison of Roman soldier-settlers, who were organized separately from Antium. The people of Antium kept local government in their own hands. While these arrangements destroyed the Latin League, they substituted the framework of a confederacy in which citizenship was granted to some and made available in time to the rest of the Latins. A loyal core of citizens and allies was formed around Rome, which remained firm in the severe test which the Romans were about to experience in the Samnite Wars.

THE SAMNITE WARS

So long as Rome was involved with the Latins, Gauls, and hill people in the region adjacent to Latium, it had been to the interest of both Samnites and Romans to remain on friendly terms. When the Latins became solidly united with Rome in the Confederacy, Roman interests enlarged to the south, to Campania, and the Samnites began to fear that they would be blocked from the plain and access to the sea. Rome established friendly relations with some Campanian towns, founded some colonies in Campania, and in 328 B.C. made an alliance with one faction in the Greek city of Neapolis (Naples), where a Samnite garrison had been established. When that garrison was forced to leave, the Samnites confronted Rome with an ultimatum to withdraw soldiers from a colony which had been placed at Fregellae in the valley of the Liris River. The Romans rejected the demand and began to attack the Samnites in their mountain valleys. The war was to prove long and difficult, for the fighting was mainly in the mountains, where the Romans discovered that their phalanx formation was too rigid and awkward to cope with the Samnites. In its later phases the war became almost a war for Italian independence against Rome, when the Umbrians, the hill people of the northern Apennines, the Etruscans, and some Gauls were drawn in. Perhaps none of these peoples regarded the conflict in this light, for their alliance was very loose, but Roman victory did make Rome the dominant power of Italy, while the grueling fighting converted the Roman soldiers into a first-rate, formidable army, able to meet the Hellenistic mercenaries of Pyrrhus, trained in the tactics of Alexander and the Successors.

During the first phase of the war, 326–16 B.C., the Romans were soundly defeated. They engaged at first in some indecisive skirmishing in the foothills, but in 321 B.C. a large Roman army was trapped by the Samnites in the valley of the Caudine Forks. The Romans tried to break out, but danger of starvation forced them into a humiliating peace on Samnite terms. The army was required to march under a yoke of crossed spears, 600 Roman cavalrymen were held as hostages, and the Romans were forced to withdraw their garrisons from the territory which the Samnites regarded as their own and to keep the peace. Rome observed the terms until 316 B.C., when a pretext was found to renew the war. Again the Romans were defeated by a Samnite army which forced its way to the coast at Lautulae, near Terracina. Although some of Rome's Campanian allies defected to the Samnite side, the Confederacy around Rome remained firm, and when in 315 B.C. the Romans won a victory near Terracina they turned to vigorous prosecution of the war. By 312 B.C. the Romans had regained their hold on Campania and started to hem the Samnites into their hills by the foundation of new colonies and garrisons. The construction of the Appian Way was authorized by the censor Appius Claudius to provide a good military road along which troops could be moved quickly from Latium to Campania.

By this stage of the war the Romans had digested their lesson in mountain fighting and converted the army into legionary formations, which gave it flexibility and speed of maneuver. The legion was made up of 4200 men, 3000 heavy-armed and 1200 light-armed troops. They were brigaded into companies of 60 men and were arranged in battle in a staggered formation with gaps between both the companies and the individual soldiers. A short javelin was adopted in place of the heavy spear, and proper age and battle experience, rather

Lucanian cavalrymen in a tomb at Paestum (late fourth century B.C.)

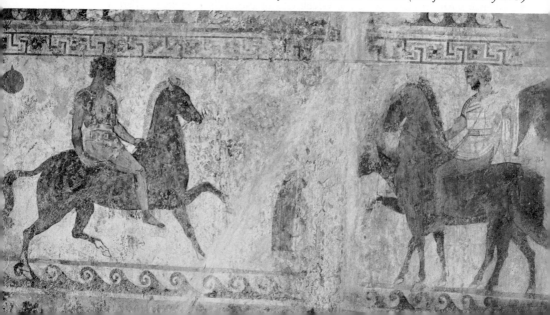

than wealth, put men in the first line of battle. Accordingly, when the Etruscans and the Umbrians joined the Samnites to crush Rome's growing power, Rome was able to deal effectively with its enemies on both the northern and southern fronts.

The Etruscans and Umbrians were defeated first, then the Samnites were rolled back and confined to their hill country. They were not finished, however, and in 299 B.C. took advantage of another Gallic thrust into Central Italy to reopen the war. When the Umbrians, Gauls and Etruscans again made common cause with the Samnites, Rome was faced with the need to make a full-scale mobilization of its own and its allies' troops. In 295 B.C. an army of forty thousand men, the largest which Italy had yet seen, was put into the field against the Italian coalition at Sentinum and won decisively. The coalition was broken, but the Samnites were not hunted out and forced into surrender until four years later. The victory at Sentinum, however, put an end to large-scale, concerted resistance. By 278 B.C. Rome had extended its network of colonies, allies and incorporated towns into the key areas of Italy from northern Etruria to the lands of the Lucanians and of the Greek colonies in the southern end of the peninsula.

The addition of the Greeks and Lucanians of southern Italy to the Roman Confederacy resulted from the defeat of King Pyrrhus of Epirus who invaded Italy in 278 at the invitation of Tarentum (p. 414). The big and wealthy city of Tarentum, founded as a Spartan colony, had gradually taken over the role of defending the Greek cities of southern Italy against the native Italic peoples. The people of Tarentum, who traded continuously across the Ionian Sea with western Greece, from time to time had called on their fellow Greeks for aid. In 282 B.C. the Lucanians attacked the Greek city of Thurii which, instead of turning to Tarentum, appealed to Rome for aid. The Romans responded and put a garrison into Thurii to hold the town. Tarentum was outraged at this interference in its own zone of influence and, when a small Roman fleet visited the waters off Tarentum, attacked the ships successfully and went on to take over Thurii. Tarentum refused to make amends to Rome and invited the assistance of Pyrrhus.

Pyrrhus quickly appeared in Italy with an army of twenty thousand men and about twenty war elephants, nominally to aid Tarentum, but, to judge from the size of the force, to acquire territory in Italy. Pyrrhus met the Romans in battle at Heraclea and won a costly, "Pyrrhic," victory with the aid of his elephants, the first which many Romans had ever seen. He marched north to Latium but was unable to take Rome and withdrew again to the south, where he defeated another Roman army at Asculum. At this point Carthage, wishing to take advantage of the general disturbance to expand in Sicily, made an alliance with Rome against Pyrrhus. Rome scarcely needed the help, for Pyrrhus had lost heavily in his battles and the Tarentines, seemingly safe, were turning lukewarm. Accordingly, Pyrrhus was glad to accept a call for help from Syracuse against the Carthaginians and moved his army into Sicily. He made a brilliant campaign there, driving the Carthaginians out of their positions, except for the big base at Lilybaeum. But when Pyrrhus expressed ideas of becoming the suzerain of Sicily himself, his Sicilian Greek allies withdrew support. In 275 B.C. Pyrrhus returned to Italy. He fought the Romans again at Beneventum but this time was unable to defeat them with his depleted forces and the limited Greek help given to him. Pyrrhus sailed back to Greece, leaving the Romans the masters of southern Italy.

Victory over Pyrrhus ushered Rome into the arena of Mediterranean political life and served notice that a strong, new power had arisen which was determined to preserve Italy for the Italian peoples under Roman leadership. The Roman Confederacy was a new type of organization among the Mediterranean powers who did not understand its strength and resiliency.

The Roman Confederacy

Although the Etruscans, Greeks and Italic peoples had established some uniformity of language and institutions in the various areas of Italy in which they had settled, Rome welded these diverse elements into a state. Italy was not to become a nation until the first century B.C., but the direction in which its peoples were to proceed was indicated by 264 B.C., when the great Roman wars of overseas conquest began. By that time Rome had developed hard and ruthless methods of war but had learned to use its victories with rare political skill. The soldiers fought with a stubborn conviction that their cause was right and with unswerving loyalty to Rome. They might, and frequently did, lose the first battles of their wars, but not the last. Rome demanded absolute surrender from its enemies and left no ground for compromise. The Romans wanted to dictate the terms of peace, even if the terms turned out to be almost what the enemy wanted in the first place, as in the case of the Latin League. The settlements were not vindictive and took the differing situations of the people with whom Rome dealt into account. The Romans had not set out with any systematic plan for conquest nor a ready-made formula for a Roman confederation, but, as in the case of their constitution, found a practical solution for the immediate issue with which they were confronted.

The Confederacy was very complex in its minute adjustments of the various members to Rome but it did exhibit certain general principles. Rome demanded military service and full control of foreign policy. The only tax which the members paid, however, was the *portoria* (customs duty) which was also paid by Romans. Although the garrisons of Rome were seldom quartered in any member community, the Romans not only insisted on peace in the Confederacy but they also protected Italy from foreign invaders. Most important was the readiness with which Roman citizenship was extended to those prepared for it and the establishment of various grades of privilege through which foreign peoples could advance to citizenship. The focus of the Confederacy was Rome, which directed its policy, but, as Roman citizenship was given, the members

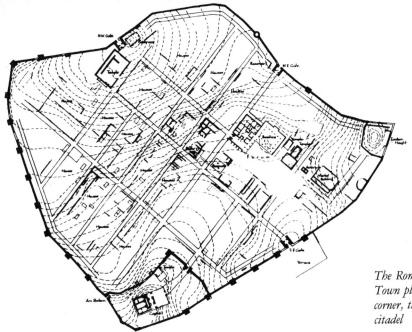

The Roman colony at Cosa. Town plan: in the lower corner, the arx, *or citadel*

acquired a share in policy-making by their enrollment into the tribes, their vote in the assemblies and eligibility for office.

In the third century B.C. there were two broad categories of members, those with full or partial Roman citizenship and those who were allied to Rome by individual treaties. The full citizens were all enrolled in the Roman tribes and exercised their political rights in Rome itself, wherever they might live in Italy. The largest group, of course, were those resident in Rome and in the land adjacent to the city, but many citizens had been granted allotments of public land elsewhere as individuals or as members of Roman colonies, so that the citizenry was scattered. The Roman colonies had been planted in the course of the wars for strategic purposes, mainly along the west coast from Tarquinii to Naples and inland along important roads northeast of Rome across to the Adriatic. The colonists were soldier-settlers, who acted as a garrison but had both local government in their colony as well as their Roman citizenship. They were sometimes placed in the territory of older towns, where they gradually mingled with the inhabitants until differences were obliterated. Some municipalities of non-Roman origin also possessed Roman citizenship as the result of political settlement, like the Latin communities in 338 B.C. Another large group of municipalities in Latium, Etruria, and Campania possessed only the private rights of citizenship (*commercium* and *conubium*) with the possibility of attaining the vote and the right to hold office when they were considered ready, that is, thoroughly Romanized. Most of these towns had their own local magistrates, councils, and assemblies, but their jurisdiction was divided with the Roman praetor in Rome or with his representative, who visited the municipalities. By 264 B.C. most of Etruria, Latium, Campania, and the mountain lands over to the Adriatic Sea had full or half-citizenship, and by 150 B.C. this

455

condition of half-citizenship had virtually disappeared, inasmuch as the holders had been promoted to full rights.

The communities allied to Rome were alien and, theoretically, independent, although the terms of the alliances varied greatly because each pact was made individually. The Romans, in fact, preferred to make alliance with the smallest unit of a people, the individual community or tribe, rather than with the people as a whole. One group of allies, however, possessed the so-called Latin Right (*Ius Latinum*) and were called the Latin Allies. These consisted of the Latin colonies, as distinguished from the Roman colonies, founded before the dissolution of the Latin League in 338 B.C., and colonies with the same rights as the earlier group but founded after that date. Their status was very similar to that of municipalities with Roman private rights. The Latin colonies not only had *commercium* and *conubium* with Rome, but individuals might also obtain Roman citizenship by changing their residence to Rome. The colonies did, however, possess complete self-government and raised and paid the troops which were required from them for Rome's service. This type of colony had been used to pen the Samnites in their hills, and after serving that purpose these colonies formed an outer ring of protection for Rome, beyond the protective cordon of Roman citizens. The other allies, such as the Greek cities of southern Italy, were bound by various types of treaties, equal and unequal, but usually possessed full local government without garrisons or Roman superintendence. They paid no tribute to Rome but were liable for military service—in the case of the Greeks, naval service—and surrendered their foreign policy to Rome's direction. Thus, by one thread or another, from full citizenship to free alliance, all of Italy was tied to Rome.

Within these political ties to Rome was woven the closer fabric of social and economic unification, which began to knit the peoples of Italy together into a nation. The Roman roads, like the Appian Way, were built primarily for military purposes, but they also encouraged commerce and ordinary travel. In the territory which they had taken over the Romans built bridges, cleared the land, and started drainage projects. In the early third century, perhaps in 269 B.C., the Romans issued their first silver coinage. It was designed primarily for Roman interests in Italy rather than in the city itself and in a few generations had replaced the local issues. Roman law and institutions were adopted gradually and a common Italian culture came into being. The physical resources of the Roman Confederacy made it potentially more powerful than Carthage or any of the Hellenistic Kingdoms. Its territory was greater than that of Macedonia, Carthage, and Egypt, while its available manpower for war was far greater. It is conjectured that in 265 B.C. the number of Roman citizens was about 1,000,000 of whom 292,000 were adult males. The allies in 225 B.C. could provide an additional 375,000 men. The Roman armies, of course, drew only a part of this pool of men for actual service, but the potential far outnumbered the supply of trained Greek soldier-settlers and mercenaries on whom the Hellenistic Kingdoms or Carthage could individually call.

XXI

The Wars of Conquest
(264–134 B.C.)

THE RESPONSIBILITIES OF LEADERSHIP in Italy, which had involved Rome in a war of defense against the invader, Pyrrhus, speedily confronted the Romans with further difficult problems and led them into the series of wars which resulted in the establishment of an overseas empire. These problems arose partly from the geographical position of Italy itself, both continental and Mediterranean, and partly from Rome's previous isolation from the political life of the other Mediterranean powers. The memory of the burning of Rome by the Gauls in 390 B.C. was still fresh in Roman memory, and some of the Gauls who remained in Italy had joined in the Samnite Wars against Rome. Since the northern Apennines were no real barrier to further inroads, in 225 B.C. Rome had to deal with another Gallic invasion. In this case Rome tried to find a solution by subjugating the Gauls in Italy and by creating the province of Cisalpine Gaul, thus extending Italy to its natural frontier of the Alps. The incorporation of the Greeks of South Italy into the Roman Confederation involved Rome in the rivalry of Carthaginians and Greeks for Sicily and for control of the Tyrrhenian Sea. Although Rome had engaged in no previous conflict of interest with Carthage, in 264 B.C. she decided on intervention in Sicily at the almost certain risk of war. The Greeks of South Italy also traded across the Ionian Sea to Greece and into the Adriatic. The piracy of the Illyrians, who operated from the Greek side of the Adriatic, provoked Roman intervention and led to the establishment of a protectorate in western Greece in the 220's. This advance brought Rome into a conflict of interest with Macedonia and speedily led to the Macedonian Wars.

Rome thus accepted the consequences of leadership in Italy and was led by a lengthening chain of circumstance into the wars of conquest. In the third century B.C. victory over Carthage in the Punic Wars gave the Romans control

The reader will find the Front Endpaper and Maps VII and XV (pages 172–73 and 416) useful as he reads this chapter.

of the western Mediterranean. In the second century Macedonia was defeated and made a province of Rome, and the Seleucids were rolled back into Syria. The more obvious causes of imperialistic expansion do not explain the Romans' willingness to emerge from their isolation and to commit themselves to lengthy wars fought overseas. Rome was not a commercial state and was not concerned in establishing overseas markets or to find colonial regions for its surplus population. In the third and early second centuries there were no financial groups in Roman society with sufficient political power to influence policy. The acquisition of territory and subject peoples for the sake of tribute is not an adequate explanation because the Romans were very slow to assert title and to assume the responsibilities of administration in the lands of their defeated enemies. Accordingly, Roman imperialism is usually explained as defensive: the Romans fought with Carthage and the Greek powers to prevent attack, or fancied attack, on themselves. While it is hardly correct to say that the Romans conquered the world in self-defense, they plainly found it impossible to live on equal terms with the other great Hellenistic powers. The Romans regarded them with extreme distrust and suspicion.

The First Punic War (264–41 B.C.)

While Rome was growing to power in Italy, Carthage had developed a commercial empire in the western Mediterranean (p. 312). The aims of each state were essentially different, and on several occasions Carthage and Rome had affirmed their friendship. In 306 B.C. the Carthaginians pledged not to interfere in Italy, while the Romans had undertaken not to interfere in Sicily. Each had promised mutual aid against Pyrrhus, although neither side had availed itself of the other's help during the war. Rome did complain, later, about the appearance of a Carthaginian fleet off Tarentum in 272 B.C., when the Romans were besieging the city, but the incident was passed over at the time. Whether the Carthaginians came in the hope of taking Tarentum themselves, as the Romans later alleged, or to help them in the siege is not clear because the fleet sailed off immediately. Perhaps the episode had some effect in rousing Roman suspicions that Carthage might move into South Italy, but the Romans themselves invited war eight years later by deliberately interfering in Sicilian affairs against the spirit, if not quite the letter, of their agreements with Carthage.

Circumstances were favorable for Carthaginian expansion into eastern Sicily in 265 B.C. The former tyrant of Syracuse, Agathocles, who had held the Carthaginians in check, had been succeeded by a young ruler, Hiero, whose hold was still insecure. Agathocles had put a garrison of Italian mercenary soldiers, the Mamertines, into the city of Messana in northeastern Sicily near the Strait of Messina. After his death the Mamertines took over Messana, killed the male citizens, married their women, and settled down to a life of piracy and collecting tolls, really protection money, on the shipping in the strait. It was to the interest of both Syracuse and of Carthage to destroy them. In 265

B.C. Hiero attacked and defeated the Mamertines, who saved their city for the moment by inviting Carthaginian help. Since Messana was too valuable a prize for the Carthaginians to give up, the garrison remained. The Mamertines, already estranged from Syracuse, invited Rome to oust the Carthaginians and to restore Mamertine independence. The Roman Senate was reluctant to accept the Mamertine request on the grounds that Rome should have no alliance with such a gang of scoundrels and pirates. The description was correct, but probably the Senate was reluctant to risk war with Carthage, which would be in violation of the treaty of 306 B.C. and would be a very difficult war to win because of Rome's lack of sea power. Also, the possibility of long campaigns strengthened popular demands for more political privilege. Accordingly, the Senate refused to decide and passed the question of alliance to the assembly. The popular leaders, including a son of Appius Claudius, the censor of 312 B.C., advocated sending help to the Mamertines, probably presenting the case as a necessary move to forestall Carthaginian expansion into eastern Sicily and ultimately into Italy.

When Rome dispatched an army of two legions to southern Italy, the Carthaginian commander, acting on his own decision, withdrew his garrison from Messana to allow a small Roman force to move in. The Carthaginian government, however, rushed troops to Sicily and made an alliance with Hiero of Syracuse to keep the "Italian barbarians," the Romans, out of Sicily. Messana was blockaded, and Rome declared war when the Carthaginians and Hiero refused to lift the blockade. Although the Romans had no fleet, except for a small force of twenty outmoded triremes and the naval aid which might be levied from the Greeks of South Italy, they succeeded in getting their army across to Sicily and set out to fight a war by land for the island. The Carthaginians put a large force into Agrigentum, planning to supply it and their other bases in Sicily by sea. They regarded the struggle as a colonial war for the defense of Sicily and made little attempt to use their sea power to attack Rome in Italy. The First Punic War, then, was essentially a conflict to get control of Sicily and the waters of the Tyrrhenian Sea.

Our sources for the war are fragmentary and preserve only episodes from its course, so that at times the motives which lie behind the moves of both Rome and Carthage are not clear. At first the Romans pressed their attack vigorously and achieved considerable success. Syracuse was besieged and Hiero, not too reluctantly, broke his alliance with Carthage and joined Rome. He was penalized by limitation of Syracusan territory to an area within a radius of thirty miles from the city and by a war indemnity of a hundred talents. The Romans took Agrigentum after a difficult siege and put its population to death or sold them as slaves. This severity, both to Syracuse and to Agrigentum, which seems to have alienated Greek and native Sicel feeling for Rome, made the land war, which Rome had envisaged, more difficult. Carthage showed no intention of coming to an agreement, and by 260 B.C. the Romans decided that they would have to become a maritime power to win a decision.

According to tradition the Romans used a wrecked Carthaginian ship as their model and built 120 vessels in two months. The model was hardly needed because both Romans and South Italian Greeks were familiar with Carthaginian ships, but the Romans did adopt the Carthaginian quinquireme as their standard warship. This was a strong, heavy vessel in which each oar was pulled by five men. To enable the boarding of enemy ships, the Romans fitted out their new vessels with a *corvus,* a sort of gangplank with a great spike in the end, by which they could make fast to the deck of an enemy. The first Roman war fleet, numbering about 140 ships, put to sea in 260 B.C. and speedily demonstrated the value of the new *corvus* by an impressive victory at the battle of Mylae. Fifty Carthaginian ships were taken, and their rams were sent to Rome to decorate the Roman Forum. Possession of a fleet opened up the war for Rome, since attack on the Carthaginian supply fleets and on Carthage itself was now possible.

In 256 B.C. a large expedition of 250 warships, eighty transports and about a hundred thousand men sailed for Cape Bon on the African coast. The fleet won a victory en route off Cape Ecnomus in eastern Sicily and landed successfully on Carthaginian territory. Although some damage was done to the farms, it was too late in the year to attack Carthage itself; therefore the consul Regulus and two legions were left in Africa to stir up the Numidian chieftains against Carthage and to await the arrival of the fleet in the following spring. During the winter the Carthaginians hired a Spartan mercenary soldier, Xanthippus, who trained their army and put the city in order for the coming action. Regulus, who had failed to rouse the Numidians, rashly advanced to meet him before the main Roman army returned and was heavily defeated by an elephant charge through his small force. Regulus himself was captured, and only two thousand Romans escaped to the coast where they waited for the fleet. The men were picked up and another Carthaginian fleet defeated, but Carthage itself was secure. The Roman fleet on its return to Italy ran into a storm and lost all but eighty ships. Apparently the Roman boarding devices were so heavy that they made the ships unseaworthy and hard to maneuver, however valuable they were for close fighting. Yet the Romans energetically built another fleet and pressed the war by land in Sicily. In 254 B.C. the big Carthaginian base at Panormus (Palermo) was taken which gave access to the western part of the island.

In the following years the war moved into a phase in which neither side could achieve a decisive victory. The Romans won minor sea battles, but lost an important engagement off Drepana, and several fleets were destroyed by storms. They settled down to a protracted siege of the Carthaginian bases at Lilybaeum and Drepana. The Carthaginians were more interested, seemingly, in extending their territory in Africa than in vigorous action in Sicily. In 247 B.C. Carthage did send an able and vigorous commander to Sicily, Hamilcar Barca, who preyed on the Roman siege lines from high in the mountains and raided the coast of Italy, but not enough men were sent to exploit the openings and to enlarge the war. Probably the Carthaginian government suffered from a divided policy. The conservative oligarchs, led by Barca's enemy, Hanno, were in control and favored action in Africa, counting on the stubborn resistance at Lilybaeum and Drepana, coupled with Barca's guerilla raids, to force Rome into an agreement which would leave them a hold on Sicily. The Romans, however, doggedly kept up their action by land and sea and finally, in 242 B.C., won a decisive naval victory off the Aegates Islands. A Carthaginian supply fleet, bringing material to Lilybaeum, was destroyed. The Carthaginian commander made terms of peace, which were later stiffened by the Romans after they had taken Lilybaeum.

The peace settlement made in 241 B.C. left Rome in full control of Sicily. The terms required Carthaginian evacuation of the island, surrender of the smaller islands between Sicily and Italy, and the payment of a war indemnity of 3,200 talents in ten years. Carthage had been broken as a sea power, while Rome emerged from the long grueling struggle of twenty-three years with a successful navy, provided that it stayed in harbor in bad weather. During the war, alliances had been made with Hiero of Syracuse and with other Greek communities. These were maintained, and the allies were placed in essentially the same category as the Greeks of South Italy. The half of Sicily taken from Carthage was put under Roman supervision and paid a tax in grain and other produce which Rome could sell in Italy or use to supply its army (pp. 484–85).

Since Carthage had been left in full control of Africa and its other possessions in the western Mediterranean, recovery from the war would have been a matter of time and careful management. The city, however, was faced with an immediate crisis. The mercenary soldiers in Carthage and in Sardinia mutinied. Rome allowed Carthage to procure supplies in Italy for the struggle in Africa, and by 238 B.C. the situation there was under control. On the other hand, the Romans accepted a request for help from the soldiers in Sardinia and took over that island and Corsica as provinces. Control of the Tyrrhenian Sea and the waters of western Italy was thus secured by the possession of the three great islands, Sicily, Sardinia, and Corsica.

This additional loss to Carthage weakened the state considerably and apparently led to the ascendancy of the Barca family in its internal politics. The Barcas seem to have suggested the intensive development of Spain as a substitute for the Tyrrhenian region, and in 237 B.C. Hamilcar Barca was sent to Spain as governor. He was succeeded in 229 by his son-in-law, Hasdrubal, who had been the popular leader in Carthage, and in 221 by Hamilcar's son, Hannibal. Under the Barcas Spain was turned into a prosperous and strong province. The silver mines of the Sierra Morena Mountains and the copper deposits of the Rio Tinto mining region were developed intensively to finance the undertaking. Carthaginian influence was extended inland in southern and eastern Spain from the trading posts on the coast, and the tribal peoples were brought into a new Carthaginian army, well trained and disciplined. A large base and trading center was constructed at New Carthage (Cartagena).

Roman tradition represented this development in Spain as the private work

Punic inscription
from Carthage

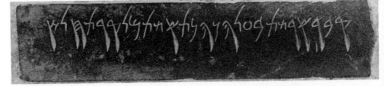

of the Barca family, dedicated to a war of revenge on Rome, but the program evidently had the continuous support of Carthage itself. Rome apparently did not allow the development to proceed without question. In 231 B.C. it is said that a Roman commission was told by Hamilcar that the development of Spain was to pay off the war indemnity to Rome. This, if true, scarcely left room for objection, but in 226 the Romans obtained an assurance from Hasdrubal that he would not lead soldiers across the Ebro River, thus setting a limit to the Carthaginian province. Roman interest in Spain was probably stimulated by the old Greek colony of Massilia. Massilia, which had become an ally of Rome, was concerned about its trade in northeastern Spain. Rome, for its part, needed to foster the alliance at this time because the Gauls in northern Italy, reinforced by their kindred from across the Alps, were preparing to strike down into Central Italy once again. Perhaps, too, Rome wished to forestall a possible alliance between Hasdrubal and the Gallic chieftains north of the Pyrenees.

The Gauls and Illyrians

The Gauls settled along the Po River had remained quiet during Rome's war with Pyrrhus and throughout the First Punic War, but in the 230's new bands of Transalpine Gauls began to move into the region. They disturbed those already there and rekindled desires to raid south of the Apennines. In 236 B.C. a group of the new arrivals and the settled Boian people struck toward the town of Ariminum on the Adriatic coast but broke up in discord before doing any serious damage. Probably to afford protection against such raids a tribune, Flaminius, carried a proposal in 232 B.C. for extensive distribution of public land south of Ariminum to the Roman poor. Because the prospect of more intensive Roman development so close to their own territory disturbed the Gauls, the tribes gathered for invasion.

In 226 B.C. a mass of about seventy thousand poured over the mountains into Etruria and headed for Rome, burning and plundering. But rather than fight down through the peninsula against the Roman armies raised to meet them, the Gauls swung over to the west coast, intending to return home. At Telamon they were trapped between two Roman armies and suffered a bloody defeat, losing about forty thousand men. The Romans decided to settle the threat once and for all by pushing the frontier of Roman Italy to the Alps. The conquest was begun in 225 and two years later Flaminius marched successfully into the heart of Gallic territory. The conquest of Gallia Cisalpina, as the new province was called, was wound up in 220 B.C. by the reduction of Istria, and development of the region was started by the founding of several Latin colonies. The Gauls, however, remained resentful and ready for revenge.

While this action was being taken against the Gauls in North Italy, a new problem was presented by Illyrian piracy in the Adriatic and Ionian Seas to the east. The Illyrians had long made a practice of sallying out from their little harbors into the adjacent waters, but about 230 B.C. the scope of their raids was enlarged. At that time the Illyrian queen, Teuta, who had extended Illyrian influence over Epirus and Acarnania to the south, was raiding shipping in the Ionian Sea and even on the coast of Italy. To protect their own communications around the end of Italy and the trade of their new Greek allies, the Romans undertook a policing action.

In 229 B.C. a fleet of two hundred ships was sent to Corcyra, where Teuta's governor, Demetrius of Pharos, surrendered to Rome. A small Roman army, put ashore on the Greek coast at Apollonia, advanced northwards with the fleet, accepting the surrender of the Greek islands and towns en route. Teuta was allowed to retain her throne but had to relinquish authority over the area which the Romans had occupied. The Romans made a protectorate of the region and avowed their friendship for its peoples. Their concern was demonstrated again in 219 B.C., when another such action was taken against Demetrius of Pharos who had resumed raiding. Because these Roman policing actions were as welcome to most Greeks as to the traders of South Italy, Rome laid up a measure of goodwill with some of the small states of Greece like Athens and with the Aetolian and Achaean Leagues. Rome, however, had raised an issue with Macedonia, traditionally an ally of Illyria, but too preoccupied in 228 and 219 B.C. to object to the Roman action. Thus Rome was introduced to the Greek states as a possible supporter of anti-Macedonian factions and to Macedonia as a threat to its influence in Greece, just at the time when Philip V had begun to rebuild the Hellenic League (pp. 389–90).

The Second Punic War (218–02 B.C.)

While the Romans, faced with a Gallic war, had formally permitted the Carthaginian buildup in Spain to continue, they evidently remained distrustful of Carthaginian intentions. The agreement made with Hasdrubal had allowed Carthage a free hand south of the Ebro River but apparently had contained no mention of the status of a native town in that area, Saguntum. By 220 B.C. Saguntum had come under Roman protection, although we do not know when this relationship was established. Presumably, if Rome had extended its protection before the treaty was made, the intention of the treaty was that Carthage should not interfere with Saguntum and that Rome should not use Saguntum to disturb Carthaginian jurisdiction. But it seems likely that Rome agreed to protect Saguntum after the treaty was signed. Thus Rome was violating the spirit of the agreement with Carthage by protecting a town in the Carthaginian sphere of influence, an action somewhat analogous to the acceptance of the Mamertine request in 264 B.C.

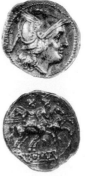

Coin of Hannibal

Saguntum, relying on Roman protection, repeatedly complained to the Senate of Carthaginian aggression and even, so Hannibal later charged, interfered with a Spanish tribe under his authority. In 220 Rome warned Hannibal not to attack Saguntum. He was thus faced with the risk of war with Rome or the continuous undermining of his work in Spain. Hannibal complained to

Rome of its interference in the affairs of Saguntum—Rome had arbitrated in favor of a faction in that city—and to Carthage of Saguntum's interference. In 219 Hannibal attacked Saguntum. The Carthaginians backed their general in a dramatic scene in the Carthaginian council before Roman envoys, and Hannibal pressed the siege. He took Saguntum in 218 and then marched his army north of the Ebro River in violation of the agreement that Rome had made in 226 with Hasdrubal.

Rome declared war on Carthage, thus entering upon the greatest and most difficult struggle in its history, in which time Hannibal was to ravage the Italian peninsula for fifteen years without defeat. Roman tradition justified the war by representing the Carthaginian development of Spain as the private revenge of the Barca family and of the treacherous Hannibal. While we do not know the Carthaginian side of the case, the sequence of events in Spain indicates that Rome forced Carthage to chose war or the disintegration of its power. The Romans had decided that Hannibal's buildup in Spain was hostile to themselves and then found that Carthage backed its general.

ROME ON THE DEFENSIVE (218–11 B.C.)

The Romans planned to strike directly at the Carthaginian bases of power in Spain and Africa. One army was concentrated in northern Italy to proceed to Massilia, where it would either await Hannibal, if he tried to invade Italy, or march into Spain from the north. Another army was to cross from Sicily to North Africa, as Regulus had done in 256 B.C. The Roman plans were designed to use their new sea power and to crush Carthage far from Italian soil. They could not, of course, realize that Hannibal was to prove a military genius, whose ability would be compared to that of Alexander and Julius Caesar by future generations. Before the Roman army was at the Rhone River in southern France to block his crossing, Hannibal was heading for the Alps to enter northern Italy. He planned to strike into Italy with his small but well-trained army, to enlist the Gauls, who were smarting from their recent defeat, and to march down through Italy, where he anticipated that the Roman Confederacy would fall apart. The plan was well conceived, for Carthage did not have the naval power or trained soldiers to move in force from Carthage itself. The chief flaw was Hannibal's false conception of the Roman Confederacy, which he envisaged as a master-subject relationship from which the Italians could be easily detached by his own victorious army. By the late third century, however, Central Italy had been welded together by grants of Roman citizenship, and Rome was able to draw on a great potential of manpower after the shock of Hannibal's early victories.

In early May, 218 B.C., Hannibal, then twenty-five years of age, started the war with an army of about forty thousand men—Africans, Carthaginians, Spaniards and Gauls—and a corps of sixty elephants. A holding force of about 25,000 was left in Spain, but Hannibal made no provision to keep communications open across southern France. In August he crossed the Rhone River, before the Romans arrived on the scene, and began his toilsome ascent into the

Alps. The army marched up the valley of the lower Durrance River, but the precise route across the mountains is unknown. The route is thought to have run between the Little St. Bernard and Mt. Genèvre. The mountain tribes were hostile, the higher mountains were covered with the first snow and ice of winter, and hardship took its toll. After almost one-third of the army and forty of the elephants perished in the crossing, Hannibal arrived with a force of about 26,000 to meet the Roman armies.

When the Romans had missed Hannibal at the Rhone, the consul Scipio sent his army on to Spain to open the planned campaign there and to cut Hannibal off from help. He himself returned to northern Italy, where he prepared to block Hannibal as he descended from the mountains. The first clash occurred at the Ticinus River, where Hannibal won a cavalry engagement and forced the Romans back across the Po River. At the Trebia, a tributary of the Po, the Roman forces were joined by the army which had been prepared for Africa, and there a full-scale battle developed in late November. Hannibal by arranging a skillful ambush defeated the Roman force with a loss of two-thirds of their men. He was safely established in northern Italy and able to recruit Gauls to bring his army up to strength.

During the winter Hannibal organized for further action. In 217 B.C. he crossed the Apennines into Etruria for what he hoped would be his decisive campaign. The adherence of the Gauls was a mixed blessing. Hannibal needed their fighting power, but fear of Gallic looting and destruction had been burned into the minds of the Italians who stiffened their resistance. Since the Roman allies did not desert to Hannibal's side, as he had hoped, the Romans were able to move their armies at will and to cover the passes through the Apennines. Hannibal emerged from the mountains and advanced through the countryside, drawing a Roman army under Flaminius in pursuit. At Lake Trasimene another ambush was prepared, into which Flaminius rashly ventured and lost his army and his life. Even so, no Roman allies came over to Hannibal, who had to turn aside from a direct attack on Rome to advance through the eastern side of the peninsula, where he ravaged and burnt as far as Apulia.

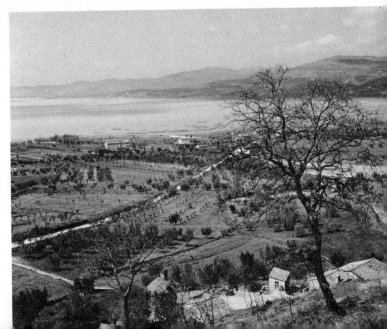

Lake Trasimene, the scene of Hannibal's victory in 217 B.C.

Flaminius had been elected consul by the people, who wanted to finish the war as quickly as possible in a decisive battle. The disasters at the Trebia River and Lake Trasimene, however, sobered the Romans sharply, and a dictator was appointed, Quintus Fabius Maximus, who advocated a very different strategy. Fabius planned a war of attrition to wear Hannibal's army down by guerilla tactics, until a favorable moment of battle could be chosen by Rome. Although these tactics were used to advantage, Hannibal continued his devastation and by 216 B.C. the patience of the people was worn out. Another great Roman army, which is said to have numbered eighty thousand men, was readied to fight under the command of Terentius Varro, the popular consul, and Lucius Aemilius Paullus, a conservative. The armies met at Cannae in Apulia. The disaster which followed was the most tragic in Roman tradition, for almost the whole force was annihilated with little loss to Hannibal's army. Roman prestige was shattered, and nearly all of southern Italy, including Campania, went over to Hannibal. The core of the Confederacy around Rome itself, however, along with Umbria and Etruria, remained loyal and Hannibal was kept from the city. Fabius' cautious guerilla tactics had been vindicated, and the aggressive strategy of the popular leaders discredited. Until Hannibal left Italy in 203 B.C. no Roman army again offered battle to him. Rome slowly recovered from its losses and fought in other theaters of war. Hannibal, thwarted in his purpose of destroying Rome quickly, turned to systematic looting and devastation in Italy, and Carthage, with the prestige of his victories fresh, extended the war by new alliances.

Until 211 B.C. Rome was on the defensive. The Carthaginians did not send aid to Hannibal in Italy, for which they are sometimes criticized, but Hannibal had demonstrated that he could win battles. Instead, reinforcements were sent to Spain and plans were made for a landing in Sardinia, to divert forces from Italy and give Carthage a base of operations near the Italian coast. In Spain there was a seesaw struggle, in which the Romans held the enemy with smaller forces until 211 B.C., when the Carthaginians won a decisive victory. Dissension among their generals, however, prevented them following it up properly. When the landing in Sardinia failed, Rome could give its attention to the new threats raised by Carthage. In Sicily, Hiero of Syracuse had maintained his alliance loyally to Rome until his death in 215 B.C. Then, after some hesitation, the new government made an alliance with Carthage. The Romans besieged Syracuse and were held at bay for three years by the fierce defense of the Syracusans and by ingenious machines invented by the scientist Archimedes. Among them was a large reflecting glass to scorch the Romans and set fire to their siege equipment. Some of the other Greek allies in Sicily followed the lead of Syracuse, but Carthage did not have sufficient sea power to move into Sicily and forcefully take over the island. Thus, in 211 the Romans were able to take Syracuse and suppress the remaining resistance in Sicily without difficulty. Syracuse was looted, and many of its citizens, including Archimedes, were killed. In the same year the Romans gained the upper hand in the war which Carthage had raised against them in Greece and were able to slacken their efforts in that theater.

In 215 B.C. Philip of Macedonia had made an alliance with Carthage, expecting that Hannibal would soon defeat Rome and that he himself could easily regain control of the Roman protectorate in western Greece. In this case, too, lack of sea power made the alliance ineffective. Carthage did not have the ships to win control of the Adriatic Sea and to ferry Macedonian troops to Italy where they could have joined Hannibal, while Philip's fleet was in the Aegean on the other side of Greece. The Romans cleverly pinned Philip in Greece by raising a Greek coalition against him, to which they sent a minimum of support. At first a Roman squadron operating in the Adriatic prevented a junction between Philip and Hannibal. In 213, however, when Hannibal captured Tarentum and Philip got control of a port on the Greek coast, the situation began to look dangerous. The Romans made an alliance with the Aetolian League, by which the Aetolians were to attack Philip and retain possession of the land and towns which they could occupy. Rome pledged limited help and, in return, was to receive all the movable plunder from the operations. In the course of the war several other Greek states joined the Roman-Aetolian coalition, notably Pergamum, which rendered valuable aid by drawing some of Philip's attention to the Aegean. Rome made no real effort to spread the war in Greece once Philip was contained and after 207 B.C. sent no further help. Aetolia dropped out of the war and in 205 B.C. Rome made peace with Philip, the Peace of Phoenice, in which Rome retained most of its protectorate. In general by 211 B.C. Sicily and Greece were in hand, some of the towns in Italy which had gone over to Hannibal after Cannae were retaken, and Rome could turn to the offensive.

ROMAN VICTORY (211–02 B.C.)

The Roman people, after five years of Fabian guerilla tactics in Italy, were anxious for more vigorous action and for victories. Their imagination was caught by a new figure in Roman political life, Publius Cornelius Scipio. In 210 B.C. he was chosen for command in Spain although he had not passed through the customary course of offices and was far younger than the usual run of Roman generals. Scipio's father and uncle had commanded in Spain, where they had served well and been killed in the fighting, and he himself was familiar with the problems of war there. Scipio was representative of a new type of young Roman just emerging in this period, well educated along Greek lines and with a broader, more international outlook than the farmer-senators, men of Fabius' type, who constituted a majority of the Senate. Scipio brought fresh confidence that the war could be won by energetic action against the bases of Carthaginian power in Spain and Africa rather than by waiting it out in Italy.

The people's confidence in Scipio was speedily justified. He took advantage of the dissension among the Carthaginian generals, who could not bear even to camp near each other and who had left the main base at New Carthage exposed. Scipio captured the town with its huge stocks of arms, supplies, and money for the Carthaginian armies. When the hostages, whom the Carthaginians had taken from the Spanish tribes to ensure good behavior, were liberated, the

Spaniards began to come over to the Roman side. In 208 B.C. Scipio fought a battle at Baecula with Hannibal's brother, Hasdrubal, to prevent him from escaping from Spain and joining Hannibal in Italy. Hasdrubal got away with an army of about 25,000 men, but Scipio, instead of pursuing, remained in Spain to methodically complete the task of wiping out the remnants of Carthaginian control. In 207 B.C. the last substantial Carthaginian forces were defeated at the battle of Ilipa. Scipio not only secured Spain for Rome, but he also improved the quality of the Roman army by loosening up the legionary formations still more, to give greater flexibility, and by adopting a Spanish type of sword, the *gladius,* which became standard Roman equipment. To the people in Rome he seemed the logical general to deal with Hannibal himself.

In Italy the Romans acted effectively to prevent a junction between Hasdrubal and Hannibal. One army was assigned to watch Hannibal in southern Italy, while another marched north to meet Hasdrubal in battle. At the Metaurus River in 207 B.C. Hasdrubal was defeated. The Romans savagely informed Hannibal of the disaster to his hopes by tossing Hasdrubal's severed head into his camp. Two years later a second attempt to reinforce Hannibal was thwarted by the repulse of another brother, Mago, near Genoa, as he tried to slip into northern Italy. Hannibal was penned in the south, and the Romans began to debate how the war should be ended.

Fabius, still cautious, wished to wait until Hannibal's army was in a thoroughly desperate condition and then finish the war in Italy. Scipio, who had returned from Spain, was in favor of an expedition to Africa to knock Carthage out. The people supported Scipio, but the Senate allowed him only two legions stationed in Sicily and as many volunteers as he could raise. Accordingly, in 204 B.C. Scipio sailed for Africa with his two legions and seven thousand volunteers. In Africa he enlisted the help of Masinissa, a Numidian prince, who hoped to get the kingship of Numidia in the event of a Roman victory. Carthage was hemmed in and asked for peace in 203 B.C., perhaps as much to gain time for Hannibal's return as for any real need of the moment. Hannibal left Italy after fifteen years, landed in Carthage and prepared for the final showdown with Scipio. In 202 B.C. the two armies met at Zama near Carthage, where Hannibal suffered some disadvantage from lack of cavalry. Scipio, well supplied in that branch of the armed forces by the Numidians under Masinissa, defeated him and brought the war to an end. A grateful people added the epithet, Africanus, to Scipio's name.

The settlement made by Rome stripped Carthage of its Empire and imposed heavy burdens on the state. The city retained its adjacent territory in Africa, roughly equivalent to about half of modern Tunisia, and some trading posts along the African coast. Numidia to the west was established as a separate kingdom under the rule of Masinissa. While Carthage retained its local autonomy, it became a dependent ally of Rome, even forbidden to defend itself against Numidia without Roman permission. Rome levied a war indemnity of ten thousand talents and demanded the surrender of the Carthaginian fleet, except

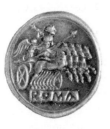
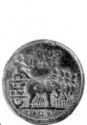
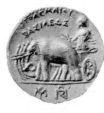
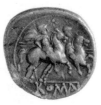

Coins of the Roman conquest

for a small squadron, and the war elephants. Hannibal, however, was allowed to remain in Carthage, and under his able administration the city began to recover financial stability and to rebuild its trade. Rome, in fact, became alarmed and in 195 B.C. demanded Hannibal's surrender. He fled to Asia where he was received by the Seleucid king, Antiochus III, and finally died in Bithynia in 182 B.C., still hounded by Rome.

Rome, as after the First Punic War, was faced with the task of administering the lands which had been won. The Romans showed no great haste or skill in taking over their responsibilities. In 197 B.C. Spain was organized into two provinces, Hither and Farther Spain, which comprised the eastern and southern coastal districts. The Romans became involved in a cruel and bitter struggle with the Spanish natives of the interior, which lasted until 134 B.C., but some progress was made in developing Spain. Roman veterans settled there, and Roman financial groups became interested in the mineral wealth and opportunities for trade. Gallia Cisalpina and Liguria in northern Italy had to be pacified and an administrative system set up. This, too, was done slowly, while Corsica and Sardinia continued to offer trouble for some years. The strip of southern France, through which the road from northern Italy to Spain lay, was made into a protectorate, with Massilia remaining a loyal ally of Rome. Although the western Mediterranean needed Rome's attention and offered ample scope for activity, this region was neglected when Rome became engaged in war with the Hellenistic Kingdoms of the eastern Mediterranean.

In Italy also urgent problems faced the Romans. Hannibal's systematic and lengthy devastation had seriously damaged the traditional system of Italian agriculture, based on the small farms of freeholding peasants. Rome was also suffering from financial exhaustion. In 215 B.C. the direct tax paid by Roman citizens had been doubled, and Rome had established a new system of supplying its armies by letting contracts for war material to private stock companies, the *societates*. Despite the need for a pause and the war weariness of the Roman people, the Roman army landed in Greece two years after Zama to fight Philip V of Macedonia.

The Wars Against Philip V and Antiochus III (200–188 B.C.)

In 200 B.C. the Romans presented an ultimatum to King Philip V of Macedonia, demanding that he stop waging war on Greek states and submit a dispute with King Attalus of Pergamum to arbitration. The demands, like those made on Carthage before the Second Punic War, forced Philip to risk war with Rome or to give up, with tremendous loss of prestige, his policy of strengthening the Macedonian position in Greece and the Aegean. If he accepted the demands of Rome, that state would have taken the position of Macedonia as the protector of Greece. The causes of Rome's sudden decision to interfere in the political affairs of the eastern Mediterranean have been the subject of a lengthy and unresolved discussion. Apparently they are to be understood partly in the light of Rome's interest in western Greece, partly because of Rome's fear that a shift in power among the Hellenistic Kingdoms, which was taking place at the end of the third century, might affect her adversely.

While the Romans and Philip had settled the First Macedonian War in 205 B.C. by the Peace of Phoenice, Philip probably seemed potentially dangerous to the Romans. He had offended them by joining Hannibal and after the Peace seems to have tampered with some of the states in the Roman protectorate in Illyria. Rome had protested but before 201 could scarcely take action because of its commitment in the war against Hannibal. Perhaps Philip had concluded that Rome would not act and so turned his attention away from western Greece to the Aegean; therefore it is primarily against the background of events there that we should understand Rome's ultimatum. The ultimatum, in fact, was designed primarily to stop Philip's activity in the Aegean and is indicative of Rome's new interest in the larger issues of Hellenistic politics.

The balance of power among the Hellenistic Kingdoms, which had been established in the third century B.C., was in process of being upset. The Seleucid king, Antiochus III (p. 382), who had made his aim the restoration of the Seleucid Empire to its original extent, from Thrace and western Asia Minor to India, returned from the borders of India in 204 B.C. with a reputation rivaling that of Alexander the Great. To round out the Empire in the west he still had to acquire Palestine, southern Syria, western Asia Minor and Thrace. In 204 Ptolemy IV Philopater of Egypt died, leaving a child as his successor. The situation seemed very favorable to the ambitions of Philip and Antiochus, and they seem to have made a secret agreement to partition the foreign possessions of Egypt. The effects became obvious in 202 B.C., while Rome was winding up the war with Hannibal. Antiochus began to take over southern Syria, and Philip seized some Greek cities in the region of the Hellespont.

Rome, then, in 202 B.C. had some grounds for complaint against Philip because of his interference in the Illyrian protectorate. The Romans also could see the beginning of large-scale disturbances in the east. The cities which Philip took over in the Hellespont were allies of the Aetolian League and of Rhodes, and his interference in this region roused the apprehensions of Pergamum. In 202 Rhodes declared war on Philip and was soon joined by Pergamum. The Aetolian League appealed to Rome for help against Macedonia, but, since Rome was still involved in war in Africa, the Senate turned the request down. When Philip's successful aggrandizement continued, Pergamum and Rhodes in their turn appealed to Rome in 201. They pictured the general disturbance in the east to the Senate, revealing and perhaps distorting the secret pact between Philip and Antiochus. It would have been obvious to Rome that, even if Antiochus were allied to Philip, he was not giving the latter much real help. Formidable as Antiochus might seem, presumably the Senate felt that they might safely take a strong line with Philip and that Antiochus would continue to pursue his own immediate interests. Despite the initial refusal of the people to vote for war, the Senate decided to force the situation to the limit.

For the time being an initial warning was sent to Philip, and the Senate worked up sentiment in Rome for a more formal ultimatum and a declaration of war. Envoys were sent to neutralize or to win over the small Greek states to Rome by picturing that state as the true protector of Greek interests, and to Antiochus in an effort to keep him out of the war. Philip replied to the final demands of Rome that his actions were none of Rome's business and that Rome was violating the agreement made with him at Phoenice. The Romans refused to argue; they insisted that Philip had committed aggression against free Greek states, and they went to war as the self-styled protectors of Greek freedom. Their envoys to Antiochus turned a deaf ear to the pleas of Egypt against Antiochus' attack in Syria and received an assurance that Antiochus would not support Philip V. Rome thus skillfully divided its potential enemies at the outset and was able to concentrate on Macedonia alone with the aid of Pergamum and Rhodes. Rome's intention was evidently to restrict Philip to Macedonia and to make him a sort of *client* king, while Greece itself would become a buffer zone between Italy and the domain of Antiochus. Conveniently for their diplomacy in Greece, the Romans could use the old formula of freedom for the Greeks, a popular slogan since the time of the Wars of Alexander's Successors. The Greeks, however, had heard their freedom proclaimed too frequently to be carried away by enthusiasm. They waited on events while the war opened between Rome and its allies—Rhodes and Pergamum—on the one side and Macedonia on the other.

The superior strength of Rome and Philip's lack of real support in Greece forced an essentially defensive war on Macedonia. The Romans could use their sea power to strike anywhere in western Greece, while the fleets of Pergamum and Rhodes provided a similar advantage in the Aegean. Almost all the Greek states, except the Aetolian League and Athens, were members of Philip's Hellenic League, but they preferred to exercise their right to remain neutral rather than to aid him. The success of Roman diplomacy in detaching members from the League waited on the success of the Roman army. In 200 B.C. Sulpicius Galba landed his troops at Apollonia and sent a naval squadron around to the Aegean to protect Athens, which had declared for Rome at the outset. After Galba penetrated through the mountains towards the frontiers of Macedonia, a slight success over Philip's army brought the Aetolians to the Roman side. Aetolia, however, proceeded to fight a somewhat unilateral war to win territory and plunder for itself.

Little more was achieved by the Romans until 198 B.C., when a new general, Titus Quinctius Flamininus, was placed in charge of operations. Flamininus proved to be an admirable choice, able to get along with the Greeks because of his genuine admiration for their culture and ability to speak Greek, but firm and determined to implement Roman policy. While Flamininus closed in on Macedonia, Philip vainly tried to negotiate a settlement which would leave him some influence in Greece. Flamininus insisted that Philip evacuate all Greece, thus driving a deeper wedge between Philip and his allies of the Hellenic League. Most were attracted by this tangible offer of Roman protection and judged Philip's attempt to negotiate a sign of weakness. The cities of Boeotia, the Achaean League, and Sparta, under its King Nabis, came over to Rome. Nevertheless, the final battle of the war, fought at Cynoscephalae in Thessaly in 197 B.C., was a Roman victory. Flamininus' veterans from the campaigns in Spain and Africa defeated the Macedonian army without great difficulty.

In the peace settlement the Roman purpose to restrict Macedonia to its own land and to cut down its power was achieved. Philip was required to give up his possessions outside Macedonia and to abstain from war against Greek states. Rome imposed a war indemnity and took over the Macedonian navy. Shortly afterwards Macedonia became a Roman ally but retained full independence because Flamininus realized, even if the Greeks did not, that some power was needed to keep the barbarian people of the Danube valley from Greece and the Aegean.

Flamininus then proceeded to arrange the affairs of Greece, Rome's new protectorate, in what the Romans considered to be their own best interests. The cities freed from Macedonian control were declared independent, not handed over to the Aetolian League, as the latter had hoped, and various territorial adjustments were made. Flamininus also engineered some internal changes of government in certain cities in favor of the wealthy upper class. With its members Flamininus and the Roman officers found a mutual understanding, and so Rome appeared to the Greeks as a supporter of the rights of property and of established governing groups. Except for the Aetolian League and Sparta, whose King Nabis was disgruntled at territorial adjustments made in favor of the Achaean League, the Roman arrangements won general favor among the Greeks. In 196 B.C. Flamininus proclaimed the new freedom of Greece at the Isthmian Games in a scene of great enthusiasm. Yet the seeds of misunderstanding had been sown. The Greeks had not understood that the Roman attitude was paternalistic and that they were expected to respect Rome's will. Even if Rome exacted no tribute, seized no territory, and actually pulled out its troops from Greece, the Romans believed that their arrangements and future requests would be fully respected.

After the victory over Philip, Rome revealed that its protectorate was to apply also to the Greeks of Asia Minor. Their inclusion in the proclamation made by Flamininus at Isthmia brought an immediate demand for clarification by Antiochus. During Rome's war with Macedonia he had almost achieved his aim of restoring the Seleucid Empire. By 196 Syria and Palestine had been taken over, and Antiochus was preparing to assert his new relationship to Egypt by a marriage into the family of the Ptolemies. In the following year Antiochus had advanced to the Hellespont and crossed into Thrace, where the big city of Lysimacheia was refortified to serve as a base.

Rome's extension of the protectorate to Asia Minor had some Greek support, for Pergamum and other Greek cities of Asia Minor had been complaining to Rome about Antiochus' aggression, but it came as a sudden shock to the king himself. He had formally established friendship with Rome and had heard no previous objections to his policy. Accordingly, Antiochus asked for clarification and got it in the form of a brusque demand to give up the cities in Asia Minor which he had taken, to refrain from attacking others, and to withdraw from Thrace. A series of negotiations protracted over the next several years followed, in which neither side would give way nor, apparently, understand the other's position. The situation was made more difficult by Antiochus' hospitable reception of Hannibal, when the latter fled from Carthage. Negotiations had reached a stalemate by 192, when Aetolia suddenly catalyzed the situation by starting war in Greece and by trying to raise a coalition of the Hellenistic states against Rome.

The Aetolians induced Nabis of Sparta to recover the towns taken from him in 195 B.C. and thus to disturb the Roman settlement. Invitations were sent to the Achaean League and to Macedonia to join the war of liberation from Rome, but they fell on deaf ears. The Achaean League was satisfied with the treatment which it had received, and Philip, who distrusted the Aetolians, had no wish for another war with Rome. Philip's suspicions were well founded, for, while the Aetolians were asking for his help, they were intriguing to replace him on the throne of Macedonia. The Aetolian appeal to Antiochus was more successful, if not much more honest, because the Aetolians pretended that the small Greek states were eager for war. Accordingly, Antiochus proclaimed that he was coming to free Greece from the effects of the Roman freedom, but he concentrated his main army in Asia Minor. He could, in fact, get only a small force to Greece, for Macedonia refused passage to the Seleucid army by land, and the fleets of Rhodes and Pergamum held the Aegean. Thus the Romans were able to separate the war into two theaters and to take on one opponent at a time. By 190 B.C. Antiochus' force in Greece, the Aetolian League and Sparta were thoroughly defeated. A Roman army was allowed by Philip to march through Macedonia and cross into Asia Minor, where Antiochus' main army was beaten in 189 B.C. at the battle of Magnesia.

Rome proceeded to readjust affairs in Greece and to make arrangements to its liking in Asia Minor. Aetolia, thoroughly plundered in the war by the Roman commander, Marcus Acilius Glabrio, was penalized by the loss of all territory outside Aetolia proper and by a heavy war indemnity. Macedonia was rewarded by the grant of some towns in Thessaly and was excused from the remainder of its indemnity from the previous war. The Achaean League was allowed to incorporate the whole of the Peloponnesus into its organization. Antiochus was excluded from western Asia Minor. His frontiers were to be the Taurus Mountains and the Halys River, and he was not to sail into the Aegean beyond the southwestern tip of Asia Minor. Antiochus' ability to wage war was crippled by the imposition of the usual large indemnity, the surrender of hostages, his war fleet, and elephants. The Greek cities of Asia Minor which had aided Rome were declared independent, while those which had fought for Antiochus were distributed to Rhodes and Pergamum. In effect, Pergamum was to control western Asia Minor north of the Maeander River, and Rhodes the area to the south. The general result of the settlements was to establish Macedonia and the Achaean League as Roman agents in Greece, while Rhodes and Pergamum played that part in Asia Minor. The effect on the Seleucid Kingdom was far-reaching. Antiochus' prestige had been seriously damaged, and the Seleucid policy of Hellenization by the founding of cities greatly impaired by exclusion from the Aegean and Asia Minor. Rome had administered a severe blow to the great Hellenistic powers, which was soon to disturb the balance between Greek and native throughout the Hellenistic world and to accelerate its fragmentation.

From Protectorate to Provinces (188–34 B.C.)

After the defeat of Antiochus, Roman troops made a successful expedition into Galatia, ostensibly in the interest of their ally, Pergamum, but were then pulled out of the East, and no specific organization for settling disputes or implementing Roman wishes was established. The Romans regarded Greece and Asia Minor as a sort of protectorate, for whose states they regulated foreign policy and in whose internal affairs they might interfere. The Roman Senate exercised supervision by remote control. A flow of envoys came from the Greek cities to Rome to air their complaints and to plead their special cases. The Senate listened, when it had time, dispatched senatorial committees and envoys to conduct hearings on the spot and to issue directives. Some states, like Pergamum, adopted an attitude of almost subservient cooperation with Rome to accomplish their purposes, while others, like Macedonia, tried to maintain their independence. The Seleucids carefully observed the settlement imposed by Rome, but assumed that they had full liberty of action south of the Aegean and Asia Minor. Rome seemed to feel that its prestige was involved in every incident and could not understand opposition and argument against its paternalistic policy.

THE THIRD MACEDONIAN WAR (172–68 B.C.)

Serious difficulty soon arose with Macedonia. Philip V and his successor, Perseus, who came to the throne in 181 B.C., were vigorous and able rulers, proud of the tradition of their state and desirous of fostering national loyalty among its people. After the war with Antiochus, in which Philip had demonstrated his cooperation with Rome, they turned to energetic campaigns against the barbarian peoples on the frontiers and to the internal consolidation of Macedonia. The mines and forests were intensively exploited, land was reclaimed for agricultural settlement, and good relations were fostered with those Greek states which were receptive, particularly with Epirus on the west. To some of Macedonia's neighbors, especially to Pergamum and the free cities of Thessaly, this renaissance seemed hostile to themselves and to the Roman settlement. As in the case of the Carthaginian buildup in Spain, we have only the Roman side of the situation in our sources for this period, but it is very unlikely that Philip and Perseus wanted to try war or to form a coalition against Rome. They did want to preserve their self-respect and to restore Macedonian prestige so far as possible. The Romans, however, seem to have swallowed the interpretation placed on Macedonian acts by Pergamum and found a cause for war in an accident which happened to King Eumenes in 172 B.C.

Eumenes had gone to Rome to urge intervention against Macedonia. On his return to Pergamum by way of Delphi he narrowly escaped death from a rock bounding down the hillside. An agent of Perseus was supposed to have dislodged it. The Romans, perhaps, were justified to some extent in feeling uneasiness about a strong Macedonia because they regarded Greece and Asia Minor as a buffer area, but there was hardly provocation to charge Perseus with planning a war on Rome and attacking Roman allies. Nevertheless in 172 B.C. the Roman armies landed once more in Greece to open the Third Macedonian War. Events revealed that the coalition which Perseus was supposed to be forming against Rome was a myth, for the only useful aid which he received came from Epirus. Even so, Roman victory was delayed for four years, partly by the stout fighting of Macedonia and partly by the incompetence of the Roman generals. In 168 B.C., however, Lucius Aemilius Paullus, commanding a first-rate Roman army, defeated Perseus with heavy casualties at the battle of Pydna.

Another series of settlements was made by Rome which further contributed to the disintegration of the Hellenistic world. In order to destroy national feeling in Macedonia, the kingdom was dissolved, and four separate republics were created in its place. Even intermarriage and ordinary business relations were prohibited among their respective citizens. The royal mines and forests, which had provided the money for the Macedonian revival, were closed temporarily. Epirus, which Rome felt had betrayed the trust reposed in it, was thoroughly pillaged and its pattern of urban life broken by the destruction of the larger towns. According to tradition, probably exaggerated, 150,000 Epirots were sold into slavery.

Rome's allies in the war came under suspicion and even heavy penalty. The Achaean League, despite its collaboration with Rome, was suspected of sympathy with Perseus. Although no documentary proof of their guilt was produced, Rome took a thousand prominent Achaeans to Rome for trial and to serve as hostages, among them the historian Polybius. The trial was delayed for seventeen years because Rome was too busy to bother with such a minor matter. Rhodes, too, had collaborated with Rome, but a small group in the state had favored Perseus. Rhodes punished them at the suggestion of a Roman general, but, nevertheless, Rome penalized the Rhodians by taking away their lands in Asia Minor and by establishing a free port at Delos, which speedily became the Aegean center of trade in grain and slaves. Even Eumenes of Pergamum was distrusted. While operating with the Romans in Macedonia, he had withdrawn his troops to winter quarters. The Roman officers, who were bungling the war, found a convenient excuse for their own incapacity in Eumenes' withdrawal and after 167 B.C. Rome began to listen favorably to the complaints about Pergamum which came from the cities of Asia Minor.

Rome extended its interest to the southeastern Mediterranean at this time and discovered a warm concern for Egypt. Antiochus IV invaded Egypt in 169 B.C. and had reached the point of victory, when a Roman envoy, Gaius Popilius, threatened him with war unless the conquest was broken off. Despite this almost obsessive desire to control affairs in the east, the Romans still annexed no territory and refused to assume the responsibilities of direct administration. The troops were taken back to Italy and indirect government, or interference, by remote control was resumed.

THE GREEK REACTION

After the defeat of Perseus there was a natural reaction by Eumenes of Pergamum and Antiochus IV to strengthen the position of Hellenism in their kingdoms. Their efforts were not directed against Rome specifically but were aimed to promote Hellenic solidarity in their own states and among the Greeks in general. Relations between the two monarchs were cordial, and Eumenes, in particular, emphasized Greek traditions. After a victory over the Galatians in 166 B.C. he erected the Great Altar of Zeus in Pergamum on which the sculptured representation of the victory of the Greek gods over the giants symbolized the triumph of Greek civilization (p. 411). Eumenes and his successor, Attalus, made many gifts to Greek cities, including the *Stoa* of Attalus given to Athens, where the king had studied as a young man.

Antiochus IV, after he was forced to withdraw from Egypt in 168 B.C., made a valiant attempt to consolidate what was left of the Seleucid Empire. As described previously (p. 384), he sent his cousin Eucratides to raise a revolt in the Kingdom of Bactria in order to restore it nominally to the Seleucids. While Bactria remained a separate kingdom, Antiochus celebrated Eucratides' success by a great thanksgiving in Babylon, in which Antiochus himself was hailed as the Savior of Asia. The selection of Babylon was not accidental, for Antiochus, cut off from the Aegean and Asia Minor, was trying to draw the native peoples into the support of his regime. His most interesting effort was a new policy of religious centralization, by which he tried to win acceptance for a universal god of the Empire, whom both Greeks and natives could worship and with whom he himself might be identified. The Greek god Zeus was identified with the Syrian Baal Shamin, and Antiochus took the epithet, Epiphanes, or the god manifest. The best-known trial of the new plan, among the Hebrews, was a failure, and it led to revolt and to the eventual establishment of an independent Jewish state, the Kingdom of the Maccabees. Elsewhere, however, Antiochus seems to have had some success but his efforts toward consolidation were cut short in 163 B.C., when he died in the course of preparations for war against the Parthians.

After the death of Antiochus IV the Seleucid state disintegrated rapidly. When dynastic quarrels continued to weaken it internally, the various native peoples split away to form separate states of their own. The Syrian Arabs set up petty sheikhdoms, the Hebrews established a kingdom in Judaea, and the Nabataeans in Arabia formed a new state. In the east, Commagene and Armenia emerged as kingdoms, while the Parthian advance to the west was resumed. Rome inherited the difficult task of reorganization a century later.

This reluctance by the Romans to assume the responsibilities of government outside of Italy, and yet interfering constantly from an obsessive anxiety about prestige and security, is perhaps to be explained in part by the nature of the wars which Rome had undertaken. They were preventive wars, and the primary purpose of the Romans was achieved when they won the wars. Yet fear continued to exist that some new threat might arise because Rome had little knowledge of the Hellenistic East and of its traditional adjustment of difficulties by diplomacy and limited war.

Even the Romans, however, should have been satisfied by the defeat of Perseus in 168 B.C. Possibly by that time another motive had become predominant. The Roman system of government had been worked out to govern a city-state. No machinery existed to administer foreign territories, and there were too few offices even for the administration of Rome itself, let alone the conduct of its wars. A workable solution for the wars had been found in the device of promagistracy, the prolongation of commands beyond their annual term, but the Second Punic War had revealed the danger latent in that system. Commanders became too independent, and some of them, like Scipio, had prolonged their power by direct appeals to the people. The senatorial class, which had come to rule Rome in the wars, had no desire to create new offices or to prolong the existing ones beyond the demands of necessity. The senators feared the rise of new men outside the existing group of great families and were apprehensive about the "great men" of their own circle. Accordingly, this very loose protectorate over the East had developed almost automatically. The system both irritated the Romans, who could not let well enough alone, and failed to achieve its purpose. Anti-Roman sentiment was fostered by interference and misunderstanding. The Third Macedonian War was the first tragic example of the protectorate's failure, and the settlements made after the war led to further difficulties in the Aegean, as well as for the Seleucids.

Macedonian nationalism was not destroyed by the partition of the kingdom.

In 149 B.C. a pretender to the throne appeared, who claimed to be the son of Perseus and rallied the Macedonians to restore his kingdom. The revolt was speedily crushed by Rome, and in 148 B.C. Macedonia was made a Roman province, placed under a governor, and required to pay tribute to Rome. The contagion of revolt, however, had spread to Greece. Despite the attempts of pro-Roman presidents, the Achaean League found that it could not live with the continuous series of Roman requests, complaints and commissions. In 148 B.C. the League revolted in a quarrel over jurisdiction. The movement was ruthlessly repressed, and in 146 B.C. the Roman general Mummius gave an object lesson to Greece by looting and destroying the city of Corinth. A general settlement was made of Greek affairs, in which individual city governments were purged, the leagues partly broken up, and Greece placed under the supervision of the governor of Macedonia.

Pergamum remained a free kingdom and ally of Rome until 133 B.C., when its last king, Attalus, died and bequeathed his kingdom to Rome. While Attalus was not subjected to the same interference as Eumenes had been, his kingdom was disturbed by social unrest as the economic effects of the wars of conquest began to make themselves felt (pp. 523–24). Since Rome supported the governing classes in the Greek city-states, the poor in both city and countryside felt no loyalty either to the Romans or to their own governments when their conditions of life worsened. Perhaps Attalus felt that the best lot for his people was to place them in Rome's hands, or perhaps he felt that he was paying Rome its just deserts. Before Rome could enjoy its inheritance, a revolt led by a pretender, Aristonicus, had to be suppressed. But in 129 B.C. the Romans formed the province of Asia out of the former Pergamene Kingdom. Asia included the rich and fertile coastal area west of the Anatolian plateau, from the Hellespont to Caria, while the remainder of the kingdom was parceled out to *client* kings, dependent on Rome in their foreign policy.

THE THIRD PUNIC WAR

In the western Mediterranean the Roman settlement made with Carthage proved as unsatisfactory as the protectorate in the East. Carthage itself did regain prosperity, which made its lands all the more desirable to Masinissa in his Kingdom of Numidia. Carthage labored under an almost impossible situation, for the state could not defend itself against Masinissa without the permission of Rome. Rome, of course, was disposed to favor the growth of Numidia rather than to protect Carthage. Masinissa, almost without Roman reproof, annexed the trading stations of Carthage along the African coast and gradually moved into the city's own territory. By 154 B.C. he had absorbed all but five thousand square miles of the original thirty thousand left to Carthage in 200 B.C. When the Carthaginians appealed to Rome for a guarantee of their frontier, the Senate sent a commission to investigate, among whose members was the Elder Cato. For some reason he became imbued with a fanatical hatred of Carthage, which was in no position to harm Rome, and instead of recommending that Masinissa be halted, demanded the destruction of Carthage, ending all his speeches in the Senate with the famous phrase, *"Carthago delenda est"* (Carthage must be destroyed).

By 150 B.C. the Carthaginians could endure no more. They declared war on King Masinissa and incurred the wrath of Rome. The Romans demanded the destruction of the city, refusing to listen to explanations or to accept any less penalty. The Carthaginians held out for three years, but in 146 B.C. Carthage was taken by Scipio, the adopted grandson of that Scipio who had defeated Hannibal. The city was looted, and most of the population killed or enslaved, as had been done with Corinth in Greece. Carthaginian territory was annexed by Rome to form a new province of Africa.

It is difficult to understand these vindictive actions of Rome, apparently the product of childish or wanton rage. Both Corinth and Carthage were important trading cities, but in the mid-second century it is still too early to explain Roman policy by commercial interest. Perhaps the destruction of Corinth was the result of a personal decision by the general Mummius, but that of Carthage was a matter of government policy. The advocates of war against Carthage had stressed the extent of Carthaginian economic recovery, but Carthage could hardly seem a real threat to Rome. Perhaps Cato feared that Carthage would soon be too strong for Numidia and would rebuild its African Empire. It has been suggested, too, that it was not so much Carthage as Numidia at which Rome wished to strike. Masinissa would be much less likely to attack the new Roman province of Africa, and it was extremely difficult for Rome to restrain the ally which had helped to win the battle of Zama. Carthage was expendable.

Obviously the Romans, whose political common sense had created the Confederacy in Italy, were failing to manage their conquests beyond its shores. They had destroyed the Carthaginian Empire in the West and the political order of the Hellenistic Kingdoms in the East. Immense damage had been done and reorganization barely started. Rome, too, had been transformed in the course of the wars, and problems were raised which led to revolution and to the breakdown of the Republic in the following century.

XXII

The Fruits of Expansion

(264–134 B.C.)

THE VICTORIES OF ROME over Carthage and the Hellenistic Kingdoms had resulted in a new order in the Mediterranean world, in which the Romans became the dominant people and established the territorial basis of their Empire. The effects on Rome were equally far-reaching. During the wars the political and social predominance of the senatorial class was so firmly established that it became almost synonymous with the Republic itself. Since senatorial direction had won the wars, the plebeian element among the Roman people had little cause for complaint, and the trend toward a more workable democracy died out.

Expansion, however, brought new problems to the senatorial government both in Rome and abroad. Some form of administrative organization had to be worked out for the new provinces, which were unprepared as yet for the methods of the Roman Confederacy in Italy. New elements appeared in Roman society and disturbed its traditional stability. A middle class of businessmen and financiers developed, whose wealth in money began to rival that of the senators and to justify their growing claim for political recognition. The thousands of slaves who came to Italy changed the economic structure of Roman society because they squeezed the small-scale farmers out of agriculture and kept them from urban employment. The cultural life of Rome was strongly affected when the Romans came into direct contact with the more highly developed civilization of Greece. A national literature came into being, which was strongly influenced by Greek models and ideas, but which emphasized Roman tradition. The education, tastes, and manners of life of the Roman upper classes were also strongly influenced, but in general these Romans were selective in their Hellenization. They took what they wanted to enrich their private lives but remained essentially Roman.

The senatorial government was reluctant to recognize change and to seek new solutions. The seeds of a revolution which was to destroy the Republic were sown, but hardly recognized by the Romans in the hectic activity of war and growth. We will look first at the system of administration in the provinces by which Rome began to link the countries of the Mediterranean to itself.

The Provincial System

ORGANIZATION

The earliest Roman provinces, Sicily, Sardinia-Corsica, and the two Spanish provinces, Hither and Farther Spain, were acquired by the Romans in war with Carthage. It was hardly possible to treat all their peoples like those in Italy, that is, by the wholesale granting of alliances and citizenship, because the provinces were alien and varied in organization from the tribal villages in the mountains of Spain to the big city-states of Sicily. The Romans reduced most of the provincials to the status of subjects. They were governed by Roman officials and paid taxes to Rome, but the senatorial government did not have the machinery to set up an elaborate administration and was reluctant to create it. Accordingly, they left a very considerable degree of local freedom to the communities within a province and were concerned mainly to keep order and to defend the provincial frontiers.

The first step in creating a province was the drawing up of the charter (*lex provinciae*) by a committee of ten senators, who usually conferred with the general who had conquered the province. The charter was then ratified by the Senate in Rome. The charter set out the rights and obligations of the provincials and provided the framework within which the governor was to work. There was considerable variation in the charters to fit the circumstances by which Rome had acquired the province and to take into account the different types of communal organization. There were, in general, three categories of relationship to Rome among the communities of a province, which expressed the freedom which each retained.

First a few communities, which were thoroughly viable and had aided the Romans, were made into free allies with individual treaties of a permanent nature, like those Rome had made with its Italian allies. These free and allied communities were called *civitates liberae et foederatae* and had full local freedom of government and immunity from taxation. Their foreign policy, of course, was subject to that of Rome and they were pledged to military aid. They were technically outside the sphere of duty (which the Latin word *provincia* means) of the governor and dealt directly with the government in Rome. A second category was made up of the free and immune communities, *civitates liberae et immunes,* which also possessed self-government and immunity from taxation, but only at the will of Rome. Their immunity might be revoked as a penalty at any time. The third category, tributary communities, *civitates stipendiariae,* by far the largest in number in any province, paid the taxes which supported the administration. These communities also enjoyed self-government but were

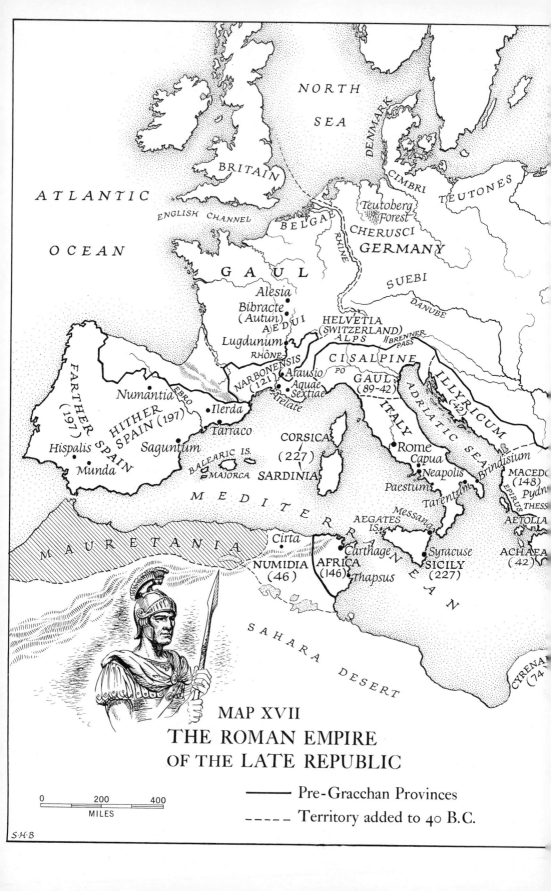

NORTH SEA

ATLANTIC OCEAN

BRITAIN

ENGLISH CHANNEL

DENMARK

CIMBRI

TEUTONES

BELGAE

Teutoberg Forest

CHERUSCI

RHINE

GERMANY

GAUL

SUEBI

DANUBE

Alesia

Bibracte (Autun)

AEDUI

HELVETIA (SWITZERLAND)

ALPS

BRENNER PASS

Lugdunum

RHÔNE

CISALPINE

ILLYRICUM (42)

FARTHER SPAIN (197)

NARBONENSIS (121)

Arausio

Aquae Sextiae

Arelate

PO

GAUL (89-42)

ITALY

ADRIATIC SEA

EBRO

Numantia

HITHER SPAIN (197)

Ilerda

Tarraco

Saguntum

BALEARIC IS.

MAJORCA

CORSICA (227)

SARDINIA

Rome

Capua

Neapolis

Paestum

Brindisium

MACEDO (148)

Hispalis

Munda

Tarentum

EPIRUS THESS

AETOLIA

MEDITERRANEAN

AEGATES IS.

Messana

ACHAEA (42)

MAURETANIA

Cirta

NUMIDIA (46)

Carthage

AFRICA (146)

Thapsus

Syracuse

SICILY (227)

CYRENA (74

SAHARA DESERT

MAP XVII

THE ROMAN EMPIRE
OF THE LATE REPUBLIC

——— Pre-Gracchan Provinces

- - - - Territory added to 40 B.C.

0   200   400

MILES

S·H·B

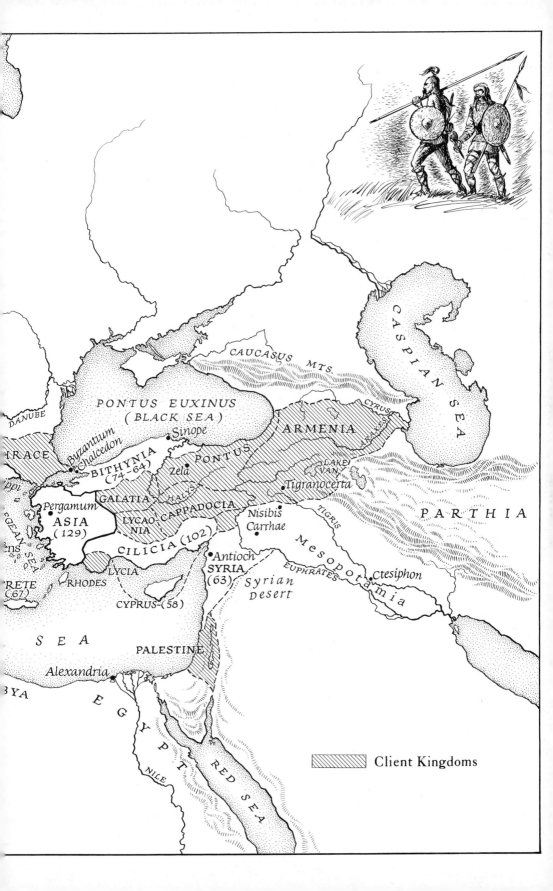

DANUBE

THRACE

PONTUS EUXINUS
(BLACK SEA)

Byzantium
Chalcedon
BITHYNIA
(74–64)
Sinope

Zela

PONTUS

CAUCASUS MTS.

CYRUS

ARMENIA

LAKE
VAN

Tigranocerta

CASPIAN
SEA

AEGEAN SEA

Pergamum
ASIA
(129)

GALATIA

LYCAO-
NIA

HALYS

CAPPADOCIA

Nisibis
Carrhae

TIGRIS

PARTHIA

Mesopotamia

Ctesiphon

CILICIA (102)

LYCIA

RHODES

CRETE
(67)

Antioch
SYRIA
(63)

EUPHRATES

Syrian
Desert

CYPRUS–(58)

SEA

PALESTINE

Alexandria

LIBYA

EGYPT

NILE

RED SEA

Client Kingdoms

liable to more supervision from the governor because of their taxable position. The Romans did not, at this early stage of their conquests, take title to all the territory of a province and declare it Roman public land, but they did claim the mines and forests. Rome might, however, confiscate a community's land as penalty for revolt, rent it back to the previous owners, then also tax them. Rome's public property in the provinces, the mines and forests as well as land, was leased for exploitation rather than administered directly by governmental agents or used for colonial settlements of Romans and Italians. If Romans moved to a province, that was their private venture.

After a brief and unsatisfactory attempt to administer the new provinces of Sicily and Sardinia-Corsica by the city praetors, the Romans in 227 B.C. began to work out a more uniform system. In that year two additional praetors were elected to serve as provincial governors, and in 197 B.C., when the Spanish provinces were organized, another two praetors were added. This trend to the creation of special officials to act as governors was halted at this point. The senatorial class was reluctant to enlarge the number of high offices in the state or to spread the plums of provincial administration beyond its own narrow circle. Accordingly, it became the regular practice to use ex-praetors and ex-consuls as governors, assigning them to provinces by lot for an annual term, although readjustments and extensions were made. The governor's staff was small. He was accompanied by a quaestor to serve as treasurer and receive the taxes. A small staff of aides (*legati*) was designated by the Senate on the governor's nomination, and a group of friends and young protégés, (the *comites*) went along to assist the governor and gain experience. No salaries were paid, but the expense allowance was very liberal, and the provincials provided entertainment and supplies at the governor's request.

The primary duties of the governor were to keep order and to protect the frontiers of his province. Accordingly, the number of troops allocated to him might vary considerably because they were not regarded as a regular garrison. The governor exercised a general supervision over the communities of his province, settling disputes among them, listening to complaints, administering justice and seeing that the taxes were duly remitted to Rome. While local courts served their own communities for the most part, the governor heard cases between Roman citizens, between Romans and provincials, and all serious and capital cases. He normally fixed his residence in the chief city of the province but traveled on a regular circuit and took charge of any military operations.

The original purpose of the tax levied on provincials was to pay the costs of administration and defense rather than to bring in vast surpluses to the Roman treasury. The taxes were, in fact, usually the same or lower than the people had paid to their previous government and were collected in the same manner. The first province, Sicily, offered a model in this respect. The tax was set at one-tenth of the grain crop, one-fifth of the orchard produce, and a sum of money on each head of grazing stock. In addition, *portoria* (harbor dues) of five per cent were paid, as by Romans and Italians in Italy. The yield of the tax, of course, fluctuated annually with the variations in the crop. To collect the tax, the Romans took over the system used by Hiero of Syracuse, which he, perhaps, had borrowed from Ptolemaic Egypt. Each community was made responsible for a census of its own produce, and the collection of Rome's share was leased by sale of contracts. The contractor could examine the census and inspect the crops before making his bid. The contracts were auctioned off in Sicily with two-fifths of one per cent as a margin for the contractor's costs and profit. In Sicily the communities usually bid in their own crops and thus eliminated a middleman in the transaction. Since Italians found it profitable to rent farms in Sicily, for which they had also to pay taxes, the tax was not excessive.

After Asia became a province, this system was extended to its taxpaying communities and unfortunately became a political football. In 122 B.C. the tribune Gaius Gracchus instituted the practice of auctioning off the tax contracts to Roman citizens in Rome, where they were bought up by stock companies, whose agents, the *publicani* (publicans), collected the taxes for remittance to the Roman quaestor. In Asia the taxes were payable in cash, equivalent to one-tenth of the crop. This change was designed to gain Gaius the support of the Roman business class which it did, but it also opened the way to great abuses. Sardinia-Corsica paid in grain as did Sicily, but in the other regions which were among the first Roman provinces—Spain, Macedonia, and Africa— another system was used by which the taxable communities paid a fixed sum in cash directly to the Roman quaestor. The grain which Rome obtained was used partly to supply the army and partly to feed the citizens of Rome, where the problem of food supply for the city became increasingly difficult as the population grew.

ABUSES

While this incipient provincial system was fair in conception and left a very considerable degree of local independence to the provincial communities, it was open to great abuse. The Roman government had no long-range policy for the provinces other than military security for their territory, and the practice of appointing governors for a short term gave them little time to develop their province, even if they had ideas and projects of their own. Too many governors saw only an opportunity for their own aggrandizement and made very considerable personal gain. They accepted or demanded gifts of money and precious objects, as well as lavish entertainment from the provincials. Little check could be exercised on the governors by the Senate, far off in Rome, and in any case the senators felt reluctant to punish a colleague. Accounts were duly scrutinized, and the governor's claims to special recognition, such as a triumph, were considered upon his return to Rome, but abuses multiplied. The provincials might complain, if they had the temerity or an influential patron in Rome to push their case, but no regular means for obtaining redress other than through the

Senate's initiative existed for a considerable time. In 149 B.C. a standing court was established (the *quaestio rerum repetundarum*) to hear suits for damages from the extortion of provincial governors. The intention was good, but the court was not very effective. Its members were fifty senators, whose verdicts were hardly impartial, the trials were lengthy, and the costs high for the complainants. The best protection which the provincials could have was an influential friend and patron in Rome, to whom they would stand in much the same relation as *clients*. Frequently the general who conquered a province or a prominent member of the commission which arranged the charter was regarded as a patron, and the provincials appealed to him and to his descendants when in need of a friend in Rome. The patron himself thus extended his own personal influence and support beyond Italy.

The system of collecting taxes through the stock companies and their publicans remained an abuse to the end of the Republic. These men had no responsibility to the provincials and none to Rome, except paying over the taxes which they had contracted to pay Rome. They were concerned more with their own personal gain and with profits for their companies. The governors did not supervise their activities properly for fear of offending Roman citizens, so the publicans often extorted more than their legitimate share and took advantage of their position to buy up goods in the provinces for their own purposes. In addition, Roman bankers and moneylenders (*negotiatores*) thronged the provinces to make investments. They offered loans at very high rates of interest to communities in financial difficulty and sometimes collected them with the governor's help. He might station Roman troops in the delinquent towns or place soldiers in the service of the moneylenders. In return the governor would get a share of the profits and support for his career in Rome. Also, upon investigation the moneylenders sometimes proved to be the front men for the senators themselves. Senators were prevented by tradition and, after 218 B.C., by law from engaging in business. The Romans had made a reasonably good beginning with their provinces, when such men as Scipio Africanus and Flamininus were in charge, but the general run of administrators was unable to resist the opportunities for private gain, and no system was devised to deal properly with the abuses.

Roman Society

THE NEW MIDDLE CLASS

The members of the Roman stock companies, whose activity we have noticed in the provinces, were representative of a new class of businessmen that began to emerge into importance in the second century. This rising middle class had found its first opportunities in local business as Rome grew to prominence in Italy, and after the war with Hannibal found the whole new field of finance open to it. The senators had dissociated themselves, officially at least, with trade and business in 218 B.C., when a law was passed prohibiting senators and their sons from owning ships of greater capacity than the small size needed to transport the produce of their own estates. The senatorial class clung to the old tradition of landed wealth and public service and, as a result, channeled the energy and ambition of the middle class wholly into business.

These businessmen continued to be active locally, particularly in supplying Rome with grain, but in the course of the wars of conquest turned more and more to taking state contracts and to banking and finance. They left the overseas trade of Italy in the hands of the Italian Greeks, who could build easily on their already established connections. In 215 B.C. stock companies had been formed, which contracted to supply the Roman army with arms and war materials. This business continued to be profitable, but in the provinces the companies entered the new business of collecting rents and taxes and undertaking the exploitation of mines and the natural resources to which Rome had taken title. From this practice it was an easy step to banking and moneylending, from which tremendous profits might be drawn both in Rome and abroad. While many members of these stock companies were men of only moderate means, who pooled their resources to make the enterprises possible, some became extremely wealthy and possessed fortunes which rivaled those of the senatorial families.

These more prosperous members of the middle class were known as *Equites,* Equestrians, or as the Equestrian Order, when their qualifications and privileges were legally defined soon after 133 B.C. This designation also included the *Equites* proper, the eighteen hundred men of the cavalry *centuries;* in fact, the name was borrowed from them. The censors had apparently found the Equestrian *centuries* a convenient place in which to register the men of new wealth. The *Equites* did not play a part in the making of Rome's policy until the latter part of the second century, but, of course, approved of the annexation of territory. They saw eye to eye with many of the senatorial class and had no conflict with the Senate itself until their own privileges in the provinces were questioned. The wealthy *Equites* also subscribed to the same social values as the senatorial class, reinvested their money in land, and became country "gentlemen" as well as urban financiers.

SLAVES

During the wars of conquest a very large number of prisoners of war were brought to Italy to be sold as slaves. They came from all the regions where fighting took place: Africa, Spain, Greece, Asia Minor, and northern Italy itself. When the wars came to an end, drying up that source of supply, the demand was satisfied partly by breeding slaves in Italy and partly by a very active slave trade with its eastern center on the island of Delos. Piracy, kidnapping, and the purchase of slaves from the barbarian fringe of the Hellenistic East supplied the Delian market.

The slaves from the Greek East who were frequently well educated, or, at least, trained as secretaries, accountants, and craftsmen, became domestic slaves in the Roman households. Some acted as tutors for the children of their owner, some as his secretaries and clerks, while others were set up in little businesses to practice their own crafts and share the profits with their masters. Many were able in time to purchase their freedom with their savings and others were freed by their owners in recognition of faithful service or by goodwill. No doubt some vanity entered into these transactions by which a Roman could advertise how many slaves he had, but the number who were freed and became citizens was considerable and began to change the character of the urban citizen body in Rome. The freedman and his descendants continued to observe a tie of loyalty to their former owner and to his family in recognition of the grant of freedom. Thus, the population of Rome was leavened by Greeks and Hellenized natives from the eastern countries. The small retail businesses, shops and craft work in Rome fell largely into their skilled hands which excluded native Romans and Italians.

The slaves from the barbarian lands, on the other hand, had a very desperate existence and seldom regained their freedom. They were bought for work on the big farms of the wealthy or in the labor gangs of the contractors who carried out the public building projects for the state. Since the supply of such slaves was large and the price cheap, their owners paid very little attention to the health and well-being of their human tools. When the slaves were worn out, replacement was easy. Those slaves who escaped fled to the mountains, where brigandage on the roads was preferable to working on a plantation. Slave revolts were frequent, and some developed into wars which required the Roman army to suppress them. In 135 B.C., for example, a slave war broke out on Sicily, which involved seventy thousand slaves and required several years to put down. In 74 B.C. the famous war of Spartacus in Italy was similarly a revolt of desperation. Because the plentiful supply of slave labor drove free men from the large farms and public work projects, Romans and Italians of the lower class consequently faced unemployment in both the country and the city.

THE PLANTATION SYSTEM (*Latifundia*)

The senatorial class and the rising middle class of Rome both improved their economic position in the wars of expansion, but the ordinary Roman soldier who had fought them found himself increasingly adrift. Hannibal's systematic devastation of Etruria and southern Italy had largely wiped out the system of small-scale farming in those regions. Owners of the farms had been killed in battle, their farmhouses and villages destroyed, and the limits or records of their property obliterated. Many soldiers who had served for long periods in the wars had little will to return to their farms on discharge or had no farm to return to. After the Punic Wars the Roman government had declared public land thousands of acres which were desolate and ownerless. It had been the traditional practice in Rome either to lease such land to bring in revenue to the state, or to settle colonies of Roman citizens on it in small lots. Since in the early second century there does not seem to have been much pressure to re-establish small-scale farming, the obvious solution was to lease the land in fairly large tracts, although a maximum limit of five hundred *iugera,* about 320 acres, to an individual, was the nominal allowance.

The availability of land, either by lease from the state or by purchase from its peasant owners, and the abundant supply of cheap labor combined to bring about a revolution in Italian agriculture. The senatorial class added to its already large holdings to develop a sort of plantation system on big estates (*latifundia*). Where the land was particularly suitable, as on the coastal plains of western Italy, specialized crops, fruit, olives, vines, and vegetables were cultivated. Also, much land which was suitable for cereal production was converted into grazing land. The owners of these ranches found it very easy to extend their holdings by allowing their cattle to graze over the proper boundaries and thus establish a title in equity to land which was rightfully that of the state. The maximum limits were disregarded, and the plantation system spread to the disadvantage of the remaining small-scale farmers. Since the latter had neither the capital nor the labor to compete, they were pushed into the hills, where the land was unfit for cereal production, or they were forced to find a living elsewhere. In the highlands of the central Apennines the old peasant system continued to survive, but many farmers emigrated from the rest of Italy into Cisalpine Gaul or moved to Rome, where they had to adjust to urban conditions, competing with the discharged soldiers, the slaves, and the freedmen.

The new system was both profitable and congenial to the senatorial class. The Elder Cato wrote a book on agriculture, *De Agricultura,* and the Senate in 146 B.C., with a rare display of cultural interest, sponsored the translation into Latin of a very technical treatise on estate management by the Carthaginian Mago. On the other hand, the dispossessed farmers resident in Rome could find little work. They did, however, have votes, which could be sold for a meagre livelihood in the *clientage* of some political leader. As we will discuss next this agricultural revolution helped to create an idle mob in Rome with serious political and military effects for the state.

NEW PEASANTS AND CRAFTSMEN

Nevertheless, other regions of Italy and other elements in the population prospered and developed rapidly. The pacification of Cisalpine Gaul threw the fertile lands of the Po River valley and the foothills of the Alps open to agricultural settlement on a large scale. The older colonies of the region, such as Verona and Patavium (Padua), grew into flourishing urban centers. Farmers moved from lower Italy to find good farms in the north, where they established the old type of small, individual holding. The settlers, clinging to their traditional Roman customs and style of living, transformed the area into a stable and sound part of Roman Italy, cherishing the traditions of the Republic and Romanizing the Gauls who were left in the region. In the first century B.C. Cisalpine Gaul produced three great figures of Latin literature, Catullus, Vergil, and Livy. It was also the chief recruiting ground for the army of Julius Caesar.

There was a marked growth, too, in the coastal towns of southern Italy, where the Greeks and Hellenized Italians profited from the new opportunities of trade and business. Campania, in particular, grew in wealth, both from the new agriculture and as a center of industry and trade. Weapons for the Roman armies and tools for agriculture were produced in Campanian workshops, and the new industry of glassmaking was introduced by immigrants from Phoenicia. Campania was also a center of shipbuilding for naval and merchant ships. As the ports of Puteoli and Pompeii grew rich on trade, the houses in Pompeii rivaled those of Rome itself at this time, exhibiting new features of plan and decoration borrowed from the Hellenistic East.

Senatorial Government

While the phrase, *Senatus Populusque Romanus* (the Senate and the Roman People) theoretically expressed the idea that the Roman government was carried on by the deliberation of the Senate and the approval of the assemblies of the people, the Senate was firmly established as the actual governing body after the war with Hannibal. The Senate, numbering about three hundred, conducted the government of Rome and made the vital decisions, curbing the power of the magistrates and skillfully manipulating the working of the popular assemblies. Foreign policy was directed by the Senate, which negotiated with envoys and foreign rulers and drew up the settlements which concluded wars. The Senate also worked out the general strategy of the wars themselves by the allocation of troops and funds to the consuls. The formal assent to war and peace given by the assembly of the people was prescribed by the Senate. In the internal government of Rome the purse strings were held by the Senate, which set revenues and expenditures, and its resolutions (*consulta*) acquired the force of law. As the Roman historian Sallust put it in the first century B.C., "kingdoms, provinces, statutes, laws, courts, war, and peace, in short, all things human and divine, were in the hands of a few." Sallust wrote with a popular bias, but the charge was close to the truth.

This assumption of authority did not rest on any constitutional change after 287 B.C., when the sovereignty of the people had been recognized by the Hortensian Law, but had been established by practice and by the changing structure of Roman society. After the First Punic War, which popular leaders had urged on the people, reforms were given a democratic appearance but actually contributed to the predominance of the senatorial class or to that of individual leaders.

For example, the structure of the Centuriate Assembly was changed, probably in 241 B.C., when two new tribes were created, making thirty-five in all, to adjust the assembly to the tribal organization. The number of *centuries* in the first class was lowered from eighty to seventy by drawing two *centuries,* a senior and a junior, from each of the thirty-five tribes. The privilege of casting the first vote was taken from the cavalry *centuries* and given to one of the first-class *centuries,* chosen by lot. These measures, of course, made the voting descend into the second class before a majority was reached and broadened the privilege of voting first. Yet this democratization was only apparent, because the seventy new *centuries* were not mixed from all the tribes as previously, but each pair of *centuries* drew its membership from the upper income group of a single tribe. There was as great an inequality in the numbers of individual voters as there was between tribes, and the urban tribes, in particular, became almost "rotten boroughs." The effect of the new system was to place the election of the higher magistrates more effectively in the hands of the upper income groups, and to make the rise of new men more difficult.

As politics became more a matter of the manipulation of certain tribes, individual leaders were able to enlarge the number of their adherents in a tribe through a speciously popular program. Gaius Flaminius, who defeated the Gauls in North Italy and lost his life in battle with Hannibal at Lake Trasimene, rose from the tribunate in 232 B.C. to become censor in 220 and was twice consul. In 232 he pushed through a bill for the distribution of public land south of Ariminum to the poor, against the opposition of the Senate. The latter argued that the land was too far from Rome for its settlers to participate properly in political life. When his land bill was passed, Flaminius enrolled the new settlers in two tribes, where they formed a solid body of support for him, and later as censor authorized the construction of a new road, the Via Flaminia, to facilitate his constituents's attendance at assembly meetings in Rome.

Popular leadership was discredited in the early stages of the Second Punic War by the disastrous defeats of Flaminius at Lake Trasimene and of Varro at Cannae. While Scipio Africanus did rise to prominence by popular support, his influence waned after the war when the more conservative groups regained the upper hand. Between 200 and 168 B.C. the control of the Senate was firmly established by its energy and success in the eastern wars. However much the effects of Roman policy on the position of Hellenism in the East may be criticized, victory and plunder marked it as successful to the Romans, and the traditional prestige of the senatorial class was confirmed.

THE NOBLES

By the time of the eastern wars the old distinction between patrician and wealthy plebeian had been virtually obliterated, and a unified senatorial class, the *nobiles,* had emerged. The members were a nobility of office holders and their descendants, men whose ancestors had held one of the *curule* magistracies from quaestorship to consulate. There was an inner circle of very great families of old patrician stock whose forefathers numbered consuls by the score, but the whole group of noble families formed a well-marked social class. They held the magistracies and places in the Senate within their own small circle and, as we have noticed, were able to strengthen their economic position by acquiring land in Italy and by plunder in war and the provinces. The nobles were practical men of affairs, managing their great estates in private life, and, in their public capacity, leading Roman armies and governing the state. They continued to represent the conservative, agricultural character of Rome and the military traditions of its early history. There was intense rivalry among the leading families for office, but, as a group, the nobility had a very strong corporate loyalty and set themselves against new men who tried to break into their circle. Leadership was in the hands of about ten great clans who were able to hold the high offices for their own members. For example, from 200 to 146 B.C., out of the 108 consuls elected, 85 came from ten families, while only four completely new men entered the charmed circle of the nobility by a public career.

The political position of a noble family rested on a wide network of connections extending through all classes of Roman society. In the center there were the members of the family and the clan to which it belonged. Beyond this the web of influence was spread by political friendships and marital alliances which might extend into the lesser nobility and into the rising middle class. Support was furnished from the lower class by the clan's rural *clientage* and by new *clients* made among the urban population of Rome. Roman political life tended to be largely a matter of rivalries among the great families in this period and focused on electoral contests for the magistracies. There were no political parties in our sense of the word, with differing principles of government, platforms, or party organization. Instead, a few great families—the Fabii, Claudii, Cornelii, Aemilii, Valerii, and Fulvii—dominated the scene by their own blocks of power and by making shifting coalitions.

A good illustration of the working of politics in Rome is the manner in which Scipio Africanus and his family were deprived of influence and relegated, in effect, to the back benches of the Senate for a time. About 200 B.C. Scipio was at the height of his prestige as a result of the victorious campaigns in Spain and Africa. In 199 he was elected censor, the crown of a successful public career. Scipio's position was very strong, for he belonged to the Cornelii and had been the general favorite of the people who backed him against the more conservative majority of the Senate led by the Fabii. Needless to say, Scipio was also a man of exceptional ability and a good politician. He saw to it that his veteran soldiers were granted land in areas where their membership in certain tribes would enlarge his voting strength. Many of Scipio's senatorial colleagues, however, not only disapproved of his political ideas but feared his popular support.

Scipio wanted Rome to stay in the East and to play a proper part among the Hellenistic states by diplomacy. Thus he opposed the withdrawal of troops from Greece in 194 B.C. as premature in the light of the worsening relations with Antiochus. His advice was disregarded and by 190 his influence was on the wane. Scipio and his brother, Lucius, were recalled from Asia Minor in that year.

The Elder Cato, narrowly Roman and conservative in outlook, took over the tradition of Fabian opposition to the Scipios and began to attack them.

After various minor members of the Scipionic group were prosecuted in the courts through tribunes, in 187 B.C. Cato felt bold enough to attack Lucius Scipio. Lucius was asked to account for five hundred talents which Antiochus had paid to him, presumably as the first installment of the war indemnity imposed after the Roman victory at Magnesia. Scipio Africanus contended that the money was the commander's private booty, for which he did not need to account, and disdainfully tore up the account books before the Senate. The matter was revived again in 184 B.C., however, when a tribune from Cato's following demanded an accounting from Lucius to the Tribal Assembly. A personal appeal from Africanus to the people saved his brother for the time being, but Lucius was later fined heavily. He refused to pay and was saved from imprisonment only by the intervention of a tribune of the Scipionic group. By this time the charges had served their purpose in damaging the reputation of the Scipios, and the case was dropped by Cato.

While Scipio's great prestige made him unusually difficult to control, most magistrates identified their own interest with that of the Senate and did not challenge its authority. The tribunes, traditional guardians of the rights of the people, had become representatives of the whole state by the end of the third century rather than of the plebeian element only. They met with the Senate, which gave some appearance of popular supervision of that body, and worked for the various groups in it to further their own careers. The office attracted ambitious young men, since it gave an opportunity to bring themselves to public attention, as in the case of Cato's henchmen, by prosecuting prominent political leaders. The other magistrates, quaestors, aediles, praetors and consuls were already in the Senate or looked forward to membership, so that they generally shared its collegiate feeling. The chief danger to senatorial control from this group was the consul who sought re-election or whose term was prolonged by a promagistracy.

After the Second Punic War, various measures were taken to guard against such excessive personal ambition: extension of commands in the field was little used; in 180 B.C. the Villian Law regulated the holding of offices by establishing a prescribed *cursus honorum* (course of office) with minimum age limits and intervals between offices. The young Roman of the senatorial class, who aspired to a public career, would spend ten years in military service and as a protégé on the staff of some provincial governor. Then, at the age of twenty-eight he became eligible for the quaestorship. He might skip the office of aedile, for which he was eligible after an interval of two years, but normally rising politicians liked to hold it, despite the expense involved. The aediles were in charge of the public festivals which could be made the occasions for lavish displays, featuring gladiatorial games and wild beast hunts. Two years later the ex-aedile was eligible for the praetorship and, if he were elected, for assignment as a provincial governor. The minimum age for the consulship was set at forty-two, and in 151 B.C. re-election was forbidden until after an interval of ten years. Even so, the consul in charge of a successful war might present a difficult problem when he regarded a war as his own personal undertaking.

A good example of such arrogant behavior is provided by Manlius Vulso, consul in 189 B.C., who was placed in charge of the war against Antiochus in Asia Minor. After the defeat of Antiochus, Manlius' command was prolonged for the following year to wind up affairs in Asia Minor. Without any authorization from the Senate, Manlius called on Attalus of Pergamum for aid and began to invade Galatia, although no war had been declared by Rome against the Gauls. En route to Galatia, Manlius sold protection from the Roman army for his personal profit and, when he actually fought the war, he collected a very large amount of booty. When Manlius was ordered home, he demanded a triumph for his services on arrival. The majority of the Senate was opposed and presented Manlius with a long list of misdemeanors: plotting to seize the person of Antiochus, planning to cross the Taurus Mountains, illegally making war on Galatia, conducting the war by wandering about in search of plunder and, finally, returning home without proper organization. Despite this military junket, Manlius' family and connections in the Senate backed his argument that subjection of the Gauls was necessary for a peaceful Asia and contrived to get a triumph for him.

Senatorial control over the assemblies was made easier by the changes in Roman society which had lessened their effectiveness as instruments for the expression of genuine popular will. As we have noticed, the Centuriate Assembly was dominated by the propertied classes as a whole; consequently it was mainly the scene of the electoral contests for the high offices. On the other hand, the Tribal Assembly, made up of the four urban and the thirty-one rural tribes, retained a tradition of real popular sovereignty from the time when Rome was small and the citizen body compact. In the second century,

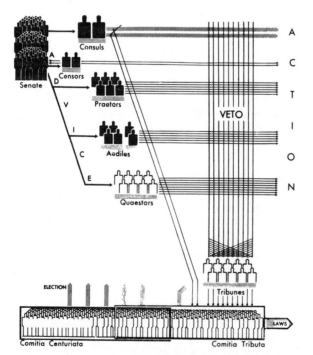

Chart illustrating the machinery of government in Rome in the mid-second century B.C.

however, Roman citizens were widely scattered in colonies and municipalities throughout Italy or absent on military service. To citizens today an obvious way of maintaining the proper tradition of the assembly would have been to make it representative. Romans, however, continued to think of their state as a city with a direct assembly meeting in Rome. Thus, although Rome had outgrown its original form, the Tribal Assembly tended to be controlled by the urban population and not the whole Roman people. The political leaders found their opportunity in this situation and were able to add compact political followings to their existing blocks of clan members and rural *clients*. Since the peasants and soldiers who had moved to the city retained their tribal affiliations by inheritance and new citizens could be enrolled in appropriate tribes, a relatively small number of voters could weight a tribal vote decisively. A majority of eighteen tribes, of course, carried the assembly.

In addition to such specific methods of vote control, the people of Rome were cultivated by new techniques of mass bribery and propaganda. The official state festivals, of which there were six in the course of a year, were made into occasions of display and advertisement for their sponsors, the aediles, as noticed above. Other politicians might make a public occasion out of the funeral of some prominent member of their family, carrying the ancestral busts in procession and marking the occasion by gladiatorial games and the distribution of gifts to the poor. The mere expense of political careers in Rome was sufficient to confine them to the very wealthy. Finally a close watch could be kept on individual voting until 139 B.C., for it remained open until that time. The Senate expressed disapproval of political bribery and corruption by a considerable amount of legislation, but its very volume indicates the ineffectiveness of the measures. Yet the votes of the people did elect officials and could pass laws. The assemblies were a potential threat to senatorial control of government because some issue might bring the genuine rural voters to Rome in sufficient numbers to upset the balance, or a demagogue among the tribunes and consuls might excite the people in his own interest.

The Greek historian Polybius, who lived in Rome during this heyday of senatorial government, made an analysis of Roman political institutions and, with other Greeks who visited Rome, began to familiarize the senatorial class with Greek political theory. To Polybius the Roman constitution seemed an ideal mixture of the best forms of government. He did realize that the Senate was in actual control, but ignored this and applied his theory somewhat mechanically. He judged that Rome was at the zenith in the cycle of change, through which all states passed, and had its political elements in proper balance and check. The consuls were supposed to represent the absolute authority of monarchy; the Senate, the high intellectual and moral quality of the best men in deliberation; and the assemblies, the collective good judgment of the people in their elective and legislative decisions. In reality the consuls were "kings" for a year only and only outside of Rome when they were conducting a war or governing a province. As noticed above, the Senate had methods of curbing those high officials who might become presumptuous. The Republic did have the machinery for an awkward, but decisive control by the people, but in practice the senatorial class was able to manipulate and direct the assemblies in its own interest.

Probably the Roman senators made their own evaluation of Polybius' analysis because they were quite familiar with the art of politics, but they found Greek theory most congenial because of the high value placed on aristocracy. The senators were pleased to discover a theoretical justification for their rule as the "best" men of the state and began to refer to themselves as *Optimates* (the best). In the political struggles of the first century B.C. convenient labels were found in the Greek political vocabulary for their opponents: tyrants for the military dictators, and demagogues for the leaders of the popular groups. The opponents of the Senate, of course, found oligarch a convenient word. While the Greeks had a word for what they saw in Rome, the machinery remained individually Roman. In the second century the senators had the practical justification of success, great ability and energy, and many of them an arrogant toughness of mind and insensibility that brooked no opposition and little argument.

Early Hellenization in Rome

The main purpose of Polybius' history was to give an account of the Romans, of Rome's wars with Hannibal and with the Hellenistic Kingdoms to his fellow Greeks. During the course of the wars, however, a reverse conquest set in, by which the Greeks began to Hellenize Rome. The Romans had been influenced to some degree by Greek civilization since the early sixth century B.C., but they did not begin to feel its direct impact until the third

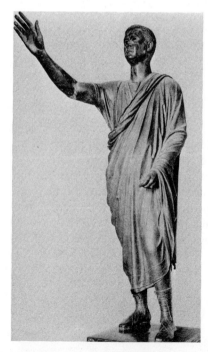

The Arringatore, or Orator. This bronze statue, found near Lake Trasimene, is inscribed with the Roman name, Aulus Metellus, in Etruscan letters.

century. In the Punic Wars two generations of Romans served in South Italy and Sicily. They saw the temples and great public buildings and became familiar with the manner of life in the large Greek cities. War, which sometimes was fought against the Greeks, was not the best way to gain a sympathetic understanding of another and more sophisticated civilization, and from the outset Roman attitudes varied from admiration to contempt. Probably the ordinary soldiers picked up a smattering of Greek and a superficial familiarity with new and exotic modes of entertainment, food and manners, while their officers learned something of Greek education and ideas from their counterparts in military alliance and negotiation.

In the course of the wars with the Eastern kingdoms, however, contacts with Hellenism were much more intense and significant. The armies served in Greece and western Asia Minor, where Greek civilization had developed, and the Roman officials were in intimate contact with highly educated Greek rulers and administrators. If the Romans did not meet these men in Greece, they heard Greek envoys in the Roman Senate pleading their city's cases. Sometimes these were distinguished rhetoricians and philosophers. For example, in 159 B.C. Athens sent a trio of philosophers to the Senate: Carneades, a Sceptic, Diogenes, a Stoic, and Critolaus, a Peripatetic. In 144 B.C. Panaetius, the foremost Stoic philosopher of the century, came from Rhodes on his city's business and remained in Rome as a guest of the Scipio family. Among the hostages and slaves brought to Rome were many highly educated Greeks who served as tutors, lecturers, and advisors for their hosts and owners. A new intellectual world dawned on the Romans of the senatorial class when they heard the dazzling rhetoric and adroit argument of their visitors.

Among the early Philhellenes were Scipio Africanus and Flamininus, but a widespread discovery of Greek intellectual achievement came after the middle of the century. At that time a very distinguished coterie, known as the Scipionic circle, was particularly receptive to such ideas. Its central figure was Scipio Africanus Minor, an adopted grandson of the great Africanus, and himself the victor over Carthage in the Third Punic War. In private life he was the patron of Polybius and Panaetius, and he encouraged Terence, the writer of Latin comedies. The other Romans of the circle, men from several of the great senatorial families, were influential and prominent in political life and interested in Roman law as well as in Greek ideas. It was through such figures as these and their children, who had been educated in both the Greek and Roman disciplines, that significant penetration of Greek ideas was made. Some men, however, like Cato the Elder, were openly contemptuous of the new Greek ways, and others, like Acilius Glabrio, who had pillaged Aetolia in 189 B.C., regarded the wars in Greece as an opportunity for personal plunder. Yet among the upper classes a steady change of education and manners set in.

The impact of Hellenization was limited mainly to the upper class because Rome had no system of public education through which new ideas might be introduced. Much of the instruction in the Greek language and in rhetoric, philosophy, and literature was limited to the family circle of the great houses although a few teachers founded private schools in which they taught for a fee. In general the Greek idea that rhetoric and philosophy fitted a man for a political career was thoroughly acceptable to the Romans of the senatorial class because of their traditions of public service. Family influences and practical familiarity with farm management, politics, and war continued to be very important in the education of the young Roman, but to an ever increasing degree, it was thought proper to add Greek training. As yet not many young men were sent to Athens or to Rhodes for training in the philosophical schools, but by the end of the century that kind of education was becoming customary.

RELIGION

Reflective Romans of the senatorial class found a congenial personal philosophy in Stoicism, with its strong emphasis on morality and responsibility to society, and they tended to remain aloof from the new religious influences from the East. The practice of identifying Roman deities with those of Greece and of incorporating Greek mythology into a Latin context continued, but the nature and practice of public Roman worship changed little. Perhaps it was impossible to change the contractual ideas and stereotyped rituals which characterized the traditional religion. The formal practices of the state religion were correctly carried on, but during the Second Punic War the government did permit the introduction of new cults from the East. The most important was that of Phrygian Cybele, the Great Mother-Goddess from Pessinus in Asia Minor. In 205 B.C., after consultation of the Sibylline Oracles, the cult was authorized in an effort to help the state in its final struggle with Hannibal.

Generally speaking, official Rome had no interest in and complete tolerance for private religious worship; consequently the new Greek and Eastern elements in the population did popularize some Eastern cults. The cult of Isis, for example, was introduced into the Campanian harbor cities. In 186 B.C., however, the spread of Dionysiac worship from southern Italy was strictly regulated because it seemed to be damaging public morality and—worse—might cloak political conspiracy. The more conservative senators disliked this orgiastic and mystical type of worship in the first place and suspected that the secret meetings of its devotees might be used for conspiracy. Accordingly, a law was passed prohibiting worship by more than five individuals in a group. This type of regulation furnished a precedent for official Roman treatment of new religions—tolerance, or rather indifference, for private belief and individual practice, but a close scrutiny and regulation for the public character of a worship.

LITERATURE

Romans had produced little imaginative literature before they came into contact with the Greeks of South Italy in the third century. The prose of their laws and oratory was simple and straightforward, and the only historical records were lists of magistrates and sacred calendars. Like other peoples they had ballads of the exploits of early heroes and folk songs for their festivals. Perhaps these would have grown into a more sophisticated native poetry in time, but contact with the developed literature of Greece was too strong. From the outset Latin literature took over Greek forms and followed Greek models almost exclusively. Although at first there was a considerable amount of translation into Latin, Roman patrons soon demanded Roman themes and the expression of Roman values; thus a national literature came into being, with Latin gradually developing into a literary language.

Among the writers of the third century the earliest was Livius Andronicus (*ca.* 284-04 B.C.), a Greek freedman from Tarentum, who made his living as a teacher in Rome and who translated the *Odyssey* and some Greek plays. His contemporary, Gnaeus Naevius, probably an Italian, sounded a more original note by writing an epic poem on the First Punic War and some satires. Because Naevius attacked prominent political personages, he landed in jail. But the poet regarded by the Romans themselves as the fountainhead of their literature was Ennius (239-169 B.C.), an Italian from the south, who was educated in Greek Tarentum. After he became a Roman citizen, he demonstrated his loyalty in a long epic poem, the *Annales,* which told the history of Rome from the settlement of Aeneas to the war with Hannibal and expressed the traditional Roman values of stability, perseverance, and responsibility. Ennius' epic, after serving as the poetic expression of Rome's new-found greatness for almost two centuries, was replaced by that of Vergil in the Augustan Age.

Interest in the history of Rome led to the writing of histories in Latin as well as in Greek. The earliest history of Rome was written about 200 B.C. by a Roman senator, Quintus Fabius Pictor. He chose to write in Greek because Latin provided no model, and he wished Greeks to read about the growth of Rome. In the following century a school of historians, known collectively as the Annalists, collected the records, legends, and early traditions of Rome and wrote their books in the form of chronicles. The style was crude, for Latin prose was in its infancy, and the accounts contained much that was not historical (pp. 429-31). Yet the Annalists are important both as a reflection of the growing consciousness of Rome's place in history and because they provided material for the voluminous history of Rome written by Livy in the time of Augustus. The Elder Cato made a more original approach to history in his *Origines,* which included accounts of the Italian peoples as well as of Rome.

It is somewhat paradoxical that the most influential and popular works of early Latin literature, the comedies of Plautus and Terence, were virtually unique and led to little subsequent development of drama. Plautus (259-184 B.C.) was an Umbrian, and Terence (195-159 B.C.) was an African slave in the household of Scipio Aemilianus. They transplanted the New Comedy of Hellenistic Greece (p. 407) to the Roman stage, but Plautus, in particular, gave an Italian stamp to his plays by developing Italian characters and situations with ribald humor. Terence's work was more polished and serious. It was closer to his Greek models and to modern taste—his *Woman of Andros* has been imitated by Thornton Wilder. Both playwrights had a very considerable influence on Renaissance comedy, but in Rome itself there were no successors worthy of note. The native taste for satire and crude comedy displayed by Plautus was carried on by the writers of satire, the most Italian of the Latin literary genres, and by ephemeral farce. Greek tragedy, too, was translated and imitated in this early period, but it did not inspire a Roman tragic drama except as a literary exercise.

LAW

The development of Roman law throughout this formative period was little affected by Greek philosophical ideas except through the medium of a few of the political leaders of Rome who made the law their private study and began to develop a theory of legal institutions. Thus the growth of Roman law, like that of political institutions, was the product of experience and of the solutions made to meet the changing condition of society. Until the publication of the Twelve Tables in 450 B.C. the interpretation of the law, through which its principles might be changed, had been entirely in the hands of the Roman priests. They "knew" the unwritten, customary laws of the community and the precise rituals and words by which cases had to be introduced and conducted before a judge. The priests were not judges themselves but gave advice, that is interpreted the law, to individuals and to the magistrates who heard the cases. The authority of early Roman law, then, was essentially religious because only the priestly college could know and change it. The publication of the Tables, however, partly detached the law from religion by making it necessary for the priests to accommodate their interpretations to the written paragraphs of the Twelve Tables.

It was not until the third century, however, that the application of law began to change rapidly. First the ritual procedures, which had remained in the priests' care, were published in 304 B.C. After that a group of men, known as jurisconsults, gradually took over the function of interpretation. These were members of the senatorial class, who felt that the law should be modified to fit the changing needs of the period. Out of their own interest and a sense of public duty they made a study of law and gave advice to individuals and to the magistrates, just as the priests had done. Their opinions were not compulsive, but their personal prestige carried great weight, so that the magistrates were continuously changing and developing the law by application of the jurisconsults' advice. At first such advice was entirely oral, but in 194 B.C. the censor, Aelius Paetus, published a book of his interpretations, the first in a long series of publications, which made the jurisconsults an important source of law.

The Romans also became aware in the third century that their own law was too rigid and local in character to settle the cases arising between Romans and foreigners. In 242 B.C. a new office, that of the *praetor peregrinus* (the alien praetor), was created to take care of such disputes. The praetor introduced the practice of issuing an edict at the beginning of his term of office in which he set out the principles by which he would assign cases to the judges who were to hear them. In these edicts the praetors departed from the rigid letter of Roman law to admit foreign practices and, most important, common-sense ideas of justice and equity. Since each successive praetor based his edict on that of his predecessor, modifying and adding where he judged it necessary, this body of law grew in response to current needs and was infused with the principles of equity. In time there developed the conception of a general law, governing all free men, Romans and foreigners alike, which became known as the *ius gentium,* or law of nations. While its conceptions sprang from practice and actual experience, later legal theorists recognized its affinity to the Greek philosophic concept of a law of nature and of an absolute principle of justice inherent in the universe. Roman law thus became a civilizing force of great importance in history during the period of the Empire, when emperors issued their edicts, based on centuries of practical experience and theoretical study, for all the provinces under Roman dominion.

The praetors also played an important part in removing the set rituals of procedure in Roman law. About 150 B.C. they were authorized to issue *formulae* (writs) which governed the hearing of a case. The praetor would conduct a preliminary hearing of the parties to the dispute and write a *formula* to the magistrate, summing up the important points to be decided and the redress to be applied. The ideas of equity embodied in these instructions were introduced into judicial decisions and modified the law somewhat in the manner of the jurisconsults. Another innovation of this period, the establishment of standing courts (*quaestiones*) the first of which was that for hearing extortion cases from the provinces, was not so effective. Others were set up to hear various types of criminal cases involving capital charges. These had been within the jurisdiction of the magistrates and had allowed appeal to the assemblies. Perhaps the assemblies were not the most suitable places for a judicial process, but the senatorial courts, whose verdicts were final, were susceptible to class interest, and their establishment infringed on an important area of popular sovereignty.

ARCHITECTURE

The most obvious effects of expansion and contact with Greece were apparent in the physical appearance of Rome and in the manner of life of the Romans. In the second century Rome was changing from a large country town into a monumental city as its population increased and large sums of money were available for building. The Forum Romanum at the foot of the Capitoline Hill took on an almost completely civic and political character, when new markets were built elsewhere for the sale of goods and produce. In the Forum three new basilicas were constructed to serve the more dignified purposes of finance and the courts of law. The basilica, adapted from Hellenistic models in the East, became a standard type of Roman building and ultimately a model for early Christian churches. The structure was long and narrow, divided by two rows of interior columns into a broad central hall and narrower side aisles. Between the

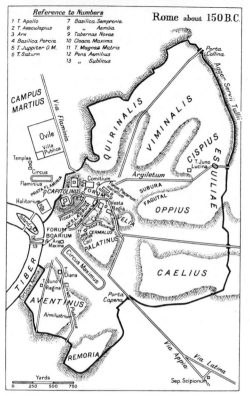

Reference to Numbers

1 T. Apollo   7 Basilica Sempronia
2 T. Aesculapius   8 „   Aemilia
3 Arx   9 Tabernae Novae
4 Basilica Porcia   10 Cloaca Maxima
5 T. Juppiter O.M.   11 T. Magnae Matris
6 T. Saturn   12 Pons Aemilius
           13 „   Sublicus

Rome about 150 B.C.

*The city of Rome about 150 B.C.,
when it was beginning to take on
the monumental form of a capital city*

Palatine and Aventine hills the Circus Maximus, where the chariot races and
other great spectacles were held, had already been laid out in the third century
B.C. New temples and colonnades were constructed at various points in the
city, and in 142 B.C. the first stone bridge, the Aemilian Bridge, named from the
prominent Scipio Aemilianus, was built across the Tiber. Yet not all the aspects
of growth in Rome were attractive, for cheap housing had to be provided for
the influx of population. Blocks of flimsily constructed apartment houses, five
or six stories in height and separated by narrow streets, were built on the lower,
less desirable ground. Since these were crowded and had no sanitary facilities or
police protection the central part of Rome soon became a dangerous slum,
where violence and fire were common. The wealthy, on the other hand, put up
luxurious houses, adapting the peristyle type, familiar from Delos (p. 396),
to the older Italian house, on the slopes of the Roman hills and constructed
villas in the countryside to avoid the bustle of life in Rome.

The Italian, or *atrium,* house consisted of a central unroofed, or partly roofed
room, the *atrium,* in the center of which was a pool to collect the rain water.
From the *atrium* a cluster of small, dark rooms opened, three of which were
arranged along the rear, somewhat in the manner of the tripartite division of the
Italian temple. Frequently the new peristyle structure, with its colonnaded central court, was added to the *atrium* house and used for the private living quarters
of the family. The *atrium* element then served the business and political life of
the owner where he met his *clients* and colleagues. The new, comfortable living

502

was on a luxurious scale. The wealthy became patrons of art, adorning their houses with fine mosaic floors, costly furniture, sculpture, and wall paintings.

Italian public architecture was improved, too, by new technical developments, as well as by the copious supply of money and by contacts with the Greeks. It had been discovered in the third century that a mixture of lime and volcanic ash made a very durable, cheap and easily handled concrete. This concrete, which was used for walls and roofs, ultimately led to the construction of large vaults, spanning great areas of space, which became characteristic of Roman building. Since concrete was drab in appearance, walls were faced with stucco and slabs of marble. Brick and mortar construction also came into wide use upon the discovery of a good lime and sand mortar. While the Romans clung conservatively to the old Italian type of temple, they began to use Greek architectural ornament on an increasing scale and made their public buildings into exhibition places for the booty brought back from the wars. New works were commissioned from Greek artists who moved to Italy and from native Italian workshops that followed the current Hellenic fashions. In Italy, just as in the countries of the Near East, the towns and cities began to take on a uniform physical appearance under the influence of Greek architecture and sculpture.

The Aemilian Bridge (left) over the Tiber in Rome; the bridge was completed by Scipio Aemilianus during his censorship in 142 B.C.

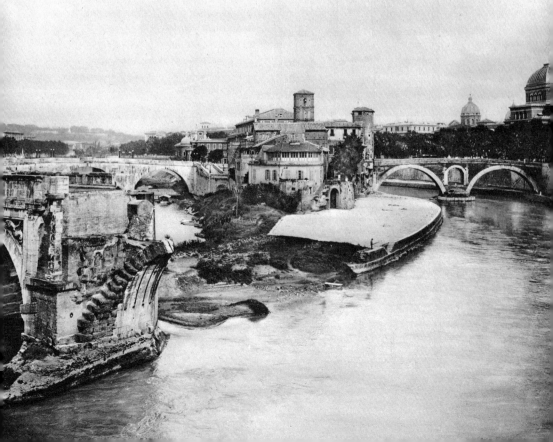

New Problems of Senatorial Government

When Polybius was writing his history, just after the Roman wars of conquest, the position of Rome seemed very secure. Roman armies had defeated all their enemies, the government had a long tradition of stability, and it had very able direction from the senatorial class. The city of Rome had become a rival of Alexandria and Antioch in size and was speedily becoming the financial, as well as the political, center of the Mediterranean. Yet Polybius judged that Rome would not continue to enjoy political stability for long. He anticipated that, in accordance with the Greek theory of cyclical change, the rivalries of Roman political leaders would break the unity of the senatorial oligarchy and lead to mob violence and demagoguery.

Rome did stand on the threshold of political breakdown, the first phase of which followed the pattern observed in the city-states of Greece, but far more complex currents of change were running. New wealth was bringing a middle class into existence in Italian society, whose political ideas and will were still unformed. The rise of the Equestrians was one manifestation, but throughout the municipalities of Italy men of moderate wealth were replacing the former peasants as the basis of society. They would not find leadership for a long time, but neither could they stand by while the senatorial nobility and the city mob of Rome, both unrepresentative of society as a whole, made a travesty of gov-

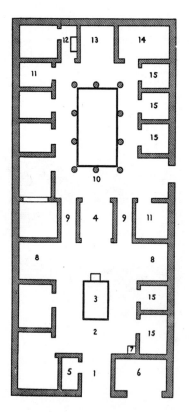

Plan of a Roman town house, exemplifying a combination of the Italian (atrium) *and Greek (peristyle) types*

1. fauces—entrance   2. atrium
3. impluvium—basin for rain water
4. tablinum—office   5. janitor—doorman
6. taberna—shop   7. lararium—altar of lares   8. alae—wings   9. andron—corridor   10. peristyle   11. triclinium—dining room   12. culina—kitchen
13. exedra—entertaining hall   14. oecus—living room   15. cubicola—bedrooms

ernment. On the wider scene, the eastern and western Mediterranean were being knit together by Roman conquest and by economic and cultural ties. In the long run the interests of the provinces had to be reconciled with those of Rome and Italy and fused into a single imperial interest, in which Rome would become a name and an idea, not merely a city. The process of revolution, which began to work rapidly in 133 B.C. with the election of Tiberius Gracchus as tribune of the people, was a lengthy, complex process which covered more than two centuries of Roman history.

Even the most percipient Romans were unaware in the decade before 133 B.C. that they stood on the threshold of a world revolution, let alone aware of the course which it would take. Some of the more thoughtful and responsible men of the senatorial class, however, were concerned about the loss of military efficiency. Being good Romans they noticed that the Roman armies operating in Spain were having unusual difficulty and suffered because of bad morale. In 143 B.C. the Numantine people, who lived in the mountains west of the upper Ebro River, revolted against Roman authority. In 137 the Roman general failed to take the fortified city of Numantia and, while returning to the Ebro River, was cut off and surrounded. He surrendered his army of twenty thousand men to the Numantines, but the Senate disgracefully broke the terms of surrender and tried to continue the war. The morale of the forces in Spain deteriorated rapidly. The men were undisciplined and enjoyed an easy life in barracks with their women and servants to wait on them. In 135 Scipio Aemilianus was placed in charge of Spain. He raised a force of volunteers and personal associates to accompany him, as much for protection from the Roman army (while he restored its efficiency) as to fight against the Numantines. Scipio reimposed discipline and in 133 B.C. reduced and destroyed Numantia. A ten-year war against a few thousand Spanish mountaineers was no credit to Roman arms, and the broken treaty of 137 stained their honor as a people.

At the siege of Numantia there were a number of young men, who were to make Roman history in the next generation: Gaius Gracchus, the brother of Tiberius Gracchus, both of whom were to bring the first serious challenges to the authority of the Senate; Gaius Marius, the first of the military dictators; and Jugurtha, a Numidian prince, whose defiance of Rome was to shake the prestige of the Senate. They were familiar with the weaknesses which had been revealed in Spain and turned them to their own purposes. The Gracchan brothers and some of the more liberal senators concluded that the decline of the small-scale farmers in Italy was crippling the efficiency of the Roman army. To them the problem of the day seemed to be agrarian and its solution the re-establishment of small-scale farming and of the sturdy Roman peasantry. Perhaps Marius learned more. When placed in charge of the war against Jugurtha in 107 B.C., he began to recruit and train a new type of army, of soldiers who became devoted to his interests. A few years later he brought his army as a personal instrument into politics. Rome was about to experience the deeper effects of its expansion.

XXIII

The Breakdown of the Republic, I

(133–78 B.C.)

AMONG THE TRIBUNES of the people elected for 133 B.C. was a young man of the senatorial class, Tiberius Sempronius Gracchus, who was backed by a small group of senators in sponsoring a new agrarian law in the Tribal Assembly. He and his supporters hoped that this measure would restore the practice of small-scale farming in Italy and thus provide more and better recruits for the Roman army. Even though the type of law was not new in Rome and even though every responsible citizen was worried about the quality of the army, yet Tiberius and his younger brother, Gaius, who continued his work, were regarded in Roman tradition as the initiators of the revolution which led to the breakdown of the Republic. In securing the passage of his law Tiberius raised issues which threatened to replace the authority of the Senate with the will of the Tribal Assembly led by a tribune.

From this beginning a struggle for power developed, which drew in all the elements of Roman and Italian society and convulsed Rome and the provinces with political strife and civil war for a century. On one side were the *Optimates,* the great majority of the senatorial class who were conservative, wealthy, and at the outset possessed the prestige of generations of successful government and war. On the other were the *Populares,* as the successors of the Gracchi were called. They were a small minority of the senatorial class who sought support among the have-nots of Rome, the poor citizens, the Equestrians, and the Italian allies. The same game could also be played by the *Optimates,* and frequently the popular leaders found the ground cut from beneath their feet. The *Populares* now welcomed the support of a new and dangerous political instrument, the army raised by Gaius Marius for war against Jugurtha of Numidia and against the Germanic peoples who threatened Italy toward the close of the second century. Again the *Optimates* learned by example, and in the late 80's

The reader will find the Front Endpaper and Maps XVII and XVIII (pages 482–83 and 544) useful as he reads this chapter.

Sulla used his army, victorious over Mithridates of Pontus, to restore the control of the Senate.

The next step, taken in the generation after Sulla, was to use the army as a means to personal power. The problems which Tiberius and Gaius Gracchus had sought to solve by constitutional reform dropped into the background when the question at issue became the form which absolute government would take. A decisive factor in the solution was the entry of hundreds of thousands of new citizens into the state, the result of the wholesale grant of Roman citizenship to the communities of the Italian allies after 90 B.C. An Italian nation was formed, which was concerned for the welfare of Italy as a whole. This ultimately found leadership in Octavius, later Augustus, the nephew of Julius Caesar and the founder of the Roman Empire. The government which he established was a unique blend of both absolute and personal control with the institutions of the Republic.

Tiberius and Gaius Gracchus (133–22 B.C.)

Tiberius and Gaius Gracchus were young Romans of the type who could look forward to a public career under distinguished patronage. Their mother, Cornelia, was a daughter of Scipio Africanus, and their father, a typical senator of the plebeian nobility, had an excellent record in Spain and had risen to the censorship. As might be expected in a family connected with the Scipios, both Tiberius and Gaius were well educated in Greek literature and philosophy. Their sister, in fact, had married Scipio Aemilianus, the founder of the Scipionic circle. Tiberius began his public career wth a quaestorship in 137 B.C., when he served in Spain with the army which the Numantines forced to surrender and on their insistance negotiated the peace later repudiated by the Senate. This repudiation of his treaty, which had saved the lives of twenty thousand Roman soldiers, probably embittered Tiberius and prejudiced his chances of a career through the usual course of office.

Accordingly, in 134 B.C. Tiberius appeared for election to the tribunate, backed by a small group of "liberals," among whom was his father-in-law, Appius Claudius Pulcher, and the jurisconsult, Publius Mucius Scaevola. They judged that a program of agrarian reform would have more chance in the Tribal Assembly than in the Senate, where strong opposition had recently compelled the withdrawal of such a measure. Tiberius, predisposed to reform by his education and personal experience with the army in Spain, perhaps saw a new opening for his career. At first he emphasized the desirability of restoring the sturdy farmers of Roman tradition and stressed the ultimate benefits to the army. That was good politics, but a current of doctrinaire humanitarianism and political theory became increasingly apparent in his speeches and conduct. Tiberius' appeal to the urban poor in Rome was an embittered call to class strife: "The savage beasts in Italy have their particular dens . . . but the men who bear arms, and expose their lives for the safety of their country, enjoy in the meantime nothing more in it but the air and the light; and having no homes or settlements of their own, are constrained to wander from place to place with their wives and children . . . They were styled the masters of the world but in the meantime had not one foot of ground which they could call their own."

THE TRIBUNATE OF TIBERIUS GRACCHUS

Tiberius' agrarian law was generous to the holders of large tracts of public land, in that their possession up to a limit of five hundred *iugera,* about 320 acres, was confirmed. Perhaps, too, an extra allowance of half that amount for each of two sons was granted. Adequate compensation was to be paid for the improvements which had been made on land above the legal allowance. The acreage above this was to be reclaimed by the state for distribution among the poor in small lots of nine to eighteen acres. The new possessors were to pay a small rent and were forbidden to sell their holdings. Thus a brake would be set on the expansion of the *latifundia* and a group of self-supporting farmers would be permanently re-established. The law, as a matter of fact, dealt only with occupied land and left untouched that used for grazing. Yet it seemed to the senatorial class to strike at the basis of their wealth, both at their actual holdings and at their control of the use of public land.

The practical difficulties in the way of implementing the law were very great. The large estates had been formed over the course of several generations, and land acquired above the stipulated limit had been transferred by sale and inheritance or pledged in mortgage. The rights of the state and the original surveys had been long forgotten. It is impossible to estimate how seriously rigorous enforcement would have really damaged the senatorial class, but the latter was dismayed and began to work for the bill's defeat. On the other hand, the prospect of a small farm caught the fancy of urban and rural poor alike. Tiberius had timed his measure skillfully for a vote in late April, when the farmers could come to Rome without serious harm to their work. As it became apparent that there would be an upset in the voting balance in the Tribal Assembly, the senators worked quietly under cover to induce another tribune, Octavius, to veto the bill.

When the time came to offer the law to the assembly, Tiberius unsuspectingly had it read and was about to call for the vote, but Octavius stepped forward and formally vetoed the proceedings. On the following day Tiberius again presented the bill. Again Octavius vetoed it. At this point Tiberius' supporters persuaded him to discuss the legislation with the Senate. He agreed to do so but was met with obstruction and abuse. Most of his supporters were prepared to give up, but Tiberius resolved to try revolutionary tactics. If Octavius obstructed the will of the people, the assembly should remove him from office. At the next meeting of the assembly Tiberius called for the deposition of Octavius in the cause of popular sovereignty and obtained his removal from the tribune's bench. A new law with no clauses for compensation was approved with implementation provided for by the establishment of a commission consisting of Tiberius himself, his father-in-law, Appius Claudius, and his brother, Gaius.

Tiberius had shifted the grounds of dispute from the agrarian law to a constitutional issue. Roman and modern scholars have argued whether the deposition of consuls, which had occurred, offered a precedent for that of a tribune. The heart of the issue, however, seems to be that Tiberius had established a precedent for terminating a magistracy at the assembly's will, and so the action threatened to transfer the dependency of magistrates from the Senate to the Tribal Assembly. Tiberius' senatorial backers were alive to this, for, with the exception of his father-in-law and a very few others, they deserted him at this point. The bill, however, had been passed, and the commission was authorized to put it into effect.

The Senate had other weapons with which to fight, and, when money was to be provided for the commission, the equivalent of thirty cents a day was granted. At this point news of the bequest of Attalus of Pergamum, by which he had left his kingdom to the Roman state, came to Rome. Tiberius seized upon the occasion to suggest using the contents of the Pergamene treasury for financing his commission's work. This would have been a blow at the Senate's traditional control of foreign affairs, and the proposal deepened the constitutional issue still more. When Tiberius, whose term as tribune was nearing its end, proposed to stand for re-election, which could be considered illegal, the *Optimates* began to apply the label of tyrant and demagogue and to prepare for violence. Tiberius' support among the people had fallen away after the passage of the agrarian law since they were not alive to the constitutional implications of his methods. During his candidacy Tiberius seems to have tried to revive interest by advocating a series of judicial and constitutional reforms but failed. Even so, the voting ran close, and, when supporters of the *Optimates* tried to block the proceedings by false religious omens, rioting nearly broke out. In this tense situation a group of senators rounded up a mob of their *clients* and slaves, broke into the assembly and beat Tiberius and three hundred of his supporters to death. Their pretext was that Tiberius aimed at kingship in Rome. The Senate gave legal color to the charge by setting up a special court to try other partisans of Tiberius for their share in his "treason."

INTERLUDE

The shock of savage violence was great and dampened the tempers on both sides. In the following months the focus of interest shifted away from Tiberius and agrarian reform after the war in Spain was concluded successfully by Scipio Aemilianus and the slave revolt in Sicily was suppressed. Discussion of Attalus' bequest occupied the Senate as they reviewed the pros and cons of establishing a new province in Asia. Tiberius had not been able to form a lasting block of support among the people and had left no aide of sufficient prominence to stir them to revenge and to carry on the attack against senatorial privilege. His father-in-law was elderly and his brother Gaius, still obscure, was at this time serving in Spain. The Senate preferred to let the situation cool and allowed the land commission to begin its work because the senators believed that the commission's work could be controlled.

At first the commission, invested with judicial authority to rule on disputed claims, began its work in Lucania and Picenum where senatorial interest was slight. But after Gaius Gracchus returned in 131 B.C. and the commission was made up of three ardent Gracchans—Gaius himself, Fulvius Flaccus, a sympathetic noble, and Carbo, a tribune—the commissioners began to move into the "protected" districts. They were speedily enmeshed in a web of technicalities and difficult suits which arose from the varied claims in equity and right of the possessors. The judicial capacity of the commission was discredited, and suspicion arose, or was planted, among the Italian allies of Rome that the commissioners might solve their problems by taking over the public land granted in time past to the allied communities. The Italians found a powerful champion in Scipio Aemilianus, who realized their military value to Rome. In 129 B.C. he succeeded in effecting the transfer of judicial power from the land commission to the consuls. The latter could be counted on to find pressing business outside of Rome, if any disturbing claims were presented. Nevertheless, the commission accomplished a considerable amount. In 125 B.C. 75,000 new names appeared on the census rolls. Not all were those of re-established farmers, for the *Optimates* had been assiduous in getting the names of their *clients* on the rolls, but a substantial improvement had been made in the position of the small farmer without seriously harming the plantation system.

The fear felt by the Italian allies about their land was symptomatic of the worsening of their relations with Rome. The allies had supplied as many troops as had Rome itself during the wars of the second century and had just cause for complaint about their share of the booty and of mistreatment at the hands of Roman officers. Allied soldiers were scourged for disciplinary offenses on military service, and their local officials were arrogantly disregarded by Roman magistrates in their own communities in Italy. The Romans, too, had stopped the practice of granting citizenship to the allies, preferring to enroll freedmen. While some individuals among the allies wanted citizenship, most communities at this time preferred protection against violation of their treaties and of their personal rights. Scipio Aemilianus had planned to do something for them in the latter respect but died suddenly in 129 B.C. on the eve of making an important speech on the subject. Suspicions of murder were current, but no definite evidence came to light. The allies were left uneasy and resentful, without a protector for their interests.

The Gracchans saw an opportunity in allied discontent to gain needed votes for their cause. In 125 B.C. Fulvius Flaccus, then consul, proposed a law that would give citizenship to those allies who wished it and would redefine the position of the remainder. The proposal ran into a wall of opposition from all classes of Roman society. The senators feared that an influx of new voters would disturb their control of the assemblies, and the urban poor did not wish to lose the value of their own votes or to share the privileges of citizenship. Flaccus withdrew his law and shortly afterwards a regulation was passed to expel the allies from Rome. There was some justification in the Roman attitude because allies had flocked to the city to join in political demonstrations, even voting if they could, but the timing of the law was vindictive. The allied town of Fregellae revolted in resentment and was destroyed by a Roman force. The other allies swallowed their anger and disappointment, but Flaccus' proposal had brought the question of citizenship and rights for the allies into the open. Rome could not postpone indefinitely the demands of a group on which its military power depended.

Other developments of this period were encouraging to the Gracchans. A bill allowing re-election to the tribunate had been proposed by Carbo and passed. There seemed to be some possibility of support from the Equestrians, who had not approved of the senatorial charter for the new province established in Asia. While Rome reserved the rich western area of Attalus' kingdom, containing the big Greek cities, large tracts in its eastern portion had been given to native kings. These monarchs were Roman allies, but remained independent in their internal administration. The Equestrians disliked the prospect of seeing such large areas kept from Roman jurisdiction and perhaps, even at this time, had begun to think of getting the tax collection of the new province into their own hands. In 124 B.C. Gaius Gracchus judged the time was proper for action and became a candidate for tribune. He was elected and so managed his program of legislation during the first year of office that he had no serious difficulty in being re-elected for the following year. Gaius' two terms as tribune were to provide the popular leaders with a "platform" and to deepen the division in the state still further.

THE TRIBUNATE OF GAIUS GRACCHUS

Gaius Gracchus proved a much more formidable opponent to the *Optimates* than his brother. Personal hatred for the men who killed Tiberius gave a depth of passion and an edge of bitterness to his program. One of Gaius' first laws was to prohibit the setting up of special courts for capital cases by the Senate, unless an appeal was allowed to the Tribal Assembly. The effect of the law was made retroactive, and Popilius Laenas, who had presided over the court which put Tiberius' followers to death, was exiled. Gaius had more sense of practical politics than his brother and understood that any leader who tried to implement fundamental reforms against the will of the Senate needed solid support among the people. He tried to effect a combination between the poor citizens and the Equestrians. When this seemed to be failing, he again raised the issue of citizenship for the Italian allies. The means chosen by Gaius to form his party was special legislation addressed to the interest of each element in it. Although most of these measures were not incompatible with genuine reform for the whole state, it was inevitable that each item of the program, whatever its merits, would become a controversial political issue. The result of Gaius' work was not so much a solution of the problems which beset Rome, as a set of issues which became the bones of contention in Roman politics for two generations. These were perhaps the proper issues, but settlement by orderly constitutional means proved impossible.

Since we do not know the order of Gaius' legislation, it is hardly possible to follow his political tactics in detail, and perhaps the program will be understood most clearly if discussed in connection with the groups whose support Gaius wished to enlist. His initial backing came from the urban and rural poor who had wanted the agrarian law of Tiberius and were familiar with Gaius' own work on the land commission. Thus agrarian settlement played a large part in Gaius' program although he was more conciliatory than his brother. Judicial power was restored to the commission, but certain districts were exempted from the latter's jurisdiction and operations were directed to marginal land. The commission seems to have coupled repossession of land with an extensive scheme to lay out and to improve secondary roads in Italy. Probably the commission's work was limited by an increasing scarcity of public land, for Gaius supplemented redistribution by new colonial foundations. Colonies of a mixed agricultural and commercial character were proposed at Capua and Tarentum in Italy, and a large settlement was planned for Carthage. The new colony there, to be called Junonia, was to consist of six thousand settlers, who were each to be granted a lot of 125 acres. The proposal ran into obstruction from the Senate who talked of the impiety of settling the land which Rome had cursed at the time of Carthage's destruction. Although the surveyors for the colony were instructed to avoid that specific area, the project was given up after Gaius' death. Yet his proposal set an important precedent. Overseas colonization speedily became a regular practice, providing a livelihood for needy Roman citizens and an instrument for Romanization in the provinces. The refounding of Carthage, however, had to wait for almost a century.

Perhaps the most controversial of Gaius' measures was the law for regular provision of grain to the needy in Rome at the state's expense, the *lex frumentaria*. While this law was partly designed to win favor from the urban poor, and succeeded so well that the practice was never abandoned, there was real need of governmental aid to procure grain. The population in Rome had increased greatly, and local production and transport were inadequate, while supplies from overseas were often delayed by storm or scarcity at their source. Near famine conditions had resulted on occasion; probably such a condition in 123 B.C. facilitated the acceptance of Gaius' law. Its provisions are imperfectly known, but it seems clear that large granaries were built to ensure a continuous supply, and that the grain was made available at regular intervals at a set price. There is controversy about the price, which, of course, affects judgment on the character of the proposal. Some scholars hold that it was near the average market price in Rome and higher than the producer's price at the source, while others consider that the grain was distributed at about half the average Roman price. Be that as it may, the law helped to assure the supply and also stabilized the market for privately imported grain in Rome. The state obtained part of its grain from the tax in Sicily, Sardinia, and Corsica. To provide the balance, contracts were leased to Roman merchants who bought wheat in Syria and Egypt. While the *Optimates* inveighed against the law as demoralizing and a grievous burden to the treasury, they accepted it, and both sides played politics with the price.

Gaius obtained the support of the Equestrians by making the collection of taxes in the new province of Asia available to the stock companies and by giving the Equestrians a recognized place and function in the state. The practice of collecting the taxes directly from the communities of the province, which had been used since 127 B.C., was changed to a contract system, somewhat like that of Sicily. The rate was to be one-tenth of the produce, but the contracts were to be auctioned in Rome by the censor exclusively to Roman citizens. In addition, the contractors were indemnified from loss through war. Because Asia was a very large and prosperous province, in a short time the collection of taxes there was greatly abused. Gaius unfortunately made abuse easier by replacing the senators in the court which heard extortion cases from the provinces by the Equestrians. The latter were thus given a sword to hold over the head of provincial governors who failed to cooperate with them, for it was very easy to fabricate some charge against the governor when he had returned to Rome. We do not know whether Gaius was fully alive to the potential misuse of his system, but the effect was to sacrifice the interests of the provincials to the enrichment of a special class in Rome and to increase the corruption in Roman government.

After re-election as tribune for 122 B.C. Gaius was an exceedingly powerful person in Rome. He retained his place on the land commission, had won the support of the poor citizens and that of the Equestrians, and the effects of his legislation were becoming visible in increased employment on the granaries and the new roads. As yet he had not raised any constitutional issue of great significance, but his career seemed to be shifting the power of government to personal leadership of the state by a tribune, backed by the people in the Tribal Assembly. Gaius felt bold enough to revive the question of citizenship for the allies. He proposed that the Latin allies be given full Roman citizenship and that other allies be raised to Latin status. The proposal met the same collective disfavor as had Fulvius Flaccus' measure in 125 B.C., and Gaius was defeated in the Tribal Assembly.

The *Optimates* felt that the time to attack, for which they had waited, was at hand. Again they worked through a tribune, Livius Drusus, but on this occasion more indirectly, in order to avoid a situation like that created in the case of Tiberius. Material for political capital was found in the charges that Fulvius Flaccus had favored the Italian allies in his work on the land commission. Drusus overbid Gaius for popular support by proposing that holders of the lots of land allocated under the agrarian law be allowed to sell them, and that twelve colonies of three thousand citizens each be established in Italy. The new farmers were pleased to have full title to their land, and the poor were delighted at the idea of colonies in Italy. There was probably not enough land for them, and the measure was never carried out, but for the moment twelve colonies sounded better than Gaius' three. Drusus quieted the Italian allies by a law protecting their soldiers from scourging at the hands of Roman officers. The ground was cut away from Gaius, and the Equestrians, in possession of their new privileges, began to find more in common with the senatorial class, men of property like themselves, than with the urban poor.

When Gaius stood for a third term as tribune, he was defeated, and the Senate proposed to annul the law authorizing the colony at Carthage. Feeling ran high in Rome in 121 B.C., and Gaius went about with a bodyguard to protect himself. In a quarrel which broke out between his men and the staff of the consul, Opimius, a member of the consul's staff was killed. The Senate declared a state of martial law by passing a final resolution, the *senatus consultum ultimum,* authorizing the consul to take whatever steps were necessary to protect the state. Opimius raised an armed force and summoned Gaius and Fulvius Flaccus before the Senate. They refused, and in the attempt to arrest them Flaccus was killed and Gaius stabbed, at his own order, by his slave to avoid arrest. To wind up the matter, about three thousand of Gaius' adherents were put to death.

The violence of the *Optimates* had enabled them to regain their hold on government for the time being, but they had made two martyrs for the *Populares* by killing the Gracchan brothers and had to accept the altered conditions of political life imposed by Gaius' legislative program. Agrarian reform, from which the Gracchan movement had started, soon took a secondary place. The land commission continued to work until 111 B.C., when a new law ended its operations. The colonists who had been granted lots in Gaius' new colonies were confirmed in possession, although Junonia was not formally founded. The grants of land made by the commission, up to five hundred *iugera,* were declared private property, and their possessors were freed from paying rent to the state and were given the right of sale. The net result had been to change over much of the public land in Italy to private ownership and to legally define the tracts which remained. Undoubtedly the law had fulfilled its purpose to some extent by restoring thousands of small-scale farmers and had hurt the senatorial class economically. Yet, after 111 B.C. the farmers could sell out and the wealthy extend their estates by buying the farms. Henceforth, if extensive distribution of land was to be made in Italy, it could be done only by wholesale confiscation of private property.

Other aspects of the Gracchan movement continued to be much more explosive than agrarian reform. The *Populares* had been given a cause, and their name was associated with distribution of grain, citizenship for the allies, and reform of the constitution. The *Equites* had tasted the rewards of political partisanship, and after the death of Gaius they continued to press for their own advantage. The way to reform by constitutional methods had been blocked by violence. In using it the *Optimates* had discovered a new tool, the "final resolution," but violence might also be returned on them as soon as the *Populares* found the means. As a solution of the fundamental issue, control of the power of government, the Gracchi had offered the Tribal Assembly as an alternative to the Senate. The fate of Gaius revealed that the assembly's lack of stability and real concern for political reform made it unsuitable. The Senate emerged from the first round with diminished prestige and shaken power. Events were soon to reveal its incapacity in foreign affairs.

Gaius Marius and the New Army (121–100 B.C.)

THE GAULS

While attention in Rome was focused on the Gracchi, the Senate had been forced to take measures for the protection of the Roman position in southern France, through which ran the road to the Spanish provinces. In 125 B.C. the Saluvii, a Celtic people who lived to the north of Massilia, invaded the latter's territory. The Romans responded to Massilia's request for help, speedily defeated the Saluvii, and improved the occasion by a campaign against the Ligurian mountaineers in northwestern Italy. Then a military road was built across the Maritime Alps to the Rhone valley and a garrison placed at Aquae Sextiae (Aix-en-Provence). About this time, 123–21 B.C., sea communications to Spain were improved by seizure of the Balearic Islands and by founding a colony on Majorca.

This Roman activity in Gaul alarmed the Celtic people who lived along the Rhone River, the Allobroges and the Arvernii. They formed a coalition against Rome, but in 121 were heavily defeated by Gnaeus Domitius Aheno-barbus near the junction of the Rhone and Isère rivers. The victory gave Rome control of southern France from the Alps to the Pyrenees, and a new province was organized, Gallia Narbonensis, often referred to simply as the Province (Provence). Three years later a colony of Roman citizens from Italy was founded at Narbo (Narbonne), probably under pressure of the *Equites,* and the new province developed rapidly as Italian traders and businessmen moved in. In defending Massilia and establishing the new province the Senate had acted with customary efficiency, but in the following years a serious threat arose with which the consular armies stationed there could not cope.

In 111 B.C. numerous Celtic and Germanic peoples who had crossed the Rhine River into northern Gaul began to press hard on the frontier of Narbonensis. These were the Cimbri and Teutones, originally from south of the Jutland peninsula, and the Tigurini from Switzerland. In the course of their movement toward Gaul, a Roman army, sent to help a friendly tribe north of the Alps, had been defeated, and so, when the Cimbri asked for permission to settle in Narbonensis, the Romans refused. The Cimbri attacked in 109 B.C. and defeated the consular army but turned back for the time being. Two years later the Tigurini defeated another Roman consular army. During this period, when the threat of mass invasion hung over Narbonensis, a crisis in North Africa created by the ambition of Jugurtha, the king of Numidia, reached its climax. Fear of a Gallic invasion helps to explain the wish of the Senate to come to some accommodation with Jugurtha, who offered no real threat to Rome, but does not excuse the vacillation, or perhaps corruption, exhibited by the senatorial envoys and Roman consuls who negotiated with him.

THE JUGURTHINE WAR

Numidia, which Rome had established as an allied kingdom after the war with Hannibal, had expanded under its able king, Masinissa, at the expense of Carthage until Rome destroyed Carthage and replaced that state with the Roman province of Africa. The formation of the province had placed a check on Numidia, which Masinissa's successor, Micipsa, had observed. In 118 B.C. Micipsa died, leaving his kingdom jointly to his two sons, Adherbal and Hiempsal, and to his nephew, Jugurtha. Jugurtha was ambitious to rule all Numidia and judged that this might be done by exploiting his connections with various Roman nobles whom he had met while serving in the Numantine War in Spain as commander of the Numidian contingent. After Micipsa's death he took over Numidia by having Hiempsal killed and driving Adherbal out of the country. In 116 B.C., when Adherbal applied to Rome for help, Jugurtha's representatives were so persuasive in the proper quarters that the Roman commission sent to adjudicate matters in Numidia allocated the larger, western, portion of the country to Jugurtha and the small eastern section to Adherbal. Jugurtha felt no scruples about encroaching on Adherbal and in 113 B.C. defeated him in battle. Cirta, the chief city of eastern Numidia was blockaded, and Adherbal appealed again to the Senate, but the envoys who came to investigate were persuaded by Jugurtha to allow the war to proceed. Cirta was taken, and its inhabitants massacred, among them a considerable number of Italians and Romans who had moved to Africa to engage in business.

The Senate might have acquiesced in this solution to the Numidian dispute, but the *Equites,* aroused by the slaughter of their associates and by the prospective difficulties of business in Africa, demanded war on Jugurtha. They were joined by the *Populares,* who were pleased to find an occasion for criticism. In 111 B.C. war was declared on Jugurtha, and the consul Bestia was sent to Numidia. Bestia seems to have arrived at an amiable understanding with Jugurtha by which the Roman army won a few slight successes, to put a good face on the war, and then he arranged a treaty which left Jugurtha in control of Numidia. When the terms became known in Rome, the opponents of the Senate suspected corruption and demanded an investigation. Jugurtha was summoned to Rome under safe-conduct to explain his actions, but in Rome he presumed too much for an alien. While bribery of two tribunes to prevent questioning might have been overlooked, the making of arrangements to have a rival for the Numidian throne murdered in Italy went too far. Even so the Senate sent the king back to Africa, but resumed the war. In 110 B.C. another Roman army was sent to Numidia. Bribery of its commanders and some actual fighting secured a victory for Jugurtha, and the consul Albinus made a treaty, once again recognizing Jugurtha's lordship over Numidia. The treaty was rejected in Rome and a full investigation demanded, which resulted in the trial and condemnation of those allegedly corrupted by Jugurtha. The Senate, badly damaged in prestige, sent a capable general and member of the great Metelli family,

Caecilius Metellus, to Africa and waited for his victory to redeem it in public opinion.

Metellus was well aware of the difficulties of war in Numidia, where the Roman legions were at a disadvantage against the excellent Numidian cavalry on its own terrain. He began a careful campaign to weaken Jugurtha by devastating the countryside and gradually taking over the towns. Jugurtha was driven into the back country of desert and mountain, but no resounding victory was won to placate opinion in Rome. The *Equites* and the *Populares* suspected that more bribery was afoot and became impatient. In this situation Gaius Marius, who had been taken to Africa by Metellus, found his opportunity to campaign for the consulship and to have the command transferred to himself.

THE CAREER OF MARIUS

Marius was a new man in politics, a wealthy Equestrian, but his career had been slow and relatively undistinguished up to this time. He had served against the Numantines in Spain and entered political life in 119 B.C. at the age of thirty-nine, when he was elected to the tribunate under the patronage of the Metelli. As a tribune Marius showed some independence of both *Optimates* and *Populares* and was defeated when he ran for aedile in the following year. He managed to obtain a praetorship in 116 B.C. but with suspicion of bribery. After a command in Spain, Marius returned to private life, until in 108 B.C. Metellus selected him as an experienced and presumably trustworthy legate. In Africa Marius played on the impatience of the *Equites* resident there by criticizing the cautious tactics of Metellus. The criticism, relayed to Rome, was exploited by Marius' Equestrian connections and won him favorable notice for the consulship of 107 B.C. In this election, since the *Optimates* labored under the disadvantage of having some of their own members under prosecution for collusion with Jugurtha, Marius was elected with the support of the *Equites* and the *Populares*. In addition, the Tribal Assembly took the assignment of provinces out of the hands of the Senate and replaced Metellus by Marius for the command in Numidia.

Marius continued Metellus' methodical campaigns against Jugurtha, who had been joined by his father-in-law, King Bocchus of Mauretania, but managed to defeat their combined forces in battle. The war was brought to an end by a quaestor in Marius' army, Lucius Cornelius Sulla, who made his way to Bocchus at considerable personal risk and played on the latter's fears that the cause of Jugurtha was lost. Sulla arranged for Bocchus to betray Jugurtha, which ended the war. Marius reaped the rewards with a triumph and re-election to the consulship for the war against the Cimbri and Teutones. Sulla, an impecunious young patrician, felt cheated of proper recognition and added personal hostility towards Marius to the natural disdain of a sophisticated young aristocrat for a middle-aged upstart. The Senate hurriedly partitioned Numidia between Bocchus and the province of Africa and turned its attention to Gaul where the situation had grown very serious.

In 105 B.C. the Cimbri and Teutones advanced down the valley of the Rhone toward Narbonensis. They were met at Arausio (Orange) by a large Roman army under the senatorial commanders Caepio and Mallius Maximus, mutually jealous and both incompetent. The Romans suffered a catastrophic defeat, which rivaled that of Cannae, since they are said to have lost sixty thousand men. The way into Roman territory lay open, but the Cimbri preferred to swing off to the west to Spain and the Teutones retired upriver. Marius made use of the time so gained to train a new army for the eventual collision. In 102 the Cimbri returned from Spain, rejoined the Teutones and the Tigurini, and the whole horde moved towards Italy. The Teutones marched through Narbonensis, intending to cross the Maritime Alps, while the Cimbri and Tigurini moved into Switzerland to enter Italy through the eastern Alps. Marius chose his ground for battle at Aquae Sextiae and destroyed the Teutones, then hurried back to Italy, where in the following year he defeated the Cimbri at Vercellae. Italy was saved and Marius became the hero of the hour. His victories were won over the greatly superior numbers of the barbarians by the fighting ability and discipline of the new army which he had created.

Marius, rather than the agrarian reforms of the Gracchi, restored the Roman army to efficiency, but at the cost of making it a double-edged weapon, which could be turned against the state. Before his time the problem of finding sufficient recruits had been solved in part by drawing on the proletarians, the men supernumerary to the five property classes from which the army was made up officially. Marius took the final step in this process by appealing for volunteers from that group and opening up a career for them. In effect, he changed the army from a citizen militia to a semiprofessional, long-service force with the prospect of civil re-establishment. At the close of his African campaign, Marius had been able to provide land grants in Africa for his veterans through his political backers in Rome. For the German campaigns he used new recruits who expected a similar reward. The effects were far-reaching. The soldiers of the post-Marian armies identified their interests with their generals, both as a matter of personal loyalty and to acquire the bonuses of land or money to which they felt entitled. The generals saw in their soldiers a potential group of *clients* to further their own political careers. The army, or rather a personal army, became the ultimately deciding factor in Roman politics. This factor might have been avoided, if the state had established a regular standing army with specified terms of service, pay, and a program of re-establishment, but that was the solution of Augustus when even the armies were tired of war. As it was, the generals were tempted to prolong wars or to find new ones in their own and the soldiers' interest.

Marius also made the army a fine fighting force by thorough reorganization and iron discipline. The legions comprised a strength of six thousand men each and were divided into ten equal tactical units, known as cohorts. The cohorts, in their turn, were divided into six *centuries*. All the men were armed alike, thoroughly drilled by methods based on those of the gladiatorial schools and infused with a new *esprit de corps* by giving each legion a silver eagle on its battle standard. Also, the legions were made more mobile and independent by furnishing each soldier with his own trenching tools and other equipment instead of transporting these for the whole force in a baggage train. The officer corps was also reorganized by assigning military tribunes as cohort commanders and sixty centurions (*century* commanders) to each legion. The centurions were the backbone of the legions, steady, battle-trained soldiers.

After his victories in 101 B.C., Marius was the most prominent figure on the Roman scene. He had defeated Rome's enemies, held the consulship for an unprecedented five terms and was in command of thousands of trained soldiers. Presumably, if he had been an *Optimate* in normal times, Marius would have retired and looked forward to election as censor and a distinguished place in the Senate, but he was a new man in a new situation. He had humiliated the senatorial generals by his victories, where they had failed, and had been the figurehead under whom the *Equites* and *Populares* had reduced senatorial prestige to a new low. Instead of retiring, Marius' ambition led him to run for his sixth consulship as the ally of the *Populares*.

The popular leaders were Lucius Apuleius Saturninus and Gaius Servilius Glaucia, both unscrupulous, violent, and devoid of ideas of reform, except for the more demagogic features of the Gracchan program. They had already helped Marius secure land allotments for his veterans in Africa and, whatever his private feelings about such colleagues, he had little choice in the matter. In 101 a slate of candidates was announced for the *Populares*: Marius as consul, Glaucia as praetor, and Saturninus for another term as tribune.

The group seems to have had no program beyond obtaining land grants for Marius' veterans. After their election, secured by Marius' prestige and the threat of force, a bill was proposed to allocate lands for the veterans in Narbonensis and to set up Latin colonies in Sicily and Macedonia. These were to include the Italian allies. A rider was added, requiring that the senators take individual oaths to observe the law within five days of its passage. Although the Senate tried to block the measure by tribunician vetoes and the urban poor were opposed to it because of the inclusion of the Italian allies, Saturninus brought Marius' veterans into the assembly to intimidate the voters and the law was approved. Marius tried to get the senators to take the oath and finally acquiesced in a subterfuge. They would take their oaths with the reservation that after the mob had dispersed, the law could be declared invalid on the grounds that it had been passed by force. Thus Marius turned against his associates and betrayed his own veterans. Glaucia and Saturninus sought re-election for 99 B.C., but in the course of the campaign, Glaucia had his rival for the consulship murdered. The Senate called on Marius to restore order, and he arrested Saturninus, Glaucia, and their chief supporters. A mob tore the roof off the building in which they were imprisoned and stoned them to death with the roof tiles. Marius had supported the Senate, the popular leaders were dead, and the brief era of popular control was terminated.

Marius' failure to use his troops, either to make a new position for himself or to support the *Populares* to the limit, naturally has raised controversy about his aims and character. He could have been Rome's first military dictator or initiated an era of popular reform, but chose the side of law and order, which in this case was represented by the Senate. Marius does not seem to have had any constructive political ideas of his own and perhaps was not much interested in politics at all, except conventionally as a means to gratify his ambition for personal prestige. As an Equestrian businessman and a good soldier, he would tend to respect tradition and the rights of property, while the spectacle of mob violence and lack of discipline would have been abhorrent. Men of his generation (he was fifty-eight at the time of his sixth consulship) had seen violence in elections and legislative assemblies but not the wholesale slaughter of civil war. At this time Marius, ambitious in the traditional fashion, probably believed that he had effected a personal reconciliation with the Senate. When he had been faced with the ultimate implications of the struggle for power, he chose as a conservative, middle-class soldier would, to support the existing order. Probably, too, the violence of Glaucia and Saturninus alienated the *Equites,* and the "solid" citizens of Rome, the *Optimates* and the *Equites,* formed a temporary coalition. Unfortunately there was no place for Marius in it.

Citizenship for the Allies (99–88 B.C.)

In the decade following the consulship of Marius, the Senate again demonstrated its failing capacity to deal with the course of change in Rome by driving the Italian allies into revolt. The allies, who had fought loyally for Rome against Jugurtha and the Germans, had been disappointed by the Senate's failure to validate the legislation which would give them a share in the projected colonies. Despite this, the Senate issued another order of expulsion from Rome in 95 B.C. Expulsion at this point proved to be a blunder of the greatest magnitude. The allies began to talk of revolt, while at the same time Rome was faced with the prospect of war in Asia Minor, where King Mithridates of Pontus had begun to encroach on the territory of the *client* kings who were allied to Rome. Warnings had deterred him so far from overt action on a large scale, but revolt in Italy would be an invitation to upset the Roman position in the East. Yet, when a proposal to grant citizenship to the allies was made in 91 B.C. by a member of the senatorial class, the Senate was still opposed. The proposal was part of a thorough plan of reform offered by a tribune, Marcus Livius Drusus, son of the Drusus who had opposed Gaius Gracchus. He is usually called the last of the civilian reformers, for after his failure reforms were made by force.

Drusus believed that broad reform was necessary in Rome and used the tribunate to launch his program, although he was regarded as an *Optimate* rather than a popular leader. To gain support in the Tribal Assembly he resorted to the now standard proposals for colonies and cheapening the price of grain. These were followed by a more controversial law to alter the composition of the standing court which heard extortion cases from the provinces. In 92 B.C. there had been a flagrant miscarriage of justice through the action of its Equestrian jurors. Rutilius Rufus, a legate of Mucius Scaevola, the jurisconsult, who had been governor of Asia, was falsely charged with extortion and found guilty. Far from extorting money, he and Scaevola had checked the abuses of the *publicani*. Drusus proposed to divide the membership of the court between the Senate and the *Equites*. He may also have proposed to enlarge the Senate by the inclusion of three hundred *Equites* but that is uncertain. These changes would have given a broader base of authority to the Senate and perhaps would have also rescued the court from its service to class interest, but the proposals met increasing opposition when it became known that Drusus planned to proceed to the question of allied citizenship. As in the past, almost all the elements of Roman society were strongly opposed. The Senate, acting on specious grounds, declared Drusus' previous legislation invalid, and some of his more intemperate opponents arranged his murder. To the Italian allies, who had been closely watching the course of events, this was the final straw. In 90 B.C. the allied communities in the hill country of Central Italy revolted and set up a new state which they called Italia.

Drusus' plan of citizenship for the allies was fully justified by the progress of unification in Italy, as well as by the specific grievances which the allies felt against Rome (p. 510). Throughout the second century Rome had acted more and more as a governing power for the whole of Italy, not merely as its leader in time of war. Despite the local independence granted to the allies by the treaties of alliance, the Romans tended to regard the latter's communities as units of the Roman state. For example, during the inquiry into the Bacchanalian scandal of 186 B.C., the Senate had investigated Italian as well as Roman towns, and Roman officials were called upon to arbitrate disputes between Italian communities. The recent extension of the secondary road system by Gaius Gracchus' commission had involved constant dealing with the Italian towns through whose territory the roads passed. In fact, generations of social and economic unification between Romans and Italians had virtually obliterated any sharp differences. The allies had ceased to feel that they were foreigners, since they behaved and talked like Romans and fulfilled the military obligations of their treaties alongside Roman soldiers. Italy was overripe for nationhood, with Rome as a capital and the various communities as its municipalities. Yet the Roman people seem to have erected a wall between themselves and the allies so far as the privileges of citizenship were concerned. The Romans were fearful of the consequences of giving the vote to thousands of new citizens. Most allies were more concerned to be treated as equal in privilege than to vote in the issues of Roman politics, but the Senate had refused to make any concessions.

In 90 B.C., when the Italian allies organized for war, they set up the nucleus of a national state. Their capital city was Corfinium, renamed Italia to symbolize this concept. A coinage was issued, bearing the image of Italy personified as a goddess. Yet, within this framework each community wished to retain its identity. The council established to conduct the war had representatives from each Italian people, and each community had its own commander in the army. The Italian idea of a state thus included both a national and a local citizenship. While the revolt was confined at first to the Oscan and Samnite peoples of the central Apennines, it was potentially very dangerous because the other allies were disaffected and many of the Italian soldiers were veterans of Marius' campaigns and had good leadership at the lower levels. The Senate was not prepared for war and was embarrassed by preoccupation with Mithridates, whose conduct became bolder when he heard of the outbreak in Italy.

In this difficult situation the Romans wisely decided to make concessions and to call on all their potential strength. Marius who was given a command acquitted himself well in the north, while Sulla performed equally well in the south. To prevent the revolt from spreading and to undermine resistance, a series of laws was passed granting citizenship. In 90 B.C. the *Lex Julia* offered the franchise to all the Latin communities and to those allies which had not revolted. In the following year the *Lex Plautia-Papiria* granted citizenship to individuals if they filed application with the praetor in Rome within sixty days. Another law, sponsored by the consul Gnaeus Pompeius Strabo, the father of Pompey the Great, granted citizenship to the towns of Cisalpine Gaul south of the Po River and Latin Rights to those north of it.

Once again the maxim "divide and conquer" won out. The heart went out of the revolt and by 88 B.C. it was virtually at an end. Grants of citizenship were extended to each community individually as it surrendered. While the allies had obtained citizenship, the Romans had retained the privilege of granting it. The Romans, too, despite their obtuseness in other matters, had an understanding of the feeling of the Italians for the individual traditions of their own towns. The idea of two citizenships was recognized, which allowed a man to participate in the local life of his community and at the same time to have the protection and privileges of citizenship in Rome, the common city of all Italy. The basis of the thriving municipal life which was to characterize Italy in the Empire was established.

The registration of the new citizens immediately became a political issue between the *Optimates* and the *Populares*. The former wished to enroll all the new citizens in a few tribes, where their votes could do the least harm, while the *Populares* were in favor of spreading them over the thirty-five tribes. The dispute continued for some years, but ultimately enrollment was made over all the tribes. In the long run the matter of where the new citizens voted was of little significance. When the time came they would follow a leader with the same broad view of Italian welfare as their own, and with the admission of the new citizens the internal political struggle in Rome began to lose its meaning.

The War with Mithridates (87–84 B.C.)

While Rome was at war with the Italian allies, Mithridates, the king of Pontus, decided to oust the Romans from the East. In 89 B.C. he began hostilities and in the following year instigated the people of the province of Asia to massacre the Romans and Italians resident there. According to tradition, which is probably exaggerated, more than eighty thousand were killed. The threat posed by Mithridates was serious and more than the mere rise of another Hellenized native king in the hinterland of Anatolia. He evidently aimed at the establishment of a powerful Hellenistic state, which could draw support from the Greeks of the Aegean region, as well as from his own semi-Hellenized and native peoples. As the massacre revealed, Mithridates could exploit the resentment felt against the Romans in the East and hoped to extend his kingdom into the Roman provinces before Rome, which was hampered by the war in Italy, could act. Not all Greeks, of course, preferred Mithridates to Rome, but the war launched by the king did represent in some degree a genuine Greek reaction against the Roman conquest.

UNREST IN THE EAST

Since the establishment of the Roman provinces of Macedonia and Asia had brought more regularity and order into that part of the eastern Mediterranean after the wars of conquest, in the latter part of the second century there was a revival of prosperity. Italy became a market for eastern products, and Italian bankers, traders, and investors moved into the new provinces. This prosperity was unequally spread, however, benefiting some regions only and contributing to the economic welfare of the middle-class governing groups rather than to that of the poor. The governing class had received the support of Rome and, in general, reciprocated by being loyal. Those areas in Greece which prospered were Delos, the center for transit trade to the west, Athens, and the fertile agricultural regions of Messenia, Central Greece, and Thessaly. Macedonia, however, although a Roman province after 148 B.C., was constantly raided and pillaged by the barbarian peoples on its frontiers, against whom the Roman consular forces were ineffective.

In Asia the Greek cities were prosperous, as shown by their building activity and the record of individual fortunes, but their social stability was precarious. Following Attalus' bequest to Rome, revolt, led by a pretender to the throne, Aristonicus, had broken out in the Pergamene Kingdom. At the outset the revolt had the character of a war of independence which was anti-Roman, but as the war developed Aristonicus had been joined by the poor and the slaves, and the struggle took on the form of a class war. Its suppression by the Roman army naturally tended to win support for Rome from the well-to-do, and at the same time it kindled hatred from the poor. Establishment of the province of Asia, however, had brought order and protection from raids.

The situation was completely different along the southern coast of Asia Minor, where there was an almost complete breakdown of authority as the Seleucid Kingdom disintegrated and Rome did not move into the vacuum. Along the coast of Cilicia, in particular, nests of pirates and adventurers were formed, who found their most profitable activity in the slave trade. The pirates kidnapped or purchased slaves for the Italian market, while slave merchants were allowed to enter the ports of Syria and Cyprus and to take their merchandise to Delos in the Aegean. So long as their piratical activity was confined to non-Italian shipping, Rome took no action to police the sea. Toward the close of the second century the pirates became bolder and carried their raids to the west where Cretans joined them. In 102 B.C. the consul, Marcus Antonius, the grandfather of Mark Antony, was assigned to the task of cleaning up Cilicia. He did so with reasonable success for the moment, but raids were soon resumed and contributed their part to the general restlessness of the Near East.

While this piratical activity disturbed the Roman provinces, the chief grievances of the provincials were laid more specifically at Rome's door. In Asia the feeling of the governing class became increasingly mixed toward Rome when the *publicani* and the moneylenders moved in. There were notorious abuses in the collection of taxes, as the condemnation of Rutilius Rufus indicates, and the *publicani* also launched out into other activities, buying land, engaging in various business enterprises, and entering the slave trade. For example, when the Romans asked for aid from Nicomedes II, the king of Bithynia, against the Cimbri, he replied that all his subjects had been carried off for the slave market by the *publicani*. The latter hardly engaged in slave raids, but they bought serfs from the great landlords and used the cities of Asia as bases for their operations. Competition from the *publicani* and the Italians in any field was ruthless and difficult because they could count usually on the Roman governor for support.

THE FIRST MITHRIDATIC WAR

Mithridates, well aware of the social unrest and the ill-feeling toward Rome, had long been anxious for a chance to expand his kingdom in Asia Minor. He had made himself sole ruler of the small Kingdom of Northern Cappadocia in 115 B.C. by murdering his mother and brother, and in the following years he extended his power across the Black Sea to annex the Greek cities in the Crimea, which had invited his aid against the Scythians. From this bridgehead Mithridates extended control westward to the mouth of the Danube and east through the Caucasus to form a link with his own territory. From this kingdom, centered on the Black Sea and appropriately called Pontus, Mithridates drew timber, grain, and manpower. To gain access to the Aegean and the Roman province of Asia, he had to take over Bithynia which was an ally of Rome.

In 89 Mithridates judged that the time was ripe to strike in full force.

Since the small Roman force in the province of Asia could offer little opposition, he speedily overran Bithynia and Asia and put his fleet into the Aegean. In Asia Mithridates was welcomed as a liberator and induced the people of the cities, probably the poor and the slaves, to massacre the Romans and Italians. He made an initial gesture of goodwill to the governing class by remitting taxes for five years, but proceeded to requisition ships, supplies, and men for an invasion of Greece. His fleet pillaged Delos en route to Athens, where the poor of the city had risen in a democratic revival against their pro-Roman government. A garrison was put in to hold the Peiraeus and Athens as a base of operations and to protect the new democratic regime. Elsewhere in Greece, Achaea and Sparta in the Peloponnesus and most of Boeotia in Central Greece declared formally for Mithridates. By 88 B.C. Rome needed to act speedily, for the whole position in the East would be lost if the rest of Greece were brought over by the initial successes of Mithridates.

The question of command against Mithridates became a political issue in Rome, where old quarrels revived again after the defeat of the Italians. Sulla, the consul for 88 B.C., was assigned to the command by the Senate, but was delayed in his departure by the siege of Nola in Campania. While Sulla was held there, Marius, whose star had risen during the war, intrigued with the *Equites* and the *Populares* to gain the command for himself. An agent was found in the tribune, Sulpicius Rufus, who had been an associate of Drusus. Rufus proposed a program by which the new citizens were to be enrolled in all thirty-five tribes, debt-ridden senators were to be removed from the Senate, and the command against Mithridates was to be given to Marius. This challenge to senatorial authority had to be carried into law by force. Sulla met it with his army. Although deprived of command, he rallied his soldiers by a personal appeal, marched on Rome, and seized the city. Rufus' legislation was revoked, Marius outlawed, and the Senate re-established in control. A law was passed to make the Senate's assent necessary before any bill was presented to the assembly.

While Sulla had won the first round in the civil war, he did not have time to arrange the elections to his liking. He counted on the consuls to hold the situation for him while he fought against Mithridates, but as soon as Sulla was well on his way to Greece, it became apparent that legislation without military backing was useless. One consul, whom Sulla had bound to himself with an oath, Cinna, joined forces with Marius, who, backed by an army of pro-Marian Romans and Samnite allies, retook Rome and annulled Sulla's laws. Sulla himself was declared an outlaw and his property confiscated, while Marius instituted a bloody massacre of his senatorial opponents until Cinna stepped in to restrain him. Sulla was thus cut off from support from Italy and left to fight Mithridates as best he could, while Cinna and the Marians organized Rome and Italy in their own interest. Marius was elected to a seventh consulship for 86 B.C. but died early in the course of his office. Probably more in the hope of damaging Sulla than Mithridates, the Marians sent another army to Greece in 86 under Valerius Flaccus with orders to supersede Sulla and to take over the war.

By the time Flaccus' army arrived, Sulla had defeated Mithridates' forces and had taken Athens and its harbor, Peiraeus. The Athenian population was decimated and the city looted, although Sulla left the public buildings standing. Flaccus' men had no desire to renew the civil war in Greece against a victorious Roman general, when there was plunder to be had, so the soldiers marched through Macedonia to invade Asia Minor from the north. Sulla himself remained in Greece awaiting the arrival of his fleet before marching after them.

Although the army of Flaccus was vastly outnumbered by the forces available to Mithridates in Asia Minor, the new Roman army won its battles without difficulty. Even a mutiny against Flaccus, in which the soldiers chose a new commander, Fimbria, did not slow their advance. The soldiers devastated and looted, sapping the enthusiasm of the provincials for war. Yet Sulla, not Fimbria, ended the war. When Sulla crossed into Asia Minor in his turn, he opened negotiations with Mithridates. Sulla's mere presence with an army influenced the soldiers of Fimbria to desert, while Fimbria himself committed suicide. Sulla thus contrived a speedy return to Italy, but the terms of his settlement fell more heavily on the people of Asia than on Mithridates himself.

Mithridates was required to abandon his conquests in western Asia Minor but was allowed to retain the Kingdom of Pontus. Eighty of his warships and two thousand talents were taken as an indemnity for the war. The terms imposed on the cities of Asia were ruthless. Sulla demanded that oligarchical governments be restored in those cities where popular revolutions had taken place, but if the offer was refused, the Romans plundered the offender systematically. A fine of twenty thousand talents was imposed on the province to be paid immediately because Sulla needed money for his return to Italy. The cities had to borrow money to pay, pledging their public buildings as security to the Roman moneylenders who turned up in the wake of the army. The Roman troops were given a holiday for the winter of 85/84 B.C. at the expense of the provincials. The soldiers were billeted in private houses, whose owners were required to provide them with daily spending money, clothes, and dinner for as many friends as the "guest" wished to invite. The *publicani* returned shortly afterwards, and Asia entered upon a trying period of maladministration and impoverishment.

Greece suffered from the requisitions made by both Sulla and the armies of Mithridates rather than from punitive measures after the Roman victories, but it did not recover for generations even the modest prosperity enjoyed before the war. The trade of Delos declined. Athens was impoverished, its trade through the Peiraeus reduced to a trickle. Sulla had removed the valuable dedications and treasures from the great sanctuaries at Olympia, Delphi, and Epidaurus. While he regarded these as loans, since an endowment was created for the shrines from confiscated lands in Boeotia, the treasures themselves were dissipated. The Mithridatic War marked the beginning of a decline in Greece and the Aegean area which was not reversed until the Empire had brought peace and stability. Mithridates retired to Pontus to bide his time for the next opportunity, while Sulla returned to Italy at the head of his veteran army, rewarded with money and loot, ready to follow their general against the Marians.

The Dictatorship of Sulla (83–79 B.C.)

Since Sulla's victories had warned the Marian leaders in Italy that they would have to continue the civil war against him in the near future, plans of reform were subordinated to the task of preparing against his return. Particular attention was paid to the new citizens and to those allies who were not yet enrolled. Registration of some of the new citizens in the thirty-one rural tribes was probably made by the censors in 86/85 B.C. Good personal relations with the leaders of the Italian communities were cultivated and preparation made for war by collecting supplies and raising troops. In the emergency the elections were suspended, and Cinna remained in office for two years, from 85 to 83 B.C. He collected an army at Brundisium (Brindisi) to attack Sulla in Greece, but on the eve of sailing the men mutinied and killed him. His associate, Carbo, however, hurriedly organized two new armies, each of which outnumbered Sulla's forces, but were untried and poorly disciplined.

Sulla tried to undermine these efforts from Greece. In a letter to the Senate he declared himself the lawful representative of Rome, who had fought the state's battles in the East and who was returning to punish the Marian rebels. The Italians were reassured that, if they remained neutral, they need have no fear of reprisal. The Senate was impressed, but Carbo overruled their desire to negotiate and continued his preparations for war. When Sulla landed in Brundisium in the spring of 83 B.C., he had an army of about thirty to forty thousand veteran soldiers, who had sworn an oath of loyalty to him. Various men of the senatorial class came in with troops which they had raised in their own districts. Among them were two young men, Pompey and Crassus, who correctly estimated that Sulla's trained army and military ability were worth more than the numbers of his opponents.

The war at first went easily for Sulla. He marched across Italy from Brundisium to Campania and defeated one of Carbo's armies without difficulty. The other lost its desire to fight and deserted. In the following year, however, the veterans of the Italian allies from Etruria and the Samnite hills joined in on the Marian side, and opposition became fiercer. Sulla had to maneuver to fight his opponents separately. The younger Marius, the son of the former consul, was beaten in Latium, which gave Sulla access to Rome. From the city he marched north into Etruria where he defeated Carbo in a hard-fought battle, only to learn that the Samnites were marching on Rome. Sulla returned just in time to defeat them at the Colline Gate outside the city. The Marians had been beaten in Italy, but their leaders fled to the provinces to organize for further war—Carbo to Africa, and Sertorius, a very able soldier whom jealousy had kept out of a command in Italy, to Spain. Sulla was free to do what he wished in Italy.

While Sulla's reorganization of government in favor of the Senate contained many sound ideas and some innovations which became permanent, the reign of terror in which he tried to liquidate the opposition both failed in its purpose and stained his reputation in Roman tradition. Some explanation for reprisal can be found in the Marian massacre of 87 B.C. and in Sulla's injured pride, but his purge was deliberately and callously allowed to extend far beyond political purposes. The terror began with the butchery of the Samnite prisoners of war taken at the battle of the Colline Gate. Thousands were tortured and killed in the heart of Rome, within hearing of the Senate. Lists of those proscribed for killing and confiscation of property were posted in Rome and throughout Italy. In addition to political enemies, the lists contained the names of men disliked by Sulla and his adherents on purely personal grounds, and of some who were guilty only of owning extensive and desirable properties and had no friend in the Sullan camp to protect them. It is estimated that about ninety senators, 2,600 *Equites* and thousands of other citizens were put to death. The Sullan vengeance was visited also on the children of the proscribed by forbidding them to hold public office in the future. Sulla and his adherents personally profited from the confiscation of property, and some, like Crassus, laid the foundation of their fortunes by buying up land cheaply. Those Italian communities which had fought against Sulla were fined and their lands confiscated. The proceeds from this wholesale confiscation of property were used to reward the veterans of Sulla's army, estimated at over a hundred thousand at the end of the war. The men were settled on the confiscated land, mainly in Etruria and the Samnite country, while the former owners were left to find a living as best they could. Sulla's power remained strong through the support of his veterans and of ten thousand slaves of the proscribed, whom he had freed. The freedmen became Sulla's *clients,* indicating their dependency by adopting his name, Cornelius, as their new surname.

Sulla took over the power of government in Rome during his reorganization by reviving the dictatorship, unused since the war against Hannibal, in a new and more comprehensive form. In 82 B.C. he was named dictator and was confirmed by the assembly for an indefinite period to issue edicts and to reorganize the government, *dictator legibus scribundis et rei publicae constituendae.* While Sulla's power was absolute, his office did have as a logical end the reorganization of the state, and Sulla did not envisage a permanent position for himself for the creation of a ruling dynasty. He began his work by allowing the regular machinery of government to function, while he restored the authority of the Senate and consolidated its position for the future.

The Senate's number was far below strength and its prestige sadly damaged. Three hundred new senators were enrolled to bring the membership up to about five hundred. The new men were drawn from the younger nobility and the wealthier *Equites* who had supported Sulla. He thus adopted the plan of Drusus, proposed in 91 B.C., to make the Senate more representative of the wealthy propertied classes of Italy, for many of the new members came from the Italian municipalities. For the future the senators were to be recruited automatically from the quaestors, thus assuring a continuous supply of vigorous young men, who would become imbued with senatorial traditions and collegiality as they rose in public office. For this purpose the number of quaestors was increased to twenty, and the censor's function of appointing senators terminated.

Strengthening of the Senate's authority over the magistrates and so, indirectly, over the assemblies was provided for by a revision of the course of office. Minimum age limits were set for the various offices: thirty for the quaestorship, forty for the praetorship, and forty-two for the consulship. A ten year interval was made obligatory for re-election to any magistracy. In this way the holding of the high offices was postponed to the years of maturity when a man should have acquired loyalty to the Senate and less inclination to stake his career on a challenge to its authority. The tribunate, which had been used by the *Populares,* was made an impotent, dead-end office, by prohibiting a tribune from offering legislation to the Tribal Assembly and from holding any other office after the tribunate.

Sulla also made changes in the system of allocating provincial governorships, presumably not so much to help the provincials as to place further checks on the high officials. To provide an annual supply of ten governors, the number of praetors was raised to eight, and the revised system sent the ten chief magistrates—the eight praetors and the two consuls—to the provinces after their term of office in Rome. The Senate, of course, was to be in charge of the allocation of provinces. The eight praetors found ample work during their year of office in Rome through a reform of the court system for criminal cases. Standing courts were set up on the model of that already established for hearing extortion cases. These were presided over by a praetor and manned by jurors from the Senate. They were to deal with extortion, treason, bribery, forgery, embezzlement, murder, and assault. The law of treason was enlarged to include such offenses of a provincial governor as starting a war without authorization and leading his army out of his province. These legal reforms proved solid and lasting and led to a rapid development of the administration of Roman criminal law, although, because no appeal was allowed to the assembly, the Senate acquired control of this whole field of justice.

While Sulla made no great innovation in political organization and was concerned to consolidate the position of the Senate, he did show considerable appreciation of the difficulty of constitutional reform in Rome. Presumably he was personally disposed to restore the power of the Senate because of his own patrician affiliations and from personal enmity to the Marians. Yet the only practicable alternative, control of government by the Tribal Assembly, can hardly be defended. The urban mob which dominated it was even less representative of the whole citizen body after the inclusion of the Italian allies as citizens than before. At least the enlarged Senate gave more voice to the propertied groups of Italy and contained the experienced, trained men who were needed to administer the provinces and to fight Rome's wars. Sulla might have continued as dictator or even tried to convert that office into monarchy with the support of his veterans and *clients,* but by 79 B.C., when he retired, his personal ambitions and the offense to his dignity were evidently satisfied. He decided to end his career in luxurious retirement. When personal rule did come two generations later with Augustus, public opinion had been prepared and the senatorial class had suffered severe attrition in the civil wars. Sulla did realize the danger to the Republic of another career like his own and had tried to guard against it by his arrangements for the provinces. He could scarcely forestall the wars which demanded special commands and enabled their holders to consolidate immense personal strength.

When Sulla retired the situation seemed reasonably secure. The Marians had been defeated in Africa by Pompey, the threat offered by Sertorius in Spain was not yet serious, and Mithridates had retired to the mountains of his Pontic Kingdom. The seeds of trouble for the new regime had been sown mainly in Italy itself. The proscriptions and confiscations left a legacy of hatred and social discontent from the relatives of those who had suffered. Even the Sullan veterans were to provide trouble when they found farming was distasteful and yearned for the action and plunder of war. Sulla himself escaped these consequences. He died in 78 B.C. on his private estate in Campania.

In the half-century between the Gracchi and Sulla the breakdown of the Republic seems to have gone beyond the possibility of repair. The issues of reform, raised by Tiberius and Gaius Gracchus, had become secondary to the struggle for power in the state. The political instruments of both "parties," the Senate of the *Optimates* and the Tribal Assembly of the *Populares,* had demonstrated their lack of capacity for government and their lack of vision to provide for the welfare of Italy and of the provinces. Personal armies had become the decisive factor in politics, but the leaders had not yet worked out a formula to express this fact in government.

Still life. Wall painting from a villa at Boscoreale. First century B.C.

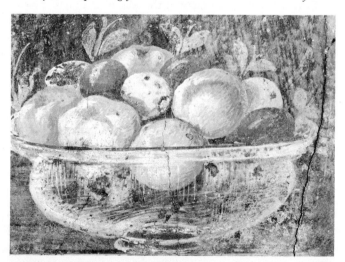

XXIV

The Breakdown of the Republic, II

(78–44 B.C.)

IN THE YEARS immediately following Sulla's death the reconstituted Senate had to deal with the results of social discontent and unfinished wars. In Italy the bitterness and suffering caused by Sulla's proscriptions were exploited by ambitious agitators, Lepidus and Catiline, and a desperate slave revolt flared, led by Spartacus. In Spain the Marian leader, Sertorius, organized a government which claimed to be the legitimate government of Rome and made an alliance with Mithridates at the other end of the Mediterranean. Mithridates himself, in alliance with the pirates of Cilicia, revived his war against Rome.

To deal with these crises special commands were created which gave their holders the opportunity to raise armies and to threaten the Republic with the very danger of dictatorship which Sulla himself had exemplified and tried to guard against. In 59 B.C. constitutional government was virtually suspended by the informal group known as the First Triumvirate, Pompey, Crassus, and Julius Caesar. Ten years later, in 49 B.C., civil war broke out between Caesar and the *Optimates,* who had brought Pompey over to their side. They were defeated, and Caesar became dictator of Rome. Yet, throughout the period from Sulla to Caesar's death in 44 B.C. Roman territory was vastly extended. Pompey organized the provinces of the East, and Julius Caesar added the whole of Transalpine Gaul. In Italy, too, the future form of government began to take shape. The *Equites* and the middle class of Italy, who supported Caesar, began to replace the senatorial governing class and even in the 50's the prestige and power of Pompey foreshadowed the eventual status of Augustus as *Princeps,* first man, of the Empire.

Pompey the Great (78–60 B.C.)

Pompey was one of the few men who started his career with the epithet "Great" rather than having it bestowed upon him by posterity. He had joined

The reader will find Maps XVII and XVIII (pages 482–83 and 544) useful as he reads this chapter.

Sulla upon the latter's return to Italy in 83 B.C. with a force raised from his own district of Picenum, where his family possessed large estates and *clients*. In recognition of Pompey's services and obvious military ability Sulla entrusted him to clean up the Marian opposition in Sicily and Africa. When this task was efficiently performed, Pompey, displaying the vanity and self-complacency which were to mark his career, demanded a triumph. This was granted because Pompey's support was too valuable to jeopardize. Sulla with some irony added the epithet "Great" to Pompey's name. The irony was misplaced for by 60 B.C. Pompey had become the most prominent and powerful figure in the Roman world and had laid a solid foundation for Rome's Empire in the East.

In 78 B.C. the Senate called upon Pompey to deal with the aftermath of a revolt fomented by the consul Marcus Lepidus in northern Italy. Lepidus, who had been a Sullan while that was advantageous, had changed his politics after Sulla's death and as consul proposed several anti-senatorial measures: cheap grain, restoration of land to those who had been dispossessed by the Sullan confiscations, and the return of exiles. These proposals were defeated, but Lepidus raised an army of malcontents in northern Italy and marched on Rome, demanding a second term as consul. Lepidus' army was defeated by his fellow consul Catulus, but Lepidus himself and a part of his force escaped to Sardinia. From there the soldiers, after Lepidus' death, crossed to Spain to join Sertorius. Pompey was entrusted with suppressing the remaining opposition in northern Italy and in the following year prevailed on the Senate to grant him a special command against Sertorius. Since the Senate had few good commanders upon whom it could call, the post was given to Pompey although he had none of the technical requirements of age and experience in office which were legally needed.

THE WAR AGAINST SERTORIUS

The task facing Pompey in Spain was formidable. Sertorius was an experienced and highly competent officer who had fought with Marius against the Cimbri and had seen service in Spain during the 90's. In addition, he displayed rare qualities of statesmanship and integrity in enlisting the support of the Spanish tribes, by which he turned Spain into a bastion of strength for the Marians. Sertorius' forces were largely made up of Spaniards from the mountain country, officered by Romans who had fled from Italy. Sertorius trained the soldiers in Roman tactics and treated all the Spaniards as potential Roman citizens, governing fairly and educating the sons of prominent families in Roman fashion. Sertorius conceived of his regime as the legitimate government of Rome, dedicated to carrying on the civil war against the Senate. Magistrates and a senate-in-exile were drawn from the refugee Marians, while Sertorius carried on intrigues with the anti-senatorials in Italy. His government also made an alliance with Mithridates, in which they took a proper Roman line by refusing the king possession of the province of Asia although granting Bithynia to his rule. All this was largely academic because mutual aid could not be implemented, but Sertorius thus provided political as well as military problems to the government in Rome.

Before the arrival of Pompey in Spain in 77 B.C., Sertorius' army had taken over most of the country and defeated both the senatorial general Metellus and the governor of the neighboring province of Narbonensis. Despite the numerically superior forces which Pompey brought, Sertorius fought with considerable success for five years. Toward the end of the struggle the Marians began to quarrel among themselves, and friction arose between the Roman officers and their Spanish soldiers, when the officers made heavier demands on the Spaniards to keep the war going. In 72 B.C. Sertorius was killed by his subordinate, Perperna, and in the following year the war was ended by Perperna's defeat. Pompey showed very considerable administrative ability and justice in the settlement of Spain. He gained the loyalty and respect of both Spaniards and Romans there, which was to stand him in good stead for the future.

LUCULLUS' WAR AGAINST MITHRIDATES

While Pompey was fighting in Spain, the Senate had to provide for war in the East where Mithridates again opened hostilities. In 75 B.C. the king of Bithynia, Nicomedes IV, had died and left his kingdom to Rome. The Senate decided to accept the bequest, but Mithridates sponsored the claim of Nicomedes' son and raised a general war against Rome. He made alliances with the Cilician pirates and, as we have seen, with Sertorius' government in Spain. The Senate assigned three generals to the work of defeating Mithridates' coalition. Gaius Aurelius Cotta, the consul, was sent to Bithynia; Marcus Antonius was to deal with the pirates; and Lucius Licinius Lucullus was given general charge of the war against Mithridates, operating from the province of Asia. Antonius made a miserable fiasco of his operations in Crete, and Cotta had to be rescued by Lucullus, but Lucullus proved himself one of Rome's great generals.

In 74 B.C. Mithridates invaded Bithynia and advanced into Asia, where he blockaded Cotta in Chalcedon and laid siege to Cyzicus. Lucullus relieved the city, despite being outnumbered about four to one, and in the next two years retook Bithynia and chased Mithridates out of Pontus into Armenia. After the subjugation of Pontus Lucullus set about repairing the financial damage done to the cities of Asia by Sulla's exactions. The debts of the cities to the Roman moneylenders had snowballed into fantastic sums, far beyond their capacity to pay and regain solvency. Lucullus set the interest rate at twelve percent, cancelled two-thirds of the accumulated interest due, and made arrangements for the payment of the debts by annual installments which the cities could afford. These sensible measures enraged the *Equites* in Rome, and when Lucullus resumed the war against Mithridates they were able to block the sending of reinforcements and worked for his replacement.

Despite the need of reinforcements, Lucullus resumed the offensive in 69 B.C. upon the refusal of Tigranes, king of Armenia, to surrender Mithridates.

Lucullus invaded Armenia with a small force of eighteen thousand men, took its heavily fortified capital city of Tigranocerta, and was pushing on through the mountains to finish the war when his men mutinied. Some of them had served with Fimbria back in 86 B.C., and all were worn out from lack of reinforcements and resentful of the severe discipline by which Lucullus kept them moving. Lucullus had to retreat into Mesopotamia, where he plundered the city of Nisibis, but was unable to resume operations against Mithridates who returned to Pontus. The pirates were then emboldened to sail into western waters and to raid the coasts of Italy. In 66 B.C. Lucullus was humiliated by an order to turn over his command to Pompey, who had emerged by that time as the favorite general of the *Populares*. Pompey had engineered a successful political turn-about upon his return from Spain by making an alliance with Crassus after the suppression of the slave revolt of Spartacus in 71 B.C.

THE REVOLT OF SPARTACUS

The revolt raised by Spartacus, a Thracian gladiator, throws a vivid light on the desperate condition of labor on the great plantations of southern Italy. The uprising began in 73 B.C. when a group of gladiators broke out of their training barracks at Capua in Campania and took refuge on the slopes of Mt. Vesuvius. They were joined by runaway slaves from the plantations, mainly Gauls, Germans, and Thracians who wanted revenge on their masters. Within a year the force had grown to seventy thousand men who were looting and devastating throughout southern Italy. Although the slaves split into two bands, one under Spartacus, the other under a Gaul, Crixus, the regular armies of the Roman consuls were unable to contain them. Crixus' band was defeated, but Spartacus fought his way up through Italy. The slaves might have escaped into Europe, but turned back to loot and devastate. In 72 B.C. the Senate was forced to assign the war as a special command to the ex-praetor, Marcus Crassus, who had fought with Sulla.

By this time Crassus was a powerful figure among the *Equites* and one of the richest men in Rome as a result of his extensive investments in land and money lending. Crassus penned Spartacus into the peninsula of Bruttium, but the slaves broke through the Roman lines and began to scatter. Crassus defeated most of them, killing Spartacus, and Pompey arrived from Spain in time to round up a small force which had fled to the north. Reprisals were cruel in the extreme, about six thousand slaves being crucified. While the Roman armies had been victorious in Spain and Italy, their success confronted the Senate with the new problem of Crassus and Pompey. Both were personally ambitious and demanded triumphs and the consulships for 70 B.C.

THE CONSULSHIP OF POMPEY AND CRASSUS (70 B.C.)

The Senate was in a very weak position. Popular demands for the restoration of the tribunate, weakened by Sulla, had already in 75 B.C. resulted in a law sponsored by Cotta, which removed the prohibition against a tribune holding further offices. Vigorous young men were elected again to the tribunate and revived the cause of the *Populares*. The senatorial courts were under criticism for some obviously partisan decisions, and a scandal of the first magnitude was looming up in the flagrant misgovernment of the *Optimate* Gaius Verres in Sicily. When the Senate was confronted by the demands of Crassus and Pompey, although those of Pompey were quite illegal, their only hope seemed to be to turn each against the other. Pompey and Crassus were rivals, but neither of them was a fool. Accordingly, they combined forces and sought support from the *Populares*. The *Equites*, of course, were annoyed already at the reforms of the *Optimate* general Lucullus in Asia Minor. The Senate withdrew its objections, and the generals were elected to their consulships, pledged to rescind the greater part of Sulla's legislation.

The right of the tribunes to introduce legislation and to exercise their veto was restored. The remainder of the new citizens were enrolled in the tribes. The composition of the court for hearing extortion cases, which had been exclusively senatorial, was altered to include one-third senators, one-third *Equites* and one-third *Tribuni Aerarii*. The latter seem to have been men of the middle class, just below the *Equites* in property rating, who had held some minor office in the tribes. This strengthening of the middle-class representation in the court was doubtless encouraged by the notorious trial of Verres in 70 B.C. by which Cicero made his reputation as a lawyer and was marked as a rising political figure.

THE TRIAL OF VERRES

Cicero, born in 106 B.C., came from the same town, Arpinum, as Marius, and also belonged to an Equestrian family of moderate wealth. He had received an excellent education in philosophy and rhetoric, partly in Italy and partly in Rhodes, which was fashionable as a "finishing school" for young Romans. Cicero had decided on a legal and political career but, as a new man, faced the usual barriers to preferment. In 70 B.C., when he was just coming to the attention of the public in Rome, he was approached by the cities of Sicily to prosecute their former governor, Verres, for extortion. Since Verres' guilt seemed plain enough and since the senatorial courts were being criticized, Cicero decided to take the case, realizing that it could help his career by bringing him to popular attention. During his tenure of office Verres had acquired about $2,000,000 in money, valuables, and works of art from the unfortunate Sicilians, asserting that he needed to make three fortunes—one for himself, one for his friends and one to bribe the jurors, if he were brought to trial. For his defense he engaged the leading lawyer in Rome, Marcus Hortensius Hortalus. Cicero skillfully blocked all the maneuvers to delay the trial and gathered such an imposing mass of evidence that, when the case was called, Hortensius did not even try to make a defense. Verres departed into voluntary exile before the verdict of guilty was handed down.

While Cicero's voluminous preparation was not needed, he published his findings in a book, the *Second Verrine Oration,* which throws a sharp light on the techniques of provincial misgovernment. Verres had made false accusations against wealthy provincials and had intimidated the judges of their cases to obtain favorable verdicts for himself. His own justice and those offices which could be brought under his patronage were for sale. He shared in the illegal profits of the tax collectors and demanded works of art and valuables from the unwilling hosts who were required to entertain him. The case deservedly brought Cicero into prominence, but Verres' friends in the Senate added dislike to the prejudice which they felt towards Cicero as a new man. Cicero's own feeling that justice should be done to the provincials was genuine, as he later demonstrated by his governorship of the province of Cilicia in 51 B.C.

POMPEY'S GREAT COMMANDS

While Crassus and Pompey retired into private life after their consulships because there were no provinces available which they felt to be appropriate to their talents, Pompey's liaison with the *Populares* soon paid a handsome dividend. In 67 B.C. the food supply of Rome was menaced by the raids of the Cilician and Cretan pirates who had even defeated a Roman naval detachment off Rome's harbor of Ostia. A tribune, Aulus Gabinius, proposed that a special command of three years duration be created to dispose of the pirate menace. The general, whom everyone assumed would be Pompey, was to be given authority over the whole Mediterranean Sea and the territories inland for fifty miles. He would be allowed to raise troops, to appoint a staff of legates of praetorian rank and to raise money in addition to the six thousand talents granted to him initially. The Senate, of course, brought out its usual political weapons in opposition: oratory, the opposition of other tribunes, and special legislation, but the danger was real and affected the people where they felt it most, in their stomachs. The Tribal Assembly passed the law and named Pompey as commander. He fully justified the choice. Within three months he had cleared both the western and eastern basins of the Mediterranean of the pirates, had destroyed their bases and had begun to settle them as colonists in the towns of Asia Minor. Since Pompey's success coincided with Lucullus' humiliating inactivity against Mithridates, in 66 B.C. a tribune, Manilius, proposed the transference of that war to Pompey. He was given overall command in the East with the right to make war or peace with whomsoever he chose. The law was again opposed by the Senate, but the *Populares* and *Equites* supported it, and Cicero spoke in favor in his oration, *Pro Lege Manilia (For the Manilian Law).* Pompey's tenure of this *maius imperium* (greater *imperium*) with authority to override that of the provincial governors placed him in a position resembling that of the later Roman *Princeps.* His prestige was immense, he held most of Rome's military power in his own hands by vote of the people, and, if he chose, he could delegate the conduct of operations to his subordinate legates, while he remained elsewhere.

Pompey again displayed his very great talent for the organization of war and administration. By 62 B.C. he had brought the East with the exception of Egypt and the Parthian Kingdom under Roman control and had laid the basis of its provincial system. Mithridates was driven from Pontus, which was divided between Bithynia and a new allied king, and took refuge across the Black Sea in the Greek Crimea, where he began to plan a grandiose thrust up the Danube valley into Europe to take Italy from the north. This plan seemed too extravagant, and in 62 B.C. Mithridates was killed by one of his own sons. Pompey advanced into Armenia from Pontus and made its king a Roman ally, so that Armenia might serve as a buffer between Roman Asia Minor and the Parthians. The native peoples between the Black and Caspian seas, to the south of the Caucasus Mountains, were also converted into nominal allies. In 64 B.C. Syria, which was in a state of political chaos after the collapse of the last Seleucid king in the 80's, was made into a province. In the adjacent area a group of native rulers was recognized as Roman allies but left to rule their own kingdoms. For example, Judaea became a dependency under its High Priest, nominated by Pompey. Pompey's work was efficient and lasting. The Roman frontier was extended to the Euphrates River, peace and order were re-established, temporarily at least, and the process of urbanization started by the Seleucids was given fresh impetus. With his work completed Pompey prepared to return to Rome in 62 B.C.

Entr'acte in Rome: Crassus, Caesar, and Cicero (67–60 B.C.)

While Pompey was in the East, Rome was the scene of feverish but essentially meaningless political activity as the various leaders and groups assessed their positions in relation to him. The real power in the state lay in Pompey's wishes, backed by the force of his armies, and he had given little indication of his views beyond a clear desire to be a great and powerful figure, rising above his contemporaries. Pompey had been a Sullan in the 80's and 70's, but backed the *Populares* when he wanted a consulship. He had received the support of the people and the *Equites* for his great command in the East, but had never appeared as an active *Popularis* in the political contests in Rome. The Senate had opposed his command for fear of the concentration of power in the hands of one man, but Pompey belonged to their class. He had been supported by Cicero, who had needed a powerful ally for his own political career, but Cicero chose Pompey, rather than Pompey, Cicero. Increasingly, however, Cicero envisaged Pompey as a protector of the state, who would guard the solid, propertied elements in it against revolutionary disturbance. Crassus was the political rival of Pompey and looked upon him as another Sulla, who might use his army to initiate a proscription. Accordingly, Crassus tried to create a counterweight of power in Rome with the help of Julius Caesar, by taking over the *Populares* and spending money lavishly to gain support for his schemes.

Julius Caesar, born in 100 B.C., was just entering upon a political career for which he needed money and support. By family connection and for the sake of opportunity he was a *Popularis*. Caesar belonged to a very old patrician family, which was impoverished and obscure in the second century, and perhaps he looked with aristocratic disdain on the newer nobility of Rome. His immediate family connections were with the Marians since his aunt had married Marius and since he himself married the daughter of Cinna. Caesar early showed some independence by refusing to divorce her at Sulla's request and some sagacity by withdrawing to Rhodes during the Sullan regime. In 68 B.C. Caesar entered politics through the quaestorship and was prepared to collaborate with Crassus for his own advancement, but, at this point, apparently did not share the personal animosity which Crassus felt for Pompey. In fact, he seems to have supported Pompey for the great commands in 67/66 B.C.

In 65 B.C. Crassus was censor and Julius Caesar aedile. Caesar used the office to make himself known to the people by underwriting the public festivals on a lavish scale and identified himself politically by prosecuting agents of the Sullan proscriptions. Crassus endeavored to find a new basis of support by enrolling the Gauls north of the Po River as Roman citizens but was blocked by his fellow censor. At least Crassus gained their goodwill for himself and Caesar. He then tried to establish a special command, presumably for Caesar, by annexing Egypt as a province. A tribune was found to disclose the astonishing news that the former king of Egypt had left his country to Rome in his will. When this patent falsehood was exposed, the proposal was defeated through the vigorous opposition of the Senate and of Cicero. Crassus, nothing daunted, tried to get the consuls for 63 B.C. in his pocket by backing the election of two impoverished and unscrupulous patricians, Sergius Catiline and Gaius Antonius. They were opposed by Cicero, who had good support from the Senate in default of a candidate more to their taste. Catiline had already failed to get a consulship in 65 B.C., when his candidacy was rejected, probably on the grounds of extortion during his term as governor of Africa. He had then conspired to kill the consuls, but the plot failed and there was insufficient evidence for prosecution. Accordingly, Crassus bought up Catiline, as he had bought many other politicians, whose family fortunes could not support the high cost of politics in Rome. Catiline and Antonius, however, proved a poor investment. Catiline lost the election, and Antonius was bribed into silence by the offer of Macedonia as a province at the end of his term of office. Cicero was the dominant consul for 63 B.C. who led the fight against the schemes of Crassus and Caesar.

The first test came with the introduction of a new agrarian bill by a tribune, Servilius Rullus. It was flagrantly conceived to set up a counterweight of power for Crassus and Caesar against Pompey. The bill proposed to establish a land commission of ten members who would be given extraordinary power for a five-year term. They were to be allowed to terminate the leases on the remaining public land in Campania, reserved by the agrarian law of 111 B.C., and to sell all the public land taken over in Pompey's war in the East. In addition, the commissioners were to have authority to confiscate land, to found colonies, and to raise troops. Cicero and the Senate fought this monstrous scheme by exposing the implications of its clauses. The bill would have sold out Italy, the provinces, and Pompey himself to the new commission, behind which stood Crassus and Caesar. The opposition was so strong that the bill did not come to a vote. Crassus and Caesar were forced to lie low for the time being, but their former tool, Catiline, a dangerous and vengeful man, precipitated another crisis by a conspiracy to seize control of Rome when he failed again to get the consulship for 62 B.C.

THE CONSPIRACY OF CATILINE

In his election campaign Catiline had called for the cancellation of debts, which appealed to distressed men of the senatorial class like himself and to the poor rural voters, among whom were many veterans of Sulla. Catiline also had a special tie with the latter as a former Sullan officer. The program, which had a dangerous sound to the wealthy *Optimates* and to the middle class, was opposed successfully by the *Optimates* and Cicero. Then Catiline turned to conspiracy with a small group of men of his own class and the Sullan veterans in Etruria. The conspirators planned to seize Rome with a band of gladiators, then throw the city open to the army of veterans who were to march on Rome. The plan was leaked by the indiscretion of one of the conspirators and came in a roundabout way to the ears of Cicero. Also, various senators received mysterious letters, warning them to be absent from Rome on a certain day. Cicero convened the Senate, alarmed the members, and was granted authority under the final resolution to protect the state. Catiline got out of Rome and joined the force in Etruria, while the conspirators left in the city planned to throw Rome and as much of Italy as they could into confusion. On December 17, when the Festival of the Saturnalia began, senators were to be assassinated, fires set in Rome, and a general appeal to revolt issued to the slaves in Rome and the countryside. It was hoped that in the widespread confusion the forces from Etruria could seize control. When this plan, too, was betrayed to Cicero by a delegation of Gauls in Rome who had been approached for cooperation, Cicero ordered the arrest of the conspirators. The other consul, Antonius, defeated Catiline and the forces of the conspirators.

The conspirators who had been rounded up in Rome were brought before the Senate for trial. There was strong sentiment for putting them to death, but Caesar, recognizing the illegality of such a penalty by the Senate, proposed that the men should be detained in various Italian towns for safekeeping. His speech seemed to have some effect, but Cato the Younger arose and made a passionate appeal for death, which swept the Senate to assent. Cato, who took such a strong line in this affair, was a singular figure in Roman political life. He was an ardent Stoic who attempted to practice his beliefs as well as to voice them. Although the former was too difficult for perfect success in the Rome of the Late Republic, the latter was easy. Cato became the very vocal conscience of the Senate and was bitterly opposed to Caesar and Crassus.

Cicero unfortunately supported the demand for the death penalty against the conspirators and obtained it. He had an exaggerated conception of the scope and danger of the conspiracy. It did reveal the reckless desperation into which a part of the population was falling, but the conspirators were few in number and without well-organized military support. If Catiline had been successful, he would have faced a civil war with Pompey, who could draw full support for such a cause from the vast resources of senators and *Equites* alike. Crassus and Caesar were both suspected of having some part in the plot, which was natural from their past association with Catiline, but they seem to have stayed clear. Crassus had everything to lose in such a movement, and Caesar perhaps had already begun to draw nearer to Pompey. In the following year a tribune, Metellus Rufus, who had been serving with Pompey, raised the question of impeaching Cicero for the illegal action of the Senate in putting the conspirators to death. As consul, acting under the "last decree," he had presided over their meetings and was responsible. The charge was dropped for the time being, but Caesar had pointed to the possibility of such action, and later, in 58 B.C., Cicero was banished from Rome on that charge. For the moment Cicero considered that he had saved the state and began to talk of a new government.

Cicero had won a victory for constitutional government by bringing together the solid, propertied classes against civil disorder. He tried to develop this temporary alliance of interest into a more permanent union, a *Concordia Ordinum* (Union of the Orders) as he styled it. At the time of the conspiracy he told the Senate that in him they had a leader who thought only of their interests, not his own, and who had brought the whole Roman people into unanimity for the first time. In his enthusiasm Cicero sadly misestimated his own position and the feeling of the Senate. He had risen to his consulship by his ability as a lawyer and orator, but to the Senate he was a new man whom they had supported for the moment but whom they could neglect after his usefulness had passed, as Marius had been neglected. Cicero, however, was a whole-hearted partisan of senatorial government, and elsewhere he spoke of his union as founded on senatorial authority. The soundest part of Cicero's dream was the idea that he might bring Pompey into the union as the protector of the state, but that factor would have had to wait on the enigmatic Pompey's return. Cicero's idea is usually criticized as born of his own vanity and miscalculation, but his conception of supporting the state by the prestige and power of Pompey anticipated the *Principate*. Perhaps that conception makes Cicero a better political theorist than politician because he could not see the Senate for what it actually was. That body soon revealed that it had no desire for compromise and went unheedingly on its own way.

Late in 62 B.C. Pompey returned to Italy with his troops and, to the pleasure of the Senate and the general surprise of all, demobilized his army. There was no reason to keep them under arms, and Pompey evidently expected that his prestige, although shorn of military power, would be sufficient to influence the Senate to cooperate in obtaining his political wishes. He brought back an immense amount of booty to be allocated between the treasury and his army: about

$10,000,000 for the treasury, $5,000,000 to his higher officers and $14,000,000 for his junior officers and private soldiers. In addition, about $7,000,000 a year were added to the revenues of Rome from the taxes on the newly acquired lands. Pompey asked the Senate for land allotments for his forty thousand soldiers and ratification of his political arrangements in the East. Cato and Lucullus, the latter embittered personally at having been replaced by Pompey, obstructed the requests. Separate discussion to each item was called for, and a land bill, proposed by a tribune friendly to Pompey, was blocked. At the same time the Senate alienated the *Equites* by refusing to modify the contracts for the Asian taxes because of a poor harvest in that province.

In 60 B.C. Julius Caesar arrived in Rome from Farther Spain, where he had served a year as governor to his own and Rome's profit. Unruly tribesmen had been put down, and Caesar had found the money to repay his debts, which amounted to well over a million dollars. Caesar wanted both a triumph and the privilege of running for consul, two grants which were technically conflicting, for he needed to stay outside of Rome with the army for his triumph and yet he had to canvass personally inside the city for the election. When his petition for waiver of the regulations was turned down by the Senate, Caesar began to canvass for his consulship. At the same time he worked behind the scenes to bring Crassus and Pompey together into an unofficial coalition, through which each would attain his desire. Out of this was born the First Triumvirate. Caesar was elected consul with the support of Crassus and Pompey, although with an *Optimate* colleague, Calpurnius Bibulus, and in 59 B.C. he used his office to obtain what the Triumvirs wanted.

The First Triumvirate (59–49 B.C.)

THE CONSULSHIP OF CAESAR

Caesar began his consulship in a conciliatory manner, attempting to gain the cooperation of his colleague, Bibulus, and of the Senate for a bill which would provide lands for Pompey's veterans. The Senate, swayed by Cato's vociferous objections, refused to sponsor the measure, and their agents blocked it in the Tribal Assembly. Tribunes applied the veto, and Bibulus indicated his disapproval by declaring the omens unpropitious for holding any assembly meetings at all. Since ordinary constitutional methods were blocked, Caesar showed his metal by turning to intimidation. Pompey's veterans were brought into the assembly meetings, and the opposition was silenced and ignored. Bibulus retired from an active part in public business, which prompted one Roman wit to declare that the consular year of 59 B.C. should be named the consulship of Julius and Caesar, not of Bibulus and Caesar.

Caesar had to provide for his own future, too, because the Senate, in anticipation of his election, had designated as his province the hills and forests of Italy. This was a petty position. Caesar wanted a foreign command for which he could raise an army. He had thought first of a Danubian project, but a new

Gallic threat presented the opportunity for a special command. Since 61 B.C. the Helvetians of Switzerland had been planning to strike across Gaul to find new homes west of the Rhone River. This would stir up the Gallic peoples and endanger Narbonensis and Cisalpine Gaul. A tribune, Vatinius, proposed that Caesar be given the province of Cisalpine Gaul for five years with three legions, which he could begin to recruit immediately. The law was passed, thus relieving Caesar of the prospect of administering the forests and mountain roads of Italy, and later the Senate, on the recommendation of Pompey, added Transalpine Gaul to Caesar's command.

Most of Caesar's legislation, however, was designed to serve the purposes of the other Triumvirs. The land bill provided generously for Pompey's veterans in Italy. Pompey's political arrangements in the East were ratified, and Crassus' purposes were achieved by granting the *Equites'* claim for a reduction of their tax returns from Asia. Caesar did have time for one very important and genuine reform measure. The right of provincial governors to accept gifts and make requisitions was carefully defined and remained the standard regulation for such matters throughout the period of the Roman Empire. All Caesar's laws, however, might be declared invalid on the grounds that they had been passed by force. Accordingly, because each of the Triumvirs had a stake in the implementation of the legislation, they continued their agreement and made arrangements to hold control of the processes of government.

The election of consuls favorable to the Triumvirate was arranged, and steps were taken to get rid of its most dangerous opponents, Cato and Cicero. Cato was rewarded by the governorship of Cyprus at the other end of the Mediterranean, a post which the Triumvirs knew his high sense of duty would not allow him to refuse. Overtures were made to bring Cicero into the service of the Triumvirate, but, true to his convictions, Cicero elected to support the Senate. Accordingly, it was arranged that Clodius, an unscrupulous member of Rome's gilded patrician youth, would be elected to the tribunate. He was already hostile to Cicero and in 58 B.C. sponsored a law banishing those who had illegally put Roman citizens to death. The reference was to the Catilinarian Conspiracy, and the target was Cicero. His property was confiscated and he left Rome for Macedonia.

While the actions of the Triumvirs had made it abundantly clear that their group controlled the government in Rome, friction existed among themselves. From the outside Pompey appeared to be the dominating figure and Crassus and Caesar his agents. Caesar and Pompey were bound together also by the marriage of Pompey to Caesar's daughter, Julia. Yet Pompey, a man who wanted to be admired, was disturbed at the coolness which had developed between himself and the Senate because of Caesar's methods. He was disturbed, too, at the banishment of Cicero, to whom he owed gratitude for support, when he had been in the East. Crassus, of course, was an old rival. On the whole, while Pompey and Crassus had satisfied their wants, Caesar, who had shown himself to be a man of resolution and adroitness in personal dealings, had grasped the opportunity to build up the real power of an army and a provincial *clientage*. When Caesar withdrew to Gaul, relations between Crassus and Pompey worsened rapidly. Pompey helped to secure the return of Cicero from exile in 57 B.C. and thus became a target for the abuse of Clodius. But mutual interest held the Triumvirs together, in name at least, until 56 B.C., by which time Caesar had made substantial progress in the conquest of Gaul.

THE CONQUEST OF GAUL

The land of Gaul, stretching from the Mediterranean through modern France and Belgium and from the Alps and the Rhine to the Atlantic, had been settled by the Celtic peoples in their westward movements from Central Europe. When Caesar's ambition marked Gaul as ripe for conquest, the country was still heavily forested, particularly in the north, but agriculture was extensively practiced in central Gaul. Towns had sprung up along the main trade routes which were mainly in the river valleys, along which traffic could move more easily. Such French cities as Paris, Lyons, Rouen, Nantes, Bordeaux, and many others had Celtic origins. Gaul had been penetrated by Greek traders from the colonies along the Mediterranean coast, who moved up the Rhone, and by Etruscans and Italians who crossed the Alps. They exchanged wine, metalware, and pottery for agricultural products or for the tin which was brought from Cornwall in England to the mouths of the big rivers on the Atlantic coast. The Celts themselves had developed several ironworking centers, such as Bourges, which produced tools and weapons of excellent quality, but in the main the people lived by agriculture and the raising of animals.

As Caesar noted in a famous remark, Gaul was divided into three parts beyond the Roman province of Narbonensis. The country was usually referred to as *Gallia comata* (the home of the long-haired Gauls). In the southwest, Aquitaine, whose population contained a large intermixture of Iberians from Spain, the raising of horses was carried on extensively and provided the mounts for an excellent Gallic cavalry. In central Gaul, from the Loire to the Seine and the Marne rivers, were the main towns and extensive clearings for agriculture. In the north the Belgae, who were mainly of Germanic origin, had been least affected by Mediterranean influences and dwelt in heavy forest and swampland.

While there was considerable similarity of social customs throughout Gaul, the various peoples had never coalesced into political unity. They were organized into many tribal states which had a very loose internal cohesion and frequently warred on one another. Among the Belgae kingship was still preserved, but the peoples of central Gaul were ruled by their clan chieftains, who vied for tribal leadership and were supported by the thousands of retainers, debtors, slaves, and serfs over whom they ruled. The Gauls were reckless individual fighters and had good cavalry forces, but their chieftains had difficulty in holding a large group together to form a disciplined, steady army. Gaul was a proper field for application of the favorite Roman device of dividing and conquering, since clan could be played against clan and tribe against tribe. The Romans had tried to

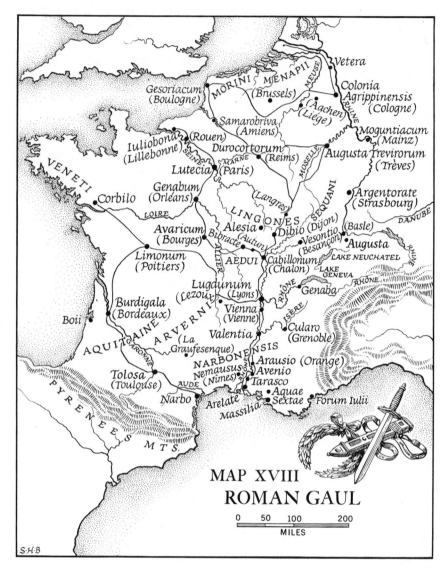

MAP XVIII
ROMAN GAUL

0   50   100   200
MILES

S·H·B

protect Narbonensis by this technique and were generally familiar with conditions in the hinterland. Towards 59 B.C. their "diplomacy" in Gaul was threatened by the arrival of a new people.

A Germanic people, the Suevi, under their king, Ariovistus, had crossed the Rhine into northern Gaul. They came to settle on land which had been promised to them by their kindred, the Sequani, in return for aid against the Aedui of central Gaul. The latter had been long allied to Rome, but in 61 B.C., when the Sequani attacked, Rome sent no aid to their Aeduan allies, who were heavily defeated. Instead, an embassy from Ariovistus was cordially received in

Rome and the king was recognized as a "friend of the Roman People." The exchange of Aeduan goodwill for the friendship of Ariovistus was of dubious value, for the latter settled far off in Alsace, while the Aedui were close to the Roman province. The Helvetians, who wished to move from Switzerland to western Gaul, were a more pressing problem. Their settlement in western Gaul would have repercussions throughout the whole land, and, what was worse, the Helvetians were talking of marching through Narbonensis. In March of 58 B.C. they began to move.

Caesar dealt with the Helvetians rapidly and effectively. Their request to cross Narbonensis was refused, and when they tried to force their way through the territory of the Sequani and the Aedui farther to the north, Caesar renewed the alliance with the Aedui and defeated the Helvetians heavily. They were compelled to return to Switzerland. This success brought in requests for alliance with Rome from many of the peoples of central Gaul, who asked for help against Ariovistus. He had begun to expand from Alsace and to invite German allies to cross the Rhine. To prevent the formation of a strong German state in Gaul, Caesar attacked Ariovistus and forced him back across the Rhine. These victories in eastern Gaul alarmed the Belgae and their neighbors in the west, so that in the winter of 58/57 B.C., they began to prepare for war. In the following year Caesar and his Aeduan allies defeated the Belgae, while his subordinate, Publius Crassus, son of the Triumvir, subjugated the peoples along the Atlantic coast. By 56 B.C. the conquest of Gaul was virtually complete, and Caesar was voted a public thanksgiving in Rome for his services. Since the work of organization and consolidation still remained, Caesar desired an extension of his command.

The Triumvirate, however, was in danger of falling apart, and Caesar's own position was under attack. Tension between Pompey and Crassus had reached such a pitch that Pompey publicly accused Crassus of plotting against his life. The *Optimate,* Lucius Domitius Ahenobarbus, stated during his candidacy for the consulship of 55 that he would ask for Caesar's recall. Accordingly, in 56 B.C. Caesar consulted with Crassus and then invited Pompey to a conference at Luca in northern Italy. The three came to an agreement to continue their cooperation and each took care to provide for his own security. Caesar was to continue in his Gallic command for five more years, while Pompey and Crassus were to be the consuls for 55 and then take over special commands themselves. Pompey was to receive Spain and Libya, and Crassus Syria, from which he planned to make war on the Parthians. Caesar retired to Gaul to plan his next moves, while Pompey and Crassus went back to Rome. They ensured their election by forcing the other candidates for the consulship to withdraw and then passed the required legislation through the Tribal Assembly.

In 55 Caesar first turned his attention to the Rhine, where some Germans were crossing. He repulsed them and made a demonstration of force on the German side of the river. This brought various German chieftains into nominal allegiance. Late in the summer Caesar made a brief preliminary campaign across the English Channel to punish the Celts of Britain for aid which they had given to the Gauls. The reconnaissance was encouraging, and in the following year Caesar invaded England with a force of about thirty thousand men. He penetrated beyond the Thames and received the submission of the British tribes of southeastern England. The invasion, however, was no more than a thrust, made partly to gain prestige and partly out of curiosity. Britain could not be held until Gaul was a settled Roman province, and the conquest and occupation of the island were not begun until about a century later by the Emperor Claudius.

After his return to Gaul Caesar was faced with a series of revolts, which required as much hard fighting to suppress as he had put into the initial conquest. In 54–53 B.C. the Belgae attacked the Roman garrisons and had to be put down by a campaign in that area. In the following year the peoples of Gaul rallied around a young prince, Vercingetorix, of the Arverni. Caesar penned him into the fortress town of Alesia, beat off the attempts at relief, and finally starved the defenders out. In the ensuing pacification Caesar showed a remarkable clemency and good sense, which turned the Gauls into his loyal adherents in the civil war against Pompey and the *Optimates*. He did not organize Gaul into a province but placed it under the governor of Narbonensis and obliged the Gauls to furnish troops and to pay tribute. Caesar had created a bastion of power for himself in Western Europe which enabled him to dominate Italy and Spain and to block the attempts of Pompey and the Senate to cause his downfall.

THE COMING OF THE CIVIL WAR

In the meantime the Triumvirate had lost its balance by the death of Crassus, and the *Optimates* were encouraged to bring Pompey over to their side and to prepare Caesar's destruction. Crassus had gone out to Syria, where he found a pretext for war against the Parthians who had advanced their territory to the Euphrates River. After a preliminary reconnaissance in 54 B.C. Crassus led a large army of forty thousand men into the Mesopotamian desert. The combination of desert war and the Parthians proved too much for the Romans, and the army was cut to pieces at the battle of Carrhae in 53 B.C. Crassus himself was treacherously killed while attempting to negotiate.

Pompey, however, had remained in Rome, governing Spain through his legates. The marriage tie with Caesar had been broken already by the death of Julia in 54, and Pompey was beginning to feel that the rise of Caesar infringed on his own prestige. As Caesar observed later in his book on the civil war, Pompey could not tolerate an equal. For the time being Pompey remained aloof from politics and let events take their course. Rome fell into political chaos. Elections for the consulship were postponed, and regular assembly meetings given up because of rioting, while rival gangs led by Clodius and another of his kind, Milo, roamed the streets fighting each other. In 52 B.C. when Clodius was murdered, the Senate called upon Pompey to restore order and to act as sole consul. His troops moved in, and the processes of government were restored.

The *Optimates* settled down in earnest to eliminate Caesar, and Pompey, while playing the great man and first citizen of Rome, was satisfied to let them have their way. A long and intricate series of political maneuvers began, until war was precipitated in January, 49 B.C.

The purpose of the *Optimates* was to force Caesar to dismiss his army and to return to private life, since, once out of office, he might be prosecuted for the illegal legislation of his consulship in 59 B.C. Caesar, of course, worked to prevent this by trying to secure his election to the consulship before he was required to give up his command in Gaul in 50 B.C., thus leaving no interval when he was vulnerable. Early in 52 Caesar received special permission to campaign for the consulship *in absentia,* but later in the year Pompey had a law passed by which candidates were required to be present in person, although Caesar was recognized as an exception. Also, a fair-sounding regulation was made, which required that there be an interval of five years between the holding of a magistracy in Rome and a governorship in the provinces. The effect of this was to enable the Senate to put loyal *Optimates* into the provincial governorships, a great advantage in the event of war. The Senate then made an overt bid for support from Pompey by extending his command in Spain so that it would considerably overlap Caesar's in Gaul. In 51 the *Optimates* moved to a direct attack on Caesar by refusing his request for extension of his own command. Also, two legions were withdrawn from him on the pretext of needing them against the Parthians, but the soldiers were kept in Italy. Caesar countered these various moves by using the tribunes in his pay to offer other proposals and to use their veto, when possible, thus giving his opposition to the *Optimates* the specious appearance of championing the people and trying to maintain himself against the governing class. At the same time he and his agents worked up public opinion in their favor by other means.

Caesar made an indirect appeal to the reading public by publishing his account of the Gallic Wars in 50 B.C. The simple, direct style of the book, in which Caesar referred to himself in the third person, skillfully conveyed the impression that Caesar was a consummate general, capable of meeting any situation, and a man who deserved well of Rome for his conquest. In Rome one of Caesar's agents, the tribune Curio, succeeded in passing a measure in the Senate by which Caesar and Pompey were to relinquish their commands at the same time. The vote in favor was heavy, which shows that anti-war sentiment was strong among the ordinary senators and which gives some validity to Caesar's later assertion that he was being attacked by a small, but powerful, faction of the *Optimates*. The consuls, however, vetoed the resolution, presumably for fear that Caesar could easily find a pretext in some Gallic uprising to hold his army beyond the fixed date. Finally the *Optimates* brought the situation to crisis. The consuls called on Pompey to protect the state and issued an ultimatum to Caesar to give up his command on a certain day. His tribunes, Mark Antony and Quintus Cassius, vetoed the decree, but the vetoes were ignored, and the tribunes fled for safety to Caesar, who had been watching events from Cisalpine Gaul.

The arrival of the tribunes faced Caesar with the most fateful decision of his career. He had to chose between war against the Republic, as represented by Pompey and the *Optimates,* or becoming a broken man. He was camped near the Rubicon River, which marked the frontier between his province of Gaul and Italy, and to cross it with his troops would be a defiance of the laws of the Republic. Early in 49 B.C. Caesar marched his small force across the Rubicon.

The Civil War (49–45 B.C.)

While neither Caesar nor Pompey was fully prepared for war because each had been trying to make the other appear as the aggressor, Caesar had the immediate advantage. He had a small force of one legion and some Gallic cavalry with him in Cisalpine Gaul and ordered two other legions to join him as quickly as possible. These were experienced, loyal troops. Pompey and the *Optimates* had only the two legions taken from Caesar and some hastily levied recruits who were untrained and barely organized. Accordingly, Caesar decided to strike down into Italy at once. He represented himself effectively to the Italians as defending the rights of the tribunes and making war to rid the state of the small faction of *Optimates* who had blinded Pompey to the true situation. To his own troops Caesar also talked of the affront to his dignity and pride as conqueror of Gaul and as commander of a loyal army. When he advanced into Italy the municipalities opened their gates, and the senatorial troops, instead of fighting, deserted their commanders and went over to Caesar. The *Optimate* Domitius Ahenobarbus tried to hold Corfinium against Pompey's wishes, but his troops deserted, and Caesar marched on to Brundisium to forestall Pompey's departure. Pompey had recognized that Italy could not be held, and so decided to concentrate his forces in Greece where he could draw on his vast connections in the Eastern provinces. Pompey made good his escape, and Caesar, for lack of a fleet, turned back to Rome and detailed his subordinate officers to get hold of Sardinia, Sicily, and Africa to secure the grain supply.

Pompey the Great

Julius Caesar

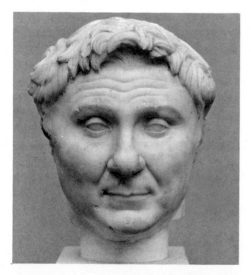

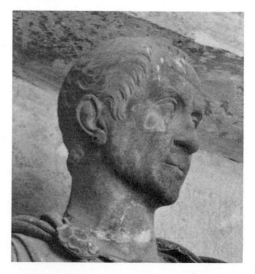

The adherence of Italy to Caesar became extremely important as the war progressed. He was able to recruit Italian soldiers to add to his trained legions from Gaul and to operate from Italy's central position in the Mediterranean, as well as to govern from Rome, thus giving his regime the appearance of legitimacy. In the long run, however, the collective strength of the *Optimates* could be very formidable, for they were able to draw upon their long-established *clientage* and connections in the provinces, as well as intrigue in Italy. But they were divided in command. Pompey regarded himself as the protector of the state, to whom its rightful government had turned and to whom it should defer. The *Optimates,* on the other hand, looked upon Pompey as their military instrument and showed a tendency not only to dispute his opinions but to engage in private operations with the troops which they could raise by their own influence. Caesar, fully aware of these difficulties among his enemies, pushed the war to obtain a decision as soon as possible.

While a fleet was being prepared to follow Pompey to Greece, Caesar attacked the Pompeian armies in Spain. En route Massilia was besieged, for the *Optimate* commander, Domitius Ahenobarbus, had taken over the city, with which he had long-standing family ties as patron. Caesar defeated the Pompeians in Spain and showed his usual clemency and good sense in his treatment of the enemy soldiers. They were dismissed from service without penalty and allowed to return to private life or to join his own forces. Many did so because Caesar had made it plain that his war was with the *Optimates,* not the ordinary soldiers of their armies. Meanwhile Pompey had established himself in western Greece, where he was concentrating the forces which his and the *Optimates'* connections with Rome's allied kings in the East could command. Although the season was late after Massilia was finally taken and the Pompeian fleet had command of the Adriatic, Caesar slipped across to Illyria with a comparatively small force and carried the war to Pompey.

Although some of the states of western Greece joined Caesar upon his arrival, his army was too small to blockade Pompey effectively for long or to crush him in battle. The Caesarian troops spent a difficult winter in the cold mountains of western Greece and in the spring crossed into Thessaly. Pompey followed from Apollonia, where he had been partially blockaded, and the two armies took up positions for battle near Pharsalus. Before the battle the *Optimate* generals tempted fate by dividing up the offices which they expected to share after Caesar's outnumbered and worn troops were beaten. Their councils were divided and their preparations were careless, despite Pompey's proper military concern. After the battle was fought, instead of returning to Rome, the *Optimates* and Pompey were in headlong flight for safety.

Pompey sailed to Egypt, followed by Caesar with a small force in hot pursuit. The young king of Egypt, Ptolemy XIV, hoping to win Caesar's goodwill, had Pompey put to death soon after he landed. Caesar, however, took the position that this was an affront to Rome and intervened in the dispute for the throne which the partisans of Ptolemy, aged fourteen, were carrying on with

Cleopatra, his wife and sister, who was about twenty years of age. Caesar supported Cleopatra, although we may assume that his reasons were not entirely political because considerable risk was involved. Her opponents roused the people of Alexandria against Caesar, and during the winter of 48/47 B.C., he was blockaded in the palace with Cleopatra. Reinforcements came in the spring, but Caesar stayed on in Alexandria, despite the growing strength of the *Optimates* in the provinces. He settled Egyptian affairs by confirming Cleopatra as ruler of Egypt and marrying her off to a still younger brother. In the meantime Roman Asia Minor was attacked by Pharnaces, the son of Mithridates. In a swift campaign Caesar marched from Egypt to Pontus, where, within five days of his arrival, he met and defeated the armies of Pharnaces at Zela and wrote to a friend: "*Veni, vidi, vici*" (I came, I saw, I conquered).

While Caesar was in the East, affairs at Rome had fallen into disorder, and Italy was experiencing a financial crisis. On his return Caesar took hold of the government by appointment as dictator once again and issued legislation to stabilize the financial situation. Caesar resisted the demands of his more impecunious friends to cancel all debts, then re-established credit by requiring that the interest already paid on loans be deducted from the principal and that prewar evaluations be accepted. He had to turn rapidly from reconstruction in Italy to war in Africa and Spain. Caesar's commander in Africa, Curio, had been defeated, and the *Optimates* who fled from Greece after Pharsalus had raised a large army. Before Caesar could even sail to Africa, he had to put down a mutiny among his own troops. Loyalty was soon restored, and in 46 B.C. the senatorial force was defeated at the battle of Thapsus. Many of the leaders were killed, and others committed suicide, following the example of Cato, who was thus established as a martyr of the Republic. Like Cicero, Cato invested the Senate with ideal qualities of virtue, wisdom, and resolution, which it was far from possessing in actuality. Cato's suicide helped the Senate also to become a symbol of the Republic, destroyed by the tyrant Caesar. Caesar, the tyrant, however, followed his usual clemency after Thapsus and pardoned those *Optimates* who survived. A group of irreconcilables, among whom were the sons of Pompey, took refuge in Spain. In 45 B.C. Caesar defeated them at Munda. After this battle the survivors were put to death, but the elder son of Pompey, Sextus Pompey, escaped and began to enlist support among his family's connections. Nevertheless, Caesar had crushed all serious opposition and after the victory at Munda dominated the Roman world.

Julius Caesar, the Dictator (47–44 B.C.)

As in the case of Alexander the Great, it is difficult to estimate Caesar the statesman as compared to Caesar the general or Caesar the political opportunist. As a general Caesar showed an amazing versatility in fighting against Gauls, Britons, Germans, and the Roman legionary armies commanded by Pompey and the experienced senatorial generals. He defeated them in almost every type of terrain and condition of war. As a politician Caesar employed the methods of his period, shrewdly and realistically sizing up his opponents and the situations with which he was confronted. Opportunist and realist are terms frequently used of Caesar, but these qualities were necessary for survival in the Late Republic. Like Alexander, Caesar had little time for any thoroughgoing reorganization of Rome before his death and is scarcely to be reproached for not doing in two years what it was to take Augustus thirty-seven years of hard, unremitting labor to accomplish with able assistants. It is more pertinent to ask whether Caesar showed any real will to grapple with the task of reorganizing the state, broken down by almost a century of political turmoil and civil war.

Until his final victory over the Pompeians in 45 B.C., much of Caesar's legislation was necessarily directed to the correction of abuses or to the repayment of old obligations. For example, the Gauls who lived north of the Po River, for whom Crassus had tried to get citizenship in 65 B.C. and who had supported Caesar, were granted citizenship. Those Romans debarred from holding political office in Rome by the Sullan proscriptions were restored to their full rights. In 48 and again in 46 B.C. Caesar restored financial stability to a debt-ridden society, and he did not aggravate its condition by a new proscription. A man of tidy mind, Caesar introduced the Julian calendar to bring the seasons and the Roman year into proper relationship. By 46 B.C. the Roman year was two months ahead of the solar year as a result of the failure of the priests to make the necessary intercalations into the lunar calendar used by Rome. Caesar introduced a new calendar based on that of the Greek astronomer, Sosigenes of Alexandria, which took effect on January 1, 45 B.C. This Julian calendar ultimately became the calendar of the Western world, with corrections by Pope Gregory XIII in A.D. 1582. It was only fitting that the Senate rename Caesar's birth month, *Quintilis,* July. Caesar also abolished most of the *collegia,* the social and trade guilds in Rome, which had become hotbeds of conspiracy in the 50's. He required that the labor force on the plantations and large ranches be made up of one-third free men in an effort to remedy unemployment, and limited the governorships of consular provinces to two years and of praetorian provinces to one.

All this, of course, was piecemeal legislation and showed no coherent plan of reform, but was useful, sensible, and tidy. In making his laws Caesar used his own discretion. As dictator he made the decisions, rejecting the pressure of his younger friends who wanted to sweep much aside, and the good advice of Cicero, who had hopes from the clemency of Caesar that the Senate might be restored to its proper place and that Caesar might protect the state from further disturbance. Cicero had been a Pompeian but had not given his support wholeheartedly, for fear that Pompey's victory would bring wholesale proscriptions.

In the last year of his life Caesar's laws were broader and more thoroughgoing and began to touch some of the fundamental needs of Rome. The grain distribution was regulated by a system of registration and continuous checking on the recipients. As a result the number was cut from 320,000 to 150,000. A municipal law was prepared although not passed until after Caesar's death and then in confused form. The law recognized some uniformity of local institutions in the Italian municipalities and provided for the upkeep of roads and regulation of traffic in Rome. While this revealed some consciousness of the unity of Italy, the law does not seem to have touched the privileges of the Italian towns or to have had the purpose of reducing Rome itself to a municipality, as sometimes stated.

Caesar's plans for the settlement of veterans followed the traditional line of making allocations of land, but Caesar also included the Pompeian veterans and settled more soldiers outside of Italy than had been the usual practice. Some were sent to Africa, but most were settled in Sicily and Narbonensis, now well Romanized. On the other hand, Caesar sponsored an extensive system of colonization for the poor Roman citizens and for freedmen. The colonies were established in Spain, Africa, and the East. Carthage and Corinth, destroyed by the Romans in the second century, were refounded, and one colony was placed as far afield as Sinope on the Black Sea coast. In the West such cities as Hispalis (Seville), Arelate (Arles), and Nemausus (Nîmes) received colonists. Through these measures Caesar seems to have aimed at the relief of social and economic distress in Italy rather than at a systematic program of Romanization. His main focus of interest was Italy, Sicily, and Gaul, which had served him so well in the civil war. In Narbonensis and Sicily, in particular, he made numerous grants of Roman citizenship, as if recognizing the almost fully Roman character of those provinces. Caesar also had numerous projects for improvement and building in Italy, some of which were under way before his death, while others were suspended in the confusion which followed it.

On the whole, Caesar followed the lines which Gaius Gracchus had laid down, placing an emphasis on social and economic reform and, as might be expected, showing a considerable regard for Italy and the Romanized areas of the West. In all this there does not appear to be any specific concern for the fundamental problem of Rome, the reorganization of government, both internally and with respect to the provinces. Rome had long since changed from a simple city to a large and complex state. Up to the time of his death Caesar continued to use the existing machinery of the Republic, in which he was dictator, and he controlled all the essential decisions. Since his last plans were for large-scale war against the barbarians of the Danube and against the Parthians, it is unlikely that he had any intentions of undertaking wholesale reorganization. Caesar was the last of the great military figures of the Republic, not the founder of the Empire.

Caesar's victory over the senatorial governing class who had staffed the magistracies, governed the provinces, and led the Roman armies, meant the end of the Republic in substance, if not in outward form. Many of the senatorial class had been killed, and those who survived through Caesar's mercy were discredited and of doubtful loyalty. Caesar's own partisans, of course, expected to be placed in positions of importance. His following was very heterogeneous.

There were a few men of the old patrician nobility, like himself, whose families antedated the Republic. Many *Equites* had joined him, as had the middle class throughout Italy. Caesar's closest and most useful aides were young men like Mark Antony, ambitious, unscrupulous, and eager to make a career under Caesar, whose chances of victory they had estimated correctly. As a group and as individuals they had small interest in political reform and limited experience in government. Caesar had little choice but to become a dictator, if merely to ensure order in Rome.

After holding temporary dictatorships in 48 and 47 B.C., Caesar was appointed dictator for ten years in 46 and then, in the following year, for life. At the same time he held a consulship and received the traditional privilege of sacrosanctity of the tribunes, which in practice had done them little good and was not to save Caesar. He had been high priest, *Pontifex Maximus,* since 63 B.C., and in 46 became "prefect of morals," a sort of perpetual censor. Apparently, however, Caesar envisaged his position as a perpetual dictatorship, with other offices to be added as they were useful for convenience or prestige. Whatever the means, he proposed to run the machinery of government in an absolute fashion without regard for the traditional functions of the Senate or assemblies. The Senate was at a low ebb after the war, and Caesar raised its membership to nine hundred, a most unwieldy body, by bringing in his own adherents. The new senators came from the Italian municipalities, even from Narbonensis, and made the Senate temporarily Caesarian in feeling. The unwieldiness did not matter because the Senate was a rubber stamp for Caesar's legislation and had no real part in policy making. Cicero complained that he received letters congratulating him on legislation of which he had no knowledge. The traditional magistracies were retained, and the number of praetors and quaestors increased, but those who held office were Caesar's nominees. In 44 B.C. he provided a slate of officials for several years in advance because he intended to be away from Rome fighting in the East. The assemblies thus retained no real elective function. The state was Caesar, but what was Caesar?

Caesar seems to have had no ambitions or plans for government other than those which have been mentioned. While he was accused by some of his opponents of planning to become a king, he stayed within the limits of Roman political institutions. The mockery which he made of the Republic gave Caesar's enemies sufficient reason to kill him. The conspiracy was planned by

The Roman Senate in session

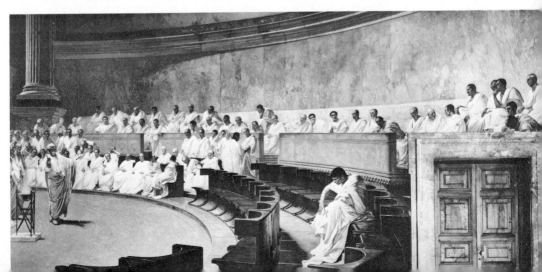

two ex-Pompeians whom Caesar had spared, Gaius Cassius and Marcus Brutus, a nephew of Cato, and was joined by Caesar's own followers, Gaius Trebonius and Decimus Junius Brutus. In all about sixty senators were associated in the plot. Although Caesar was informed that a conspiracy was being prepared, he ignored the warning, and on the fifteenth of March, 44 B.C., he entered the Senate without a bodyguard. The conspirators clustered around him near the statue of Pompey and stabbed him to death. Their plans had gone no farther than Caesar's death, and they speedily found that the state could not exist without a personal ruler. Thirteen more years were required to decide whether the ruler would be Octavius or Mark Antony and whether the Empire would be organized along Roman lines or as an Eastern monarchy. The traditional Republic, however, was as dead as Caesar:

"Liberty! Freedom! Tyranny is dead!
Run hence, proclaim, cry it about the streets . . .
. . . ambition's debt is paid."

The Revolution in Society

The political breakdown of Rome, which culminated in the death of Caesar, was, of course, a part of the more complex transformation of the Mediterranean world which the rise of Rome had brought about. The process of change had been painful. Italy had become a nation by the revolt of the Italian allies. The destruction of Carthage, of the Hellenistic Kingdoms, of Numidian kings, and Gallic chieftains had focused the life of their peoples on Rome. Outwardly Rome dominated and ruled her new Empire, but Roman and Italian well-being had become increasingly dependent on the provinces. It remained for Octavius to work out a satisfactory political form to express these relationships although by the time of Caesar's death the new ties were already strong. In Italian society the senatorial ruling class had been discredited and largely destroyed, but the middle class of Italy was ready to take its place. We will look first at the relation between Rome and the provinces and then at the change of society in Italy.

ROME AND THE EMPIRE

Rome and other large Italian cities had become dependent on external sources for their staple food supply and for many of the luxuries and needs of material life which prosperity and a more cosmopolitan taste demanded. At first the grain was brought from the provinces of Sicily and Sardinia as part of the taxes demanded by Rome, then the supply was increased by importation from Africa. Ultimately, when the East became wholly Roman, much of the grain was imported from Syria and Egypt. The supply of grain was largely an operation of the Roman government which was only a part of the network of trade which linked Italy and the provinces.

In war the Romans had stolen objects of art, expensive luxury goods, and money, but their taste for such things and for less costly exotics could only be satisfied by trade after the wars were won. The market in Italy was large because the senatorial class, middle class and common soldiers, who had served abroad, were alike affected. The growth of trade and the migration of Greeks and Hellenized Eastern natives to Italy, which had begun in the second century, continued throughout the first. In its turn Italy began to export special products on an increasing scale: wine, olive oil, metalwork, pottery, and other manufactured goods. They were sent to Spain, Africa, and Narbonensis, as these provinces became urbanized. Roman moneylenders and bankers had made Rome the financial center of the Mediterranean, not only by lending money to cities whom Roman wars and governors had ruined, but also by investing in contracts to work the mines, buying land, and engaging in business ventures of their own.

The provinces, particularly in the East, which had been the scene of the Mithridatic and civil war and which were to be fought over again by Octavius and Mark Antony, were hard hit in the first century B.C. Their capital resources were impaired by continuous requisitions of supplies and money, by levies of men for the Roman armies, and by the damage and looting of war. Yet this damage was speedily repaired when peace and order returned under Octavius after 31 B.C. In the course of the wars the provincials had been brought into the internal political life of Rome by the ties of *clientage* which had been established between their leading citizens and the Roman political leaders who acted as provincial patrons. Pompey had drawn Spain, Africa, and the East to himself. Caesar was in the course of replacing Pompey as the grand patron of the provinces at the time the conspirators killed him. These ties were real, for the provincials were generally loyal and responsive, as the continued Pompeian resistance in Spain to Caesar indicates. The provincials in their turn were receiving some benefits. Both Pompey and Caesar made many grants of citizenship, and Caesar inaugurated a policy of provincial colonization in which old centers such as Carthage and Corinth were rebuilt. Octavius, who recognized the validity and meaning of these ties which had been established between Italy and the provinces, contrived to direct this vast *clientage* to himself and to Rome as a state in order to give the Empire a focal point of loyalty.

ROMAN SOCIETY

In Italy the small-scale farmer, typical of the old Republic, who had grown grain for himself and sold his small surplus in the market of the neighboring town, had not been restored by the agrarian laws of the Gracchan Period. Further damage had been done by the large-scale confiscations of private land by Sulla. The farmers were to be hard hit again in 43 B.C. when Octavius and Mark Antony made further confiscations for their troops. The veterans who were settled as farmers proved restless and discontented. They sold out to wealthier proprietors and drifted to Rome or were ready to re-enlist in the armies and to join movements like that of Catiline. Italian agriculture continued to be diversified and enriched by the growth of the plantations and big estates, but this growth did not favor the senatorial class, however, as much as it did the wealthy *Equites* and businessmen of the middle groups. There were immensely rich, landed men of the senatorial class in the first century B.C., like Pompey and Domitius Ahenobarbus, who could raise private armies from their own tenants and slaves, or Lucullus, who retired from his campaigns against Mithridates to his private estate. Ownership of land, traditionally respectable, remained so and attracted the investment of the middle class. The new "farmers" managed their estates well and made money, while at the same time they acquired the badge of respectability which ownership of land and villas conferred.

The general economic growth of Italy brought a tremendous advance to the middle class, from the wealthy *Equites* with their greatly diversified investments, to the publicans and traders who followed the armies, doing business with the Roman soldiers and settling in their wake. The conditions of business were chaotic and bustling and brought wealth to all types, from the illiterate parvenu to highly educated and influential men who became the friends and confidants of the political leaders.

A good example of the latter is Titus Pomponius Atticus, born in 109 B.C. in Arpinum, where he was a schoolfellow of Cicero. Since Atticus' family was well off, he received an excellent education. After the Mithridatic Wars he bought up large tracts of land in Greece and lived there until the late 60's. Upon his return to Rome Atticus became a very close friend of Cicero, with whom he carried on a voluminous correspondence. He knew Pompey, Caesar, and others of the politically great, and skillfully maintained his friendships without compromising himself politically. His business interests ranged from banking to the training of gladiators. Atticus' own family and others of his class rose in the social scale by alliance with the great. For example, Atticus' daughter, Vipsania, married Agrippa, who became the right-hand man of Octavius. Octavius' own grandfather was a banker. As the senatorial class declined in wealth and power, the able and vigorous families of the middle class moved into their places, at first indirectly, then by the deliberate choice of Caesar and Octavius, who made them senators and administrators.

In the course of the first century B.C. the senatorial nobility were broken as a governing group. Their fortunes were dissipated by the high cost of life and politics in Rome, and only a few individuals, like Sulla and Caesar, were able to recoup them on a grand scale. Preoccupation with public life often resulted in neglect and mismanagement of estates. When such estates were mortgaged and sold to the middle class, the children of these noble families dropped in the social scale, to disappear or turn to violence, like Catiline. Many senators were killed, of course, in the proscriptions and wars dating from the massacre of Marius to the defeat of Mark Antony. Among the upper class, in particular, the close family life of the old Republic, characterized by strong patriarchal authority, died out rapidly. Divorce and remarriage, often for political purposes, were frequent. Accordingly, the birth rate was low, but women came to play a much greater role in society, even political life, than previously. A woman had considerable influence as the mistress or the wife who brought new support to her husband's political position. Her way of living was also emancipated. Clodia, for example, the sister of the tribune Clodius, was the center of a brilliant group in Rome, which lived a bohemian and reckless life which shocked the propriety of the more conservative and older members of society.

Despite the political failure of the senatorial nobility, the stamp which it imprinted on the cultural tradition of Rome in the Late Republic was lasting. In the first century B.C. it had become the regular practice for the children of wealthy families to receive a thorough education in Greek literature, rhetoric, and philosophy. Young men, like Cicero and Julius Caesar, frequently went abroad to Athens or to Rhodes for rhetorical training, while many Greeks came to Rome to teach in private schools or to act as the tutors in both the upper- and middle-class families. While some of the young went overboard in their enthusiasm for sophistry and the devices of rhetoric, like the young men of classical Athens, Roman tradition was not swamped. Instead, a balance of classical humanism was attained which is exemplified in particular by Cicero. He gave his name to the age in which he lived, the Ciceronian Period, and became perhaps the most influential figure in Latin literature. After a brief eclipse in the Early Roman Empire, because of his political opposition to Caesar, Cicero was read and his ideas were used by the Christian writers of the Middle Ages and by men from the Renaissance to the present time.

THE LITERATURE OF THE LATE REPUBLIC

Cicero's work was voluminous and almost forms a library in itself. For the historian his private letters and his legal and political speeches, from the trial of Verres to the First Triumvirate and again against Mark Antony after the death of Caesar, make this period the best documented in Roman history. Cicero also created a Latin prose style, which was rhythmic and fluent, magnificent and rich without ornamental emptiness, and which became a model for the Latin of the Vatican and, by imitation in English, for such writers and orators as Burke and Winston Churchill. While Cicero took the somewhat deprecating view of a practical-minded Roman to his own rhetorical and philosophical works—that they were to occupy his leisure and to distract his mind— they were of great significance for the education of his own and subsequent generations. Cicero enlarged the resources of Roman education by transferring to Latin and discussing the technical methods of Greek rhetoric in works like the *De Oratore* (*On Oratory*). His philosophical treatises, such as the *De Officiis* (*On Obligations*), the *Republic* and *Laws,* not only gave Latin a philosophical vocabulary and popularized Platonic and Stoic ideas, but gave a particularly Roman emphasis to classical humanism through their discussion of the functions of law and justice in society. The *De Officiis* was studied by the Church Fathers, and its ideas of the moral obligations of man became a part of Christian ethics.

The *Republic,* put in the form of a dialogue, like Plato's *Republic,* raised questions which were as pertinent to Cicero's own age as to Plato's. What was

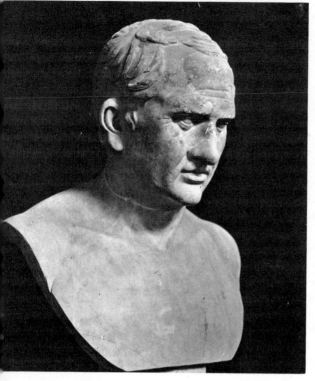

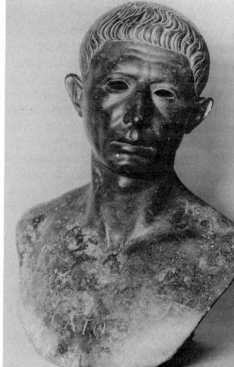

Cicero   *Cato the Younger*

the best form of government, and what was the function of the ideal states-man? The speakers in the dialogue, the members of the Scipionic circle of the previous century, placed great emphasis on the Law of Nature, the idea that the universe is ruled by reason, which God possesses and man can apprehend. This universal principle of justice might be expressed to varying degrees in the laws of actual states, the government of which should be in accord with the principle of justice. In his picture of an ideal society Cicero stressed tradi-tional Roman practices and institutions. The family should be of the old Roman type, with strong patriarchal authority and discipline. Education was to be largely a matter of family training with a strong emphasis on ethics. Religion, too, should have the political function of keeping society stable and of instilling respect for authority. At a time when society and the state were collapsing Cicero idealized the past in a search for stability.

In his own political life Cicero had been a good constitutionalist, with a profound respect for law, order, and authority. In the *Republic* he argued that law was the common denominator of society because it affected all men alike, regardless of their class. It could ensure liberty by safeguarding the positive rights of the citizen to participate in political functions. Cicero, of course, found his ideal organ of government in the Senate, which would be a model and guide to the state by the high ethical quality of its conduct of government.

The thought of Cicero and the martyrdom of Cato did much to idealize and to preserve the principles of the Republic at the time when its institutions were in danger of destruction. Octavius found that he could not escape this legacy and had to set his own rule in a framework of Republican traditions.

The other major writers of the Ciceronian Period reflect other aspects of the age as these touched their own lives. The feverish intensity of life in Rome in the sixties and fifties is shown in the lyric poetry of Gaius Valerius Catullus (*ca.* 84-54 B.C.), who came from Verona to live in Rome and worship for a time at the feet of Clodia, the thinly veiled Lesbia of his poems. Catullus introduced Greek lyric metres and the genres of Alexandrian poetry to Latin literature, but his freshness and intensity of feeling were individual and Italian. The beauty of the countryside, his affection for his family and for Italy, his love (and later his hate) for Lesbia, all his personal thoughts and feelings, were expressed in language which indicates that Latin literature was fast coming to maturity.

Lucretius (*ca.* 94-55 B.C.) in his didactic poem *De Rerum Natura* (*On the Nature of Things*) showed profound concern for the spiritual crisis of his age, afflicted by war and death and faced by a collapse of tradition. Lucretius found the Epicurean philosophy particularly congenial for himself and for his period. He was an aristocrat who lived in seclusion and took no part in political life. Epicureanism was the tool which would free men from the fear in which they lived, above all from superstitious fear of the gods and of death. Lucretius explained Epicurus' mechanistic theory of the universe and the rise of man from savagery to civilization with prophetic fervor and a sense of mission. Man, not the gods, had created civilization, and the exercise of human reason could free men. Through reason men would recognize that death was simply a release from the miseries of the human condition and could understand and accept the facts of existence.

Because the chief historians of the Ciceronian Period were engaged in making history, they exhibited considerable bias in their expression of their own or that of their party's position. We have already noticed Caesar's books on the Gallic and Civil Wars. They were written as military memoirs, a literary form which had been popular since King Ptolemy I of Egypt wrote an account of the campaigns of Alexander the Great. Caesar not only provided a factual account of his campaigns and skillfully presented his own achievements, but by implication he also presented the case against the *Optimates* in a straightforward, convincing style. Sallust (86-36 B.C.) was also a Caesarian. He served under Caesar and then retired to a magnificent villa to write and live at ease. Sallust's most important work, the *Histories,* describing the period from 78 to 67 B.C., has not survived, but his monographs on the Jugurthine War and the Catilinarian Conspiracy are preserved. While not entirely uncritical of the *Populares,* Sallust's bias against the *Optimates* greatly affected his explanation of the decay of the Republic as the result of their corruption. He is scarcely cognizant of the fact that Rome had outgrown its own institutional framework and was groping towards a reorganization of society.

X X V

The Reorganization of Augustus

(44 B.C.–A.D. 14)

THE MEN WHO KILLED Julius Caesar expected that by his removal they would restore freedom of political life in the Republic and leadership to the Senate. Their miscalculation speedily became apparent. Caesar's successful war against Pompey and the *Optimates* had been more than a military victory. He had been supported by the people of Rome and Italy, and at the time of his death, his prestige was replacing that of the senatorial leaders in the provinces. Ordinary men throughout the Empire who had little interest in the political life of Rome, so cherished by the senatorial class, had hoped that the wars were over. Caesar's power, too, had been very real and personal. His subordinates, like the consul Mark Antony and the Master of Horse, Marcus Aemilius Lepidus, were in key positions, while in the background were the veterans and the great army groups. While many veterans were in Rome and Italy waiting for their land grants, the armies were massed in Spain, the Gallic provinces, and Macedonia. The soldiers proved loyal to Caesar's name. When the senatorial and Caesarian leaders attempted to gain control for their own purposes, it became apparent that the decisive factor in the situation was the wishes of the soldiers. They forced the Caesarian leaders, Lepidus, Antony, and Caesar's heir, Octavius (Augustus), despite their personal rivalry, to make common cause against the conspirators and the Senate. The latter were defeated, and the dictatorship of Caesar was replaced by that of the Second Triumvirate.

When Octavius was struggling with the problem of settling veterans in Italy, he apparently began to realize that power had to be founded more broadly than on military support alone. The assassination of Caesar and the persistence of loyalty to the Republic among the educated classes of Italy had demonstrated that five hundred years of tradition could not be wiped out. Yet Octavius owed his own survival to the soldiers of Caesar, and the past century of civil conflict had shown that the state would lapse into anarchy without a strong

The reader will find Map XIX (page 576) useful as he reads this chapter.

leader. Octavius began to identify himself as the protector of Roman tradition. Antony, however, chose to carry on the plans of Caesar for the conquest of Parthia. After his invasion failed, he turned more and more to Cleopatra's dream of making Egypt the center of the Roman Empire. The victory of Octavius over Antony and Cleopatra at the battle of Actium in 31 B.C. marked the end of the struggle for power.

Octavius then began to reconcile the traditions of the Republic with the need for strong, personal leadership. As the restorer of peace and order to the state and the commander of seventy legions, his wishes could hardly be disputed. Fortunately for Rome, Octavius was an adroit and shrewd statesman, who saw the need of reorganization and had the will and power to act. Octavius' reorganization initiated the era of the Roman Empire and endured much as he created it for almost two centuries. It is called the Principate from the position of the ruler, who was the *Princeps* or first man of the state. The position of the *Princeps* rested on a unique blend of legal power, military autocracy, and personal prestige. Octavius began his career as a military dictator and ended it as one of the great constructive statesmen of history.

The Contest for Empire: Octavius and Antony

REPUBLIC OR DICTATORSHIP?

In the hours following Caesar's death both the Senate and Mark Antony were uneasy and played for time. While many of the senators owed their positions to Caesar, leadership came from the former Pompeians and Republican constitutionalists who hailed the conspirators as Liberators. These men distrusted Antony; they thought him ambitious and unscrupulous and feared that he would try to take Caesar's dictatorship for himself. Antony did not know how much support the Liberators and the Senate could muster or how the other Caesarian leaders would view his ambitions. Lepidus, the Master of Horse, was near Rome with a legion under arms. For the time being the Senate and Antony came to terms and tried to pass the situation off. It was agreed that the conspirators were not to be punished, but that Caesar's acts should be ratified and that he should be given a public funeral.

This compromise did not work. Antony made the formal speech of praise at Caesar's funeral, probably not the skillful incitement to violence which Shakespeare adapted from Plutarch, but a sober account of the dictator's career. The reading of Caesar's will was sufficient to rouse the people to demand vengeance on his killers. Caesar left his private gardens along the Tiber as a public park and a legacy of three hundred sesterces (about fifteen dollars) to each Roman citizen. Caesar's main heir, whom he adopted in his will as his son, was his great-nephew, Octavius, a relatively unknown young man of eighteen, who was at Apollonia in Greece at this time. Antony and one of the conspirators, Decimus Brutus, were named as minor heirs. Upon the reading of the will the mob in the Forum took over the funeral. They surged out to look for the Liberators, who escaped, but returned to cremate Caesar's body in the Forum and to light the proceedings by firing the Senate House, which stood conveniently nearby.

Since this popular demonstration for Caesar strengthened Antony's hand, he moved to make himself master of the government. A personal bodyguard of six thousand men was raised from Caesar's veterans in Rome and the backing of Lepidus was secured. Antony put a number of useful arrangements into effect for which he claimed to find authority among Caesar's papers. Above all, Antony needed to concentrate military power in his own hands; therefore he shuffled the provincial governorships as much to his own advantage as possible. Lepidus was repaid by election as *Pontifex Maximus* in the place of Caesar and departed for Spain to make a deal with Sextus Pompey, who was stirring up revolt once again. For the moment Antony had to allow Decimus Brutus to go to Cisalpine Gaul, which Caesar had designated as a province for him. Cassius and Marcus Brutus, for whom Rome was not safe, were removed by being assigned to the grain supply and later to the provinces of Cyrenaica and Crete. They went to the East, not to govern their provinces, but to raise armies which would enable them to make a stand for the Senate against Antony and the Caesarians.

Antony himself had been slated for Macedonia after his consulship, but he realized that the key to power lay in the armies concentrated in the Gallic provinces. Accordingly, he had Decimus Brutus transferred to Macedonia and himself to Cisalpine Gaul, to which he added Transalpine Gaul and extended his term for five years. In addition, he arranged for the transfer of four legions from Macedonia to his own command. Antony's fellow consul, Dolabella, who had been granted Syria as a province, was mollified by a similar extension of tenure. While Antony would probably have to fight Decimus Brutus to remove him from Cisalpine Gaul, he was in the process of setting up the situation to his liking within a few months after the death of Caesar. The Senate had been cowed into acquiescence, and Cicero, who strenuously opposed Antony, was preparing to join the Liberators in the East. The arrival of Octavius, however, who came to Italy to claim his inheritance, complicated the situation.

Octavius showed that even at the age of eighteen he was a worthy heir to Julius Caesar in more than name. He first approached the minor Caesarian leaders for support and found in Balbus, Caesar's secretary, a mine of useful information. Then he called on Cicero, who rather fatuously saw in himself a political guide to the young Octavius, and in Octavius a tool who could be used to split the Caesarian support from Antony. Octavius, however, made his own political future. When Antony refused to give him his inheritance from Caesar, probably because he was spending it for his own purposes and because he regarded Octavius as negligible, the latter recruited a private army. The appeal of his new names, Gaius Iulius Caesar Octavianus (Octavian), and funds from wealthy *Equites,* with whom he had family connections or a recommendation from Balbus, were effective among the veterans. Even two of the legions from Macedonia, summoned by Antony, came over to him.

Antony had to act quickly to acquire a large army and to save his dwindling power. He marched north against Decimus Brutus in Cisalpine Gaul and besieged him in Mutina, but the Senate dispatched the consuls for 43 B.C. and Octavian to relieve the town. They raised the siege and forced Antony to retreat across the Alps. As the Senate's star was on the rise, Cicero fulminated against Antony in the Senate with his famous series of *Philippics,* so-named to recall Demosthenes' struggle against the tyrant, Philip of Macedonia. In the meantime Cassius and Marcus Brutus had defeated Dolabella in Syria and were raising a large force, ultimately about eighty thousand men, in the Eastern provinces. The Senate declared Antony a public enemy, placed Decimus Brutus in charge of Italy, and granted Cassius and Marcus Brutus an overall command in the East.

Octavian, of whom Cicero had written in a letter that he was to be praised, honored, but repudiated for office, was virtually ignored. He demanded a triumph, a consulship, rewards for his soldiers, and marched on Rome. The legions brought by the Senate from Africa to fight against Octavian deserted to him, and Octavian took over Rome. The senators had forgotten that the Caesarians had a common cause against the Liberators and the Senate, and that Caesar's troops were loyal to the dictator and not to be cheated of the rewards of their victory. The sequel was swift. Octavian rescinded the decree against Antony. Antony and Lepidus made common cause when their troops fraternized and soon were joined by the army of Plancus, the Caesarian leader in Gaul. Twenty-two legions marched into Cisalpine Gaul, where the army of Decimus Brutus deserted to them. Brutus was killed by a Gallic chieftain. Octavian, with his own army of eleven legions, met the other Caesarian leaders near Bononia (Bologna) and combined forces with them. Out of this situation developed the dictatorial commission of the Second Triumvirate, consisting of Antony, Lepidus, and Octavian. They commanded a huge force of veteran soldiers who wanted vengeance on the Liberators and bonuses for themselves.

THE SECOND TRIUMVIRATE

The Second Triumvirate, instead of operating behind the scenes like its predecessor, obtained authorization for its existence for five years from the assembly and ruled dictatorially. Its first purpose was to crush opposition in Italy and then to defeat Cassius and Brutus in the East and Sextus Pompey in the West. The Triumvirs inaugurated their regime by a bloody proscription. Several thousand lesser men and about a hundred senators were killed, among them Cicero, who had particularly offended Antony. In addition to confiscating their victims' property, the Triumvirs levied heavy taxes on Italy and designated the territory of eighteen Italian towns for allocations of land to the troops.

In 42 B.C. Antony and Octavian landed their forces in Greece to meet the armies of the Liberators, which had been joined by refugees from Rome. The last battles for the Republic were fought near Philippi in Macedonia and won for the Caesarians largely by Antony, for Octavian had fallen sick. Cassius and Brutus committed suicide upon their defeat. While Sextus Pompey had raised a fleet in the western Mediterranean and held Sicily, the victory of the Triumvirs placed most of the provinces at their disposal, and the administration was divided.

Antony, who had emerged as the strongest figure in the coalition, got the lion's share. He received the Eastern provinces and, in addition, Transalpine Gaul, which he administered through a legate. Octavian obtained the Western provinces but inherited the war with Sextus Pompey and the invidious problem of settling the veterans in Italy. He was weakened, too, by the impotent jealousy of Lepidus and the recognition of Cisalpine Gaul as a part of Italy, that is, neutral ground. The unfortunate Lepidus, suspected of collusion with Sextus Pompey, was virtually squeezed out, retaining only the promise of Africa when conditions might warrant it.

At first Antony found the East most congenial. Cleopatra came to Tarsus in Cilicia to meet him and to explain the interests of Egypt in the new situation. Antony followed her to Alexandria, putting the affairs of Syria and Palestine in order en route. While Antony spent the winter of 40 in Egypt, his interest in Cleopatra at this time seems to have been much the same as Caesar's had been. The result, too, was the same—each had a son by Cleopatra. In the spring when the cares of office became pressing, Antony had to return to Italy. The Parthians had raided Syria in force, while Antony's agents in Italy, his brother Lucius and his wife Fulvia, had provoked Octavian to war and had been defeated. The Triumvirate was threatened by collapse. When Antony landed at Brundisium, some fighting broke out, but the Caesarian soldiers saw little profit to themselves in mutual destruction and forced their leaders into a reconciliation. By the Treaty of Brundisium a new bargain was made, in which Octavian improved his position by the acquisition of Transalpine Gaul, where Antony's legate had died. The death of Antony's wife also opened the way to forging a personal tie between Octavian and Antony. The latter married Octavian's sister, Octavia, and the prospects for concord seemed good.

Three years later, in 37 B.C., the unity of the Triumvirate was again strained, but Octavia, with whom Antony had been living congenially in Athens, was able to bring her brother and husband into a reaffirmation of the Triumvirate for five years. Each needed the other's help. Octavian wanted some warships to attack Sextus Pompey, and Antony, who had been preparing for war on Parthia, needed more Roman troops. The pact was sealed by a pledge of mutual help, which Antony honored by sending 120 ships, but Octavian ignored the pact. With the aid of Antony's warships Sextus Pompey was crushed in Sicily. He fled to Asia Minor, where he was put to death by Antony two years later. Lepidus, who had aided Octavian in the war against Pompey, tried to take over Sicily upon its conclusion, but his troops deserted and Octavian relegated him to obscurity by detention in an Italian town. Lepidus died in 12 B.C., retaining his title of *Pontifex Maximus* and the memories of being an aide to Caesar as the sole fruits of his former career.

Octavian, thus left in sole control of the West, began to create a new image of himself as he engaged in the difficult problems of settling the veterans and of coping with the political obstruction of Antony's agents and supporters in Italy. Gradually the despotic Triumvir gave place to the protector of Roman tradition and the champion of Italy. In 36 B.C. Octavian was granted the sacrosanctity of the tribunes and the right to sit on the tribune's bench in the Senate as a mark of honor. Julius Caesar had held a similar privilege, and Octavian was concerned at this time to stress his position as the adopted son of the great man whom the Triumvirs had designated in 42 B.C. as a god. Octavian surrounded himself with very able aides, drawn from the *Equites*. Marcus Vipsanius Agrippa, who was later to be one of the principal helpers of Octavian in reorganizing the state, had defeated Sextus Pompey. Maecenas, a wealthy Equestrian of Etruscan origin, a man of refined artistic taste and a patron of literature, began to discover young writers. He encouraged Vergil (p. 584), whose family had lost land in the confiscations of the Triumvirate, to work on the *Georgics,* a poem of praise for the land of Italy and its farmers. Vergil introduced another young poet, Horace, to Maecenas. Horace had fought for the Republic at Philippi, but he was later to support Octavian's policy for the regeneration of Roman society. Thus, by various means a feeling of confidence in Octavian as the leader of Rome and Italy was encouraged.

In contrast Antony seemed more and more to become a protagonist of the Hellenistic East or was made to appear so by the supporters of Octavian. In 36 B.C. Antony set out to attack the Parthians who were raiding Syria and to win fresh laurels for himself and Rome. Antony avoided the Mesopotamian desert and struck inland through Asia Minor and Armenia. The king of Armenia, upon whose cooperation he counted, played him false and betrayed the Roman supply train to the Parthians. Although Antony skillfully saved a large part of his army, he was forced to retreat and got back to the Mediterranean with the loss of over twenty thousand men and considerable damage to his prestige. The legions promised by Octavian had not been sent, and the rift between the two was made wider by Antony's refusal to see Octavia. He had already affronted her by marriage to Cleopatra, although that was not recognized as valid by Roman law.

Antony thus had to rely more on Egypt and on the East than previously, and it is a moot point whether he was used by Cleopatra for her schemes of empire or whether he contemplated using her for his. Our knowledge of their relationship is drawn mostly from the propaganda of Octavian, which naturally represented Antony as a weak-willed pawn of Cleopatra, and the war which developed as a conflict with Cleopatra and Egypt. In any case, the plans of Antony and Cleopatra were revealed in a festival held at Alexandria in 34 B.C., where the two presided on thrones of gold. Antony made a speech to the Alexandrians in which he divided up the Roman provinces of the East among Cleopatra and her children. Cleopatra was proclaimed Queen of Egypt, Cyprus, Crete, and lower Syria, to rule along with her son by Caesar, Ptolemy Caesarion. The sons of Antony and Cleopatra were given Armenia, Media and Parthia (still to be conquered) and the Roman provinces of Syria and Cilicia. Antony had been charged with the reorganization of the Roman East, but he appeared to be giving it away to his bride and to her family, as if he were the personal ruler of the Roman Empire. While he did not claim kingship for himself, he acted as if he were establishing a dynasty of the Hellenistic type, in which Egypt, not Rome, was to be paramount.

This spectacle played into the hands of Octavian, and events moved rapidly to an open break and to war. To gain support in Italy Antony wrote to the Senate, asking for approval of his actions in the East and offering to restore the old constitution of the Republic when the Triumvirate expired. One of Antony's supporters introduced a motion calling for the resignation of Octavian, but the latter blocked the measure through a tribune's veto. Octavian himself appeared in the Senate with a bodyguard, took over the government, and publicized Antony's will which was deposited in the Temple of Vesta for safekeeping. The will confirmed, perhaps by forgery, the Alexandrian Donations, as they are called. Octavian secured an oath of loyalty to himself from those senators who remained in Italy and from the Italian towns and the provinces of the West. As the champion of Rome and Italy he terminated Antony's command and declared war on Cleopatra.

The preparations for war on both sides were impressive. Cleopatra financed an army of ninety thousand men and a fleet of five hundred ships from the resources of Egypt. In 32 B.C. the armada moved to Actium in western Greece, preparatory to attacking Italy, but waited over the winter. In the spring of 31 B.C. Octavian sailed with an army of equal size and a fleet of four hundred warships. The morale of Antony's and Cleopatra's troops was low, for many of the Romans objected to Cleopatra's presence. Octavian's admiral, Agrippa, blockaded the Egyptian fleet, and his army cut the communications of Antony's force in Greece. As time passed Antony's men began to desert to Octavian, and the eventual sea battle of Actium was little more than a breakout by Antony

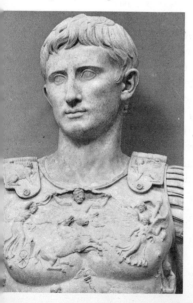

Augustus as imperator

The Empress Livia

Agrippa

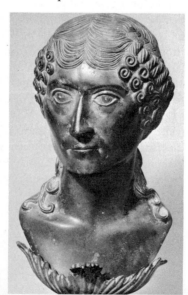

and Cleopatra to the open sea, where they ran for Egypt. The battle, which propaganda magnified into a hard-fought and glorious victory for Octavian, really ended the war.

Octavian followed the royal couple to Alexandria, where Antony attempted another stand. His troops deserted, and Antony himself, on a rumor of Cleopatra's death, committed suicide. The queen had been taken prisoner and rather than grace a Roman triumph she, too, killed herself. Octavian put young Caesarion and Antony's elder son to death, in order to dispose of their possible claims to the throne of Egypt, and annexed the country to the Roman Empire. The century of conquest and civil war, which had begun with the tribunate of Tiberius Gracchus, was ended. The next forty-five years of Octavian's life were to be devoted to restoring peace to Rome and the Empire.

The Principate of Augustus

THE PRINCEPS

Upon his return from Egypt in 29 B.C., Octavian began to encourage reconciliation and the hope of a new era in Rome's history. His victory was celebrated by a great triumph which lasted for three days, but the end of war was symbolized in traditional fashion by closing the doors of the Temple of Janus for the first time in two hundred years. The war booty from Egypt allowed arrears of taxation to be forgiven. Large numbers of men were demobilized, and an amnesty allowed the supporters of Antony to return to Rome. In 28 B.C. Octavian and his aide, Agrippa, were elected as censors and prepared the Senate for the coming reorganization of government. The membership of the Senate, which had grown to about a thousand, was cut down to eight hundred by the removal of unsuitable senators. The scene was set and Octavian began the establishment of the Principate.

In his official autobiography, the *Res Gestae,* published toward the end of his life, Octavian described his action in 28 and 27 B.C. in these words:

> In my sixth and seventh consulships after I had extinguished the civil wars, having gained possession of all power by the consent of all men, I transferred the state from my own power to the judgment of the Senate and the Roman People. For this meritorious action of mine I was named Augustus by a decree of the Senate . . . after that time I surpassed all in authority (prestige) but had no more power than the others who were my colleagues in each magistracy.

About a century later the historian Tacitus commented: "Augustus concentrated in himself the functions of the Senate, the magistrates, and the laws."

The new government was publicized as a restoration of the Republic, and outwardly that was the case, for all the familiar institutions were retained: the Senate, magistrates, assemblies, and provincial governorships. Yet, the personal ruler was brought into the government by successive stages as an indispensable element. From the outset the ruler, the *Princeps,* held the sources of real power: command over the armies, special political privileges, and the incalculable weight of personal authority. The chief Republican element, the Senate, did have a large share in administration and possessed the prestige of tradition, but the partnership, or dyarchy, was unequally weighted. As the Principate was consolidated, the position of the *Princeps* became increasingly stronger, until the office was greater than the man who held it. A return to the Republic was impossible, as Tacitus acknowledged, despite his condemnation of the early rulers as tyrants.

When Octavian indicated that he would transfer the Republic to the Senate and People, neither he nor they considered his retirement seriously. He had not spent seventeen strenuous years to retire at the age of thirty-five and to leave his various projects up in the air. Octavian's gesture was the prelude to a shift of important powers of government to himself. He recognized the Senate and People (through their assemblies) as the source of sovereignty in the state, and they delegated powers to him by proper legal processes and by free consent. The Principate was founded in law.

The first grant which Octavian received in 27 B.C. was most important because it concentrated military power in his hands. He was given a special command, a proconsular *imperium,* for a period of ten years over the block of provinces in which the organized armies were stationed: Spain, Gaul, Syria, and Egypt. Octavian was to administer these provinces and command their armies directly while the Senate continued its traditional administration of the rest of the Empire. Government in Rome and Italy would proceed as usual, but Octavian retained his consulship. There was, of course, precedent for such a grant in the special commands of the past, particularly those of Pompey. Octavian was also honored in 27 B.C. by the title of Augustus, a word with the religious overtones of "the revered and majestic one." He was thus set off from other men in an indefinable area of prestige. Augustus truthfully said that he surpassed all in this respect, but his statement that he had no more power than his colleagues was only formally correct. There were other provincial governors, but Augustus held the command of the army groups. The creation of a separate administration had begun and in the following years was rapidly extended.

Four years later, in 23 B.C., Augustus' proconsular *imperium* was enlarged to become a greater command, a *maius imperium*. This enabled him to overrule the authority of the governors in the senatorial provinces and was effective in the city of Rome, but he did not take over the administration of either. It was enough to be able to interfere legally, if he judged it necessary. At the same time Augustus resigned the consulship, which he had been holding for successive years, but was granted certain consular powers: the right to convoke the Senate and to introduce business first. He was also given the full powers of the tribunate. Augustus prized these very highly, for the remaining years of his reign were dated annually by reference to the beginning of his tribunician authority. Augustus had thus contrived to blend the revolutionary, popular tradition of the tribunes of the people with the discipline and authority inherent in the *imperium*. He was the head of state in both a military and civil capacity.

In the following year, 22 B.C., Augustus began to take over certain important areas of administration and to encroach on the activity of magistrates and Senate. This was a year of near famine in Rome, in which the Senate had been unable to provide grain for the people. By popular demand Augustus was entrusted with the *cura annonae* (the provision of grain). He established a government department by the appointment of a prefect, responsible to himself, although the actual distribution of grain was still carried on by the Senate.

In 12 B.C. Lepidus, Augustus' old colleague in the Triumvirate, died, and Augustus was elected to the office of *Pontifex Maximus*. As High Priest he was able to proceed directly with the reorganization of public religion in Rome. This office completed the formal powers by which Augustus acted in government, but he was granted many other titles and honors.[1] For example, in 18 B.C. he received the right to use the formal symbols of the consulship, the *fasces* and the *curule* chair of ivory. In 2 B.C. Augustus became the *pater patriae,* the father of the fatherland, an honor which expressed the traditional discipline and responsibility of the father in Roman life.

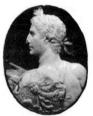

An Augustan cameo

Throughout this whole process Augustus had obtained his powers of government and titles of honor as a person by resolutions of the Senate and votes of the assembly. Some honors like the tribunician power and the high priesthood were held for life, but the military command had been renewed for successive terms. In 18 B.C. it was extended for five years and thereafter for five and ten year periods. At no time was there any question of the command not being renewed, but theoretically the Principate was a parcel of separate, special items, limited in tenure and granted to an individual, to Augustus himself. He could not automatically transfer his powers to a successor at death because they reverted to the Senate and People. The latter might redelegate all or a part of the powers to one or several men or decide to administer the whole government by itself. In short the Principate was not automatically hereditary.

Yet Augustus' long and successful reign, his hold on the army, and the

---

[1] The complex character of the Principate is indicated by the fact that there was no proper title for the ruler which indicated his whole office. *Princeps,* or prince, was an old term of Republican usage, which designated a man of surpassing prominence among his fellows and had been applied regularly to the senior senator, the *princeps senatus. Imperator,* or emperor, ultimately became the usual title for the ruler, and so "emperor" is generally used to refer to the Roman rulers. At first, however, *imperator* was an honorary military title, given by acclamation of the army after victory and by approval of the Senate. Augustus received the title after the victory at Mutina and in the 30's, while he was emphasizing the military aspect of his position, made it a personal name, his *praenomen.* He was *the imperator.* After Actium he chose to stress the civilian character of the Principate, and *imperator* did not become a regular part of the imperial titulature until after 69 when Vespasian, who owed his position to the support of the army, adopted it. *Caesar* was the family name of the Julian line, but was transferred to the Flavians, who succeeded them, to bolster their legitimacy. *Caesar* thus began its long history as a royal title, which culminated with Kaiser and Czar. From the outset Greek writers who regarded the Principate as a hereditary office called the *Princeps, Autokrator,* and referred to his *basileia,* or kingdom. Augustus is said to have expressed the ideas involved for the Romans: "I am master of the slaves, *Imperator* of the army, and *Princeps* of the rest."

establishment of large areas of government, for which administrative services responsible to him were set up, made a *Princeps* indispensable. Augustus invented a method for transferring the succession but had very great difficulty in selecting a person from his own family circle, as he wished to do. His difficulties gave upper-class society in Rome considerable material for gossip and speculation until his choice came finally to rest on his stepson Tiberius (pp. 590–93). The latter was brought forward to a public position of responsibility and power. Well before Augustus' death in A.D. 14, Tiberius had been granted the tribunician power and a special proconsular command, so that he seemed the natural and inevitable candidate. When Augustus died, the Senate and People invested Tiberius with the other necessary powers and legally created a new *Princeps* from the Julio-Claudian family.

Augustus deliberately emphasized the continuity of his Principate with the traditions of the Republic and so appealed in particular to the people of Italy and of the Romanized provinces of the West: Sicily, Sardinia-Corsica, Narbonensis, Spain, and Africa. The Eastern provinces, however, were infused with the traditions of Hellenistic monarchy, while the new European provinces, Gaul, and those which Augustus added along the Danube, were Celtic and Germanic in tradition. To link these regions to the *Princeps,* a different tie of sentiment was needed. For this purpose Augustus and his successors made use of the device of ruler cult, the formal and public worship of the ruler in association with Rome.

In the Hellenistic East the practice of ruler cult needed no encouragement but rather judicious control. From the time of the Macedonian Wars various Roman generals, from Flamininus to Mark Antony, had been honored by the establishment of cults in Greek cities as a token of recognition and gratitude. They had stepped easily into the place of the Hellenistic kings. Augustus' restoration of peace and order was hailed by a spontaneous outburst of enthusiasm in the East, and he received many requests to establish cults for his worship. In general Augustus set the policy of allowing the cities to do as they wished. Sometimes he gave their municipal cults prestige by his express approval, but, when existing league organizations or whole provinces wished to establish his worship, he judged that it was preferable to regulate the cult carefully. These larger associations were politically significant and could be of use to the central government as a gauge of feeling in the province, apart from the normal channels of provincial government. In the provincial cults delegates were chosen by the members of the organization and met for an annual festival at a designated center. While the main purpose of the assembly was to celebrate the worship of the ruler, matters of general concern to the province were discussed and might be referred to the *Princeps* for his personal attention. Augustus allowed such provincial cults to be formed in Asia Minor in the 20's, and they were rapidly extended.

The value of ruler cult for the new European provinces was recognized in 12 B.C., when the governor of Gaul, Drusus, a stepson of Augustus, sponsored the building of altars to Augustus and Rome at Lugdunum (Lyons). The Gallic tribal chieftains met there in assembly and later a temple was constructed to link even more closely the personal worship of the *Princeps* and the annual meeting of the Gauls. In this period, too, a similar cult was established in Cologne to facilitate Roman control of the Germanic peoples along the Rhine.

Extension of the cult to the Romanized provinces of the West, however, did not take place until the 70's of the first century after Christ. At first upper-class Roman sentiment was opposed to deification of the living ruler, and the emperors not only made no deliberate attempt to establish the cult but discouraged requests which came to them from the provincials. A similar practice obtained in Italy, of course, where the Senate preferred to pass judgment on the ruler after his death. A precedent for deification had been set in 42 B.C., when worship was established for Julius Caesar. After Augustus' death he, too, was duly deified by the Senate as a mark of approval, and thereafter deification became standard for the "good" emperors. In fact, a cynic might say that this was the only opportunity which the Senate had to pass judgment freely on its partner in the administration.

THE SENATE

Although the senatorial nobility of the Republic had been broken as a governing class in the civil wars, Augustus took considerable pains to revive the Senatorial Order and to make the Senate an important part of government. Since the senators as a whole were representative of upper-class educated society in Italy, it was important to secure their cooperation. By family tradition or as a result of their own careers, they still had influence in Italy and, to some degree, in the provinces. Some old and distinguished families of the Republic survived who were the social equals or the superiors of Augustus himself. These families not only formed a living link to the Republic but could also be of very great use to the *Princeps*, for these men were proud and eager to maintain the traditional prestige of the Senate and of their class. Augustus was able to effect a reconciliation with them, and in some cases restored the financial resources of old families at his personal expense. Many senators, of course, were new men who had been rewarded for their services by Julius Caesar, by the Triumvirs, and by Augustus himself. The latter were favorable to the Principate, but they, too, were quick to absorb the traditions of their class and to cherish the standing which senatorial rank conferred. Accordingly, Augustus and most of his successors were careful to keep the senatorial class in good order and to deal carefully with the Senate as an organ of government.

After his initial "purge" in 28 B.C. Augustus made several other revisions of senatorial membership, all of which were carried out by proper censorial authority and were based on the regular qualifications for the Order. For entry and the retention of membership in the Order, it was necessary to have a good record and a property rating of at least a million sesterces, or about fifty thousand dollars. Entry continued to be through the quaestorship as in the past, but like Caesar, Augustus recognized talent and brought in deserving men, so that the senatorial class did not remain a closed group as it had under the Republic. By the exercise of tact and good sense he was able to win cooperation and to set a pattern of proper procedure for his successors in this respect. The senators knew that the *Princeps* had the force to coerce them and that he controlled their advancement by his patronage, but Augustus was careful to conceal these realities. He guided the Senate by suggestion rather than command, consulted it frequently, and gave a lead when he sought advice. The dignity and self-esteem of the body were preserved, and its members responded to the new opportunities which the *Princeps* could provide.

The patronage of the *Princeps* could affect a senator's career at several points. As in the past, the young Roman of senatorial family began his career with military service, but now began as a junior officer in the army of the *Princeps* in one of the imperial provinces. Again, when the senator became a candidate for the praetorship or consulship, the good will of the *Princeps* was valuable and by A.D. 8 almost necessary. Through his consular power Augustus had the right of approving the list of candidates for higher offices (*nominatio*), and he might even endorse certain names (*commendatio*). At first Augustus used this right of recommendation sparingly, but, as the need for experienced administrators increased, he recommended candidates more frequently to provide a supply of governors and high officers in the army. By A.D. 8 it had become the practice to publish a slate of candidates filled by names of his own choice. Ambitious men were eager for this notice because the governorships of the *Princeps'* provinces were of indefinite tenure and good service might lead from the minor to the major provinces. Augustus, too, increased the stock of potential governors by appointing *suffecti* (substitute consuls) who were given the rank of consul and served part of a year. These practices, of course, made election by the assembly an empty convention, and in Augustus' own reign the hectic activity of the electoral contests died out. After A.D. 19 the elections were transferred to the Senate by his successor, Tiberius.

The governmental work of the Senate was closely scrutinized by the *Princeps,* partly because Augustus chose to work with that body, and partly because his *imperium* allowed interference in the senatorial provinces and in Rome. His office remedied the Republic's lack of some central authority to take an overall and continuing view of the needs of Empire. The Senate and the higher magistrates were responsible for the administration of the unarmed, senatorial provinces, for Rome and for Italy, but in all these there was a gradual erosion of senatorial independence, resulting from the growth of the *Princeps'* own administration.

The system of government for the senatorial provinces remained essentially the same as under the Republic, but its quality improved considerably. The governors were appointed from the ex-consuls and ex-praetors after a specified interval beyond their tenure of office in Rome—ten years for the consuls and five for the praetors. The important provinces of Asia and Africa, in the latter of which there were a few troops for protection against the nomads of the desert, were consular provinces, the remainder, praetorian. The governors were assigned by lot to their provinces for an annual term. Taxes were collected by *publicani* for the stock companies which had taken up the contracts, but their behavior and that of the governors were sharply watched, and maladministration was severely punished. It was rarely necessary for Augustus to interfere, but when he did so, it was with his usual tact and care for the Senate's feelings. For example, when it was necessary to establish a panel of judges in Cyrenaica, a senatorial province, Augustus directed the governor to observe certain procedures "until the Senate deliberates on the question, and I have devised a better plan." The close association of Senate and *Princeps* is apparent, too, in the making of laws and in the administration of justice.

While Augustus could convoke the Senate and introduce the first business, he tended to avoid such an overt control because it might seem offensive and also because he was a very busy man and away from Rome for long periods. To establish a link between himself and the Senate a "cabinet" (*consilium*) was set up through which business was regularly channeled. The "cabinet" consisted of the *Princeps,* the consuls, one from each of the other colleges of magistrates, and fifteen senators selected by lot who served for six months. Most legislation thus went through the regular channels, even if it originated from the *Princeps*. The Senate debated measures, with freedom of speech tempered by discretion, and passed resolutions, which the consuls or tribunes could introduce into the proper assemblies for approval.

Yet this apparent freedom of action and full collaboration were really illusory. The important decisions were not made by the "cabinet" but by the *Princeps* and a small group of advisers. These were trusted and experienced men of the type of Agrippa and Maecenas who had long been connected with Augustus and who could be entrusted individually with particularly important administrative or military assignments. The *Princeps,* too, by virtue of his *imperium,* was continually issuing directives, deciding questions, and instructing his subordinates in the administration of his own provinces and on important matters brought to him. Augustus was not yet in legal terminology a proper "source of law," but this activity pointed to the time when the edicts of the Emperor would come to be the sole source of law for the Empire. Even so, the reality of popular legislation, just as of the electoral process, dwindled away.

A similar trend of encroachment by the *Princeps* on the traditional preserves of the administration of justice was apparent. As in the Republic the various magistrates in their proper spheres, and the special courts established by Sulla, continued to function, but the more important cases were diverted from them. The *Princeps,* through his *imperium,* was a final court of appeal for cases from his own provinces and from Rome. To judge them he presided over his *consilium* as a court and delegated his judicial power to legates in the provinces and to an important new official in Rome, the city prefect (*praefectus urbi*). The prefect combined the duties of a chief of police, who commanded a corps of 4500 military police, the urban cohorts, and city magistrate, who gradually replaced the praetors' courts.

In a somewhat similar fashion the Senate itself became a high court of justice, which heard cases of maladministration in the provinces and, towards the end of Augustus' reign, cases of treason. At what point maladministration by a provincial governor became treason it was difficult to decide, for the state was injured by either. In fact, the whole area of treason to the new regime, ranging from disrespect and insult to the *Princeps* as a person to conspiracy against his life or the state, needed to be clarified. Augustus' own reign was relatively free from conspiracy, but, as the Principate developed, certain rulers provoked opposition by their conduct, and the problem remained thorny throughout the first century after Christ.

THE IMPERIAL ADMINISTRATION

Although the Senate and the regular magistrates were responsible for a large part of government, Augustus began to form an imperial civil service directly responsible to himself which would not only serve his own provinces, and the various new departments, such as the grain supply and the policing of Rome, but also help him personally. The imperial bureaucracy, once established, followed the rapid growth of officialdom which characterizes centralization of government. For provincial governors and army commanders, the *legati Augusti pro praetore,* Augustus used trustworthy and experienced consuls and praetors of the senatorial class. He could offer them long tenure and promotion when they proved their caliber. In general this arrangement satisfied the ambitions of these men who would have been the potential Caesars, Sullas, and Pompeys in the Republic. They were too few in number, however, and too valuable to be wasted on routine or specialized posts, which Augustus was to fill from the ranks of the middle class and the freedmen.

The *Equites* were taken in hand by Augustus and made into a distinctive order of society with strict qualifications and special privileges of their own. The minimum property rating for the Equestrian Order was 400,000 sesterces, about twenty thousand dollars, and its members were distinguished by the right of wearing a special costume and by their own privileges at ceremonies. The Order was hereditary but was strengthened by bringing in ex-centurions from the legions and men from the country towns of Italy and the Romanized provinces. While the *Equites* continued to engage in their traditional business and financial enterprises, Augustus opened new careers to them in the imperial services as procurators and, at the top, prefects of the government services. Financial experience made the *Equites* valuable in the imperial provinces where procurators were used to administer the direct taxes. The traditional contract system was used at first by Augustus for the collection of indirect taxes, but procuratorial duties were expanded eventually into this area also. While no fixed system up the steps of a civil service career came into existence for some time, Augustus did shift and promote his procurators to fill certain difficult and specialized posts. These were in small districts with special problems. For example, the Alpine regions of northern Italy, peopled by mountaineers living in small villages, and Judaea, where religious nationalism caused trouble, were made into procuratorial districts.

The important prefectures, which were the plums of a procuratorial career, were of as much importance in government as the posts open to senators. A prefect, directly responsible to the *Princeps,* was in charge of the procurement of grain, another commanded the praetorian guard which protected the *Princeps,* and another administered Egypt. The latter commanded a small legionary army, but no men of senatorial rank were allowed to visit the country without special permission. Presumably Augustus wished to prevent any potential rival from using Egypt as a base of operations. The land, of course, was easily defended and provided a large part of the grain supply to Rome.

The freedmen of Roman society, large numbers of whom were trained for secretarial and clerical work, were employed by Augustus in his own household and on his estates. Almost automatically they developed into the personal secretariat of the *Princeps.* His correspondence, of course, was voluminous, and the detail of administration continuously increased. At a later date, in the reign of the Emperor Claudius, the freedmen of the palace were to become important and influential figures in their capacity as confidential secretaries.

ROME AND ITALY

Although Rome had grown into a great city in the last two centuries of the Republic, the municipal administration and services had been haphazardly conducted. The magistrates, originally created to look after the affairs of a city-state, had been engaged in conducting wars, governing provinces, and promoting their own careers. Much of the routine work of city administration had fallen upon the young aediles, and the services for protection against fires and for policing were woefully inadequate. For example, the public slaves, who acted as police under the direction of the magistrates, had been completely unable to check the rioting and gang warfare of the 50's. The flimsy frame apartments in the slums were swept periodically by fires with which private fire brigades vainly tried to cope. It is said that Crassus made considerable profit from his brigade by refusing its services to the owner of a building until a satisfactory bargain was struck for the purchase of the property in flames.

Augustus transformed Rome into an imperial capital, not only by large-scale building projects, but by providing proper administration and services. By A.D. 6 the city had been divided into fourteen regions and 265 wards for purposes of local administration. Each ward elected its own *magister* (mayor), usually a freedman, who had a part in the distribution of grain, in fire protection, and public religion (p. 583). A special force of firemen and night police (the *vigiles*), seven thousand in number, was set up under the direction of the prefect of the watch and allocated among the regions of the city. The distribution of grain was systemically regulated by a system of registration and provided for

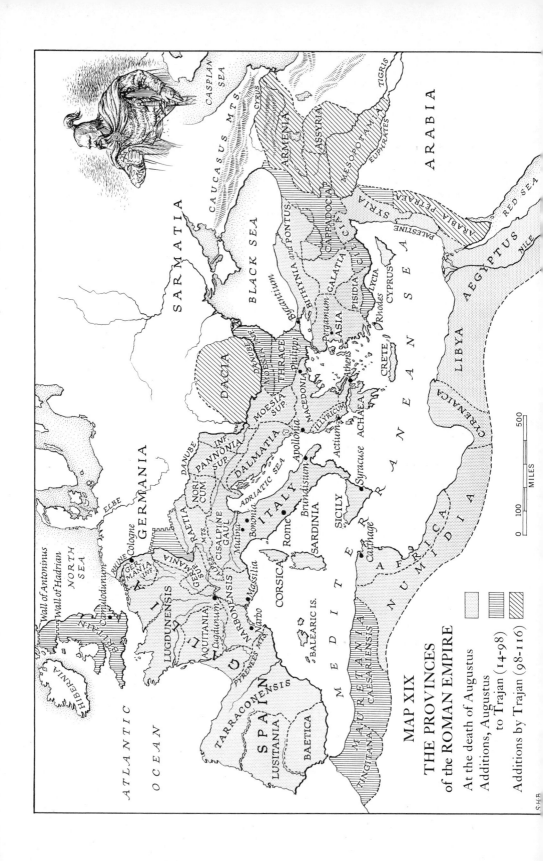

MAP XIX

THE PROVINCES
of the ROMAN EMPIRE

At the death of Augustus

Additions, Augustus
to Trajan (14-98)

Additions by Trajan (98-116)

about 200,000 people. The recipients were not completely indigent, for some had part-time work, and the charge, while necessary, was no great part of the whole budget of the Empire. Commissions, composed mainly of senators, were set up to look after the water supply, through the construction and maintenance of aqueducts and fountains, to supervise public building, and to provide protection against the periodic flooding of the Tiber. The commissioners were technical experts and liberal funds were provided by the *Princeps.*

Italy had become a nation by the time of Augustus, a fact which he had recognized and capitalized on in the struggle with Antony. All the privileges and opportunities of Roman citizenship were available to the people of the Italian towns, just as they were to the citizens who lived in Rome itself. Those Italians who met the qualifications for membership in the Senatorial and Equestrian orders could enter upon imperial careers, while the ordinary townsmen and farmers were encouraged to volunteer for service in the army, which Augustus preferred to keep largely Italian. The Italians showed little concern about voting in the Roman assemblies, which had become largely perfunctory and meaningless, but had a healthy municipal life in their own towns by which they satisfied a modest political ambition.

The institutions of the towns were increasingly patterned on those of Rome. Each had two or more magistrates and a local senate, for which a property qualification was set. While the administration and political honors of the community thus fell to the middle and upper classes, the whole community met in assembly to elect the town officials and to discuss matters of general concern. The towns were prosperous and their citizens public spirited, so that buildings and public services were well maintained. The central government in Rome, however, necessarily took measures for Italian development as a whole, and the *Princeps* paid for the construction and maintenance of roads, harbor development, and large-scale projects of land reclamation. In general, Italy continued to develop along the lines already started. Small-scale farming made some comeback as a result of Augustus' careful program of veteran settlement, but around Rome and along the west coast of Italy below the city, villas and estates multiplied. Ambitious building projects brought employment and developed a larger market for the products of Italian industry and for imported luxuries. Italian prosperity reflected the favored position of Italy as the center of the Empire.

THE ARMY AND FOREIGN POLICY

Augustus' command of the armies in the provinces along the frontiers of the Empire meant that the making of Rome's foreign policy was in his hands. In general, his aim was defensive, that is, to provide a broad territorial basis for the Empire with easily tenable frontier lines. This policy did involve considerable fighting and enlargement of territory, particularly in Europe, where he wished to expand to the Elbe and to the Danube rivers. Augustus conducted some of the wars himself, but most were entrusted to subordinates, particularly to Agrippa and to the *Princeps'* stepsons, Drusus and Tiberius. For the first time an overall plan for the defense of the Empire was worked out, and the army was converted into a regular establishment adapted to that purpose. To some Romans this seemed a denial of the aggressive wars of conquest which had characterized the Republic, but Augustus' policy was accepted by most of his successors. Claudius was to add Britain and Trajan was to thrust into Central Europe beyond the Danube, but, in the main, the Empire attained its territorial limits and was able to settle down to internal development through the work of Augustus.

After the battle of Actium, Augustus had first to demobilize both his own and Antony's huge forces. The veterans were settled in Italy on lots of land obtained by purchase, as Augustus boasted, and in colonies located mainly in Spain, Africa, and Gaul, where the soldiers were in a congenial Roman environment. Augustus' goal seems to have been an army of twenty-eight legions, which was achieved by 13 B.C. Until the reign of Septimius Severus (192–211) the legionary forces were to vary from twenty-five to thirty legions, or from 150,000 to 180,000 men. In addition to the legions there were the auxiliaries and the praetorian guard of about nine thousand men for the protection of the regime in Italy. The auxiliaries, about equal in number to the legionaries, were recruited from the most warlike of the subject peoples and were brigaded into small infantry and cavalry units, cohorts and *alae*. The auxiliaries replaced the Italian allies and provincial levies of the Republican Period. This total force of about 300,000 men, deemed sufficient by Augustus to protect the Empire, was a very large establishment by ancient standards, and the cost of their maintenance was high. To provide the money a special treasury, the *aerarium militare*, was set up and funded by the receipts from a new five percent tax on inheritances and a one percent sales tax.

The legions were a well-trained, professional force of long-service troops, loyal to the *Princeps* and commanded by able soldiers rather than political careerists. The men were recruited by voluntary enlistment from Roman citizens, at first mainly Italians, and in A.D. 6 their term of service was set at twenty years. The pay was low and the conditions of service hard, which caused some dissatisfaction, but the veterans were granted a gratuity upon discharge and were settled in veterans' colonies in the provinces where they had served. In many cases they had married native wives, although these unions between Romans and natives were illegal. Despite Augustus' wish to keep the army Italian, this proved impossible. From the outset the auxiliaries were recruited from provincials, and the non-Italian element in the legions was large and steadily increased. Most Italians, of course, wished to enjoy the benefits of peace and had all the privileges of Roman citizenship, but for the provincials the army was an avenue to citizenship and possible entry to a career in government service. The recruits for the legions were drawn mainly from the middle class of the provincial towns, and if they were not already Roman citizens on enlistment, they were made citizens after they enlisted. The auxiliary forces came from the countryside and automatically obtained their citizenship upon discharge.

While Augustus thus established a professional army, he was concerned to preserve the traditional link between civilian and military careers at the officer level. Young Equestrians usually served as commanders in the auxiliaries or as tribunes in a legion before proceeding to a career in the procuratorial service, while the junior officers of the legions were young men of the senatorial class, putting in their military service. To most officers the ultimate goal was a civilian, not a military, career. As we have noticed, Augustus brought the ex-centurions, the regular service officers, into the civilian Equestrian service. While Augustus gave long-term commands to his generals, these were men of his own choice, of whose loyalty and ability he felt sure. They remained generally loyal although the long tenure did result in a bond of attachment being formed between legionary soldiers and generals, just as it permitted the growth of an *esprit de corps* in the separate army groups. The *Princeps,* however, made special efforts to maintain his own military position to keep the loyalty of the soldiers. The men swore an oath of loyalty to him, and he made frequent tours to visit the armies and saw to it that even in time of peace there were border exercises and minor raids to keep up morale. The praetorian guard offered a special problem by its proximity to Rome and by the fact that it was the only military force in Italy. The soldiers had to be pampered because they and their prefects could exercise an undue influence on government and on the succession. Augustus' successor, Tiberius, neatly described the military position of the *Princeps* by observing that it was like holding a wolf by the ears.

Nature had provided convenient frontiers for the Empire in Africa by the Sahara Desert and in Western Europe by the Atlantic Ocean, and so needs of defense were relatively simple in those regions. In northwestern Africa Augustus annexed Numidia and recognized a *client* kingdom in Mauretania under King Juba. Control over the nomadic desert tribes was exercised by stationing a legion in the Roman province of Africa. Egypt, as in times past, remained open to the south through the Nile valley. Augustus defeated the Ethiopians, who had raided Egyptian territory, and extended the limits of the Roman province to the First Cataract. Defense against both the Ethiopians and the possible ambition of fellow Romans was ensured by a force of three legions under the Equestrian prefect. In Western Europe the northwestern area of Spain, from which the mountain tribes raided the Roman provinces, was subdued and a new province, Lusitania, organized. Augustus devoted much time and energy to Transalpine Gaul, where the former organization by tribal communities (*civitates*) was continued and the Gallic chieftains were won over to Rome. Lugdunum (Lyons) was made the center for the Gallic districts, with the frontier being fixed on the line of the Rhine River and the Alps.

The eastern frontiers of Gaul and the general continental position of Italy in Europe, however, provided Augustus and his successors with very difficult problems. The Germanic peoples, who had threatened Italy twice in the past century, had to be contained or conquered. Conquest of Germany and Central Europe, a vast territory of mountain, forest, and swamp, unurbanized and peopled by predatory tribes who shifted and fought for land and plunder, was an immense and endless task. Ultimately Augustus had to settle on a defense system based on the Rhine and the Danube rivers and to leave an awkward gap between the two.

The Alpine region north of Italy, whose peoples raided into the fertile land of Cisalpine Gaul and controlled the high passes into eastern Gaul and Switzerland, was occupied in hard fighting. Then Augustus established a broad belt of Roman territory between the head of the Adriatic Sea and Macedonia up to the Danube River. While he himself did not complete the organization of the whole area, new provinces, Raetia and Noricum, were established on the upper Danube and Pannonia and Moesia in the central portion along the south bank of the river. Between Macedonia and the Danube the *client* kingdom of Thrace was recognized under a king, Cotys. These acquisitions protected Italy and allowed the development of land communication from the Adriatic to Asia Minor, but the new provinces in their turn were exposed to the peoples of Germany and of Central Europe north of the Danube.

Augustus attempted to remedy the situation by conquest of Germany as far east as the Elbe River. His first thrust was successful, but in A.D. 9 the Germans revolted under their king, Arminius, and wiped out a Roman army of three legions under Varus in the Teutoberg Forest. This first great battle of German national history rolled the Romans back to the Rhine. Augustus decided that the price of conquering Germany was too high and, instead, protected the Rhine frontier by holding a narrow belt of land on the German side. Threat of barbarian raids, however, necessitated the construction of fortified bases and posting the bulk of the Roman armies on the Rhine and the Danube. Under Tiberius fifteen legions were stationed on the two frontiers, along with most of the auxiliaries.

In the East Augustus chose to follow the general lines of organization which Pompey had marked out and did not emulate the plans of conquest which Crassus, Caesar, and Antony had entertained. The Roman frontier ran along the line of the Euphrates River and the Arabian Desert, and concerning this area Augustus conducted relations with Parthia by diplomacy, not war. In inner Asia Minor, Galatia was made into a province, while Cappadocia was recognized as a *client* kingdom and Armenia as a buffer state between the Empire and Parthia. As such, Armenia became a field for diplomatic struggle, in whose internal life both Rome and Parthia interfered, with the advantage oscillating from one to the other.

Augustus correctly judged that the Parthian Kingdom was not a serious threat to the Roman provinces of the East. Like the Persian and the Seleucid empires of the past, Parthia was torn by dynastic rivalry for the throne and by the rise of minor princes to temporary independence. Concerted use of its great manpower was almost impossible in these circumstances, and, while Parthia might raid occasionally and interfere in Armenia, its general role during the Principate was that of an intermediary for the luxury goods of the East.

The caravan trade flourished, and centers like Palmyra and Damascus began to rise to importance. Augustus judged that Syria could be protected by an army of five or six legions, less than half the force which was needed for Europe. He did make an attack against the Nabataeans in Arabia, presumably to gain control of the important caravan route along its west coast, but the invasion failed, and therefore Egypt and Syria remained the chief centers for the Eastern trade.

The Mediterranean Sea became a Roman lake after the provinces which bordered it were restored to peace, and naval defense on a large scale was not a matter of concern. Fleet bases, however, were developed at Misenum and Ravenna in Italy, and flotillas were posted at Alexandria and other strategic harbors. Augustus' generals also made effective use of a fleet along the coast of the North Sea and the Baltic in their operations against the Germans. River patrols on the Rhine and Danube too were a regular part of the system of defense. The Romans, however, preferred land to sea communications, and the "life lines" of the Empire were the road systems, not the seaways.

Romanitas

SOCIAL AND RELIGIOUS REFORM

The desire for peace and stability felt by all classes of Roman society, which had resulted in the acceptance of Augustus' political organization, was conducive also to his social and religious reforms. In the Late Republic there had been a breakdown of tradition. Individuals had turned to scepticism, to Greek philosophy or, like Cicero, to an idealized Roman past. In society among many signs of breakdown the most significant were the disintegration of the family, particularly among the upper class, and personal irresponsibility, which ranged from the irresponsible pursuit of material wealth and pleasure to ambitious career building, where law and constitutionality were flouted. The formal religious life of Rome, the political value of which had been recognized by Polybius and Cicero, whatever their personal beliefs, had fallen into neglect. A reform of society, which could provide new values and restore personal responsibility, was needed to breathe life into Augustus' political reorganization.

While moral reform by legislation and governmental propaganda might seem futile, Augustus was able to achieve a very great deal in this respect. His program was designed to recreate a society imbued with Roman ideals and traditions and to make Roman Italy a solid core for the Empire. He did not aim at the Romanization of its peoples, yet the regeneration which he sponsored became a preliminary to that. The name, Rome, grew into a concept, which we might call *Romanitas,* the summing up of Rome's function in history as a political and moral force. This achievement resulted partly from the deliberate policy of Augustus, partly from the spontaneous expression of writers, artists, and their patrons, but above all it was made a reality by the genuine enthusiasm for the new order in society as a whole.

The reformation of the Senatorial and Equestrian orders formed a large part, of course, of Augustus' plans for reforming society, but it affected only the upper and middle classes. The ordinary people of Italy were thoroughly Italian in tradition, but Augustus felt that the new Roman citizens of slave origin were too alien and too great in number to be readily assimilated. Throughout the first century B.C. thousands had been set free by their owners. The latter were motivated frequently by vanity, to show how many slaves they possessed, rather than by humanitarian considerations, and the processes of emancipation were easy.

To protect the Roman traditions from too much dilution, Augustus set a series of legal brakes to slow down the making of citizens from slaves. A half-way stage to full citizenship was set by the Junian Law. Those slaves freed by informal manumission, a process which merely required written or oral notification to the slave before witnesses, were classed as Junian Latins. These men were restricted in their property rights by a prohibition on receiving inheritances and by reversion of their property to their patrons. The children of Junian Latins, however, automatically became full citizens. Other legislation regulated the number of slaves who might be freed by the owner's will and checked the freeing of slaves by owners still in their minority.

Considerable legislation was passed to safeguard the family. Adultery was made a criminal offense. Inheritance laws were tightened up to prevent property from going outside the family circle when heirs existed because legacy hunting, by flattery and obsequious attendance, had been widespread among the wealthy. Premiums were placed on marriage and the birth of children in wedlock. For example, age limits for political office were lowered in accordance with the number of children which a candidate possessed, and, in the case of an equal vote, the father with the larger number of children was declared the winner. Sumptuary legislation was also tried to regulate expenditures on funerals and other social occasions. All this provoked many witty remarks, as such legislation does, and it is difficult to estimate the efficiency of the laws. There was improvement, but that was to be expected with the betterment of social conditions and with

Scene from the Altar of Peace (Ara Pacis) *of Augustus, dedicated in 9 B.C. to symbolize the general peace of the Augustan era. Priests and members of the imperial family in procession*

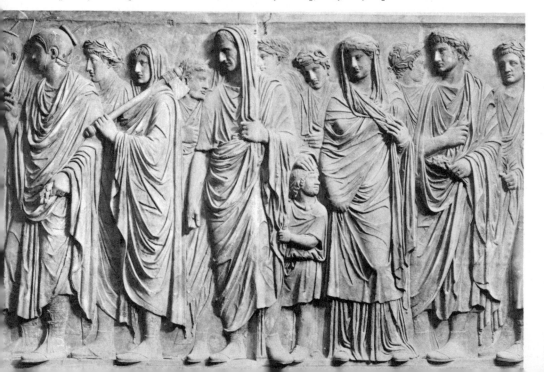

public knowledge of the *Princeps'* views and of the example which he himself set. The court of Augustus was a relatively simple one in which hard work and efficiency brought notice. His own daughter Julia was banished from Rome because of her notoriously dissolute and extravagant behavior. Those men who wished advancement in their careers did well to become at least public models of propriety.

After 12 B.C. Augustus as *Pontifex Maximus* could proceed directly and officially with the reform of public religion to make it once again a meaningful part of the political life of the state. These reforms can be dismissed too easily as purely formal and political in intention, for belief in the old gods of Rome could not be legislated. Yet religious reform was intimately associated with the genuine feeling of nostalgic pride in the gods under whose auspices Rome had risen to empire. The pomp and circumstance of the state religion once again became impressive in itself. More than eighty temples and shrines were built, repaired, or enlarged in the city of Rome, including the great temples of Jupiter Capitolinus and of Quirinus, the deified Romulus, who had founded Rome. Particular attention was paid to the gods connected with the Julian family, into which Augustus had been adopted, Venus, Mars, and Apollo. The old priestly colleges were reorganized and given fresh dignity when Augustus and members of his family served as priests in them. Old cults, which had originated in the days of the kings and of the Early Republic, were revived and liberally endowed, while new foreign worships, such as that of Isis from Egypt, were officially prohibited in the city. In short, the formal religion of Rome became an integral part of both the political and conceptual character of the new order which Augustus was creating.

Augustus himself, while he was not worshipped as a living god, became intimately entwined in religious practice and tradition. Roman writers, particularly Vergil, emphasized the legendary connection of the Julian family to Venus by descent from Aeneas, while Horace, perhaps as a literary conceit, referred to Augustus as the incarnation of Mercury. More significantly, Augustus himself was associated with religious practices in which the people of Rome participated. When the city was divided into wards, an old custom of worshipping the Lares of the crossroads, who protected wayfarers, was revived. Altars were erected by the roadside, and the people of each ward were represented by their mayor in the administration of the worship. Augustus' Genius, his "double," was linked in prayer with the Lares, so that he became a protector of the ordinary freedmen and slaves who worshipped at the shrine. In the latter part of Augustus' reign the practice of worshipping his Genius, along with the major gods, began to spread to the Italian towns. A board of priests, the *Seviri Augustales,* was elected to look after the worship. Upon posthumous deification, of course, Augustus joined Julius Caesar and the great gods of Rome and was worshipped by a state cult and a special priesthood.

LITERATURE AND ART

The conception of Rome as a proud imperial state whose citizens were destined by fate to rule the world through their qualities of courage, justice, and duty, is due mainly to the major writers of the Augustan Period—the Golden Age of Latin literature. Most of them had grown to manhood in the closing years of the Republic, and some had suffered indirectly from the acts of the Second Triumvirate. Nevertheless, they were genuinely responsive to Augustus' policies, although some regret was felt for the freer political life of the Republic. As a group, with the notable exception of the poet Ovid, the Augustans expressed the social ideals for which Augustus worked. At the same time they were men of genius, who wrote with a full mastery of style and material at a time when the Latin language had come to maturity. The Augustan Age was Rome's counterpart to the Classical Period of Greek literature.

Vergil (70–19 B.C.) was the most important Augustan writer. He came from Mantua in northern Italy, where his family's land had been confiscated by the Second Triumvirate, and found a patron first in Asinius Pollio, a good Republican, and then in Maecenas, the aide of Augustus. Vergil's first work of importance, the *Eclogues,* was a set of ten pastoral idylls in the Hellenistic manner of Theocritus, but thoroughly Italian in feeling. In the fourth eclogue he heralded the dawn of a new era through the birth of a child, probably the son of his patron Pollio, but in a later age Christians suggested that Vergil had prophesied the birth of Christ. This skill in pastoral poetry perhaps prompted Maecenas to suggest to Vergil the theme of the *Georgics,* modeled on the *Works and Days* of the Greek writer Hesiod, but aptly called a hymn of praise to Italy. Vergil's laudation of the Italian farmer coincided with the settlement of veterans by Augustus, but the poem is free from any overt propaganda.

The *Aeneid,* too, was in accord with Augustus' policy, but in its universal humanity it has passed far beyond idealization of Rome's history and as an epic has become a part of the great literature of the world. It tells the story of Aeneas, the Trojan prince, who left Troy with his infant son and aged father to make an odyssey to Italy. Aeneas was prompted by fate and by his own *pietas* to leave the Phoenician queen, Dido, despite her offer of marriage and the throne of Carthage, for the higher destiny of establishing his line in Italy. Aeneas' vision of the future greatness of Rome, pictured in Book Six, and of the glorious destiny which awaited his progeny, encouraged him to fight for a place in Italy. On his deathbed Vergil is said to have asked that the unfinished *Aeneid* be burnt. The request was refused, and the poem became the national epic of Rome and the most widely read work of Latin literature to the present day.

Horace (65–8 B.C.) was also a protégé of Maecenas, to whom he was introduced by Vergil, when the latter saw the promise of the early *Satires.* Horace fought for the Republic at Philippi and later found work in Rome, where he

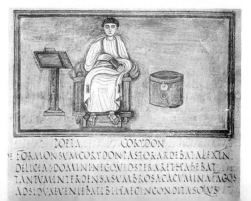

Vergil. Latin manuscript illumination

lived in poverty until Maecenas provided encouragment and a better living. Eventually Maecenas gave Horace a villa in the Sabine Hills, where the poet spent much of his time and wrote the *Odes,* the four books of lyric poetry for which he is best known. These were skillful adaptations of Greek lyric metres to Latin verse and on a variety of subjects, from love and friendship to politics. The Roman odes, as the first six poems of Book Three are sometimes called, were concerned with the traditional Roman virtues, courage, justice, and *pietas,* which had made Rome great. After the death of Vergil, Horace, who virtually became the poet laureate of Augustus, wrote the *Carmen Saeculare,* a hymn sung by a choir of boys and girls at the festival of the Saeculum in 17 B.C., which symbolized the opening of a new era. The mellow geniality and urbanity of Horace's poetry reveal a quality of Roman life, its mature, civilized character, which is too easy to ignore in the period of war and politics.

The other poetry of the Augustan Period was of a different order from that of Vergil and Horace. Propertius (47-15 B.C.) and Tibullus (55-19 B.C.), who wrote love elegies, showed some feeling for Roman tradition and love of the Italian countryside, but their work was too sophisticated in artistry and too slight in subject matter to have a general appeal. Ovid (43 B.C.–A.D. 18) mirrored the tastes of high society in Rome and wrote light, facile poetry for entertainment. His *Metamorphoses,* a sort of mythological epic, is one of the most popular works of Latin literature because of its vividly told stories from the cycle of Greek myth. His *Art of Love* and *Remedy of Love,* both light and immoral in tone, apparently were very popular. Ovid exemplified the type of life and interest which Augustus was trying to curb, and in A.D. 8 the *Princeps* found an excuse to send him into exile to Tomi in the Black Sea. He died there

From Augustus' Altar of Peace. Italy or Mother Earth, in the center, presides over the fruits of the earth, air (left) and water (right).

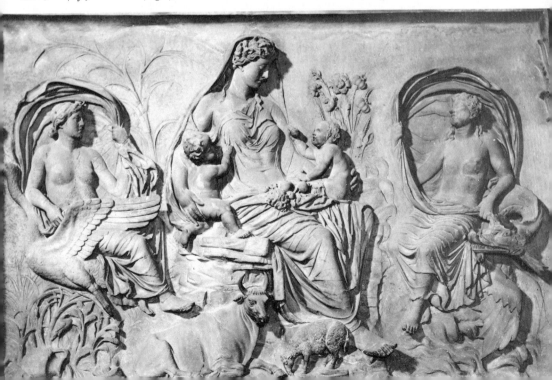

in A.D. 18, writing copious laments on his hard life at the other end of the world from Rome.

Livy (59 B.C.–A.D. 17), who came from Patavium (Padua) in northern Italy, was the most important prose writer of the period. His *History of Rome* from the origins to 9 B.C. became the standard history of the Republic, replacing the earlier works of the Annalists. The history was very lengthy, consisting of 145 books, of which Books I–X, covering the period to 293 B.C., and Books XXI–XLV, which described the Second Punic War and the eastern conquests to 167 B.C., still survive. An epitome of the remainder helps to make some of the missing material available. Livy's history was an editorial rewriting of his source material in a dramatic and colorful style rather than a critical and original account. He was aware of the difficulties of writing a history of early Rome and wisely did not try to sift the legends because only partial truths would have emerged. Instead, his work has the importance of representing the national myth of the Roman Republic, which was of more importance to Augustan Rome and to the Empire than the historical truth.

Art, like literature, was given a new purpose in the Augustan Age when it came under the patronage of the *Princeps*. Artists, of course, continued to serve private patrons and individual interests, but the rulers wanted, in addition, to popularize their programs and the majesty of Rome in another medium. Accordingly Augustus sponsored great building projects. Architects and sculptors represented the significance of Roman history and the achievements of the *Princeps* in symbolic form. As in literature, Greek influence was strong and, significantly enough, the dignified idealism of fifth-century Greek art was revived in portrait sculpture to represent the new *Princeps* and his family.

One of the best-known statues of Augustus, the statue found in the villa of his wife Livia at Prima Porta, depicted the ruler in his military aspect. The *Princeps* was represented as the *Imperator*, clad in armor and with hand outstretched, like that of an orator, to address his troops. The richly decorated body armor was highly symbolic. On Augustus' shoulder was the Sphinx, his personal seal. In the center the Parthian standards were shown, lost by Crassus and recovered by Augustus in negotiation with the king of Parthia. The sun represented the new day which had dawned for Rome. Even the dolphin, by which the statue was supported, hinted at the connection of the Julian family with Venus, born from the sea. The portrait busts of Livia pictured the empress with a cold severe dignity. Like Augustus himself, the family of the *Princeps* was removed from ordinary men, and a new image of imperial dignity was created by displaying their portrait statues in "authorized" types throughout Rome and the important cities of the Empire.

The most significant monument of the new regime was the Altar of Peace, dedicated in 9 B.C. to mark the general pacification of the Roman world. The altar was set in the center of an open enclosure, whose walls were covered with a relief, reminiscent of that which encircled the colonnade of the Parthenon in Athens. A procession moved in two parts, one representing the *Princeps* and his

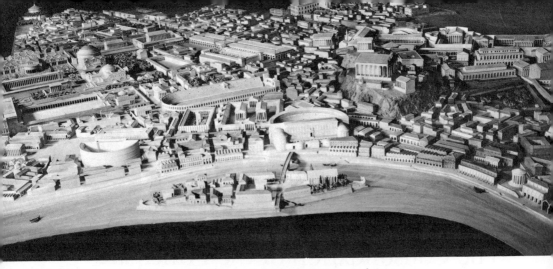

Imperial Rome. The city which started to come into being in the Principate of Augustus

family, and the other the Senate and People of Rome. On the door of the enclosure were symbolic representations of the universe, of Italy with its fruits and grain, of the air, and the sea. The historical pageant symbolized the history of Rome as culminating in Augustus. The figures were dignified and relaxed, conscious of their high place in the world, and fully assured that they and Rome would continue.

Augustus, too, provided for the perpetuation of himself and his family in majesty after death by the construction of a huge mausoleum, which was begun as early as 28 B.C. It was constructed outside the *pomoerium,* the sacred boundary of the city, in the Field of Mars. The mausoleum was built in the moundlike form of the old Etruscan *tumuli* at Tarquinii and consisted of a great drum of concrete, 290 feet in diameter and 143 feet in height, with four tiers of corridors and rooms around a central chamber destined for the body of the *Princeps.* The whole structure was covered with earth and planted with cypress trees, and at the entrance, engraved on bronze plates, was the *Res Gestae,* or autobiography of Augustus.

Augustus also began the architectural transformation of Rome into an imperial capital by large-scale building projects throughout the city. The old Roman Forum was regularized into a roughly triangular shape and adorned by new buildings, among them the temple to Julius Caesar, the rebuilt Aemilian Basilica, a new Senate House, the Curia, and a house for Vesta and her attendant Vestal Virgins. Augustus also constructed a new forum of his own, typical in plan of the Imperial Fora, as they are called (pp. 649–50) and designed to serve as a hall of fame for the Julian family. At its end stood a temple of Mars Ultor, the Avenger, who had brought victory to Augustus. Elsewhere in Rome colonnades, libraries, a theater, and numerous other monuments were erected. The victory at Actium was fittingly commemorated by the construction of an arch, on which were engraved lists of the consuls and of the generals who had won triumphs since the founding of the Republic. The concept of Eternal Rome had emerged showing its link to the legendary past and its promise of a new era.

XXVI

The Consolidation of the Principate

(A.D. 14–96)

DURING THE FIRST CENTURY after Christ the Principate continued to develop along the lines marked out by Augustus although the ruling family which he established, the Julio-Claudians, collapsed in 68, when Nero committed suicide. Nero lost the support of the generals of the army, and upon his death a competition for the Principate resulted among them. The winner was Vespasian, who became *Princeps* in 69 and established the Flavian dynasty. Its last representative, Domitian, was murdered in 96 by a palace conspiracy. Although Vespasian had gained power by military support, he retained the civilian character, rooted in law, which Augustus had given to the Principate, and returned the armies to their function of frontier defense. Throughout the whole period the power of the *Princeps* and of his imperial administration grew steadily at the expense of the Senate. Yet each emperor—Gaius, Nero, and Domitian—who showed a tendency to autocracy and a desire to convert his office into a monarchy of the Hellenistic type, was removed.

There was little real sentiment for a return to the Republic, and the governing classes in general felt that the Augustan form of the Principate should be preserved. Yet opposition to autocracy, based on Stoic philosophical theory, crystallized among some members of the senatorial class. The philosophers condemned the autocratic rulers as tyrants, exalted Marcus Brutus and Cato as martyrs, and recognized the cause of tyranny in the practice of hereditary succession. But after the death of Domitian, the philosophers were able to find a compromise for their views in the circumstances of the succession. None of the "good" emperors of the second century, except Marcus Aurelius (161–80), had a son of his own. Each theoretically chose the best man in the state as a successor, adopted him as a son, and invested him with the essential powers of

The reader will find the Back Endpaper and Maps XVIII and XIX (pages 544 and 576) useful as he reads this chapter.

office. This reasoned choice of a successor seemed to the philosophers to convert the Principate from a potential tyranny into a benevolent kingship.

Throughout the first century the people of Italy retained that primacy in the Empire which Augustus had won for them, but as the provinces gained ground in the general condition of peace and order, Italy began to recede in importance. Men from the provinces, particularly from the more Romanized Western part of the Empire, played a larger part in government. Some became senators, many entered the imperial service, and the army was recruited to an increasing degree from the provinces. In general, the emperors paid more attention to administration and to internal development, following the lead of Augustus, than to territorial expansion. The only notable addition to the territory of the Empire was that of Britain by Claudius. On the whole the people of the Empire accepted Roman rule enthusiastically, and Romanization and urban growth were rapid. There were minor revolts among the people newly brought under Roman authority, and the Romans found the Jews particularly troublesome. They ultimately removed the problem of Jewish religious nationalism by force, rather than trying to solve it. Yet the achievement of the Empire was apparent in the civilizing of Europe and in the development of a government satisfactory and helpful to the people of the provinces.

Nevertheless, the rulers of Rome in the first century were given an almost uniformly black reputation in Roman historical tradition. The historian Tacitus (pp. 656-58) and the biographer Suetonius, in his *Lives of the Twelve Caesars*, focused their interest on the *Princeps* in Rome and on his relations with the Senate and with his own palace circle of family and advisers. They tended to ignore, or take for granted, the larger picture of the Empire. Tiberius (14-37) was pictured as a cruel hypocrite, Gaius (37-41) as a lunatic, and Claudius (41-54) as a fool under the thumb of his palace freedmen and wives. Nero (54-68) was granted an initial good period of five years while he was advised by the Stoic philosopher Seneca, but thereafter he was shown as an extravagant, pleasure-seeking tyrant. The first Flavian emperors, Vespasian (69-79) and Titus (79-81), fared considerably better, but Domitian (81-96) was described as cruel and bloodthirsty, purging the Senate of its best men in a Reign of Terror. Despite the alleged succession of villains, fools, and despots, the whole Empire grew markedly in material wealth and population, while thousands of inscriptions from the provinces recorded the gratitude and loyalty of their people to the emperors.

In contrast to the Roman writers, modern historians of Rome emphasize that the significant history of the Empire lies in the growth of the provinces and in the concept of Empire, not in the court and the city of Rome. The distortion and bias in the accounts of the Roman historians are explained by the writers' sympathy and connections with the senatorial class in Rome, whose conflict with the *Princeps* was almost implicit in the system of divided government. Augustus had put an end to the free political life of the old governing class of the Republic, that is, he destroyed "Liberty," as its proponents charged. This fact became starkly clear in the reigns of his successors when the *Princeps* became more and more the center of government. Also, despite Augustus' insistence on Italian primacy, the restoration of peace automatically involved a gradual shift in gravity from Italy to the provinces, as their resources in wealth and population were developed. But the traditions of the senatorial class of the Republic persisted for a century in upper-class society. Until that society itself was transformed in the second century after Christ, these traditions made the position of some members of this group very painful.

The Julio-Claudian Rulers (A.D. 14–68)

TIBERIUS (14–37)

In the course of his own long reign, Augustus had outlived most of the members of his family who might have succeeded him, and only in the later years of his rule had he settled on his stepson Tiberius as a belated, last choice. Augustus' attempts to arrange the succession left a legacy of dissension in the family, of which Tiberius reaped the harvest. Augustus himself had no sons and only one daughter, Julia, despite three marriages. His third wife, Livia, had brought him two sons, Tiberius and Drusus, by her former husband, a member of the patrician Claudian house, thus combining the Julian and Claudian families. While Augustus used his stepsons in imperial service, he attempted to secure the succession in his own family line by using Julia as a pawn in dynastic marriages.

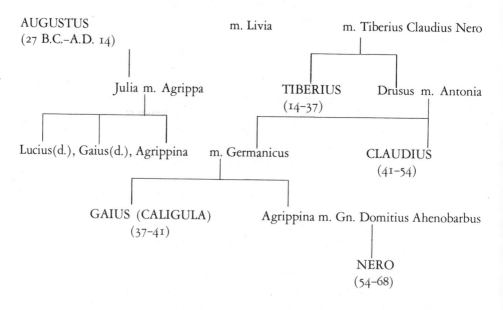

THE JULIO-CLAUDIAN EMPERORS

First, in 25 B.C., Augustus married Julia to his nephew Marcellus, who died two years later. While this marriage proved childless, Julia did have two sons, Lucius and Gaius Caesar, by Agrippa, Augustus' chief aide on whom she was bestowed in 21 B.C. Agrippa himself died in 12 B.C. Soon afterwards Julia was married to Tiberius, which may have raised his hopes of the succession, although the marriage was reportedly much against Tiberius' will. Augustus continued to use Tiberius in his service. His chances for the Principate appeared even brighter in 9 B.C. upon the death of his brother Drusus, who was killed by a fall from his horse. However, Augustus spoiled the prospect by cultivation of the young Lucius and Gaius. Finally, in 6 B.C., Tiberius withdrew to private life on the island of Rhodes without consulting Augustus. Perhaps he did so because Julia's notorious marital indiscretions were still unofficially unknown, or perhaps because of the favoritism shown to Lucius and Gaius. Their deaths in A.D. 2 and 4, however, left Tiberius the only mature man of ability and experience in the family. The breach between Tiberius and Augustus had to be mended. The Empress Livia used her influence with each, and in A.D. 4 Tiberius was brought out of retirement and associated in active rule with Augustus.

Despite Tiberius' obvious ability and good record, he had certain difficulties of temperament which may have influenced Augustus to pass him over previously. He was austere and aloof, terse and brusque in speech, and without Augustus' tact in personal relations. Nevertheless, Tiberius served Augustus faithfully and even accepted the additional slight of being required to accept his nephew Germanicus as a potential successor, rather than his own son, the younger Drusus. Inasmuch as Germanicus had married Julia's daughter Agrippina, Augustus probably hoped to combine both branches of the family by this maneuver. In 14, when Augustus died, Tiberius seems to have been genuinely reluctant to accept the full responsibility of the Principate and made a futile effort to get the Senate to accept a larger share. He came to office at the age of fifty-six, embittered by his unhappy private life and the public knowledge that he and his own family were Augustus' last choice. Germanicus and his ambitious wife Agrippina seem to have been waiting for the day when Tiberius would step aside.

At the outset of the reign, Tiberius was faced with mutinies in the army on the Rhine, which was under Germanicus' command, and among the troops of Illyricum, which were under his own son Drusus. The soldiers were not hostile to the Principate or to Tiberius, but judged that the beginning of a new reign was an appropriate occasion to remedy their grievances. Many had been kept in service beyond their proper time of discharge, and there was general resentment at the low pay and at the hard conditions of service on the frontiers. Germanicus, who was concerned to remain personally popular and who made hasty and unnecessary concessions to bring his troops into line, was unwilling to take the responsibility for punishment of the ringleaders. On the other hand, Drusus settled the Illyrian mutiny firmly with regard to the needs of discipline and to the legitimate grievances of the soldiers. Tiberius, however, remained loyal to Augustus' arrangements and continued to promote the career of Germanicus.

Germanicus, spurred by the driving ambition of his wife for her husband and children, sought the limelight and began to act independently. His infant son Gaius received the nickname of Caligula (Little Boots) in the camps of the Rhineland, where Agrippina dressed the child in a legionary uniform complete with military boots to cultivate popularity among the soldiers. In 14, after the suppression of the mutiny, Germanicus embarked on the conquest of Germany without asking permission from Tiberius. In several campaigns he penetrated deeply, damaged farms and villages, but incurred heavy losses and did not hold the territory. Tiberius called off the invasion two years later as too costly and mollified Germanicus' feelings by a triumph and the assignment of an overall command in the East to settle the affairs of Armenia in the interest of Rome. Tiberius judged the time proper for reorganization in Gaul and established three provinces corresponding to the natural divisions of the land, Aquitania, Lugdunensis, and Belgica, while along the Rhine new provinces of Upper and Lower Germany were organized.

In the East Germanicus settled the Armenian kingship to Roman satisfaction, but regarded his tour of duty as an opportunity to impress the provincial peoples. He paid a visit to Egypt, again without permission from Tiberius, and interfered in the prefect's administration by making a distribution of grain in Alexandria. In Syria he quarreled with the governor, Piso, who resented Germanicus' intrusion into his own province. When Germanicus suddenly died in 18, Piso was accused of poisoning him and was recalled to Rome for trial. Before the case was properly aired, Piso committed suicide and thus gave some color of veracity to the charge of Agrippina that Tiberius had been ultimately responsible for Germanicus' death. In disappointment and anger at the check to her ambitions, she began to intrigue to get the Principate for her children.

Tiberius' son, Drusus, became the apparent successor and was promoted by his father until he, too, suddenly died in 23. Tiberius, without a congenial helper and disturbed at the plotting of Agrippina, began to use Sejanus, the prefect of the praetorian guard, as an aide and in 26 left Rome for the seclusion of his villa on the island of Capri. Popular imagination, fed by the gossip of Tiberius' enemies, pictured this retreat as the scene of unnatural orgies, but withdrawal from the uncongenial society of Rome and a hostile family circle at the age of sixty-eight seems quite understandable. Unfortunately Tiberius' absence from Rome made him lean more heavily on Sejanus, whom he used as a go-between to the Senate. This action alienated the older members of that body who were initially favorable to Tiberius but gained Sejanus some following among the younger men who wished to promote their careers. Sejanus himself seems to have succeeded in having Agrippina and her two older children arrested and exiled.

In 31, however, Sejanus was tripped up. He was in a very powerful position since he was consul with Tiberius, the holder of a proconsular command, and engaged to marry Tiberius' granddaughter. Officially Tiberius accused Sejanus of conspiracy to make himself *Princeps,* but the latter might reasonably expect that or at least the regency of Tiberius' grandson upon the emperor's death. The reasons for Tiberius' action are obscure, but if the story that Tiberius' sister-in-law provided him with proof that Sejanus had seduced the younger Drusus' wife and poisoned Drusus was correct, Tiberius had reason enough. The emperor acted decisively to secure Sejanus' condemnation and to investigate the ramifications of the alleged conspiracy.

At least until his withdrawal to Capri, Tiberius had made a serious personal effort to make the Senate a responsible partner in government. He worked closely with it as Augustus had done, and much of the legislation during his reign took the form of resolutions of the Senate. Its functions were increased by the transference of elections from the assembly and by the enlargement of its duties as a court to hear cases of extortion and treason. Hearing such cases was by no means congenial to most of the senators because they had to deal with cases which involved their own colleagues, members of the *Princeps'* family, and close associates. In general, the senators declined to accept all of their responsibility where the *Princeps* was concerned and lost the opportunity to acquire the greater power in government which Tiberius seems to have sincerely offered.

Tiberius' own personality was partly to blame for this. He perhaps had trouble in arriving at a clear decision in his own mind and certainly was diffident about expressing his opinion. Instead of using the cabinet for liaison as Augustus had done to give a tactful lead, Tiberius had an uncomfortable habit of remaining noncommittal in the Senate too long and then coming to the point. Feelings were hurt, and there were many awkward moments. When he moved to Capri and directed by remote control, by letters, or through Sejanus, the dependency of the Senate was clearly exposed, and humiliation was added to incomprehension. Nevertheless, Tiberius did win the general cooperation of his contemporaries, the older members of the Senate, some of whom were from ancient Republican families like his own. He promoted them to high offices and to the important commands. It is also noteworthy that his reign was not marked by the defection of the generals or by disturbances in the army after the initial mutinies. These older men, however, were alienated by the favor shown Sejanus, whose downfall came too late to remedy the situation. The reign closed in 37 in an atmosphere heavy with suspicion and fear, caused by the activity of informers laying their charges of treason. Tiberius made no proper provision for a successor. His personal heirs were the youngest son of Germanicus, Gaius, who had received little training for public office, and Tiberius' own grandson, Tiberius Gemellus, who was still a child.

Tiberius' administration had been carefully conservative and sound, following the precedents of Augustus closely. The provinces were well governed and the frontiers were successfully guarded. Tiberius, too, was frugal and personally disinclined to indulge the people in Rome with spectacles and frequent appearances in public. He left a surplus in the treasury, but died feared by the Senate and unpopular with the people of Rome.

GAIUS (37–41)

After Tiberius' death the Senate, able to administer a posthumous rebuke, denied him deification and made Germanicus' son, Gaius, *Princeps* at the age of twenty-five. Within a short time the senators discovered that they had acquired a ruler who wished to reign autocratically and to be worshipped as a living god. At first Gaius made a good impression by pardoning political offenders of the previous regime and by spending lavishly—he seems to have run through Tiberius' surplus within a year. Then he removed his cousin, Tiberius Gemellus, to whom he had shown favor at first, and became arrogant and insulting toward the Senate. Demands for the deification of his sister and of himself were pressed. Construction of a temple for his own worship, combined with that of Jupiter, was authorized but the projected worship had not started before his assassination. Gaius also made grandiose plans for invasions of Germany and of Britain, but these ended with military exercises on the Rhine and on the Gallic side of the English Channel. More practically he annexed Mauretania to restore his finances with the treasury of its king and then turned to increased taxation and to the prosecution of conspirators, by which he might confiscate his victims' property. In 41 Gaius, his wife and infant daughter were put to death by a small group of senators and officers of the praetorian guard who had been insulted by Gaius and who feared for their own lives.

The charitable verdict of Roman tradition, that of the senatorial class, was that Gaius was a lunatic. His overindulgence had brought on a serious illness which perhaps resulted in mental derangement, but Gaius may have looked at the Principate from the Greek rather than the Roman point of view and over-estimated his power in his efforts to change the character of that office. He had been brought up in the household of his great-aunt Antonia, Mark Antony's daughter, where he met many Easterners and made a friend of Herod, the *client* king of Judaea. Before becoming *Princeps* his only experience with Roman political life had been a single term as quaestor and an honorary priesthood.

CLAUDIUS (41–54)

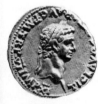

A coin portrait of Claudius

The behavior of Gaius had been a shock to the practice of hereditary succession in the Julio-Claudian family, and for a brief time after his death the Senate talked of restoring the Republic. In a sense the situation was not unfavorable. The only males of the Julio-Claudian line were Claudius, a younger brother of Germanicus who was now over fifty years of age, and the future emperor Nero, aged four. Claudius had been ignored by Augustus and Tiberius, for he appeared to be a bumbling, scholarly pedant, content with the leisure to write a history of the Etruscans. The Senate debated the restoration of the Republic, with appropriate references to tyranny and freedom and the assassination of Julius Caesar, but it soon became apparent that the chief advocates of freedom among the senators were those who wanted to become *Princeps*. The praetorian guard, on the other hand, acted as well as talked. The soldiers are reported to have discussed the political situation in a meeting in which they concluded that a re-stored Republic would be incapable of rule, and, if it were restored, they would be out of work. Accordingly, they decided that the choice of a new *Princeps* was theirs. The guards sought out Claudius and presented him to the Senate as their choice. Neither Claudius nor the Senate was in a position to refuse, and the will of the guard was duly approved. The guards were rewarded with a generous donation and the Senate was presented with an unexpectedly competent and firm-minded ruler.

Despite Claudius' lack of practical experience in government, he had read widely in the history of the Republic and had absorbed some of its traditions. He respected the dignity of the Senate and encouraged the members to debate and to criticize his proposals. Claudius also understood that Rome had grown not only by military conquest but by the political flexibility which had extended citizenship to Latium and ultimately to all of Italy. His own reign marked the first important break in the practice of Italian primacy in the Empire. Unfor-tunately the Senate's own views did not match the breadth of Claudius' idea that provincials should be brought into government. They opposed him in a pro-posal which he made as censor in 47 to enroll some prominent Gallic nobles into the Senate. Claudius, however, had his way. Some were enrolled in the Senate, while the Roman magistracies were made available to Roman citizens of Gaul. In addition, Claudius promoted a vigorous policy of Romanization by extending citizenship to provincials, using them in the imperial service, found-ing colonies, and improving the status of provincial cities (p. 610). His grants of citizenship probably accounted in considerable degree for the increase in the number of Roman citizens recorded by the census of 48. The total was 6,994,000, up about one million from the end of Augustus' reign.

While the members of the Senate were encouraged to show initiative, Claudius also enlarged the *Princeps'* administration by the establishment of some-thing like regular departments of state. These had been shaped to some extent by Augustus' and Tiberius' use of household freedmen, but Claudius created regular bureaus for the secretarial and financial services: a secretariat to deal with correspondence (*ab epistulis*), an office to handle petitions (*a libellis*), a bureau of the treasury (*a rationibus*), and an office for judicial records (*a cogni-tionibus*). The freedmen who headed them were in close contact with the em-peror, and several came to exert considerable personal influence on Claudius. These appointments provoked acrid criticism from the senatorial class in Rome, who resented the inclusion of Greeks in important offices. They resented, too, Claudius' conversion of several technical senatorial commissions—those in charge of roads, the water supply, and harbor development at Ostia—into pro-curatorial services directly responsible to the *Princeps*.

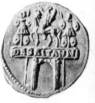

Reverse of the coin shown on page 594

Rather surprisingly Claudius showed that he was aware of the military as-pect of the *Princeps* and of the possible disgruntlement of the legions at his liberality to the praetorian guard. He cultivated the goodwill of the soldiers by frequent visits and by taking a personal part in the closing phases of the invasion of Britain. This project could be justified by the fact that a free Britain stirred unrest among the Celts of Gaul, but its chief attractions were probably an exaggerated idea of the mineral resources of the island and Claudius' need to strengthen the army's loyalty. In 43 his armies crossed the Thames and brought the southeastern part of England under Roman control. The town of Camulodunum (Colchester) was made the capital, and a ruler cult was established there to focus the loyalty of the Britons on Rome. Claudius' generals extended Roman authority to the Humber River on the north and into southern Wales, but the occupation of the whole of England was not completed until the Flavian period. Claudius also put down revolt in Mauretania and divided the former kingdom into provinces. The defenses of the Danube were strengthened by the conversion of the *client* Kingdom of Thrace into a province. The provincial administration of Claudius was firm and shrewd and is exemplified, in particular, by his settlement of the difficult problem of Jewish agitation for the citizenship of Alexandria (pp. 611–12).

It is difficult to judge the real nature of Claudius' private life in the palace. Tradition represents him as dominated by the personal influence of the freedmen, secretaries, and of his successive wives, four in number. Certainly the freedmen secured appointments for their fellows in the imperial service and brought Greeks into the Equestrian Order. This, however, was in accordance with Claudius' general practice of using men of non-Italian origin in government. But the emperor's personal life does seem to have been dominated by his intimates. His last wife, Agrippina, the daughter of Germanicus and the mother of Nero, seems to have forced out Claudius' son Britannicus in favor of her own Nero. Like her mother, the younger Agrippina was an ambitious, unscrupulous woman in the promotion of her family interests. She arranged Nero's marriage to Claudius' daughter and influenced her husband to put young Nero, aged thirteen, in position for the succession by a grant of the proconsular *imperium*. Then in 54 she hastened Nero's succession by poisoning Claudius.

NERO (54–68)

Nero succeeded to the Principate at the age of sixteen, and for a beginning announced his intention of preserving the place of the Senate in government. Some visible evidence of this assertion was furnished by the rehabilitation of several impoverished senatorial families at the emperor's personal expense. In the main Nero kept, or was kept, to good administration during his first years in office by the influence of his tutor, the philosopher Seneca, and of the praetorian prefect Burrus. But as he grew older, Nero chafed under their restraint and that of his mother, who wanted to be the power behind the throne. As early as A.D. 55, however, Nero had removed Claudius' son, Britannicus, to get rid of a possible rival and by 59 was in complete rebellion.

About the remainder of Nero's reign there is little good to be said, except that his conduct hastened its end. He repudiated his wife Octavia, married his mistress Poppaea, and had his mother murdered. Under the sinister influence of a new praetorian prefect, Tigellinus, Seneca's influence waned completely, and the senators acquired more cause for dislike to add to their outrage at Nero's public behavior. The upper classes, senatorial and equestrian alike, were offended by the emperor's blatant display of Greek tastes and his excessive vanity. Nero introduced Greek musical contests into the Roman public festivals and departed from the imperial dignity to compete personally. It is fair to suspect that he owed his victories as much to his rank as to his ability.

Distaste and dislike soon passed into fear and hate. Some senators began to absent themselves ostentatiously from the meetings of the Senate and by 65 a series of conspiracies and prosecutions developed which led to Nero's isolation. In 65 the conspiracy of Piso, a prominent senator, was revealed and its ramifications were traced among the Stoics to Seneca himself. While the philosophers felt some desire for a restoration of the Republic, their chief criticism turned on Nero's tyrannical rule. He was held to exemplify the selfish, evil qualities of despotism. Piso's conspiracy, however, was poorly organized and ended in a fiasco. Seneca was executed for complicity along with his nephew, the epic poet Lucan, in whose poem, the *Pharsalia,* the worthies of the Republic were praised and Julius Caesar, the founder of the Julian line, was condemned. Another Stoic senator, Thrasea Paetus, was put to death and his son-in-law, Helvidius Priscus, was exiled. The more reputable members of the Senate were alienated from Nero, and, what was more important, their fellows, the high officers of the army, lost confidence in the *Princeps.*

A coin portrait of Nero

The conspiracy of Corbulo, one of Rome's best generals of the century, was symptomatic of the feeling among the generals. Corbulo had been assigned to operations against the Parthian King Vologases, who had pulled Parthia together in the fifties and put his brother, Tiridates, on the throne of Armenia. After a lengthy and difficult war, Corbulo forced Vologases to acknowledge Rome's authority in Armenia and compelled Tiridates to come to Rome to receive his crown from Nero's hands. Four years later, in 67, Corbulo organized a conspiracy against Nero, in which the governors of Upper and Lower Germany were implicated. Upon its disclosure the emperor invited the conspirators to commit suicide, which was the polite way out for traitors of rank. Nero also slighted his general Vespasian, who was in charge of the suppression of revolt in Judaea when the emperor went to Greece in 66 to compete in the musical events of the Olympic Games. After Nero won first prize, he preferred to tour Greece rather than to visit the army in Judaea.

In Rome the people suspected Nero of setting the famous fire of 64, which raged for nine days and destroyed a large part of the slum quarters of the city, where Nero later built his new palace, the Golden House. The charge was probably untrue, but Nero diverted attention from himself by making scapegoats out of the Christian community in Rome who were apparently more disliked by the general populace than the emperor himself. This episode, the first official prosecution of Christians by the Roman government, involved only trial before the city prefect and did not lead to any persecution outside Rome. Nero's punishment of the Christians was a particularly unpleasant spectacle, and Tacitus, who reported the event, evidently felt that the punishment, burning at the stake, was as degrading as the social behavior of the Christians. When the chain reaction of revolt, started by Corbulo's conspiracy, spread to other generals, Nero had nowhere to turn for support. He had alienated responsible Roman society, the Senate, the generals, the armies, and the people of Rome itself. The last of the Julio-Claudians committed suicide and left the Principate to be won in civil war.

The Year of the Four Emperors (A.D. 68/69)

While Augustus had founded the Principate in law and by the universal consent of the people of the Empire, as he put it, he had obtained his supremacy by military force and had been careful to preserve the military aspect of the Principate. Despite long periods of relative peace and routine defense, the *Princeps* could not forget that he was commander-in-chief of the army. The fact that the ultimate basis of power was military had emerged after the death of Gaius, when Claudius was nominated by the praetorian guard. Claudius, unmartial as he was, sensibly took care to cultivate the generals and the army.

While it is scarcely possible to credit the army as a whole with developed political views in the crisis of government in 68/69, the soldiers evidently felt that the Principate should be maintained and showed a will to support their own particular commanders. The Roman system of holding the legions and their generals in one region for a long period of time had contributed to the re-entry of the army into politics. An *esprit de corps* had grown up in the separate armies of the Rhine, the Danube, and of Syria, so that each could be moved as a unit by its commander, to whom the soldiers felt personal loyalty. Augustus, Tiberius, and Claudius had each contrived to center the loyalties of the commanders and of the soldiers on himself as the apex of the military pyramid. Nero had neglected to do so. Thus, in 68 a chain reaction set in when the ambition of each commander in turn was fired to fill the vacuum of the Principate. Precedent could be found, if the commanders thought of it, for military acclamation to the Principate in the nomination of Claudius by the praetorian guard. The problem for the generals was to enlist the support of all the army groups, as the Julio-Claudians had done until Nero's failure.

The process was set in motion by the revolt of Vindex, the governor of Gallia Lugdunensis, who demanded freedom from the tyrant Nero and autonomy for Gaul. The demand for freedom was designed to enlist support among the Gauls, some of whom were chafing because of their taxes, and perhaps was not meant very seriously by Vindex. He himself, believing that the Senate should choose a new *Princeps,* favored Galba, the governor of Tarraco in Spain. Vindex' revolt was regarded as dangerously nationalistic, however, by Verginius Rufus, the governor of Upper Germany, who acted speedily to suppress it. In the meantime Galba was acclaimed by the praetorian guard, who betrayed Nero, and was accepted by the Senate as *Princeps*.

Galba was a man of civilian outlook, congenial to the senators, and, as Tacitus put it, "equal to empire, if he had never been emperor." Tacitus also credited Galba with various theoretical views on the Principate, which, if not strictly Galba's, do give some idea of how the senators were thinking about the office. Galba sought legitimacy for his new position among the more intangible concepts of the *Princeps* as a champion of the human race. When Galba picked as successor another senator, Lucius Calpurnius Piso, he talked of his selection as that of the "best" man and wistfully acknowledged that there could no longer be a Republic: "You have to reign over men," he told Piso, "who cannot bear either absolute slavery or absolute freedom." Galba, however, lost both the potential support of the Rhine legions by recalling Rufus, and of the guard by failing to pay them a bonus. A fervid harangue by Piso to the guard on the merits of selection of the best man as opposed to hereditary succession did nothing to change their minds. The guard put Piso and Galba to death and nominated Otho, a former husband of Nero's wife, Poppaea, as *Princeps* in exchange for a substantial bonus. The guard, however, did not speak for the armies, which began to move.

The troops on the Rhine had acclaimed their commander, Vitellius, as *Princeps*. With the support of the other provincial governors in Western Europe he marched on Italy to oppose Otho, who had been recognized by the army groups of the Danube and the East. Otho chose to fight Vitellius at Cremona in northern Italy without awaiting the arrival of help from the Danubian troops and was defeated. Vitellius occupied Rome and was duly recognized by the Senate who had to bow to force. Vitellius soon proved his incapacity as *Princeps* by allowing his soldiers to plunder in Italy and by sacrificing the potential support of the Danubian legions by putting some centurions to death and assigning the soldiers to labor details. He himself showed a notable enthusiasm for elaborate banquets.

In the meantime Vespasian, who had gone about his business of suppressing the Jewish revolt, had recognized the various nominees for the Principate, each in his turn. In July of 69 he acted. The fifteen legions in Egypt, Syria, and Judaea, the greater part of the Roman army, acclaimed Vespasian as *Princeps,* and he set about winning the Principate by a military operation. He assigned the command in Judaea to his son, Titus, and sent off his subordinate, Mucianus, through Asia Minor to Europe. Vespasian himself held Egypt and thus controlled the grain supply to Italy. The Danubian army came over to him and advanced on Italy from the north. The fleet at Ravenna deserted Vitellius, but his troops remained loyal. The war was terminated only by a victory over the Vitellians at Cremona and the capture and partial pillage of Rome by the Danubian forces. After recognition by the remaining troops in the West and by the Senate in December of 69, Vespasian came to Rome to begin his Principate.

The Flavian Rulers (A.D. 69–96)

VESPASIAN (69–79)

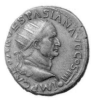

A coin portrait of Vespasian

Although Vespasian had acquired the Principate by the acclamation and support of his soldiers, he was in no sense their tool, nor, like Gaius and Nero, did he think of the Principate as a Hellenistic monarchy. He was an Italian of Equestrian family who had risen to senatorial rank and an army command in a lengthy career which had taken him to Britain under Claudius and to most parts of the Empire. Thus Vespasian brought to the Principate a considerable knowledge of the provinces. He had a hardheaded common sense, as well as the judgment and experience to deal realistically with men and situations. During his ten years of rule the Principate was re-established on the Augustan model, its finances were put into sound order, and the administration and frontier defenses were restored to efficient working.

Before the armies could be reorganized, Vespasian had to suppress revolts in Gaul and Judaea (pp. 612–15). Both were terminated in 70 and the Empire returned to peace. The mutinous legions on the Rhine who had joined in the revolt were disbanded and reformed, but the bulk of the army merely needed replacements and discipline. Vespasian set the total force at twenty-eight legions and about as many auxiliary troops. Several steps were taken to correct the dangers which had come to light in the civil wars and the Gallic revolt. The auxiliary units were made less homogeneous in character by mixing recruits of different localities and assigning more Roman officers. Probably for reasons of economy, Vespasian continued to station the legions for long periods of time in a single area, but he did rotate their commanding officers more frequently. A new praetorian guard of nine thousand men was recruited to replace that which Vitellius had drawn from his own legionary troops, and Titus was made its commander. Vespasian, however, had to accelerate the practice of enrolling legionary soldiers from the Roman citizens of the provinces because the Italians, after almost a century of peace, had lost their military traditions and were not suited for the conditions of service on the frontiers. Vespasian and his successors kept the armies active by extending the limits of the Roman province in Britain into Scotland, by occupying the weak salient in the frontier between the Rhine and the Danube, and by establishing new base camps and garrison points along the Danube and Euphrates.

Vespasian began his reign with an empty treasury because of Nero's extravagant spending and because of the expense of having four emperors in a single year. He is said to have estimated that forty billion sesterces (about two billion dollars) would be necessary to repair the war damage and to restore the state to a sound financial condition. This is the largest single sum mentioned in ancient history, and unfortunately we do not know how Vespasian arrived at it or very much about his operations for raising and spending the money. He did increase taxes throughout the Empire, he did shift provinces between his own and the Senate's jurisdiction, and he did cancel the immunities from taxation which some provincial cities had enjoyed since they were made Roman allies in the Republican wars of conquest. Evidently the Empire could well afford the new levies because economic growth continued without check, and the Flavians, after some initial frugality by Vespasian, spent lavishly on building programs in both Rome and the provinces. Apart from the new defense installations on the frontiers, the Flavian Period saw much road building and construction of aqueducts and other public facilities. In Rome a new temple was built for Jupiter on the Capitoline Hill to replace the former building which had been damaged in the fighting with Vitellius. This temple, which burnt down during the reign of Titus, was replaced by Domitian. The great Colosseum of Rome was also erected by the Flavians to house the gladiatorial combats, contests between man and beast, and wild beast hunts.

Vespasian was dignified and firm in dealing with the Senate, granting its members respect and courtesy but holding the reigns of government securely in his own hands. As censor in 74 he continued the policy of Claudius, when he came to fill the vacancies caused by the war and by expulsions. Provincials were enrolled, mainly from the more Romanized provinces of Spain, Gaul, and Africa, but some also from Asia Minor. Vespasian and his successors promoted Romanization vigorously (p. 610). In general, the Senate responded to Vespasian's methods and administration with approval and support, but a few small groups proved uncooperative or even disloyal.

The opposition was led at first by Helvidius Priscus, who returned from an exile imposed by Nero and who was elected praetor for the year 70. Before Vespasian arrived in Rome, Priscus endeavored to persuade the Senate to show its independence of the new *Princeps*. For example, in a discussion about the appointment of delegates to meet Vespasian, Priscus insisted that the members should be selected from the "best" men of the Senate, not chosen by lot. Again, he wanted the Senate to control finance and to direct the restoration of buildings damaged in the war, while the *Princeps* paid the costs. Both proposals were turned down, but Priscus persisted in his opposition and took a more specifically Republican line when Vespasian came to Rome. He called the emperor by his personal name and refused to use the official titles on the documents which he himself issued as praetor. While such discourtesy might have been overlooked in a private individual, Priscus was a senator and a praetor. His conduct was close to treason, and Vespasian had him exiled and later put to death. Vespasian also banished the Cynic philosophers who orated on the street corners against the Principate as a tyranny and against civilization in general.

TITUS (79–81)

Titus, who had been closely associated in administration by Vespasian, succeeded his father in 79, but died of a fever two years later. His brief reign gave promise of a genial and popular ruler as well as an efficient one, but was marred by a devastating fire in Rome and the great eruption of Vesuvius in 79 which

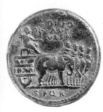

covered the towns of Pompeii and Herculaneum with volcanic ash and mud. The excavation of their houses, streets and public buildings, thus suddenly sealed over, has revealed the generally prosperous and comfortable conditions of life in the Italian towns of the early Empire.

DOMITIAN (81–96)

A coin of Titus

Unlike Titus, his younger brother Domitian, who succeeded to the Principate in 81, again departed in the direction of autocracy and absolutism. Domitian was an energetic and able ruler, among the best administrators which the Empire knew, but his handling of the Principate was far more dangerous to its Roman traditions than that of Gaius or Nero. He controlled membership in the Senate much more rigorously than any of his predecessors since Augustus and held a perpetual censorship from 85 until his death. Domitian also dominated the consulship by holding that office seventeen times. To exalt the Flavian dynasty he established a priestly college, the *Flaviales,* which administered the worship of his deified father and brother as did the *Augustales* for the Julio-Claudians. In addition, temples were built for Vespasian and Titus and for the Flavian family. Domitian welcomed flattering comparisons of himself to Jupiter from the court poets and liked to be referred to as *dominus et deus* (master and lord). Although he did not use that title officially, Domitian was clearly working to the end of deification as a living god in Rome and to the exaltation of the *Princeps* above ordinary men and above his nominal colleagues in government. In this connection several prosecutions for atheism were launched, apparently directed against individuals refusing to participate in the ruler cult. Atheism was, in effect, a charge of treason. Among the prosecuted were a cousin of Domitian, Flavius Clemens, and the latter's wife, Domitilla, who may have been a patroness of the Christian community in Rome.

Until 89, however, Domitian did not engage in a wholesale attempt to silence and remove the opposition which his conduct provoked. Then his suspicion and anger were aroused by a revolt of Aulus Saturninus, the governor of Upper Germany, who counted on aid from the Germans east of the Rhine and from his fellow commanders. Since the Germans were unable to cross the river and since the other generals remained loyal to Domitian, the revolt was easily suppressed. Domitian, however, began a series of investigations, listened to informers, and traced the threads of conspiracy and opposition into the upper ranks of the Senate. Some provincial governors, the proconsul of Asia and a legate in Britain, were ultimately involved, and Domitian proceeded to a purge which extended to the philosophic opposition. This group had again become vocal. Helvidius Priscus' son wrote a mythological farce about Paris and Oenone, which Domitian interpreted as political satire, and panegyrics were published on Thrasea Paetus, the martyr of Nero's reign. In 95 the philosophers were again banished from Rome. The situation became so difficult that able men were afraid to undertake public office, and in 96 a conspiracy of palace officials and senators murdered Domitian and ended the Flavian dynasty.

The governing classes would not accept the conversion of the Principate into absolutism, but, because there was no constitutional method of removing the *Princeps,* they had to resort to assassination. However, since Domitian had held the loyalty of the army generals and soldiers, there was danger of a repetition of the events of 68/69. The conspirators and the Senate selected an elderly and sickly senator, Nerva, as *Princeps.* He had little military reputation and only averted military revolt and civil war by choosing Trajan, a general of ability and experience, as his colleague and successor. Nerva's action, born of necessity, provided a new formula for succession to the Principate. The principles of selection of the best man and of hereditary transmission of the office were combined to usher in the era of the Roman Peace in the second century after Christ.

The Empire

FINANCE AND TAXATION

The rapid growth of prosperity in the Empire during the first century was facilitated by the basic reforms which Augustus made in the issuance of Roman currency and in the tax system. His monetary reorganization provided a free and plentiful circulation of money within the Empire and a sound gold and silver currency which circulated beyond its frontiers.[1] About 19 B.C. Augustus reopened the Roman mint under new officials, and he and his successors coined both in Rome and in provincial mints, sharing this function, too, with the Senate. The *Princeps,* however, took most of the minting and issuance of money under his own care, particularly that of the gold and silver. Money was issued mainly through the expenditures of the *Princeps* and thus permitted some control of the market to be exercised. Yet in the Early Empire this did not extend to any systematic regulation of business and finance. The coinage was of good quality and the gold coins became a world currency, used even in Parthia and India, where they had been exported by merchants for the purchase of luxuries

---

[1] The Romans used coins of copper, bronze (the *aes* coinage), of silver, and of gold. The pieces were called the *as* (copper), *sestertius* (bronze), *denarius* (silver), and *aureus* (gold), and were issued both in fractional and whole values. The *as* was originally a Roman pound of copper, a heavy weight, but as a coin it was of small value and was referred to contemptuously. The scale of values was as follows:

1 *aureus* = 25 *denarii*
1 *denarius* = 4 *sestertii* (the *denarius* had been equated with the Athenian *drachma ca.* 187 B.C.)
1 *sestertius* = 14 *asses*

The *aureus* was worth about five dollars in bullion value, so that the large sums given in *sestertii* (sesterces) may be roughly equated to dollars by dividing by twenty. Just as in the case of Greek money, it is virtually impossible to give the modern equivalents in purchasing power because of the variables (p. 256, n. 1).

The gold coins circulated throughout the Empire, but the silver was used mainly in the Western provinces and in Italy. Local issues of bronze took its place in the East, where the emperors allowed the old Greek cities and leagues to preserve their traditions of independence by operating local mints. All the coins, however, were minted according to Roman standards. The government marketed money through payments to the army and for other imperial purposes or through banks. For example, in 33, Tiberius put 100,000,000 sesterces into circulation through the banks by giving them the money from his own funds to make loans without interest. In the Early Empire the standards set by Augustus remained fixed until the reign of Nero, when a ten percent depreciation was made. Trajan, early in the second century, made a similar devaluation, but the coinage remained sound and of good quality until the early third century.

(pp. 638–39). No control was exercised by the government over this outward flow of gold, although Roman writers were critical. Their concern, however, was more with the moral problem of the extensive use of luxuries than with the fiscal soundness of the practice.

The government was, in fact, as much concerned with the use of the coinage as a vehicle of propaganda, like postage stamps in our own day, as with the financial problems involved in coining. The imperial coins usually bore a portrait of the emperor, as he wished to appear to his subjects, and the legend on the coin emphasized some characteristic quality of his reign or of Rome itself. For example, the emperor's "benevolence" or his "foresight" might be stressed, while military victories and other signal events were commemorated. In fact, this propaganda effect of the coinage was so carefully pursued that the coins afford a valuable clue to the policies of the emperors in developing their conception of the Principate.

The taxation system of the Republic was transferred to the Empire by Augustus, but, as might be expected, there was considerably more regulation of its incidence and care in collection. Italy remained a privileged area in this respect. The Italians had paid no direct taxes since 167 B.C., a privilege which came to be known as the Italian Right, the *Ius Italicum*. On occasion this was granted to municipalities in the provinces as a mark of favor. The Italians, however, had paid indirect taxes: the *portoria,* or customs dues up to five percent on the value of goods, and a five percent tax on the manumission of slaves. These were continued, and Augustus added to them a five percent tax on inheritances, and a one percent sales tax, both earmarked for the military treasury, the *aerarium militare.*

Augustus inaugurated his reign by a careful census of the provinces, which came to be repeated every five years. The number and legal status of the inhabitants of the Empire were recorded, as well as the amount and sources of their wealth for tax purposes. The main source of revenue was a direct land tax, the *tributum soli,* which fell on all provincial land, whether in private ownership or rented from the public land of the Roman state. Rome did not regard itself as the owner of all provincial land although both the state and the *Princeps* had title to immense tracts, which had been confiscated from the private estates of previous rulers or of rebels against Roman authority. Other forms of property than land were subject to a levy known as the *tributum capitis.* This sounds like a poll tax, but poll taxes were used only in Egypt, always an exception, and for regions of the Empire where the evaluation of property was difficult.

The government also requisitioned grain for the army, hay for its animals, and lodging for troops, but the regular establishment of the frontier defenses and the normal absence of civil war made such requisitions relatively infrequent. The taxes as a whole were not heavy, and, through the budgeting which the regular census allowed, and the carefully supervised collection, a considerable surplus was left to individuals for profit and investment and to cities for their own financial needs. The rapid economic growth of the Empire, which culminated in the second century (pp. 640–54), attests the generally high quality of the imperial administration.

When the Principate was established, the state treasury of the Republic, the *aerarium Saturni,* so-called because its monies had once been kept in the temple of Saturn, was retained. All the revenues from the provinces were paid into it, and Augustus had been authorized to make withdrawals as needed. There was, however, little movement of cash, for the *Princeps* set up separate chests (*fisci*) for each of his imperial provinces and only balances were transferred from the provinces to Rome. The same practice probably prevailed in the senatorial provinces. There was actually very little surplus from the provinces, if any, and the *aerarium* was frequently in difficulties. Augustus had paid sums into it from his private property (the *patrimonium*), which he used extensively to establish his position as patron and benefactor of the state. Theoretically the *aerarium Saturni* continued to be the repository of all revenues and bore all state costs, but as the imperial treasury (also called the *fiscus*) grew and encroached on senatorial preserves, the *aerarium* was brought more and more under the *Princeps'* control. As noted above, in the reign of Claudius the *fiscus* emerged as a bureau of the treasury, organized as a separate department of government. Vespasian's fresh start in financing probably entailed the merger of the *aerarium* with the *fiscus,* and the success of Flavian financial policies established the *fiscus* as the chief treasury of the state. When the *aerarium* was disentangled by the emperors of the third century, it was used mainly as the municipal treasury of the city of Rome.

The initial impetus to this process of centralization was given by the immense personal wealth of Augustus, who was not only the richest individual in the Empire, but whose wealth almost equaled that of the state itself. He inherited the property of Julius Caesar, not all of which Antony could spend, and that of his father, and acquired great wealth from the wars by plunder and confiscation. The wealth of the Egyptian monarchy, which largely owned Egypt, came to Augustus as the victor over Cleopatra. In Italy and the provinces he held estates which had been acquired by confiscation, purchase, or were left to him through bequest. The *Princeps* and the members of his family, both men and women, invested in business as well as in land. From his store of private wealth, Augustus purchased land for his veterans, financed the construction of buildings for public use and works projects, and made distributions of money to the people of Rome at festivals and as gifts to individuals. The successors of Augustus continued these practices, and, despite the extravagance of Caligula and Nero, it is likely that Vespasian took over a large *patrimonium* from the Julio-Claudian house, to which the succeeding emperors added.

THE FRONTIERS

The most notable exception to Augustus' defensive policy for the Empire was the invasion of Britain by Claudius in 43 (pp. 595–96). While Claudius' armies occupied much of England, the organization of the territory proceeded with difficulty and met resistance. In 59, during Nero's reign, the Britons rose in revolt under the leadership of the warrior-queen Boudicca, whom Roman officials had insulted and whose people were angered at the maladministration of the Roman procurators. The towns of Camulodunum (Colchester), Verulamium (St. Albans), and Londinium (London), which had become Roman centers, were destroyed, and thousands of Romans were massacred. Nero's general Paulinus put down the revolt by 62, with little thanks from Nero, and the pacification of the island continued. The conquest had been virtually completed under the Flavians, when Agricola, Tacitus' father-in-law, was governor from 77 to 84. He reduced the Druid stronghold on the island of Mona (Anglesea) because the Druids had encouraged resistance, occupied northern England, where Eboracum (York) became a Roman military base, and penetrated into Scotland as far as the highlands. A projected invasion of Ireland was given up when Agricola was recalled, but his fleet circumnavigated Britain, as Pytheas of Massilia had done four centuries before. Under Roman government military roads were laid out, towns gradually developed, and a villa, or manorial, system of farming came into use as the land was cleared and new fruits and crops were introduced.

The Flavian rulers strengthened and improved the defenses on the other frontiers and encouraged the exploitation of the land behind them. In Mauretania the limits of the desert were pushed back as more land was brought under cultivation by irrigation. The nomads were policed and prevented from raiding the new fields and towns. In the East Vespasian was able to build on Corbulo's work by enlarging Roman territory and founding new garrison posts at the chief crossings of the Euphrates. Galatia and Cappadocia in Asia Minor were combined into a single large province, while the Syrian boundary was extended by the incorporation of the *client* kingdoms of Commagene and Palmyra on the fringe of the Syrian Desert.

Both Vespasian and Domitian attempted to correct the weak point which Augustus had left in the area between the upper Rhine and the Danube rivers by advancing into the salient and constructing fortifications. Communications were thus shortened between the two army groups of Europe to facilitate defense on both frontiers. As the Roman frontier provinces were settled and increased in wealth they naturally became more attractive to the German tribal peoples, who tried to raid across the rivers for booty. The Germans, who became familiar with Roman weapons and tactics, were pushed into coalescence by Roman pressure, so that something like a competition in growth developed. The better the Roman defenses became and the wealthier the provinces grew, the heavier became the German pressure. Both Vespasian and Domitian made extensive raids across the Rhine to punish and repress the Chatti (as the chief people of western Germany were called), and Domitian had difficulty in merely holding the line of the Danube.

All along the Danube River powerful peoples pressed against the frontier, particularly the Marcomanni of Bohemia in the west, and the Dacians who lived in what is now Hungary and Rumania. The Dacians were very formidable after they had been united into a kingdom by ambitious King Decebalus. In 85 they crossed the Danube into Moesia, defeated the Roman army there and killed the governor. Although the Dacians were pushed back, they defeated another army sent across the river after them, and their success set the Marcomanni and other peoples farther to the west in motion. To free his hands for action against these, Domitian made an agreement with Decebalus, by which he paid the king a subsidy to stay north of the river and supplied him with Roman engineers to help develop the kingdom. Domitian defeated the Marcomanni in 93 and held the line of the Danube, but Decebalus' strength had increased and posed a problem to Domitian's successors.

Behind the screen of the river frontiers the Empire's lines of communication in Europe were devloped with the head of the Adriatic as the hub between Western Europe and the Balkans. The old route to the East by the Egnatian Way, across the Adriatic Sea from Italy to Illyricum, thence by road over the mountains to Thessalonica (Saloniki) in Macedonia and eastwards through Thrace to the Bosporus, continued in use, but a new land route was added. From Aquileia, at the head of the Adriatic, a road ran to Emana, then down the Save River to the Danube, and along the south bank of the river to branch off, either to Thessalonica, or, farther eastward, to Byzantium. These routes became literally the life lines of the Empire, for along them the legions could be shuttled from the Euphrates by way of Asia Minor and the Danube to the Rhine or vice versa, when they were needed in one area or the other. While the emperors of the first century did not have to face heavy pressure on two fronts at the same time, they were presumably aware of the contingency. It spurred the extensive road building and Romanization which was undertaken in the European provinces.

ROMANIZATION

During the Roman wars of conquest and in the Late Republic, Roman citizens had begun to migrate from Italy to the provinces. Some had been sent as colonists to found organized colonies, some had developed towns of their own, while individual settlers had moved into native communities to do business or to invest in land. This emigration had gone mostly to the older provinces close to Italy, to Narbonensis, to southern and eastern Spain, to Sicily, and Africa. The result had been an early start in the cultural Romanization of these provinces as the natives learned Latin, imitated Roman customs, and traded with the Roman merchants.

While Julius Caesar and Augustus continued the practice of sending out groups of colonies from Italy, mainly composed of veterans, they also began the more significant practice of recognizing the desire of the provincials to become Roman citizens. Wholesale grants of citizenship were made, and the status of native communities was raised to approach that of the self-governing Roman colonies. After the Augustan Period the migration of Italians to the provinces was slight, not only because Italy was a desirable place in which to live, but also because the veterans usually settled in the provinces where they had served. For a time the process of Romanization by deliberate government policy also slackened, but under Claudius and the Flavians it began to acquire an increasing momentum. The culmination was reached in A.D. 212, when the Emperor Caracalla issued an edict conferring Roman citizenship on virtually all the peoples of the Empire. This was not a grand gesture of generosity, but rather the recognition of an accomplished fact. By that time most of the inhabitants of the Empire had become Roman citizens, and distinctions of privilege and status from the point of view of citizenship had ceased to exist.

The Empire, however, was cosmopolitan in culture—Roman, Greek, and Oriental—for Rome did not demand or try to impose cultural uniformity on its subjects. Romanization, in the broad sense of the term, was a complex process and is perhaps easier to understand if we regard it in two ways. First, there was cultural Romanization, in which the native peoples learned Latin, imitated Roman customs, and absorbed the traditions of Rome through their education and way of life. Second, there was the extension of legal privilege, of Roman citizenship and its nexus of legal, social, and political obligations and rights. Native peoples were free to accept or to reject Roman culture as they wished, providing they accepted Roman authority, but the conferment of citizenship, which became the common denominator of the Empire, was a matter of government policy.

Generally speaking, the Western part of the Empire, the European and African provinces, became Romanized in both senses of the term. The Romans, who came to conquer and to organize, brought the appeal of a higher, privileged culture to which the native peoples aspired. Before the Roman establishment of provinces, there had been only a fringe of Carthaginian and Greek trading posts and small cities along the coasts, while behind them the Numidians, Iberians, Celts, and Germans had lived in village settlements. Among these native peoples the desire to Romanize was strong and proceeded spontaneously. Individuals and communities became Roman, as their native speech and customs were gradually forgotten and those of Rome adopted. When the Roman armies went in, roads were built, legionary camps were constructed near which new native settlements sprang up to do business with the soldiers, and the process of Romanization started. It was accelerated when Roman traders, businessmen, officials, and colonists followed the soldiers. The Roman government, as their predecessors of the Republic had done in Italy, took advantage of the situation. When the government judged the time was ripe, it extended the privileges of citizenship to individuals and to whole communities, which became self-governing units, like the Roman colonies and towns. The same methods were employed which Rome had used to form the Roman Confederacy in Italy—Latin Rights, municipal status, and special privileges.

The Eastern provinces, however, remained Greek or Greco-Oriental in culture. The Romans and Italians who migrated to the East speedily became bilingual, if they were not already so, and in a few generations they adapted to the culture of their environment. The Roman colony authorized by Julius Caesar at Corinth in Greece is a case in point. At first the official inscriptions of the town were in Latin, but in the second century Greek had taken over. The same is true of the other Roman colonies in the East, which were relatively few in number. In the unurbanized areas of the Eastern provinces, such as inner Asia Minor and parts of Syria, however, a process of urban growth, like that of the West, was encouraged by the conditions of peace and order and stimulated by the Roman government. Nomads settled down, villages grew into towns, and the towns grew into cities. But the cities were Greek cities, and the whole process was essentially a continuation of that which the Hellenistic kings had started. Egypt, as ever, remained the exception. Alexandria was its only great city, while elsewhere in Egypt the people continued to live in their time-old manner.

As a result Romanization in the East consisted mainly in the extension of legal privilege. Although individual Greeks and Orientals were made Roman citizens, and although their communities might be granted self-government or made into municipalities, or retained as such, if Rome had already made them free allies during the Republic, nevertheless throughout the East the culture remained Hellenic. As we have noticed, the upper classes in Italy, despite the Hellenization of Roman art, literature, and even thought, remained somewhat hostile to the Greeks and Orientals as individuals during the first century after Christ. A more genuine homogeneity of feeling between East and West, a common classical culture, was the product of the second century.

With these distinctions in mind, it is useful to review the methods and progress of Romanization in the West, where it was particularly marked in the first century. A good example of the self-governing Roman colony, which became a model of municipal organization for the native communities, is afforded by one of Julius Caesar's foundations in Spain. It was located in the province of Baetica and called Colonia Genetiva Julia (Urso). The original charter indicates that the colony was organized like an Italian municipality, a little model of Rome itself. The magistrates were called duovirs, aediles and quaestors, and there were boards of priests to administer the civic religious worship. Since the colonists had brought their Roman gods, Romanization therefore involved a very considerable extension of Roman religion, just as the Greek settlers of the Hellenistic East had carried their worships to the lands of the Persian Empire. A council, the *curia,* whose members were drawn from the upper class and were called *decurions,* directed the administration of the colony. Councilors and magistrates were elected, however, by an assembly of all the citizens, which had legislative powers similar to the Roman assemblies. The colonists were assigned lands in the nearby countryside, and law, education, festivals and the general manner of life in the whole district were Roman.

The native communities, however, could only attain to this by stages. When a native community, a tribal village or small settlement, had grown into a town or city and attained a degree of Romanization by its own efforts, it

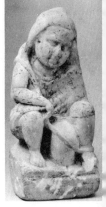

Figurine of a Roman slave waiting for his master

might be started on the way by the grant of Latin Rights. After the Latins of Italy had attained full Roman citizenship in 89 B.C., this expression had become a legal term to denote a parcel of privileges which the Roman government could bestow on a community: *commercium* and *conubium* (p. 456) and access to full citizenship for the ex-magistrates and their descendants. Year by year in these communities possessing Latin Rights, the number of Roman citizens increased among the upper class, and the community become more Romanized by example and deliberate effort of its own. Julius Caesar marked the partial Romanization of Narbonensis by granting Latin Rights to all the towns and cities of that province. Claudius made a similar grant to many individual communities in the provinces, and Vespasian conferred the Latin Rights on the Spanish provinces as a wholesale grant.

The next stage up the ladder of status was the recognition of the town with Latin Rights as a self-governing municipality, a *municipium,* in which all the inhabitants were Roman citizens and possessed an organization for self-government similar to that of a Roman colony. Finally, the title of colony might be given to such a community as a mark of prestige by the *Princeps*. The first titular colony, as they are called, was the city of Vienne in central France, so designated by Claudius. Thus a ladder of privilege was built, for which the first condition was urbanization. By the late second century after Christ, the Empire had become a vast aggregate of self-governing cities, whose people were Roman citizens.

The chief exceptions to this general picture of municipalization were provided by the Gallic provinces and Egypt. In Gaul Augustus had allowed the continuance of tribal units, each controlled by its native nobility. Towns and cities grew rapidly, but a general pattern of municipal self-government was not established until the third century, when the chief towns of each Gallic tribal commune were made self-governing municipalities. In Egypt the organization established by the Ptolemies was followed (pp. 372–75). The Egyptian peasantry lived in villages, and the land was divided into nomes for administrative purposes. Alexandria, because of its turbulent population, was governed by an imperial official, but the old Greek cities of Naukratis and Ptolemais had self-government, as did a new foundation of Hadrian, Antinoopolis. In the third century, however, even Alexandria was allowed to have the council for which its citizens had long clamored.

Roman citizenship, of course, carried with it very tangible privileges and, in the Early Empire, few oppressive obligations. Theoretically every citizen was liable to military service, but in practice the armies were recruited by volunteer enlistment and, to an ever increasing degree, from the frontier provinces. Roman citizens in the provinces enjoyed the protection of Roman law and had the right of appeal to the governor, and in theory, to the *Princeps* himself. At the same time, of course, they were liable for the taxes and obligations imposed by their own communities. Through the policy of the emperors, the imperial services were thrown open to the Roman citizens of the provinces, from the lowest grades of the freedmen and Equestrian careers to the Senate, and eventually to the office of *Princeps*. Trajan, for example, belonged to a Roman family in Spain.

Throughout this whole process the initiative came from the *Princeps* rather than from the Senate, which tended to stand for the principle of Italian primacy. The result, of course, was that the provincials looked on the *Princeps* as the fount of their privileges, and they expressed their loyalty to him and to Rome through the ruler cult. There was little opposition of a nationalistic type to Rome throughout the period from Augustus to the Flavians, except for sporadic revolts in the new provinces of Mauretania and Britain, and the special cases of the Gauls of the Rhineland and the Jews.

THE JEWISH OPPOSITION

The Romans had inherited the difficulties created by Jewish religious exclusiveness for any governing power when they organized the Eastern provinces out of the former domains of the Seleucids and the Ptolemies. In Palestine the Jews predominated in population and many of them cherished traditions of a national state, derived from the Kingdom of Solomon and the more recent rule of the Maccabees. There, too, was their religious capital, Jerusalem, with the temple and High Priesthood, the center of the traditions of Jewish history. Living outside of Palestine were the Jews of the Diaspora, the Scattering, who had moved into the Greek cities of the Near East. The group at Alexandria was especially large and influential and had been established since the third century before Christ. In the Greek cities the Jews were aliens who lived in a quarter separate from the Greeks and kept themselves distinct by their religious life and education which was centered in the synagogues. They acknowledged the religious leadership of Jerusalem and paid a monetary contribution to the temple. The whole Hebrew community formed a sort of theocracy, without political organization, but with its religious privileges traditionally established by the Hellenistic rulers. For the Jews of the Diaspora the price of religious freedom was separatism and non-participation in the political life of the cities. Their problems were of a different kind than those in Palestine, and we might look first at the situation in Alexandria. Both the situation and the Roman policy, implemented there by Claudius, were typical.

At the time of the wars of Julius Caesar and Augustus against Pompey and Antony, the Alexandrian Jews had supported the victors and, in return, their privileges had been confirmed. They were allowed the free exercise of their own religion, exemption from the civic religious rites of the Greek citizens, including the ruler cult, the right of not appearing in court on the Sabbath, and permission to pay their contribution to the temple. The privileges were a source of irritation to the Greek citizens who resented such an island of exclusiveness in their city. For their part the Jews both wished to retain the privileges and to be reckoned as citizens of Alexandria, with freedom to live outside their own quarter. They were not, of course, prepared to participate in the civic religion, which was just as much a function of citizenship as the obligations of government and society. To the Greeks citizenship was only to be obtained by the training given to *ephebes*, their young men, in the gymnasium, and by registration in the *demes* and tribes upon which the civic organization was based.

During the reign of Tiberius and his immediate successors, the friction between Jews and Greeks came to a head when the Jews began to spread beyond their own quarter and to press for citizen rights. The Greeks felt that they should have civic control over the Jews, presumably wishing to confine them to their own region and to prevent Jewish attempts to petition the emperor in the name of the city of Alexandria. During the reign of Gaius his friend Herod Agrippa, the ruler of the *client* kingdom of Judaea, visited Alexandria and was warmly welcomed by the Jews. Upon his departure the Greeks staged a parody of the proceedings, and then, to avert Gaius' anticipated displeasure, they made an attempt to install the emperor's statue in the Jewish synagogues. Refusal of the Jews to worship would, of course, divert Gaius' anger from themselves to the Jews. The scheme seems to have worked, for, when the Greeks looted in the Jewish quarter, Gaius ignored a Jewish petition for redress.

The prefect of Egypt then enflamed the situation by directing the Jews to return to their own quarter of the city, while the Greeks indulged in rioting and the looting of Jewish property. Both sides appealed to Claudius, who issued a stern directive outlining his imperial policy: citizenship in Alexandria was limited to the Greeks, but they were ordered not to coerce the Jews in any manner; the Jewish privileges were reconfirmed, but they were ordered not to agitate for citizenship or to send delegations to the *Princeps* in the name of Alexandria; further, they were ordered not to encroach on the Greek sections of the city and not to bring in more Jews. In short, Claudius was interested only in keeping order in Alexandria in accordance with the original scope of the Jewish privileges and restrictions. He regarded the matter as essentially a local problem, which was already regulated, and had no interest in the religious issue involved nor in a change in the regulations.

The Roman purpose in Judaea was similar, to keep order, but there the problem was far more complex. The Jews were themselves divided on religious issues of their own faith, in their attitudes to Hellenization and by social conflict between the farmers and shepherds and the rich landowners and the merchants of the cities. The Romans worked with the wealthy Hellenizing Jews, supporting that element in the Sanhedrin and for the High Priesthood. Accordingly, the Jews of the lower class, hostile to their own administrators, automatically transferred their hatred to the Romans. In Judaea the Romans had made other concessions to Jewish religious scruples, in addition to allowing their traditional organization to function freely. The coinage used there did not bear the emperor's head because the Jews were iconoclastic, the standards of the legions were bare of pagan insignia, and the Jews were exempted from military service. Also, while Judaea was a procuratorial district, the Sanhedrin administered justice. The procurator, Pontius Pilate, might have saved Christ from crucifixion at the time of his trial, but he would have incurred the charge of religious interference from the Jews. The Romans thus found great difficulty in administering Judaea

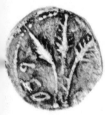

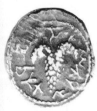

Jewish coins of the first century after Christ

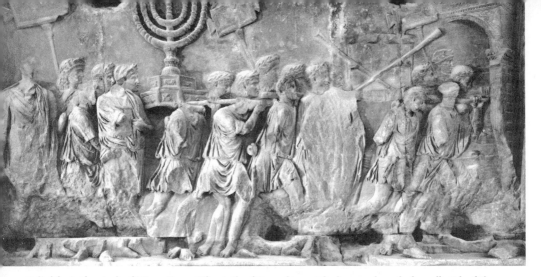

Relief from the Arch of Titus, Rome. The spoils of Jerusalem, with the seven-branched candlestick of the Hebrew temple, being carried in triumph

and alternated between the *client* kingship of the Herods and a procuratorial district. They finally settled on the latter in 44, but in the following years disorder increased. Jewish fanatics turned to brigandage and assassination, economic difficulties aggravated the religious and cultural clashes, and Rome was unfortunate in its choice of procurators.

By 64 the taxes from Judaea had fallen into arrears, and the governor confiscated seventeen talents from the temple to make them up. When the Jews rioted, the Roman soldiers were allowed to plunder in reprisal. Such reprisals merely had the effect of spreading revolt, and Nero therefore sent in an army under Vespasian. The revolt, interrupted momentarily by Vespasian's drive for the Principate, lasted until 70. Jerusalem was captured, the temple was plundered and the city was largely destroyed. Titus celebrated a triumph in Rome, where his victory was commemorated in the Arch of Titus at the lower end of the Roman Forum. Its vault bears a relief showing the plunder from the temple being carried in triumphal procession. Much of Judaea was declared public land and used for colonization or rented to the Jews, while Jewish towns were destroyed and the prisoners of war were sold as slaves. The theocratic organization was dissolved, and worship or restoration of the temple in Jerusalem was forbidden. Freedom of worship, however, was confirmed to the Jews as individuals upon the payment of a charge of two drachmas per person. Judaism thus became a licensed religion in the Roman Empire, but revolt flared again in the second century (pp. 621–23).

THE GALLIC OPPOSITION

The revolt against Roman authority in Gaul was partly nationalistic and partly a mutiny of the legions stationed along the Rhine, whose rebellion originated in the disturbance of administration and the shift of troops in the civil war of 68/69. Since the Gauls themselves had little cause for revolt, it did not spread widely. Gaul had become the richest province of the Empire, and the chief city, Lugdunum, was the busiest and largest city in the West after Rome itself. Augustus had started this vigorous growth by founding colonies and towns and by sponsoring the erection of commemorative arches, temples, theaters, and other public buildings on an impressive scale. The pleasing little Roman temple in Nîmes, the Maison Carrée, and the great aqueduct near the city, the Pont du Gard, were both built in Augustus' period. The Gauls themselves followed the Roman example, and villages grew rapidly into towns as the pattern of urbanization spread. The land was cleared and careful surveys made to start an agricultural development which continued through the Roman Empire into the Middle Ages.

The Roman government, however, had preserved the tribal communities of the Gallic peoples and kept their chieftains in authority. Although the latter had become Romanized and had been encouraged by such privileges as Claudius made available, some still cherished a tradition of complete independence. This was particularly true of the Rhineland, where connections were close between the Gauls and their Germanic kindred east of the Rhine. There the Romans recruited Germans as well as Gauls in the legions and auxiliaries and had stationed the troops in their native districts with their own chieftains as officers. The men were discontented at being shifted from their homeland in the course of the civil wars, and in 69 serious revolt broke out.

The Roman forces stationed in the Rhineland were depleted by Vitellius for his march on Italy, and, when the Danubian army of Vespasian was advancing westwards in 69, the latter's supporters in Italy had been concerned that the troops remaining in the Rhineland might attack. To deal with the situation a Romanized German officer, Civilis, of the Batavian people who were allied to Rome, was persuaded to declare for Vespasian and to open hostilities. Civilis drew support from others of his kind, Romanized German and Gallic officers who had seen service in the auxiliaries and were able to bring over their tribesmen. Civilis played his part for Vespasian successfully, but, despite the latter's

The Pont du Gard, perhaps the most impressive of Roman aqueducts. Rising in three lofty tiers above the Gard River, it carried water to Nemausus (Nîmes). Built in the Augustan Period

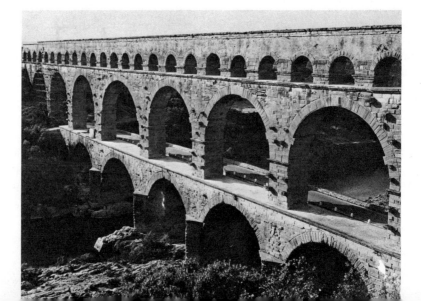

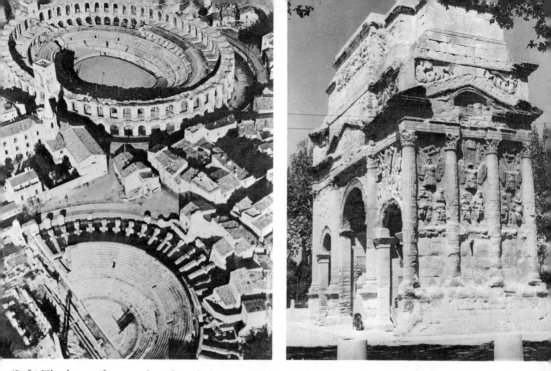

(Left) The theater (foreground) and amphitheater at Arles. These are among the earliest surviving buildings of Roman Gaul and indicate the flourishing condition of the province during the Empire. The amphitheater seated about 20,000 people, the theater about 7,000. (Right) The Arch at Arausio (Orange). The reliefs commemorate the victories of the Second Legion, whose soldiers fought for Julius Caesar against the Gauls and at the siege of Massilia in 49 B.C. Veterans of the legion were settled at Arausio.

victory in Italy, held his force together and solicited help from the rest of Gaul. A national state was to be founded, an *Imperium Galliarum,* with its capital at the city of Trèves. The invitation to independence had some local effect, and the revolt took a serious turn when it was joined by the four Roman legions left on the Rhine. The soldiers, who had supported Vitellius, probably calculated that they would be safer as citizens of a new Gaul than in the hands of Vespasian. The revolt, however, remained local. When a force was sent from Italy by Vespasian's general Mucianus, it rapidly dwindled. The rebellious legions were returned to Roman service, and Civilis fled into Germany. Since the penalties were light, Gaul rapidly returned to the internal development by which it was to become almost more Roman than Italy itself.

By the end of the first century after Christ, the Empire was in a flourishing condition. The *Princeps* and the Senate were on harmonious terms since Trajan, an able and popular ruler, had replaced the weak and ailing Nerva. After the Flavian reorganization of the army, the troops were in good condition and their morale high. The finances of the state were sound, and the processes of Romanization and urbanization in the provinces were proceeding steadily. The Empire was on the threshold of the era known as the Roman Peace, characterized by the historian Gibbon as the happiest and most prosperous period in the history of mankind. Yet there were also signs of stagnation and even of decline.

XXVII

The Roman Peace
I: Government

(A.D. 96–192)

FROM THE ACCESSION OF NERVA to the Principate in 96 until the death of Commodus in 192, the Roman Empire was at the height of its territorial extent and prosperity. This era is often called the Roman Peace, *Pax Romana,* because of the general condition of peace, order, and stability which prevailed. The government ruled over about three and a half million square miles in Europe, Africa, and western Asia, and perhaps as many as seventy million people. Peace was by no means absolute because at the outset Trajan revived the aggressive imperialism of the Republic and added Dacia in Europe and Armenia and Mesopotamia in the East to the Empire. Towards the end of the period Marcus Aurelius had to fight very difficult frontier wars, both in the East where Trajan's conquests had been given up, and along the Danube River. There were sporadic revolts in the more unsettled provinces and rioting by the turbulent populations of the big Eastern cities, like Alexandria, but in general internal peace reigned.

Since the emperors of this era were from the provinces, they naturally devoted much attention to the provincial peoples. Hadrian, in particular, made extensive tours of inspection and spent more time away from Rome than in the city. Little friction existed between the *Princeps* and the Senate because the latter had become representative of the Empire as a whole. The senators acquiesced in the growth of an imperial bureaucracy which took over virtually complete administration of the Empire, but the *Princeps* was not an autocrat in the manner of Nero and Domitian. The educated opinion of the Empire, shared by the rulers themselves, demanded that government be kept to the principles which Augustus had worked out.

Under this harmonious rule the processes of Romanization worked rapidly, and the concepts of the Empire were expressed by both Latin and Greek citizens. Already in the first century after Christ the Roman writer Pliny the Elder (23–79) had stated Rome's mission: "To unite scattered empires, to make man-

The reader will find the Back Endpaper and Map XIX (page 576) useful as he reads this chapter.

ners gentle, to draw together in converse by community of language the jarring and uncouth tongues of so many nations, to give mankind civilization, and in a word to become throughout the world the fatherland of all the races." In the mid-second century a Greek rhetorician, Aelius Aristides (*ca.* 117–85), in a formal address entitled *To Rome,* developed the idea: "You have caused the word Roman to be the label, not of membership in a city, but of some common nationality, and this not just one among all, but one balancing all the rest." To Aelius the world consisted of the Roman Empire, which blended its peoples in common loyalty, and an outer limbo of anarchic barbarism.

The Emperors

NERVA (96–98) AND THE REFORMED PRINCIPATE

Nerva

Before the assassination of Domitian, the senators had picked out a prominent colleague, Marcus Cocceius Nerva, as their candidate for *Princeps.* Nerva was sixty years of age and had had a distinguished senatorial career, but was of unstable health and had little military experience. The Senate accepted him enthusiastically, the praetorian guard was kept quiet by a gift of money, and for the time being the armies acquiesced. Nerva reversed the policies of Domitian. He granted an amnesty to the political offenders of the previous regime and suspended the laws of treason. Various relief measures put into effect in Italy heralded the generally humanitarian character of the Principate in the second century. Loans were made to farmers at low rates of interest, and a welfare program, the alimentary system, as it was called, provided aid for the children of the poor. Nerva, however, proved to lack firmness, and even in his brief reign there was a rash of extortion scandals in the senatorial provinces which the Senate was reluctant to investigate. More significantly, he failed to maintain discipline in the praetorian guard and to gain the goodwill of the legionary soldiers. When his health was failing, Nerva had the good sense to select Marcus Ulpius Traianus, the commander of the army in Upper Germany, as his colleague and successor, a soldier of proven experience who was also acceptable to the Senate. Trajan was adopted by Nerva as his son, given the title Caesar by the Senate and granted tribunician authority and proconsular *imperium.* After three months of association in rule, which kept the armies quiet, Trajan succeeded early in 98 on Nerva's death to the Principate. Selection and adoption of a successor, born of necessity, became standard practice until Marcus Aurelius regrettably chose his own son Commodus to succeed him.

The emperors of the Roman Peace, Nerva, Trajan, Hadrian, Antoninus Pius, and Marcus Aurelius, are generally referred to as the Five Good Emperors. The epithet not only marks the approval of their method of selection by the senatorial class, but also reflects the constitutional nature of their government and the high personal quality of the men as administrators and individuals. By contrast with Domitian who preceded them and Commodus who followed Marcus Aurelius, they excelled.

A conception of the ideal *Princeps,* whom these emperors seemed to approach, had been developed in the course of the preceding century. This concept of the ideal ruler had been elaborated partly by the philosophers, including the Stoics of the Senate, who considered the theoretical aspects of the Principate, and partly by the emperors themselves who emphasized the responsibility of their office in caring for the welfare and safety of the Empire. The rulers had propagandized their service to the state by slogans stressing their foresight and paternal benevolence. In theory the good *Princeps* was selected by divine providence, which ruled the universe, and thus he was not a living god himself but the servant of society, a man who used his power with a high sense of duty to his people. The senators, the best men of the regime, were regarded as the *Princeps'* friends and associates who shared in government and from whom the best was selected as the *Princeps'* successor. The device of adoption had satisfied the desire for a hereditary succession, which was particularly strong in the Eastern part of the Empire and, of course, had been a long-standing practice of Roman upper-class society to maintain the continuity of the family.

The *Princeps* and the eternal city, *Aeterna Roma,* had become symbols of permanence and stability. The long and successful reign of Augustus had firmly associated *Princeps* and state as part of the divine dispensation made by providence for the place of Rome in history. That is, the gods had provided the Empire with a ruler who brought peace and stability and protected the state from danger. Augustus' successors continued to emphasize these functions of the ruler, and Vespasian, in particular, had restored confidence in the Principate. While Domitian damaged the concept, the good emperors confirmed the associated ideas of Rome's eternity and the function of the *Princeps* as its guardian.

TRAJAN (98–117)

The reign of Trajan brought a fresh surge of confidence to the peoples of the Empire, and posterity ranked him almost on a par with Augustus. The senatorial class, of course, contrasted him with the hated Domitian, and to posterity Trajan seemed to have revived the great days of Roman conquest. There was also very solid ground for Trajan's good reputation in the firm and energetic government which he provided for the Empire. Trajan, who came from a prominent Roman family of the Spanish province of Baetica, was the first provincial citizen to become *Princeps.* With this background, and his long and distinguished military career which had begun under Vespasian and taken him to most of the frontiers of the Empire, Trajan had a thorough knowledge of the provinces and wide administrative and military experience. In addition, he was a genial and dignified man in vigorous early middle age at the time of his succession, who inspired friendship and respect among civilians and soldiers alike. At the outset he gave an indication of his quality by speedily clearing up the scandals of provincial government, permitted by Nerva's laxity, without any display of autocracy or cavalier treatment of the Senate.

The relief measures which Nerva had inaugurated in Italy were developed by Trajan. Apparently by the turn of the century Italian farming and industry had begun to show signs of weakness as a result of the competition offered by the Western provinces. There was poverty in the towns and probably a falling birth rate in society when purchasing power declined. The alimentary program was organized to make loans to farmers at a low rate of interest, and the receipts from the interest payments were turned over to the municipalities for child welfare. In the city of Rome poor children were included in the distribution of grain to the public.

The financial affairs of those municipalities in both Italy and the provinces, which were in difficulty, were regulated by the appointment of imperial officials, known as *curators*. They visited the municipalities, inspected the accounts and suggested remedies. The financial stress of the cities arose partly from mismanagement by local, amateur magistrates and partly from the too ambitious building schemes in which they indulged. Trajan also took the municipal affairs of the whole provinces of Greece and Bithynia in hand. His governor in Bithynia, Pliny, carried on an extensive correspondence with the emperor, which reveals Trajan's firm and thorough patience in dealing with the minutiae of provincial government. While the measures taken seem to have been beneficial to the municipalities for the time being, they also marked the first stage of interference by the central government in local autonomy.

In Bithynia Pliny was harassed by the friction between the Christian communities and the Greek citizens in some of the cities of his province. Dislike of the Christians arose mainly, as in the case of the Jews, from their religious exclusiveness and their refusal to participate in civic religious life. Pliny sought guidance from the emperor, and the ruling which Trajan gave set the general policy of the emperors toward Christianity until the mid-third century: "It is not possible to lay down any general rule. . . . No search should be made for these people; when they are discovered and found guilty they should be punished; with the restriction, however, that when the party denies himself to be a Christian, and shall give proof that he is not (that is, by adoring our gods) he shall be pardoned. . . . Information without the accuser's name subscribed must not be admitted against anyone. . . ." That is, the Roman officials were to take no notice, unless an accusation was brought into court against a Christian as such. A test of loyalty might be applied, which consisted of prayer to the emperor and to the gods. Refusal to pray might be construed as guilt, and the offender was to be punished. As in the case of the Jews, the interest of the Roman government was to ensure order. Accusations which were brought by the fellow townsmen of the Christians were to be investigated properly. Evidently the government was not engaged in deliberate persecution or an attempt to stamp out the Christian faith and communities. Local friction produced some martyrs, but Christianity was able to spread through the Eastern part of the Empire and to become an organized church in the general condition of internal peace.

The most significant features of Trajan's imperial policy were the ambitious conquests undertaken against the Dacians and Parthians. The unsatisfactory agreement which Domitian had made with Decebalus, by which Rome contributed to the development of the latter's kingdom, rankled, and the existence of gold mines in the Carpathian Mountains added inducement. In 101 Trajan found a pretext for attack and led the Roman army across the Danube. The terrain was difficult and the resistance of Decebalus skillful and stubborn. Two campaigns were necessary to reduce him to the status of a Roman vassal. To ensure his good behavior Roman garrisons were placed in Dacia, and a permanent stone bridge was built across the Danube near the Iron Gate. Trajan thus followed at this time the standard Roman policy of establishing a subservient *client* kingdom along the frontier.

Three years later, however, in 105, Decebalus broke the arrangement and attacked the Iazyges in Hungary, who were allies of Rome, and massacred the Roman garrisons in his own country. Trajan led a great army of thirteen legions into Dacia, took over the land and made a new Roman province north of the river. Decebalus himself committed suicide, and fifty thousand prisoners of war were taken to Rome to be sold as slaves, ten thousand of them to fight to the death in gladiatorial combats. To repopulate and develop Dacia, Trajan brought in thousands of new settlers from elsewhere in the Empire, from as far afield as Syria and Africa. Romania, the land of the Romans, was born. The gold mines were developed intensively and a new defense system was installed along the Dacian frontiers. The conquest thrust a great triangular salient of Roman territory into Eastern Europe which did protect the provinces south of the Danube and did provide a base for controlling the barbaric tribal peoples to the east and west of the new province, but the lengthening of the frontier imposed additional expense on the Roman military establishment. The armies were brought into contact with more aggressive and ruder people than the semi-Romanized Dacians.

Trajan's aggressive policy towards Parthia was probably motivated in large part by this new concept of defense in great depth, but the initial weakness of the Parthians led the emperor too fast and too far. Chosroes, the king of Parthia, furnished a pretext for invasion by altering the arrangements for Armenia which had been in effect since the settlement made by Corbulo in Nero's reign. At that time it had been provided that the king of Armenia was to be a member of the Parthian royal house but was to receive his crown from the Roman emperor; that is, he was subject to Rome's approval. Chosroes put a relative of his own on the throne but neglected to ask for Roman assent. Since Chosroes and Decebalus had been in amicable negotiation at the time of the Dacian wars, Trajan seized the occasion to lead his armies into Armenia in 113.

At first the conquest went very rapidly, for Trajan had chosen the time well. Chosroes was tied down by the revolts of vassal kings and of the great landholders in the eastern part of the Empire beyond the Tigris River. Trajan overran Armenia in a single campaign and advanced into northern Mesopotamia, apparently with the aim of complete conquest. Perhaps the prospect of success where Crassus and Antony failed was in his mind. Probably, too, the prospect of new territory and control of the caravan routes, by which goods from the Far East were brought to Roman Syria, made the conquest seem profitable. Already in 106 Trajan had found the time to send a successful expedition to the land of the Nabataean Arabs and had formed the province of Arabia. The advance into the Parthian Kingdom was easy and rapid. The Parthian vassal kings in northern Mesopotamia came over to Trajan or fled to the east, and a new province of Mesopotamia was set up. In 116 Trajan crossed the Tigris into the land of Adiabene and called it the province of Assyria. Another thrust carried him down the Tigris, where the capital city, Ctesiphon, was taken. The conquest was rounded off by a voyage down the Tigris to Charax, the port for trade from India at the head of the Persian Gulf.

At the height of his victorious advance Trajan's conquests suddenly crumbled. Since he had taken no time for consolidation, revolts broke out in his wake. Chosroes, who had pulled the eastern part of his kingdom together, advanced to the west. Incited in part by the king's agents, revolts flared among the Jewish population in the Eastern cities of the Empire. The rebellion spread from Cyrene to Egypt and Palestine. Where the Jews gained the upper hand, the Greek population was tortured and put to death. Trajan's attention was diverted from the war against Parthia, and he had to assign one of his most competent, and cruel, generals, Lucius Quietus from Numidia, to suppress the Jews. Quietus ruthlessly restored order in the cities, and Trajan tried to salvage what he could in Parthia. Southern Mesopotamia was made into a vassal kingdom, nominally ruled for Rome by a Parthian prince. Assyria was given up and part of Armenia lost, but Trajan held on to northern Mesopotamia from which he could launch another campaign. The emperor withdrew to Antioch in preparation for a trip to Rome, and then another try against Parthia, but in 117, worn out by the hardships of the past four years, Trajan died in Cilicia on his way back to Rome.

Trajan's reign was remembered not only for his conquests but for one of the most extensive building programs yet to be carried on by an emperor. In Rome Trajan's architect, Apollonius, built the most magnificent of the Imperial Fora, the Forum of Trajan, and celebrated the Dacian conquest by erecting the famous Column of Trajan, which still stands at the end of the emperor's Forum (p. 661). A great archway at the city of Beneventum in southern Italy gave a review of the reign in the relief sculpture on its arches (p. 662). In a more practical vein, four new harbors were constructed in Italy, the most important of which was at the port of Ostia. Throughout the Empire Trajan sponsored an ambitious program of road building, aqueducts, and bridges. In addition to the bridge over the Danube, the handsome stone bridge spanning the Tajus River in Spain, near Alicantara, still recalls Trajan to its present-day users. More land on the desert fringe of Numidia was reclaimed for agriculture, and the large city of Thamugadi (Timgad), whose buildings still dominate the surrounding desert, was begun.

HADRIAN (117–38)

Publius Aelius Hadrianus, the Emperor Hadrian, had had to wait upon Trajan's death for assurance of his adoption and definite selection as successor. Hadrian was in many ways an obvious choice. He was thoroughly experienced, first as a civil magistrate in Rome and then as Trajan's associate in the Dacian and Parthian campaigns. He was also a Spanish Roman, a relative of Trajan, and the emperor's ward from the age of twelve. Perhaps towards the end of his reign Trajan suspected that Hadrian felt little sympathy for continued conquest and so had delayed his decision. In any case, Hadrian was selected by those in attendance on Trajan at his death and was informed of his adoption. He took speedy steps to assure his hold on the Principate. He was acclaimed by the army in Syria and invested with all the proper powers by the Senate in Rome. Before Hadrian arrived in the city in 118, the Senate dealt with an alleged conspiracy of some of Trajan's generals, among them Lucius Quietus, by putting the men to death. Whatever Hadrian's share was in this action, he acted quickly to gain general favor. Liberal gifts were given to the soldiers and to the people of Rome,

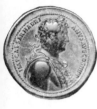

Hadrian

while the Italians and provincials were gratified by a remission of tax arrears for the past fifteen years, at a cost of about $45,000,000.

Hadrian, more than any other emperor of the second century, was responsible for the form of the Empire at its height. He was a skilled general and well liked by the soldiers although he put many of them to work on building the defenses of the frontiers, which began to acquire a permanent form in his reign. His model in administration was Augustus, whom he rivaled in shrewd and wise statesmanship, and the goals of the reign were peace and internal consolidation to restore the Empire after the strenuous wars of Trajan. Accordingly, the imperial bureaucracy was formalized and enlarged, and a tremendous program of building and development was launched in the provinces. Hadrian's legal experts undertook the first great codification of Roman law, to bring it into accord with the increasing complexity of administration.

While these achievements were sufficient for one emperor, Hadrian had a complex and restless personality which demanded an intense, individual life. As well as an expert in military fortification, he was an enthusiastic and highly gifted amateur architect. Presumably the Pantheon in Rome, the Mausoleum of Hadrian, now called the Castel San Angelo, and his own villa at Tibur (Tivoli), the most magnificent of Roman villas, owed much to his own conception and detailed planning. A Greek education, which had taken him to Athens as a young man, and his personal taste for literature and art predisposed him to appreciate the Hellenic provinces of the Empire. His official patronage encouraged the renaissance of Hellenism which characterized the intellectual life of the second century. Hadrian, however, was no absurd dilettante like Nero but a highly versatile and percipient man, who could turn from the problems of the frontiers to the minutiae of civil administration, or from both to the composition of poetry and aesthetic enjoyment of Greek literature and art. He shared the humanitarian interests of his age and passed legislation to protect the personal rights of children and slaves from abuse by their fathers and masters. He also had a statesmanlike vision of humane civilization for the Empire. He founded or endowed schools of rhetoric in the Eastern cities and granted exemptions from taxation to doctors and professors.

In pursuance of his goal of peace Hadrian abandoned the conquest of Parthia and made a treaty with Chosroes, by which Rome gave up all but a small part of northern Mesopotamia and returned to the previous arrangements for Armenia. The Parthians showed no disposition to break the treaty even when the Roman forces in the East were tied down by Jewish revolt in Palestine. Dacia, however, was retained, and Hadrian himself fought skillfully and courageously along the lower Danube in the early part of his reign to check the barbarian attacks in that region.

The most strenuous war of his reign was hardly of Hadrian's own seeking. It was fought from 132 to 135 in Palestine against the Jews who rose in revolt at the emperor's plan to found a new Roman city, Aelia Capitolina, on the site of Jerusalem which was still in ruins from the destruction of Titus. Bands of Jewish patriots, the Zealots, harassed the Roman officials and troops by assassination and raids until war flared up under the leadership of Bar Kochba, the Son of the Star, a self-proclaimed Messiah of the Jewish people. For three years the Jews fought the Roman army in the difficult terrain of Palestine, taking and holding Jerusalem in the process. They were finally defeated and broken as a nation for the rest of antiquity. Many towns in Palestine were destroyed and looted, the prisoners of war and their families were sold into slavery, and the land was reorganized as non-Jewish territory. Jerusalem became a new Roman city and the Jews were forbidden to use it for their religious purposes. As individuals in the cities of the Empire, the Jews were granted the same privilege that they had under Vespasian—practice of their religion under license—but revival of religious nationalism in Palestine was made impossible.

Hadrian's care for the provinces and his own restless energy took him on two lengthy tours of inspection from 121 to 125 and 128 to 133, in the course of which he traveled from Britain to the Syrian Desert and visited almost every province of the Empire. The provinces of Greece and Asia were favored above all because of his personal interests. In Athens Hadrian completed the building of the Temple of Zeus Olympios, begun by the tyrant Peisistratus about six hundred years before, added a new suburb to the city, constructed a large library, and was himself initiated into the Eleusinian Mysteries. In the rest of the Empire his building program was also extensive. A new city rose in Thrace, Hadrianopolis (Edirne), whose settlers were drawn mainly from the veterans of his Danubian campaign. In Egypt Hadrian built a Greek city, Antinoopolis, far up the Nile to commemorate his favorite, Antinous, a handsome Greek boy from Bithynia, to whom he was attached by erotic idealism. The emperor himself planned its civic and religious organization, the latter designed to worship Antinous as a god.

While Hadrian began his reign on good terms with the Senate and continued until his death to accord senators both respect and dignity, after his death it required all the persuasiveness of Antoninus, his successor, to secure deification for his predecessor. The long absences from Rome erected a barrier to understanding, and with all but close intimates Hadrian was aloof and cool. While the senators hardly expected to take an increased part in government, Hadrian's enlargement of the bureaucracy cut into their remaining prerogatives. For example, the administration of justice in Italy, formerly the care of the Senate and praetors, was taken from them. Italy was divided into four juridical districts which were administered by judges of consular rank appointed by the emperor. The arrangement particularly offended the Senate's dignity and later was canceled by Antoninus.

During Hadrian's reign, too, the issuance of legislation was shifted markedly from the Senate to the imperial side of the government. Hadrian seems to have made his *consilium* on legal matters, the group of men whom he consulted for such purposes, into a more formal body by including several recognized jurisconsults. Experts had been consulted by emperors previously, but this group invited by Hadrian formed a sort of nucleus which was regularly included in meetings with his associates. The whole council helped him to frame legislation which was issued in the form of an imperial edict, rather than a resolution of the Senate. That body might still be called to legislate, as a matter of courtesy, but from the time of Hadrian the emperor became a regular source of law and the legal experts increasingly important. One of Hadrian's experts, Salvius Julianus, was charged with a formal revision of the praetors' edict, to purge it of contradictions and obsolete rules and make a Permanent Edict (*Edictum Perpetuum*).

Towards the end of his reign, in 136, Hadrian dealt swiftly and surely with a small conspiracy, engineered by his brother-in-law, the latter's son, and several men of senatorial rank. This action raised the old bogey of treason trials, although Hadrian made no move to extend prosecution to those who merely might have talked indiscreetly, or to change his general attitude of cool courtesy to the senators.

In 136, when Hadrian became seriously ill of a heart ailment, he began to plan the succession. He himself was childless and by no means well disposed toward most of his relatives. Although he lived on terms of distant politeness with his wife, a niece of Trajan, the conspiracy of his brother-in-law had alienated that connection from consideration. The emperor's first choice was a young man of senatorial rank, Lucius Ceionius Verus, who seems to have resembled Hadrian in temperament and had long been a favorite. Verus, however, became ill and died during the year after his adoption as the emperor's son. Hadrian's next choice was a middle-aged senator, Titus Aurelius Antoninus, a man of almost blameless reputation. In the manner of Augustus, Hadrian tried to control the future succession also. Antoninus was requested to adopt both the infant son of the dead Verus and Hadrian's own nephew, Marcus Aurelius.

Hadrian spent the last two years of his reign awaiting death in his villa at Tibur, where he had surrounded himself with reminders of his career and personal tastes. Villa is scarcely the term to apply to Hadrian's estate, for it was a great complex of buildings, parks, and gardens. In addition to a palace and administrative offices, there were private retreats, baths, exercise areas, a theater, library, and colonnades. Nearby the emperor built a replica of the sanctuary of Serapis at Alexandria which he called the Canopus and in which he placed a statue of his favorite, Antinous, sculptured in the Egyptian style. Some of the buildings were called by names famous in the intellectual history of antiquity: the Academy, the Lyceum, and the Painted *Stoa*. Hadrian died in 138 and was buried in the great mausoleum where he had already placed the body of Verus, his adopted son. The emperor had written his epitaph sometime before, with characteristic and studied insouciance:

> Little soul, gentle and drifting, guest and companion
> of my body, now you will dwell below in pallid places,
> stark and bare; there you will abandon your play of yore.

Despite his play, Hadrian had found time to be a distinguished ruler, a highly remarkable individual, and to die with proper forethought for the succession.

ANTONINUS PIUS (138–61)

Antoninus Pius

The epithet Pius, which the Emperor Antoninus shared with Vergil's Aeneas, was given to him for his filial devotion in securing Hadrian's deification from the Senate. That was only proper, for Antoninus reaped the fruits of Hadrian's hard work and modeled his reign on that of his predecessor. Antoninus was himself representative of the best in the upper-class society of the period, wealthy, well educated, and with a wide experience in administration and an interest in improvement of the law. He had been governor of Asia and a member of Hadrian's *consilium*. Since Antoninus came to the Principate at the age of fifty-two and was naturally a conservative, stable individual, he made few changes and innovations. His particular contribution to the growth of the Principate was in the administration of law, where the use of equity and humanitarian considerations was further developed. Antoninus governed efficiently from Rome, partly from a disinclination to travel, partly because the machine of government functioned well, and the Empire was almost free from revolts and attacks along the frontiers. He did extend the frontier of Britain to the north and was troubled by Parthian encroachment in Armenia, but, on the whole, the reign of Antoninus marked the culmination of the Roman Peace, and the emperor received an accolade of praise from senators, provincials, and cities alike. Upon Antoninus' death in 161 Marcus Aurelius, whom he had adopted at Hadrian's request, succeeded and associated his adoptive brother, Lucius Verus, with himself as a colleague. For the first time two emperors (*Augusti*) shared the rule.

MARCUS AURELIUS (161–80)

The general peace which had prevailed during the period of Antoninus was disturbed in the reign of Marcus Aurelius and Verus by almost continuous warfare along the frontiers. In the East the Parthians invaded Syria and devastated its lands. Along the Danube the Marcomanni and the other peoples west of Dacia broke through the defenses and reached Aquileia at the head of the Adriatic. Along the lower Danube other barbarians crossed the river and devastated the frontier provinces. The legions fighting in the East were struck by a plague, possibly smallpox, which spread from Syria through the Eastern provinces and into Europe. When the costs of war temporarily bankrupted the imperial treasury, Marcus Aurelius had to sell his family jewels and plate to tide over the situation.

We know Marcus Aurelius, who faced and resolved these crises, more intimately than other emperors for he wrote down his thoughts in the latter years of the fighting along the Danube. They were published in a book called the *Meditations.* As a young man Marcus Aurelius had become a Stoic and had made its principles into his personal religion. In the *Meditations* he revealed an almost fatal acquiescence in his lot as *Princeps:* "Now to set a certain time to every man's actions, belongs unto him only, who as first he was of thy composition, so is now the cause of thy dissolution. As for thyself, thou hast to do with neither. Go thy ways then well pleased and contented, for so is he that dismisseth thee." While this mood might not seem to be the best in which to deal with a military crisis, Marcus Aurelius was unflinching. Under his direction Roman generals invaded Parthia, and he himself pushed the barbarians back across the Danube. At the time of his death the emperor was engaged in organizing new provinces north of the river to serve, like Dacia, as a bulwark against fresh invasions.

The long years of peace under Antoninus had bred slackness and inefficiency in the Roman armies and served as an incubation period of revolt for the peoples across the frontiers. The Parthian King Vologeses III had pulled his kingdom together and felt strong enough to attack. The Germanic peoples north of the Danube, the Marcomanni, Quadi, and Iazyges, had coalesced into strong kingships, like that of the Dacians a century earlier, and the Roman provinces south of the river offered a richer field for plunder. Behind the semi-Romanized peoples along the river, new tribal peoples in Eastern Europe were pushing against their backs and forcing them toward the Roman lands.

In 162 Vologeses III took over Armenia and broke into Syria . Marcus Aurelius himself remained in Rome and sent his co-ruler, Lucius Verus, to organize the defense. Legions were shifted from their bases on the Danube, but Verus, apparently somewhat indolent by nature, allowed the field command to be exercised by his generals, Statius Priscus and Avidius Cassius. Priscus recovered Armenia, while Cassius, a strict disciplinarian, restored morale and efficiency in the Syrian legions. Then Cassius was given general command over Cilicia, Syria, and Palestine, and struck back at the Parthians along the lines of attack which Trajan had used. The Romans advanced from Armenia into northern Mesopotamia and crossed the lower Euphrates. They took the great Parthian cities of Ctesiphon and Seleucia on the Tigris and in the winter of 164/65 were preparing for an advance into Media. At this point the plague struck the army which forced a general retreat into Syria. From the camps in Syria the disease spread into Egypt and Asia Minor, followed the line of communication up the Danube, and hit northern Italy and Gaul. In 166, however, the Roman armies in Syria returned successfully to the offensive. Part of northern Mesopotamia was permanently occupied, and Armenia was made into a *client* kingdom. The Parthians had not only been rolled back, but Rome had improved its defensive position.

While the plague was raging and the Parthian War unfinished, the barbarians along the western Danube broke through the weakened defenses. In 167 a large group entered Raetia and penetrated to the head of the Adriatic, where they besieged Aquileia and started to spread into northern Italy. This was the first serious threat to the heart of the Empire since the days of Marius, almost three hundred years earlier. The Empire's communications between Western Europe and the Balkan provinces were imperiled, but the generals on either side of the corridor in Raetia and Pannonia reduced the peril with their forces, while Aurelius and Verus marched north from Italy, rolling the main group back. The success was temporary. Two years later the barbarians raided again in force, while on the lower Danube the Costobacci broke through.

Marcus Aurelius began to develop a solution for the problem along the lines which Trajan had marked out by the conquest of Dacia. Instead of merely pushing the Germans back across the Danube, he planned to set up two new provinces in Hungary, Bohemia, and Moravia, to the west of Dacia. By this action he would have shortened the northern frontier and made a deep defensive zone. By 175 the emperor was on the point of achieving his aim after hard fighting when news came that Avidius Cassius had been acclaimed *Princeps* by the Syrian armies. Perhaps Avidius was too ambitious, but a report had been re-

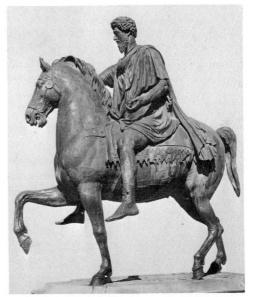

Marcus Aurelius. Equestrian bronze statue in Rome. The emperor as imperator *addresses his army and people.*

ceived in Syria that Marcus Aurelius was dead. The situation was potentially serious because Egypt had declared for Avidius and the grain supply of Rome was threatened. As soon as news came that the emperor was alive and on the point of setting out to the East to recover control, the troops had a change of heart and some of Avidius' officers killed him.

The interruption, however, had forced Marcus Aurelius to make a premature settlement with the Danubian peoples. Although they agreed to withdraw from the north bank of the river for five miles, to leave a neutral zone, they were granted trading rights through Dacia. Barbarian peoples were brought in to restore the population of the ravaged frontier provinces. In return for land the new settlers were made liable for military service or enlisted as mercenaries in the Roman formations. Germans were thus employed to fight Germans, and a mass of non-Romanized people was introduced into the Empire. While this temporarily solved the military situation, a new process of assimilation and Romanization had to begin.

Marcus Aurelius, however, returned to the idea of setting up new provinces and in 177 launched a third war against the Marcomanni. His colleague Verus had died in 169, and taking warning from the acclamation of Avidius Cassius, Marcus named his own son, Commodus, co-ruler at the age of sixteen. Their campaigns were successful, but just as Aurelius had begun to organize the new provinces, he died at Vindobona (Vienna) in 180, and Commodus succeeded. The damage done by barbarian raids, plague, and the excessive costs of war was considerable, but Marcus Aurelius had protected the frontiers and won a period of peace from external attack. The Empire needed another Vespasian or Hadrian, but in Commodus it got another Gaius.

COMMODUS (180–92)

Commodus hastened to conclude an agreement with the barbarians on the general lines of his father's previous arrangement. The new provinces were given up and the Roman troops were withdrawn to the old frontiers. Peace was restored at the price of renewed attacks in the future, while Commodus returned to Rome. The new emperor was a handsome young man, inexperienced in administration, and largely untrained for rule. The latter was no fault of his own, but Commodus was indolent, colossally vain, and perhaps vicious to the edge of lunacy. For several years some appearance of conscientious administration was maintained through the efforts of Marcus Aurelius' advisers, but Commodus soon began to leave decisions to his favorites and to treat the Senate with contempt. A conspiracy against his life in 182 was the prelude to ten years of prosecutions against reputable senators whom Commodus disliked. Commodus himself seems to have had no political ideas other than his self-glorification. His last announced intention was to appear before the Roman people on New Year's Day to assume the consulship in a gladiator's lion skin, in which guise he conceived of himself as the earthly incarnation of Hercules. But the Romans were not yet ready for divine monarchy, and Commodus' own intimates could not

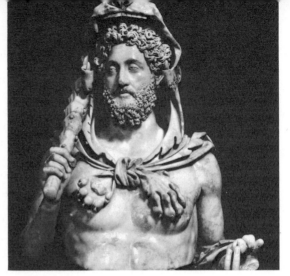

Commodus. The emperor wears the attributes, a lion skin and club, of Hercules, patron of his gladiatorial exploits.

live with him in safety. In 192, through the connivance of one of his current mistresses, the emperor was strangled. Fortunately for the Empire Commodus had stayed in Rome and concentrated on his gladiatorial training instead of interfering with provincial government. The chance for orderly reorganization had been lost, and on Commodus' death the Empire was torn again by civil war. The Roman state could endure a great deal, but its character was transformed by the crises of the third century. It is time to discuss the structure and society of the Empire at its height, before examining the breakdown.

The Empire

THE IMPERIAL BUREAUCRACY

Although theoretically, and even in outward appearance, the Senate remained the *Princeps'* partner at the height of the Empire, virtually all the functions of government had come under the emperor's direction. The prestige of the Senate remained very high, not only because of the continuous tradition of seven hundred years of government, but also because of the social position of the members. They were recruited from the great landowners of Italy and of the Empire and from the eminent Equestrians who had risen to the highest posts in the emperor's administration. While senators from Italy probably predominated in number until the third century, the body was genuinely representative of the Romanized Western provinces and to an ever increasing degree of the Empire as a whole. Republican sentiment had almost died out, except as a reminiscence —in the time of Hadrian there seem to have been only about thirty members from families which had survived from the Republic. The idea of Italian primacy still had some strength but largely as a matter of tradition and because of the position of Rome as capital. In general, both Senate and *Princeps* shared the same broad views of Empire, and, with the exceptions which we have noticed, relations between them were harmonious. The emperors not only tried to make them so, but the emperors themselves were more genuinely representative of the Senate than they had been in the past.

629

Yet the trends to full direction of government by the *Princeps,* which Augustus and his successors had set in motion, culminated in the time of Hadrian and the Antonine Emperors. The prefects and the commissions appointed by the *Princeps* had taken the government of the city of Rome and of Italy almost entirely out of the hands of the magistrates. The right of election, which the assembly had lost to the Senate in the reign of Tiberius, became meaningless after the mid-first century as a result of the emperor's nominations and recommendations of all candidates. The magistrates, if they were ambitious and energetic, looked forward to a career under the *Princeps* rather than in their traditional duties of office, except, of course, as the governors of senatorial provinces. The process of legislation was kept in the hands of the *Princeps* by the controlled resolutions of the Senate and from the time of Hadrian through the recognition of the emperor's edicts and legal verdicts as the source of law. The jurisconsults of the emperor explained the new source of law by the theory, developed from the nature of the office, that the *Princeps* was the representative of the whole people. The source of decision and action in government, then, was the *Princeps* and his advisory councils, *consilia,* rather than the *Princeps* and the Senate.

This centralization of government was accompanied by the growth of a complex and formalized imperial bureaucracy. It was divided into great departments of state, the heads of which consulted with the *Princeps,* while the staff rose up a fixed ladder of promotion and salary scale. The bureaucracy was established as an imperial service by the final conversion of the household offices, which Claudius had developed from his own freedmen, into true departments of state by the multiplication of imperial prefectures and commissions. It was staffed in the middle and upper grades by Equestrians, who followed what is called a procuratorial career. The career service was made truly imperial by drawing men from the upper classes of the provinces as Roman citizenship was extended. In the lower grades freedmen were employed as clerks and secretaries, and soldiers were assigned to administrative work by the governors of imperial provinces. This junior personnel tended to remain fixed, but the careerists would hold a variety of offices in different parts of the Empire until the most efficient and aggressive obtained the important prefectures and were enrolled in the Senate by the emperor. In a sense the Senate itself was drawn into the bureaucracy by the overall direction of government by the *Princeps* and by his use of ex-consuls and praetors for special posts. While the Equestrian career was open to talent and its followers were mobile, it must be remembered that a sizable personal property of about twenty thousand dollars was necessary to qualify as an Equestrian. Deserving and qualified freedmen and officers of junior grade in the army might be promoted to Equestrian rank, but the imperial government was largely a government by the upper classes and was confined to them.

The functions of the bureaucracy had been widely extended to include

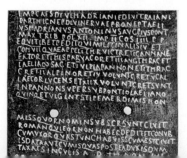

Military diploma granting citizenship to honorably discharged soldiers (reign of Antoninus Pius)

operations which had been previously under senatorial control, and those which had once been private to the *Princeps* or under the local government of the cities. For example, the taking of the census, which had been carried out by the cities of the Empire in their own districts, was placed under imperial procurators. The appointment of imperial *curators* from the time of Trajan infringed on the municipalities' control of their own finances. The tax-collecting functions of the procurators were enlarged to collect the inheritance taxes in all the provinces, as the Roman citizens who were liable for them increased in number. By the time of Antoninus the use of the contract system to collect taxes in the senatorial provinces had been assigned to the procurators of the imperial service. Hadrian established new officials, the *advocati fisci,* who had the power to prosecute individuals for recovery of tax arrears. The vast private estates of the *Princeps* also were placed under the direction of imperial procurators. Imperial communications, to relay the government's orders to the various parts of the Empire, were at first administered by freedmen, but in Trajan's reign came to be supervised by a special department headed by a prefect who administered from Rome. In each province a subordinate official arranged the staging posts, the supply of horses, and accommodations for the messengers. The imperial orders flew along the roads of the Empire, but private communications were left to the individual's own arrangements.

Within the bureaucracy the offices were classified in four categories marked by their differing pay scales. In the lowest grade were the *sexagenarii,* who received 60,000 sesterces a year, then the *centenarii,* at 100,000, the *ducenarii* at 200,000 and at the top the *trecenarii* at 300,000. Among the latter were the imperial prefects. In this system, status titles came into being which were used for senators and for the upper grades of Equestrians. The senators were called *viri clarissimi* (most illustrious). The Equestrian titles were *egregius* (distinguished), *perfectissimus* (most perfect), and *eminentissimus* (most eminent), the latter being reserved for the prefects. All these were titles of office and were not hereditary in character.

The members of the civil service were very proud of their careers. We know of the civil service in detail mainly through the thousands of inscriptions which record honors paid by a grateful community to a distinguished bureaucrat or those honors which family pride recorded on a tombstone. The following inscription gives the career of one Gaius Junius Flavianus, who started as a tribune in the Seventh German Legion and became prefect of the grain supply: "In honor of Gaius Junius Flavianus, son of Gaius, prefect of the grain supply (his highest post), procurator of the treasury, procurator of the provinces of Lugdunensis and Aquitania (in Gaul), procurator of the inheritance tax in Hither Spain for the districts of Asturia and Callaecia, procurator of the Maritime Alps, department head in the office of the inheritance tax (his first civil office), tribune of the soldiers in the Seventh German Legion, a minor priest." The inscription was paid for by a group of grain and olive oil merchants, who subscribed to it in honor of the prefect for some service which he had done for them.

PROVINCIAL ADMINISTRATION

The government of the Empire during the first and second centuries after Christ exhibited a remarkable blend of carefully supervised central administration and of local freedom in the urban communities, the characteristic units of the provinces. The result was the tremendous growth in urbanization and prosperity which the remains of cities attest, from the Atlantic to the Middle East, and from the Sahara to the Rhine and the Danube. While it will be more convenient to discuss the organization of the cities in the following chapter in connection with the society of the Empire, we might look here briefly at the general picture of administration.

There was little formal change in the system from the time of the Republic (pp. 481–84), but the provinces were markedly more prosperous and contented. As before, the governors were responsible for administration, justice, and, in the imperial provinces, for their armies and for military protection. Already in the last century of the Republic there had been a growing concern about the abuses which the provincials suffered. Cicero had spoken out against them, and Sulla and Julius Caesar had passed carefully framed laws to check them. Caesar's law of 59 B.C. remained the basis for curbing extortion throughout the whole period of the Empire and was developed and refined. Although extortion and malpractice by governors and procurators were certainly not rare in the Empire, the standards of provincial administration improved under the emperor's supervision. The best of the rulers, however, were very busy men and the Empire was very large. Probably the imperial provinces fared best, but it remained difficult for all provincials to bring their grievances to the emperor's attention. The provincials were timid about charging their governors and prosecuting them before the Senate.

The means of bringing cases of extortion to the emperor's attention were improved to some extent by the creation of the provincial assemblies which had originated in the spread of ruler cult. Yet these had to get general agreement among their delegates for such a complaint, and they met only once a year at the annual festival. But the emperors did listen to and investigate these official complaints and the petitions of individual cities. Perhaps more than any very great improvement in the quality of administration, the benefits of peace and the gradual raising of the status of the provincials themselves to the same level as the Romans, facilitated the material well-being of the people of the Empire.

The provincial assemblies were the chief instrument of provincial self-government, but they could scarcely develop beyond a certain point because of collision with the trend to centralized administration. They were useful in that they provided a personal tie between the *Princeps* and the provincials of the upper class. Their presidents, elected annually, were figures of great importance in their own provinces and came to hold membership in the assemblies for life, perhaps by imitation of the life membership in the Roman Senate. They were known as high priest, *archiereus,* in the Greek East, and *flamen,* or *sacerdos,* in the

Romanized West. The religious title indicates the main function of the president: to preside at the sacrifices and annual assembly for the worship of the ruler. The enthusiasm of the delegates and high priests for their association is indicated by the lavish gifts, both money and buildings, which individuals made to supplement the small contributions of the member-cities of the assembly. Although they often represented the provinces to the *Princeps,* the role of the assemblies was sometimes reversed. The *Princeps* used them to publicize his edicts to the cities of a province. The assemblies, however, possessed no coercive control over their membership, and the regular channel of administration was through the governor and the imperial officials.

The administrative picture which the provinces presented was extremely varied. By the time of Hadrian there were forty-five provinces in contrast to the fourteen of the Late Republic, and the Romans had adjusted administration to the character of each when it entered the Empire and as it developed. Some new provinces, like Britain, had been added by conquest; others formed from former *client* kingdoms, while some were made by splitting up large provinces into smaller units. The basic element in each was the local community (*civitas*) which might vary from a native village, town, or city under the governor's administration, to the self-governing tribal communes of Gaul and the municipalities and Roman colonies in other provinces. As we have noticed, the policy of the Empire was to encourage self-government, which at least cut down the costs of administration.

In many provinces there were also vast imperial estates belonging to the *Princeps* and administered by imperial procurators. Africa in the second century, and Asia Minor in the third, held many of these. In the case of Africa the land had been acquired largely by Nero through confiscation of the property of his enemies in the Senate. The estates in Asia Minor were obtained in the same manner by the Severan Emperors in the early third century. The estates were called *tractus,* or *regiones,* and consisted of thousands of acres of land. They were subdivided into separate large farms, the *fundi* or *saltus.* An imperial procurator was assigned to administer a tract, on which he leased the large farms to tenant contractors, the *conductores.* These worked part of the land themselves and sublet the remainder in small parcels to tenant farmers, the *coloni.* These latter might be immigrant Italians, as in Africa, but more usually were natives who lived in villages on the estates. The *colonus* was a sharecropper, who paid part of his rent in a fixed proportion of the crop and, in addition, performed some work on the land of the contractor. The latter thus solved his own labor problem, but the obligation was a sore point to the *coloni.* The latter were encouraged to occupy and to develop vacant land, and by the time of Hadrian had come to be regarded as life possessors. They were not, however, tied permanently to the land or placed in a serflike status until the Late Empire.

In addition to the imperial estates, there were also great private estates owned by Roman senators and wealthy Equestrians or by the wealthy natives of the provincial upper class. These, too, were usually worked by tenant farmers although the owner might maintain a villa on the estate, while he himself spent most of his time in a city or in imperial service. The temple estates in Asia Minor and Syria, a legacy from the past, were managed by priests and worked by temple serfs. The Roman government seldom attempted to change their character and was satisfied by the payment of rent. The mining properties of a province, like the imperial estates, were also directly managed by imperial procurators. Spain, whose mines provided the west with gold, silver, copper, and tin, is especially well-known in this respect from the survival of some of the regulations drafted for its mining towns.

THE DEFENSE OF THE FRONTIERS

In the reign of Hadrian the conversion of the frontier defense lines into permanent form, already begun by the Flavians in southern Germany, proceeded rapidly. Because Hadrian's policy was that of peace and internal consolidation, the army adopted a defensive role. On the frontiers he built walls of stone and timber which stretched for hundreds of miles, giving the Empire a strong outward appearance, while internally it remained peaceful and unarmed.

The ramparts were built in regions where no natural barriers existed, such as broad rivers and desert, and where barbarian pressure was continuous. In England the Wall of Hadrian, about eighty miles in length, was constructed from Newcastle on Tyne to the Solway Firth, to help protect the land from the predatory Caledonians of the Scotch Highlands. In Northumberland, where local stone was available, the wall was built of stone blocks over a core of rubble and mortar, ten feet in thickness. Elsewhere it was of turf and timber. The height was uniformly twenty feet, and before the wall was a ditch, thirty feet in depth. The wall linked a series of seventeen forts, each designed to hold a garrison of about a thousand men, and incorporated in it were mile-castles and signal towers for

The Wall of Hadrian, which guarded northern England from Newcastle-on-Tyne to the Solway Firth

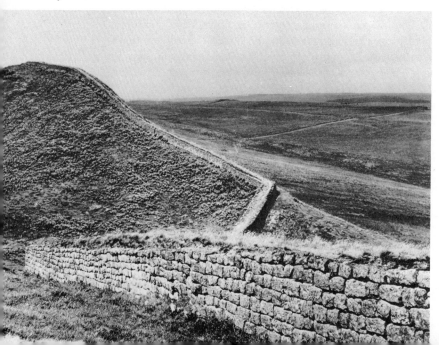

the patrolling sentries. There were gates at intervals to permit peaceful traffic, and considerable trade developed with the Scotch Lowlands.

The wall was an obstacle to smugglers, seeking to avoid the customs offices at the gates, and to raiding parties of moderate size, but the Romans deployed their forces to check large-scale attacks by battle in the field rather than turn them back from the wall. The auxiliaries who garrisoned the forts were counted on to engage the enemy in front of the wall in order to enable the legions to prepare an organized campaign if a breakthrough was made. The soldiers of the legions were quartered in large base camps, such as Eboracum (York), well behind the wall to give them room for maneuver. When the Scotch Lowlands became partially Romanized, Antoninus Pius enlarged the area of Roman territory by building another wall of turf from the Firth of Forth to the Clyde. This wall, however, was abandoned in the early third century, and Roman Britain retreated to Hadrian's Wall.

The frontier region between the upper Rhine and the Danube known as the German *Limites* was somewhat similarly protected. Domitian had already constructed fortifications which were reorganized and given permanent form by Hadrian and his successors. The term *limites,* used in reference to the frontier fortifications, originally designated the system of military roads in a frontier area, and as forts and guard houses grew up along them, the term was applied to the whole complex of installations along the frontier line. The German *Limites* stretched for about 345 miles, from Rheinbroll to Heinheim on the Danube. Hadrian's soldiers put in a palisade of split-oak trunks, nine feet in height, along the whole line and protected it by a shallow ditch. Forts of timber and earth were constructed near the wall. At a later date these were converted into stone, and in the early third century the Emperor Caracalla rebuilt the Raetian section of the wall, 105 miles, in stone. As in Britain, the wall was designed primarily to control the border traffic and to discourage small raiding parties, while the real defense was provided by the auxiliaries on the line and the legions behind it. Elsewhere in Europe the Rhine and the Danube rivers, both formidable obstacles, were the defensive lines. The rivers were held by fortifications near the weak points, where crossings were possible, by river patrols and by large, permanent base camps.

The *limites* in Asia and Africa never acquired the permanent form which those of Europe had, and protection from raids was provided by an excellent road system, patrolled by soldiers stationed in small forts. Strategic communication points in the rear, through which full-scale invasion would have had to pass, were held by legionary bases and, where possible, by quartering the legions in cities. In some regions, like the Libyan plateau to the south of Cyrene, the landholders lived in fortified farms and formed a sort of border militia. As we have noticed, few troops were needed for the African frontier; consequently the great army groups were stationed behind the Rhine, the Danube, and the Euphrates rivers.

The army was deployed again, after Trajan's aggressive campaigns, for a permanent role in the new defenses. Extensive changes were made in organization by which the practical distinctions between legions and auxiliaries were obliterated. The auxiliaries were given the same training and weapons and were stationed along the frontier lines, while the legions were kept in the big base camps to the rear. They might be shifted from time to time, but the auxiliaries tended to become a fixed frontier guard. Both, however, were recruited locally, often from the same families, for sons tended to follow their father's profession. Close to the permanent forts and the legionary bases civilian settlements (*canabae*) sprang up, where the soldiers found wives and where they usually settled after their discharge. Hadrian raised many of the towns which served as legionary headquarters to municipal status and honored them with his visits.

In the place of the auxiliaries, which had become heavy-armed infantry, like the legions, Hadrian developed other units, the *numeri,* which had appeared in the army during the Flavian Period. These were recruited from the same areas and the same rural section of the population as the auxiliaries, but were named from their place of origin and referred to collectively as foreign troops. They were, however, a regular part of the Roman army and worked closely with the auxiliaries as light-armed troops and cavalry. Apparently, they were also subject to the same conditions of service and, because they used Latin as a common language, became Romanized like the auxiliaries.

The effects of this military development on the Empire were far-reaching. The establishment of such an organization added considerable cost to the already expensive imperial bureaucracy and yet did not really solve the problems of defense. When a major breakthrough was made, as in the reign of Marcus Aurelius, much time was required to concentrate the scattered legions from their bases and to get them moving in a concerted campaign. War on two fronts simultaneously had strained the resources of the Empire almost to the breaking point. The system also restored the potential danger, which Vespasian had sought to correct, of the growth of an *esprit de corps* in the separate groups of legionary soldiers and auxiliaries.

There were also psychological effects on both civilians and soldiers. The citizens of the long-settled and peaceful provinces showed little inclination to serve in the army. The security provided by the seemingly impregnable ring of defenses gave no stimulus, and ordinary citizens had no knowledge of the cares of imperial government. In short, they saw no need for their own services in the army and became temperamentally unfit for it. This same feeling, of course, tended to pervade the thinking of the more recent citizens of the frontier provinces once the privileges of citizenship had been secured. Accordingly, the government recruited more and more from the rural and less Romanized elements, who found soldiering congenial or who hoped to improve their status. Since the burden of defense was borne by the ruder peoples of the frontier provinces, one of the apparent privileges of citizenship was freedom from military service. The very concept of Empire, in fact, was affected by the defensive ring. The frontiers shaped the form of the Roman Empire, called the Circle of the Lands (*Orbis Terrarum*). Behind these walls was the home of civilized men.

THE EMPIRE AND THE OUTER WORLD

While the lasting influences of Roman civilization were felt almost wholly within the provinces of the Empire, directly under Roman administration and affected by the processes of Romanization, Roman interests extended far beyond the frontiers. Much of the concern, of course, was political and a part of the policy of defense. Diplomatic missions were sent to make allies and to play on the divisions existing among the barbarian peoples close to the European frontiers. As we have seen, diplomacy, rather than war, was also the preferred policy towards Parthia. But since the wealthy upper class of the Empire was anxious to acquire certain foreign luxury goods, the government took a limited part in commercial expansion. The exchange of expensive gifts was a recognized part of diplomacy with foreign peoples. The emperors entertained missions from states as far afield as India, which expressed a desire to trade with the Empire. Revenues were drawn from the customs levies imposed at the Roman termini of the Eastern caravan routes, such as Palmyra and Damascus, and at the entry gates on the European frontiers. Part of this trade was carried on by traders from the Empire; part of it, across remote regions, was indirect and through the medium of foreign traders. While there was little mutual influence on the institutions and ideas of either party, the range of trade and the variety of articles exchanged are surprising.

In Europe Roman trade extended into the Scandinavian countries, across Germany into Poland, into the regions north of the Danube, and around the Black Sea. First Italy, then the Western provinces of the Empire, exported silver plate, bronze vessels, pottery, and coins, the latter regarded as bullion or jewelry. One trade route led from the head of the Adriatic to the Danube and through the lands of the Marcomanni, where trade was carried on with both purchasers and middlemen. Another route was from Gaul across the Rhine into western Germany or by sea along the coast of Denmark into the Baltic. Most of the

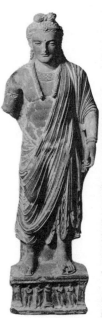

Right: Gandhara (India) sculpture, showing Greco-Roman influence in the pose and the details of hair and drapery

Below: Roman craft products: millefiori glass bowl and silver dish

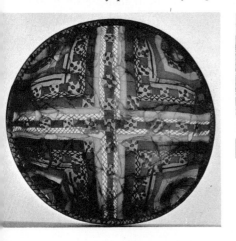

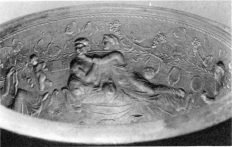

articles found in archaeological excavation seem to be trade goods although some are presumably diplomatic gifts to win the favor of tribal chieftains, while others are from the plunder obtained in raids. In return, the Romans probably received slaves, hides, furs, cattle, horses, and amber from the Baltic. Close to the frontier this exchange was accompanied by a cultural Romanization, which became less intense as the distance from Rome increased. Thorough Romanization of the tribal peoples could be accomplished only when they were inside the frontiers. The Empire, however, became known as a source of wealth which stimulated and attracted movement. Very often we are not sure what forces propelled the barbarian peoples from the hinterlands, but they at least knew in what direction to move. The Empire was a magnet which drew the warlike, migrating peoples to itself.

The Roman trade with Africa and Arabia was a natural continuation of trade carried on in the Hellenistic Period by the Ptolemies from Egypt (pp. 392–93). It reached into the desert for such luxuries as ostrich feathers, gold dust, animals for the wild beast hunts, ivory, and slaves which were brought by native traders. The volume of trade in the Red Sea increased greatly. Metal tools and weapons, glass, and wine were sent to east Africa and to southern Arabia for the tropical exotics of ivory, palm oil, tortoise shell, slaves, spices, and incense. A large part of this activity in the Red Sea, however, was the result of regular, direct trade with India.

Probably from the time of Augustus the traders to India made regular use of the monsoons, starting out in early summer and returning in the fall. The volume of trade was great, for the geographer Strabo told of 120 ships clearing each year from the Red Sea port of Myus Hormus, and a book, the *Periplus* (Navigation Guide) *of the Red Sea,* which specifically described the Eastern trade as far as the Malay Peninsula was probably compiled in Trajan's reign. The author's impression of Malaya was vague, but he had some knowledge of Chinese trade into India. The merchants who gathered on the border of India were described as "having short bodies and broad flat faces and a peaceable disposition." Most significant, however, is the existence of Arikamedu, a Roman trading station on the Bay of Bengal, in which a considerable amount of Italian-made Arretine pottery has been found. Traders from the Empire evidently resided permanently in Indian coastal cities, because the Indian literary sources tell of the Yanvan, probably Egyptian Greeks and Syrians, who brought gold and took pepper.

The gold coins which the Romans used in trade were treated as bullion, although the native gold coinage of the Kushan Empire in northwest India was struck on the Roman standard. When the Roman coinage was devalued by Nero and Trajan, the Roman traders seem to have used more manufactured articles like fine textiles, glass, silver plate, copper, and tin. In return, the Romans seem to have wanted pepper above all, but also they bought spices, muslin, pearls and other precious gems. In northwest India, however, they were less interested in the products of India than in Chinese silk, which had been brought along the Silk Route that led from Honan in China to Bactra (Balkh) in Afghanistan. The caravans were diverted south when the Parthians refused to permit goods for Roman Syria to cross their territory or when the Parthians' tolls were too heavy. By this route, too, turquoise and furs from Siberia could be obtained.

To judge from the flourishing condition of the caravan cities on the eastern fringe of the Roman Empire, trade with Parthia was also extremely profitable. The Parthians, established in the territory of the former Seleucid Empire, were in a position not only to act as middlemen for the luxury goods from the East and from Arabia, but also to purchase Roman goods for themselves. Since the profits were high, the Parthians were determined to exploit the transit trade to their own advantage. Although the Romans knew of China and the Chinese knew of the Roman Empire, there was no really direct intercourse or mutual influence. One enterprising merchant from the Roman Empire, the Marco Polo of his time, arrived at the court of the Han Emperors in the reign of Marcus Aurelius. He seems to have represented himself as an envoy from the Emperor Antoninus, whom the Chinese annals called An-Tun. He gave a very favorable impression of the Romans as coiners of gold and silver, honest traders with India and Parthia, who sold without double-dealing. The Chinese were told, too, that Rome had always wished to trade with China for silk but had been prevented by the Parthians.

In general, the Eastern trade supplied the wealthy upper class of the Empire with costly luxuries for which they had acquired a taste and for which they had the means to pay. The Emperor Trajan, when he stood on the shore of the Persian Gulf in 116, expressed a wish to go to India, like Alexander the Great, but since only the traders went, the great civilizations of the ancient world remained apart. Some scholars have suggested that the fluctuations of history in Rome and China were affected by the trade relations or that a factor in the breakdown of Rome was the flow of gold to the East. Neither hypothesis seems very cogent because the trade was in very costly exotics in relatively small quantities. Each civilization had little real knowledge of the other beyond its name.

Nevertheless, a tangible impact was evidently made by Greco-Roman art of the Early Empire on the Buddhist sculpture of northwestern India. It is perceptible in the art of Gandhara. Statuettes were imported into the region from the eastern Mediterranean, probably from Alexandria, and stylistic influence was strong on the Buddhist work. In fact, it is probable that Greek craftsmen actually taught their techniques to Indian workmen. The Buddhists evidently felt some affinity in their own aesthetic needs with those of the people of the Hellenic part of the Roman Empire and seized on Western modes of expression as more satisfactory than their own. While it is sometimes suggested that Greek artistic traditions had survived in India from the Hellenistic Kingdom of Bactria, that seems unlikely because the stylistic influence is that of the Early Roman Empire rather than of the Hellenistic Period.

From Gandhara. A Greco-Roman triton

XXVIII

The Roman Peace
II: Society

IT IS SCARCELY POSSIBLE to give more than a very general impression of the economic and social character of the Roman Empire because of its vast extent and regional variations. Even if we were to ignore the older lands around the Mediterranean Sea, which Rome had taken over at an advanced stage of urban development, there would still be much to discuss: almost half the continent of Europe, the land between the coastal cities and desert in Africa, a part of the similar region in Syria and of inner Asia Minor. These were raised to a point of development, which, once lost, was not regained, except for Europe, until modern times. These hitherto backward regions were converted into farming land, studded with urban communities, and brought to the level which Italy and the older provinces had reached previously. Each province, moreover, had its own character and rate of growth, and there were a few regions which never attained the characteristic pattern of urban life. Britain, for example, was not urbanized to the same degree as Spain or central and southern Gaul. London became a thriving commercial city, but the general pattern of growth in Britain was that of the manorial farm, rather than of the municipality with its adjacent territory. There were, however, certain general factors which shaped and limited the internal growth of the Empire.

Economic Organization

GENERAL FACTORS

While the Empire was knit together by a centralized government, it never achieved a thoroughly interdependent economic unity. There was a remarkable road system which linked the centers of each province together and the provinces to one another. In fact, the Roman roads, which are straight and so well engi-

The reader will find the Back Endpaper and Map XIX (page 576) useful as he reads this chapter.

neered that some (along with their bridges) are still in use, dictated the communications and patterns of settlement in some regions for centuries. The Mediterranean, freed from pirates, connected the inner provinces by sea, and Roman shipping used the Red Sea, the Black Sea, the Atlantic and the Baltic coasts. Yet economic development during the Empire tended towards regional, even local, self-sufficiency, without significant exchange of basic commodities over wide areas. This condition did enable some regions to remain relatively prosperous when others were overrun by invasion or struck by natural disasters. But this also meant that, when the limit of growth was reached—the locally sufficient municipality, with its adjacent rural territory—the economy became static.

A number of factors contributed to this condition. Despite the numerous and excellent roads, transport was slow and goods had to be carried by animal pack or by cart. Thus the cost of articles carried over long land routes was greatly increased, and the land transport of staple and bulky commodities, like grain, wine, and olive oil, was rare. These goods, of course, could be carried by sea, and there was considerable trade between the older, more developed lands around the Mediterranean and the port cities of the new provinces in the initial stages of their growth. Yet the new regions rapidly became self-sufficient in their food supply. Agriculture was always the basic activity throughout the Empire and generally provided sufficient food for local needs. The importation of grain to Rome was an important exception, but that trade was organized and subsidized by the government. Because the coastal and island cities of the Aegean Sea also needed to import grain as regularly as they had in the past, they were supplied from Egypt and the Black Sea region, but elsewhere the trade in grain was sporadic, trade that was carried on to relieve temporary local shortages.

There was an extensive trade in luxuries and certain types of small manufactured articles: metalware, fine textiles, glass, precious and exotic goods of various kinds. These, however, came from special centers of production and were purchased by the wealthy. In general, trade was limited by the conditions of transport and employed relatively few of the inhabitants of the Empire. Like the trade across the frontiers with the Far East, the variety and the organization of inter-regional trade are interesting, but it is easy to overestimate its impor-

Roman transport. Ship in port, represented on a mosaic of ca. A.D. 200. Cartage by land; the transport of bulky goods over long distances was very costly.

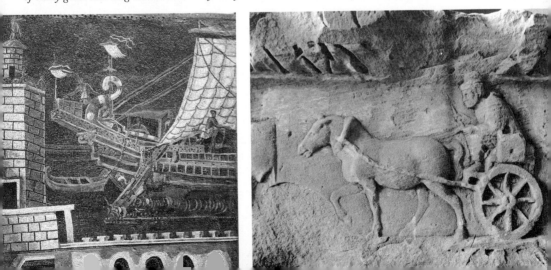

tance in the economy. The corollary, of course, was that industry, too, tended to be organized on a relatively small scale for the supply of local markets. The Roman Empire, like the more ancient civilizations of the Near East and of Greece, had no mass market for the consumption of industrial goods. Wealth was concentrated in the relatively small upper and middle classes, and the mass of the population lived close to the level of subsistence.

ITALY AND THE WESTERN PROVINCES

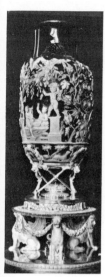

Amphora from Pompeii decorated with a cameo of cupids gathering grapes

Perhaps the best illustration of these conditions is offered by the relation of Italy to the new Western provinces. In the first century after Christ, Italy, which had remained basically agricultural, was able to supply the people with food grown on Italian farms, with the exception of Rome. Italian agriculture, in fact, seems to have flourished. The big plantations were still in existence, and ranching was developed on the hill slopes and in the south, where pasture was plentiful. The plantations were almost self-sufficient because, in addition to their special crops, they grew grain to feed their workers, made clothing, and manufactured and repaired some of their tools. There was also an increase in the number of moderate-sized farms, those from about thirty to two hundred acres. Some were genuine farms, but some were resorts whose owners made farming a profitable side line by selling their surplus on the local town markets. The small-scale farmer, too, had made some comeback in the Augustan Period.

During the first century, however, a change in the condition of labor was perceptible, when tenant farmers (*coloni*) like those on the big imperial estates appeared. In some cases ex-soldiers, to whom land had been allocated, would rent their holdings to tenants rather than work them, and on the large plantations, too, *coloni* began to replace slave labor. The abundant supply of slaves was cut off by the end of the wars of conquest, and domestic population did not supply the deficiency. Also, the humanitarian feeling and specific legislation of the Early Empire did not permit the abuse and waste of slaves as human tools.

During this same period the growth of industry noticed in the Late Republic continued for a time. It was organized to supply both Italy and the undeveloped European provinces. A handsome molded pottery, decorated with pictorial vignettes, was produced in great quantity at Arretium (Arezzo). This was the tableware for those who could not afford silver plate. Bronze articles were manufactured at Capua in Campania and glass was made in the factories of that region. Textiles were manufactured for export as well as for local consumption. Great stimulus was given to the production of lead pipes, of tiles and bricks, and to the marble- and stone-working industries by the tremendous building programs of the emperors. In fact, the *Princeps* himself was in the brickmaking business.

Yet these terms—industry, factory, and manufacture—need to be qualified and put in perspective. Even with the provincial markets and the great consumption in Rome and the large Italian towns, industry, with the exceptions noted above, did not grow beyond the craft stage. The standard type of establishment is well revealed in Pompeii. There, workroom, retail shop and living quarters were all combined. The "factories" for tile and brick production, and for pottery and glass did produce in quantity, but the largest (and they were few in number) employed workmen by the hundreds, and most plants only by the score. The owners of the "factories" were wealthy men, but industry as a whole was of the craft type, and the owners belonged to the freedman class. As in the case of trade, opportunities for employment and the growth of capital were not available on a large scale. Further, the techniques of industry were not significantly improved by new inventions or by the practical application of scientific knowledge.

Various explanations may account for this failure to develop new techniques and to expand the organization of industry. Labor, whether slave or free, was cheap, and some emperors felt concern about providing employment. Vespasian was said to have refused to use a newly invented hoist for the building trade, observing, "I must feed my poor." Most cogent, perhaps, was the lack of a mass market, as noticed before, and the lack of interest and initiative by the wealthy. No prestige was attached to industry, while ownership of land continued to be held in esteem and was profitable for the big landholders.

In the latter part of the first century both farming and industry declined in Italy. As we have seen, the emperors inaugurated a program of loans to farmers and of welfare for the poor children in the Italian municipalities. The decline of purchasing power which made these measures necessary is to be ascribed in part to the exhaustion of Italian land but mainly to the economic growth of the Western provinces. Olive groves had been planted in Spain and southern France. Vineyards had developed in Gaul and along the Rhine and the Moselle. There was no need to import wine and olive oil from Italy since the provinces were, in fact, sending their best products of this type to Rome. A striking record of this importation is to be seen in Monte Testaccio in Rome, a hill three thousand feet in circumference and 140 feet high, built up of the fragments of oil and wine jars, mainly from Spain. Industry, too, was exported on a considerable scale to the provinces and supplied their market. In Gaul large pottery kilns had been established at La Grafausenque and Lezoux. Lugdunum was a thriving business and industrial center, and Trèves and Cologne were centers of industry. Their products not only cut out Italian goods in Gaul but replaced them in the barbarian lands. Thus Italy dropped behind in prosperity as the provinces became self-sufficient and began to export. Rome, of course, remained an important market for luxury products because of the wealth of the upper classes. Rome provided employment because of the building programs, but a decline in business had begun which neither the emperors nor private men of wealth attempted to check by economic measures. In the new provinces, too, growth beyond the stage exemplified by Italian organization was scarcely possible, for they were also subject to the same limitations on distribution and technology and served a restricted market.

These same observations are generally true of the Empire as a whole. Agriculture, however organized in different regions, was basic to the economy. Industry was adapted to the local market, except for luxury goods. Trade was carried on in luxury goods and in a small range of manufactured items from special centers. The chief exceptions were the government-controlled transport of grain by sea and some inter-regional shipping of grain, olive oil, and wine to special markets and to relieve temporary shortages. The typical unit of the Empire was the municipality, self-governing and largely self-sufficient.

The Provincial Cities

In the Western provinces of the Empire the growth of cities was a part of Romanization, and the form which they assumed was modeled on that of the self-governing Roman colony, which in itself was a small-scale imitation of Rome (page 609). In the Hellenized lands of the Near East, however, a strong tradition of city life and local autonomy persisted from the past. Throughout the Empire, both East and West, the organization of the cities was essentially similar: each was the urban center of a large tract of rural territory which it administered directly. The government of the city was in the hands of a public-spirited middle class, usually referred to by modern historians as a bourgeoisie. In economic organization the city tended to be a local market, depending on its adjacent territory for well-being. First we will examine the political organization of the Greek cities and then discuss the city as a type.

THE CITIES OF THE EAST

When the Romans moved into the East in the second and first centuries before Christ, they found that the governing class in the cities of their new provinces was the middle group of landowners and businessmen (page 523). The Romans gave their support to this element in society, aiding where necessary in the suppression of lower-class revolt and of nationalistic native movements. The governing groups, in their turn, supported the Roman government and, after the victory of Augustus, registered their approval of the new *Princeps* by the establishment of ruler cults and by congratulatory honors and affirmations of loyalty. The Romans had a ready-made instrument of administration at hand which they grasped. For a considerable time each city was used as a means of taking the census of its own territory, and the city became the unit on which imperial taxation was levied. In return, local autonomy was respected, except for occasional judicial interference by the governor of the province.

Accordingly, the Romans planted few colonies in the East and did not push a deliberate policy of Romanization. The purposes of colonization were to restore devastated areas, as, for example, at Corinth and in Epirus in Greece and at Jerusalem in Palestine, to hold territory which was initially restless, as in Galatia in Asia Minor, and to develop Roman public land which had been confiscated from the previous owners. The Roman army in the East was quartered in the existing cities, when that was practicable, or in legionary camps on the unurbanized frontiers, like that of the upper Euphrates. Because the troops were recruited locally, the soldiers were Greek in speech and culture, and the Roman army was therefore not an instrument for Romanization as it was in Europe.

In general, then, cultural Romanization was slight and the granting of Latin Rights was infrequent. On the other hand, many cities achieved municipal status or were raised from that rank to the position of a titular colony. Most of the immunities from taxation, which the free allied cities of the Republican Period had possessed, were canceled in the Flavian Period, but local autonomy was preserved. Titular colonies were made by allowing the use of new names taken from the ruling dynasty. Thus we find names with a Roman sound, Juliopolis, Caesarea, Hadrianopolis, which cloak a Hellenized population. This nomenclature, of course, was a natural development from the Hellenistic practice which had produced the Philippi's, Alexandria's, and Antioch's. The Romans, too, encouraged urbanization in the districts which Seleucid policy had not touched, such as eastern Asia Minor, remote parts of Syria, and Nabataea.

The municipalities of the East continued Greek traditions in their local institutions. Each city had a popular assembly (an *ecclesia*) a council (the *boule*), and chief magistrates called *archons* or *strategoi*. The most important addition was a priesthood for the ruler cult. The original powers of the assembly had dwindled, and the name "democracy" which the governments liked to be called was simply a fashionable title. The right to initiate legislation had passed to the magistrates although the popular assemblies still elected the latter. The right to elect councilors gradually lapsed. For example, in Bithynia in the second century council members were enrolled for life by a censor, and at a later date each councilor nominated his successor. For both councilor and magistrate a property qualification was necessary. Effective government was in the hands of the wealthy, and the council had come to be the chief legislative organ of the city.

THE *CURIAL* CLASS

In both East and West the members of the council, the magistrates, and their families formed a privileged group, known as the *curial* class. It was marked by prestige of social position, by wealth, and by certain privileges in law. *Curials*, for example, were not to be punished by the ignominious penalty of flogging, and, if condemned to death, could appeal to the *Princeps*. It was from this group that the Equestrian order was recruited as Roman citizenship was extended into the provinces.

The *curials* were the backbone of society. They were not, for the most part, as well educated and articulate as the upper class, but we know about them from the numerous inscriptions in which their communities paid them honor. As a group they were conservative in outlook and tradition, observed a conventional morality in their behavior, and condemned those who did not behave in this manner. They had a sense of individual worth and pride in their status, and while their wealthier and more prominent members might rise to the Senatorial Order, these were relatively few in number.

During the second century there seems to have been an increase in the number of very wealthy men in the provinces. We hear of individuals who were princely patrons of their cities, like Herodes Atticus, who built the Odeum of that name for his native city, Athens. These men were known throughout their province and were often friends of the *Princeps* himself. Their money was sometimes made by business and inter-regional trade, more often by investment in land. In the West they were frequently descendants of early Roman settlers and of the native nobility of the time before the Roman Conquest. In the East some great families had survived from the Hellenistic Period, but many were new. Their founders had discovered their opportunity in the wars of conquest and the conditions of peace and rapid growth in the first century after Christ. It was from this group that the provincial senators came, and their great wealth marked them off from the *curials* of their own cities.

THE ECONOMY AND SOCIETY OF THE CITIES

The city included both the urban center and its adjacent rural territory, which might take in hundreds of square miles and various villages, where the peasants and tenant farmers lived who tilled the land. The government of the city collected taxes, administered justice, and kept order for the whole district. The citizen class was composed of the free inhabitants of the city and the free, landowning peasants in the rural areas. The latter group was often small in number. There was some upward movement into the citizen body from the people of the dependent villages, the *perioeci* or *attributi,* as they were called in East and West respectively. When these became sufficiently Hellenized or Romanized, as the case might be, they were incorporated into the citizen class. While the society of the city was not closed, the peasants were definitely less privileged than the city dwellers. They did not share in the amenities and services which the city provided since they lived too far away or were for the most part tenants, rather than landowners and citizens.

The city depended for its revenues primarily on the local resources available in its own district. These were rents from public property, such as land and fishing waters, tolls on goods crossing the local borders, local taxes, fees, and the fines levied in the courts. Although administrative costs were low because the city officials were unsalaried, the municipal expenditures were very high. Each city felt that its dignity demanded an extensive public building program and a multitude of services. Accordingly, theaters, arenas, temples, baths, water systems, market places, civic buildings, educational facilities, and even limited medical care were provided. In time of food shortage the city undertook to provide grain for its people, which was costly because of the expense of transport. For all these amenities and services, considered necessary even for cities of moderate size, the municipal revenues were insufficient.

Sometimes the *Princeps* donated buildings as a mark of special favor, but the extra burden was carried largely by the *curial* class. Quite voluntarily and as a matter of public duty at first, the *curials* underwrote the cost of buildings, of services, and of festivals to commemorate their period of office in the council or as a magistrate. Voluntary generosity came to be customary and ultimately obligatory. Instead of receiving a salary for office, the magistrate paid a fee, and in place of civic office, he might be elected to a *liturgy*. The latter device, a capital levy on the rich to maintain some public service, had a long history in the Greek city-state, from the time when citizens of Periclean Athens outfitted triremes to the Late Roman Empire when horses were provided for the imperial post. When incomes were reduced and the costs of government rose, the *liturgies* came to be a grievous burden, but in the second century after Christ they were passing from the customary to the obligatory stage and were still tolerable and in most cases an occasion for pride.

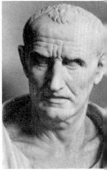

A Roman of the first century after Christ

As we have noticed, some cities began to fall into financial difficulties in the time of Trajan. When this was the result of amateur financing, it was correctable, but too frequently civic ambitions outran local resources. Since the provincial cities were local markets, there was little that could be done to gain new wealth. The city absorbed the produce of its territory without surplus for export and provided the goods for its own population and for the peasants of its countryside. The spending power of the unit could hardly be increased. This was not true of all cities, but the exceptions were specialized and became fewer in number. Such exceptions were the cities which produced the luxuries and special manufactured goods for trade, and the important shipping centers, like Alexandria, and the big port cities of Syria, Asia Minor, Italy, and Spain. Others, like Palmyra, were transit centers for the caravan trade. Some, too, were used extensively by the imperial government, like Antioch, where the emperors used the palaces of the Seleucid rulers when they were in the East. There were a few centers of learning, like Athens, which attracted wealthy young students and tourists. But, in the main, the provincial cities of the Empire were local markets which reached the limit of their potential growth and began to suffer strain in the second century.

The *curial* class was also limited in its capital resources. Most of the individuals who composed it were landowners, whose fields lay in the city's territory and were worked by tenant farmers. Those who drew a living from professional fees—doctors, teachers, and architects—were few in number, as were the businessmen and traders. The latter, of course, tended to be concentrated in the port cities and the termini of the caravan routes. Accordingly, the land was the source of wealth for the middle class in the cities, just as it provided most of the revenue for the imperial government through the land tax.

While the peasants who worked on the lands of the municipalities had some share in the city's amenities when they went to town, those peasants in Egypt and on the great imperial and private estates had only their village life. Throughout the Empire the freeholder was giving way to the sharecropping *colonus,* whose position was tending to become permanent. In the conditions of peace in the Early Empire the peasants were reasonably secure and were encouraged to develop land. Generally speaking, however, they had no opportunity for education and no chance to break away from their occupation. There was a deep gulf between city and country.

While the position of the lower classes in the cities was better than that of the peasants, a gulf also existed between them and the middle class. The poor man of the city was provided with public services and recreational facilities denied to his counterpart in the country, but his opportunities for wealth were limited by the narrow market in which he worked. Occupations were few: retail trade in small shops, peddling, and the various crafts. The lower positions of the municipal services and domestic employment were taken by slaves.

In these restricted conditions of life the lower classes of the cities, free and slave alike, turned to the formation of social clubs, the *collegia*. Some were entirely religious in nature, formed by men and women who grouped together to worship a foreign god whose cult was not included in the civic religion. The Christian communities in the cities are to be regarded in this category in their early stages. Many *collegia* were burial societies, formed to ensure a decent burial and a day of remembrance for their members. These might be solitary individuals or might belong to families too poor to provide burial except by pooling their resources through small fees.

Most numerous, however, were the *collegia* formed by workers in the same trade. These bear a superficial resemblance to trade guilds and to labor unions, but their common work was only a stimulus to form social associations. The *collegia* did not try to regulate their own trades by the establishment of rules for apprenticeship or to gain advantages from bargaining as a group. We do know of one case where the porters of Rome obtained a government order to exclude "non-union" labor, but that was rare. For its social activity the organization usually acquired a meeting place and centered its activity around a religious cult, of which the annual festival was a red letter day for the members. The *collegia* were organized in much the same way as the municipalities themselves, with an elected *magister,* a mayor or master, and a council. It had always been Roman practice to take official notice of the *collegia* because the latter had sometimes become cells for political agitation. Accordingly, in the Empire the *collegia* were licensed. The government could requisition labor or supplies from them, but until the third century this practice was not regular, except in time of war.

The City of Rome

The great city of the Empire, of course, was Rome, built into an imperial capital by the emperors, each of whom emulated and tried to surpass his predecessor. Probably in the second century after Christ the population was about 1,000,000. Although the provincial cities could not hope to rival Rome's basilicas, palaces, temples, forums, and huge recreational buildings which were made possible by the vast sums spent by the emperors, they tried, and some came very close. Rome was a model of the monumental grandeur and richness of Roman architecture which characterized the Empire. In the older Hellenic cities of the East new public buildings were erected and new quarters were added, while scores of new cities were built in the hitherto unurbanized regions. The Italian towns and the provinces of the West and of Africa followed suit. In general the inspiration of the architecture was Hellenic, but the spirit was thoroughly Roman, and new types of buildings were developed to satisfy the needs of Roman urban life. The simplicity of plan and the perfection of proportion and finish, which had characterized classical Greek architecture, gave way to baroque richness and to sheer size. Complex and grandiose structures were made possible by new materials, brick and concrete, and by the techniques of vaulting which the architects had developed for their use. The buildings were sheathed and floored with marble and richly decorated with sculpture and luxuriant ornament. Since there was very considerable uniformity throughout the cities of the Empire in the type and style of buildings, perhaps a brief description of Rome, to which the other cities aspired and where the most talented architects worked, will suggest a picture of the cities of this period.

In the center of Rome where space had to be provided for large crowds, there were the imperial forums, for which the Forum of Augustus provided a model. Its original inspiration was the rectangular market place of the Hellenistic cities surrounded by colonnades, but in Augustus' Forum a temple of Roman type with a deep porch, dedicated to Mars the Avenger, was erected on a high base at the end. The whole plan was axially symmetrical, and on either side of the temple was an *exedra*, a semicircular open area decorated with

View across the Roman Forum. On the left, the Temple of Saturn and, appearing through its columns, the Temple of Antoninus and Faustina, his empress

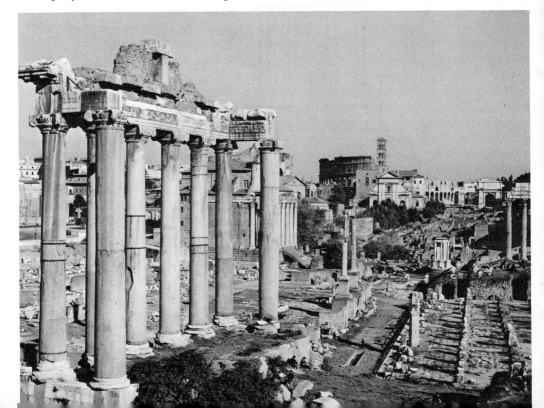

statues to form a Hall of Fame. Other forums were built for Julius Caesar, Vespasian, and for Trajan (a passageway, the *Forum Transitorium,* was built for Nerva).

Trajan's huge Forum was one of the important monuments of Roman architecture. The open area of the Forum was enclosed on each side by a double colonnade, behind which were *exedras.* That on the east rose to a height of six stories. The central element of the complex was the Ulpian Basilica, the largest and most ornate of the Roman world. Its central hall was flanked by two aisles, at the ends of which were apsidal chambers, each the size of a large theater, designed for the law courts. On the central axis of the Forum, directly behind the Basilica, was Trajan's Column, encircled by a spiraling band of relief sculpture which narrated the events of the Dacian War. The reliefs, impossible to follow from the ground, could be viewed from the balconies of the Latin and Greek Libraries on either side. Hadrian completed the design by a temple to the deified Trajan at the end of the Forum.

Although Tiberius started the series of imperial palaces with an elaborate mansion on the Palatine Hill, and Claudius converted into monumental form several of the important gates of Rome, among them the Porta Maggiore, the fire in Nero's reign provided the first real opportunity to remodel the heart of the city. It burned out much of the old slum quarter, the *Subura,* which had grown up in the low central part of Rome. Nero constructed his Golden House there, a combined palace and country estate. Pavilions, parks, lakes, fountains and retreats made it a forerunner of Versailles. Here in the Golden House the emperor's artistic genius might be enshrined. Public opinion and the more commonplace taste of the Flavians, however, converted the Golden House to

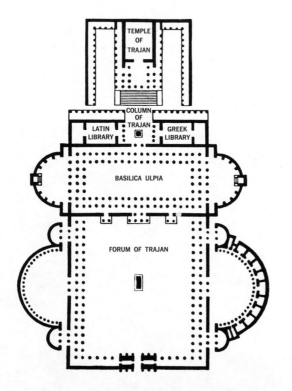

Plan of the Forum of Trajan, Rome: in the foreground, the market square with its great exedras; in the center, the Ulpian basilica (law courts); the temple at the far end was built for the deified Trajan by Hadrian.

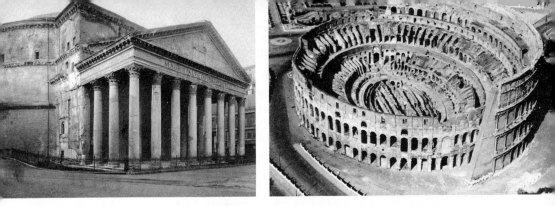

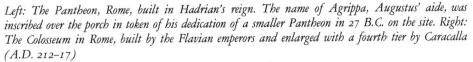

Left: The Pantheon, Rome, built in Hadrian's reign. The name of Agrippa, Augustus' aide, was inscribed over the porch in token of his dedication of a smaller Pantheon in 27 B.C. on the site. Right: The Colosseum in Rome, built by the Flavian emperors and enlarged with a fourth tier by Caracalla (A.D. 212–17)

public use at first and then removed it entirely. Apartments and arcades of shops at street level, the Colosseum and the imperial forums, mentioned above, covered the ground which it had occupied.

A new feature of the religious life of Rome was the series of temples for the deified emperors, built in various quarters of the city. Vespasian and Antoninus Pius managed to squeeze theirs into the old Forum Romanum. Most striking, however, was the Pantheon (Santa Maria Rotonda), built by Hadrian to replace the original structure of Agrippa, which was erected in 27 B.C. and destroyed by fire in the reign of Titus. As the name implies, the Pantheon was for worship of all the gods, but tended to be used mainly for the deified predecessors of Hadrian. Later it became the burial ground of Christian martyrs and of the kings of Italy. The building is an architectural masterpiece, the type of which is reproduced in St. Peter's in the Vatican and in Monticello. The main element, the rotunda, is a drum of concrete, 145 feet in diameter, with eight hollow piers supporting the dome. The opening in the top of the dome, to admit light, is 145 feet from the floor and twenty-seven feet in diameter. The floor was paved with slabs of variegated marble and the interior was richly decorated with niches, statues, and columns. The building was given a conventional temple front with columns in the Corinthian style, almost universally used for Roman public structures.

The recreational buildings constructed by the emperors for the festivals and leisure of the people of Rome were among the most grandiose structures of the city. Among them the theaters took a secondary place, for drama had lost popularity to the more spectacular and savage sports of the arena, and in its own genre had been replaced with pantomime and farce. Rome's best-known theater, that of Marcellus, built by Augustus in memory of his nephew and son-in-law, is still partly standing, for it was converted into a palace in the Medieval Period. It seated about fourteen thousand in contrast to the fifty thousand of the Colosseum and the 140,000 of the Circus Maximus, where chariot races were held. Roman theaters, unlike their Greek prototypes, had a high stage with a towering architectural backdrop, decorated with niches, pilasters and statues. The former *orchestra* circle was converted into a special seating area, and the action of the plays was carried out entirely on the stage.

Rome had two circuses, the well-known Circus Maximus, which had been first built in the third century B.C., and a smaller one, constructed by Gaius. They were primarily for the chariot races, although they were used also for wild beast hunts when a particularly large spectacle of that type was arranged. In its final form the Circus Maximus seated an estimated 140,000 people on rows of seats supported by three tiers of arcades erected around the half-mile track. From the front the Circus resembled a great fortress with towers and a battlemented façade. The track was divided by the *spina,* a long pier of masonry, decorated by obelisks and statues, around which the chariots turned to make their full course. The four racing syndicates of Rome were distinguished by their colors, red, white, blue, and green. Each had its clique of fans, and successful charioteers were the idols of the people of the city.

For the gladiatorial fights and wild beast hunts, which had long since lost their original character of funeral games and developed into bloody spectacles, the Romans invented the amphitheater. It was similar to a modern arena, circular or oval in shape, with the seating supported by tiers of arcades and vaulting. The Colosseum, although now stripped of its original stonework and marble, is still an impressive structure. It was erected by the Flavian emperors with three tiers of arcades and enlarged by a fourth in the reign of Caracalla in the early third century. The seating was by social class, with the dignitaries and the emperor in the first three rows and with the seats of the poor higher up. The audience was protected by a wall, fifteen feet in height, and the arena was serviced by underground corridors and counterweighted elevators, through which the gladiators and beasts made their appearance. Perhaps the most spectacular of the gladiatorial shows were those staged by Trajan, who had ten thousand Dacian prisoners of war fight to the death. The usual performers were trained gladiators and wild animals from the forests of Germany or Africa. The savagery was deplored by philosophers and discouraged by some of the emperors, but the spectacles remained popular to the end of the Empire. While the ordinary people of Rome did not live entirely on free bread or spend all their time at circuses, it was fortunate for the Empire that they no longer retained a voice in its government.

A better use of leisure was provided by the public baths of Rome. The city had 176 baths, both private and public, in 33 B.C., and nine hundred in the early fourth century after Christ. The largest, the baths of Diocletian, covered thirty-two acres of ground, and several others approached these in size. The structures were, of course, much more than simple bathing pools. In addition to hot, tepid, and cold baths, there were exercise and training facilities, parks, great halls for lounging, libraries, and gardens—in short, the baths were "athletic" clubs on the grand scale, to which the emperor also resorted on occasion to show himself to the public.

The most remarkable service which Rome provided to its people was the public water supply, administered by an imperial commission of experts. The

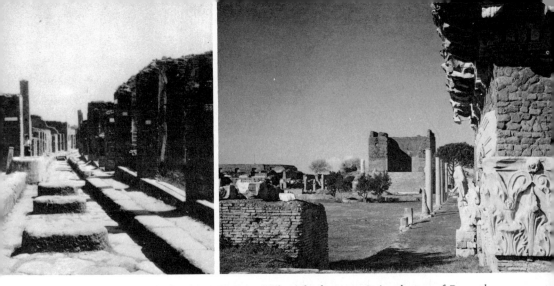

Left: A street in Pompeii showing stepping stones. Right: The forum at Ostia, the port of Rome; the form is typical of the cities of the Empire; the forum was bordered with colonnades and at the end was the Capitolium (Temple of Jupiter Capitolinus).

water was brought to the city from the hills by aqueducts, numbering eleven in the time of Trajan, to be held in reservoirs or distributed directly throughout the city. Water was provided for the baths and public fountains, or piped to the houses of the wealthy for their pools and gardens. One of the interesting technical books of the Early Empire is a treatise on the *Waters of Rome* by Frontinus, Trajan's *curator* of the water commission.

The character of the towns and smaller cities of Italy is well illustrated by the remains of Pompeii and Herculaneum, covered over in the eruption of Vesuvius in 79, and of Ostia, the port of Rome, which was silted in by the Tiber in late antiquity. Since we have already noticed the type of house used by the well-to-do at Pompeii (pp. 502–03), we might turn to Ostia which has preserved the best examples of the apartment houses, *insulae,* in which the lower classes were housed. The population of Ostia and its neighborhood was cosmopolitan and polyglot, as befitted the harbor through which Rome obtained its grain and exotic luxuries from overseas. While some wealthy merchants lived in the town, most of the population consisted of laborers who worked at the docks and warehouses, and government employees of the lower grades who worked in the grain supply. An interesting feature of the town were the shrines to foreign gods and the offices of the merchants—the olive oil and grain dealers, the traders of Alexandria, and the like—who formed *collegia* according to their trade or place of origin. Yet the layout and civic buildings of Ostia were Roman. Two main thoroughfares crossed at right angles to form the axes of the grid on which the blocks for residence and for the public buildings were laid out. In the center of town was the Forum, colonnaded on three sides and with a Capitolium, an imposing Temple of Jupiter Capitolinus, at the end. For the leisure of the citizens there were the usual buildings: a theater, colonnades, baths, and parks, in addition to the warehouses and granaries for the storage of grain.

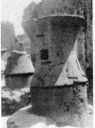

Stone mills for grinding grain (Pompeii)

653

The *insulae* were built of brick, several stories in height, and occupied a complete city block. The more elaborate were in the form of a quadrangle around a central garden area for common use by the residents. At the street level on the exterior there were shops and workrooms for retail business and crafts. The individual apartments were small in size, where life must have been very crowded, but the inner courtyards and public areas in the city offered escape. This type of building, combining living and working areas, had a long architectural history in the cities of Western Europe, and may be seen in the older quarters to the present day.

Society and Intellectual Life

While there was much in the social life of the Empire that was brutal and ugly—the gladiatorial combats and wild beast hunts, the lax morality, vice, and gluttony, which Roman satirists and moralists singled out—society was also humane and civilized. Possession of great wealth was marked by abuse, but the wealthy also demonstrated their civic spirit. Individuals were generous in supporting the services of their cities, even if they were ostentatious about it. Humanitarian legislation, which protected children and slaves from abuse, characterized the Roman Peace, and the interest in the law shown by Hadrian and Antoninus benefited society as a whole. Their jurists took equity and humane considerations into account, worked out legal procedures more carefully, and improved them by seeking expert opinion in evidence. No doubt prosperity made it easier to be humane, but both upper- and middle-class Roman society demonstrated a sense of social responsibility.

In Rome, the seat of imperial government, a court and high society had come into existence which was affluent, cosmopolitan in its tastes, and relaxed in its morals. As the role of the senatorial class in government declined, members of this group filled their time by "going into society" and pursuing their private interests. This upper-class society had an outer decorum and traditional etiquette which might mask a variety of private tastes and indulgences. To some men and women (women moved in it freely) a successful literary séance with a visiting Greek "lion" or the pleasure of reading their own compositions was

Apartments (insulae) *at Ostia. A reconstruction and the surviving brickwork*

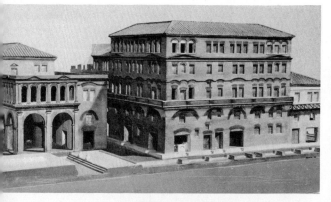
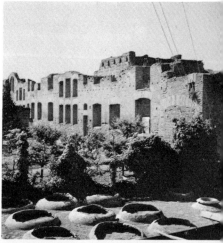

highly important. To others an elaborate dinner party, not an orgy, or the planning of their country villa seemed as significant as holding office. Many pursued a relatively quiet life of luxurious and sensible leisure, while a few indulged in a hectic career of debauchery that extended beyond sowing the wild oats of youth. It was an old, civilized, and complex high society, whose *grandes dames* and *dilettanti* set the tone and dictated tastes and fashions. It also condemned and dropped those who made public displays of their vices and gluttony. Naturally the frothier elements and public exhibitions attracted attention since the Roman satirists of the period singled out the abnormal and found the typical dull.

The creed professed by this upper-class society was Stoicism, and, as we have seen, outspoken criticism of the emperors cost some of its members their lives in the first century after Christ. While this political aspect of philosophy terminated with the reconciliation between Senate and *Princeps* in the reigns of Nerva and Trajan, Stoicism remained a personal creed. We know its character, in particular, from the works of Seneca (4–65), whom Nero executed, and from the *Meditations* of Marcus Aurelius. Seneca wrote a series of moral essays, packed with terse maxims for proper behavior in the vicissitudes of life, and nine plays for recitation rather than performance on the stage. Their heroes and heroines show an almost unrelenting desire to meet their death like Stoic martyrs. (While the plays are usually criticized for their bombastic and melodramatic character, they had a very great influence on Renaissance drama.) The Roman Stoics believed in the government of the universe by an all-wise Providence to whose will they fatalistically subjected themselves with unflinching duty. It was *his* will since the Stoic Providence was almost a fatherly god who loved and protected all people. However, the main emphasis of Roman Stoicism was on an upright and just life, in which patience and duty were virtues. The religious aspect of Stoicism was developed in particular by the Greek philosopher Epictetus (*ca.* 55–135), a Greek freedman who taught first in Rome until Domitian expelled the philosophers in 90, then in Nicopolis in Epirus. His works, the *Discourses* and the *Enchiridion,* stressed the brotherhood of man and man's share in the divinity of god.

The Younger Pliny (*ca.* 62–113) was a prominent senator of the Empire as revealed in his *Letters*. The correspondence covered a variety of subjects, from a vivid account of the eruption of Vesuvius in 79 to a series of official communications with the Emperor Trajan while Pliny was governor of Bithynia. Pliny had a distinguished public career, becoming a consul and *augur,* as well as provincial governor. He had, in fact, been selected to deliver the official speech of praise at Trajan's succession. Despite all this, Pliny found time to put his letters in literary form and to lead the social life of a cultured man of affairs in Rome. He was punctilious and fussy in behavior, vain of his family and career, but generous, conscientious as an administrator, and happy in his personal life. He was devoted to his wife and to the arrangements of his country villa on the coast south of Rome.

LITERATURE

It is easy to forget that Rome was not the only city of the Empire, for the capital was the literary and artistic center, where the taste of its society and that of the *Princeps* set the fashion. Yet in Alexandria the work of the Museum and the Library, started by the Ptolemies (pp. 402, 406), was continued under the patronage of the emperors. The schools of philosophy in Athens were popular, and in many of the large Greek cities of the East new schools of rhetoric were founded. Under the favorable conditions of peace there was a renaissance of Greek literature, the Second Sophistic Movement, which the philhellenism of Hadrian encouraged. Neither science nor philosophy produced original discoveries or new systems of thought to rival those of the past, but useful syntheses, which were to serve the Western and Arabic world for centuries, were compiled.

The Latin literature of the Silver Age, as the period of the Early Empire is called, while developing a new style of expression, generally looked back to the Augustan Period and to the writers of the Republic. The Greek literature, too, was essentially a continuation of classical and Hellenistic forms. The intellectual traditions of the Greco-Roman world were beginning to crystalize and to fuse together. Such a process, of course, seems to lack originality and invites the terms, decay and decline. How properly applicable they are is a matter of viewpoint. It is salutary to remember that Roman architecture achieved its rich, monumental grandeur at this time and that periods of Western culture other than our own have found more inspiration in the literature and art of the Roman Empire than in those of classical Greece.

Tacitus, who was Rome's most original and significant historian, lived during the Silver Age and stamped his disparaging estimate of the Julio-Claudian emperors upon Roman tradition (page 589). He was born into a good family during the reign of Nero and improved his social position by marrying into a prominent senatorial family. His father-in-law, Agricola, whose biography Tacitus wrote, was governor of Britain from 77 to 84 and played a useful role in the early development of the province. Tacitus himself became a praetor in 88, when Domitian began his so-called Terror against the senators. Thus Tacitus was very much alive to the relations of *Princeps* and Senate, both as an official and as a man whose colleagues and friends were struck down by Domitian.

Tacitus wrote his chief works, the *Annals,* which covered the reigns of the Julio-Claudians, and the *Histories,* an account of the Flavian dynasty, under Trajan and Hadrian. Then it was both safe and proper to criticize the previous regimes. Tacitus' writing was consummately skillful. By rhetoric and color, innuendo and emphasis, although not by actual omission and falsification of fact, he wrote an "inside" account of the intrigue, private life, and government of the emperors. In an earlier work, the *Orators,* Tacitus had implied that the Principate was responsible for the destruction of liberty and thus accountable for the general decline of morality and creativity which he pessimistically found in imperial Rome. His great historical works developed this theme, but from his own experience and knowledge Tacitus conceded that the Principate was necessary and that the Senate, except for individual members, was not fitted to rule. Tacitus' distaste for the society of Rome appeared also in his *Germania,* where he contrasted the effete society of the capital with the rugged, primitive virtues of the Germans.

The satirists and moralists of the Silver Age, along with Suetonius (the biographer of the Caesars), Seneca, and Pliny, provide vivid material for the social history of the Early Empire. Persius (34–62) wrote six satires in verse, filled with Stoic maxims and literary obscurity. Juvenal (55–*ca.* 130) was one of the great figures of Latin literature, who savagely attacked the depravity of upper-class society and was scathingly hostile to the Hellenized Orientals who formed a very large part of the lower class of Rome by the second century. Juvenal's Third and Tenth satires were imitated by Samuel Johnson in his *London* and *The Vanity of Human Wishes.* A lesser figure of the same period, Martial (40– *ca.* 102), the writer of epigrams, was talented, witty, and spiteful.

In the reign of Nero one of the most interesting books of Latin literature, the *Satyricon* of Petronius, was written. The author is probably to be identified with a well-known senator of the period, Petronius Arbiter, whose elegance is said to have excited Nero's jealousy and to have provoked an invitation from the latter to Petronius to commit suicide. Petronius was presumably involved in one of the senatorial conspiracies. The book was a prototype of the picaresque novel and narrated the misadventures of a pair of freedmen, one of whom, Encolpius, told the story. It is best known for its classic picture of the parvenu Trimalchio, who was satirized in the account of a fantastic banquet. A century later Lucius Apuleius wrote a novel, *The Golden Ass,* in the form of a fictitious biography. For the historian it is valuable for its treatment of superstition and exotic religious worships which monopolized the mind of the lower classes. Of value for the history of literature and education is the book on rhetorical method and literary criticism by Quintilian (35–100), who had a just estimate of the excessive emphasis on rhetoric and epigrammatic expression which characterized the style of Silver Age Latin.

Several important questions call for attention in a consideration of this literature. The major writers were pessimistic in tone, and some of them painted a very black picture of Roman society. Tacitus blamed the Principate for the loss of liberty which the senatorial class had enjoyed during the Republic, and Juvenal was savage in his indignation. The epic poet Lucan, put to death in 65 by Nero, conceived of Julius Caesar as a satanic figure in his *Pharsalia,* an epic poem on the civil wars. Even a writer favorable to the Principate, the minor historian of Tiberius' reign, Velleius Paterculus, recognized a decay in literary creativity after the great Augustans of the Golden Age. Very few of the Latin writers, except the timeservers and the official panegyrists, were impressed by (one might even say conceived of) the achievement of Rome in the provinces. Few could accommodate themselves happily to the times in which they lived.

The writers themselves have various explanations for this condition. Seneca found the cause of decay and of his own dissatisfaction in the growth of luxury and vice. Tacitus, himself a student of oratory, blamed the decline on the loss of political freedom. Velleius did not consider the regime tyrannical, but found an explanation in the sterile imitation of past models. Roman literature had developed from imitating, or to put the case patriotically, in rivaling Greek literary forms. The Augustans, particularly Vergil, had achieved the ultimate and left nothing for their successors. It is true that even the new blood from the Spanish provinces—Seneca, Martial, and Quintilian— were absorbed also in the cult of tradition.

After the reconciliation between Senate and *Princeps,* Tacitus and Suetonius could write freely about the emperors of the first century, and Juvenal about the society of Domitian's reign, but they and their successors were discreetly silent, except by implication, about the political regime of their own periods. Freedom of thought and speech had been nominally restored, but the will to oppose openly seems to have vanished. Perhaps the explanation lies in the combination of factors already mentioned. The traditions of the Republic, both political and literary, were so strong among the upper class who wrote and patronized literature, that they automatically applied its values to their own age. The literature which they read and imitated stressed the days of senatorial freedom and extolled idealized heroes of the Republic. The present seemed to be filled with lesser men, who used cheap tricks to realize their ambitions and pleasures. When the senators made comparisons, criticized, or conspired, autocratic emperors proceeded to purges, and even Vespasian banished the philosophers from Rome. Opinion, publicly expressed, was not free under the early emperors, and spies and informers made private utterance dangerous.

The emperors not only relied on informal sources of information, but also had developed an organized secret service by the end of the first century. Domitian was probably its chief creator. Before his time the rulers relied mainly on the centurions and tribunes of the praetorian guard, their own freedmen, and on the ubiquitous informers for reports in Rome. For information in the provinces they used the procurators. Domitian, however, set up a regular agency made up of the junior officers of the supply service for procuring grain, the *frumentarii.* They were in a good position to spy, for their business brought them into contact with members of the public, bureaucrats, and the officers of the army. Perhaps creative genius could accommodate itself to these conditions and find a politically harmless outlet, but it did not do so in Rome. The traditions of Latin literature, as established in the Republic and Early Empire, virtually end in the mid-second century.

While the Greeks had long since lost their political freedom and were not embittered (and then resigned) as were the Romans, the Second Sophistic Movement also is criticized for lack of freshness and originality. It did build on the past and tended to ignore Roman literature, but some of the writers were impressed and genuinely enthusiastic about the imperial achievement of Rome, like

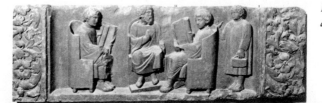

Relief of a teacher and his pupils

the rhetorician Aelius Aristides (quoted p. 617) and Plutarch. Nearly all the prominent writers were invited to display their talents in the capital, and many lesser lights came of their own accord, but for most, pride in their own heritage seems to have smothered curiosity. Thus the higher Greek culture of the second century had a curiously artificial nature, without much cognizance of Rome or roots in the mass culture of the people. In the West the Greek renaissance mainly affected the educated Romans of the upper class. And only a few of the emperors could be included. For example, the Greek rhetorician Dio, whom Trajan favored by invitations to dinner, remarked to the emperor on one occasion, "Socrates, an old and poor Athenian, of whom you, too, have heard."

The most publicized, if not the most important, literary figures were the rhetoricians who taught in the rhetorical schools and gave public lectures in the cities of the East and to small groups in Rome. The emperors gave them gifts of money and sometimes endowed their schools, while the public in the Eastern cities flocked to hear their declamations. Many of these were on stock themes, which the speakers made attractive by rhetorical devices, by color, and bizarre turns of phrase and vocabulary. A few were more seriously concerned with the conditions of their period. Dio Chrysostomus, the Golden Mouthed, from Prusa in Bithynia was expelled from Rome by Domitian for his political criticism and wandered through the Eastern cities making a living as best he could. He became concerned to preserve the traditions of Hellenism which, he observed, were being swamped by oriental influences. In later life, as we have seen, Dio dined at the table of the *Princeps*. Aelius Aristides (*ca.* 117–85) was more representative of the new Sophists and of some historical significance for his fervent expression of the achievement of Rome in uniting the peoples of the Empire. Among the most interesting of his works are a series of essays which record his cure from illness at the sanctuary of Asclepius, the healing god, at Pergamum.

The most significant and influential writer of the Greek renaissance was Plutarch of Chaeronea in Central Greece (42–126). Plutarch had been trained in philosophy rather than in rhetoric, but during the earlier period of his life taught in the Greek cities and in Rome, where he had many friends. He returned to his native Chaeronea, where he became a priest of the oracle of Delphi, wrote his books, and took part in the political life of his community. Plutarch's writing was voluminous, and his *Parallel Lives of the Famous Greeks and Romans* is one of the most widely read books of Greek literature. Plutarch saw some value in Roman history, and the arrangement of the *Lives,* in which a famous Greek and a famous Roman are paired, may have been designed to impress his Greek readers with the fact that Rome, too, had a history worthy of their attention. Since the material for the biographies was drawn from the whole range of classical Greek and Hellenistic historical and biographical writing, Plutarch's *Lives* are a valuable source of information. The material, however, is only as good as its source because Plutarch's concern was to moralize about life by referring to the virtues and vices of his subjects. However psychologically and historically deplorable this may seem to our own age, Plutarch was and is eminently readable and ever popular. It is through adaptations of his material that Romans like Julius Caesar and Mark Antony, and Greeks likes Pericles and Alexander the Great, have made their popular impression. Plutarch's *Moralia,* although less well known than the *Lives,* is a large, miscellaneous collection of essays, characterized by the same humanity and wide range of interest.

The most original writer of the Sophistic Movement was Lucian of Samosata in Syria (*ca.* 120–180), who made the traditional philosophic dialogue of Greek literature into a comic form. Lucian was a witty and acute debunker of the great and the solemn, clever and frothily entertaining for a single reading only. He was essentially out of place in a serious age, whose philosophers were concerned with moral conduct and whose masses were caught in a welter of superstition and exotic religious worships. Pausanias of Lydia, on a more pedestrian level, wrote a guidebook to Greece which is of more interest to modern classical archaeologists than it was of service to tourists of his own period. Although Pausanias was interested above all in religious antiquities and curiosities, he presented the cult of the antique in a humdrum and involved fashion.

Much of the higher culture of the Early Empire was thus sterile and artificial because it lost touch with the contemporary scene and sought its inspiration in the models and traditions of the past. When writers cared about their own period, they were moved to bitterness and resignation or to an almost empty self-congratulation. Most people were engrossed by the amusements offered by the cities and by their own personal and family problems. For spiritual and emotional satisfaction, they turned to superstition and to the excitement and warmth of the more exotic Eastern religious worships of the period. These forms of worship had moved into the Western part of the Empire and were making their way upwards into the higher classes. The rationality of the classical Greek tradition and the vigor of Roman life alike were being vitiated. This conquest became almost complete in the third century, and it will be more appropriate to consider it when we discuss the decay of Rome in that connection (pp. 676–82).

ART

The imperial patronage of art, used successfully and on the grand scale by Augustus to propagandize his regime, was also regularly practiced by his successors for the same purpose. Almost every type of monument, from the imperial portraits on the coins to the grandiose buildings of Rome, was affected. Architecture perhaps received the greatest stimulus, but the individual imperial tastes are more perceptible in sculpture. The fashions were set by the imperial household and by the great families of Rome who could employ the most skilled artists for their portraits, for the sculpture on monuments and buildings, and for the furniture and decoration of their houses. Under this patronage significant new developments were made. The achievements of the emperors were represented in great pictorial themes, in which the problems of narrative and of composition caught the interest of the artists. They did not try to exploit the human body for its own sake, as had the artists of Greece, but represented crowds of people, soldiers in battle, and the landscapes in which they moved.

The scenes on Trajan's Column, commemorating the Dacian conquest, are an excellent example of Roman sculpture. The relief was cut low and flat, and the figures picked out by color and metal accessories, but the impression of crowded movement and the development of the story were the important innovations. The artist did not attempt to give a chronologically accurate and factual account of the campaigns but represented an ideally conducted war. The emperor gave speeches to the troops at the proper moment, sacrifices were offered to the gods, embassies were sent and received. The troops were shown on the march, crossing the Danube, assaulting towns, and fighting on the field of battle. The enemy surrendered, and pitiful throngs of prisoners, old men, women, and children, marched in the victorious wake of Trajan. Yet the masses of men and the landscapes in which they move were skillfully handled, and if the relief is followed in detail, by walking twenty-two times around the column with the head thrown back, there is no confusion in following the action.

On the Arch of Beneventum in southern Italy, the whole Principate of Trajan was reviewed in the sequence of paneled scenes. His conquests, acceptance of the surrenders of his enemies, and his reception by the people of Rome are commemorated. Trajan's alimentary measures were recorded by scenes of the children of Italy, while the series culminated in the emperor's apotheosis in heaven, where he was received by the Roman triad of Jupiter, Juno, and Minerva. These works commissioned by Trajan were only two of the hundreds of arches, columns, altars, and other monuments which commemorated the emperors in Rome and the provinces.

The changing styles of sculpture, as set by the *Princeps,* are best illustrated by the portraits of the emperors. The severely cold, idealizing heads of the Julio-Claudian Period, which Augustus had made fashionable, were replaced in the Flavian Period by a return to a realism more native to Italian tradition. The vitality and directness of the best work can be seen in the portraits of Vespasian

Scenes from the Column of Trajan. These relief bands, at the butt of the column, show the start of Trajan's campaigns: the god of the Danube watches the Roman army crossing on a pontoon bridge of boats, and, above, the soldiers are building a walled camp.

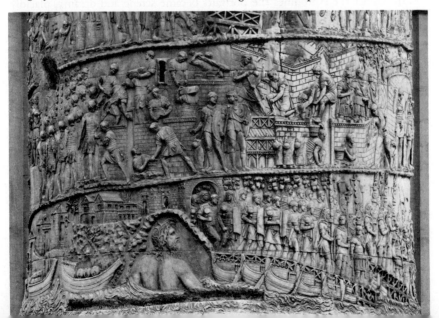

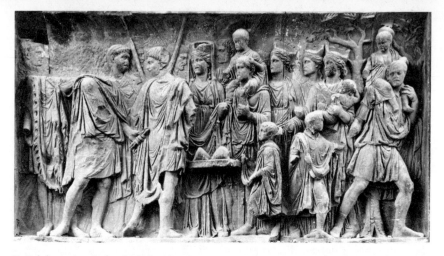

Relief from the Arch of Trajan in Beneventum. The emperor is distributing alms to the children of the town (the alimenta*).*

himself, whose earthy, middle-class temperament had little sympathy for the idealistic Hellenism of Nero whom he replaced. The quality of Flavian workmanship was high and the artists exhibited a remarkable observation of their subjects. The great ladies of the court seem to anticipate their counterparts at the courts of eighteenth-century Europe. The elaborate, tiered hairdressing apparently represented wigs or masses of hair built up by switches and such devices.

Flavian realism swung back to Greek idealism under Hadrian. By his reign the Greek literary renaissance had been in progress for several generations and had begun to affect Roman upper-class education strongly. Hadrian's adornment of Athens, the center of classical Greece, was symptomatic of its nature. He looked back to the Greece of the fifth and fourth centuries B.C. and set a vogue for the imitation of classical art. Hadrian himself cultivated a beard in proper Greek philosophical style. Perhaps this was intended to cover a scar on his chin, but the Roman upper class, clean shaven for centuries, took to beards. More seriously, Hadrian's ideal and the ideal of his period was apparent in the numerous statues of Antinous, the emperor's favorite. The boy was usually represented in Pheidian style, with a serious, thoughtful face, heavy eyes, and sulky mouth. Under the Antonines the portraits became serene and dreamy, placidly dignified, but touched with effeminacy, mirroring the contented comfort of the Antonine Empire.

Thanks to the eruption of Vesuvius in 79 which covered Pompeii and Herculaneum (and to the excavation of numerous Roman villas) our knowledge of tastes in painting and new developments in that art during the first century after Christ is considerable. The walls of the rooms were decorated with murals which date from the second century B.C. to the year of their engulfment. Some of the paintings were copies of major works of Greek art which are unknown to us, but many represent the fashion of the generation or so before the eruption. The most striking development of the Roman Period was the use of techniques of impressionistic painting. As in the relief sculpture, human figures in themselves have ceased to be the focus of interest. The landscapes stretch away into unlimited space and in them the figures are subordinated as an element of the whole scene. The atmosphere is hazy, and illusion is created by the subtle color hues, reminiscent of the skies in Campania. Essentially the same technique of narrative was used as in relief sculpture which may be seen in the series of episodes from Homer's *Odyssey,* called the "Odyssey Landscapes." The action is viewed as if through a window into a far-off landscape. Akin to these in feeling are the so-called villa landscapes, derived from Syrian and Alexandrian proto-types, which represent the great Roman villas, with temples, gardens, sculpture, and walks.

Some idea of ethnic types, at least among the population in Egypt, may be gained from a group of about four hundred painted portraits from the Fayoum. This area had been reclaimed for agriculture and settled by the early Ptolemies, and in the course of time a remarkable mixture of Greeks, Italians, Jews, Syrians, and Egyptians had come to live there. The inhabitants had adopted the Egyptian practice of mummification. A realistic portrait of the dead person was painted on wooden boards and then wrapped into the mummy casings. The portraits were done by local artists while the subject was still alive and were kept until the person died. While of no great artistic merit, the portraits are "speaking like-nesses," and we can contrast the ruddy-faced, thick-necked Italian with the East-erner, who was dark-skinned, oval-faced, with large liquid eyes and a prominent nose.

The Roman Peace: Signs of Weakness

During the Roman Peace the Empire was obviously prosperous and gener-ally well governed. The frontiers had been successfully defended. Yet the hopes for Rome's eternity, expressed by the emperors, were belied by signs of potential weakness and of breakdown, which we can observe in the light of knowledge after the event. The emperors themselves, with the exception of Commodus, were aware of some weaknesses and worked hard and conscientiously to keep the Empire in order.

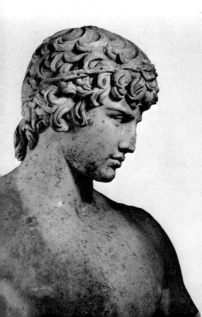

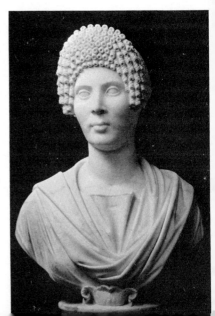

Antinous.
Idealized portrait
of Hadrian's favorite

A Roman lady of
the Flavian Period

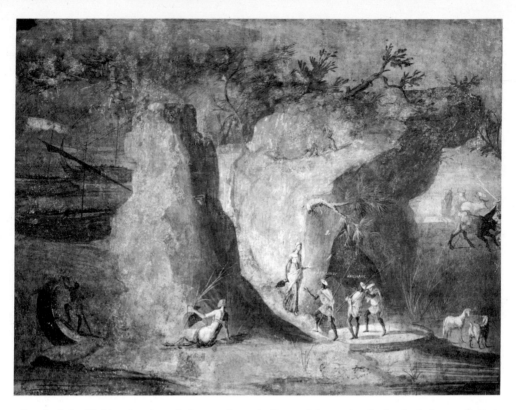

Panel of the "Odysey Landscapes" from a house in Rome. Odysseus in the land of the cannibalistic Laestrygones

The military situation was potentially dangerous. The army and the civilian population of the inner provinces were growing farther apart in feeling and tradition. In the reign of Marcus Aurelius, war on two fronts had demonstrated that, large as the army was for the Empire's resources, it had been barely large enough to hold out against simultaneous heavy attack on the European and Eastern frontiers. During his reign Aurelius had scraped the bottom of the financial barrel. The revenues were not large enough to support the growing administrative system, the ambitious building programs, and war. The barbarian invasions had been thrown back, but they left looted cities and devastated fields. The Roman armies had weakened the provincial cities by requisitions of supplies and the materials for war. We do not know how many people died of the plague in Aurelius' reign, but it was at least a severe temporary shock. An ancient writer tells of the death of two thousand people in a day, and a recent modern estimate places the total loss at about a million.

In the cities of the Empire, signs of financial instability had been apparent from the beginning of the second century. Pliny found in Bithynia that the number of *curials* was too small for the burdens which they had to carry in the administration of their cities. Throughout the reigns of Hadrian and Antoninus, although conditions were generally peaceful, the emperors had received an increasing number of petitions from the cities, some for financial help and some

664

for guidance and advice. Imperial interference, marked initially by the appointment of *curators,* was undermining the desire for self-government. The emperors had responded to the difficulties and to the petitions for help, but their remedies were political in character. *Curators* were appointed, and the imperial bureaucracy was increased in size and complexity, yet the cause of the malaise was economic and was implicit in the economic organization of the Empire itself. The emperors had inherited and did little to interfere with the practice of *laissez-faire.*

Throughout the Empire there was a very sharp cleavage in wealth and privilege between the dwellers in the cities and the peasants of the countryside and between the upper and lower classes of the cities. The governing class was showing obvious signs of resignation and a lack of creativity. Its members found their lives easy and comfortable, so why should they change? The machine of government, which had been organized by the persevering work of the emperors over two centuries, was very strong and could run on its own momentum for a long time. Given a responsible and strong ruler after the death of Marcus Aurelius, the immediate damage of the wars and the plague might have been repaired, and the transformation of the state might have proceeded without breakdown and violence. The Empire, however, was unfortunate in Marcus Aurelius' very human choice of his own son. Commodus' reign is usually regarded as the turning point in its history. Twelve years of frivolous inertia did not matter so much perhaps, but upon Commodus' death the continuity of sensible, orderly succession was broken. As in 68/69, after the death of Nero, contest for the Empire and civil war resulted. In 192, however, the Empire was weakened and had moved too far from its original Augustan character to be restored as Vespasian had restored it.

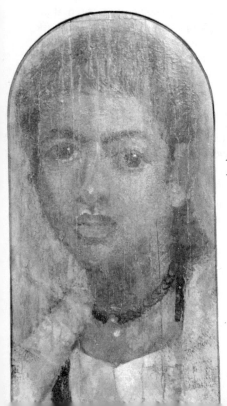

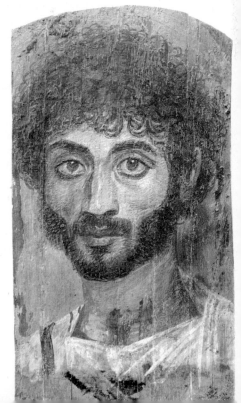

Portraits from the Fayoum in Egypt. These realistic pictures were painted on wooden boards and wrapped into the mummy casings at the time of burial.

XXIX

Crisis and Revolution

(A.D. 192–285)

IN THE THIRD CENTURY after Christ the Roman Empire passed through a crucial period of internal anarchy and foreign invasion which transformed its nature. The death of Commodus in 192 was followed by civil war, from which Septimius Severus, the commander of the Danubian legions, emerged as victor and established the Severan Dynasty of rulers. The Severan regime was transitional between the constitutional Principate of Augustus and his successors and the religious and military autocracy of the Late Empire in the fourth century. The Severan emperors founded their rule directly on the support of the army and sought legitimization for it in religious concepts. The last of the family, Alexander Severus, forfeited the loyalty of the soldiers and was killed in 235. For almost fifty years the Empire was plunged into military anarchy and exposed to invasion. During the Severan Period new and strong peoples had arisen along the frontiers. In the East the Sassanid Persian kings founded an Empire on the ruins of the Parthian Kingdom. In Europe new hordes of barbarians, the Goths, appeared, and Rome's older German enemies raided the Western provinces in ever increasing force. From 268, however, a series of soldier-emperors from Illyria —Claudius, Aurelian, and Probus—brought the situation under control. The army was disciplined, lost territory was regained, and the frontier defenses were re-established.

Political anarchy was accompanied by a reorientation of thought which had been long in the making. Men tended to reject the rationality of Greco-Roman civilization and moved into a world dominated by superstition and religion. A mark of this was the popularity of the Eastern religions which had been spreading from Asia Minor, Syria, and Egypt to the West. Most of these were easily accommodated in the political structure of the state, but Christianity stood apart and, as it gained converts and developed its doctrines, it came into open political and ideological conflict with paganism. When the fortunes of the Empire were

The reader will find the Back Endpaper and Map XIX (page 576) useful as he reads this chapter.

at their lowest ebb, in the mid-third century, and the emperors demanded a mass demonstration of loyalty to the gods of Rome, the Christians refused to participate and were hounded by widespread persecution. When the attempts to stamp out Christianity failed and the faith gained converts rapidly as the pagan cults declined, a fundamental issue had been raised.

The Severan Dynasty (A.D. 192–235)

CIVIL WAR

After the murder of Commodus in 192 the Senate and the praetorian guard concurred in the selection of the city prefect, Pertinax, as emperor. Pertinax, a man of good ability and administrative experience, lasted not quite three months. His economies in government and his attempt to impose strict discipline offended the guard, spoiled by the extravaganzas of Commodus. The soldiers put Pertinax to death and took the selection of a new emperor into their own hands. An auction was held, in which the winner was an elderly senator, Marcus Didius Julianus, whose only qualifications for rule were great wealth and ambition. The cost was a promise of twenty-five thousand sesterces, about $1250, to each guardsman. At this point the commanders of the army groups on the frontiers stepped in, and the play in Rome came to an abrupt end.

Even the people of Rome, who seldom felt a flicker of political responsibility, were angered at the death of Pertinax and in a mob meeting issued an invitation to the commander of the Syrian army, Pescennius Niger, to become emperor. Niger was acclaimed by his troops and speedily got control of Egypt and Asia Minor. A crossing point to Europe was secured by the occupation of Byzantium on the Bosporus. Niger had need of haste because the governor of Upper Pannonia, Septimius Severus, was closer to Rome and announced that he would avenge the death of Pertinax. Eleven legions of the Danubian army and four on the Rhine, half the Roman army, gave him their support. Septimius marched on the capital and took over with his seasoned troops.

Before Septimius arrived in Rome, the Senate had found the courage to deify Pertinax, and the praetorian guard, turning on Julianus, put him to death. Septimius, however, showed no inclination to be indebted to anyone. The guard was demobilized and replaced by fifteen thousand legionary soldiers to give Septimius control of Italy, while he dealt with his rivals. For the time being he remained in accord with the Senate and pledged not to put any of its members to death without trial.

Another rival, in addition to Niger, was Clodius Albinus, the governor of Britain, who was on good terms with many influential senators. To gain freedom of action Septimius agreed to Albinus being named Caesar and recognized as his successor. Then he marched against Niger. In 194 Niger's army was defeated at Issus in Cilicia, and Septimius confiscated vast estates from the private individuals who had supported his enemy and penalized the rebellious cities. Antioch was deprived of its position as capital of Syria, and Byzantium, taken after a siege of two years, was destroyed. Septimius pushed on into Parthian territory because the Parthian king, Vologases IV, had offered aid to Niger and had tampered with the loyalty of one of Rome's vassal kings. Septimius overran northern Mesopotamia and had crossed the Tigris when news came that Albinus had landed in Gaul with an army from Britain.

Albinus, supported by his British troops and senatorial friends from the Western provinces, established himself at Lugdunum (Lyons) and awaited Septimius' advance. In 197 a battle was fought near the city in which Septimius inflicted a crushing defeat on his enemies. Lugdunum was looted and partly demolished, a blow from which it never recovered. Again, as in Asia, Septimius confiscated the property of his opponents and made a virtual purge of the Senate. He then returned to the invasion of Parthia, penetrated as far as the Tigris, where Ctesiphon, the capital, was burnt. The Parthian rulers, already tottering precariously on the throne, were seriously weakened by the Roman thrust, and Septimius was able to organize a new province in Mesopotamia. He appointed an Equestrian bureaucrat as governor, rather than a senator.

SEPTIMIUS SEVERUS

In Septimius the Empire acquired a new type of ruler after the Antonines, a ruthless, able general of Trajan's caliber, who acted decisively and brooked no opposition. He was of Carthaginian descent, born in 146 in the city of Leptis Magna in Africa, Romanized in general culture and well educated, but essentially provincial rather than Italian in point of view. Septimius had risen from the Equestrian bureaucracy, starting as a lawyer for the treasury, to senatorial rank and the governorship of central Gaul and Pannonia. His wife, Julia Domna, was from a prominent, wealthy family of Syria, talented, well educated and in-

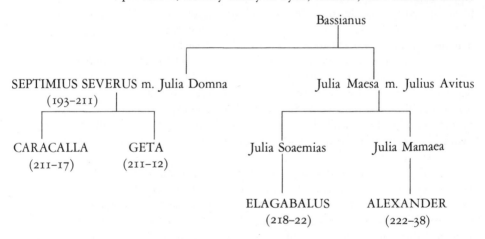

THE SEVERAN EMPERORS

tensely ambitious, like the other women of her family, a sister and two nieces. They were all to play an important part in the history of the Severan Dynasty, which Septimius was determined to establish through his two sons, Caracalla and Geta. When the civil wars were over and Parthia cowed, Septimius proceeded to the organization of his Principate as efficiently as he had fought to get it.

Septimius, a "new man" of relatively obscure origin, like Vespasian, made a place for his family among the deified Roman emperors. In the course of the war against Niger he had himself adopted as the son of Marcus Aurelius and even insisted on the deification of Commodus. Since the army accepted this, the Senate had no choice in the matter. In 198, following Albinus' defeat, Septimius named his elder son, Caracalla, co-ruler, and later promoted Geta to the same position. Both succeeded when Septimius died in 211. The practice of selection of the best, which had governed the choice of emperors from Nerva to Marcus Aurelius, was set aside again, and Septimius founded his rule on the army and on the accumulated prestige of the deified emperors of Rome.

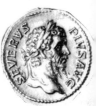

Septimius Severus

The reign of Septimius visibly demonstrated the culmination of the process by which the Senate had been subordinated continuously to the government of the *Princeps*. Septimius had no reason even to show the courtesy which had been customary from the Antonine Emperors because in the struggle for power many senators had compromised themselves by supporting Albinus. They were put to death and their places were filled by provincials who came mainly from Syria and Africa. The Senate was rarely consulted as a group, and as individuals the members were usually passed over in favor of Equestrian bureaucrats and military careerists. The latter were made governors of some senatorial provinces, given high commands, and appointed to other posts of importance. The praetors' courts were abolished, and the city prefect was given jurisdiction over Rome and the territory for a hundred miles from the city. Beyond that limit the praetorian prefect administered justice. This reduction of Italy to the semblance of a province was accentuated by stationing a regular legion at the Alban Lake near Rome.

Septimius' most important innovation, however, was in the enlargement of the prefects' areas of administration. The praetorian prefect became the emperor's second in command, in charge of the military forces in Italy and able to convoke the emperor's council when the latter was absent. In addition, the praetorian prefect was placed in charge of the procurement of grain for Italy although the actual distribution was left in the hands of the prefect of the grain supply. The latter acquired the unenviable task of supplying the armies as well. The praetorian prefect's most important duties, however, were legal. He heard the appeals from the provinces and was expected to develop the principles and administration of law in accompaniment with the rapidly expanding bureaucratic administration.

Septimius' first appointment to the office was a fellow African, Fulvius Plautianus, who became so powerful and arrogant that he incurred the enmity of

Julia Domna and of Caracalla—no difficult matter in either case. They intrigued to have Plautianus killed in 205, and Septimius replaced him by two prefects. One was the famous jurist Papinian, who was followed in office by Paul and Ulpian, who are equally well known for their development of the law. These jurists were Hellenized Syrians, well educated not only in the law of Rome and of the Eastern cities, but in the humane traditions of Greek thought. They followed the line of legal development laid down by Hadrian's lawyers, admitting humanitarian considerations and principles of equity into their decisions and interpretations. It is likely that at this time, too, certain Eastern administrative practices and conceptions came into Roman law. The general tenor of Severan legislation was in favor of the underprivileged. The government's policy was liberal toward the formation of *collegia* by the poor and zealous for the protection of their rights against the upper, governing classes. Nevertheless, such measures required also that a sharp distinction be drawn between the more worthy (*honestiores*), the senators, Equestrians, *curials,* and soldiers and the lower classes (*humiliores*). The Severan jurists also provided a rationale for the increased authority of the emperor by advancing the theory that the Senate had surrendered, not delegated, its rights of government to him.

Septimius amply paid his debt to the army and held its loyalty by improving the conditions of service. The soldiers' pay was raised by a third, but perhaps that only kept abreast of inflation. The men were allowed, however, to contract legal marriages while in service and to live in the civilian settlements near the

The Arch of Septimius Severus in the Roman Forum, dedicated in A.D. 203 to the emperor and his sons, Caracalla and Geta, by the Senate and the people of Rome

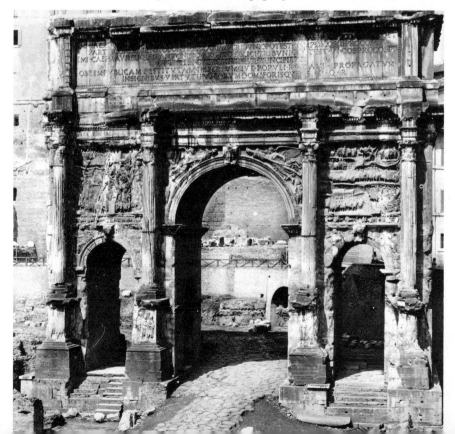

camps. The noncommissioned officers were allowed to form *collegia,* mainly social in purpose, but some were also mutual insurance societies. The army was increased in size from thirty to thirty-three legions, bringing the total force up to about 400,000. It was an efficient, well-trained army, but the soldiers were very conscious of their part in the making of the emperor, and their appetite had been stimulated by the taste of rewards and privileges.

The cost of this enlarged bureaucracy and army to the Empire was very great. A generation earlier Marcus Aurelius had told his troops that an increase in pay could come only from the suffering of their own relatives in civilian life. Septimius and his successors drove the point home. While much of the initial cost was borne by the wholesale confiscations of property made by Septimius, these were on such a scale that, along with the damage of the civil wars, there was an economic upheaval and serious inflation. The state finances had to be reorganized. A new department of the treasury was set up to administer the confiscated properties and was supported for the future by the income from the emperor's private estates rather than by taxation. It was called the *res privata.* The *patrimonium,* which passed from one emperor to the next, had come to be regarded as crown property and it remained, along with the revenues from taxation, in the *fiscus.* Inflation was countered by a twenty percent devaluation of the standard silver coin, the *denarius,* and by a further slight depreciation in the reign of Caracalla, who issued a new coin, the *Antoninianus.*

Most of the seemingly progressive and liberal policies of the Severan regime were motivated by financial urgency. For example, the city of Alexandria and the large native towns of Egypt were made into proper municipalities by permitting them to elect governing councils. These municipalities, however, as elsewhere in the Empire, were made responsible for the full amount of imperial taxes from their city, as well as for the usual municipal services. Caracalla's grant of Roman citizenship to the free inhabitants of the Empire, the climax of Romanization, apparently was made to allow the government to collect taxes, like the inheritance tax, for which only citizens were liable. While Severan policy was liberal in the formation of *collegia,* at the same time compulsory services were imposed on them. The *curials* of the cities were obliged to fulfill *liturgies,* and in almost every city of the Empire the central government required a *curator.* Again the soldiers were favored. Veterans were exempted from civil *liturgies* and the responsibility of holding office in the cities where they elected to live.

The Severan Dynasty, with its mark to make in imperial tradition, engaged in large-scale building programs and provincial development. Some projects were designed only to repair the damage of the civil wars, as in Byzantium and Antioch, but Africa and Syria were particularly favored. Septimius' own city of Leptis Magna was granted immunity from taxation and large sums were lavished on its buildings. The frontier defenses were put in order; Septimius effectively intimidated the Caledonians by leading a campaign into the Scotch Highlands. Hadrian's Wall across northern England was repaired, and Britain entered on a period of peace, which lasted throughout the third century.

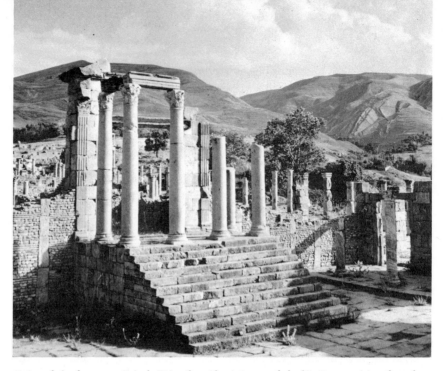

Ruins of the forum at Cuicul (Djemila, Algeria), one of the big Roman cities of northern Africa

While Septimius himself was busied with the political and military tasks of reorganization, his empress, Julia Domna, held a brilliant court for Greek men of letters. One of her protégés, Philostratus, wrote a life of Apollonius of Tyana, a Syrian miracle-worker, whom the pagans later set up as a foil to Christ for his pure and upright life. Another member of Julia's circle, the physician Galen, wrote a synthesis of medical science and philosophic thought on the nature of the human body and mind which was continued by his followers. These writings as a whole form the most important body of medical literature which has survived from antiquity. On the lighter side, the best-known romantic novel of antiquity, Longus' *Daphnis and Chloe,* belongs to the Severan Period. In the tradition of Theocritus' pastoral poetry it told a story of lovers who wander through an idyllic countryside, populated by nymphs and satyrs and decorated with rustic shrines of Pan—an agreeable escape from the increasingly uncomfortable realities of life.

In 211 Septimius died in Eboracum (York). In Rome his reign was commemorated by the great arch which stands today at the entrance to the Roman Forum. To his successors Septimius left a mixed legacy. His hard and efficient administration had pulled the Empire together after the reign of Commodus and the civil wars, but the army had been recognized outwardly as the basis of power. Septimius at least ensured its loyalty to his family for almost a generation. The soldiers were prepared even to accept petticoat government in the palace so long as favors were continued and until they needed another military emperor to lead them in war.

CARACALLA

When Septimius died, his sons, Caracalla and Geta, succeeded as joint rulers, according to their father's plan. Their mutual hostility made the arrangement unworkable, and within a year Caracalla had Geta murdered. Caracalla was despotic and arrogant, even brutal, but by no means without ability as a soldier and with some statesmanlike concern for the Empire. In general, he left internal government to his mother, Julia Domna, and to his officials, while he cultivated the army and fought on the frontiers. He won the goodwill of the soldiers by giving them a raise in pay, and their respect by a successful campaign against the Alemanni on the German border and by a successful thrust into Parthia. The most notable event of Caracalla's reign, in perspective at least, was the extension of Roman citizenship in 212 to all the free inhabitants of the Empire. In actuality this act was little more than a recognition of an accomplished fact, but it did mean that Roman law became the binding force throughout imperial society. Caracalla also seems to have had some idea of making an alliance with Parthia since he proposed marriage to the daughter of the Parthian king. Both the proposal and his invasion of Parthia were left as unfinished business in 217 when he was killed as the result of a plot engineered by the praetorian prefect, Macrinus.

Macrinus, the first Equestrian to become *Princeps,* held the loyalty of the army for a brief time by taking the name, Severus, and by directing the Senate

Roman lady of the Severan Period, sometimes identified as Julia Domna, the wife of Septimius Severus   *Caracalla*

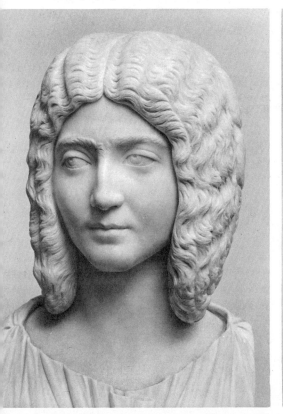

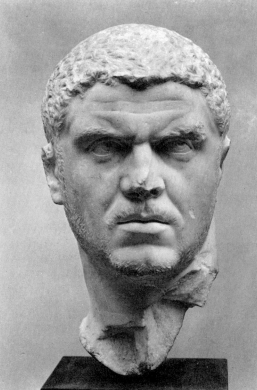

to deify Caracalla, but the relatives of Julia Domna in Syria—she herself had died—conspired to get the throne into their own branch of the family. When Macrinus was defeated in battle by the Parthians and paid them off with a subsidy, he lost the loyalty of the soldiers. The Severans defeated the remnants of his army, and the troops acclaimed their candidate as emperor.

ELAGABALUS

The moving force in the intrigue against Macrinus was Julia Maesa, the sister-in-law of Septimius Severus. Her candidate for emperor was her young grandson, sixteen years of age, Varius Avidius Bassianus, son of Julia Soaemias and a Syrian senator. Maesa, however, set a rumor going that Bassianus was really the son of Caracalla, which helped to win over the soldiers. The new emperor was a priest of the sun-god Elagabal of Emesa in Syria, and so is usually called Elagabalus or Heliogebalus. He was entirely Syrian in habit and thought, devoted to his priestly duties and to debauchery, which was by no means incompatible with the worship of a Baal who was supposed to reside in a black fetish stone and whose cult practice included temple prostitution. In 218 Elagabalus came to Rome and for four years amazed the capital by one of the Empire's more fantastic reigns.

Elagabalus rewarded his Syrian clique of priests, members of the family, and expectant hangers-on with high administrative posts and honors, and he promoted his god Elagabal to a share in Empire. Elagabalus' own priestly title was added to the usual Roman titles of the emperor. The fetish was brought to Rome, where a wife was found for it in Minerva and, since the Baal did not object to bigamy, it was married also to Tanit, the Phoenician moon-goddess. This heavenly union of East and West was paralleled on earth by Elagabalus'

Baalbek in Syria. Reconstruction of the interior of the Temple of Bacchus, an example of the rich, baroque architecture of imperial Rome

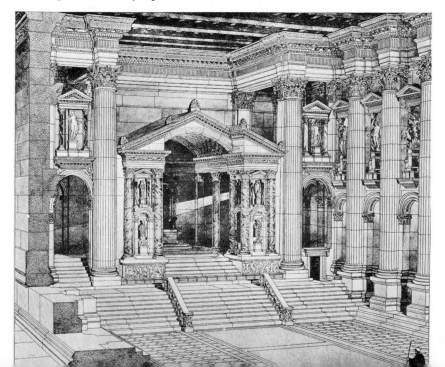

own marriage to a Roman vestal virgin. Roman upper-class opinion could endure a great deal from an emperor, but all this, compounded with temple prostitution, circumcision, and ritual taboos against eating pork which the Romans liked, was too much. Elagabalus himself had neither the knowledge to rule nor the interest and ability to learn. Julia Maesa, well aware of the disgust of most of the high officials and of the Senate, persuaded Elagabalus to adopt his cousin Alexander as heir and then intrigued to have Elagabalus and his mother killed. This accomplished, the Baal was sent home and Alexander succeeded as emperor.

While Elagabalus' conduct seemed fantastic and irresponsible to the Roman upper class, as it does to us, it was of considerable significance for the future. Elagabalus evidently conceived of the Roman emperor in the fashion of oriental kingship in which the king was the servant of the Empire's god, appointed and protected by him to rule the state. Fifty years later, the Emperor Aurelian, a man of very different stamp than Elagabalus, established the sun as a universal deity of the Empire and regarded this god as his patron.

ALEXANDER

Since Severus Alexander was only fourteen when he succeeded in 222, his rule could scarcely be direct. The power behind the throne was first his grandmother, Julia Maesa, and then his mother, Julia Mamaea, who made an alliance with the Senate and the high officials of the bureaucracy, which gave the regime a more civilian character. Alexander himself seems to have been an intelligent, serious boy, who followed Roman traditions carefully. The prestige, if not the governing power of the Senate, was restored. A council of sixteen senators was set up to advise the emperor, and the *consilium* was enlarged to seventy, twenty of whom were legal experts and fifty, men of distinction. Relations between the Senate and the praetorian prefect were smoothed over by making the latter a senator while in office. Under this direction governmental policy was generally humanitarian, if excessively bureaucratic, and much money was spent on the provinces. An elementary-school system was extended, and useful building projects, aqueducts, roads, and baths, were sponsored. Taxes were reduced and the alimentary programs enlarged.

The army, however, had made the Severan Dynasty, and towards the end of Alexander's reign pressure on the frontiers compelled the emperor to take a belated interest in military affairs. Mutinies had forewarned him that morale among the soldiers was unsatisfactory. In 228 the praetorian guard killed their prefect, the jurist Ulpian, and the Mesopotamian army put their commander to death. Action and victories might have saved the throne, but Alexander failed to rise to the occasion. A well-conceived plan of attack in 231 against the Persians, who had invaded Syria, failed for lack of good generalship in the field. The Persians were driven across the frontier, but Roman losses were heavy. At the same time the Alemanni broke through the defenses on the upper Rhine, and Alexander, instead of fighting as his generals wished, followed his mother's advice and bought them off. In 235, under the leadership of Maximinus, a tough Thracian peasant who had risen from the ranks to the governorship of Pannonia, the legions mutinied. Alexander and his mother were killed, and Maximinus was acclaimed emperor. The determination of the soldiers to have emperors to their liking plunged the Empire into fifty years of civil war, anarchy and disintegration.

Religious Change in the Empire

THE SPREAD OF EASTERN RELIGIONS

During the Severan Period there were many other indications of the emergence of a new mentality in addition to the glaring example of Elagabalus. As we have noticed, the educated upper class focused its interest on the cultural traditions of the past, while the popular culture of ordinary people revealed itself more clearly. Older native languages and institutions began to reassert themselves, and in remote regions of the Empire knowledge of Greek and Latin was no longer necessary to hold governmental posts and to issue official documents. The mass culture was exemplified, in particular, by the spread of Eastern religious worships, which penetrated into the Western provinces and into the upper class itself. While orientalization was most obvious, the process of change was more complex, for Celtic influences reappeared in Gaul and Britain, and Germanic customs crossed the frontiers. These changes indicate the weakening of the classical traditions which had been the driving force in the Empire since the time of Augustus.

Most noticeable in religious life was the search for a god who would help his worshippers in the current difficulties of their life and assure their welfare in the hereafter. As the present grew more painful, men at least wanted a happy future. Almost equally apparent was the syncretism between the traditional Greco-Roman worships and the Eastern cults, not merely by the old practice of making mutual identifications among their gods, but in thought as well. The attitude of Plutarch was symptomatic. He found some truth in all the religions with which he was familiar—Greek, Roman, and Oriental. Ordinary men, too, were both eclectic and catholic. A man might select one religion as his favorite, but by no means excluded others from his attention. Christianity, of course, was not immune. Its educated leaders shared in the tradition of Greek thought, while its practice admitted or shared ritual from pagan worships. Above all, however, the individual wanted a personal god of his own, for he could no longer find satisfaction in the old, established religious practice of his city or of the state. Security and immortality seemed the most desirable goods when traditional values were disappearing.

The public worships of the Empire were, of course, fundamentally political in character and origin. In the old Greek cities of the East the civic cults had come into existence when the cities were independent states and when the citizen's identification with his city and with the gods who protected it was strong.

In the Hellenistic Period these civic cults had been transferred to the new cities, and identifications were made with native gods, while some Eastern practices and beliefs were absorbed by the Greeks. Although the Hellenized natives had accepted Greek religion to a considerable degree, the mass of the people had kept their traditional beliefs. A state of balance had been achieved which persisted into the Empire. In Italy and the culturally Romanized cities of the West the formal and political religion of Rome had been established with its apparatus of priestly colleges and worship of the triad, Jupiter, Juno, and Minerva. The public cults of both East and West were supported by the cities, and the people worshipped in these cults as an integral part of civic life. Such worships appealed through traditional prestige, time-honored festivals, and ritual, but the worshippers had little personal participation.

On the other hand, the minor pagan religious practices had retained a genuinely personal appeal. Closest to ordinary men were the intimate little gods of their household and locality, of their crafts, and of the fields. Men worshipped these divinities in their family and in the *collegiate* associations. Yet these gods were petty and their power was limited. The only properly universal worship of the Empire was the ruler cult, which did have genuine religious qualities in the recognition and worship of the attributes of the idealized ruler—his foresight, benevolence, and patience. Observance of ruler cult, however, was mainly an expression of political loyalty, and its ritual was carried out by a priesthood, while the emperor himself was almost as remote as the great gods. Since none of these traditional worships was exclusive, men could observe them and at the same time turn to the foreign religions of the East and find a different kind of satisfaction in each.

Some of the mystery religions, like the worship of Cybele, the Great Mother-Goddess of Asia Minor, and of Isis of Egypt had already made their way to Italy at the time of the Roman conquest of the East. Cybele was officially installed in Rome in 205 B.C., and her worship had been carried to the Roman cities of the Western provinces by colonists. The other cults, however, had a more difficult time and were spread largely by personal media. They were brought by slaves who continued to worship their chosen gods when they became freedmen and citizens, by traders to the port cities and to the market towns, and by the legionary soldiers. The initial policy of the government had been to stamp out the cults or, at least, to limit worship to small, private groups. But in the Empire the cults won official recognition, as well as many private followers. For example, Augustus and Tiberius prohibited the building of a temple to Isis in Rome, but Gaius seems to have allowed it, and Domitian indicated his favor by using symbols of Isis on his coinage.

In the second and third centuries after Christ these mystery cults grew rapidly in popularity in Italy and spread to the Romanized provinces of the West. Their appeal lay in the universal and at the same time intensely personal nature of worship. Anyone, rich or poor, free or slave, and of any race might become a worshipper. The traveler from Egypt or Syria would find a welcome

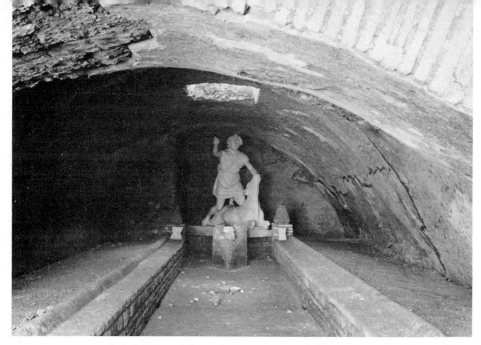

A Mithraeum at Ostia. The shrines were in the form of a cave with the cult statue of Mithras at the end.

among his fellows in Rome or London. Common to most of the cults was the myth of a god who suffered, died, and was resurrected. His story was re-enacted in an impressive pageant in which the worshipper shared the god's experience by vicarious identification. Most cults, too, had impressive and elaborate rites of initiation, although in some cases these were limited by the assessment of a substantial fee. Men were given a feeling of warm security and the hope of immortality by the rites of purification, by observance of a moral code, and by a sense of community with their fellow worshippers. They could pray directly to the god themselves and hope confidently for a personal vision and for a miracle. Thus the gods were brought close to men.

MITHRAISM

The religion of Mithraism, frequently referred to as the chief rival of Christianity, was rather later in making its way to the West than the mystery cults and differed from them in several important respects. Mithras was the Persian god of light in the old Persian religion (pp. 163–64), but the form of the cult which spread through the Roman Empire originated in Asia Minor among the Iranian elements of the population. The soldiers carried it back to Italy and to the frontier provinces, to Britain, and to the camps along the Rhine and the Danube. In London a Mithraeum, as the shrines were called, was discovered in the heart of the modern city, revealed by the bombing of World War II. Mithraism is, in fact, known from the shrines rather than from any surviving scriptures.

The shrines reproduced a cave, at the end of which was a sculptured relief showing Mithras killing a bull. On the walls other reliefs represented the story of the god's life, but the ceremonies did not include a dramatic reenactment of the myth. The bull was a symbol of the source of life, and Mithras was depicted as chasing and capturing it. When the bull was put to death, Mithras received the homage of the sun-god for his exploit and shared a sacred meal with him. The worshippers passed through an elaborate initiation, in which they rose to the grade of *pater* (father) of the group. The fathers administered the cult, since there was no priesthood or official hierarchy. The worship thus stressed a community of feeling among the members, symbolized by a common, sacred meal. Only men could become members and the cult was particularly popular with the soldiers.

Mithraism never became a Roman state cult like that of Cybele, but it was spread by its own vitality and the specific appeal of Mithras, a cosmic god who had helped to make the world and who would return at the millennium. Mithras protected his worshippers in this life and ensured their welfare in the hereafter if they observed his moral demands. He was not the only god of the religion, however, since Ahura Mazda, the remote and aloof Persian sun-god and Ahriman, a former god of evil opposing him, also existed. Mithras, too, had his angelic helpers in the struggle to aid mankind. The religion was not exclusive, and therefore worshippers might participate in other cults and, of course, in the worship of the emperor, which the soldier's military oath required. Women were excluded, however, and this imposed a definite limitation on the number of converts. Despite its label as a rival of Christianity, Mithraism was most popular in those regions of the Empire to which Christianity did not spread until very late.

THE RISE OF CHRISTIANITY

By the third century Christianity was becoming a perceptible social force in the Empire. It had spread widely through the Eastern provinces and passed to Rome and other Italian cities and into Africa, but was still very weak in the newer provinces of Europe. We cannot estimate the number of Christians at that time, but the religion had acquired strength through its church organization and was attracting able and well-educated men. The officials of the church could exert discipline and insist on orthodoxy, for the experiment and variety of early Christianity had been systematized in the second century by St. Irenaeus (*ca.* 125–202) in his book, *Against Heresies*.

The appeal of early Christianity is to be understood in the same historical context as that of the mystery religions. In fact, Christianity had much in common with them: a God who had suffered, died, and had been resurrected; the rites of baptism and of the eucharist were mystical and shared by initiates; and not the least in that age were its miracles and visions. Men could find in Christianity the secure intimacy of a small group and a strong supernatural protector, Jesus, who would help them in their present distress and assure them of immortality. They could gain courage and assurance from the revelation and the common performance of the rites of worship.

There were also essential differences in Christianity from the mystery religions which added to its appeal and helped in its establishment. At the outset Jesus' teaching had enlarged the concept of God as a loving father; he had stressed the brotherhood of man and insisted on faith and personal goodness. As the Dead Sea scrolls have recently revealed, not all of this was peculiar to Jesus, but the Essene communities which shared much with early Christianity had taken to the desert, while Christianity developed an apostolic mission. The Christians retained a forceful code of conduct based on the Old Testament but, largely through the work of St. Paul, discarded the letter of the Mosaic Law. Some of its taboos and ritual practices, such as circumcision, were offensive to Gentiles. Thus, from the mid-first century Christianity had grown rapidly beyond its matrix of Judaism and had attracted Gentiles by its own qualities and by the zeal of its missionaries. In contrast to the mystery religions, Christianity developed the discipline and unity of a hierarchical organization, knit by political as well as religious ties.

Because Christianity was at first regarded as a schismatic sect of Judaism and originated in the East, conservative, upper-class Roman society condemned it automatically and showed no interest in its ideas. We have already noticed the remarks of Tacitus in connection with Nero's attempt to fasten guilt on the Christians of Rome for the fire of 64. The Christians were "men hated for their abominations . . . a most mischievous superstition." Pliny had the curiosity to investigate the behavior of the Christians in Bithynia and found that they disavowed crime, adultery, and perjury, ate ordinary food, and got up before sunrise to sing hymns to their God. Yet social prejudice had resulted in the Christians being regarded as hostile to the state and open to prosecution. The government's policy in that respect remained that of Trajan well into the third century —Christians were to be tolerated, unless specific charges were brought against them as individuals before the magistrates. Their guilt was determined by refusal to worship the gods of the state.

As it was with Judaism, the prejudice against Christians seems to have arisen from their religious exclusiveness in a society to which this idea was foreign. The Christians met in small groups in private houses and did not participate in the civic religious life of their communities. Imagination, always ready to supply such details, pictured the secret meetings as orgies of vice and cannibalistic feasts, evidently a misinterpretation of the eucharist. The Christians of the first century expected that the present world order would end speedily and awaited the imminent return of Christ. Accordingly they were not particularly concerned with the ordinary values of society but leveled distinctions of property and of status and regarded marriage as unimportant. Christians, of course, could scarcely hold civic office and serve in the army where religious ceremonies to worship the Roman gods and the emperor were required. Because Christians were different, society rejected them and, because failure to join in the state religion was disloyalty, they were regarded as hostile to the state.

But as the Christians grew in numbers and confidence, defenders of their position appeared, notably Justin Martyr (*ca.* 100–65) who wrote in Greek, and Tertullian of Carthage (160–220), a brilliant Latin stylist, who is regarded as the founder of church Latin. Tertullian wrote a defense addressed to the provincial governors, under whose jurisdiction prosecutions might be made. He protested that the Christians were social beings, like the pagans. They engaged in the ordinary business of life, used the legal and commercial institutions of society and were loyal. What was more, the Christians paid their taxes honestly. The only point of difference was that they did not join in the worship of the Roman gods. In short, Christians could worship their own god and still be good Roman citizens. In practice the government had agreed in this by its policy of toleration, but in theory it could not do so, for the state and its political religion were indissolubly connected.

By the third century, when the difficulties of the Empire began to multiply, pagan society was readier to find fault with the Christians' disloyalty. From the time of Marcus Aurelius there were more individual prosecutions, and in some cities large-scale rioting broke out against the Christian communities. At least one educated Roman, the philosopher Celsus, published a pamphlet, the *True Discourse,* in which he attacked Christianity on ideological grounds and issued an appeal to the Christians to cooperate in the defense of the Empire. Ideological battle, however, was scarcely joined before the late third and fourth centuries and, until that time, the chief feeling against the Christians seems to have been that of Celsus, that they were not pulling their weight at a time of danger for the Empire.

A clash was implicit in the situation. The Christians had not only begun to assert their convictions publicly, but the church was growing into a state within the state, a phenomenon which the Roman government could hardly ignore. At first the Christian communities had been small independent groups, much like the *collegia.* They were linked by their common faith, although with much local variety, and by the exchange of visitors and letters. Each group elected its own officials. We hear of bishops, elders, teachers, miracle-workers, and prophets. The apostle who founded a congregation did appoint deacons to handle the business affairs, but there was no central head or chain of officials. In the second century, however, most of these minor offices disappeared, and in each city a single bishop became supreme and exercised disciplinary power. In the regions where Christians were numerous they tended to regard the bishop in the provincial capital as their metropolitan. Around him a hierarchy of officials coalesced to administer, and a clergy developed whose function it was to preach. No real distinction in authority was made as yet between the various metropolitans of Antioch, Alexandria, and of Rome, but the bishop of Rome assumed, and was sometimes granted, recognition as chief officer. Thus the Roman government began to see an organization patterned on the regional divisions of the Empire, among whose groups connection and discipline existed. Public opinion and the law regarded the members of this organization as intrinsically disloyal.

As we have noticed above, the Severan emperors were themselves moving toward an absolutism which sought legitimation among the pagan gods, rather than in the constitutional, legal ground of the Augustan Principate. In an increasingly religious age, which was to be convulsed by political and economic breakdown, it was natural that a clash would occur. The great persecutions made against the Christian church coincided with the acute distress of the Empire in the mid-third century and with the change in the nature of the Principate.

The Military Anarchy (A. D. 235–85)

With the acclamation of Maximinus, the Thracian general, in 235 by the army on the upper Rhine, the soldiers again began the dangerous practice of emperor-making. Maximinus defeated the Germans decisively but could not cope with the problems of financial administration, and within three years his exactions provoked a revolt in Africa. The Senate made an attempt, successful for a brief time, to hold back the rising tide of military anarchy, but the soldiers were too conscious of their power. Revolt and civil war became the normal pattern of political life from 238 until 285. It is almost impossible to follow the changes of rule and the challenges to rule which took place. Scores of aspirants to the throne appeared in brief scenes, which lasted only a few days or weeks. Occasionally their drive for power stretched into a lengthy and difficult civil war. In the reign of Gallienus (253–68), when the disintegration of the Empire reached its climax, eighteen rivals were suppressed. In this period the central government lost control of many of the Eastern provinces and of Gaul, Spain, and Britain in the West, while at the same time the Danubian provinces were overrun by the Goths. Even nature did not spare the people of the Empire, for plague arose in Egypt and spread through the other provinces, and great earthquakes shook Italy and the East. It is estimated that by the time the Empire was pulled together again in the 270's, the population had been reduced by a third.

The causes of the disintegration are complex and, of course, involved in what is usually referred to as the "decline and fall" of the Roman Empire. Decline was certainly evident, but it was arrested, and before discussing the larger problem, it might be useful to gain perspective by reviewing the crisis and the resulting transformation of the state and of society. The breakdown in the third century did change the character of the Empire profoundly, but after the reorganization of Diocletian and Constantine, it was still Roman and still very much alive. The most obvious factor in the breakdown was the behavior of the army and its inability to protect the frontiers against the Persians and the Goths. Accordingly, we will begin with that aspect of the crisis.

THE ARMY

Throughout the period it seems to have been the soldiers themselves, the rank and file of the army, who stirred up military anarchy, not the generals and the provincial governors. Some generals and governors did take advantage of the situation to further their private ambition, but in the main the generals were reluctant to accept the acclamation of their troops because they feared for their personal safety. Those who ruled as emperor for a sufficient length of time to permit us to form any judgment of their conduct proved to be sincerely devoted to restoring order and to defending the Empire as best they could. On the other hand, the soldiers of the separate army groups, or even of a few legions engaged in a campaign, made and unmade emperors, dividing their time between fighting each other and fighting off barbarians. The internal anarchy, of course, tended to invite barbarian invasion, and successful invasion accelerated the anarchy in turn.

It has been suggested that the unrest of the soldiers was really a revolution of the lower class, specifically of the peasants of the countryside from whom the army was recruited, against the upper and middle classes of the cities. Yet the soldiers oppressed peasant and city-dweller alike. In the end, although the middle class of the cities was severely damaged and many senatorial proprietors were destroyed, the peasants were worse off. Even when the generals of peasant origin had the opportunity, they made no change in the system of land tenure, which was the only real way to better the position of the peasants. No doubt the lower class in both city and country took some satisfaction in the distress of their "betters," but the army's behavior seems to stem from the soldiers' greed and lack of loyalty to the concept of Empire.

While it had been traditional practice for emperors to gain favor with the soldiers by liberal gifts of money at the outset of their reign or to mark some special occasion, the Severan emperors had almost bought their continuance of rule by raises in pay, very large gifts, and the granting of privileges. These may have been deserved, but the army became a privileged group in the population. The soldiers, of course, recognized that the rule of the Severans rested directly on their support and that they were also indispensable to the Empire because of the increased pressure of the barbarians on the frontiers. The soldiers were able to demand favors and to take them by force.

Perhaps the lack of responsibility to the interests of the Empire as a whole is to be explained by the type of soldier recruited by the Severan emperors. Roman citizenship had been an inducement to the more responsible type of recruit who wished to secure its privileges for the advancement of his own career and for his family. Caracalla's virtually universal extension of citizenship removed this inducement and made it necessary to recruit among the more violent and uncivilized groups of the population or outside the Empire altogether. The men were attracted by the improved conditions of service in the Severan army and expected opportunities for action and plunder. The historians of the Severan Period commented on the savage and uncouth character of the soldiers, often drawn from men who would normally live by banditry. The anarchy of the third century gave them full scope for recklessness and plundering, and the chief motivation of the soldiers seems to have been the realization of the advantages to be obtained by use of their power.

There were other factors, too, which made it difficult for the generals to maintain a good morale. The armies were handicapped by the need to fight simultaneously on two fronts against heavy odds. They discovered that, when the barbarians had broken through the fixed frontier defenses, their legionary formations and standard weapons were not able to cope with a fast-moving war of pursuit. The soldiers were good fighting men, and if the legions could force an action on a field to their liking, they won handily, but against the large formations of mounted archers and mail-clad cavalry, which the Persians had, they were at a disadvantage.

The main pressure from new enemies came on the Eastern and European provinces and these were seriously damaged. Africa was raided to some degree by the desert tribes, but the provinces there were held without difficulty, while Britain enjoyed the unique privilege of suffering only occasional piratical raids on the coastal towns.

THE LOSS OF THE EASTERN PROVINCES

In the East the Romans were aware that a new and formidable power had risen against them when Alexander Severus' carefully planned offensive failed to achieve its purpose in 231/32. The Romans drove the Persians back across the Euphrates but failed to penetrate deeply, as Septimius and Caracalla had done. Those expeditions, in fact, had played a part in weakening the Parthian kingship and in permitting the rise of the new Sassanian Persian Empire. The Sassanid kings built on the foundations of Parthian rule and controlled the whole of the Middle East until it fell to Islam in the seventh century after Christ.

The rise of the Sassanian Empire was strikingly like that of the Persian Empire of Cyrus the Great and of Darius (pp. 160–70), to which the Sassanid kings looked back for nationalistic inspiration. The kings of Persis, the heart of the old Persian Empire, had been vassals of Parthia, ruling in the city of Stakhr, near Persepolis. In 208 King Ardashir came to the throne of Persis, and in the following years he reduced the neighboring princes of Iran and seized some of the adjacent Parthian provinces. When the Parthians tried to suppress Ardashir, he defeated them in battle in 224 and was crowned King of Kings. The avowed aim of the Sassanids was to restore the Achaemenid Empire of Darius, which had stretched from the Mediterranean to India and to central Asia. Ardashir was successful in the East, and in 231 attacked Roman Mesopotamia as preliminary to the conquest of Asia Minor, Armenia, and Syria.

While the Sassanian Empire was outwardly just a replacement of the Parthian Kingdom, the Persians were fired with the energy of a successful beginning and with nationalistic zeal. They made Stakhr a holy city, where the kings were crowned in the fire temple of Anahita, for a religious revival accompanied the political and military renaissance. The monarchs ruled, however, from Ctesiphon, the Parthian capital, which was the center of communications in the Middle East, and rebuilt Seleucia, just across the Tigris from Ctesiphon. Seleucia had lain in ruin since its destruction at the hands of Avidius Cassius during the reign of Marcus Aurelius. In place of the loosely organized vassal kingdoms which had made up the Parthian state, the Sassanids developed a more centralized system of government, whose provincial governors were called kings (*shahs*), but who were subordinated to the King of Kings. While the old feudal system of social organization was maintained and the bulk of the army fought in levies around the great nobles, a formidable mail-clad cavalry was organized from the lesser nobility. The official religion, in effect a state church, was based on Zoroastrianism, and King Shapur I, the son of Ardashir, encouraged the priesthood to produce a canonized version of the Persian scriptures, the Zend-Avesta. Shapur, however, was tolerant of Judaism and Christianity, when these were spread by missionaries and prisoners of war, who had been taken into Persia.

After the death of Alexander Severus, the Persians again advanced to the west in 237 and took over Roman Mesopotamia. From there in 241 Shapur struck into Syria and threatened Antioch. The Roman government was able to organize an effective counterattack, led by Timesitheus, the praetorian prefect and father-in-law of the boy emperor, Gordian III. Timesitheus recovered Roman Mesopotamia but died on the eve of further campaigns, and the emperor fell into the hands of a desert prince, Philip the Arab. Philip put Gordian out of the way and became emperor in his place. To hold his position Philip had to return to the West, and so concluded a peace with Shapur which kept Roman territory intact for the time being.

When the Gothic raids along the Danube tied Rome's hands in the 250's, however, Shapur struck again. The occupation of Armenia in 252 secured his northern flank, and Shapur could move along the whole frontier. Mesopotamia was reoccupied, and raids were mounted into Cappadocia and Syria. The Roman emperor, Valerian, left his son Gallienus in charge of Italy and moved to Antioch to organize the defense of the Eastern provinces. Valerian won an initial success against the Persians, but the plague struck his army, forcing him to negotiate. It is not clear whether Shapur treacherously took Valerian prisoner in the course of the negotiations, as the Parthians had once seized Crassus, or whether he was defeated in a minor battle. In any case, the Roman emperor was taken back to the heart of the Persian Empire, and Shapur commemorated the feat by having cut on the cliffs of Persis five separate sculptural representations of Valerian kneeling before him. The remainder of the Roman army retreated into Asia Minor, and Shapur thrust on to take Antioch and Tarsus and to raid in Asia Minor.

Despite the capture of the emperor and the overrunning of Roman territory, Shapur failed to add the Roman East to his Empire. His warfare against the urbanized provinces followed the age-old pattern of Eastern *razzias,* raids for devastation and plunder, rather than a deliberate plan of conquest and occupation. His excessive plundering alienated the provincials, and so prevented the exploitation of anti-Roman sentiment. Most important, Shapur estranged the powerful ruler of Palmyra, the desert caravan city, by cutting off its trade with the Arabians and the Persian Gulf. As the Persian campaign broke up into plundering forays, Shapur retreated back into Persian territory, harassed by guerilla warfare and by the stiff resistance put up by the walled cities in the Roman provinces.

When Rome proved unable to hold the East, the rulers of Palmyra, King Odenathus and his wife, Zenobia, took over the task and set up a virtually independent Palmyrene state from the Bosporus to Egypt. The city of Palmyra had grown immensely wealthy on the profits of the desert caravan trade, but its rulers had been loyal allies of Rome, contributing effectively to frontier defense along the fringe of the desert. Odenathus was able to gather up some of the remnants of Valerian's army and to meet the Persians successfully with his own mounted archers and armored cavalry. He sent help to the northern cities of Asia Minor, harassed by Gothic sea raids, and extended his influence through Syria and Palestine into Egypt. Since Valerian's son Gallienus could not bring an army to the East, he loaded Odenathus with complimentary titles and maintained the fiction that the king was an ally of Rome.

Odenathus acquiesced in this, but on his death Zenobia plainly demonstrated that she wanted an Eastern Empire on full terms of equality with the Roman West. Zenobia was one of the most remarkable women of antiquity, beautiful and ambitious like Cleopatra, and also intellectually talented and a patroness of Neoplatonist philosophers. She later charged them with whetting her political ambitions, but their advice was hardly needed. Zenobia watched her opportunities carefully and in 270 refused to acknowledge the current and very weak Roman emperor. She occupied western Asia Minor and Egypt with military force and took the title of Augusta for herself and Augustus for her son.

The Emperor Valerian kneeling in submission to Shapur I of Persia. A rock-relief at Naqsh-i Rustam, Iran

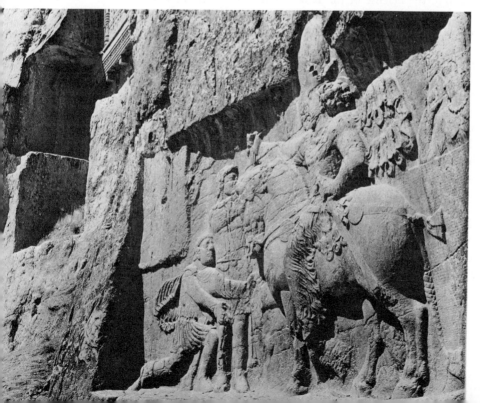

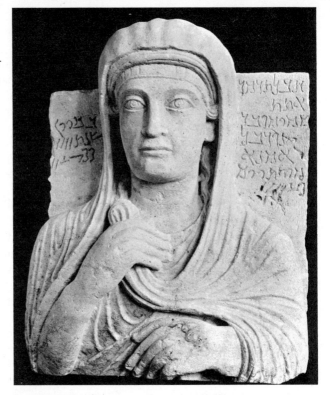

*Grave monument of
a Palmyrene lady*

When Aurelian, the restorer of the Roman Empire, came to the throne in 270,
he had to reconquer the East from Zenobia.

THE DISINTEGRATION OF ROMAN EUROPE

While the Eastern provinces were being devastated by Persian attacks and
given over to Palmyrene rule, the European frontier defenses were broken all
along the river lines from the Black Sea to the lower Rhine. The most serious
damage was done by a Germanic people, the Goths. Their original homeland
had been around the Baltic Sea and in east Germany, but for some time they
had been moving in migratory bands into south Russia. As reports of growing
Roman weakness filtered through to them, the Goths began to move to the
lower Danube, first appearing there in the reign of Alexander Severus. They
were a warrior people of the old Celtic type, bent on looting and destruction
rather than on permanent settlement, and they fought in kinship or local territorial groups, not in organized tactical formations. Before a walled city the
Goths were impatient and unskilled and speedily broke up after a defeat, but
their great numbers and mobility would have made it difficult for the Roman
legions to deal with them under the best of circumstances. It proved impossible
when the Danubian armies were weakened by diversion to other fronts and
when Rome was in a state of anarchy.

Throughout the 230's and 240's the Goths probed and raided along the
lower stretches of the Danube, but the emperors, busy with war in the East and
in defending themselves against rivals, fought only minor engagements or paid

687

the Goths subsidies in gold to stay on the north side of the river. In 249, however, when much of the Danubian army had been withdrawn to Italy, large numbers of Goths broke through into Moesia and Thrace, and into Dacia from the east. The emperor Decius, an able and loyal soldier, made a valiant effort to drive them back, but after an initial success was killed in battle. In 251 when the barriers were swept aside, the Goths poured over the frontiers to loot and devastate, attracting more of their kindred from the north.

For almost twenty years, in an ebb and flow of warfare, the Balkan provinces were overrun. At times the Romans bought peace with subsidies, at times they defeated and turned back the invaders briefly, but the damage was severe and lasting. The Goths around the eastern and northern shores of the Black Sea made piratical forays on the great coastal cities of Asia Minor from Trapezus to Ephesus. In Greece, Gothic bands penetrated to ancient Sparta and attacked Athens. The people of Athens dismantled the public buildings in the lower city and hastily threw up a defensive wall with the stones. This saved a part of Athens, including the Acropolis, but the remainder was burnt and never fully rebuilt. Thousands of provincials were killed or carried off as slaves, and in sheer joy of destruction, buildings were damaged and crops and orchards burnt. Where the Goths did not devastate, the Roman armies sent to fight them had to requisition supplies and food and put the civilian population to work on roads and fortifications. In 267/68, however, the Emperor Gallienus inflicted heavy defeats on those Goths who had raided into Greece but had to leave the war unfinished while he hurried back to Italy. Gallienus was assassinated in 268, and the Gothic wars, too, were left for the Illyrian Emperors to fight.

Farther to the west, in the region between the upper Rhine and the Danube, the Alemanni and the other German peoples west of the Elbe River took advantage of the Empire's weakness. Raetia was overrun and for a time lost to Rome to become a sort of no-man's land. Thrusts were made into Italy, even approaching Rome, and in 258 Gallienus fought a full-scale battle near Milan in an attempt to throw the invaders out. But operations against the Alemanni and against the Franks along the lower Rhine were made even more difficult when a separate Gallic Kingdom was formed in 260 which resisted the central government of Gallienus.

Along the lower Rhine the Franks, whose name was applied to the confederation of Germanic peoples in that region, had taken advantage of the confusion of the 250's to step up their raids. The Roman army was weakened by withdrawals to other fronts, and Gallienus was unable to protect the Gallic provinces, despite a frantic combination of counterattacks and attempts to sow dissension among the Frankish chieftains. In 260 the Roman army of the Rhine, after a victory over the Franks, acclaimed one of the generals, Postumus, as emperor and killed the son of Gallienus, their nominal commander. Postumus set up his capital at Trèves and established a Gallic Kingdom with the general assent of the provincials, as well as of the army. He appointed a senate, issued a coinage, and even began some reconstruction to repair the damage of the Frankish raids. The latter were checked, and Postumus repelled an attack of

Gallienus to recover Gaul. He added Spain and Britain to his kingdom, but the soldiers were unhappy at the prospect of an orderly regime in which they would be returned to garrison duty and to hard labor. Rivals to Postumus appeared, and in 268, when he refused to allow his soldiers to plunder Mainz, the soldiers turned on the emperor and put him to death. The Gallic Kingdom was held together for a few years with considerable difficulty by Tetricus, the governor of Aquitania, but when Aurelian came to Gaul in 274, Tetricus gladly deserted his own unstable army and joined the emperor. The rebels were defeated and the Gallic Kingdom was recovered.

THE RESTORATION OF THE EMPIRE

While the ordinary soldiers of the Roman army bear much of the blame for the anarchy of the third century, the military achievement of the soldier-emperors who whipped the men back to discipline and recovered the lost provinces within a few years can scarcely be overpraised. These were the tough generals of the Danubian frontier, the emperors, Claudius, Aurelian, and Probus, who reigned from 268 to 282. They were able to build on the work of Gallienus (253–68), who experienced the most disastrous years of the crisis, but who still found time to establish new formations in the army and to originate a new plan of frontier defense.

Gallienus was a versatile, even learned man, of Hadrian's temperament, who encouraged Neoplatonist philosophers, although his career was a frantic scramble to hold what he could and to defeat the barbarians where he found them. He realized that the old legionary formations and infantry tactics were not successful, and he therefore developed a new military arm, cavalry formations, which would act quickly and independently of the infantry. A light cavalry armed with javelins was formed from the Moors of Africa, while mounted archers and heavy, armored cavalry (the *cataphractarii*) were modeled on the Palmyrene and Persian units.

The failure of the fixed frontier defenses led Gallienus to devise a deep and mobile system behind the frontier lines. In this scheme northern Italy became the pivot of the European defenses, and its important cities, Verona, Milan and Aquileia, were turned into great army bases. Large forces were stationed in them, which could move out rapidly to east or west, arms factories were established, and the imperial mints moved from Rome. Elsewhere, cities deep behind the frontier line were heavily fortified to serve as bases for detachments of troops. Because the emperor had to be where the important army units were stationed, the new military bases became governmental centers as well, and Rome diminished in importance.

The first of the Illyrian Emperors, Claudius (268–70), drove the Germans out of North Italy and then entered the Balkan provinces to complete Gallienus' campaign against the Goths. He defeated them heavily south of the Danube and was awarded the epithet Gothicus for his victories. Upon his death, unusual in that the plague and not violence was the cause, another Illyrian officer, Aurelian, succeeded to the throne.

Aurelian (270–75), in his brief career of five years, restored the lost territory of the Empire and was recorded in history as the *Restitutor Orbis,* the Restorer of the World. He was an iron disciplinarian and among the soldiers was known as *manu ad ferrum* (hand to sword). First, Aurelian cleared northern Italy of the Germans who had returned to the area by inflicting a heavy defeat on them near Milan. Then, the future safety of Rome was assured by starting construction on a wall around the city, the first which Rome had needed against foreign enemies since the invasion of Hannibal, about five hundred years before. The circuit was built of brick, twelve miles in circumference, twenty feet in height, and twelve feet in thickness. For the labor the brickmakers' and masons' *collegia* of Rome were pressed into service. Aurelian's Wall is still one of the picturesque landmarks of the city, which now extends far beyond it.

When construction was started, Aurelian marched eastward to deal with the Goths along the Danube and to fight against Palmyra, reserving an attack on the Gallic Kingdom for the future. After the defeat of their kindred by Claudius, other Goths gathered. Aurelian defeated them also in battle north of the river, and reorganized the Danubian defenses. He decided to give up Dacia as too costly to recover and to hold, while the East and Gaul were still independent. The province had suffered terribly, and parts of it were under the control of Gothic and German bands. Accordingly, the remaining Roman troops were utilized to guard the vital crossing points along the Danube, while the transfer of the civilian population to the provinces south of the river started. In Dacia and the region to the east, Gothic kingdoms began to coalesce and the processes of trade and assimilation, interrupted for twenty years, began once more. The victories of Gallienus, Claudius, and Aurelian were to ensure relative peace in the region for a century.

Aurelian marched on down the Danube, across Asia Minor, where he restored imperial authority, and came upon the main Palmyrene army near Antioch in Syria. The army was defeated in a difficult battle, and Aurelian pressed on to Palmyra where Zenobia, her son, and her philosophers were taken. Some of the philosophers, whom Zenobia charged with advising her to break from Rome, were put to death, but Zenobia and her son were sent to Rome to grace Aurelian's triumph. When the emperor was on his way back to Europe, news came that Palmyra, which had been well treated, had revolted. The revolt was speedily suppressed, and Aurelian in reprisal allowed his soldiers to plunder and partially destroy the city. Zenobia, however, was given a villa near Rome in Italy where she spent the remainder of her life in peace.

Despite the recovery of the provinces, the position of Rome in the East had become more difficult. Shapur I died in 272, but the Sassanian Empire remained a strong and militant power, against which Roman and Byzantine emperors had to contend. The caravan trade, however, was resumed, and Persian influences began to affect the Eastern provinces strongly.

In 274, as noticed before, Aurelian invaded the Gallic Kingdom of Tetricus and recovered the lost provinces of Gaul, Spain, and Britain. The territorial restoration of the Empire was virtually complete when Aurelian was assassinated in 275. A group of officers, whom the emperor's treacherous secretary had misled into thinking that they were slated for punishment, were the culprits. After a brief and unsatisfactory interlude under a senatorial emperor, Tacitus, the third of the Illyrian generals, Probus, came to the throne.

Probus (276–82), who restored the frontier defenses and completed the internal pacification of the provinces, was known as the *Pacator Orbis,* the Pacifier of the World. His reign opened with a fresh invasion of the Franks into Gaul, but they were speedily defeated and chased back across the Rhine. On the east bank of the stream, opposite the Roman cities, Probus built a series of big forts to hold the crossings and to serve as bases for strong garrisons. He then moved over to the Danube, ridding Raetia and Pannonia of barbarians, and resettling the depopulated lands with groups which had been dislodged from their own homes by the Goths. In southern Asia Minor colonies of veteran soldiers were planted. Probus' tour of the Empire was completed in Egypt, where he drove African marauders from the Sudan back into their own land. Probus then began the task of agricultural reconstruction by planting vineyards in Gaul and the Danubian provinces and by putting the soldiers to work at ditching, road-building, and drainage projects. In resentment the troops mutinied and killed him, but Probus had virtually completed the work of military restoration.

During the military anarchy the Romanized and semi-Romanized manpower of the Empire had been largely used up. Gallienus and the Illyrian Emperors had found it necessary to use barbarians extensively both for their field armies and for frontier defense. The practice, of course, was traditional, but the scale on which the emperors of the third century had to work almost completely changed the personnel of the Roman military establishment. Sections of the European frontier line were taken over by barbarian allies, and great numbers were settled as soldier-settlers to help defend and repopulate the ravaged provinces. In addition, barbarians were hired as individual mercenaries or brigaded into the regular army as whole new units. They came at different levels, as ordinary soldiers and officers, and some rose to prominence very rapidly. For example, a Frankish general played a prominent part in Aurelian's war against Palmyra. While a new reservoir of manpower was tapped, the costs were very high and the processes of assimilation had to begin once more.

THE CHRISTIAN PERSECUTIONS

At the height of the crisis through which the Empire had passed, the implicit hostility between the Roman government and the Christians developed into wholesale persecution. The pagan population and the emperors tended to find the cause of the Empire's suffering in the lack of faith and disloyalty which the Christians showed to the pagan gods. For example, during the reign of Maximinus the people of Cappadocia held the Christians responsible for a severe earthquake and lodged charges against them with the governor. In this same period some of the Christians, like the church father Origen of Alexandria, became more aggressive. He wrote an elaborate reply to Celsus' charges (p. 681), and boldly looked forward to the day when the pagan cults would disappear. Actually, there was no specific fault to be found in the loyalty of the Christians to the Empire because some served in the army and at no time did the church try to betray Rome to an enemy. Yet, when the existence of the state was in danger, any group whose "loyalty" was questionable, was considered dangerous.

The first large-scale persecution was made by Decius during his struggle with the Goths about 250. He himself was conservative and conventional in his thought, and the troops which he commanded were mainly from the upper and middle Danubian provinces where Christianity had made little headway against the older Roman religious worships. In his struggle with the Goths, it seemed obvious to Decius that the help of the gods must be invoked, so an order was issued throughout the Empire for a mass demonstration of loyalty. Everyone was to sacrifice to the Roman gods. The Christians were not required to abjure their own faith, but to make this gesture. As good Christians they could not do so. The administrative machinery of the state was used to register those who made the necessary sacrifices and to issue certificates of compliance. Some Christians saved their lives and property by sacrificing, and many suffered death and imprisonment. Some magistrates were lenient, however, since Decius could not control the whole Empire as efficiently as he would have done in time of peace. In 251, when Decius and his son were killed in battle, the pressure was relaxed.

In 257, however, when Valerian was embarking on his war against Persia, new edicts which struck at the organization of the church were issued. Christian leaders were arrested and a scale of penalties was set for the clergy, varying from death to forced labor in the mines and the confiscation of property. Meetings for religious purposes were prohibited, and entry into the cemeteries for burial of the dead was forbidden. It was in the 250's, in particular, that the Christians made their greatest use of the catacombs in Rome for secret meetings and burial. This persecution lasted until 260, but diminished in intensity while Valerian was engaged in war with Shapur. Since his son Gallienus was reluctant to persecute, the church on the whole did not suffer as much as might have been expected. Enforcement of the orders by local Roman officials varied considerably, while the Christians who had suffered martyrdom became an example to their fellows and to converts. For those who apostasized, a formula of absolution was worked out between the martyrs and the regular clergy, and the apostates were brought back into the church.

The advent of Gallienus as "sole" emperor, if that adjective can be used for his reign, brought a very different treatment of Christianity. Gallienus saw the need for unanimity in the Empire as strongly as had his father and Decius, but his own philosophical education suggested intellectual rather than political attack. Freedom of worship was restored to the Christians, while the Neopla-

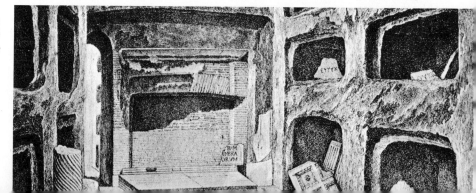

A Christian catacomb in Rome

tonist philosopher Porphyry took up the work of Celsus and attacked the Christians on ideological grounds. Such an attack, however, could scarcely appeal to the masses, but it was the real beginning of the intellectual war between Christian churchmen and pagan philosophers, which lasted well into the fourth century. The Christians, too, considered that they had a share in the intellectual heritage of the Greco-Roman world, and the Christian writers not only expressed their own theology in Greek philosophic terminology, but developed their defense of the Christian position on a philosophical basis.

During the remainder of the century the emperors made no further moves against the Christians, and the church gained considerable strength. The pagan cults, which depended on local and state funds for their festivals and maintenance, were weakened by the economic crisis of the period. The statements of the Christian leaders, too, were considerably stronger than the actions of the laity. Public service might be strictly incompatible with Christianity, but Christians did enter the army and the administration. Many, of course, felt as strong a responsibility to the Empire as did the pagans and were no longer disposed to reject society. Probably in many communities both Christians and pagans deliberately avoided difficult situations. Yet the fundamental difficulty in the Christian position was still unresolved. Since they had been declared hostile to the state, it rested with public opinion and the will of the emperors to turn juridical hostility into direct persecution. In fact, the development of the Principate into autocracy based on a religious sanction made another clash almost unavoidable.

The ill-conceived experiment of Elagabalus was tried again by Aurelian in a different and more acceptable form. He is said to have been conscious of divine help in the course of his battle with the Palmyrenes and to have attributed it to the sun-god Elagabal of Emesa. On another occasion Aurelian is reported to have told his troops that god, not they, made emperors. When he returned victoriously to Rome in 274, he introduced the cult of the unconquered sun, Sol Invictus, as a formal state worship for the Empire. A new temple was built for Sol, and the god's birthday, December 25, became a national festival, while his day, Sunday, headed the week. Worship of the sun-god was easy for the members of many other cults, with whose gods he had been long identified, with Apollo among the Greek and Roman gods, and with Mithras, the god of light. The cult of Sol in Rome, of course, was in a proper Roman tradition. Its chief temple was in the capital, and a college of priests was drawn from the senatorials, the highest social class of the state. Aurelian conceived of himself as the protégé and companion of the sun, a position which his godlike role in the ruler cult easily permitted. The idea of universal solar monotheism and of the emperor as the god's companion might have led to renewed persecution of the Christians by Aurelian, but the issue was postponed for a generation by his sudden death.

THE ECONOMIC DISTRESS OF THE EMPIRE

The anarchy and invasions of the third century brought financial collapse and, ultimately, economic absolutism to the Empire, for the treasuries had no reserves and no system of credit financing, like the war loans and bonds of modern times. Even in the second century, as we have noticed, the Empire was financed on a hand-to-mouth basis. The increased military and administrative establishment of the Severans had been paid for initially by confiscations and then by the impositions of many additional burdens on cities and individuals. The emperors and generals of the period of crisis had no alternative but to requisition labor, food, supplies, and money from the civilian population and to use the coercive force of the state for collection.

The taxable resources of the Empire were, of course, seriously damaged by war. Land went out of use through devastation and subsequent neglect, trade was disrupted, cities were destroyed, and individual fortunes were lost. At the same time the central and local governments were faced with the extraordinary expenditures of continuous warfare. Even if the emperors had plans for betterment, there was no time or opportunity to put them into effect. In this situation the exaction of compulsory labor from individuals and *collegia,* compulsory transport of supplies, demands for imperial taxes from the local city councils, the *liturgies* imposed on civic officials, and capital levies—all became a regular feature of life.

The effects were catastrophic. In the 250's the hard metal currency of the Empire was given up, destroyed by inflation and scarcity, and the state issued the *denarius* with only a two percent silver content. The coins were used by the sackful for purchases. The requisitions of the government were made in produce and in service, and in some parts of the Empire barter of goods began to replace the monetary economy. Aurelian temporarily closed the mint and devalued the coinage eight to one to bring money into line with the rise in prices. The distribution of grain in Rome was changed to a distribution of bread, baked by the bakers' *collegia* under state control, and meat, olive oil, and salt were also distributed. While these emergency measures saved the situation, many of them hardened into regular practice and became a part of the new order of Diocletian and Constantine in the following century.

The effects on society were far-reaching and permanent. Some of the upperclass held on to their estates and were joined by new members from the high officers of the army and the upper ranks of the civil services. The middle class of the cities, the *curials,* was very severely damaged, for its members were the easiest for the authorities to get at and by tradition were liable for municipal services and imperial tax money. Many families were wiped out and those who remained had to bear added burdens. The lower classes of the cities labored under compulsion for the state. The peasants did not profit because the trend from small-scale free farming to the *colonate* was accelerated as men sought security on the large estates. The *coloni* themselves began to change from free tenants with life possession to the status of serfs, as they worked under the compulsory burdens of production and service. Breakdown was averted by Diocletian and Constantine, but the price was a totalitarian state ruled by an autocrat.

X X X

The Reorganization of Diocletian and Constantine

(A.D. 285–395)

THE RULERS OF THE ROMAN EMPIRE in the fourth century after Christ had to grapple continuously with the task of holding the Empire together under a single, centralized authority. At the outset, Diocletian and Constantine thoroughly reorganized the institutions of government and society between 285 and 337, and Constantine sought a new basis for imperial unity in religion by favoring Christianity. Their reforms remained basic well beyond the final split between the Latin West and the Hellenic East which followed the death of Theodosius the Great in 395. Yet the forces of disintegration, set in motion by the breakdown of the third century, were too great to be overcome. The Empire had to repair its own internal weakness and to resist a stronger and more restless barbarian world with greatly diminished resources in wealth and manpower. The new Persian Kingdom in the East could be contained by war and diplomacy, but in Europe the great folk migrations of the early Middle Ages were set in motion in the 370's. At that time the Huns, a people of Mongolian origin from central Asia, broke up the Kingdom of the Eastern Goths in the Ukraine and pushed on into Central Europe. The Western Goths were pushed against the Roman frontier and were taken into the Empire as a separate, and virtually independent, people. The West and East each became engrossed in its individual problems of survival, and imperial unity could no longer be maintained.

The society and intellectual life of the fourth century revealed the impending end of the Greco-Roman era and the start of the Middle Ages. The shape of Medieval Europe could be seen in the growth of vast estates, self-contained and worked by peasants attached to the soil; in the shrinkage of the open cities into small, walled towns; and in the general changeover from urban civilization to rural existence. In the literature and art of the period there was a striking mixture of older, classical traditions and of new conceptions, as ancient culture was transformed.

The reader will find Maps XIX and XX (pages 576 and 704) useful as he reads this chapter.

Diocletian (A.D. 285–305)

Before Diocletian became emperor, his career was very similar to those of the soldier-emperors from Illyria who had preceded him. He was of lower-class origin, born in Dalmatia about 245, and rose to high army command by his ability as a soldier and his tough, overbearing personality. His immediate predecessor, Numerianus, was murdered by the praetorian prefect, Aper, but the generals of the Eastern army chose Diocletian as emperor instead of supporting the prefect. In 285 Diocletian defeated Carinus, Numerianus' brother, who marched against him from the West, and became sole ruler. Once he had become emperor, Diocletian began to prove himself a statesman. He was concerned about preserving the Empire and was able to guard his own position by a wise selection of colleagues.

Diocletian

Rather than entrust important commands to subordinate officers whose success would only encourage their soldiers to oust him as emperor, Diocletian decided to share the responsibilities of military command by elevating his best generals to the position of partners in rule. In 286 he selected another Illyrian soldier, Maximianus, a capable general whom Diocletian judged to be a man without excessive political ambitions. Maximianus was made Caesar and thus designated as a potential successor. He was entrusted with operations in Gaul where revolt had broken out among the peasants, the *Bagaudae,* who were in despair at the failure of Rome to protect their lands from German raids and resentful at the combined exactions of their landlords and of the government. Maximianus quickly settled the rebellion and drove the Germans back across the Rhine, but proved less fortunate in his choice of an admiral, Carausius. The latter had been stationed in Gesoriacum (Boulogne) to clear the coasts of pirates. He did so, but took over Boulogne, crossed the English Channel to Britain, and declared himself Augustus. Maximianus, himself elevated to the rank of Augustus for his earlier successes, failed to defeat Carausius and, for the time being, Diocletian had to acquiesce in an independent Britain and an unwanted colleague.

The divided command between Diocletian and Maximianus, apart from the defection of Carausius, worked out satisfactorily. Maximianus looked after the West from Milan, and Diocletian ruled the East from Nicomedia. In 293 Diocletian extended his collegiate system by the creation of the Tetrarchy, as it was called, a fourfold division of military responsibility, in which Diocletian was senior. Two Caesars were picked to assist Maximianus and Diocletian, the Augusti, with the implicit understanding that they would succeed their superiors in due time. The Caesars were Galerius, who assisted Diocletian, and Constantius Chlorus, the father of Constantine the Great, to help Maximianus. Both were experienced and able Illyrian generals. The Caesars were further bound to their senior Augusti by marriage with the latters' daughters, so that the new college of rulers was tied closely together by family ties, a mutual share in administrative responsibility, and the prospect of an orderly succession. The arrangement was, in effect, a return to the old practice of selection of the best man, a practice which had been employed in the second century.

The Empire was divided into four regions for military defense although it was treated as an administrative unity, and Diocletian acted as the senior ruler. Maximianus protected Italy, Spain, and Africa, operating mainly from Milan to keep an eye on the vulnerable area between the upper Rhine and the Danube. Constantius was placed in charge of Gaul and Britain, which had to be regained from Carausius, and had his headquarters at Trèves. Galerius, at Sirmium on the lower Save River, defended the middle and lower Danube, while Diocletian continued to take charge of the East from Nicomedia. This arrangement involved the maintenance of four "courts" and, of course, relegated Rome to the background. That city was the ceremonial capital, so to speak, but the real business of government was done where the rulers resided. More than ever Rome was a kept city, its Senate a social ornament, and its people were fed and entertained at the imperial expense.

While Diocletian could not prevent some personal friction and mutual jealousy among his colleagues, he did make the new system work by his own dominating personality. The Tetrarchy solved the military problems of the Empire for the time being. Constantius recovered Britain in 296 and protected Gaul very efficiently from German raids. His capital at Trèves developed into a flourishing city, while Gallic agriculture and the frontier defenses were improved by the settlement of barbarians captured on his campaigns. In the East Galerius engaged in a similar program along the Danube, while Diocletian put down a rebellion in Egypt and rid the country of invaders from the Sudan. Diocletian's preoccupation with Egyptian affairs, however, encouraged King Narses of Persia to attack Armenia and Syria in 297. At first his invasion was successful, and Galerius, who had marched down from the Danube to counter it, was defeated. But in 298 the latter won a smashing victory over Narses in Armenia. The resulting settlement provided a much deeper defensive buffer than previously for Roman Asia Minor and Syria, and this area was not seriously disturbed for almost fifty years. Rome acquired Mesopotamia and some territory beyond the Tigris River as provinces, while Armenia and the region south of the Caucasus Mountains were placed under Roman protection.

Diocletian ruled as an autocrat by edict and fiat, and very speedily the difference between the emperor and his subjects was marked by a stately ceremonial, borrowed in part from that of oriental kings. The emperor was remote and unapproachable, hedged in by palace functionaries and rigid etiquette. Those who were admitted to audience had to prostrate themselves, while the privileged few were permitted to kiss the border of the emperor's robe. He wore a special costume for state occasions, a jeweled diadem and dress of purple with threads of gold. All this, of course, exemplified the new conception of the ruler which had been developing throughout the third century. Diocletian expressed it by calling himself Jovian, the earthly representative of Jupiter, while Maximianus was Herculius, a mighty laborer for the Empire, like Hercules. The power of the emperor was considered to be derived from the gods and no longer by either delegation or transfer from the Roman citizens. In contrast to the Principate when the emperor had been the foremost among citizens, the Late Empire derived the name Dominate from the new title *dominus,* master or lord, which came into use. The emperor, however, was not a god and was not referred to as such officially although flatterers might have used the term in speaking of him.

The emphasis placed by Diocletian on the divine origin of his power carried the implicit threat of persecution for the Christians, but for almost twenty years, until 303, the emperor made no move against them. Since Gallienus' edict of toleration issued in 260, the church had grown in numbers and strength, and Christians were playing a responsible part in society. Yet Diocletian suddenly reversed the practice of toleration and issued a series of edicts which were plainly designed to destroy Christianity. His motives are obscure, but, if the idea was Diocletian's own, perhaps the most plausible explanation is that he had waited until the military situation was in hand. Then he decided to promote religious unanimity in the state. Perhaps, however, as Christian tradition explains the persecution, Diocletian was influenced by Galerius. The latter's position was very strong as a result of his great victory over the Persians, and, judging from Galerius' continuance of the persecution after Diocletian's retirement in 305, he felt that Christianity should be eradicated. Whatever the cause, the persecution was the most severe and lasting which the church had undergone.

Three edicts were issued in 303. One confiscated church property and destroyed the churches; a second called for the arrest of the clergy; and a third forbade private assembly for worship and made Christians outlaws to be dismissed from public office and denied access to the courts and the protection of the law. In the following years, after outbreaks of violence and arson in Syria which were blamed on the Christians, sacrifice to the Roman gods under the penalty of death was demanded. The edicts were stringently enforced by Diocletian, Galerius, and Maximianus in their sections of the Empire, but Constantius seems to have done little in Gaul and Britain except to pull down some churches. In 311 the persecutions were suddenly terminated by an edict of toleration from Galerius, then senior ruler, who was fatally ill. Perhaps this was the indifference of an old, sick man, or as Christian tradition explained it, Galerius' wife Valeria, herself sympathetic to Christianity, influenced him. While no compensation was made for the losses sustained, freedom of worship, at least, was restored to the Christians.

In 305 Diocletian, who seems to have suffered a stroke, decided to retire from rule and to end his days in the great fortified palace which he had built for himself at Salonae (Split), near his birthplace. He was able to influence Maximianus, his fellow Augustus, to retire, so that the Tetrarchy was reconstituted. The Caesars, Constantius and Galerius, moved up to the position of Augusti, although Constantius was made senior. Two new men were also

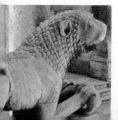

Lion from the Palace of Diocletian

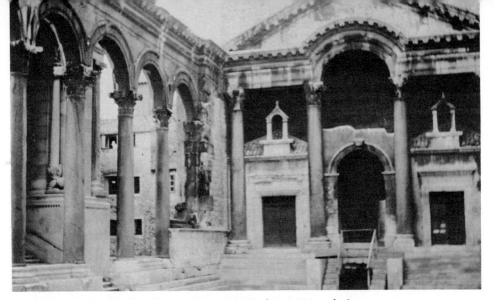

Ruined colonnade in the Palace of Diocletian at Split (Salonae) in Jugoslavia

brought in as Caesars, Severus and Maximinus Daia—the latter to aid Galerius in the East. Since the sons of the new Augusti, Maxentius and Constantine, had been passed over, both were resentful, and since old Maximianus had retired under protest, the situation was explosive. The Empire was nevertheless held together by Diocletian's moral authority.

In 306 Constantius was killed in battle in northern England fighting against the Picts and Scots, and his army acclaimed Constantine as Augustus. The situation was smoothed over by Galerius, who recognized Constantine as Caesar and promoted Severus to the rank of Augustus. Yet the arrangements for succession had been broken by the army in Britain, and Constantine had won a position from which he might drive on to complete rule over the Empire. We need not follow the complicated moves and countermoves by which the Tetrarchy broke down and was repaired in the next few years, except to notice the personnel in 311 when the senior Augustus, Galerius, died. He was replaced by an able and conservative general, Licinius, who continued to administer Asia Minor and the lower Danubian provinces. Constantine still ruled in Britain and Gaul and Maximinus Daia in Syria and Egypt. Maxentius, however, had acquired Italy and controlled the other Western provinces. Serious civil war had been averted, but Constantine had already begun to move for the whole Empire.

Constantine and the Christian Empire (A.D. 312–37)

THE RISE OF CONSTANTINE

Constantine, although without much administrative and military experience before he became a Caesar in 306, proved an astute and conscientious governor and a good general. He protected his provinces successfully and won the good will and support of both the provincials and his own soldiers. In 310, when the Tetrarchy was obviously weakening, Constantine began his move to take over the Empire by announcing that his father was an illegitimate son of Claudius Gothicus, who had died in 270, and that his own patron deity was Sol Invictus, the unconquered sun. The first implied that Constantine had a hereditary claim to the whole Empire and ignored Diocletian's arrangements, and the second that he was turning from Jupiter and Hercules who had supported the Tetrarchs, to the god of Aurelian, the Restorer of the World.

Constantine began military operations with the annexation of Spain and in 311, when Galerius died, came to an understanding with Licinius against their seniors, Maxentius and Maximinus Daia. In 312 he marched with an army of about forty thousand men against Maxentius in Italy, leaving the bulk of his forces in Gaul. Near Turin Constantine inflicted a heavy defeat on Maxentius' army, and despite his own losses, decided to drive on to Rome. Instead of remaining in safety behind Aurelian's Wall, Maxentius led his troops out of the city to hold the crossing of the Tiber at the Milvian Bridge. Before the battle, according to Christian tradition, Constantine had a vision in which he was instructed to place the monogram of Christ, a Greek Rho superimposed on a Chi, on the shields of his soldiers. He is also said to have seen a flaming cross in the sky and below it, written in Greek, the words, "By this sign, you will conquer." Accordingly, Constantine went into battle at the Milvian Bridge in 312 under the auspices of Christ, and the resulting victory was regarded by the Christians as a vindication of the power of their god. Constantine himself was rather more ambiguous, if not modest. His commemorative arch in Rome attributed victory to the inspiration of an unknown divinity and to Constantine's own greatness of mind. With the defeat of Maxentius Constantine gained possession of the West.

In the following year Constantine met Licinius in Milan and entered into an agreement by which Christians were granted complete freedom of worship and the churches were guaranteed in their property rights. This was not publicized in the form of an edict (the so-called Edict of Milan), but Licinius put the terms into effect in his own domain and strengthened his alliance with Constantine by marrying his daughter. While Constantine gave no indication of sending military help to Licinius, Maximinus Daia regarded the alliance as hostile to himself and attacked Licinius. He was defeated, and Licinius took over control of the Eastern portion of the Empire. Each Augustus ruled individually in his own area, but at least the fiction of imperial unity was preserved by their alliance, while each sought to undermine the other.

For ten years tension continued to grow as Constantine's actions revealed that his aim was to control the whole Empire. At first he tried to set up a buffer area between himself and Licinius, ruled by a subordinate Caesar, but Licinius countered by tampering with the loyalty of Constantine's troops. In the resulting war Constantine acquired all of the European provinces of Licinius except Thrace, but recognized the independence of his fellow Augustus in administration. Then, in 317, the two made an arrangement for the succession, by which the two elder sons of Constantine, Crispus and Constantine II, and Licinius' son,

Licinianus, became Caesars. This unequal bargain was soon strained by religious difficulties. Constantine favored Christianity in his part of the Empire, which made it almost imperative for Licinius to take the opposite course and to engage in petty persecution. When war again broke out in 324, the Christians, who were more numerous in the East, regarded it almost as a crusade for their protection although the immediate cause was political. Constantine had entered Thrace, Licinius' province, in the course of some operations against the Goths and forced the war by rejecting Licinius' very proper protest. The two met in battle at Adrianople, where Constantine defeated Licinius' army, while Crispus won a naval victory near the Hellespont. Since the road was then opened to Asia Minor, shortly afterwards Constantine defeated the remnants of Licinius' forces at Chrysopolis near the Bosporus and took Licinius prisoner. After six months Licinius was put to death, and in 326 his son Licinianus was removed. Constantine had become sole emperor and secured the succession for his own family.

Constantine immediately began the construction of a new imperial capital, Constantinople (Istanbul), which was built on the site of the old Greek colony of Byzantium on the Bosporus. The choice of the site was admirable for strategic needs and had been foreshadowed by the shift of gravity in the Empire. A location at the crossroads of Europe and Asia, with ready access to the Danubian and Euphrates frontiers, was needed as a nerve center for both East and West. Constantine gave his new city the same privileges which Rome enjoyed, freedom from direct taxation and a subsidized food supply. A second Senate was created, which drew its members from the great landowners and dignitaries of the East but which was ranked in dignity below the Senate of Rome. The population was mainly Greek, made up of the former inhabitants of Byzantium and families from the imperial estates in Asia Minor. At first Constantinople had a superficially Latin character because Latin was used for official purposes, but use of that language disappeared in the sixth century when Constantinople had become the capital of the Byzantine Empire. It became, of course, one of the great cities of the world, outshadowing Rome and the cities of Western Europe, a center of trade between Asia and Europe, and influential in the development of the Slavic states of Russia.

CONSTANTINE AND CHRISTIANITY

After his victory over Maxentius, Constantine began to refound the unity of the Empire on the orthodox Christian religion. Not only Christian historians of his period, but Constantine himself, represented the war against Licinius as a religious war to recover the East and to restore unity. Constantine's momentous decision, of course, made his reign one of the pivotal periods of ancient history. While an eventual settlement betweeen Christianity and the imperial government had to come, Constantine was the revolutionary emperor who broke with tradition by seeking unity through Christianity rather than by its suppression. For the future his decision meant a fundamental, if gradual, change in the institutions and values of society.

There was no obvious reason for Constantine's decision in 312. He was opposed to his pagan colleagues in the Tetrarchy, but he had already issued a religious challenge to them by supporting the sun-god. He was not rescuing Christianity from persecution because it was tolerated by Galerius' edict. He did enlist Christian help for himself, but the position of the church could scarcely have seemed very strong at that time. It had just passed through a long persecution in which Christians had been purged from political office. Also, Constantine's troops were devoted to the worship of the sun-god as he himself professed to be. Christianity had spread to every province of the Empire, but it was still much weaker numerically than paganism, perhaps numbering no more than a fifth of the inhabitants of the whole Empire. In perspective, of course, Christianity appears as a vital, dynamic force, unified and disciplined in its church organization. Presumably Constantine had some appreciation of this fact in 312, but few of his contemporaries in government would have shared his view.

Constantine's decision presented no difficulties to his Christian contemporaries. His was regarded as a genuine conversion by divine inspiration in which they saw the hand of God at work in history. Constantine also presented his position to his Christian subjects in this manner, although he delayed baptism until his death bed. Christianity, however, was not made the state religion in an official sense. The emperor remained *Pontifex Maximus,* accepted the formal worship of the ruler cult, and used the Roman ceremonies of *augury* and divination. He continued to display the symbols of sun worship on his coinage for some time after his "conversion," but in 317 adopted the Christian *labarum* as a standard, a gold wreath encircling the monogram of Christ.

The legislation of Constantine's reign showed an increasing tendency to favor Christianity. For example, while the Empire was divided between him and Licinius, Constantine issued edicts exempting the Christian clergy from the municipal *liturgies,* as pagan priests were exempted. Slaves could be freed in churches as in pagan temples. The judicial decisions of bishops, who tried legal cases at the request of both litigants, were declared as valid as those of the civil courts. After the defeat of Licinius, the emperor supported Christianity much more emphatically, and it began to pass into a favored position. All personal and private rights were restored to Christians throughout the Empire, and in an edict Constantine made a strong recommendation to pagans to become Christians. State support was gradually withdrawn from pagan temples, while money was given for the construction of churches. Constantine, however, never went to the extreme of persecuting paganism as some of his successors did. Throughout his reign the religions were in a state of balance, in which the emperor tipped the scales in favor of Christianity. His own children were brought up in that faith, so that the Empire looked forward to the succession of a Christian dynasty. Constantine could scarcely go farther without disturbing the hard won unity which he had achieved, for the bureaucracy, the army, and most of the upper classes were still predominantly pagan until well on in his reign.

Constantine found no difficulty in accommodating his Christianity to the contemporary conception of the ruler. He regarded himself as the earthly representative of the Christian God, by whose grace he ruled the Empire, and he expected that his Christian subjects would obey him as God's representative. This conception of his office was charged with great significance for the future relations of church and state and was demonstrated by Constantine on several occasions. Constantine decided in favor of the orthodox clergy when Donatus, leader of the heretical Donatists of Africa, competed with Caecilius, an orthodox candidate, for the bishopric of Carthage. In 314 the emperor wrote to the synod of Arles that it was wrong for the clergy to conceal disagreement from him because God had entrusted him with the direction of human affairs. When the Donatists refused to obey the decision of the synod, Constantine used military force to suppress them. When this failed, he left the heretics to the judgment of God—the first, but not the last emperor to impale himself on the thorny question of church discipline.

Constantine also felt it proper to intervene in the Arian controversy about the nature of Christ's divinity. At the imperial expense and under the emperor's auspices, bishops from all parts of the Empire attended an ecumenical meeting in 325, the Council of Nicaea, at which the Nicaean Creed was formulated. The controversy was not terminated, but Constantine at least obtained a statement of orthodoxy. In his dealings with the church, Constantine exhibited a typical Roman attitude. As ruler he was concerned to ensure unity and order in the Empire.

While all historians are agreed on the significance of Constantine's decision to support Christianity by his imperial authority, his motives have been explained in various ways. To some the explanation is as simple as it was to Constantine's Christian contemporaries. The emperor was converted and acted in accordance with his principles. The ambiguities of his reign are explained as necessary to avoid violent upheaval because Constantine could scarcely plunge the Empire into fresh religious controversy and disunity by a sudden and complete repudiation of paganism. At the other extreme is the view that Constantine was essentially a nonreligious figure in a religious age, who assessed its character correctly and divided his interest astutely between a dynamic Christianity and a faltering paganism. Certainly the emperor's aims were imperial unity and stability, and his religious program was only one means of attaining them.

Political and Social Reorganization

Just as imperial unity and defense were the primary political aims of Diocletian and Constantine, stability was their goal in internal reorganization. Since the work of the two emperors was complementary, it is convenient to describe it as a unit. In general, Diocletian initiated financial reform and the methods by which society was pressed into the service of the state, while Constantine solidified the social structure. Their reorganization remained basic, and

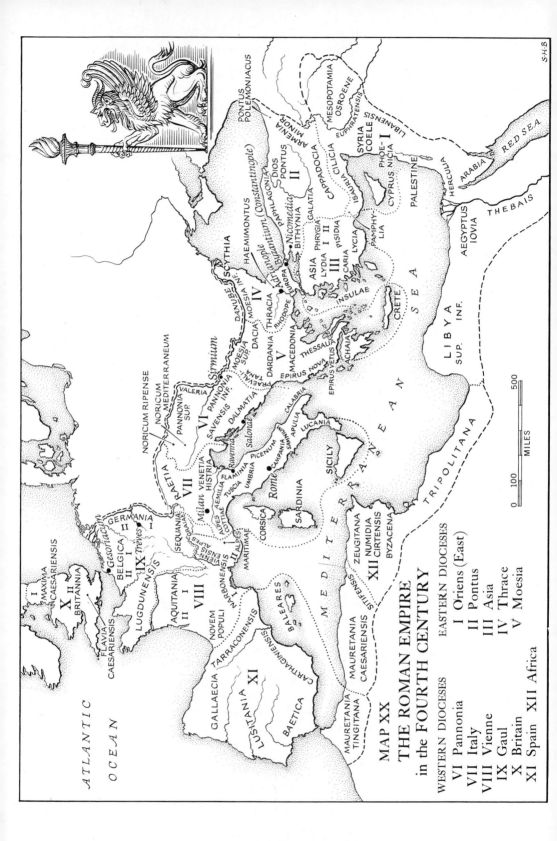

ATLANTIC
OCEAN

MEDITERRANEAN SEA

RED SEA

MAP XX
THE ROMAN EMPIRE
in the FOURTH CENTURY

WESTERN DIOCESES   EASTERN DIOCESES
VI   Pannonia   I   Oriens (East)
VII Italy   II   Pontus
VIII Vienne   III   Asia
IX   Gaul   IV   Thrace
X   Britain   V   Moesia
XI   Spain   XII Africa

0   100   500
MILES

their successors did little more than elaborate upon it. The result was a thorough regimentation of society in which the people of the Empire were controlled and used for the state. The free enterprise and social mobility which had characterized the Principate almost vanished, but the Empire was preserved.

GOVERNMENT

In the Late Empire the emperors ruled by edict through an elaborate civilian bureaucracy which was kept separate from the military establishment. No distinction was made between Equestrian and senatorial careers because the civil administration formed a single system, culminating in the praetorian prefects and the high officials of the palace and of the various governmental departments. The Senate had no share in rule, although the social prestige of its members was very high, and the emperor used them as individuals in various posts. The former council, the *consilium,* was replaced by a new advisory group, known as the *consistorium* (the consistory) appointed by the emperor. It was made up of the high dignitaries of the state, including such officials as the secretary of the palace, the controller of the offices and the head of the secret police. The latter was used very extensively to observe the emperor's colleagues, to check on the conduct of the bureaucracy, and to watch the loyalty of the army and of the people. The totalitarian state, of course, needed constant supervision for the maintenance of government.

While the praetorian prefects were relieved of their military duties, they were still the most important officials of state and administered the four great prefectures into which the Empire was now divided. These were Gaul, Italy, Illyricum, and the Orient. Even for military campaigns the generals had to draw upon the prefect's administration for supplies. Specifically, the most important duties of the prefect were the supervision of the tax collection in his prefecture, of the imperial post and of the administration of justice. In 333 the prefects became the final court of appeal for cases in their prefectures. Within each, the provinces were grouped into large territorial units known as dioceses, twelve of them in the whole Empire. Each was governed by a *vicarius* (a vicar) who was responsible to the prefect. The provinces themselves, as the result of subdivision, were much smaller than those of the Principate and numbered about 120 at the end of the fourth century. For example, the former province of Asia was divided into seven new provinces and Egypt into three. Each province was administered by a provincial governor and in effect replaced the municipalities as the characteristic link between the central government and the individual subject. The power of the provincial governors had shrunk drastically with the size of their provinces and their subordination to the vicars and the prefects.

The army was enlarged and organized along the lines drawn by the soldier-emperors in the previous century. While Diocletian and Constantine cut down on the large cavalry corps formed by Gallienus, they maintained his general plan for imperial defense. A border guard, the *limitanei,* was stationed on the frontiers, and a large mobile field force was quartered in fortified cities deep behind the frontiers. To facilitate distribution of the field force, Diocletian reduced the legions to about a thousand men each, thus forming small mobile regiments which could be deployed easily and widely. The border soldiers were mainly soldier-settlers, who worked their own farms and were drawn from the barbarian element of the frontier population. They were paid less and served longer than the field troops, who made up a highly efficient and privileged professional army.

It was difficult for the government to obtain manpower for the army in the fourth century because the population was declining steadily and the essential occupations of the economy had to be maintained. Peasants were needed for agriculture, workers for transport and essential building operations, and the civilian population of the cities was unsuitable for military service. Accordingly, the rulers recruited barbarians, hired mercenaries, invited volunteers, and occasionally conscripted peasants. Ultimately the profession of soldiering became largely hereditary, and the sons of soldiers were automatically directed into the army. Among the population as a whole the army formed a privileged group, exempted after discharge from municipal *liturgies* and office, receiving good pay, partly in money and partly in kind, and the generals had a prominent voice in the emperor's council and policy making.

The costs of government in the fourth century were excessively high in relation to the Empire's taxable resources. The bureaucracy, of which we have indicated only the broad outline, contained thousands of officials in its various grades. The army numbered over 400,000 men at first although it seems to have declined sharply in the latter part of the century. Most of the emperors and their colleagues maintained an extremely expensive court life and continued to indulge their tastes for extensive building. To pay for all this, Diocletian attempted to restore the commercial life of the Empire by reform of the currency and a new system of taxation. The government collected its taxes in produce and paid the army and the bureaucracy directly in kind. Nevertheless, commerce remained at a low ebb, and throughout the century the emperors were harassed by financial difficulties. The new system, however simplified and efficient from the government's point of view, ultimately defeated its purpose by destroying the taxpayers.

THE TAX SYSTEM

Diocletian began currency reform in 286 by issuing a new gold coin still called the *aureus,* a new silver piece (the *argentius*), and three new bronze coins for small change. His evaluations were apparently too high because by 301 a monetary crisis had developed, with widespread distress from high prices, inflation, and profiteering. Instead of correcting the currency, Diocletian tried to fix maximum prices. In 301 he issued the famous Edict on Prices, one of the most interesting documents of ancient history. The Edict was apparently designed for application throughout the Empire, although copies of it have been found only in the Eastern provinces and in Italy. The document began with a sharp warning to profiteers and a plea for the welfare of the ordinary citizens and soldiers who were hurt by their actions. Ceilings were set for well over a thousand items, on both commodities and wages. Penalties for violation were severe, but the Edict seems to have had a limited success and was given up in a few years except for the purpose of government purchases. Such a regulation was too rigid for the Empire's economy in which there were great regional variations, and there was no correspondingly complete control of production. The reform of the currency, however, did have some stabilizing effect on which Constantine improved.

In 324 Constantine modified the coinage standard by issuing the gold coins at seventy-two, rather than sixty, to the Roman pound (327 grams), and by scaling down the value of the bronze pieces. Constantine's gold coin, known as the *solidus,* had a very wide circulation and helped to restore the Eastern trade to some degree. The coins are found in Persia and India, and the standard lasted well into medieval times. In the Late Empire money was largely an imperial instrument rather than an article of commerce. Since its issuance was strictly limited to the imperial mint, the supply of money was plentiful only in those regions where the government spent on a large scale and in a few special trading centers. The Empire never returned to its former free flow of money, and as imperial authority broke down, barter of natural products became established over large regions, except for the most important transactions.

Diocletian's system of taxation swept away the former land tax and the indirect taxes which had been paid in money and substituted payment in natural produce and compulsory services. This system was not so much an innovation, geared to the new needs of government, as the regularization of the practice of requisitioning supplies and labor which had been born of necessity in the third century. The tax was known as the *annona,* and the system was called *capitatio.* It was based on an elaborate census of the landowners of the Empire, recording the types and quality of the land which they owned and the labor used to work their properties. Italy lost its once privileged status. Northern Italy was treated like the other provinces, while the south was made liable for the provision of food, wine, olive oil, and firewood for Rome.

Throughout the Empire all the productive land and the labor used on it were divided into theoretically equal units of production on which the tax was levied. The unit of land was called a *iugum,* and, of course, varied in size with the productivity and the type of crop grown. The unit of labor, a *caput,* was a full day's work for one man or two women, a "man day." The categories and methods of equalization were very complicated and differed for various parts of the Empire, but the purpose of the system everywhere was to provide the government with the needed amount of produce to supply the army and the bureaucracy. The soldiers received a part of their pay in produce and were able to convert it into money, but the system was essentially designed to channel the produce of the land directly into payment of the major expenses of administration. Such a plan, of course, protected the government from inflation, but it also prevented the producers from selling their products in a high market and saddled the state with an immense and complicated system of tax administration.

Each year the praetorian prefect made an announcement of the needs of his prefecture and an assessment on the provinces to supply them which was known as an indiction. The overall needs for the Empire were calculated every five years, later every fifteen, and the interval, too, came to be called an indiction. In the Late Roman Empire, as well as at other times, taxes were as certain as death, and so the indictions came to be used as the basis for a system of chronology by which events were recorded as happening in a certain year of a particular indiction. Collection centers were designated to which the produce was brought and from which the government distributed it as needed. In each municipality the collection was carried out by the *curials,* who gathered the produce from the landowners and were held responsible for the full amount. The whole system was riddled with corruption and illegal bargains between government officials and *curials* and between *curials* and landowners. In addition to the *annona,* which provided the greater part of the tax revenue, owners of property other than land paid a tax in money, which was used by the emperors for the distribution of alms. Members of the various *collegia* were made liable for regular service to the state. The appropriate groups supplied the transport and services for the *annona* and troop movements, labor for building and animals for the imperial post.

Successful operation of the system required that the number and character of the productive units be fixed as firmly as possible. Compulsion was used from the outset to ensure that the *annona* was paid to the government and the various services duly rendered. The heaviest burden fell on the *curials* of the cities, the former bourgeoisie who had supported the municipal life of the Empire. The class was defined by a minimum property qualification of about fifteen acres of land, and so included men of very modest wealth. Yet the *curials* were held responsible for the collection of the *annona* from their district, as well as for their own municipal *liturgies.* The odious task of collection and the frequent need to make up deficits from their own resources drove the *curials* to evade their responsibilities as best they could. In 325 Constantine made membership in the *curial* class hereditary and permanent. They were forbidden to sell out and were prohibited from moving into the more privileged groups of the army and clergy. The attrition of the middle class proceeded rapidly and contributed much to the decline of the cities.

Obviously the market, which the cities had provided for craftsmen and laborers, shrank as the purchasing power of the middle class declined and the municipalities made fewer expenditures for maintenance and renewal of their facilities. Local industry tended to shift from the cities to the big estates, whose owners maintained craftsmen and specialized workmen as well as tenant farmers. Thus, urban craftsmen and laborers worked for a relatively small market in the fourth century and were responsible in addition for the production and services required by the government. In Constantine's reign, too, the process of making membership in the *collegia* hereditary and permanent began.

In the early part of the fourth century, however, the economic picture was by no means entirely dark because relative peace and political stability did stimulate some recovery. The luxury trade with the East and within the Empire supplied the market offered by the wealthy governing class. Certain specialized industries, the making of the luxury items, glass, and war materials, continued to bring some prosperity to their places of manufacture. In those parts of the Empire which enjoyed relative peace—Egypt, Syria, Asia Minor, Britain, and Gaul—agriculture revived and cities became active and bustling as imperial headquarters and provincial centers.

Also, throughout the Empire a new economic system was growing to replace that founded on the municipalities. Already in the second century the cities had shown signs of distress, and the transformation to a new type of rural economy had been apparent in the growth of large estates worked by tenants. The tempo of change was increased after the death of Constantine when the impact of barbarian pressure on the frontiers and the impact of civil wars for the throne were felt once again.

The owners of the big estates, as well as the emperor himself, were the high officials in the government, the army and the clergy. They felt little obligation or need to support the cities but lived in princely style in large fortified villas, surrounded by their tenant farmers and workmen. The tenants, the *coloni*, increased rapidly in numbers during the third and fourth centuries. The estates had weathered the storms of the third century better than the cities and had attracted tenants for the sake of the protection offered by the great landholders. In the fourth century, since small-scale freeholders found it very difficult to carry the new tax burdens, they turned again to the patronage of the landlords. Individual peasants and even whole villages were taken over. Until 322 the *colonus* was free to try another landlord or, if completely despondent, to wander, but in that year the *coloni* on both the imperial and private estates were attached to their lots of land and made into a hereditary *colonate*. They became serfs who were sold with the land but could not be sold separately.

In some respects it was convenient for the government to deal with these great estates as units, represented by their owners, but vigorous owners might also defy the government from the security of their holdings. The owners gradually acquired legal rights over the persons of their tenants for whom they acted as magistrates and tax collectors. The estates became quasi-legal units in themselves, exempted from the jurisdiction of the cities and of the provincial governors. Entrenched in their fortified villas, which we know from the remains in Italy, Gaul, North Africa, and Asia Minor, the great lords achieved an independence which the central government had to take into account. Against this background of decline and transition, the successors of Constantine tried to cope with the centrifugal tendencies of the Empire and the renewed barbarian pressure on the frontiers.

The Struggle for Unity

The form of rule which Constantine had established, a single family reigning as the representative of the Christian God, with the support of the army and the bureaucracy, proved very difficult to maintain. There was rivalry among the male members of his family for seniority, and, as in the past, the army was ready to take matters into its own hands. The victory of Christianity proved in the event to have been won, but at the time of Constantine's death the mass of the population in the big cities and countryside, as well as many of the governing class, were still pagan. The Christian emperors had to devote time and energy to the establishment of the church and, in addition, attempt to heal schisms among their Christian subjects. Above all, the Persians on the Eastern frontier and the barbarians along the Danube and the Rhine had to be fought off. Yet the rulers of the fourth century held the Empire together until the death of Theodosius the Great in 395.

THE DYNASTY OF CONSTANTINE: CONSTANTIUS AND JULIAN THE APOSTATE (337–63)

Constantine, like Diocletian, realized the need for divided responsibility in the administration of the Empire, but had shared rule among the members of his family under his own direction. None of his sons, however, Constantius, Constantine II, and Constans, had been clearly marked for seniority, which was as necessary for order as the division of administrative cares. Thus Constantine's death in 337 was followed by an uneasy lull for four months. Then the army took matters into its own hands, perhaps at the instigation of Constantius. The soldiers in Constantinople simplified the problem of rule by recognizing Constantine's three sons and putting the other members of the family to death. Two boys were spared, Gallus and Julian, nephews of Constantine, who were too young to be of concern. As the result of the army's action Constantius ruled in the East and Constantine II in the West, while Constans occupied the middle ground of Italy, Illyria, and Africa, nominally under the authority of Constantine II.

This divided administration, in which no clearly recognized overall authority existed, was an invitation both to the outbreak of civil war and to the renewal of barbarian attacks. In 338 Shapur II of Persia invaded Armenia and Roman Mesopotamia, tying Constantius down in a long and costly war. In the West Constans defeated his brother in 340, but was himself replaced by a usurper, Magnentius, an army general. Not until 353 was Constantius able to defeat Magnentius and to bring the Empire under his single rule. By that time, however, the Franks and the Alemanni were raiding heavily along the Rhine and the upper Danube. Beset by war on several fronts, Constantius turned first to his cousin Gallus, named him a Caesar and sent him to the Eastern frontier. Gallus proved untrustworthy and vicious and had to be removed in 354. Then the emperor appointed his other cousin Julian as Caesar, married him to his own daughter and sent him to Gaul to fight the Franks. Outwardly the family of Constantius seemed to be firmly established, but Constantius and Julian were incompatible.

Constantius worked hard and zealously at the tasks of government but seems to have been a man of mediocre ability, very much under the influence of palace functionaries. For example, the chief historian of the period, Ammianus Marcellinus, observed sarcastically that Constantius had considerable influence with the master of his bedroom, the eunuch Eusebius. Constantius, however, was unflagging in his efforts to stamp out paganism and issued a series of edicts, more remarkable for their language than their effect, "Let superstition give way, the madness of sacrificial ceremonies be wiped out." The chief obstacle to wiping out the sacrifices was that the mass of the population in the big cities, Alexandria, Antioch and Rome, liked the spectacles and festivals of pagan religion. There was too much risk of riot and disturbance to enforce the emperor's edicts, but he did cut off financial support from some of the pagan cults, seized temple property, and strengthened the Christian element in the administration. Constantius' standing with the army, however, was not high, for he had made little headway against Persia. Accordingly, the emperor was reluctant to bring Julian to command and surrounded him with spies. Perhaps the rumor that Julian was a pagan seemed worse to Constantius than his potential rivalry.

Although Julian had had no previous administrative or military experience, he rapidly developed into a good governor and general, defeating the Alemanni and the Franks and restoring the defenses on the Rhine. In 360 Julian received an order from Constantius to send a large part of his best troops to the East, where Shapur II had broken into Mesopotamia again. The soldiers refused to march and, instead, acclaimed Julian as Augustus. Despite Julian's offer to divide the rule, Constantius left the Persian war unfinished and marched to the West to oppose him. He died in Tarsus in 361, but named Julian as his successor.

The rumor that Julian was a secret pagan was entirely true. As sole emperor he tried to suppress Christianity and to establish a pagan church, for which the Christian tradition has labelled him Julian the Apostate. Julian, born in 332, had been kept in seclusion until he was fifteen. During this time he read avidly in classical Greek literature and philosophy and began to idealize the traditions of Greece but remained a Christian. Upon his return to Nicomedia and to society Julian came under the influence of the famous Greek rhetorician, Libanius of Antioch, and a pagan miracle-worker, Maximus. He became a Neoplatonist but had to keep his paganism hidden until, as emperor, he could throw off the mask.

The Neoplatonism which took Julian's mind by storm was a far cry from the thought of Plato. The new philosophy, which had been developed in the mid-third century by Plotinus and his followers Porphyry and Iamblichus, remained the possession of a small, esoteric group of scholars. Plotinus led a simple, ascetic life, and his thought, known through his book, the *Enneads,* was obscure and tended to reject human reason as a means to explanation. It emphasized instead intuition and mystical experience. Neoplatonism, in fact, was as much a religion as a philosophy. It drew a sharp distinction between the soul and body and insisted that the liberation of the soul from the material body was through a mystical experience. By the time of Julian the philosophy had come to represent a refined syncretism of pagan religious and philosophical ideas in which a place could be found for almost any god, including Christ. The Christians themselves were condemned for their exclusiveness, and Porphyry and Iamblichus had carried on an intellectual war with the fathers of the church. Neoplatonism was too abstract and difficult to understand except for a few highly educated scholars, and so Julian had to find a less theoretical approach and to use the power of the state for his religious revolution.

Julian did not persecute Christianity but stripped away the privileges to which the church had become used. Rather artfully, he allowed bishops, whom Constantius had banished in the interests of church unity, to return and told the clergy that they might teach whatever doctrines they wished. He tried to divorce Christianity from the Hellenic intellectual heritage by forbidding Christians to teach in schools where Greek and Latin literary works were used, although Christian children might attend. The economic position of the church was damaged by the requirement that all lands confiscated from pagan temples should be returned, by the withdrawal of public money for the Christian poor and by the withdrawal of the privileges of immunity from *liturgies* and taxation from the clergy. Christians were turned out of the administration, so far as possible, and into their places flocked the philosophers, pagan priests, and sudden converts to paganism.

To make some link between the rarefied tenets of Neoplatonism and the common man, Julian encouraged solar monotheism, the worship of the sun-god, in which the sun was regarded as the visible manifestation of the Divine. Julian himself wrote a treatise on sun worship and hoped that the universality of the cult would unite all paganism and draw Christians to it. This pagan church was to be administered by a hierarchy of priests, modeled on the Christian organization, while Julian, as *Pontifex Maximus,* would be a sort of pagan pope and emperor combined. A start was made, but little enthusiasm was generated except in Julian and his advisers. Solar monotheism, like Neoplatonism, was too abstract for a pagan world which liked the mystery religions and the familiar festivals. Then, in the intellectual world of paganism there was an awful quietness. The scholars wished to be left in peace or, if that could not be, at least to argue, but not to administer or to preach.

Julian was called from religious reform to the practical need of taking the field against Persia. In the spirit of Alexander the Great he prepared a campaign to conquer Persia and to place a Roman ruler on the throne of the Sassanids. An alliance was made with the king of Armenia, and Julian drove deep into the Middle East in 363, defeating a Persian army under the walls of Ctesiphon, the capital. When he turned north along the Tigris, however, to meet his ally from Armenia, he was killed in a minor battle, and the army acclaimed Jovian, the commander of the king's bodyguard, as emperor. The death of Julian marked the real end of paganism as a political force in the Empire. The observation of the Christian bishop Athanasius on Julian's program, "It will pass," was true. It did, leaving scarcely a trace of opposition to the succeeding Christian emperors.

Julian's successor, Jovian, was both an unambitious general and a good Christian. He made a hasty treaty with Shapur II of Persia by which he saved his army but had to give up Roman territory east of the Euphrates, including the great fortified city of Nisibis and the protectorate over Armenia. Jovian hurried back to Asia Minor where he repealed Julian's anti-Christian legislation and issued an edict of toleration for the pagans. He died within eight months.

VALENTINIAN AND VALENS (364–79)

At the time of Jovian's death the situation of the Empire was critical. The peace with Persia had been costly, and the Franks and the Alemanni had taken advantage of Julian's activity in the East to renew their attacks along the Rhine and the upper Danube. Along the lower course of that river another great storm of destruction was gathering. The Goths were restless under the pressure of great migratory movements set in motion by the advance of the Mongolian Huns westwards into Europe. The Huns had destroyed the Kingdom of the Eastern Goths, the Ostrogoths, in the Ukraine, and refugee bands of the latter were pushing against their western kindred, the Visigoths, in the lands north of the middle and lower Danube.

Military considerations were paramount in the choice of an emperor, and so the high military and bureaucratic officials selected Valentinian, a choleric soldier of considerable experience from Pannonia. He proceeded to establish a family dynasty by appointing his brother Valens to rule in the East from Constantinople and making his son Gratian, a boy of nine, a third Augustus. Valentinian himself operated from Milan against the Franks and Alemanni. For ten years, from 365 to 375, he fought them successfully and rebuilt the forts along the Rhine, winning a generation of peace for the province of Gaul. At the same time his general Theodosius drove the Picts and Scots from northern England and put down a rebellion in Africa. In 375 Valentinian died in a burst of rage, while negotiating with the barbarians in Pannonia, and was succeeded by Valens as senior ruler, while Gratian took over the West.

The brief reign of Valens was momentous in the history of the Empire, for his failure on the Danubian frontier brought a mass of Goths into its lands. In 377 the Western Goths, who were partially Romanized and converts of the Christian missionary Ulfilas asked Valens for permission to reside in Thrace. Permission was granted on condition of surrendering their arms. The Goths bribed the Roman officials to overlook their weapons, and then the officials foolishly tried to exploit the refugees by charging high prices for food. The Goths turned to plundering and were joined soon by other groups from north of the Danube. Valens decided to expel the whole people and risked battle at Adrianople, before his colleague Gratian could arrive with help. The Roman army was almost annihilated, Valens was killed, and the Goths fanned out to ravage the provinces from the head of the Adriatic to the Bosporus, as they had done a century previously.

Gratian was unable to cope with the situation and in 379 appointed an experienced general as co-ruler, Theodosius, the son of Valentinian's general of that name. He was placed in charge of the East to deal with the Goths.

THEODOSIUS THE GREAT (379-95)

Theodosius was the last emperor of an effectively united Roman Empire and won his title to greatness by his strenuous efforts to hold the East and West together. At the time of his appointment he was an energetic, experienced officer of thirty-four, living in Spain. He marched at once to the East and, by a mixture of diplomacy and limited war, he exploited the divisions among the Goths and was able to quiet them down. He was too weak, however, to drive them back across the Danube and in 382 came to an agreement with their chieftains. The Goths were to reside in the Empire, retaining their own laws and organization, but were pledged to defend the frontiers under the command of their own chieftains. Thus they formed a virtually independent, barbarian enclave in the territory of the Empire. Theirs was not the first, for groups of Franks had been admitted previously to Gaul on similar conditions, but the Goths were very numerous and were settled astride the road linking the Eastern and Western parts of the Empire.

While Theodosius was dealing with the Goths, Gratian lost control of the Western portion of the Empire to Maximus, the commander of the troops in Britain. Theodosius had to devote much of the latter part of his reign to its reconquest, first from Maximus, then from one of his own generals, Arbogast the Frank, who proved disloyal. Unity of rule was restored in 394, but in the following year Theodosius died in Milan. He had provided for the succession by making Arcadius, his elder son, Augustus in 383 and installing him in Constantinople. He made his younger son Honorius ruler of the West. Both, however, were under the influence of their chief officials, able and ambitious barbarian generals. Arcadius' guardian was Rufinus, the praetorian prefect of Illyricum, and Honorius' guardian was Stilicho, a Vandal, who had married the niece of Theodosius. The mutual rivalry of these men meant that the unity of Empire under Theodosius' dynasty was nominal and, in effect, East and West were divided, each preoccupied with the problems of its own survival.

The Intellectual Life of the Fourth Century

PAGANISM AND CHRISTIANITY

The reign of Julian had seen the last political effort of paganism to reassert itself, and under Theodosius orthodox Christianity was firmly installed as the state religion. Until the 370's an anomaly had continued to exist in the Roman government. The emperors were Christian, the church was strong, but the official religion of the state was pagan. The emperor was *Pontifex Maximus,* in Rome the worship of the pagan gods had been officially continued, and the holy days of the year were the festival days of the old gods. Gratian, a devout Christian, even if a poor ruler, set about to remove the anomalies. Upon becoming emperor in 375 he refused to take the title of *Pontifex Maximus* and several years later cut off the funds for the pagan festivals.

Gratian's final act was to order the removal of the altar of the goddess Victory from the Senate House. In the controversy which followed the altar became a symbol of Roman history. The pagans of Rome were led by Symmachus, a learned senator, and the Christians by Bishop Ambrose of Milan, one of the most trenchant and strong-minded leaders of the church. Their correspondence on the issue has survived. Symmachus argued in a letter to the emperor that worship of the goddess had resulted in the Roman conquest of the world and that she had defended Rome from Hannibal and the Gauls. To the Christians, however, the Christian Roman Empire was a fulfillment of God's universal planning. Ambrose could reply in the name of progress that worship of Victory was outmoded and should be cast aside with other childish practices. The worship of Victory was discontinued, but the controversy lasted for ten years more. The pagan senators enrolled in the priesthoods, paid for sacrifices themselves and hoped for support from Theodosius' general Arbogast. Their efforts were futile. In 394 Theodosius prohibited the pagan religious rites and abolished the pagan religious calendar. More than a thousand years of continuous religious tradition had come to an official end in the city of Rome.

Yet the cults did not all terminate abruptly, nor did Greco-Roman literature and philosophy cease to be an intellectual force in society. Pagan religion experienced a long drawn-out decay as the revenues of its cults were cut off and the number of worshippers declined. Christianity, however, adopted what it wanted from pagan thought and preserved what its monks and clergy found intrinsically useful and interesting in literature and scholarship. Christian education, apart from specifically religious instruction, used the educational methods of Roman and Greek rhetoric, based on Cicero and Quintilian in the West and on the writers of the New Sophistic Movement in the East. The Christians justified their use of the classical intellectual heritage by recalling that the Hebrews had used the spoils of Egypt to make the vessels for their temple in Jerusalem. Why should the Christians not take what was good from the pagans? The practice caused some qualms to the early fathers of the church but was soon taken for granted. St. Jerome (345-420), who was devoted to Vergil and Cicero, felt doubts about his admission to heaven on this score, but overcame his scruples and used Cicero's books on law and ethics to reinforce his own doctrinal writings. Yet, just as the Empire had split politically, it soon began to split intellectually. Knowledge of Greek disappeared in the West in the fifth century, and Latin, never highly regarded by the Greek intellectuals of the East, went out of use there in the sixth century.

Apart from the Neoplatonist philosophy on the pagan side and the work of the Christian fathers in doctrine, the most interesting writing of the fourth century was in historiography. Ammianus Marcellinus (*ca.* 330–400), a pagan from Antioch, wrote a continuation of the history of Tacitus, but only the latter part, treating the reigns of Constantius from 353 and of Valentinian and Valens, has been preserved. Ammianus was an army officer, well acquainted with conditions in the Empire and a historian of good judgment. He worked carefully and produced a sound and readable history, remarkably objective in an age of religious controversy. He is generally ranked with Livy and Tacitus as one of Rome's important historians.

More important from the point of view of historiography was the development of the Christian view of history, most notably by Eusebius in the East and by St. Augustine in the West. Eusebius (*ca.* 263–339) was an extremely erudite scholar, familiar with Latin, Greek, and Hebrew, who worked at Caesarea in Palestine. He suffered to some degree from the persecution of Galerius, but was in high favor during the reign of Constantine, when he delivered the opening speech at the Council of Nicaea. His works developed the view that by God's design Christianity had taken over the heritage of the past. The Roman Empire itself had been created to smooth the way for the Christian mission, while the culmination of God's purpose had been reached in the victory of Constantine. Henceforth the destiny of Empire and church was bound together. In addition to his history of the church, the *Ecclesiastical History,* and a brief sketch of world history, Eusebius compiled chronological tables of Greek, Roman, and Eastern events from the time of Abraham to the year 325. The tables were widely translated into the Near Eastern languages and remained the basis for ancient chronology for centuries.

Constantine found a Christian spokesman for his reign in Lactantius (256–330), who began his career as a teacher of rhetoric in Nicomedia but was converted to Christianity and became the tutor of Constantine's children. Lactantius' most important work was the *Institutiones Divinae* (*Divine Institutes*), a treatise on Christian teaching for educated pagans, but in his *De Mortibus Persecutorum* (*On the Deaths of the Persecutors*) the Christian apocalyptic view of history appeared.

The most important intellectual figure of the period, and for centuries to come, was St. Augustine (354–430). Like Lactantius, Augustine had been trained as a teacher of rhetoric and was converted from Manichean and Neoplatonist ideas to Christianity. He was baptized by Ambrose in Milan in 387 and served as the bishop of Hippo (Bône) in his native Africa until 430. Augustine died there in that year while Vandal armies were besieging the city. He wrote an account of his life and spiritual growth in the *Confessions* and a large number of important theological works, but his view of human history appears in the *De Civitate Dei* (the *City of God*).

In form the book was an answer to the pagan charge that the sack of Rome by Alaric the Visigoth in 410 was the penalty for disbelief in the pagan gods. The Christian community needed reassurance in its feeling of despair that the Christian Empire, so recently established, could perish. God's purpose in history, explained with such facility by the writers of Constantine's period, needed further explanation. Augustine wrote: "God, the author and giver of felicity, because He alone is the true God, Himself grants earthly kingdoms both to good and bad. Neither does He do this rashly, and, as it were, fortuitously,— because He is God, not fortune—but according to the order of things and times, which is hidden from us, but thoroughly known to Himself. . . . The cause, then, of the greatness of the Roman Empire is neither fortuitous nor fatal. . . . Human kingdoms are established by divine providence." To Augustine man's history was a conflict between good, the City of God, and evil, its earthly counterpart, in which the good will ultimately triumph. God was purposive in history, but its events were sometimes paradoxical, and the heavenly and earthly cities intermingled. As well as emphasizing the optimistic viewpoint of Christian historiography, Augustine did his faith the good service of separating it from identification with the temporal fortunes of the Roman Empire.

ART

The quality and character of the fourth century can be seen clearly in the late classical art of the period. Mingled with the formal classical traditions of the past there appeared strong Eastern influences in design and ornament and the signs of folk art, both of which pointed forward to the Medieval Period. Workmanship was frequently crude and unskilled, in contrast to the sophisticated techniques of the Roman Peace—an obvious result of the decline of patronage in the anarchy of the third century. Yet sculptors achieved a primitive strength in some of their portrait heads, and builders were able to express the

Life on a great estate of the Late Roman Empire; in the center, the fortified manor and, in each corner, typical activity of one of the four seasons. A mosaic from Carthage

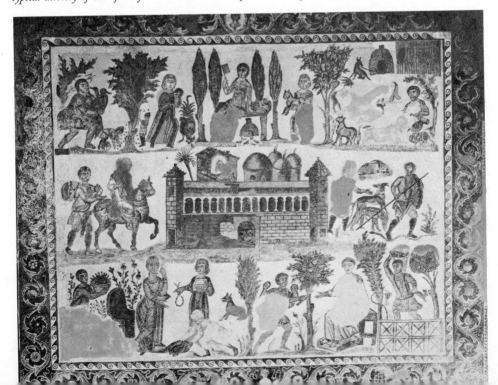

character of the Dominate in such structures as Diocletian's Palace at Salonae (Split), in his Baths, and in the great Basilica of Maxentius in Rome. These were massive structures, bold and original in conception, like the political acts of the emperors who tried to reorganize the structure of the Empire.

The Palace of Diocletian on the seacoast at Split in Dalmatia was built on the model of a Roman military camp, transformed into monumental form. It was a large quadrangular fortress, one wall of which rose sheer from the sea, while the others were protected by corner and gate towers. In the interior the roads, which bisected a camp at right angles, were preserved to mark off the elements of the palace. In place of the usual military tribunal, placed before the headquarters, were Diocletian's Mausoleum and a temple set in a walled garden. Such a dwelling was a far cry from the luxurious villa at Tivoli which Hadrian had built for his retirement, and it is an eloquent commentary on the changed conditions of life in the Empire.

The Baths of Diocletian (Terme Museum and Santa Maria degli Angeli) and the Basilica of Maxentius in Rome both exhibit a massive, unified central- ization, despite their tremendous size. The Baths were the largest ever con- structed in the Empire, able to accommodate about 3200 bathers, but the architect was able to draw the great central rooms together into a unified com- plex. The planning of the Basilica of Maxentius was equally original. Its large central hall, an element borrowed from the Baths, was a unit in itself, terminat- ing in an apse and opening out into side rooms between the piers which sup- ported the vaulting, rather than dividing into the conventional central nave and side aisles.

The construction of temples, of course, ended during this period, and in their place the Christian church began to develop as a new type of religious architecture. The most usual church type in the fourth century was an adapta- tion of the Roman basilica to the needs of the Christian service, where clergy and congregation were separated. The basilica was modified by placing a transept across the end of the aisles and the central nave, thus interposing quiet

Reconstruction of the fortified Palace of Diocletian at Split (Salonae) in Jugoslavia

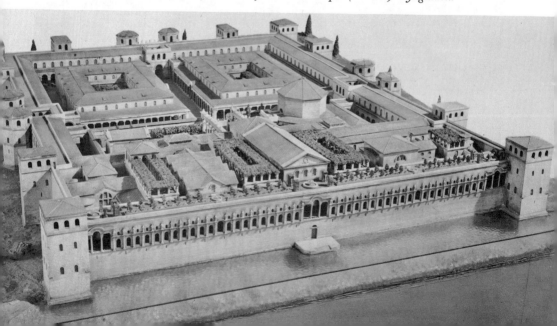

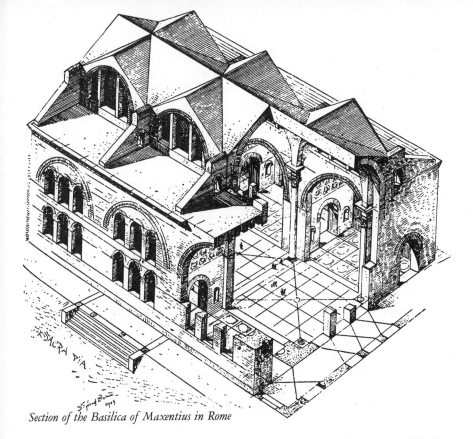

Section of the Basilica of Maxentius in Rome

order between the congregation and the more sacred area of the apse. The interiors of the churches were decorated with mosaics and paintings which preached to the congregation as eloquently as did the clergy by their portrayal of scenes from the Christian mythology of the Old and New Testaments. A new field of religious art grew rapidly, the results of which we can see in the Byzantine churches at Ravenna in Italy and at Hagia Sophia in Istanbul.

Although the demand for sculpture and the number of trained artists dwindled in the fourth century, their work shows new conceptions which form a striking contrast to the classicizing style of the second century. The technique was crude, but the sculpture had strength and a refreshing originality. Sculpture in the round was used mainly for the statues of the emperors, now objects of awe and veneration. Some, like the head of Constantine, were on a gigantic scale. The features are exaggerated and simplified, primitive in appearance, but with a massive strength that the most facile work of the Hadrianic and Antonine periods could not attain. Even more instructive is the Arch of Constantine, still standing in Rome near the Colosseum. Built into it are sculptured medallions of the Antonine Period, which contrast strongly with the relief friezes of Constantine's own era. The motifs of the latter are traditional: lively scenes from the emperor's battles and representations of his acts of administration. But the human figures are individualized by touches of folk interest and reveal different types of character with an almost sly interest in personality. It is

719

useful to contrast the scenes on Constantine's arch, where the emperor is larger and set apart from his subjects, with those on the Altar of Peace of Augustus, in which the Roman citizens and their *Princeps* move together in quiet and thoughtful dignity, and all alike are the focus of interest.

The Divided Empire

In the fourth century we can begin to discern clearly the forms of another world. The emperor regarded himself as the representative of the Christian God, whose faith had become the state religion. The city, which had been characteristic of Greek and Roman civilization, was being replaced by big estates, reminiscent in organization of those of the ancient Near East. There was an obvious and striking decline in material well-being, security, and individual freedom. If we look back at the fourth century from our own time, it seems that the Middle Ages were coming into being and that men were making a fresh start. Much that had been familiar and cherished in the past had been destroyed or would vanish in the near future. But much that seemed useful was preserved, and there was freshness in the new concepts of history and of human society which were being worked out by Christian thinkers. The fourth century was the midpoint in an age of transition, but the scale of change was immeasurably greater than any other of ancient history, for the whole of the ancient world which had come into being over the course of three thousand years, was being transformed and history reshaped.

THE WEST: THE GERMANIC KINGDOMS

In the Western part of the Empire the break with the past seems fairly rapid and decisive, for in the fifth century Roman rule was replaced by separate

Left: Colossal head of Constantine the Great. The portrait expresses the new concept of the emperor's position: the vicero
of God aloof from his subjects in contrast to the Princeps, *the first among his fellow citizens. Right: scene from the Arch o*
Constantine in Rome. The relief shows the emperor giving alms to the poor of Rome. The medallions above were reuse
in the arch from a monument of the Antonine Period.

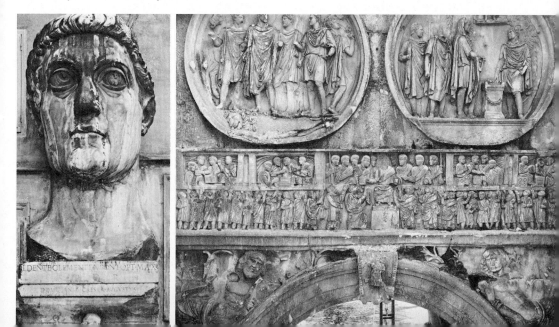

Germanic kingdoms, and the Roman population was mastered by barbarian peoples from across the Rhine and the Danube. There was no sudden avalanche of destruction, however, and barbarian attitudes to the Empire varied widely, but there were simply too many barbarians to be assimilated once the barriers were down. Some of the warlike leaders, like Stilicho at the beginning of the fifth century, worked for the union of Romans and barbarians, while others, like Alaric, saw only an opportunity for extortion and plunder. Many large groups of barbarians came into the provinces as the Goths had come, as allies (*foederati*) pledged to defend the lands on which they settled. Goths and Franks in Gaul joined the Romans in turning back Attila the Hun in 451 near Troyes.

Yet the Romans had to depend on the barbarians for protection, and the real rulers in the West were the barbarian generals who served the Roman emperors. In 476 the last Roman emperor of the West, named significantly enough Romulus Augustulus, was forced to abdicate by the German Odoacer, the leader of bands of mercenary soldiers in Italy. By that time most of the former provinces had become the seats of Germanic kingdoms, although there was considerable variation in their organization and relations with the Roman population.

In Britain virtually all traces of the Roman regime had vanished. The Romans had pulled their troops out of the island for service on the continent early in the fifth century. Angles, Saxons, Jutes, Picts, and Scots followed up their previous raids by settlement. Romanization had been superficial in Britain, and when the soldiers and the officials left, native Celtic speech and institutions reasserted themselves, along with those of the newcomers.

In Italy, on the other hand, Roman institutions were preserved almost intact. In 493 Odoacer was replaced by the Ostrogothic king, Theodoric, who was sponsored by the Roman emperor in Constantinople. Both Odoacer and Theodoric retained the Roman system of administration. While the Roman population of northern Gaul was almost obliterated by the Salian Franks, the Visigoths and Burgundians lived side by side with the Romans as a separate people. The Roman population in the Rhone valley and in western France below the Loire River and in Spain retained their own institutions under the German regime. These Germanic regimes in Western Europe, however, were short-lived and unstable because they depended primarily on the military success of their rulers who warred with one another and the new groups of barbarians who thrust against them.

In Africa, however, the Vandals established a strongly centralized kingship and founded a small empire, reminiscent of that of Carthage in the past. In the early fifth century they had swept through Gaul and Spain, selling their military services or plundering, as the occasion offered and in 429 they crossed to North Africa. There the Vandal chieftains took over the big estates, sometimes retaining their former owners as stewards and transferring the services of the *coloni* to themselves. By 442 their kingdom had formed, and in the following generation the Vandals became a sea power. The islands of the western Mediterranean were taken over and forays were made against Italy and into the eastern Mediterranean. The Western part of the Empire had fragmented, but the rulers of the East in Constantinople continued to regard themselves as rightful rulers of the whole, and in the sixth century, the Emperor Justinian was able to make good the claim to a considerable degree.

THE EAST: THE BYZANTINE EMPIRE

The Byzantine Empire seems to evolve logically and naturally out of the era of Constantine and his successors. Until the end of the fifth century there was danger that the government at Constantinople might come under the control of Gothic generals and the state disintegrate into regional kingdoms. The Eastern emperors, however, contrived to use the manpower of Asia Minor, particularly the hardy Isaurian mountaineers of southern Anatolia, and therefore avoided the experience of their contemporaries in the West. They skillfully played one barbarian general against another and hired small groups of mercenary soldiers instead of whole peoples. The main impact of the migrations, of course, fell on Europe rather than on Asia Minor. In Persia the Byzantine rulers had an enemy whom they knew and whose resources were limited. But in the long run the survival of the Empire was its ability to draw on the wealth and manpower of Asia Minor. When the southern and eastern provinces were lost to Islam in the seventh century and much of the Balkans to the Slavs, the Empire was concentrated in its homogeneous Greek area and the bastion of Asia Minor.

The Byzantine emperors preserved and added to the legacy of Roman law as the basis for their administration. In 438 the Emperor Theodosius II (408–50) published the Theodosian Code, in which the edicts of the emperors from the late third century were collected. It served for both the East and for those areas in the West where Roman law was used. In the reign of Justinian the great codification known as the *Corpus Iuris Civilis* was compiled and published. The emperor's aim was to collect all the sources of law in effect, and the *Corpus* came to be the fundamental summation of Roman law by which its practice was carried on and its principles transmitted. The work was issued in three parts: the *Code,* which collected all the previous imperial constitutions; the *Digest,* which abstracted the interpretations of the great jurists of the Roman Empire; and the *Institutes,* which was a handbook for students of law. Future emperors added their own edicts in the *Novels.*

Justinian (527–65) may be properly called the last of the Roman emperors and the founder of the Medieval Byzantine Empire. He was a Roman from the province of Moesia along the Danube and used Latin as his native tongue. He came to the throne in 527 with the aim of recovering the West and restoring that imperial unity which the Byzantine emperors claimed. This was to be both a unity of secular administration and of Christianity under his own imperial authority, for Justinian conceived of the emperor's position as an autocracy over state and church. His rule was a model for the absolute Byzantine regime in which the state was controlled through an elaborate bureaucracy and the church through an ecclesiastical hierarchy headed by the patriarch of Constantinople. First, Justinian made an accord with the Western church to obtain the support of its clergy and to give his conquest the form of a crusade to unite the Christian world and the Roman Empire. The use of Christianity as a unifying factor for the West had validity, of course, because most of the barbarian peoples had been converted. Justinian could find pretexts for interference in their kingdoms through the claim that the rulers were his vassals, and in 532 the reconquest of the West began through his general, Belisarius.

Justinian had two excellent generals in Belisarius and Narses and a good fighting army of mercenary soldiers. Although the officers and men were unruly and eager for plunder, they were skilled, tough fighters. Among them the mailed horsemen were particularly effective. Yet the army was small and Byzantine resources were limited for great military projects. As well as planning conquest in the West, Justinian had to guard his eastern frontier against the Persians and defend the Danubian lands against the Slavic inroads, which were continuously increasing in scale. Persia was held off, and in 562 a peace was made for fifty years by which the territory of the Empire remained largely intact. Since the Balkan provinces, however, could not be defended, the Empire in southeastern Europe was reduced to the extremity of Thrace.

In the West Justinian was more successful, although the wars were lengthy and much of the territory recovered soon had to be given up. The Vandal Kingdom in Africa and the big islands of the western Mediterranean were retaken in 533 and 534 by Belisarius. In the following year Moorish revolt was suppressed, and Africa remained a possession of the Byzantine Empire under Roman forms of administration until the Islamic conquest. The whole peninsula of Italy was taken by Belisarius and Narses between 535 and 554, but was lost to the Lombards in the latter part of the century, except for Ravenna, Rome, and the extreme south. From Italy, Narses made an attempt on Spain in 554 but was able to take only a few coastal towns, and these were soon lost again to the Visigoths.

Nevertheless Justinian had succeeded in restoring a semblance of imperial unity and in making the Byzantine state the chief power of the Mediterranean. This was not to last for long, but at a critical time he gave fresh life to the Greek and Roman traditions. The heritage of law had been embodied in the codes and in the administration. The intellectual heritage of Rome was a part of the church in the West, and that of Greece a living force in Byzantine culture. Byzantine art, rooted in classical and Eastern traditions, had come to an early maturity by the construction of the great Church of Hagia Sophia in Constantinople and those at Ravenna in Italy. The people of the Byzantine Empire were to be known as "Romans" until the crusaders from Western Europe and the Turks from Asia dismembered its lands. Until 1453, when the Turks moved into Constantinople, the political form of the Byzantine Empire was preserved in some fashion. Well before that time Western Europe had rediscovered the humanism of Greek and Roman civilization, and the men of the Renaissance were making it a vital force in modern history.

Epilogue

IN THE LONG STORY OF THE ANCIENT WORLD we have seen the rise and decline of many states and empires, each of which left some mark on the life of its successor. Ancient civilization was cumulative and enduring, even if the political organizations of its peoples were transitory. Similarly, those institutions and ideas of the Roman Empire which men of the Middle Ages felt useful for themselves were preserved and transmitted. If we consider the classic question of the "decline and fall" of the Roman Empire from this point of view, the terms of the question seem incorrect. There was a long drawn-out process of change from the second to the seventh and eighth centuries after Christ. After the rise of Islam and in the full bloom of the Middle Ages, the Roman Empire seems to have disappeared, but its disappearance, like those of the Sumerian city-states and of classical Athens in the course of ancient history, was illusory. Roman civilization had been absorbed, partly for immediate use, partly to lie dormant and to reappear as a vital force at a later and more congenial era of history.

Obviously, however, there was a breakdown of political stability and of military efficiency in the third century. The character of the Empire in the fourth century was very different from that of the second, farther from classical Greece and Rome, closer to the Middle Ages. The Empire could be reorganized as a whole at the outset of the fourth century, but the unity of administration could not be maintained and the Western, or Roman, part soon fragmented. There, the framework of Roman government and social organization collapsed. It is usually in these terms that the "decline and fall" of Rome has been discussed as an historical question. Why did the Roman Empire in the West weaken and ultimately collapse?

During the crisis of the third century, pagan Roman society assigned the cause of its suffering to the failure of the Christians to worship the gods of Rome. Several generations later, when Christianity had become the favored religion of the state, popular Christian thought confidently assumed that God's

724

purpose was being worked out in history and that the Empire was secure. Thus the people of the Late Empire interpreted their history in the framework of religious reference which characterized their age. Men of the Renaissance found a military explanation—barbarian invasion. The barbarians have not been absolved entirely, for some present-day historians still explain the collapse of the Roman Empire by this external factor. Yet the Empire showed a remarkable ability to absorb and use barbarians until the fifth century, by which time its internal character had already changed radically. Sometimes a facile single explanation is advanced: the moral degeneracy of the Romans, soil exhaustion, racial mixture, the export of gold to the East in trade. But with a little reflection, these explanations may be dismissed with equal facility.

Most modern historians of Rome tend to seek the explanation in the internal structure of the Empire and in a complex of symptoms, causes, and effects. They have found it difficult, however, to assign satisfactory emphasis, for symptom may be mistaken for cause, cause passes into effect, and effect into further cause. It has been easier for each successive discussion to point out the inadequacy of previous arguments than to establish its own. In short, the discussion has raised questions about human history which should be asked, but which the historian of ancient times, working with scanty source materials over a broad period, can scarcely answer satisfactorily. Perhaps the value is in the dialogue and not in the answers.

Many of the factors which seem to have contributed to the decline of the Empire have been mentioned in the course of the narrative, and it would be useful to review them briefly. The earliest signs of weakness seem to have appeared at the time when the Empire was outwardly very strong and stable, in the second century after Christ. There was at that time an obvious falling off of creative originality in literature, thought, and art, as if classical civilization had worked out the resources inherent in its own intellectual forms and methods of expression. There seemed to be some signs of weakness in the social and economic organization, indicated by the financial difficulties of certain cities and the decline of prosperity in Italy, the heart of the Empire. It has been suggested that these signs of weakness may have resulted from two main factors: the limitations set by the economic organization itself—the pattern of local and regional self-sufficiency—and the tendency of industry to export itself from the older regions to the newer. Also, the wealth of the Empire supported the upper- and middle-class urban groups at a high standard of material well-being and leisure, but did not extend down to the lower class in city and countryside. That is, the limit of expansion in terms of internal organization had been reached, and the processes of development had begun to reverse themselves. The decline of the cities had begun, and the *coloni* were growing in numbers as the large estates developed.

In terms of political organization, the achievement of the Empire in extending citizenship and legal privilege was counterbalanced by the tendency towards absolutism and centralization of government. Citizenship opened up participation in administration of the Empire to many, but not to participation in government. By the Antonine Period the Senate and the bureaucracy were representative of much of the Empire, and became more so, but the power of government had passed to the emperor and his advisers. The self-governing cities were becoming more restricted in their operations as they turned to the central government for assistance and direction. Political freedom in its various aspects (of which both the conceptions and implementations had been worked out) had disappeared in all but tradition and name.

The army, except for its assertion of power in 68/69, had been kept as an instrument of the state and not a source of political power for almost two centuries from Augustus to Marcus Aurelius. But during that period most of the Empire's peoples had lost their military traditions, and the soldiers had been drawn from the ruder elements of the population. At the same time the army became an efficient, well-organized machine, able to perform its function of defending the Empire well. When the soldiers became conscious of themselves as a source of power in the state under the favored treatment of the Severan emperors, they became the destructive element which triggered the breakdown.

The anarchy and breakdown of the third century were further aggravated by the natural disasters of plague and a falling birth rate—the latter encouraged by insecurity and poverty. The breakdown severely eroded the wealth of the Empire, but repair was sought along the lines of increased governmental efficiency. There was a reconstruction of society, but it seems to have proceeded almost automatically from the economic trends which had already started in the second century: the decline of the cities, the growth of the large estates, and the continuous shrinkage to local and regional self-sufficiency. The government recognized the new society and attempted to solidify its classes, but could not reorient it.

The real end of the Roman Empire, then, seems to have come in the breakdown of the third century, and the causes of the breakdown to lie in a complex of forces inherent in the character and organization of the Empire itself. Such forces worked at different speeds, interacted in various combinations, and their individual force is estimated in different ways by historians. One may find a primary cause in the loss of individual freedom and tend to regard the whole ancient world as in decline from the time of classical Greece. Another may stress the failure of the Empire to extend the material privileges of civilization to the mass of the people and so to prevent the reinforcement of society. The reverse, too, has been suggested: classical culture was extended so far that it became shallow and simplified beyond the possibility of deliberately changing its processes. Almost each generation has found the reflection of a particular concern of its own contemporary life in the termination of an ancient civilization. That fact in itself has a significance which makes it important. If this book can stimulate such a concern and if it can provide the material for discussion and comparison, its purpose will have been achieved.

Bibliography

The following bibliography is intended to suggest some easily accessible books in English for use by students. Paperback editions are indicated by an asterisk.

General Reference

The American Historical Association Guide to Historical Literature. New York, 1961.
Cambridge Ancient History. Ed. by J. B. Bury, S. A. Cook, F. E. Adcock, M. P. Charlesworth. 12 vols. Cambridge, England, 1923-39. From 1961 chapters of a revised edition of Vols. I and II have been published separately.
Cary, Max. *The Geographic Background of Greek and Roman History.* Oxford, 1949.
Kraeling, E. G. *Bible Atlas.* Chicago, 1956.
The Oxford Classical Dictionary. Ed. by Max Cary, Alfred Nock and others. Oxford, 1949.
van der Hayden, A. A. M. and H. H. Scullard. *Atlas of the Classical World.* London, 1960.

The Ancient Near East

*Albright, W. F. *The Archaeology of Palestine.* Harmondsworth, England, 1949 (Pelican book).
*———. *From the Stone Age to Christianity: Monotheism and the Historical Process.* New York, 1957 (Doubleday).
Aldred, Cyril. *The Egyptians.* New York, 1961.
Braidwood, R. J. *The Near East and the Foundations for Civilization.* Eugene, Oregon, 1952.
Breasted, J. H. *Ancient Records of Egypt.* 5 vols. Chicago, 1906-07. Source material in English translation.
Bright, John. *A History of Israel.* Philadelphia, n.d.
*Childe, V. Gordon. *Man Makes Himself.* New York, 1952 (Mentor book).
Contenau, G. *Everyday Life in Babylonia and Assyria.* Tr. by H. R. and A. R. Maxwell-Hyslop. New York, 1954.
Driver, S. R. *Introduction to the Literature of the Old Testament.* New York, 1956.
*Edwards, I. E. S. *The Pyramids of Egypt.* Rev. ed. Baltimore, 1961 (Pelican book).
Erman, A. *The Literature of the Ancient Egyptians.* Tr. by Aylward M. Blackman. London, 1927.
Finegan, Jack. *Light From the Ancient Past.* Princeton, 1959.
*Frankfort, Henri. *Before Philosophy.* Harmondsworth, England, 1949 (Pelican book).
*———. *The Birth of Civilization in the Near East.* New York, 1956 (Doubleday).
Gardiner, Sir Alan. *Egypt of the Pharaohs.* Oxford, 1961.

Gelb, I. J. *The Study of Writing*. Chicago, 1952.

*Ghirshman, R. *Iran*. Harmondsworth, England, 1956 (Pelican book).

Granville, S. R. K. (ed.) *The Legacy of Egypt*. Oxford, 1942.

*Gurney, O. R. *The Hittites*. Harmondsworth, England, 1961 (Pelican book).

Hayes, William C. *The Scepter of Egypt*. 2 vols. New York, 1953, 1959.

*Kramer, S. N. *History Begins at Sumer: Twenty-seven "Firsts" in Man's Recorded History*. New York, 1959 (Doubleday).

———. *The Sumerians: Their History, Culture and Character*. Chicago, 1963.

*Lloyd, Seton. *The Art of the Ancient Near East*. New York, 1961.

*———. *Early Anatolia*. Harmondsworth, England, 1956 (Pelican book).

Luckenbill, D. D. *Ancient Records of Assyria and Babylonia*. 2 vols. Chicago, 1926. Source material in English translation.

*Moscati, Sabatino. *The Face of the Ancient Orient*. New York, 1962 (Doubleday).

Neugebauer, O. *The Exact Sciences in Antiquity*. Princeton, 1952.

Oppenheim, A. Leo. *Ancient Mesopotamia*. Chicago, 1964.

Pritchard, James B. (ed.) *Ancient Near Eastern Texts Relating to the Old Testament*. Rev. ed. Princeton, 1955. Source material in English translation.

Saggs, R. W. F. *The Greatness That Was Babylon: A Sketch of the Ancient Civilization of the Tigris-Euphrates Valley*. London, 1962.

Steindorff, George and K. C. Seele. *When Egypt Ruled the East*. Chicago, 1957.

*Wilson, John A. *The Culture of Egypt*. Chicago, 1956 (Phoenix book).

Greece and the Hellenistic Age

Andrewes, A. *The Greek Tyrants*. London, 1956.

Botsford, G. W. and Ernest Sihler. *Hellenic Civilization*. New York, 1915. Source material in English translation.

*Bowra, Sir Cecil M. *Ancient Greek Literature*. New York, 1960 (Oxford University Press).

Burn, A. R. *The Lyric Age of Greece*. New York, 1960.

Burnet, J. *Early Greek Philosophy*. New York, 1957.

Bury, J. B. *A History of Greece to the Death of Alexander the Great*. Rev. by Russell Meiggs. 3rd ed. New York, 1951.

Cary, Max. *The Legacy of Alexander: A History of the Greek World from 323 to 146 B.C.* London, 1932.

Chadwick, John. *The Decipherment of Linear B*. Cambridge, England, 1959.

Cook, J. M. *The Greeks in Ionia and the East*. London, 1962.

*Farrington, B. *Greek Science*. Harmondsworth, England, 1949 (Pelican book).

Finley, M. I. *The Ancient Greeks: An Introduction to Their Life and Thought*. New York, 1963.

———. (ed.). *The Greek Historians: The Essence of Herodotus, Thucydides, Xenophon, Polybius*. New York, 1959.

———. *Slavery in Antiquity*. Cambridge, England, 1960.

———. *The World of Odysseus*. New York, 1954.

*Fustel de Coulanges, Numa. *The Ancient City*. New York, 1956 (Doubleday).

Glotz, G. *The Greek City and Its Institutions*. Tr. by N. Mallinson. New York, 1930.

Graham, J. W. *The Palaces of Crete*. Princeton, 1962.

*Guthrie, William K. C. *The Greeks and Their Gods*. Boston, 1951.

Herodotus. *History*. Tr. by George Rawlinson. New York, 1927 (Everyman's Library).

Hignett, C. *The Athenian Constitution*. Oxford, 1952.

Huxley, G. E. *Early Sparta*. Cambridge, Mass., 1962.

Jones, A. H. M. *Athenian Democracy*. Oxford, 1957.

*Kitto, H. D. F. *Greek Tragedy: A Literary Study*. New York, 1954 (Doubleday).

*Lawrence, A. W. *Greek Architecture*. Harmondsworth, England (Pelican book).

Mackendrick, Paul. *The Greek Stones Speak*. New York, 1962.

Michell, H. *The Economics of Ancient Greece*. Rev. ed. Cambridge, England, 1956.

*Murray, Gilbert. *Five Stages of Greek Religion*. New York (Doubleday).

Mylonas, George. *Ancient Mycenae*. Princeton, 1957.

Nilsson, M. P. *Homer and Mycenae*. London, 1933.

Plutarch, *Lives*. Tr. by Dryden; rev. by H. H. Clough. New York, 1932 (Everyman's Library).

*Rostovtzeff, M. I. *Greece*. Oxford, 1964.

———. *The Social and Economic History of the Hellenistic World*. 3 vols. Oxford, 1941.

*Snell, B. *The Discovery of the Mind*. New York, 1960.

Starr, Chester. *The Origins of Greek Civilization*. New York, 1961.

Tarn, William W. and G. T. Griffith. *Hellenistic Civilization*. 3rd ed. rev. London, 1952.

*Tarn, William W. *Alexander the Great*. Boston, 1956 (Beacon).

*Taylor, A. E. *Socrates: The Man and His Thought*. New York, 1953 (Doubleday).

*Thucydides. *The Peloponnesian War*. Tr. by Richard Crawley. New York, 1961 (Doubleday).

Vermeule, Emily. *Greece in the Bronze Age*. Chicago, 1964.

Wilcken, U. *Alexander the Great*. Tr. by G. C. Richards. New York, 1932.

Woodhead, A. G. *The Greeks in the West*. London, 1962.

Wycherley, R. E. *How the Greeks Built Cities*. 2d ed. New York, 1961.

*Zimmern, Sir Alfred. *The Greek Commonwealth: Politics and Economics in Fifth Century Athens*. 5th ed. rev. New York, 1931 (Oxford University Press).

Rome

Abbot, Frank F. *History and Description of Roman Political Institutions*. 3rd ed. Boston, 1911.

Arnold, Edward V. *Roman Stoicism*. Cambridge, England, 1911.

Bailey, C. (ed.). *The Legacy of Rome*. London, 1923.

Baynes, Norman H. *Constantine the Great and the Christian Church*. London, 1931.

Boak, Arthur E. R. and William G. Sinnigen. *A History of Rome to A.D. 565*. 5th ed. New York, 1965.

Boethius, C. Axel. *Roman Architecture*. Göteborg, Sweden, 1944.

Brogen, Oliver. *Roman Gaul*. Cambridge, Mass., and London, 1953.

Buchan, John. *Augustus*. Boston, 1937.

———. *Caesar*. London, 1932.

Carcopino, J. *Daily Life in Ancient Rome*. Ed. by H. T. Rowell; tr. by E. O. Lorimer. New Haven, 1940.

Charlesworth, Martin P. *The Roman Empire*. Oxford, 1951.

Charlesworth, M. P. *Five Men: Character Studies From the Roman Empire*. Cambridge, Mass., 1936.

*Cochrane, C. N. *Christianity and Classical Culture: A Study of Thought and Action from Augustus to Augustine*. New York, 1944 (Oxford University Press).

*Cowell, F. R. *Cicero and the Roman Republic*. Harmondsworth, England, 1956 (Pelican book).

*Dill, S. *Roman Society From Nero to Marcus Aurelius*. New York, 1956 (Meridian book).

*Duff, J. Wight. *Literary History of Rome From the Origins to the Close of the Golden Age*. 3rd ed. Rev. by A. M. Duff. New York, 1963.

———. *A Literary History of Rome in the Silver Age*. 2d ed. Rev. by A. M. Duff. London, 1960.

Fowler, William W. *Social Life at Rome in the Age of Cicero*. New York, 1909.

———. *The Religious Experience of the Roman People*. London, 1911.

Frank, Tenney. *An Economic History of Rome*. 2d rev. ed. Baltimore, 1927.

———. *Life and Literature in the Roman Republic*. Berkeley, 1930.

*Grant, M. *Roman Literature*. Harmondsworth, England, 1958 (Pelican book).

Hammond, Mason. *The Augustan Principate in Theory and Practice During the Julio-Claudian Period*. Cambridge, Mass., 1933.

Hill, H. *The Roman Middle Class in the Republican Period*. New York, 1952.

*Kagan, Donald (ed.). *Decline and Fall of the Roman Empire.* Boston, 1962 (Heath).

Laistner, M. L. W. *The Greater Roman Historians.* Berkeley, 1947.

Lewis, Naphtali and Meyer Reinhold. *Roman Civilization.* 2 vols. New York, 1951, 1955. Source material in English translation.

Maiuri, Amedeo. *Roman Painting.* Lausanne, 1953.

Marrou, H. I. *A History of Education in Antiquity.* Tr. by G. Lamb. New York, 1956.

Marsh, F. B. *The Founding of the Roman Empire.* 2d rev. ed. Oxford, 1927.

———. *The Reign of Tiberius.* London, 1931.

Mattingly, H. *Roman Coins.* London, 1960.

Momigliano, Arnaldo. *Claudius, the Emperor and His Achievement.* Tr. by W. B. Hogarth. Oxford, 1939.

Mommsen, Theodore. *History of Rome.* Tr. by W. P. Dickinson. Rev. ed. 4 vols. London and New York, 1911 (Everyman's Library).

———. *The Provinces of the Roman Empire, Caesar to Diocletian.* Tr. by W. P. Dickinson. 2d ed. 2 vols. London, 1908.

Nash, Ernest. *Roman Towns.* New York, 1949.

*Pallottino, M. *The Etruscans.* Harmondsworth, England, 1955 (Pelican book).

———. *Etruscan Painting.* Lausanne, 1952.

Parker, H. M. D. *A History of the Roman World from A.D. 138 to 337.* London, 1935.

Robathan, D. *The Monuments of Ancient Rome.* Rome, 1950.

Rostovtzeff, M. I. *Caravan Cities.* Oxford, 1932.

———. *The Social and Economic History of the Roman Empire.* Rev. by P. M. Fraser. 2d rev. ed. 2 vols. Oxford, 1957.

Salmon, Edward T. *A History of the Roman World from 30 B.C. to A.D. 138.* 4th rev. ed. London, 1963.

Schulz, Fritz. *Principles of Roman Law.* Oxford, 1936.

Scullard, Howard H. *A History of the Roman World from 753 to 146 B.C.* 4th rev. ed. London, 1963.

*———. *From the Gracchi to Nero: A History of Rome from 133 B.C. to A.D. 68.* 2d ed. London, 1963.

Stevenson, G. H. *Roman Provincial Administration.* 2d ed. New York, 1949.

*Syme, Sir Ronald. *The Roman Revolution.* New York, 1960 (Oxford University Press).

Taylor, L. R. *Party Politics in the Age of Caesar.* Berkeley, 1949.

*Wheeler, Sir Mortimer. *Rome Beyond the Imperial Frontiers.* Harmondsworth, England, 1955 (Pelican book).

Chronological Tables

PREHISTORY

All dates are approximate

Pleistocene (Age of Glaciation)	1,000,000–10,000 years ago
Appearance of man and tools	700,000–600,000 years ago
Appearance of new man	100,000 years ago
Upper Palaeolithic cultures	30,000–10,000 years ago
Holocene (Recent Geological Age)	10,000 years ago
Neolithic Age	8000–3000 B.C.
Transition to agriculture	8000–7000 B.C.
Formation of farming villages	7000–6000 B.C.
Developed Neolithic cultures	6000–4000 B.C.
Chalcolithic Period	4500–3000 B.C.
Civilization	*ca.* 3000 B.C.

MESOPOTAMIA

All dates are B.C. and most approximate

Sumerian Civilization	3200–2000
Sumerian Settlement	3500
Civilization (organization)	3200–2800
Royal burials of Ur	2750–2650
Kingdom of Lagash	2500–2340
Akkadian Empire (Sargon)	2340–2150
Gutian Domination	2200–2135
Third Dynasty of Ur	2135–2027
Amorite Invasion	*ca.* 2000
Kingdoms of Isin and Larsa (rise)	2000–1960
Babylonian Empire	1792–1550
Hammurabi	1792–1750

Hurrian Infiltration	1650
Hittite raid on Babylon	1595
Kassite Rule (Babylonia)	1550–1000
Kingdom of Mitanni (northern Mesopotamia)	1500–1370
Aramaean Infiltration	1000–800
Assyrian Rule	*ca.* 800–612
New Babylonian Empire	612–539
Persian Conquest	539
Alexander's Conquest	331
Parthian Conquest	100

EGYPT

All dates are B.C. and most approximate

Agricultural villages	4500
Gerzean Culture (rise)	3600
Unification of Egypt-Menes	3100
Civilization—Archaic Period	3100–2686
Old Kingdom (Dynasties III–VI)	2686–2180
Great Pyramids	2600–2500
First Intermediate Period—Anarchy	2180–2080
Middle Kingdom	2080–1640
Eleventh Dynasty—Thebes	2080–2040
Twelfth Dynasty—"Classical Egypt"	2040–1785
Hyksos "Invasion"	1720–1570
New Kingdom or Empire (Dynasties XVIII–XX)	1570–1075
Ahmose I—Expulsion of Hyksos	1570–1546
Thothmes III—Establishment of Empire	1482–1450
Amenophis III—Height of Empire	1417–1379
Akhnaton—Religious reform	1379–1365
Rameses II	1298–1232
Battle of Kadesh (Hittites)	1287
Treaty with Hittites	1268
Repulse of Peoples of the Sea	1225–1187
Division and weakness in Egypt	1085–650
Assyrian Conquest	671
Saite Kingdom (Dynasty XXVI)	663–525
Persian Conquest	525
Alexander the Great's Conquest	332
Ptolemaic Egypt	306–30
Roman Annexation	30

ANATOLIA

All dates are B.C. and most approximate

Formation of farming villages	7000
Bronze Age	3000–1200
Arrival of Luwians, Hittites (I.E.)	2500–2000

Assyrian Colonies	1900–1800
Old Hittite Kingdom	1650–1500
Hittite Empire	1500–1200
Shuppiluliumash	1380–1335
Destruction of Hittite Empire	1200
Invasions and Dark Age	1200–800
Greek Settlement in Ionia	1050–900
Kingdom of Urartu	900–700
Kingdom of Phrygia	850 (?)–696
Cimmerian Invasion	705–650
Kingdom of Lydia	685–547
Gyges and the Cimmerians	668 and 652
Invention of Coinage	650–625
Treaty between Lydia and Media	585
Croesus	560–547
Persian Conquest	547–540
Alexander's Conquest	334–333
Greek Cities, Native Kingdoms, Seleucids	3rd and 2nd centuries
Kingdom of Pergamum	263–129
Roman defeat of Antiochus III	189
Roman Province of Asia	129
Mithridates VI of Pontus	121–63
Roman organization of Asia Minor	1st century

SYRIA AND PALESTINE
All dates are B.C. and most approximate

Semitic Infiltration	3500 and 2000
Hyksos Occupation	1800–1600
Egyptian, Mitanni and Hittite Rivalry	1500–1200
Ugarit (height)	1500–1200
Peoples of the Sea	1200
Philistine Settlement	1180
Hebrew Settlement	1250–1100
Aramaean Settlement	1200–1000
Phoenician Cities (height)	1100–700
Hebrew Amphictyony	1100–1000
Hebrew Kingdom	1000–922
Kingdom of Israel	922–721
Kingdom of Judah	922–586
Assyrian Conquest and Empire	850–612
New Babylonian Conquest	605–539
Persian Conquest and Rule	539–332
Alexander's Conquest	332
Ptolemaic and Seleucid Rivalry	3rd century
Seleucid Empire	3rd and 2nd centuries
Maccabaean Revolt	150's
Roman organization	1st century

ASSYRIA

All dates are B.C.

Assyrian Colonies in Cappadocia	1900–1800
First Assyrian Empire	1365–1250
Assyrian Revival	911–745
Ashur-nasir-pal II	883–859
Assyrian Empire	745–612
Tiglath—Pileser III	745–727
Defeat of Urartu	714
Conquest of Egypt	671
Ashurbanipal (height of Empire)	669–627
Destruction of Nineveh	612

PERSIA

All dates are B.C.

Arrival of Medes and Persians	*ca.* 1000
Kingdom of Media	650–550
Persian Empire	550–330
Cyrus' Conquest of Media	550
Cyrus' Conquest of Lydia	547
Cyrus' Conquest of Ionia	546–540
Cyrus' Conquest of Babylonia	539
Cambyses (Conquest of Egypt)	525
Darius	522–486
Darius' Scythian Expedition	513
Darius' Foundation of Persepolis	512
Ionian Revolt and Invasion of Greece	499–490
Xerxes	486–464
Xerxes' Invasion of Greece	481–479
Peace with Greece (?)	449/8
Intervention in the Peloponnesian War	411–404
Expedition of Cyrus and the "10,000"	401
King's Peace with Greece	387
Alexander's Conquest	334–323
Destruction of Persepolis	330
Seleucid Control	3rd century
Parthian Kingdom (rise)	247

GREECE

All dates are B.C.

Bronze Age Civilization	3rd and 2nd millennia
Minoan Civilization (height)	2000–1500
Mycenaean Civilization (height)	1400–1200
Destruction of Homeric (?) Troy	1250
Destruction of Mycenaean Civilization	1200–1100

Dark Age Greece	1100–750
Dorian Settlement	1100–1000
Ionian Migration	1050–900
Homeric Greece	900–700
Hesiod	750–700 (?)
Archaic Period	750–480
Colonization Movement	750–550
Spartan Conquest of Messenia	750–700
Spartan Revolution	750–650
Age of the Tyrants	675–500
Athenian *Eupatrid* Government	750–600
Draco	621
Solon	594
Peisistratid Tyranny	560 (546)–510
Peloponnesian League (rise)	550–500
Persian Conquest of Ionia	546–540
Cleisthenes and Democracy	508
Ionian Revolt	499–494
Themistocles' Archonship	492
Marathon	490
Themistocles' building of navy	483/2
Xerxes' Invasion	481–479
Battle of Himera	480
Classical Greece (5th and 4th centuries)	480–323
Hellenic League	479–461
Delian League (established)	477
Cimon's victory at Eurymedon	466
Ostracism of Cimon	461
Athenian Empire (establishment)	460–445
Rise of Pericles	460–450
Death of Cimon	450
Peace with Persia (Callias?)	449/8
Peace with Sparta	445
Building on the Acropolis	440's–404
Athenian Empire (organization)	445–431
Peloponnesian War	431–404
Archidamian War	431–421
Death of Pericles (plague)	429
Cleon	428–421
Peace of Nicias	421
Alcibiades' career	420–404
Destruction of Melos	416
Sicilian Expedition	415–413
Revolution of the "Four Hundred"	411
Restoration of Democracy	410
Fall of Athens	404
Spartan Empire	404–371
Revolution of the "Thirty" in Athens	404/03

War against Aetolia and Antiochus	192–189
Perseus of Macedonia	179–168
Antiochus IV Epiphanes	175–163
Third Macedonian War	171–168
Maccabaean Revolt	160's
Roman Province of Macedonia	148
Roman Province of Asia	129
Roman Province of Cyrene	96
Mithridatic Wars against Rome	87–63
Roman Province of Syria	63
Roman Province of Egypt	30
Roman Province of Achaea (Greece)	27

ROME

All dates are B.C. through the Republic

Neolithic Age in Italy (height)	*ca.* 2500–2000
Bronze Age	*ca.* 2000–1000
Terremare Culture	*ca.* 1500
Indo-European Settlement	*ca.* 1200–1000
Early Iron Age (begins)	*ca.* 1000–800
Phoenician Colonization	9th and 8th centuries
Etruscan Colonization	9th century
Greek Colonization	8th and 7th centuries
Founding of Rome (traditional)	753
Etruscan Expansion	6th century
Expulsion of Kings from Rome	*ca.* 500
Early Roman Republic	509 (traditional)–264
Servian Reforms	6th–5th centuries
Twelve Tables	451/50
Capture of Veii	396
Gallic capture of Rome	390
Licinian-Sextian Laws	367
Revolt of Latin League	340–338
Samnite Wars	326–290
Censorship of Appius Claudius	312
Hortensian Law	287
War with Pyrrhus and Tarentum	281–272
Wars of Conquest (Middle Republic)	264–134
Senatorial Government (height)	264–134
First Punic War	264–241
Reform of Centuriate Assembly	241
Acquisition of Sardinia and Corsica	238
First Illyrian War	229–228
First Province organized (Sicily)	227
Acquisition of Gallia Cisalpina	225–219
Second Illyrian War	220–219
Second Punic War (Hannibalic War)	218–202
Battle of Zama	202

Tiberius	14-37
Death of Germanicus	19
Tiberius' retirement to Capri	26
Conspiracy of Sejanus	31
Gaius (Caligula)	37-41
Claudius	41-54
Conquest of Britain (begins)	43
Nero	54-68
Great Fire at Rome	64
Jewish Revolt	66-70
Seneca, Lucan, Petronius	Neronian Period
Civil War (Galba, Otho, Vitellius, Vespasian)	68-69
Flavian Emperors	69-96
Vespasian	69-79
Titus	79-81
Destruction of Pompeii and Herculaneum	79
Domitian	81-96
German *Limites* (beginning)	81-96
Five Good Emperors (Roman Peace)	96-180
Nerva	96-98
Trajan	98-117
Dacian Conquest	101-02, 105-06
Parthian Conquest	114-117
Hadrian	117-138
The British *Limites* (beginning)	117-138
Antoninus Pius	138-161
Quintilian, Martial, Pliny the Younger, Juvenal, Tacitus, Plutarch, Lucian, Epictetus, Dio Chrysostom, Aelius Aristides	1st and 2nd centuries
Marcus Aurelius	161-180
Lucius Verus	161-169
Parthian Wars	162-175
Danubian Wars	166-180
Plague	166
Commodus	180-192
Pertinax and Didius Julianus	192
The Severan Dynasty	192-235
Septimius Severus	192-211
Defeat of Niger	194
Parthian War	195-199
Defeat of Albinus	197
Caracalla	211-217
Geta	211-212
Grant of Citizenship to Empire	212
Macrinus	217-218
Elagabalus	218-222
Severus Alexander	222-235
Sassanid Kingdom (Persia)	227
Persian Wars	230-232

German Wars	235
Assassination of Alexander	235
The Military Anarchy	235–285
Maximinus	235–238
Decius	249–251
Persecution of Christians	249–250
Valerian	253–260
Persecution of Christians	257–260
Gallienus	253–268
Gallic Kingdom	260–274
Palmyrene Kingdom	260–272
Claudius Gothicus (defeat of Goths)	268–270
Aurelian (restoration of Empire)	270–275
Probus (pacification)	276–282
Persian, Gothic, German attacks, plague, anarchy	235–285
The Late Empire (Dominate)	285–5th century
Diocletian	285–305
Maximian	286–305
Tetrarchy established	293
Edict on Prices	301
Persecution of Christians	302–311
Constantine the Great and Licinius	307–324
Battle of the Milvian Bridge	312
Constantine, sole Emperor	324–337
Foundation of Constantinople	330
Constantius	337–360
Julian the Apostate	360–363
Valentinian I	364–375
Valens	364–379
Valentinian II	375–392
Battle of Adrianople	378
Theodosius the Great	378–395
Division of Empire	395
Ammianus Marcellinus, Eusebius of Caesarea, Lactantius, Ambrose, St. Augustine	4th–5th centuries
The Western Empire	
Honorius	395–423
Sack of Rome by Alaric	410
Vandal Invasion of Africa	429
Death of Attila the Hun	453
Romulus Augustulus, last Roman Emperor	475–476
Foundation of Germanic Kingdoms	5th century
The Eastern Empire (The Byzantine Empire)	395–1453
Arcadius	395–408
Theodosius II	408–450
Theodosian Code	438
Justinian	527–565
Code of Justinian	528–535
Closing of the Schools of Philosophy	529

Picture Sources

PHOTOGRAPHS

Aleppo Museum, Syria: p. 21
American Friends of the Hebrew University, New York: p. 135
American Museum of Natural History, New York: pp. 11, 38
American Numismatic Society: pp. 166 (margin), 187 (middle), 188 (except bottom right), 239, 315, 332, 369 (left and right), 469 (second from right), 594, 595
American School of Classical Studies, Athens: pp. 247 (right), 325
Antikensammlungen, Munich: pp. 413 (bottom), 647, 673 (left)
Archaeological Expedition of the University of Cincinnati: pp. 115 (bottom), 118 (bottom right)
Archives Photographiques: pp. 10, 16, 31, 43 (right)
Art Reference Bureau:
    Alinari: pp. 354, 410 (bottom), 412, 413 (top), 423, 424 (margin), 426, 427 (right), 428 (left), 436, 452, 503, 553, 582, 585 587, 613, 641 (left), 642, 654 (left), 658, 661, 662, 664, 670, 718, 720 (left)
    Anderson: pp. 334, 345 (bottom), 377, 496, 627, 629, 692, 720 (right)
    Foto Marburg: pp. 53, 86 (right), 89, 149, 641 (right), 651 (left)
Atkins Museum of Fine Arts, Kansas City (William Nelson Rockhill Gallery of Art): pp. 235, 636, 663 (right)
Bardo Museum, Tunis: pp. 461, 717
Bibliothèque Nationale: pp. 617, 622, 625
Bologna Museum, Italy: p. 255 (right) (Photograph by Mr. A. Stanzani)
James H. Breasted (from page 79, *A History of Egypt*): p. 60
British Information Services: p. 634
British Museum, London: pp. 28 (margin), 34, 142, 144, 147, 152, 161, 187 (right), 232, 252, 255 (left), 271, 272, 300, 424 (bottom left), 463, 469 (extreme left and right)
Brooklyn Museum, New York: pp. 72, 170
Chicago Natural History Museum: p. 17
The Cleveland Museum of Art (Purchase from the J. H. Wade Fund): p. 177
Directorate General of Antiquities, Baghdad, Iraq: p. 43 (left)
Dumbarton Oaks Collections, Washington, D.C. (Bliss Collection): p. 258
Editions "TEL," Paris (Photograph by André Vigneau): p. 150

Fototeca Unione, Rome: pp. 558 (right), 653 (right), 654 (right), 678
Alison Frantz: pp. 109, 111, 112 (right), 114, 115 (middle right margin), 226 (right), 247 (left), 270, 274, 331 (right)
French Embassy Press and Information Division: pp. 9, 615 (right)
French Government Tourist Office: p. 615 (left)
Ewing Galloway: pp. 58, 445, 672
Giraudon, Paris: p. 163 (right)
Department of Archaeology, Government of India: p. 41 (margin)
Israel Government Coins and Medals Corp. Ltd., Jerusalem: p. 612
Israeli Information Services: p. 125
Italian State Tourist Office: p. 651 (right)
Lick Observatory, Mt. Hamilton, California: p. 2
Louvre, Paris: p. 99 (right) (Photograph by Maurice Chuzeville, Paris)
Metropolitan Museum of Art:
> pp. 66, 71, 85, 187 (left), 188 (bottom right), 229, 231, 530, 566 (right), 609, 630, 637 (left)
> (The Cesnola Collection; purchased by subscription, 1874-1876) pp. 221 (top left), 395 (left)
> (Edith Perry Chapman Fund, 1952) p. 566 (middle)
> (Dodge Fund, 1930) p. 228
> (Gift of David Dows, 1945) p. 25 (top)
> (Gift of Joseph H. Durkee, 1899) pp. 597, 669, 696
> (Fletcher Fund, 1930) p. 220 (right); 1940, p. 637 (left)
> (Gift of the Greek Government, 1930) p. 220 (left)
> (Gift of Edmund Kerper, 1952) p. 189 (left)
> (Samuel D. Lee Fund, 1940) p. 673 (right)
> (Gift of J. Pierpont Morgan, 1905) pp. 189 (right), 369 (middle), 398
> (Purchase, 1942, Joseph Pulitzer Bequest) p. 569
> (Rogers Fund) pp. 25 (right) (Joint Expedition to Nippur, 1959), 52 (1912), 66 (1920), 73 (1924), 166 (bottom, 1955), 220 (middle, 1906), 221 (margin, 1921), 222 (right, 1917), 344 (left, 1920) (right, 1911), 395 (right, 1908) (middle, 1906), 427 (left, 1903), 469 (second from left, 1908), 600 (1908), 602 (1908), 630 (1923), 637 (right, 1919), 639 (1913), 665 (right, 1909)
> (Museum Excavations, 1920, Rogers Fund and contribution of Edward S. Harkness) p. 67
> (Purchase, 1902, Funds from various donors) p. 687

La Mission Archéologique de Mari: p. 20 (Photograph by Maurice Chuzeville, Paris)
Monkmeyer Press and Photo Service: pp. 269 (Engelhard), 465 (Davidson)
The Montreal Museum of Fine Arts: p. 665 (left)
Musei Communali, Rome: p. 428 (right)
National Museum of Athens: p. 115 (top)
National Tourist Organization of Greece: pp. 104, 105, 119, 216, 243, 273, 275, 331 (left), 663 (left)
Ny Carlsberg Glyptotek, Copenhagen: p. 548 (left)
The Olympia Museum: p. 345 (top) (Photograph by Dr. Walter Hege, Karlsruhe, Germany)
The Oriental Institute, University of Chicago: pp. 36, 39 (bottom), 54, 70 (right), 81, 148, 163 (left), 164, 167, 169

Paul Popper Ltd., London: p. 686
Mary Roebuck: pp. 118 (left), 221 (top right), 328
Jean Roubier, Paris: p. 614
Royal Consulate General of Greece, Press and Information Division: pp. 175, 226
    (left), 265, 663 (left)
Royal Ontario Museum, University of Toronto: p. 329
Claude F. A. Schaeffer (from Ugaritica III): pp. 96 (margin), 99 (left)
Staatliche Museen Berlin: pp. 39 (top), 86 (left), 409, 410 (top)
Trans World Airlines, Inc: p. 649
Turkish Information Office: pp. 46, 93, 96 (bottom), 97, 136, 137
The University Museum, Philadelphia: pp. 24, 28 (top), 41 (bottom), 42, 138, 139
The Vatican Museum, General Direction of: pp. 548 (right), 558 (left), 566 (left), 584
Joan Wall: pp. 652, 653 (left), 699
Hamilton Wright: pp. 69, 80
Yugoslav Information Bureau: p. 698

PLANS AND DIAGRAMS—PAGE REFERENCES REFER TO PAGES IN THIS BOOK

American School of Classical Studies at Athens: p. 326
Archaeological Expedition of the University of Cincinnati: p. 116
Cook, J. M., *The Greeks in Ionia and the East.* Frederick A. Praeger, New York.
    Thames and Hudson, London. 1962: p. 181
Cowell, F. R., *Cicero and the Roman Republic.* Sir Isaac Pitman & Sons, Ltd. London,
    1948 and courtesy Max Parrish & Co. Ltd.: p. 494
Dinsmoor, W. B., *The Architecture of Ancient Greece.* B. T. Batsford, Ltd. London,
    1950: pp. 223, 346
Durm, J., *Die Baukunst der Romer.* Alfred Kroner. Stuttgart, 1905: p. 719
Ecole Française d'Athènes: p. 397
From *Art Through the Ages* by Helen Gardner, copyright © 1926, 1936, 1948, 1954,
    1959, 1964, by Harcourt, Brace & World, Inc. and reproduced with their per-
    mission: pp. 179, 224, 650
Graham, J. Walter and Robinson, David M., *Excavations at Olynthus.* Johns Hopkins
    University Press, Baltimore, 1938: p. 329
Courtesy of Jean-Philippe Lauer: p. 56
From Ernest Nash, *Roman Towns,* 1944: p. 507
From Pendlebury, J. D. S., *Handbook to the Palace of Minos at Knossos.* Macmillan,
    London, 1933: p. 110
Perkins, J. B. Ward, *Town Planning Review.* October, 1955. University of Liverpool:
    p. 455
Scullard, H. H., *A History of the Roman World.* Methuen & Company Ltd., London,
    1961: p. 502
Reprinted by permission of the publishers from J. I. Sewall, trans. by Morris H.
    Morgan *Vitruvius.* Cambridge, Mass.: Harvard University Press, 1914: p. 427
    (right)
Wiegand, Theodor, *Baalbek,* Vol. II. Verlag von Walther de Gruyter & Co. Berlin,
    1923: p. 674

Index

The index is designed also to serve as a brief glossary through the insertion of definitions for technical terms and to be of some help in the pronunciation of ancient names by the indication of accentual stress.

745